Technological Advances in Surgery, Trauma and Critical Care

Rifat Latifi
Peter Rhee
Rainer W.G. Gruessner
Editors

Technological Advances in Surgery, Trauma and Critical Care

Foreword by David B Hoyt

Springer

Editors
Rifat Latifi, M.D., F.A.C.S.
Professor of Surgery
Division of Trauma, Critical Care, Burn and Emergency Surgery
Co-Director Trauma Research Institute
Department of Surgery
University of Arizona
Tucson, AZ, USA

Peter Rhee, M.D., F.A.C.S.
Chief of Division of Trauma, Critical Care, Burn and Emergency Surgery
Professor of Surgery
Martin Gluck Endowed Chair
Co-Director Trauma Research Institute
University of Arizona
Tucson, AZ, USA

Rainer W.G. Gruessner, M.D., F.A.C.S.
Professor of Surgery
Department of Surgery
University of Arizona
Tucson, AZ, USA

ISBN 978-1-4939-2670-1 ISBN 978-1-4939-2671-8 (eBook)
DOI 10.1007/978-1-4939-2671-8

Library of Congress Control Number: 2015942924

Springer New York Heidelberg Dordrecht London

Printed on acid-free paper

Springer Science+Business Media LLC New York is part of Springer Science+Business Media (www.springer.com)

To all past, present, and future innovators in surgery.

Foreword

This new book *Technical Advances in Surgery, Trauma, and Critical Care* edited by Rifat Latifi, Peter Rhee, and Rainer Gruessner is truly a unique contribution. The editors have assembled a work that champions new technology and innovations that have recently occurred throughout surgery. Reading the chapters is like taking a trip to a world's fair and being exposed to the frontiers of surgical practice. I will never forget going to the GE Exhibit at the World's Fair in Flushing, New York, in 1964 with my parents and feeling I had glimpsed into the future. I had that same feeling reading many of these chapters 50 years later.

This book explores a vision of a new hospital, the use of performance improvement techniques, and new concepts such as taking the injured patient directly to the operating room. The importance of nanotechnology, genomics, and proteomics for disease staging, treatment selection, and individualized surgical treatment is covered. A modern academic department to support this kind of innovation and care delivery is also described.

A significant part of the book is dedicated to specific aspects of the biology of surgery, including genetics, tissue repair, rejection, immunosuppression, resuscitation end points, and damage control resuscitation.

A majority of the text brings us up to the date on what is new with head and neck cancer, neurosurgery, endocrine surgery, and innovations in pulmonary, cardiac, and abdominal surgery. The innovations accompanying the use of robotic surgery and natural orifice surgery are highlighted in each of these areas, and exciting, evolutionary themes are addressed for each.

Telepresence is reviewed for what it currently is and can be in the future, and the ethics of surgery are discussed with appropriate emphasis.

Surgery is going through a continuous evolution, emphasizing more precise, less invasive, more organ specific, and less painful procedures. At a time when it is often popular to complain about health care in general and the economic challenges we face, this book celebrates our remarkable success and will challenge your imagination about the bright future of surgery and the benefits we can provide to patients. This will stimulate your recommitment to the best profession of all.

The opportunity and responsibility we owe our patients to know what is new and possible makes this book particularly timely and important.

Congratulations to Drs. Latifi, Rhee, and Gruessner and to all the chapter authors for this wonderful contribution!

David B. Hoyt, M.D., F.A.C.S.

Prologue

The young man involved in a major car crash is brought to the trauma with blood pressure barely readable and pulse barely palpable. Until yesterday, trauma surgeons across the world would open his left chest and clamp his aorta. Morbid procedure, some called it exercise in futility. Today, the surgeon approaches his femoral artery, puts a balloon in and inflates it, and occludes the aorta at any level that he or she wishes from the inside. The almost dead patient now is alive, perfusing his heart and his brain, and resuscitation continues. During the same procedure, his almost destroyed liver get embolized and bleeding stops. All this occurs in the new, hybrid operating room without moving the patient from floor to floor through various departments. This may have been a dream of the trauma surgeons for a long time. This is not a dream anymore! This is a reality today.

This is just one of the new advances that we deal with on a routine basis, and the rest of them are part of this book, 50 chapters written by 111 authors from many institutions and spread out on five continents. Yet, chances are that by the time you finish reading this introduction, something new will happen in surgery, and your inbox will alert you to a new message about news of technological advances.

Throughout their careers, the editors of this book have been on the forefront of both developing and implementing many of these new technologies and are keenly aware of their impact on clinical practice, surgical education, and research. However, the continued subspecialization makes it almost impossible for any surgeon to be fully aware of all the technological advances in surgery, trauma, and critical care.

Thus, we thought that a book like this may at least attempt to bring together in one tome the most important technological advances that continue to impact our patients' lives and change the future of medicine. To this end, we asked the Who's Who in the field of these advances to bring to the readers the latest and the newest. The process of selecting the contributors for this book was not an easy task. We did not want to compile just another run-of-the-mill surgery textbook. There are a number of outstanding surgeon researchers around the world that have made or are in the process of making significant contributions to the science and technology of surgery. We selected those whom we thought are the true stars in their fields and asked them to help us.

And they did. Now we have an outstanding collection that we hope will shed true light on the progress that has been made in technologies in surgery, trauma, and critical care.

Anyone who has ever worked on a book similar to this one knows first-hand what is involved. Each of us is a busy practitioner, researcher, or leader of a department; some lead medical schools or major health care systems. Some are clinicians *par excellence* and spend most of the day in the hospital, clinic, and the operating room, caring for the patient. That is what we all love to do. Most of us, however, do not have enough time for family, friends, and our hobbies (if we have any). Stopping all of that and sitting down to write a chapter for a book is, at times, the last thing that we can find time to do. Yet, 110 surgeons from around the world did just that. And what we have in hand is their outstanding contributions.

Organizing the book was another major issue. We went though many versions, and, finally, we settled on this one. The first part of the book set the stage. The chapters on genomics and nanotechnologies are brilliantly written and truly represent the *crème de la crème* of technological advances. Part II of the book focuses on trauma, resuscitation, and nutrition and summarizes the latest directions of caring for these patients from the moment of arrival in the trauma room to the development of multiorgan failure. Part III of the book is dedicated to system-oriented advances, from head and neck, chest, and to intra-abdominal organs. Some outstanding chapters in these sections describe truly revolutionary changes and advances in each field. Part IV of the book discusses transplantation of heart and valves, and intra-abdominal organs including small bowel and islet cells to face and limb transplant. Part V brings some of the newest advances in abdominal wall and limb reconstruction and pediatric surgery to center stage.

We are thankful to each of the contributors for the hard work and time that was put into this book. Without their efforts, we would not have been able to describe all the technological advances in surgery, trauma, and critical care.

Finally, we hope that we have been able to convey the message regarding how much our field has been transformed, from the individual surgeon to the department of surgery to the care that we provide for the same diseases that we have been caring for centuries. These changes are truly remarkable, and more changes are to come. As we dissect the genome of human body, as we enter part of the anatomy with cameras that are smaller than what the naked eye can see, the revolution in surgery is apparent.

Despite all the technological advances in surgical techniques and in approaches to surgical diseases, the decision made by the surgeon to operate or not to operate is still the most important element. No technological advances can decide when to take out the diseased gallbladder or when should we *reoperate* in a patient with a visibly hostile abdomen.

In summary, we believe that, as a result of this endeavor, a unique collection of chapters on new surgical technologies in surgery, trauma, and critical care is provided, and we hope that this textbook will become the standard textbook on surgical technological advances for practicing surgeons, fellows, residents, and medical students. The ultimate judge regarding the quality of this book, however, will be you—our peers. Whether already practicing or still in training, we hope that the information that this book provides will not only help you to further advance surgical care but also motivate you to further advance the field of surgery by developing other innovative technologies.

There are many people who have made this work possible. In particular, we would like to thank Liz Tilley, Ph.D., research assistant to Rifat Latifi, for her contributions at the earlier stages of the book, and Liz Corra and Richard Hruska from Springer Science for their outstanding assistance during this process.

Rifat Latifi, M.D., F.A.C.S.
Peter Rhee, M.D., F.A.C.S.
Rainer W.G. Gruessner, M.D., F.A.C.S.

Contents

Contributors

Mahmoud A.Z. Abdelaal, M.D. Department of Surgery, University of Arizona Medical Center, Tucson, AZ, USA

Kareem R. AbdelFattah, M.D. Department of Surgery, Parkland Memorial Hospital, University of Texas – Southwestern Medical Center, Dallas, TX, USA

Hassan Al-Thani, M.D. Department of Surgery, Trauma Surgery Section, Hamad General Hospital, Doha, Qatar

Russell J. Andrews, M.D. Center for Nanotechnology, NASA Ames Research Center, Moffett Field, CA, USA

David G. Armstrong, D.P.M., M.D., Ph.D. Department of Surgery, University of Arizona Medical Center, Tucson, AZ, USA

Horacio J. Asbun, M.D. Department of General Surgery, Mayo Clinic, Jacksonville, FL, USA

Mohammad Asim, Ph.D. Department of Surgery, Clinical Research, Hamad General Hospital, Doha, Qatar

Juan P. Barret, M.D., Ph.D. Department of Plastic Surgery and Burn Center, Hospital Universitari Vall d'Hebron, Barcelona, Spain

Shuntaye D. Batson, M.D. Department of Surgery, The University of Mississippi Medical Center, Jackson, MS, USA

David W. Birchley, M.B.B.S., F.R.C.S., M.Sc. Department of Vascular Surgery, Royal Devon and Exeter NHS Foundation Trust, Exeter, UK

Christoph Bode, M.D. Department of Cardiology and Angiology, Heart Center of Freiburg University, Freiburg, Germany

Kenneth D. Boffard, M.B. F.R.C.S., F.A.C.S. Department of Surgery, University of the Witwatersrand, Johannesburg, South Africa

Milpark Hospital, Johannesburg, South Africa

Robert S. Boffard, BJOURN(Rhodes) Vancouver, BC, Canada

Gerald Brandacher, M.D. Reconstructive Transplantation Program, Department of Plastic and Reconstructive Surgery, Johns Hopkins University School of Medicine, Baltimore, MD, USA

Jonathan D. Braun, M.D. Division of Vascular Surgery, Department of Vascular and Endovascular Surgery, Arizona Health Sciences Center, University of Arizona Medical Center, Tucson, AZ, USA

Fernando Carbonell-Tatay, M.D. Department of Abdominal Wall Surgery, Faculty of Medicine, University of Valencia, La Fe University Hospital, Valencia, Spain

Napoleon E. Cieza, M.D. General Surgery Residency Program, University of Arizona, Tucson, AZ, USA

Raul Coimbra, M.D., Ph.D., F.A.C.S. Division of Trauma, Surgical Critical Care, Burns and Acute Care Surgery, Department of Surgery, UC San Diego Health Sciences, San Diego, CA, USA

Todd W. Costantini, M.D., F.A.C.S. Division of Trauma, Surgical Critical Care, Burns and Acute Care Surgery, Department of Surgery, UC San Diego Health Sciences, San Diego, CA, USA

Laurent Coubeau, M.D. Department of Abdominal and Transplantation Surgery, Starzl Unit of Abdominal Transplantation University Hospitals Saint Luc, Université Catholique de Louvain UCL, Brussels, Belgium

Marion E. Couch, M.D., Ph.D., M.B.A. Department of Otolaryngology – Head and Neck Surgery, Indiana University School of Medicine, Indianapolis, IN, USA

Elias Degiannis, M.D., Ph.D., F.R.C.S., F.C.S.(SA) Department of Surgery, Chris Hani Baragwanath Academic Hospital, University of the Witwatersrand, Johannesburg, South Africa

Matthew J. Delano, M.D., Ph.D. Division of Acute Care Surgery, Department of Surgery, University of Michigan Health System, Ann Arbor, MI, USA

Fernando Dip, M.D. Department of Surgical Oncology, Hospital de Clinicas Jose de San Martin, Buenos Aires, Argentina

John M. Draus Jr., M.D. Division of Pediatric Surgery, Department of Surgery, Kentucky Children's Hospital, Lexington, KY, USA

Stanley J. Dudrick, M.D., F.A.C.S., F.A.C.N. Department of Clinical Sciences, The Commonwealth Medical College, Scranton, PA, USA

Department of Surgery, Yale University Medical School, New Haven, CT, USA

David T. Efron, M.D., F.A.C.S. Division of Acute Care Surgery, Department of Surgery, Johns Hopkins Hospital, Baltimore, MD, USA

Manuela Elía-Guedea, M.D. Department of Surgery, Clinic University Hospital of Zaragoza, Zaragoza, Spain

Ayman Ahmed El-Menyar, M.D., F.R.C.P(Glasg). Department of Surgery, Clinical Research, Hamad General Hospital & Clinical Medicine, Weill Cornell Medical College, Doha, Qatar

Marcie Feinman, M.D. Department of Surgery, Sinai Hospital of Baltimore, Baltimore, MD, USA

Alberto R. Ferreres, M.D., Ph.D., J.D., M.P.H., F.A.C.S. Department of General Surgery, Hospital Dr. Carlos A. Bocalandro, University of Buenos Aires, Buenos Aires, Argentina

Kiyotaka Fukamachi, M.D., Ph.D. Department of Biomedical Engineering, Lerner Research Institute, Cleveland Clinic, Cleveland, OH, USA

Carlos A. Galvani, M.D. Department of Surgery, University of Arizona Medical Center, Tucson, AZ, USA

Farid Gharagozloo, M.D. Department of Surgery, University of Arizona, Arizona Cancer Center, Tucson, AZ, USA

Nicholas A. Giovinco, D.P.M. Department of Surgery, University of Arizona Medical Center, Tucson, AZ, USA

Jose Antonio Gracia-Solanas, M.D. Department of Surgery, Clinic University Hospital of Zaragoza, Zaragoza, Spain

Rainer W.G. Gruessner, M.D., F.A.C.S., F.I.C.S. Department of Surgery, University of Arizona Medical Center, Tucson, AZ, USA

Gabriel Gruionu, M.S., Ph.D. Division of Trauma, Emergency Surgery, and Surgical Critical Care, Department of Surgery, Massachusetts General Hospital, Boston, MA, USA

Alison Guy, M.B.Ch.B., M.R.C.S. Department of Vascular Surgery, Royal Devon and Exeter Hospital, Exeter, UK

Monika E. Hagen, M.D., M.B.A. Department of Surgery, University Hospital Geneva, Geneva, Switzerland

ByoungJun Han, B.S. Department of Neurosurgery, New York University School of Medicine, New York, NY, USA

Jacqueline S. Hebert, M.D. Department of Medicine, University of Alberta, Edmonton, AB, Canada

William W. Hope, M.D. Department of Surgery, New Hanover Regional Medical Center, Wilmington, NC, USA

David A. Iannitti, M.D., F.A.C.S. Department of Hepatopancreatobiliary Surgery, Carolinas Medical Center, Charlotte, NC, USA

Whitney Sheen James, M.D., M.H.S. Division of Neurosurgery, Department of Surgery, University of Arizona Medical Center, Tucson, AZ, USA

Tun Jie, M.D., M.S., F.A.C.S. Department of Surgery, School of Medicine, University of Arizona, Tucson, AZ, USA

Timothy G. Johnson, M.D. Department of Surgery, New Hanover Regional Medical Center, Wilmington, NC, USA

Masato Kanzaki, M.D., Ph.D. Department of Surgery, Tokyo Women's Medical University, Tokyo, Japan

Jamshid H. Karimov, M.D., Ph.D. Department of Biomedical Engineering, Lerner Research Institute, Cleveland, OH, USA

Santosh Kesari, M.D., Ph.D. Department of Neurosciences, UC San Diego, Moores Cancer Center, La Jolla, CA, USA

Soroosh Kiani, M.D., M.S., M.A. Department of Internal Medicine, University of Virginia, Charlottesville, VA, USA

Russell C. Kirks Jr., M.D. Department of General Surgery, Carolinas Medical Center, Charlotte, NC, USA

Leslie Kobayashi, M.D., F.A.C.S. Division of Trauma, Surgical Critical Care, Burns and Acute Care Surgery, Department of Surgery, UC San Diego Health Sciences, San Diego, CA, USA

Rifat Latifi, M.D., F.A.C.S., F.I.C.S. Department of Surgery, University of Arizona, Tucson, AZ, USA

W.P. Andrew Lee, M.D. Reconstructive Transplantation Program, Department of Plastic and Reconstructive Surgery, Johns Hopkins University School of Medicine, Baltimore, MD, USA

G. Michael Lemole Jr., M.D. Division of Neurosurgery, Department of Surgery, University of Arizona, Tucson, AZ, USA

Luis R. Leon Jr., M.D., R.V.T., F.A.C.S. Pima Heart, PC, Department of Vascular and Endovascular Surgery, Tucson Medical Center, Tucson, AZ, USA

Jan P.M. Lerut, M.D., Ph.D., F.A.C.S. Department of Abdominal and Transplantation Surgery, Starzl Unit of Abdominal Transplantation University Hospitals Saint Luc, Université catholique de Louvain - UCL Brussels, Belgium

Ronald V. Maier, M.D., F.A.C.S. Department of Surgery, Harborview Medical Center, University of Washington, Seattle, WA, USA

Paul D. Marasco, Ph.D. Department of Biomedical Engineering, Cleveland Clinic, Cleveland, OH, USA

Advanced Platform Technology Center of Excellence, Louis Stokes Cleveland Department of Veterans Affairs Medical Center, Cleveland, OH, USA

Shinichi Matsumoto, M.D., Ph.D. Department of Pancreatic Islet Cell Transplantation, Research Institute, National Center for Global Health and Medicine, Tokyo, Japan

Ronald C. Merrell, M.D., F.A.C.S. Department of Surgery, Virginia Commonwealth University, Richmond, VA, USA

Nader Moazami, M.D. Department of Thoracic and Cardiovascular Surgery, Kaufman Center for Heart Failure, Cardiac Transplantation and Mechanical Circulatory Support, Miller Family Heart and Vascular Institute, Cleveland Clinic, Cleveland, OH, USA

Miguel Montero-Baker, M.D. Pima Vascular Group, Department of Vascular and Endovascular Surgery, University of Arizona Health Sciences, Tucson, AZ, USA

Philippe Morel, M.D. Department of Surgery, Geneva University Hospital, Geneva, Switzerland

Giuseppe Orlando, M.D., Ph.D. Section of Transplantation, Department of General Surgery, Wake Forest Baptist Health, Wake Forest Institute for Regenerative Medicine, Wake Forest School of Medicine, Winston-Salem, NC, USA

Beth M. Orzell, B.S.M.E. Prosthetics and Sensory Aid Service, Louis Stokes Cleveland, Department of Veterans Affairs Medical Center, Cleveland, OH, USA

Mehmet Mahir Ozmen, M.D., M.S., F.A.C.S., F.R.C.S. Department of Surgery, Hacettepe University Medical School, Ankara, Turkey

Mihir R. Patel, M.D. Department of Otolaryngology – Head and Neck Surgery, Winship Cancer Institute of Emory University, Atlanta, GA, USA

Frank Plani, M.D., F.C.S.(SA), F.R.A.C.S. Department of Surgery, Chris Hani Baragwanath Academic Hospital, Johannesburg, South Africa

John M. Porter, M.D., F.A.C.S. Department of Surgery, Cooper University Hospital, Camden, NJ, USA

Marian Porubsky, M.D., F.A.C.S. Department of Surgery, School of Medicine, University of Arizona, Tucson, AZ, USA

Robert S. Poston, M.D. Department of Cardiothoracic Surgery, St Francis Medical Center, Trenton, NJ, USA

Riaan Pretorius, M.B.Ch.B., F.C.S. Department of Surgery/Trauma, Chris Hani Baragwanath Academic Hospital, University of the Witwatersrand, Johannesburg, South Africa

Jose Manuel Ramírez-Rodríguez, M.D. Department of Surgery, Clinic University Hospital of Zaragoza, Zaragoza, Spain

Timothy M. Rankin, M.D., M.S. Department of Surgery, University of Arizona Medical Center, Tucson, AZ, USA

Jochen Reinöhl, M.D. Department of Cardiology and Angiology, Heart Center of Freiburg University, Freiburg, Germany

T. Elizabeth Robertson, M.D., F.A.C.S. Department of Surgery, The University of Mississippi Medical Center, Jackson, MS, USA

Sanziana A. Roman, M.D., F.A.C.S. Department of Surgery, Duke University, Durham, NC, USA

Alexander Rosemurgy, M.D., F.A.C.S. Florida Hospital Tampa, Tampa, FL, USA

Sharona Ross, M.D., F.A.C.S. Florida Hospital Tampa, Tampa, FL, USA

Uzma Samadani, M.D., Ph.D. Department of Neurosurgery, Psychiatry, Physiology, and Neuroscience, New York Harbor Health Care System, New York University School of Medicine, New York, NY, USA

Julia Samamé, M.D. Department of Surgery, University of Arizona, Tucson, AZ, USA

Norio Sato, M.D., Ph.D. Department of Primary Care and Emergency Medicine, Kyoto University Hospital, Kyoto City, Japan

Randall P. Scheri, M.D. Department of Surgery, Duke University, Durham, NC, USA

Brian J. Scott, M.D. Tufts University School of Medicine, Boston, MA, USA

Lahey Hospital and Medical Center, Burlington, MA, USA

Ramanathan M. Seshadri, M.D. Department of Hepatopancreatobiliary Surgery, Carolinas Medical Center, Charlotte, NC, USA

Masayuki Shimoda, M.D., Ph.D. Department of Pancreatic Islet Cell Transplantation, Research Institute, National Center for Global Health and Medicine, Tokyo, Japan

Jaimie T. Shores, M.D. Department of Plastic and Reconstructive Surgery, Johns Hopkins University School of Medicine, Baltimore, MD, USA

Diego Sinagra, M.D. Department of Surgical Oncology, Hospital de Clinicas Jose de San Martin, Buenos Aires, Argentina

Marvin J. Slepian, M.D. Department of Surgery, University of Arizona Medical Center, Tucson, AZ, USA

Julie A. Sosa, M.D., M.A. Department of Surgery, Duke University, Durham, NC, USA

Michael E. Stadler, M.D. Department of Otolaryngology and Communication Sciences, Medical College of Wisconsin, Milwaukee, WI, USA

John A. Stauffer, M.D. Department of General Surgery, Mayo Clinic, Jacksonville, FL, USA

Robert J. Stratta, M.D. Department of General Surgery, Wake Forest School of Medicine, Winston-Salem, NC, USA

Prashant Sukharamwala, M.D. Florida Hospital Tampa, Tampa, FL, USA

Takeshi Takahara, M.D., Ph.D. Department of Surgery, Iwate Medical University School of Medicine, Morioka, Japan

William M. Tauxe, M.S.T. Emory University School of Medicine, Atlanta, GA, USA

Masako Toyoda Princeton University, Princeton, NJ, USA

Yasuhiro Toyoda University of Pittsburgh, Pittsburgh, PA, USA

Yoshiko Toyoda, B.A. Weill Cornell Medical College, New York, NY, USA

Yoshiya Toyoda, M.D., Ph.D. Department of Surgery, Temple University Hospital, Philadelphia, PA, USA

George C. Velmahos, M.D., Ph.D., M.S.Ed., F.A.C.S. Division of Trauma, Emergency Surgery, and Surgical Critical Care, Department of Surgery, Massachusetts General Hospital, Boston, MA, USA

Go Wakabayashi, M.D., Ph.D., F.A.C.S. Department of Surgery, Ageo Central General Hospital, Ageo, Saitama, Japan

Craig Weinkauf, M.D., Ph.D. Division of Vascular Surgery, Department of Surgery, University of Arizona Medical Center, Tucson, AZ, USA

Catherine E. Western, M.B.B.S., B.Sc. Department of Vascular Surgery, Royal Devon and Exeter Hospital, Exeter, UK

Steven E. Wolf, M.D., F.A.C.S. Department of Surgery, University of Texas – Southwestern Medical Center, Dallas, TX, USA

Baris Dogu Yildiz, M.D. Department of General Surgery and Transplant Surgery, Ankara Numune Teaching Hospital, Ankara, Turkey

Manfred Zehender, M.D. Department of Cardiology and Angiology, Heart Center of Freiburg University, Freiburg, Germany

Angel Zorraquino González, M.D. Department of General Surgery, Abdominal Wall Surgery Unit, Faculty of Medicine at the Basque Country University, Basurto University Hospital, Bilbao, Basque Country, Spain

Part I

Surgical Science and Practice: The New Direction

The New Surgeon: Patient-Centered, Disease-Focused, Technology-Driven, and Team-Oriented

1

Rifat Latifi, Stanley J. Dudrick, and Ronald C. Merrell

Introduction

The first question that we need to address is: How did the new surgeon evolve? There are a number of major events that happened and that are responsible for the new surgeon. For example, the surgeon trained 50 years ago was not taught endoscopy or even the use of staplers. The antibiotic formulary had not quite yet added cephalosporins. Also, ICU was a very primitive matter, and use of ventilators was generally fatal if you could not wean in a week. For the transition, we are struck that the older surgeons not only became the new surgeons but also radically changed their practices by adding knowledge of the staplers, laparoscopes, lasers, endoscopes, and imaging. The EVOLVING surgeon became the new surgeon. In the interim, infection in the ventilated patient became a black mark of poor management. Antibiotics went from profligate use of too many to highly targeted use, and prophylaxis got some sense.

The 2014 Clinical Congress of the American College of Surgeons (ACS) theme was "The Surgeon of the Future." This topic was very timely and leads us to ask: What will the surgeon of the future look like? There is much to consider when we attempt to envision the surgeon of the future, but in order to explore this topic meaningfully, we need to have a foundational knowledge of the surgeons of the past and understand our current status as surgeons. While a comprehensive historical description of the surgeon is beyond the scope of this chapter, it is clear that much has changed in the practice of medicine overall, and, particularly, in surgery, so much so that trying to describe these changes in one chapter or even in one volume would be an impossible task to complete, even for medical historians.

Yet, in order to discover what has occurred in the continuum of transition and transformation of surgery and what has changed during the last century or so, we do not really need to go very far. One only has to look back within our own practices and recognize the changes in surgery within our own lifetimes in order to realize how much surgery has been reinvented and how much surgeons have been transformed. If we do this, perhaps we may begin to understand the

R. Latifi, M.D., F.A.C.S. (✉)
Department of Surgery, University of Arizona Medical Center, Tucson, AZ, USA
e-mail: latifi@surgery.arizona.edu

S.J. Dudrick, M.D., F.A.C.S., F.A.C.N.
Department of Clinical Sciences, The Commonwealth Medical College, Scanton, PA, USA

Department of Surgery, Yale University Medical School, New Haven, CT, USA
e-mail: sjdudrickmd@comcast.net

R.C. Merrell, M.D., F.A.C.S.
Department of Surgery, Virginia Commonwealth University, Richmond, VA, USA
e-mail: rcmerrel@vcu.edu

R. Latifi et al. (eds.), *Technological Advances in Surgery, Trauma and Critical Care*,
DOI 10.1007/978-1-4939-2671-8_1

complexity of the process and the magnitude of adaptation required to stay current with surgical science. This chapter does not address whether we are better or worse, but merely acknowledges that we have become different surgeons, and that the stage on which we practice surgery has been utterly transformed. Nonetheless, when one briefly reviews the entire spectrum of technological advances, one cannot help but conclude that we have become better surgeons, at least if this definition is based on surgical outcomes of many operative procedures that we perform today, which have significantly lowered morbidity and mortality rates and produced much better quality of life for patients.

What Kind of Surgeons Have We Become?

The metamorphosis of surgery and surgeons is due to the combination of intuitivity, ingenuity, and courage of surgeons and other professionals involved in advancing medical technologies around the world, medical industry explosions in a variety of fields, patients becoming better educated consumers and expecting better outcomes, and hospitals undergoing major transformations by embracing and integrating technological advances. These are just a few of the factors which provide evidence that surgery, trauma, and critical care medicine have undergone an amazing evolution. The best consequence of this evolution is that the care of the patient has been greatly improved; outcomes are significantly better; and, most importantly, the development and appreciation of surgical science has progressed immensely. To be a student of surgery today requires that one must embrace the technological advances and the "new surgery world order" in addition to becoming a master of the anatomy, physiology, and pathology of the disease.

Patient-Centered

This phrase is representative of a new trend used by hospital administrators and the media, but it does not take into account or consideration that surgeons feel that they have been patient-centered all along. Indeed, many discussions have been more about the "surgeon's ego" rather than "the quality of their work and results."

While the concern has always been for the welfare and outcomes of the patient, the new phrase "patient-centered" care refers to the shift in focus on who determines what is necessary and who can provide input on outcomes. Patient-centered models incorporate the perceptions and needs of the patient [1]. Recent systematic review of 14 studies (seven of which were randomized clinical trials) on laparoscopic repair of ventral hernia (LVHR) [2] found that LVHR improved the overall health-related quality of life of patients (HRQoL) in 6 of the 8 studies. These authors found that LVHR demonstrated improved pain scores and improved functionality (in 12 studies). Return to work ranged from 6 to 18 days postoperatively in 50 % of studies, while the physical function scores were improved in the remaining 50 % of the studies. Overall patient satisfaction improved after LVHR in all studies assessing patient satisfaction, including improving mental and emotional well-being (in 6 of the 7 studies).

The phrase "patient-centered" is a new model of care and a specific metric that has now been incorporated into how surgeons and physicians assess results and interact with patients. Using a patient-centered focus has broadly changed the environment in which surgeons work. To this end, patients' satisfaction with an operation has become a common theme and a focus in many important scientific deliberations and peer-reviewed journals [3].

Technology-Driven

Technology has become a major component of surgical care, and much of it is industry supported; however, technology has not always been seen as a positive influence in the surgical sciences. When the first author of this chapter was a junior resident and suggested to one of his professors that surgeons needed to learn laparoscopic cholecystectomy, since this may become the "new standard of care," the professor's negative reaction caused the resident to fear that he would be dismissed from the service.

Furthermore, at Yale New Haven Hospital, as a junior resident in trauma service, when he (RL) brought an article to the journal club on the use of CT scans to screen patients suspected to have suffered an aortic injury instead of using a formal aortogram [4], the article was not well received despite the fact that similar articles on the subject had been published long before that year [5].

Every resident on trauma services remembers countless hours spent in radiology looking after trauma patients undergoing a formal aortic angiogram, an expensive and toxic procedure to their kidneys. But for any patient who had any serious trauma and was "at risk for aortic injury," this technique was once considered the gold standard of care. Today, CT angio is the new gold standard of care. Perhaps in the future something much less invasive will become the standard as technology continues to advance.

Serious doubt accompanying surgical innovations is not a new phenomenon. In 1959, there were serious doubts that Total Parenteral Nutrition (TPN) would actually be able to sustain life [6]; yet, since 1968, TPN has become the standard of care for all patients who cannot or should not be fed and will not be able to maintain their nutritional status by oral or enteral means [7].

When Dr. "Barney" Crile Jr. of Cleveland Clinic suggested that, "we do not need to perform radical Halstedian mastectomy" [8], he was expelled from the Cleveland Academy of Surgeons [9, 10]. He was not the only one rejected by his peers for innovative thinking. Prof. Dr. Med Erich Mühe of Böblingen, Germany, performed the first laparoscopic cholecystectomy (LC) on September 12, 1985 [11]. When he reported this accomplishment in 1986 to the German Surgical Society, he was rejected from the group. Yet, in 1992, he received their highest award, the German Surgical Society Anniversary Award, and, in 1999, he was recognized by SAGES for having performed the first laparoscopic cholecystectomy. Now LC is a standard of care throughout the world.

Specialized Surgeons: Disease-Based

We have become highly specialized surgeons. Patients undergoing complex surgical procedures at high-volume centers have been shown to have improved outcomes. A relevant example is aortic procedures [12]. In-hospital mortality correlates to center volume ($P = 0.014$) with low, intermediate, and high-volume centers having mortality rates of 23.4 % ($n = 187$), 20.1 % ($n = 62$), and 12.1 % ($n = 15$), respectively. This relationship persisted when controlling for severity of comorbid illness ($P = 0.007$). The number of complications per patient varied significantly by center volume ($P = 0.044$) as well. Other examples of surgical excellence in high-volume centers that perform pancreatectomy have been clearly documented [13]. In a study performed in one of the major American institutions, all 1,000 pancreaticoduodenectomies performed between March 1969 and May 2003 by a single surgeon reported an unprecedented mortality rate of 1 %. In addition, the median operative time decreased significantly over the 5 decades, with 8.8 h reported in the 1970s and 5.5 h during the 2000s. Postoperative length of stay dropped from a median of 17 days in the 1980s to 9 days in the 2000s. Overall 5-year survival was 18 %; for the lymph node-negative patients, it was 32 %; and for node-negative, margin-negative patients, it was 41 %. Another report from the same institution [14] has demonstrated that patients who have cancers with favorable pathological features have statistically significant improved long-term survival.

Team-Oriented

A team-based approach has become the new model for delivering surgical care. There has been a shift in the focus on how the surgical group works as a team, how they communicate, how they collaboratively make decisions, and how they manage tasks. While the surgeon has always worked with a team, the need for communication and group decision-making has recently been emphasized. In essence, the surgeon is required to master the competency to work in a team. All members of the surgical team are required to focus on working together toward better proficiency. Maximizing the potential of how a team works together has been assessed as well. Recently, an opinion piece in JAMA Surgery titled "Evolution of Surgery: The Story of Two Poems" summarized wonderfully the transformation of surgery and the surgeon [15]. The message is clear: it is not all about the surgeon and his or her kingdom. Rather, it is about the patient, the team, the quality, the outcomes, and seeking new ways of providing the best possible care.

Hospitals That Look Like Space Shuttles

Standards have changed, and some standards are changing rapidly, so that there is a need for surgeons to be well informed at all times. While the need to be informed is imperative to the success of surgeons and for optimum results, acquiring and retaining this new information can be overwhelming. Recently, the first author of this chapter spent 2 days learning about electronic health records in a new hospital, and it was difficult to understand the process.

Intensive care units are now so complex that one needs a week of orientation to learn the environment, and often you cannot see the patient among all the computers and other hardware and technology. This is not always an easy milieu in which to work, but it is an improvement in many aspects. An intensive care unit (ICU) room can be transformed into a dialyzing unit or into an operating room within minutes. These are "All In One" ICU models where virtually anything can be done. You can see intubated patients walking through the corridors of hospitals hooked to cardiac devices while waiting for new hearts. The trauma room has an angio suite, an operating room, CT scan, MRI, and everything needed to care effectively for the patient.

Military Transport of Critically Ill and Injured Patients

One group of patients who have benefited greatly from advances in technology are those involved as military casualties [16, 17]. Now, a critically ill and severely injured military patient can get care in three different continents, all while flying above 10,000 m, attached to and supported by some of the most sophisticated machines that man has ever conceived and invented [18]. A retrospective review of Critical Care Air Transport Team (CCATT) of 975 of injured individuals from Iraq and Afghanistan transferred to Germany demonstrated a mortality of 2.1 % and inflight mortality of 0.02 %. The evacuation of the injured patients from the war zone is part of the damage control [19]. All this occurs while the patient is being continuously monitored from the ground somewhere in North America.

New civilian hospitals have video conferencing equipment and basic telemedicine ability in their patient's room, while the operating room looks more like the cockpit of the airbus 380 than anything else. All of this is ergonomically and functionally friendly.

Coping with Technological Changes

In a recent conversation with medical students, the first author of this chapter told them that, despite all the changes and perhaps what some might call "difficult times," he would choose again and again the same profession with the same training. Yet, handling the technological transitions and adapting to new metamorphosis is not simple. This transformation has not been without a huge toll on surgeons [20–28]. Practicing physicians and surgeons as well as medical students and medical and surgical residents dedicate their lives to providing optimum patient care, but doing so places them at significant risk for personal and professional stress and, ultimately, burnout. The unrecognized stress and unmanaged burnout are more prevalent among residents than previously believed [21]. Overwhelming physical and emotional exhaustion, feelings of cynicism and detachment from the job, a sense of ineffectiveness and lack of accomplishment, over-identification with work due to the exclusion of other activities, and irritability and hypervigilance have been identified as characteristics of burnouts [24]. When things go wrong [25] and bad things happen to good surgeons [26], surgeons and other physicians have been identified as the "second victim" [27].

It is important to acknowledge the high rates of burnout among surgeons and residents and to take preventive measures against risk factors for burnout and suicide. We as surgeons must remember to take care of ourselves and each other. Perhaps we need to remember a mundane rule that we have heard many times on an airplane: "to put the oxygen mask first on yourself before assisting others." We need to take care of ourselves and, in doing so, may become more helpful to others who are in the same position. Risk of anxiety, depression, stressed or broken relationships, substance dependence, and possibly suicide as a result of these stressors affect up to 75 % of surgeons [24].

Various strategies have been suggested to avoid burnout and help surgeons deal with stress and the new environment [24]. In a study of 3,911 surgeons who responded to a survey, 55.0 % of surgeons participated in aerobic exercise and 2,611 (36.3 %) in muscle-strengthening activities. More than 46 % participating surgeons saw their primary care provider within 12 months, and those who had seen their primary care provider in the last 12 months were more likely to be up to date with all age-appropriate health care screening and had superior overall and physical QOL scores (all $P<0.0001$). When authors did multivariate analysis, they found that surgeons placing greater emphasis on finding meaning in work, focusing on what is important in life, maintaining a positive outlook, and embracing a philosophy that stresses work/life balance were less likely to be burned out (all $P<0.0001$).

Respecting the Past, Leading the Future

As new surgeons, we must continue to respect the past, which includes the professors and teachers who gave us the skills to perform surgery, with which we not only make a rewarding professional, intellectual living, but which also enables us to save lives and lead an amazing profession. The surgeon of the present is not only a surgeon but also a successful executive and leader of a major organization [29], yet only a handful of surgeons have had, or have, a chance to build new hospitals or transform the current establishment as physician chief executives.

Summary

It is difficult to imagine how a professor of surgery of the last century would react if one would have told him that one day we would be removing the appendix though the vagina or the mouth or that we would be using nanotechnology to deliver tiny tubes in places that only the greatest anatomist would know existed.

The patient, the public, and the hospitals expect the highest quality of care and best outcomes, which includes published individual and institutional results. Nationally, ACS and other groups have created a number of programs that measure quality (NSQIP, NTDB) and that have become models for the rest of the world.

Despite all technological advances, today's surgeon has multiple challenges which are encountered while using exciting technology that has changed the quality of care and allowed surgeons to enhance their patient-centered practices. These challenges include rapidly changing technology, increasing bureaucratic logistics, and revisions in hospital design that enhance the quality of care, while incorporating more complexities. Because of these changes, the new surgeon is required to be informed, alert, up to date, and ready for change, incorporating new knowledge of disease and technology, all the while jumping over the multiple hurdles that have always been present, and always keeping the patient foremost in mind.

References

1. Rickert J. Patient centered care: what it means and how to get there. Health Affairs Blog. http://healthaffairs.org/blog/2012/01/24/patient-centered-care-what-it-means-and-how-to-get-there/ Accessed 19 Nov 2014.
2. Sosin M, Patel KM, Nahabedian MY, Bhanot P. Patient-centered outcomes following laparoscopic ventral hernia repair: a systematic review of the current literature. Am J Surg. 2014;208:677–84.
3. Liang MK, Clapp M, Li LT, Berger RL, Hicks SC, Awad S. Patient satisfaction, chronic pain, and functional status following laparoscopic ventral hernia repair. World J Surg. 2013;37(3):530–7.
4. Durham RM, Zuckerman D, Wolverson M, Heiberg E, Luchtefeld WB, Herr DJ, Shapiro MJ, Mazuski JE, Salimi Z, Sundaram M. Computed tomography as a screening exam in patients with suspected blunt aortic injury. Ann Surg. 1994;220(5):699–704.
5. Brooks AP, Olson LK, Shackford SR. Computed tomography in the diagnosis of traumatic rupture of the thoracic aorta. Clin Radiol. 1989;40:133–8.
6. Moore FD. Metabolic care of the surgical patient. Philadelphia and London: W. B. Saunders Co; 1959.
7. Dudrick SJ, Wilmore DW, Vars HM, Rhoads JE. Long-term total parenteral nutrition with growth, development, and positive nitrogen balance. Surgery. 1968;64:134.
8. Lerner BH. The breast cancer wars. Fear, hope, and pursuit of a cure in 20th century America. New York: Oxford University Press; 2001.
9. Hermann RE. Three unforgettable surgeons. Surgery. 2004;135:1114–7.
10. Saxon W. Dr. George Crile Jr, 84, Foe of unneeded surgery dies. New York Times. http://www.nytimes.com/1992/09/12/us/dr-george-crile-jr-84-foe-of-unneeded-surgery-dies.html. Accessed 19 Nov 2014.
11. Reynolds Jr W. The first laparoscopic cholecystectomy. JSLS. 2001;5(1):89–94.
12. Iribarne A, Milner R, Merlo AE, Singh A, Saunders CR, Russo MJ. Outcomes following emergent open repair for thoracic aortic dissection are improved at higher volume centers. J Card Surg. 2015;30(1): 74–9.
13. Cameron JL, Riall TS, Coleman J, Belcher KA. One thousand consecutive pancreaticoduodenectomies. Ann Surg. 2006;244(1):10–5.
14. Winter JM, Cameron JL, Campbell KA, Arnold MA, Chang DC, Coleman J, Hodgin MB, Sauter PK, Hruban RH, Riall TS, Schulick RD, Choti MA, Lillemoe KD, Yeo CJ. 1423 pancreaticoduodenectomies for pancreatic cancer: a single-institution experience. J Gastrointest Surg. 2006;10(9):1199–210. discussion 1210-1.
15. Freischlag JA, Kibbe MR. The evolution of surgery: the story of "Two Poems". JAMA. 2014;312(17): 1737–8.
16. Pruitt Jr BA. Combat casualty care and surgical progress. Ann Surg. 2006;243(6):715–29.
17. Blackbourne LH, Baer DG, Eastridge BJ, Kheirabadi B, Bagley S, Kragh Jr JF, Cap AP, Dubick MA, Morrison JJ, Midwinter MJ, Butler FK, Kotwal RS, Holcomb JB. Military medical revolution: prehospital combat casualty care. J Trauma Acute Care Surg. 2012;73(6 Suppl 5):S372–7.
18. Ingalls N, Zonies D, Bailey JA, Martin KD, Iddins BO, Carlton PK, Hanseman D, Branson R, Dorlac W, Johannigman J. A review of the first 10 years of critical care aeromedical transport during operation Iraqi freedom and operation enduring freedom: the importance of evacuation timing. JAMA Surg. 2014;149(8):807–13.
19. Palm K, Apodaca A, Spencer D, Costanzo G, Bailey J, Blackbourne LH, Spott MA, Eastridge BJ. Evaluation of military trauma system practices related to damage-control resuscitation. J Trauma Acute Care Surg. 2012;73(6 Suppl 5):S459–64.
20. Shanafelt TD, Balch CM, Dyrbye L, Bechamps G, Russell T, Satele D, Rummans T, Swartz K, Novotny PJ, Sloan J, Oreskovich MR. Special report. Suicidal ideation among American surgeons. Arch Surg. 2011;146(1):54–62.
21. Bittner 4th JG, Khan Z, Babu M, Hamed O. Stress, burnout, and maladaptive coping: strategies for surgeon well-being. Bull Am Coll Surg. 2011;96(8): 17–22.
22. Balch CM, Freischlag JA, Shanafelt TD. Stress and burnout among surgeons: understanding and managing the syndrome and avoiding the adverse consequences. Arch Surg. 2009;144(4):371–6.
23. Balch CM, Shanafelt T. Combating stress and burnout in surgical practice: a review. Adv Surg. 2010;44:29–47. Review.
24. Shanafelt TD, Oreskovich MR, Dyrbye LN, Satele DV, Hanks JB, Sloan JA, Balch CM. Avoiding burnout: the personal health habits and wellness practices of US surgeons. Ann Surg. 2012;255(4):625–33.
25. Sakran JV, Kaafarani H, Mouawad NJ, Santry HP. When things go wrong. ACS Bull. 2011;96(8): 13–6.
26. Luu S, Leung SO, Moulton CA. When bad things happen to good surgeons: reactions to adverse events. Surg Clin North Am. 2012;92(1):153–61.
27. Wu A. Medical error: the second victim. the doctor who makes the mistake needs help too. BMJ. 2000; 320:726–7.
28. Wallace JE, Lemaire JB, Ghali WA. Physician wellness: a missing quality indicator. Lancet. 2009 ;374(9702):1714–21.
29. Look FD. Leadership and medicine. Gulf Breeze, FL: Fire Starter Publishing; 2009.

The Ever-Changing Departments of Surgery: The New Paradigm—The Roadmap to a Modern Department of Surgery

2

Rainer W.G. Gruessner

The Different Types of Surgery Departments: The "Old" and "New" Schools

Departments of surgery are not isolated islands; they are and need to be aligned with their respective institution's mission, vision, and goals. This basic requirement defines the type of a specific department of surgery. As a result, different types of departments of surgery exist:

- *First,* the department of surgery can be part of an academic institution within a medical school or part of a nonacademic healthcare organization with little interest in academic tasks such as research and education. For academic departments, clinical programs are not only revenue-generating units but also essential components for the advancement of research and education; for nonacademic departments, the focus lies primarily on financially solid clinical programs with excellent patient outcome and satisfaction but usually without an authentic interest in research and/or education.
- *Second,* the department of surgery can represent an "old-school" department in which all surgery services and subspecialties are bundled together or a "surgery-core" department which includes general surgery and a few other specialties which are usually not represented in independent departments; this may include cardiothoracic, pediatric, reconstructive, transplant, and vascular surgical services in different combinations. The former allows one to build noncompeting clinical programs and avoids competition for the same patients because of only one departmental leadership structure; the latter almost invites the development of competing clinical programs under multiple departmental leadership arrangements because of the substantial overlap between the different surgical services. One such example is whether the surgical director of a kidney transplant program should be a transplant surgeon or an urologist.

Historically, all surgical services were frequently concentrated under one departmental roof: this included such different specialties as orthopedic surgery, gynecology and obstetrics, ophthalmology, urology, ENT, and neurosurgery. In the 1960s and 1970s, depending on the institutional vision and goals, some of the surgical specialties were organized as independent departments because of strong clinical and academic performance, continued subspecialization, and/or in order to attract

R.W.G. Gruessner, M.D., F.A.C.S., F.I.C.S. (✉)
Department of Surgery, University of Arizona Medical Center, Tucson, AZ, USA
e-mail: rgruessner@surgery.arizona.edu

R. Latifi et al. (eds.), *Technological Advances in Surgery, Trauma and Critical Care*,
DOI 10.1007/978-1-4939-2671-8_2

some of the brightest faculty and residents. Over the next few decades, this splitting off of the "old-school" department of surgery continued, and, at most institutions, orthopedic surgery, gynecology and obstetrics, ophthalmology, urology, ENT, and neurosurgery have become independent departments. But even "surgery-core" departments have become smaller with cardiothoracic, reconstructive, pediatric, and/or vascular surgical services sometimes splitting off into independent departments. Only more recently, this trend seems to have stopped and some institutions have now begun to reintegrate surgical subspecialties into "old-school" or "surgery-core" departments. As always, financial considerations commonly dictate the setup of institution-specific departmental structures. Due to the explosion of surgical knowledge and techniques over the past decades, the "surgery-core" departments have also substantially grown in their own right and frequently include the following subspecialties: surgical oncology (e.g., breast, colorectal, HPB [hepato-pancreatico-biliary], skin, and soft tissue surgery), endocrine surgery, minimally invasive surgery (MIS, further divided into laparoscopic and robot-assisted services), transplant surgery, trauma, critical care surgery, and, most recently, acute care surgery. Of note, "general surgery" is hardly mentioned as an independent specialty: at many institutions it has been integrated into and absorbed by the different subspecialties.

- *Third,* surgery departments may also be defined by other factors: is the department's basis only one hospital, is there an additional VA association, or is it embedded in a system-wide, multiple hospital encompassing health system? What is the vision of the institutional leadership—to draw patients primarily from the community or to also attract patients regionally or even nationally? It is important to point out that extremely prosperous clinical programs offered by surgery departments frequently help to define the role and success of the entire institution. One such example is the transplant program that Dr. Thomas Starzl built at the University of Pittsburgh in the 1980s: he almost single-handedly created the largest transplant program of its kind not only in the nation, but in the world, which allowed his institution in years to come to grow into a multibillion health network by purchasing many others hospitals.

Institutional Reporting Structures

The reporting structures are obviously different for academic versus nonacademic institutions.

As surgery departments are solidly embedded into their respective institutions, the chair of an academic department usually reports directly to the dean of the college/school of medicine who appoints the chair and has the power to remove him/her from office as well. However, there are also "dotted" reporting lines to the CEO/president of the hospital or health organization and to the CEO/director of the practice plan. Thus, multiple reporting lines exist and strong alignment among the three entities is absolutely crucial for the success of the institution and the surgery department. If this alignment does not exist—sometimes called the "3-headed monster"—failure and turmoil are almost certain. Although it is rare at academic institutions that the college of medicine, the hospital(s), and the practice plan are united under one leader (usually the vice president of the academic health center), this structure clearly shortens and, in theory, improves the decision-making processes and strategic planning. More often, the hospital and the practice plan are united as one entity, and the college of medicine remains separate; this structure typically results in two separate leadership positions, and close collaboration between the two leaders is the key to success.

In contrast, nonacademic institutions have a different reporting structure. Here, the chair of the nonacademic department usually reports only to the CEO/president of the health organization or to his/her designee. This makes decision-making processes and strategic planning easier. However, nonacademic institutions are not infrequently associated with medical schools and both residents and students may spend rotations away from their academic institutions. In this case, the department chair may interact with the dean of the medical school but is usually not appointed by the dean and does not report directly to him. In case of an independent residency program at a nonacademic institution, a reporting structure to a dean may not exist at all.

At both academic and nonacademic institutions, the surgery chair reports to the institution's senior administrative leadership. While the surgery chair is in charge of departmental matters, he/she holds only a mid-level management position within the whole organization. Thus, the leader of the surgery department may help to influence key decisions but usually has no final say.

Involvement of the chair or his/her designee in strategic planning, contract negotiations with insurance providers, and other key organizational committees, task forces, etc. is of mutual advantage and benefits the whole organization.

The interaction between the chair and his/her supervisors (dean/hospital CEO) should be of mutual respect and requires the chair's ability to closely cooperate and to compromise with his/her supervisors. Consensus building and a clear understanding of the issues that the dean and hospital CEO are dealing with (beyond individual departmental matters) are additional attributes to a successful tenure as chair.

Departmental Structure and Organization

The department chair is ultimately responsible for all clinical, academic, financial, and administrative activities within the department. The chair should appoint a strong and loyal deputy chair who will represent the chair in his/her absence. The deputy chair is "primus inter pares" among the vice-chairs. In academic institutions, due to the size of surgery departments, several faculty members may serve administratively as vice-chairs. While there is no definitive number as to how many vice-chairs are required, the following positions are advisable: vice-chair for clinical affairs, vice-chair for academic affairs, vice-chair for financial affairs, vice-chair for education, and vice-chair for research. Other vice-chair positions, such as vice-chair for financial affairs, vice-chair for HR issues, etc. may also be reasonable. The chair, the various vice-chairs, and the division/section chiefs form the departmental "cabinet," the senior leadership group; it is not unusual that residency director(s), the surgery service chiefs at satellite hospitals, and the administrative director of the department join this group. Sharing responsibilities among the departmental leadership group fosters team work and consensus building.

The vice-chairs are usually in charge of their respective committees which should ideally consist of faculty members from different departmental divisions/sections. The committees should meet on a regular basis and a report should be generated at least twice per year for the chair's review.

The chair should meet individually and on a regular basis with all faculty members; this is usually mandated by most institutions in order to complete the annual faculty member evaluation. Depending on the size of the department, the chair may have the division/section chiefs meet with their junior faculty, but the chair should be responsible for the evaluations of his/her vice-chairs, division/section chiefs, and senior faculty. Since most academic institutions mandate a departmental mentoring plan for faculty, the evaluations should be based on expectations and benchmarks as defined by the individual mentoring plan. In most departments, division/section chiefs are responsible for mentoring of their junior faculty.

All faculty members should be encouraged to not only be members in their respective societies but also seek leadership positions. Equally important are membership in NIH study sections, national committees, and task forces. These engagements benefit the faculty member, the division/section, and the entire department. Representation of surgical faculty in institutional (college/university) or local community committees is equally significant.

Departmental faculty meetings or retreats should be conducted semiannually. It is important that all faculty members have access to key departmental information including departmental finances—the willingness of the chair to share "sensitive" financial information frequently results in faculty "buy-in" if unpopular measures (most commonly to balance the budget) need to be taken. The more transparent and accountable the chair acts, the greater the support of his faculty. "Cabinet" support for the chair is also essential. The chair has the obligation to be the best departmental steward possible and recognized as such—once the faculty members realize that the chair works diligently and honestly in his/her own and the department's best interest, support for the chair comes naturally.

The chair depends on the expertise of his/her financial team. Most chairs know relatively little about how to run a mid-size company such as a surgery department financially until they are on the job. Having the departmental financial team work with the college/hospital financial teams in close collaboration is the key to departmental and institutional success.

The chair should be fair and objective in distributing the scarce resources among the different divisions. Although it is the prerogative of the chair to set departmental priorities, it appears prudent to support his/her programs in an equal fashion. It frequently helps the chair's overall reputation if he/she is still clinically active and operates on patients. That way, the chair remains in the loop with regard to issues in the clinics, operating rooms, etc. In contrast to nonsurgical disciplines, surgeons develop a high degree of respect for their leader if the clinical programs that he/she directs are successful and if the faculty knows of the chair's excellent technical skills. Given the background of great clinical accomplishments, the chair should ordinarily be the one who runs the departmental morbidity and mortality conferences as well as grand rounds.

In contrast to departmental chairs, system chairs overseeing surgical services at several hospitals within a large health network tend to be mostly administrators with little or no clinical responsibility. The role of a system chair is more frequently found in nonacademic institutions and focuses on developing smooth algorithms and operations within the organization to ensure an effective and productive work environment for all surgeons that are affiliated.

Being a chair can be very satisfactory, but you have to pick your battles wisely and always remember that the average chair survival is no longer than 10 years. A chair should steadfastly stand by his principles and moral convictions and realize when the time has come that he is no longer a good fit for the organization that he serves. Ultimately, despite the power and authority that the chair enjoys in his/her department, the position of a chair is that of a mid-level administrator. Rarely does a chair have final say in institutional matters; it is important for the chair to realize his/her limitations with regard to extra-departmental issues and the willingness to cooperate and compromise with his/her supervisors and peers.

Departmental Infrastructure and Resources

Provision of adequate space has become a top priority and top concern for departmental leadership; basically, there is never enough space to accommodate all departmental needs. Space is needed for faculty offices, administrative support staff, residency quarters, and laboratories. Conference rooms and auditoriums are usually shared between departments within the college of medicine.

The number of support staff depends on the department's financial circumstances and that of individually funded faculty. The administrative assistance to faculty ratio can range from 1 to 10.

Additional administrative support staff is required for residency, clerkship, and fellowship programs.

Due to the close interaction, the chair's office(s) should be in close proximity to the administrative offices—the chair meets regularly and frequently several times per week with the department's administrative director who oversees all financial matters and reports directly to the chair. In contrast to the administrative offices, coding and billing offices are frequently no longer departmental units, but rather centralized. Unfortunately, this is a shift towards less departmental autonomy and commonly dictated by financial considerations.

To fulfill the educational mission, academic support staff is essential. Depending on the funding opportunities, financial support for a (bio-) statistician, research nurses, data manager, and an editor is desirable. Sometimes these resources need to be shared with other departments. Because innovative and rare surgical procedures have a high PR effect, the recruitment of a departmental PR manager/director and a fundraising director will enhance the department's regional/national reputation and increase the number of donation and gifts. In times of financial tightness, the role of the latter two positions is controversial; however, financial analyses commonly show that a successful departmental fundraiser generates enough income through donations to justify his/her salary. A PR manager or marketing director is not only responsible for disseminating departmental news (through newsletters or the departmental web site) but also coordinates meetings with both established and newly referring physicians. Both fundraiser and PR manager are crucial in developing good relationships with the local/regional communities and can frequently establish new national connections.

IT support staff is essential for the various faculty, resident, and staff needs and is usually shared with other departments within the college of medicine or the hospital. Advertising on Google, Twitter, Facebook pages, etc. has become important departmental tools to connect with physicians, patients, and communities.

Departmental resources are usually scarce; major recruitment or retention packages (see below) are generally not possible without hospital/college/university support. Many surgery departments have little or no financial reserves. Interest from endowed chairs is ordinarily used to support faculty salaries rather than research endeavors. Successful fundraising and other departmental activities as described below have become increasingly important avenues to accrue additional revenue.

Financial Requirements

Financial stability of any surgery department is pivotal to its academic and clinical success.

By and large, surgery departments depend on the following types of income: (1) clinical revenue as generated by faculty, residents, mid-level providers etc.; (2) financial support from the hospital and the college of medicine/university; (3) grant funding and research dollars; (4) donations, gifts, departmental reserves, and interest (endowed chairs); (5) patents, device development, telemedicine services, and industry support.

Clinical revenue usually contributes the most to departmental income. However, most surgery departments cannot rely on clinical income alone: faculty salaries, specifically in competitive markets and recruitment of highly qualified staff, require additional hospital and/or college/university support; depending on the institution, additional support may add another 25–50 % to the department's budget. Strong funding of grants and research is important to the department's national reputation and to attract highly talented faculty and residents, but departments themselves usually do not profit financially from research funding unless some of the indirect costs are redistributed to the department. Donations and gifts can add substantially to a department's bottom line if successful departmental fundraising is accomplished. Interest from endowed chairs usually contributes little to the overall bottom line; the same is true for income from patents or device development.

On the downside, departments are facing increased taxation specifically from the college of medicine (e.g., dean's tax) and the practice plans (e.g., for central coding and billing). Close interaction between the departmental administrative/financial director and the hospital and college CFOs is crucial to establish a balanced budget. Since surgical services attract a high-margin, elective patient clientele the downstream effect that surgery generates is not only substantial for the hospital itself but for many other departments such as anesthesiology, pathology/laboratory medicine, radiology, medicine, etc.

It is important to educate hospital and university administrators about the downstream effect generated by the surgery department particularly for surgical programs that at first sight appear not to be profitable (e.g., surgical breast cancer or wound healing programs). If the downstream effect is taken into consideration, a money-losing surgical program may still be an essential part of a multidisciplinary and financially profitable program and should not be closed. Under these circumstances, the chair may ask for additional support from the institution for such programs in order to avoid a (potentially steep) salary cut for the affected faculty member and growing faculty frustration and dissatisfaction.

Providing financial information to individual faculty members on a regular basis (preferably monthly) regarding their billings and collections is essential to keep faculty members up-to-date and educated as to their individual financial performance. Regular information about the individual faculty member's financial performance also allows for his/her timely adjustment(s) of clinical activities or for coding/billing corrections. It also provides the basis for salary alterations based on clinical activities or funded support for research, education, and administrative duties. It is important to emphasize that the financial support for educational and administrative responsibilities is unfortunately the weakest of all due to the scarce financial resources of most surgery departments.

Faculty Recruitment and Retention

Successful recruitment of excellent faculty at academic departments and successful recruitment of outstanding surgeons at nonacademic departments is critical to the mission and vision of most surgery departments and institutions. Recruitment efforts have to be aligned with the existing infrastructure and the strategic objectives of both department and institution. It is usually easier to recruit a new faculty member or a surgeon to an already existing and established clinical program. Recruitment(s) for new clinical programs is more complex and frequently requires flexibility, patience, and persistence on part of the recruited faculty/surgeon as well as on the hospital side. To make new clinical programs successful, market and pro-forma analyses need to be performed: they are essential to define clinical, financial, and academic expectations and benchmarks. New clinical programs may require costly investments in cutting-edge devices (e.g., daVinci robot) or expensive renovation and expansion of operating rooms (e.g., construction of hybrid ORs). Appropriate funds (usually from the hospital) have to be available before the recruitment commences.

How can the best faculty/surgeons be attracted? It is usually easier to attract outstanding faculty/surgeons to institutions that have an established track record of high performance, stimulating work environment, and financial stability. Outstanding recruitment candidates are usually attracted by the presence of like-minded and similarly performing faculty/surgeon(s), nationally reputed departments, and prestigious institutions. But an attractive recruitment package and a grand organizational vision may sway reluctant but exceptional candidates to even less reputable institutions: such enticements may include above-average AAMC salary, salary guarantee for several years, strong program support (e.g., mid-level providers, administrative assistance, etc.), sign-on bonus, incentive payments, and/or additional administrative responsibilities.

In general, recruitments should be pursued in such a way that all stakeholders within the department, the hospital, and the college of medicine are involved in the interview process and the candidate selection. The broader the consensus is between the different stakeholders, the greater the chance is of successful recruitment and buy-in from all sides. Broad initial support is also necessary if the program fails eventually. In that case, it is not the "fault" of the surgery chair alone (or whoever is in charge of the recruitment) but of everyone who was involved and agreed to the recruitment.

Consensus in faculty recruitment is important to pick the "right" candidate: this may not necessarily be the one with the most outstanding CV but an individual who understands the importance of teamwork and his/her role within the system.

The recruitment of exceptional faculty and building/expansion of excellent clinical programs have an important ripple effect: it facilitates the department's recruitment of top medical students, residents, and fellows alike and it allows other departments to recruit faculty of similar caliber.

Retention of respected or key faculty is as important as is recruitment—and, in most cases, it is usually financially more prudent to retain a valued faculty member than to recruit a new one. Retention packages frequently include salary increases, additional program support, and/or additional administrative responsibilities and titles.

In contrast to whole departments, individual faculty members in this day and age are no longer "triple-threats" because of the complex and time-consuming challenges in clinical, research, and educational activities. At most academic institutions, faculty members are "dual-threats." Beyond the traditional big "3 s," administrative duties represent now an independent yet equally important and demanding field.

Clinical Services and Programs

Like with faculty recruitment, expansion of existing and development of new clinical programs has to be aligned with the institutional goals and infrastructure. First and foremost, the institutional goals should be defined by the needs of the local/regional community and are frequently in competition with other hospitals. As programs or centers of excellence develop, regional or even national recognition may result in further expansion. Institutional support is critical to provide the necessary infrastructure which may include additional personnel, additional space (clinics and/or operating rooms), and/or purchase of new, and frequently expensive, surgical equipment. Institutions tend to more readily support multidisciplinary programs or programs that generate substantial downstream revenue. The key to institutional support is the development of a robust financial model and broad consensus among the program stakeholders which should include the department chair(s) and the institution's senior leadership. A market analysis needs to be the basis for expansion or development of new programs. There also needs to be an institutional willingness to invest into PR activities, ranging from TV commercials and advertisements to education of referring physicians and patients. At regular meetings, the clinical service or program director has to provide updates to his administrative partners and/or supervisors within the hospital and college. These status reports are important to let the stakeholders know about potential issues, additional needs or modifications of benchmarks, and financial projections or adjustments. Finally, the success of financially viable programs is also measured by patient outcome and satisfaction—these factors usually determine a program's future.

Education

In academic departments, residency and fellowship programs as well as the education of medical students are essential components of the academic mission. All departmental faculty members must have a sincere interest in education and enjoy their involvement in educational activities. A solid clinical training experience is the foundation of any residency program. This includes sufficient and adequate operating experience, excellent patient care and management, as well as participation in all types of teaching activities. Residents expect valuable feedback from faculty, and faculty expect a genuine interest in all aspects of surgical care from their residents. Faculty evaluations and annual in-service tests are critical tools for resident assessment.

Departmental compliance with residency requirements is essential for continued program accreditation. Although the work hour limitations are not infrequently questioned by both faculty and residents (e.g., residents not being able to participate in an operation despite their interest and willingness because of possible duty hour violations), the regulations have to be honored and individuals who violate against them have to be reprimanded and/or face other consequences.

What elements make a specific residency program more attractive than others? In their interviews, resident candidates tend to focus on excellent training, a friendly and collegial climate, a productive and successful work environment, and a reliable and honest interaction between faculty and fellow residents. Without doubt, these factors are important but so are the residents' academic accomplishments which only few at that early stage in their career fully understand. To get residents started in their academic endeavors, there should be a departmental policy that within the first year each resident has to identify a faculty mentor. There should also be a requirement that each resident has to author or coauthor 1 scientific manuscript per year. This ensures that each resident at the end of the residency has at least five publications to his/her credit which positions any resident very competitively when applying for a fellowship or a junior faculty/staff position. Residents should also be encouraged to present their research at local, regional, and national meetings specifically if departmental resources are available. If possible, academic departments should make ongoing research opportunities available to residents. For those residents that are interested in basic science research, under optimal conditions, a 1–3 years laboratory experience to obtain an MS or PhD degree is preferably offered after the third year. Acceptance into such a departmental research program should be considered an extraordinary achievement in itself: it requires the resident to work with the academic mentor in such a way that a resident research grant within the first 2 years should be submitted. Depending on the funding opportunities, the resident may then pursue a scientific career aside from the clinical training. Departmental honors and awards for clinical or research accomplishments create further incentives for the residents to excel.

Another attraction to residents and resident candidates is a functioning departmental animal lab. Such facilities allow residents to acquire for example minimally invasive or robotic techniques in large animals and help to avoid technical unpreparedness in the clinical setting. It is preferable to offer these courses to residents 1 week at a time and relieve the residents from all clinical duties during the course duration. A decrease in operating times, a decrease in cost, superior clinical resident training, etc. are commonly the results of these animal lab courses.

Fellows are usually attracted by strong clinical programs and should be encouraged by their faculty to engage in clinical and translational research. As mentioned below, easy access to databases as well as biostatistical and editorial support are crucial ingredients for fellows to become academically prolific.

Medical students need to be engaged in the field of surgery. All too often, faculty and residents are not genuinely interested in time-consuming training of medical students because they are still so early in their career. However, to get them interested in applying for a residency in surgery, they should not only do H&Ps and busy work but also participate in the operating room and learn basic surgical tasks (e.g., skin closure, placement and removal of drains, etc.). Because the quality of life of surgeons is frequently considered to be lower than that of other specialties, it is important to demonstrate to students the great personal satisfaction that comes from the surgical profession. Getting medical students interested in all aspects of surgery and convincing them to apply for a surgical residency is crucial for our profession since our nation will face a critical shortage of surgeons in the near future.

Presence at morbidity and mortality conferences, didactic sessions, journal club meetings, and grand rounds should be mandatory for all residents and medical students on surgery rotations. The results of the annual resident in-service exams provide a tool to the residency leadership to identify weak performers and to focus on improving their results.

Surgery departments should regularly organize meetings and conferences for educational purposes where faculty and residents present. Such activities help to expand ties with the local community and attract referring physicians specifically if CME credits are awarded.

Research

For academic departments the research component is of fundamental importance as it, more than almost anything else, defines the department's national reputation. The recruitment of researchers has to be aligned primarily with the vision and goals of the college of medicine. The development of new research programs should be coordinated in such a way that interdepartmental or even intercollegial cooperation is accomplished. This approach usually increases the chances of extramural funding.

A department's national research ranking is a reflection of the overall research money that is available from all types of grants but specifically from NIH funding. For clinically active surgeons, it has become increasingly difficult to obtain NIH funding. The right choice of co-investigator(s) (Ph.D., biostatistician, etc.) is a crucial decision that frequently determines if funding is obtained or not. Junior faculty with research support as part of their recruitment package should be encouraged to seek collaboration across the college of medicine or across campus, specifically with college of science faculty. Junior faculty funding is usually provided by the department or the college of medicine for 1–2 years, with benchmarks attached and the expectation that continued funding will be obtained. This puts tremendous pressure on junior faculty who, at an early stage in their career, are also expected to become increasingly clinically active.

Each academic department should have a few well-funded laboratories in place, also to provide research opportunities to residents and medical students. Individual laboratories should be aligned with core facilities and laboratories to avoid costly duplication of services and to foster collaboration. A sore subject to all researches has been the topic of high indirect costs; a solution to this problem is not on the horizon.

Aside from basic science research, surgery departments need to be engaged in translational and clinical research as well. Not infrequently, clinical trials may generate additional income to the department if effectively conducted. Sharing of research nurses and administrative staff when multiple clinical trials or studies are conducted at the same time is one such way that can contribute to greater cost-effectiveness.

Challenges

It is evident that the challenges for surgery departments are multiple and frequently not easy to overcome. Departments of surgery are expected to be leaders in generating hospital income and downstream revenue for other departments and the organization. With dwindling reimbursement rates, diminished institutional support, etc. it is all but impossible to fulfill these expectations particularly in light of absent financial resources within the department. The chair's negotiation skills, additional institutional support, and a strong chair recruitment package are all necessary to provide a positive bottom line. Ongoing institutional support remains the key to departmental growth and success.

Centers and multidisciplinary programs frequently weaken departmental positions by tapping into their resources and increasing their financial burden. One such example is the department's responsibility for faculty salaries but income generated from clinical services staying with centers or programs. Another example is open-staff hospital policies that may cause issues when surgeons that are associated with the department and/or a single practice plan compete with private practice surgeons for operating room availabilities and capacities. Hospital directorship positions are frequently not standardized in terms of financial support and may cause friction among faculty. And a high faculty turnover is definitively not wanted as it indicates departmental instability and volatility. All these challenges require a high degree of persistence, determination, and perseverance on part of the chair and the departmental leadership to stay course and lead the department successfully.

Finally, on a personal level, an advice to future chairs: it is lonely at the top. You have to almost constantly compromise: usually, if both sides are equally happy or unhappy with your decision(s), you are "leading from the middle," using common sense. You will notice that no one ever comes to your office to tell you that he/she is absolutely happy, has no requests whatsoever, and is not interested in a salary increase. And no one will honestly tell you that you are doing a great job. You, the chair, are constantly challenged, in the middle of controversies, and forced to make unpopular and difficult decisions. The chair has to be guided by objective, transparent, and reproducible decisions based on facts and evidence and be documented as such. Strong support for the chair's decisions should come from the cabinet after appropriate consultation, from task forces, special investigators, and various committees.

Summary

Surgery departments have evolved remarkably over the past century from relatively simple constructs providing primarily clinical services to "triple-threat" (clinical, educational, and research) units and ultimately to complex, multi-matrix-embedded entities that must withstand, and adapt to, the numerous challenges of our constantly changing health system. The financial survivability of surgery departments has added yet another dimension that severely impacts the traditional departmental tasks both in positive and negative ways. What has not changed over time is that the departmental reputation continues to depend on the quality of surgeons/faculty which in turn determines the quality of the residents. Departments remain the foundation of progress in surgical research and education and the place to train the next generation of surgeon leaders. Clinical service lines, multidisciplinary programs, and center designations have not eliminated the need for surgery departments which remain the "home" to surgeon faculty. Most surgery departments can no longer survive on clinical income only, and financial support for research and education is dwindling. Nowadays departmental leadership is forced to attract new sources of income in form of industry collaboration, gifts and donations, patents, device development, and other creative activities. Most importantly, surgery departments are not isolated islands but important components of healthcare-providing institutions; surgery departments have to be aligned with the institutional vision, mission, and goals in order to successfully provide the highest service to both the institution and the community that they serve.

Genomics in Surgery, Trauma, and Critical Care: How Do We Control the Future?

3

Matthew J. Delano and Ronald V. Maier

Introduction

Deoxyribonucleic acid (DNA) microarray technology evolved from the initial reports published in the 1970s indicating that labeled nucleic acids could be incorporated to monitor the expression of nucleic acid molecules attached to solid state support scaffolds. Over the next 20 years, genomic analysis methods continued to evolve until 1995 when the first article describing the application of DNA microarray technology used for genomic expression analysis was published.

Over the last two decades the manner of application of genome-wide expression analysis at the cellular level has exploded. Microarray technology has made dramatic advancements since its development and gained an increasing popularity among scientist, researchers, biologist, oncologist, statisticians, and physicians. The broad array of technological advancements and biological applications that comprise the field of human genomic analysis has solidified microarray technology indispensable as a research methodology and robust diagnostic tool.

The prevalence of DNA microarray technology along with its ubiquitous adoption by industry, medicine, and research laboratories has fostered the ability to quickly and accurately perform simultaneous analysis of thousands of genes or proteins. A single human microarray provides the ability to analyze the entire human genome from a single peripheral blood or tissue sample providing extensive and valuable information on gene expression, interaction, and function in a disease-specific manner. In this chapter our aim is to give a brief overview of cDNA microarray technology and how its application has contributed to the evolution of surgical diseases from oncology, to trauma, and critical care.

DNA Microarray Technology

DNA microarray technology in its simplest sense is a high-throughput, versatile technology used for prokaryotic and eukaryotic gene expression analysis of thousands of known or unknown genes in a simultaneous fashion. A more precise and accurate definition of DNA microarray technology is an orderly arrangement of thousands of identified sequenced genes printed on an impermeable solid support scaffold, usually glass, silicon chips, or nylon membrane.

M.J. Delano, M.D., Ph.D.
Division of Acute Care Surgery, Department of Surgery, University of Michigan Health System, Ann Arbor, MI, USA
e-mail: mjdelano@umich.edu

R.V. Maier, M.D., F.A.C.S. (✉)
Department of Surgery, Harborview Medical Center, University of Washington, Seattle, WA, USA
e-mail: ronmaier@uw.edu

R. Latifi et al. (eds.), *Technological Advances in Surgery, Trauma and Critical Care*,
DOI 10.1007/978-1-4939-2671-8_3

Basics of Microarray Technology

DNA microarray analysis is an efficient, flexible, and versatile approach to achieve high-throughput explorations of genome structure, expression, and function at the cellular and organism levels. This capability provides researchers and clinicians alike with a powerful tool to discern between, confirm diagnosis, and make predictions in various disease states. DNA microarray analysis is a complex multistep process involving numerous and specific pieces of scientific instrumentation and strong multidisciplinary expertise in various scientific and medical specialties including molecular biology, image analysis, statistical computing, and medical genetics.

Scientists use DNA microarrays to measure the expression levels of large numbers of genes simultaneously or to genotype multiple regions of a genome. A DNA microarray (also commonly known as DNA chip, biochip, or gene chip) is a collection of microscopic DNA spots attached to a solid surface. Each DNA spot contains a specific DNA sequence, or probes (probe sets, reporters, or oligos). These can vary between a short section of a gene or other DNA-based target elements that are used to hybridize a strand of cDNA (complimentary DNA) synthesized from a purified, tissue-specific mRNA (messenger ribonucleic acid) template in a catalyzed reaction using reverse transcriptase and DNA polymerase reactions. Probe-target hybridization is usually detected and quantified by detection of a fluorochrome, silver, or chemiluminescence, labeled targets to determine relative abundance of nucleic acid sequences in the target.

Once the experimental tissue is processed and hybridized to the gene chip, the gene chip fluorescence is quantified with a specific gene chip scanner that transposes the fluorescence values at each target probe into specific gene or probe set expression levels. Using an ever evolving cadre of powerful statistical analysis packages the genomic expression levels can be compared between groups of patients, tissues, cells, or normal controls to discover genomic differences between control and test groups. A schematic of the methodology involved to process an experimental tissue, hybridize the target cDNA to the gene chip, and then analyze the chip for meaningful genomic expression values is summarized in Fig. 3.1.

In addition to high-throughput genomic analysis, another complimentary tool for the analysis of proteins and other physiologic biomarkers is based on multiplex technologies intended to detect low levels of multiple protein types from a single tissue, blood, or urine sample. Multiplex technology is bead-based multiplexing, where beads are internally dyed with fluorescent dyes to produce a specific spectral or fluorescence address. Biomolecules, such as antibodies, can be conjugated to the surface of inert beads to capture physiologic molecules of interest. This technology uses flow cytometric or other imaging technologies for characterization of the beads as well as detection of the light emission due to target molecule presence. Luminex™ (Austin, TX) technology enables up to 500 proteins to be detected in each well of a 96-well plate, using very small starting sample volumes. Common applications include cytokines, chemokines, metabolic markers, autocrines, and phosphorylated proteins. A schematic representation of the tissue processing through data readout using a multiplex approach to cytokine analysis is depicted in Fig. 3.2.

Affymetrix GeneChip® Arrays (Santa Clara, CA)

Affymetrix makes quartz chips for genome-wide analysis called GeneChips. Affymetrix's GeneChips enable researchers to quickly scan for the presence of particular genes in a variety of biological samples. Moreover, Affymetrix is uniquely focused on oligonucleotide microarray technology. These specific microarrays are incorporated to determine which genes exist in a biologic sample by detecting precise pieces of mRNA.

Each gene on an Affymetrix microarray Gene Chip is typically represented by a probe set consisting of 11 different pairs of 25-bp oligos covering features of the transcribed region of that gene.

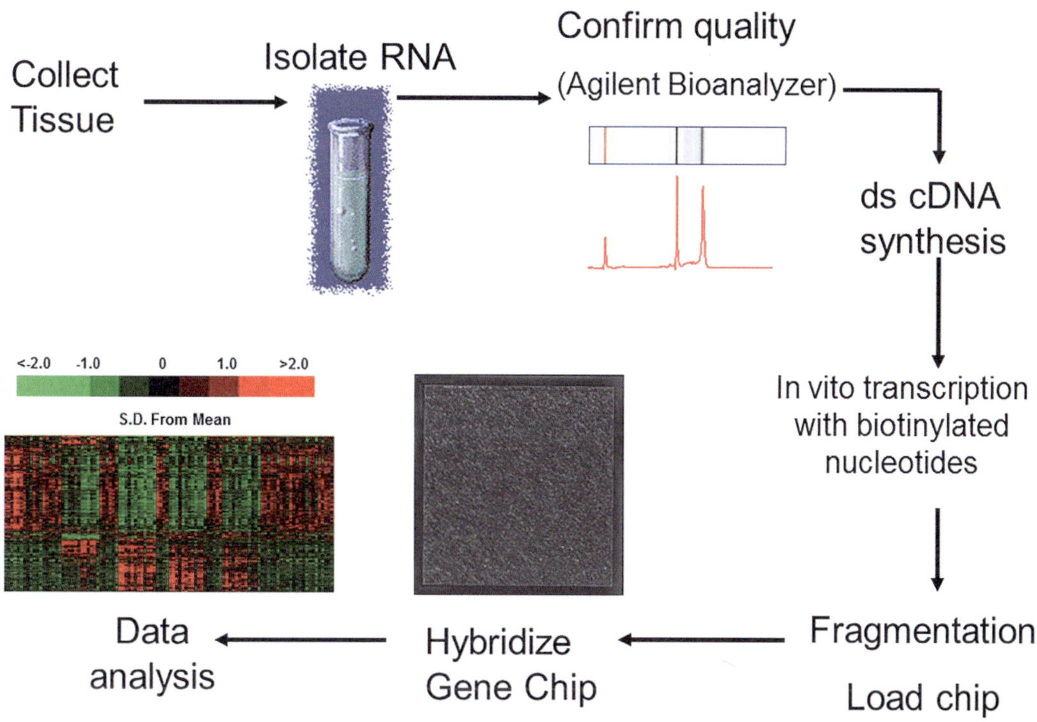

Fig. 3.1 Schematic of sample processing to gene chip analysis. A schematic of the methodology involved to process an experimental tissue, hybridize the target cDNA to the gene chip, and then analyze the chip for meaningful genomic expression values

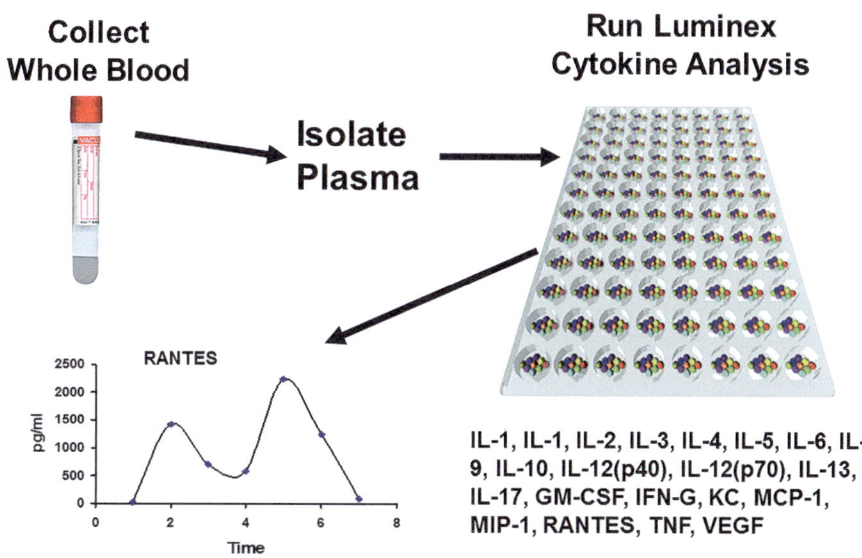

Fig. 3.2 Multiplex cytokine analysis. A schematic representation of the tissue processing through data readout required using a multiplex approach to cytokine analysis

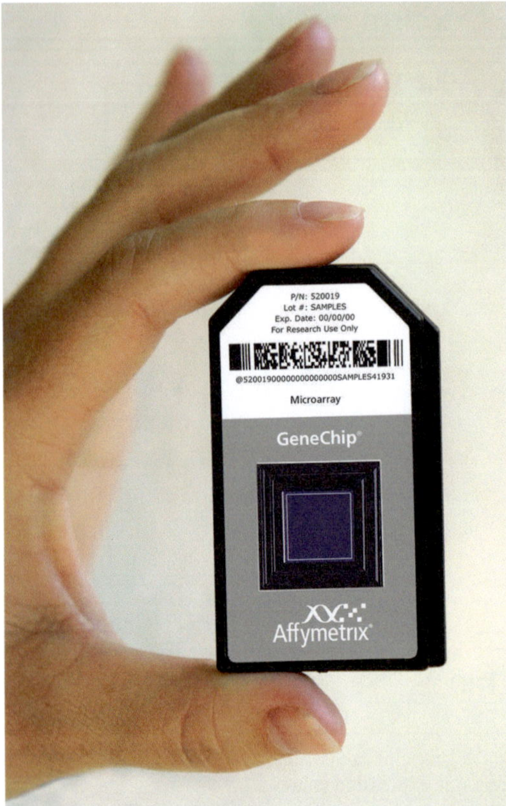

Fig. 3.3 Affymetrix U133 2.0. This is an actual Affymetrix U133 2.0 human GeneChip®. A single gene chip packed with fragments from each of the 35,000 known genes that make up the human genome. (Courtesy of Affymetrix, Inc., Santa Clara, CA, USA)

Each pair consists of a perfect match (PM) and a mismatch (MM) oligonucleotide. The PM probe exactly matches the sequence of a particular standard genotype, often one parent of a cross, while the MM differs in a single substitution in the central, 13th base. The MM probe is designed to distinguish noise caused by nonspecific hybridization from the specific hybridization signal. Affymetrix GeneChip microarrays are the most popular high density oligonucleotide gene expression arrays and have become an invaluable tool in genomics studies worldwide. Figure 3.3 represents an actual Affymetrix Human Gene Chip U133 plus 2.0.

Microarray Technology Impacts Surgical Care

Each human cell contains approximately three billion DNA base pairs that are estimated to encode approximately 30,000 genes that are responsible for maintaining the structural and functional integrity of a cell. These genes encode the RNA and proteins that produce the cell phenotype. A neoplastic phenotype develops out of an aberration or alteration in the normal expression of genes. A variety of specific mechanisms have been implicated in the transformation process including chromosomal rearrangement, deletions, amplification, methylation, and mutations of genes. Elucidating the fundamental molecular mechanisms that are involved in the stepwise progression from normal tissues to malignant tumors, organ-specific inflammation or systemic inflammation is essential in our knowledge of the development of cancers. This would ultimately lead to improved methods of detection, treatment, and cures for cancers. Comprehensive analyses of cancer genomes promise to better inform prognoses and improve precise cancer treatments improving patient-centered and specific cancer care and chemotherapeutics [1].

Melanoma

Malignant melanoma is a highly aggressive disease accounting for a majority of the deaths from skin malignancies with patient survival dependent on early detection and diagnosis. Although some promising new therapies have recently emerged, a better understanding of the molecular alterations involved in melanoma progression, particularly from localized tumors to metastasis, such as genomic and epigenetic aberrations, will aid in early detection and development of biomarkers and future targeted treatment strategies.

Melanoma, like other solid tumors, is thought to arise from a series of genetic and epigenetic events. Genetic aberrations have been identified in the past decade and have potential utility as biomarkers. Multiple studies have revealed that epigenetic events, such as genomic promoter region methylation of CpG islands, histone modification, and microRNA (miRNA) expression, have been shown to be important regulators of melanoma progression, and that these epigenetic changes can potentially serve as molecular biomarkers in tumor tissues and in blood as circulating DNA, for diagnosing disease and predicting disease outcome and progression [2].

Epigenetics refers to heritable changes in gene expression that are not caused by changes in the genomic DNA sequence. DNA methylation is one of the hallmark epigenetic events most studied in cancers. DNA methylation involves the addition of a methyl group to the 5′ carbon of a cytosine ring located 5′ to a guanosine base in a CpG dinucleotide and is catalyzed by DNA methyltransferases. Methylation events of promoter regions have been strongly implicated in cutaneous melanoma progression. Many of these genes are involved in cell cycle control, cell signaling, migration and invasion, apoptosis, angiogenesis, and metastasis. Comparing the methylation status of melanoma primary tumor and metastasis, an increase in hypermethylation of WIF1, TFPI2, RASSF1A, and SOCS1 was seen with increasing clinical tumor stage. Despite advances in this field and development of multiple platforms for studying genomic methylation, uniformity and standardization remain significant issues in evaluating and comparing results.

miRNAs are evolutionarily conserved, endogenous, noncoding RNA transcripts of 22 nucleotides in length that serve to temporally and spatially regulate biological function. miRNAs are considered an epigenomic mechanism that can have normal regulatory function but also can have negative influence when dysregulated, particularly in cancer progression as in melanoma. They are derived from noncoding intergenic or intronic regions of DNA that, once in their mature form, interfere with protein translation from mRNA transcripts. miRNA can preferentially bind with mRNA transcripts to inhibit translation or degrade the mRNA transcript before translation can take place. miRNA can modulate biological functions such as cell cycle, proliferation, apoptosis, and angiogenesis, which, if aberrantly regulated, can lead to malignancy. As an example miR-221/222 was found to interfere with c-KIT and p27, causing dysregulation of the cell cycle during the progression of melanoma. miRNA regulation may influence the microenvironment and can contribute to tumor cell invasion, migration, and metastasis. miRNA regulation of protein coding genes is, therefore, an essential regulatory element in biological development and function [2]. Lastly, deregulated miRNA expression may serve as diagnostic or prognostic biomarker in cutaneous melanoma.

By collectively assimilating the ever evolving cadre of miRNA, biomarkers, epigenetic phenomena, and small molecule expression markers, genomic expression finger prints can be developed that serve to stratify malignant melanoma metastatic risk, responsiveness to therapy, and even long-term survival odds prospectively and prior to therapeutic intervention. No more will the responsiveness to therapy be the clinicians best guess and experience but rather based on individualized genetic and biomarker-specific expression matrix gathered from each patient.

Prostate Cancer

Prostate cancer is the most common type of cancer in men and the second leading cause of cancer death in men in the United States. The recent surge of high-throughput sequencing of cancer genomes has supported an expanding molecular classification of prostate cancer. Translation of these basic science studies into clinically valuable biomarkers for diagnosis, prognosis, and biomarkers that are predictive for therapy is critical to the development of precision medicine in prostate cancer. Many recent genomic applications are aimed at improving screening specificity in prostate cancer by differentiating aggressive versus indolent prostate cancers. Over the past decade a host of candidate gene biomarkers have been centered on three distinct groups involving

ETS gene rearrangements, *PTEN* inactivation, and androgen receptor signaling. These and other putative biomarkers may provide a rationale for matching patients with molecularly targeted therapies in clinical trials [3].

One of the major barriers prohibiting scientist, oncologist, and clinicians from better understanding comprehensive analyses of prostate cancer genomes is the inaccessibility of metastatic tissue. A potential solution is to characterize circulating prostate tumor cells (CTCs). In the past this has required overcoming the challenges of isolating rare and metastatic prostate cancer cells and sequencing low-input material. However, recently investigators have reported an integrated process to isolate, qualify, and sequence whole exomes of prostate CTCs with high fidelity using a census-based sequencing strategy. The authors' data support the notion that CTC sequencing can reveal early mutations in tumor evolution and those that could be shared among metastatic sites. The genomic technology involved provides a minimally invasive window into the mutational landscape of metastatic prostate cancer and will provide investigators and clinicians with more robust tools to better tailor prostate cancer chemotherapeutics in cases of metastatic disease [4].

Breast Cancer

Cancer genomics has already revolutionized our knowledge of breast cancer molecular pathology, fostering the development of new and more effective clinical protocols. The most recent advances in the field of cancer genomics and epigenomics include DNA alterations and driver gene mutations, gene fusions, DNA methylation, and miRNA expression [5].

Genome-wide association studies have allowed the discovery of only a portion of genomic alterations associated with hereditary breast cancer risk. The genes BRCA1, BRCA2, TP53, PTEN, STK11, and CDH1 with high-penetrance mutations account for only 20–25 % of all cases of hereditary breast cancer. It has been speculated that the majority of breast cancer may be explained by the accumulation of low-penetrance and acquired genetic alterations, interacting together in a polygenic model, associated with a modification of the epigenetic component. The exact definition of the patient-specific occurrence and interaction of genomic alteration is expected to be the greatest contribution that next generation sequencing will provide to breast cancer management. Until the identification of these low-penetrance genomic influences is completed, treatment of breast cancer will continue to depend on the level of expression of receptors for estrogen, progesterone, and epidermal growth factor type 2 receptor (HER2/neu) [5]. However as the genomic expression profiles evolve new chemotherapeutics and chemotherapeutic combinations will be tailored to treat individual patients with breast cancer.

Inflammatory Bowel Disease

Inflammatory bowel disease (IBD) affects over 2.5 million people of European ancestry, with a rising prevalence in other countries. There is overwhelming evidence for the role of genetics in IBD as evidenced by initial reports of familial clustering. The last 15 years have seen a tremendous degree of progress regarding the identification of genetic loci involved in IBD. This has happened in part because of technological advances and growth in the genetic approaches used to identify these genes. Although other variations do exist, Crohn's disease and ulcerative colitis are the two most common forms of inflammatory disease and continue to confound investigators and clinicians [6].

Genome-wide association studies and meta-analyses of patients with these two diseases have implicated a sundry of previously unsuspected cellular mechanisms, such as autophagy, in their pathogenesis. Furthermore these findings have shown that some IBD loci are shared with other inflammatory diseases like ankylosing spondylitis. Meta-analysis of Crohn's disease and ulcerative colitis combined a total of more than 75,000 cases and controls in genome-wide association scans. The investigators found 71 new genomic associations for a total of 163 IBD loci that met genome-wide significance thresholds. The authors found that most of the discovered loci contribute to both IBD phenotypes. In addition many of the IBD-associated loci were also implicated in other immune-mediated disorders such as ankylosing spondylitis and psoriasis. An additional and unexpected finding was that there is considerable overlap between susceptibility loci for IBD and mycobacterial infection. Gene co-expression canonical pathway and network analysis emphasize this relationship, with pathways shared between host responses to mycobacteria and those predisposing to the development of IBD [7]. The findings suggest that either mycobacteria directly or the immune processes involved in mycobacteria eradication cause immune dysregulation which potentiates IBD development.

As a consequence of the ability to simultaneously scan and catalog thousands of genomic expression patterns for a disease state, biomarker panels with a high level of diagnostic sensitivity and specificity have been developed to more quickly and accurately identify patients with IBD. One such panel used in the diagnosis of Crohn's disease is the PROMETHEUS® Crohn's Prognostic test (Prometheus Labs, San Diego, CA). This technology combines proprietary serologic and genetic biomarkers in a logistic regression model to provide individual patients with probabilities for developing disease complications after diagnosis with Crohn's disease. The test enables physicians to stratify patients according to their risks of developing complications and develop patient-centered treatment plans rather than a blanket therapeutic approach.

Microarray Technology in Trauma and Critical Care

The *Inflammation and the Host Response to Injury* collaboration is a large-scale research program centered on the immune-inflammatory response in trauma and sepsis. The mission of the multi-institutional collaborative effort funded by the National Institute of Health is to understand key regulatory elements that drive the host's response to traumatic injury and its accompanying systemic inflammation response. The participating investigators used a discovery-driven approach to acquire large amounts of new human genomic data to try and identify genomic expression patterns that may serve as new targets for therapeutic development. In an effort to streamline the clinical sample processing and analysis, the investigators were able to develop novel genome-wide microarray technologies and introduce high-throughput proteomics to clinical medicine. These efforts have culminated in the identification of novel genomic and proteomic markers that predict patient outcomes and serve as new therapeutic targets for basic and clinical research and pharmaceutical development.

Human survival from traumatic injury whether penetrating or blunt requires an appropriate inflammatory and immune systemic response. Until recently, the immune cell genomic expression patterns underlying the systemic inflammatory response to traumatic injury were unknown. Investigators from the *Inflammation and the Host Response to Injury* have described the circulating leukocyte transcriptome after severe trauma and burn injury and have shown that severe injury produces a global reprioritization affecting greater than 80 % of the cellular functions and pathways in a manner they termed a "genomic storm." Early after severe traumatic injury, the investigators found that the leukocyte genomic response is consistent with a simultaneously increased expression of genes involved in the systemic inflammation, innate immunity, and the compensatory anti-inflammatory response with concomitant suppression of genes involved in adaptive immunity; see Fig. 3.4a–d. Moreover, complications such as nosocomial pneumonia and organ failure were not associated with any genomic evidence of a physiologic second hit phenomenon that has been historically postulated in the literature and clinical reports. The similarities in gene expression patterns between the various injury models investigated reveal a fundamental human genomic signature to

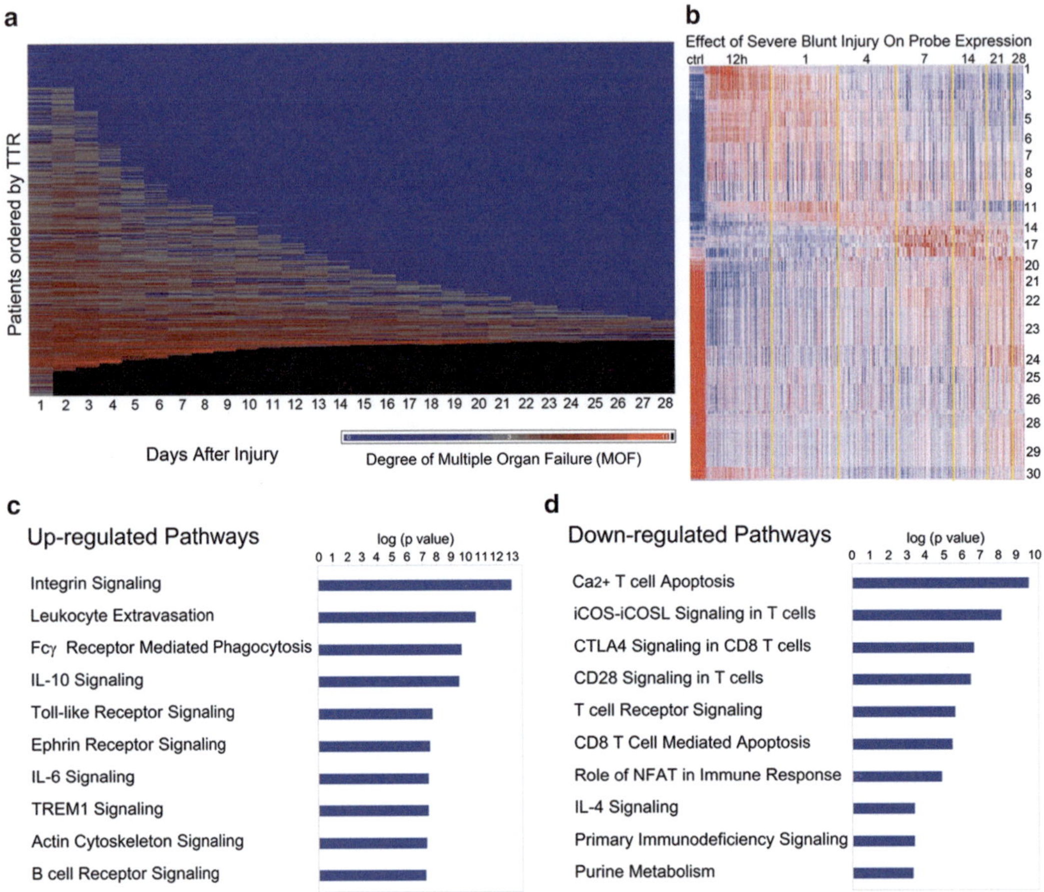

Fig. 3.4 (**a**–**d**) Immune cell gene expression in trauma. Organ injury and genomic changes associated with severe blunt trauma. (**a**) Whole blood was taken from severe blunt trauma patients, leukocytes were isolated, and total cellular RNA was extracted and hybridized onto an HU133 Plus 2.0 GeneChip® (Affymetrix, Santa Clara, CA). The continuum of clinical responses to severe blunt trauma in the 1,637 total patients from which the 167 sampling trauma patients were drawn is shown graphically. Each row represents an individual patient ordered by time to recovery (TTR), and the *x* axis represents time from injury in days. Patients are sorted from least to most severe organ injury and mortality. The presence and severity of organ injury is represented by colors from *blue* (least severe) to *red* (most severe). *Black* indicates death. (**b**) K-means clustering of the genes into 30 clusters based on patterns of expression over time. *Red* indicates increased and *blue* indicates decreased expression relative to the mean (*white*). Five thousand one hundred and thirty six genes were differentially expressed between patients and controls (ctrl; FDR <0.001 and at least twofold change). (**c**, **d**) Summary of the canonical pathways that are most affected by trauma. The graph shows the log10 (*p* value) of the enrichment of the pathway. (**a**–**d**: Copyright © Xiao et al. 2011. Originally published in Xiao W, Mindrinos MN, Seok J, Cuschieri J, Cuenca AG, Gao H, et al. A genomic storm in critically injured humans. The Journal of Experimental Medicine. 2011;208(13):2581–90)

inflammatory stress that are far more common than different [8]. This notion explains why simplistic models of inflammation based on one or several overexpressed biomarkers have simplistically failed over the past 40 years. Moreover, the data suggest a complex cellular system-based approach toward therapeutic intervention targeted at optimizing the patient's individualized inflammatory response may be more beneficial than the current single-agent interventions.

Class Prediction and Outcome of Sepsis in Trauma

Despite the advances in medical sciences, the morbidity and mortality due to sepsis in severe trauma patients remains high and thus there is a need for early and accurate identification of those patients that are genetically predisposed to develop severe sepsis or other complications that predispose the patient to poorer outcomes. Over the past three decades a vast amount of resources have been dedicated to determining a prediction model sensitive and specific enough to reasonably prognosticate which patients will develop severe sepsis and which will not. Using a high-throughput genomic strategy several recent reports show promise in being able to differentiate the groups of patients that will develop complications based on their genomic signature.

Complicated and Uncomplicated Outcomes in Trauma

Many patients have complicated recoveries following severe traumatic injury due to the development of end organ injury. Physiological biomarkers and prognosticators to date have had limited success in predicting patient clinical trajectories. Recently investigators from the *Inflammation and the Host Response to Injury* collaboration developed a retrospective validation of a simple genomic composite score that shows promise to rapidly predict clinical outcomes. Microarray-derived genomic data obtained from 167 severely traumatized patients over 28 days were assessed for differences in messenger RNA abundance among individuals with various clinical trajectories.

Once a set of genes was identified based on differences in expression over the entire study period, messenger RNA abundance from these subjects obtained in the first 24 h was analyzed using a rapid multiplex platform, and the genomic expression data reduced to a single metric. The researchers identified development of a genomic metric that can be rapidly used to predict clinical outcome in severely injured trauma patients; see Fig. 3.5a, b. The group then developed a composite score that showed good discriminatory capacity to distinguish patients with a complicated outcome which was significantly better than the predictive power of either Acute Physiology and Chronic Health Evaluation II or new injury severity score scoring systems. The excitement surrounding the study stems from the fact that clinicians can now obtain a rapid genomic composite score after trauma that can identify trauma patients who are likely to develop complicated clinical trajectories rather than the wait and see approach that is now used. The ability to accurately predict patient complication patterns would enable clinicians to develop new strategies to prevent rather than treat complications [9].

Gram-Negative Bacteremia and Outcomes

Trauma patients that develop bacteremia during their hospitalization have a higher risk of death than their non-bacteremic counterparts. However, the role that trauma altered immunity plays in the development of bacteremia was unknown until a recent report further elucidated the subject. Total leukocyte gene expression was used to compare trauma subjects in whom Gram-negative bacteremia developed and those in whom it did not develop. The results showed that Gram-negative bacteremia was found to be an independent risk factor for death.

The investigators went further to show that as hospitalization time progressed to 96 h after injury, 102 probes of genes were differentially expressed. Twenty probe sets represented fifteen innate or adaptive immunity genes. Some of the noteworthy genes discovered were a downregulation of *IL1B* and an upregulation of *IL1R2* which reflect suppression of innate immunity in patients developing Gram-negative bacteremia. In addition downregulation of adaptive immune genes in Gram-negative bacteremia subjects was also observed. The authors concluded that by 96 h after injury, there are differences in leukocyte gene expression associated with the subsequent development of Gram-negative bacteremia, reflecting suppression of both innate and adaptive immunity; see Fig. 3.6a, b. Importantly, Gram-negative bacteremia after trauma is, in part, the consequence of host immunity failure and

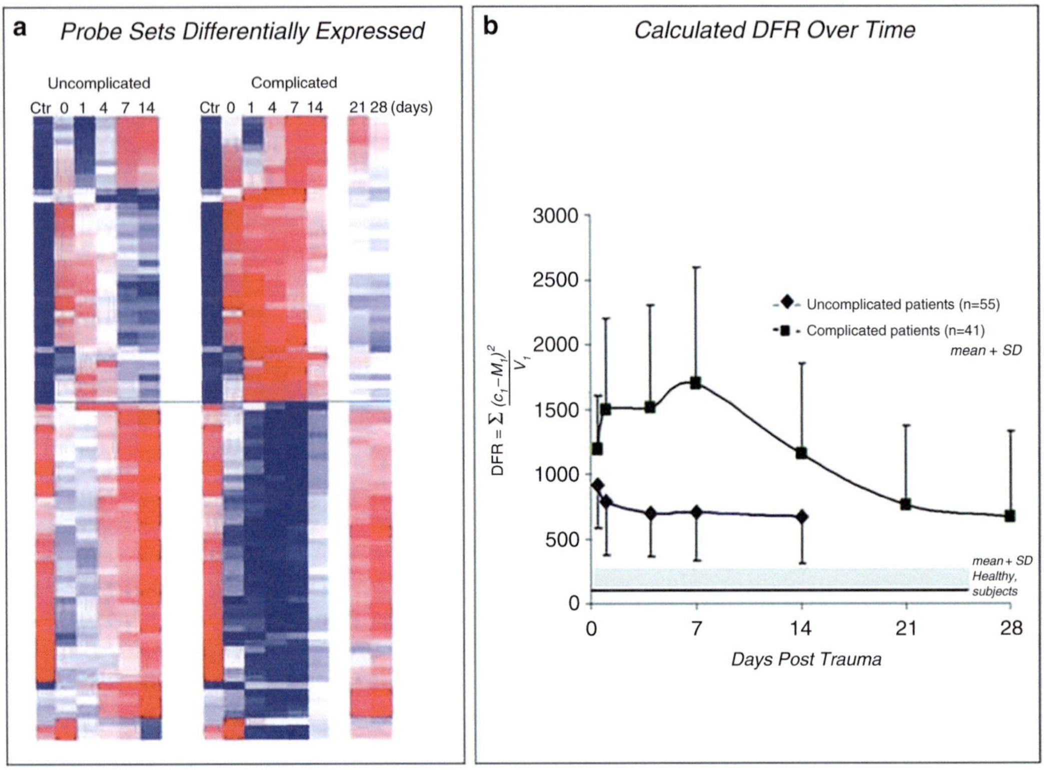

Fig. 3.5 (**a**, **b**) Heatmap and calculated difference from reference (DFR). These are the 63 genes that were found to distinguish clinical trajectory. Using a false discovery adjusted probability of less than 0.001 and a twofold difference in expression, the temporal pattern of expression of 63 genes that differed between patients with the two clinical outcomes is presented. (**a**) Cluster analysis of the two cohorts. (**b**) Summary of the difference from reference score calculated for each patient in the uncomplicated and complicated cohorts at each time point. Statistical analysis at each time point (0, 1, 4, 7, and 14 days) revealed significant differences in difference from reference (DFR) between complicated and uncomplicated patients ($p<0.05$, Mann-Whitney rank analysis). (**a**, **b**: Used with permission from Cuenca AG, Gentile LF, Lopez MC, Ungaro R, Liu H, Xiao W, et al. Development of a genomic metric that can be rapidly used to predict clinical outcome in severely injured trauma patients. Critical Care Medicine. 2013;41(5):1175–85)

may not be completely preventable by standard infection-control techniques.

The above report highlights the unique ability offered to scientist and clinician alike to more precisely identify patients that may be predisposed to developing hospital acquired infections while recovering from their primary injury. Not only is the genomic identification of subsets of immune compromised patients valuable in its own regard but also gives us genetic insight into how subtle variations in human genomic expression can predispose patients to develop life-threatening infections. As further genomic signatures are acquired and linked to human diseases and patient outcomes, improved, more proactive solutions and treatments will evolve to better serve select subgroups of patients of high risk within a disease group [10].

Ventilator-Associated Pneumonia and Outcomes

Ventilator-associated pneumonia is a prevalent complication in the critical care setting and predisposes many patients recovering from traumatic injury to unnecessary death. A microarray study of ventilator-associated pneumonia (VAP) patients suggested that 85 leukocyte genes can be used to diagnose VAP. Furthermore a validation

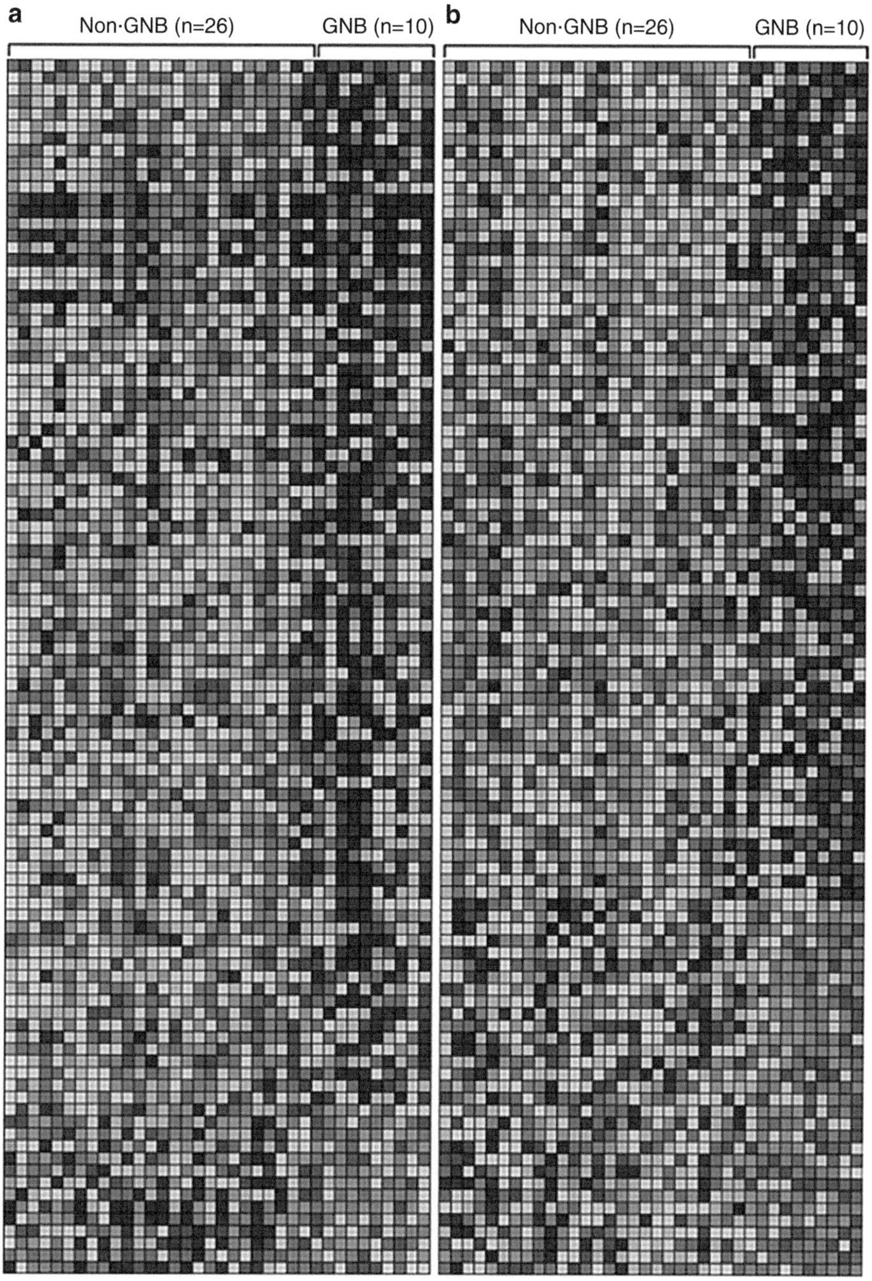

Fig. 3.6 (**a**, **b**) Trauma patients may be predisposed to develop bacteremia. (**a**) Heatmap of top 100 ranked differentially expressed probe sets from within 12 h after injury. (**b**) Heatmap of top 100 ranked differentially expressed probe sets at 96 h after injury. The lighter *gray* colors represent decreased expression, and the darker *black* colors represent increased expression with the darker colors indicating a greater degree difference. GNB = subjects in whom Gram-negative bacteremia developed, non-GNB = subjects in whom Gram-negative bacteremia did not develop. (**a**, **b**: Used with permission from Thompson CM, Park CH, Maier RV, O'Keefe GE. Traumatic Injury, Early Gene Expression, and Gram-Negative Bacteremia. Critical Care Medicine. 2014 Jun;42(6):1397–405)

of this gene set to detect VAP was tested using data from an independent patient cohort. Circulating leukocyte GeneChip U133 plus 2.0 expression values were measured over a 28 days time period after injury. Leukocyte transcriptional profiles were analyzed using repeated measures logistic regression. A compound covariate model based on leukocyte gene transcriptional profiles in a training subset of patients was tested to determine predictive accuracy for VAP up to 4 days prior to clinical diagnosis in the test subset. Using gene expression values measured on each study day 27 of the 85 genes were associated with the diagnosis of VAP 1–4 days before diagnosis. However, the compound covariate model based on these 85 genes did not predict VAP in the test cohort better than chance ($P=0.27$). In contrast, a compound covariate model based upon de novo transcriptional analysis predicted VAP better than chance 4 days before diagnosis with a sensitivity of 57 % and a specificity of 69 % [11].

The Future of Microarray Technology in Trauma, Sepsis, and Critical Care

Although high-throughput genomics and proteomics have revolutionized the ability of clinicians to diagnose disease prognosticate patients outcome, the science is hampered by genetic variation within a disease group and with the technicalities of tissue analysis which require large amounts of patient-derived RNA. Affymetrix, in association with the *Inflammation and the Host Response to Injury* collaboration or "Glue Grant," has attempted to solve the problem by the development of a new gene chip technology minimizing the amount of initial patient RNA used while maximizing the amount of genomic information recovered.

The new gene chip is a 6.9 million-feature oligonucleotide array of the human transcriptome [Glue Grant human transcriptome (GG-H array)] that has been developed for high-throughput and cost-effective analyses in clinical studies. This array allows comprehensive examination of gene expression and genome-wide identification of alternative splicing as well as detection of coding SNPs and noncoding transcripts. The authors tested the performance of the array with mRNA sequencing results over multiple independent replicates of human tissue samples; see Fig. 3.7a, b. The GG-H array is highly reproducible in estimating gene and exon abundance while requiring minimal amounts of patient tissue samples. Affymetrix, in conjunction with the *Inflammation and the Host Response to Injury* collaboration, has implemented the GGH gene chip in a multicenter clinical program and has generated high-quality reproducible data. Considering the clinical trial requirements of cost, sample availability, and throughput, the GG-H array has a wide range of applications [12].

This technology will offer a robust platform from which to analyze all the variations of human disease genetic targets with very little starting material. Now not only can disease diagnosis be made rapidly and early, but also the known genetic variability within a disease process explored and treated. These microarrays will be the future of multicenter disease-focused collaborative efforts that are aimed at genetic prognostication for diseases in general and select patients in specific.

Microfluidics and Point of Care Genomic Prognostication

Francis Collins, one of the fathers of the Human Genome Project, clarified his vision for the future of "personalized medicine," where the fruits of the Human Genome Project would ultimately influence not only human biology and medicine, but human society as well. The goals of individualized gene-based medicine are, for the most part, still beyond the capabilities of most healthcare centers because of several remaining technical challenges, only some of which have been addressed by the Human Genome Project. Technologies have recently become available to cost-effectively conduct genomic analyses such that previously unobtainable questions have become technically possible. However, several

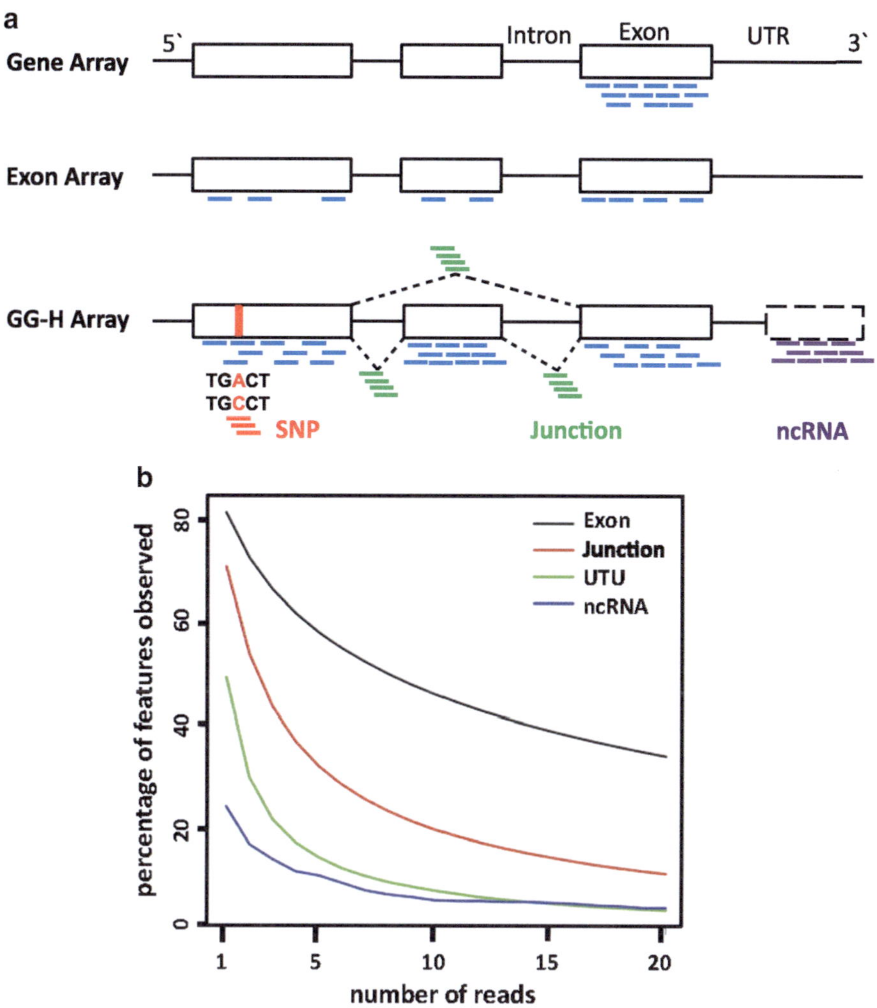

Fig. 3.7 (**a**, **b**) Affymetrix glue grant human transcriptome (GG-H array) (Santa Clara, CA). Design of the GG-H human transcriptome array for comprehensive examination of gene and exon expression, alternative splicing, and additional contents of the human transcriptome. (**a**) On a 3′ gene array, such as the Affymetrix HU-133 Array, 11 probes were designed for the 3′-end exon(s) of each gene. On an exon array, such as the Affymetrix Human Exon 1.0 ST Array, there are two to four probes for each exon of the gene. In contrast, the GG-H array uses, on average, ten probes for each exon/PSR and four probes for each exon–exon junction; in addition, six pairs of probes were designed for each coding SNP, and ten probes were designed for each noncoding RNA transcript. (**b**) Comparison of the GG-H array contents with mRNA sequencing data on multiple tissues. The percentages of exons, junctions, UTUs, and ncRNAs (*y* axis) supported by at least a specified number of sequencing reads (*x* axis) are shown. (**a**, **b**: Copyright © National Academy of Sciences. Originally published in Xu W, Seok J, Mindrinos MN, Schweitzer AC, Jiang H, Wilhelmy J, et al. Human transcriptome array for high-throughput clinical studies. Proceedings of the National Academy of Sciences of the United States of America. 2011;108(9):3707–12)

technical challenges still remain that prevent widespread use of these technologies in the clinical setting, including rapid sample accrual, large sample volumes, lengthy processing times, and complex data analysis.

Gene expression analysis can be a powerful tool in predicting patient outcomes and identifying patients who may benefit from targeted therapies. However, isolating human blood polymorphonuclear cells (PMNs) as well as other human immune cells for genomic analysis has been challenging. Several investigators have thrust their efforts into providing a platform from which human neutrophils can be rapidly isolated from peripheral blood. Using a novel microfluidic technique that isolates PMNs by capturing CD66b^{+} cells, the authors use bronchoalveolar lavage (BAL) samples of patients with acute respiratory distress syndrome (ARDS) to evaluate PMN genomic alterations secondary to pulmonary sequestration. Blood and BAL fluid PMNs were also isolated using microfluidics from seven hospitalized patients with ARDS. Gene expression was inferred from extracted RNA using Affymetrix U133 Plus 2.0 GeneChips. Patterns of gene expression from blood and BAL PMNs differed significantly from each other in the patients with ARDS. The authors further demonstrate the cost savings, alacrity, and ease that can be gained by using a microfluidics approach to point of care cell separation and testing rather than using traditional isolation and analysis methods [13, 14].

The ability to rapidly isolate circulating blood PMNs for diagnostic and laboratory evaluation arms physicians with a powerful tool to more efficiently and accurately predict which patients are at risk for the development of ARDS. Early stratification of those at risk for the development of ARDS will allow for the development of better ARDS prevention strategies.

Final Conclusions

As we better understand the genomic etiologies of more diseases states, our focus will inevitably shift from reaction to prevention. Patient treatment plans will be based on the sets of complications that may hinder their recovery progress. Rather than focus on generalized disease prevention, we will focus on patient-centered disease identification before the symptomatology and sequel are apparent. By applying genomics and other high-throughput technologies, clinicians and researchers will have a robust platform for using the human transcriptome as a diagnostic tool in the clinical setting.

The technical, statistical, and methodological challenges of handling human genomic information and translating it into reliable tools applicable in clinical decision-making will overcome one major hurdle preventing the widespread use of genomics in clinical medicine, and that is translating basic science discoveries into new and better treatments. Over the past 30 years a cadre of clinicians and researchers alike has described the genomic and proteomic response to inflammation and severe injury in leukocyte populations from humans. Now is the time to take advantage of the large scientific database of information and use it to implement a diagnostic test for predicting outcome and appropriateness for therapy in the critically ill trauma patient, cancer patient, or acute care surgery patient.

Advances in the treatment of critically ill trauma, cancer, and acute care surgery patients have stagnated over the past decade. The enthusiasm in the 1990s for new therapeutics to treat surgically oriented diseased patients has been stymied by an inability to identify those patients who would benefit from such therapies. Current stratification and diagnostics to identify patients who will have an adverse clinical trajectory or outcome are imprecise. The future of improved outcomes is rooted in new genomic diagnostics that can accurately identify patients who may benefit from therapies aimed at disease prevention and not reaction.

References

1. Kristensen VN, Lingjaerde OC, Russnes HG, Vollan HK, Frigessi A, Borresen-Dale AL. Principles and methods of integrative genomic analyses in cancer. Nat Rev Cancer. 2014;14(5):299–313.
2. Greenberg ES, Chong KK, Huynh KT, Tanaka R, Hoon DS. Epigenetic biomarkers in skin cancer. Cancer Lett. 2014;342(2):170–7.
3. Roychowdhury S, Chinnaiyan AM. Advancing precision medicine for prostate cancer through genomics. J Clin Oncol. 2013;31(15):1866–73.
4. Lohr JG, Adalsteinsson VA, Cibulskis K, Choudhury AD, Rosenberg M, Cruz-Gordillo P, et al. Whole-exome sequencing of circulating tumor cells provides a window into metastatic prostate cancer. Nat Biotechnol. 2014;32:479–84.

5. Previati M, Manfrini M, Galasso M, Zerbinati C, Palatini J, Gasparini P, et al. Next generation analysis of breast cancer genomes for precision medicine. Cancer Lett. 2013;339(1):1–7.
6. McCauley JL, Abreu MT. Genetics in diagnosing and managing inflammatory bowel disease. Gastroenterol Clin North Am. 2012;41(2):513–22.
7. Jostins L, Ripke S, Weersma RK, Duerr RH, McGovern DP, Hui KY, et al. Host-microbe interactions have shaped the genetic architecture of inflammatory bowel disease. Nature. 2012;491(7422): 119–24.
8. Xiao W, Mindrinos MN, Seok J, Cuschieri J, Cuenca AG, Gao H, et al. A genomic storm in critically injured humans. J Exp Med. 2011;208(13): 2581–90.
9. Cuenca AG, Gentile LF, Lopez MC, Ungaro R, Liu H, Xiao W, et al. Development of a genomic metric that can be rapidly used to predict clinical outcome in severely injured trauma patients. Crit Care Med. 2013;41(5):1175–85.
10. Thompson CM, Park CH, Maier RV, O'Keefe GE. Traumatic injury, early gene expression, and gram-negative bacteremia. Crit Care Med. 2014;42(6): 1397–405.
11. Cobb JP, Moore EE, Hayden DL, Minei JP, Cuschieri J, Yang J, et al. Validation of the riboleukogram to detect ventilator-associated pneumonia after severe injury. Ann Surg. 2009;250(4):531–9.
12. Xu W, Seok J, Mindrinos MN, Schweitzer AC, Jiang H, Wilhelmy J, et al. Human transcriptome array for high-throughput clinical studies. Proc Natl Acad Sci U S A. 2011;108(9):3707–12.
13. Kotz KT, Xiao W, Miller-Graziano C, Qian WJ, Russom A, Warner EA, et al. Clinical microfluidics for neutrophil genomics and proteomics. Nat Med. 2010;16(9):1042–7.
14. Warner EA, Kotz KT, Ungaro RF, Abouhamze AS, Lopez MC, Cuenca AG, et al. Microfluidics-based capture of human neutrophils for expression analysis in blood and bronchoalveolar lavage. Lab Invest. 2011;91(12):1787–95.

Nanotechnologies in Surgery: The New Paradigm

4

Russell J. Andrews

Introduction

> ...it would be interesting in surgery if you could swallow the surgeon. You put the mechanical surgeon inside the blood vessel and it goes into the heart and "looks" around. ...It finds out which valve is the faulty one and takes a little knife and slices it out. Other small machines might be permanently incorporated in the body to assist some inadequately-functioning organs.
>
> Feynman RP (attributed to AR Hibbs) [1]

> What I want to talk about is the problem of manipulating and controlling things on a small scale. ... It is a staggeringly small world that is below. In the year 2000, when they look back at this age, they will wonder why it was not until the year 1960 that anybody began seriously to move in this direction.
>
> Feynman RP [1]

The twentieth century saw the surgeon become a master at precision excision and minimally invasive tissue manipulation and repair. About the time of Feynman's famous lecture at CalTech quoted above, 1960, the operating microscope began to revolutionize operations for neurosurgeons, otolaryngologists, ophthalmologists, and other surgeons. Over the following decades, techniques such as endoscopy and laparoscopy made minimally invasive surgery a reality—the length of both incisions and postoperative hospital stays decreased dramatically. Sophisticated microendovascular techniques have come close to realizing Feynman's "mechanical surgeon inside the blood vessel" not only for cardiac disease but also for more peripheral arterial disease and various vascular malformations such as cerebral aneurysms.

Feynman's mechanical endovascular surgeon was not a true "nanosurgeon" but rather a miniaturized twentieth century endovascular surgeon separated from the catheter controlled by the "full-size" human surgeon. The twenty-first century "nanosurgeon" was envisaged four decades later in 1999 by Richard Smalley, the Nobel Prize-winning chemist who discovered the C^{60} buckyball:

> Twenty years ago, without even this crude chemotherapy, I would already be dead. But 20 years from now, nanoscale missiles will target cancer cells in the human body and leave everything else blissfully alone. I may not live to see it. But I am confident it will happen.
>
> Smalley R [2]

Although Smalley died 6 years later, in 2005, of non-Hodgkin's lymphoma, his prediction regarding "nanoscale missiles" for targeting cancer cells is very much "on target." Numerous other nanotechniques for surgery are being developed, many of them much more subtle than nanoscale missiles or endovascular micro- or nano-robotic surgeons.

R.J. Andrews, M.D. (✉)
Center for Nanotechnology, NASA Ames Research Center, Moffett Field, CA, USA
e-mail: rja@russelljandrews.org

R. Latifi et al. (eds.), *Technological Advances in Surgery, Trauma and Critical Care*,
DOI 10.1007/978-1-4939-2671-8_4

It would be remiss to look toward the future of nanotechniques in surgery without acknowledging the past. The Damascus blade of medieval Muslim blacksmiths was never replicated by Western blacksmiths—much to the chagrin (and likely loss of life) of the Crusaders. The extraordinary mechanical properties and sharpness of the Damascus blade have recently been attributed to carbon nanotube "impurities" in the blade [3]. It appears that ores from India used in the forging process were responsible for the formation of carbon nanotubes—resulting in the unique characteristics of the Damascus blade. The loss of supply of these ores during the eighteenth century led to the demise of this chemical skill amongst the blacksmiths of Damascus, relieving the world of an instrument capable of atrocities with surgical precision.

A single chapter can only provide an overview of nanotechniques being developed for surgery. Recent books on nanosurgery and related topics have appeared [4, 5]. The US National Nanotechnology Initiative web site is an extensive resource (www.nano.gov).

The Nanorealm and Nanomaterials

One nanometer is 10^{-9} m (Fig. 4.1) [6], *nanos* being Greek for dwarf. The nanorealm is typically considered to be particles, devices, or techniques less than 100 nm in size, although practically speaking less than 1 μm (1,000 nm) is more appropriate. One micron is roughly 1/10 the diameter of a red blood cell, or 1/100 the diameter of a human hair.

Equally important to small size for nanotechnology is the concept of constructing or manipulating materials atom-by-atom or molecule-by-molecule. This concept was expressed—and the term "nanotechnology" coined—by Norio Taniguchi in 1974. Two quite different techniques for nanofabrication include (1) "top-down" methods such as nanolithography (Greek "small writing on rocks") and (2) "bottom-up" methods such as self-assembly (of atoms, molecules, proteins, etc) and chemical vapor deposition (e.g., to produce carbon nanotubes—Fig. 4.2a, b) [7].

Three types of nanomaterials important for nanomedicine and nanosurgery include nanoparticles (NPs), nanoscaffolds (NSs), and nanotubes/nanofibers. Several types of nanoparticles and nanotechniques for tumor targeting are depicted in Fig. 4.3a–j [8]. Another important nanoparticle is the quantum dot (QD) [9, 10]. QDs (Fig. 4.4a–c) have the unusual property that they fluoresce with a different color depending on their size. QDs are therefore extremely useful for multiple tagging—drugs, tumor cells, receptors, etc.—to follow the various tagged moieties over time and space [11].

NSs are typically self-assembling arrays such as the peptide NS illustrated in Fig. 4.5a–c [12]. Peptides composed of charged amino acids self-assemble into scaffolds in the presence of physiological salt solutions and body fluids

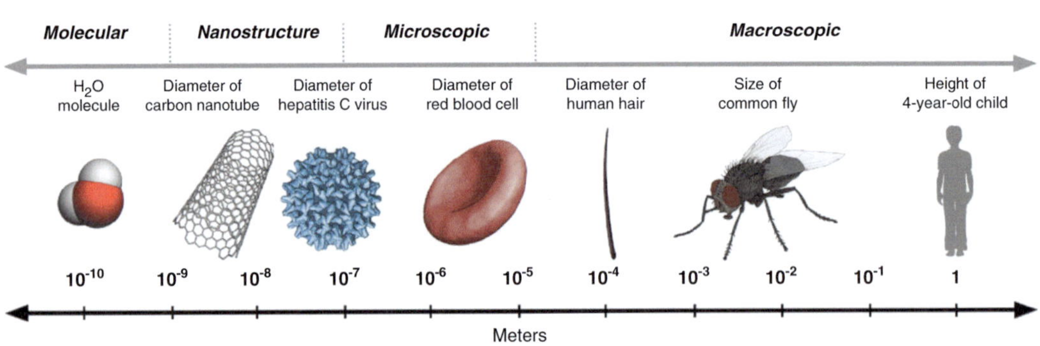

Fig. 4.1 Comparison of size of objects from 10^{-10} to 1 m. (Used with permission from Kateb B, Chiu K, Black KL, et al. Nanoplatforms for constructing new approaches to cancer treatment, imaging, and drug delivery: what should be the policy? Neuroimage 2011;54:S106–S124)

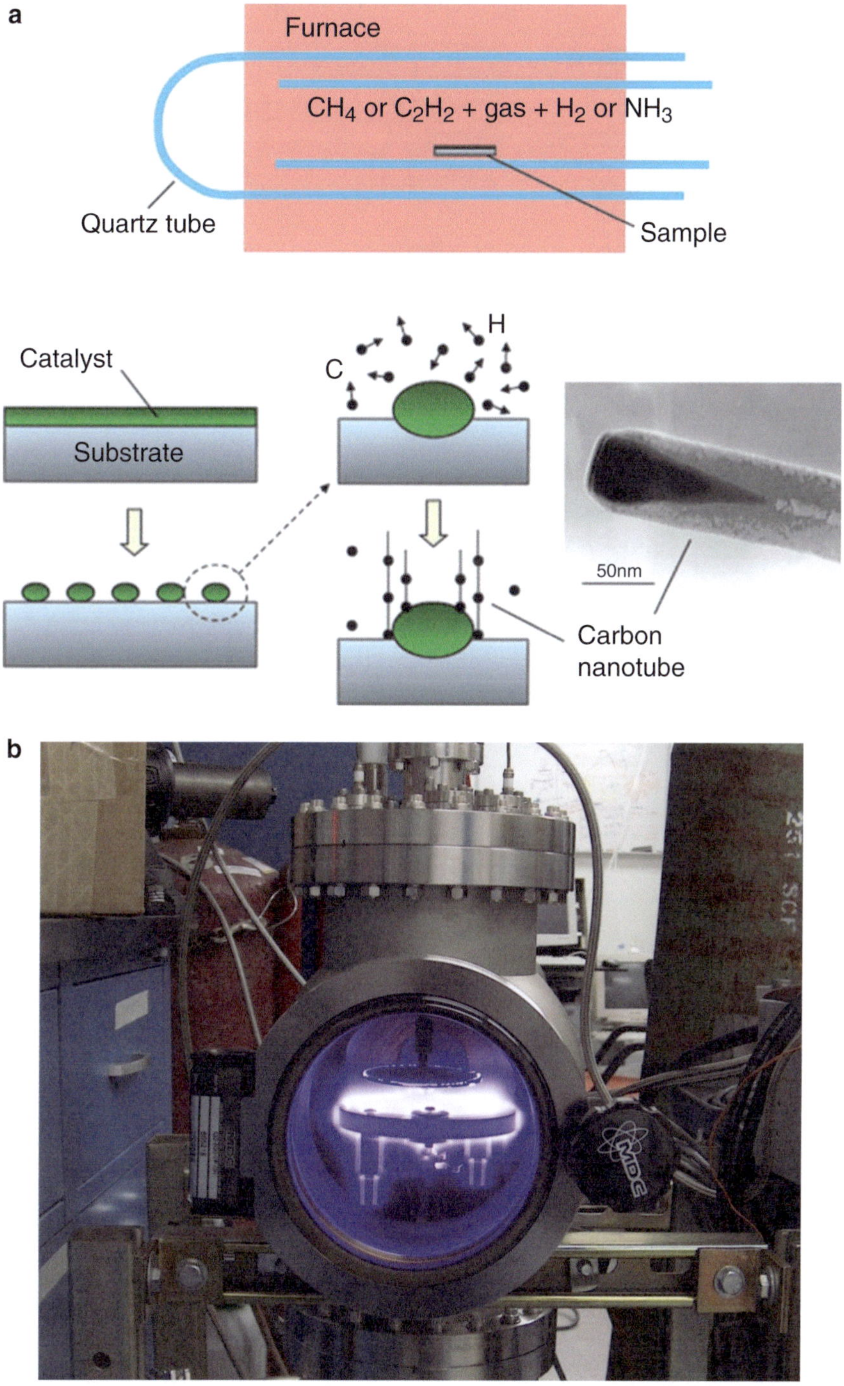

Fig. 4.2 (**a**, **b**) (**a**) Schematics of a chemical vapor deposition reactor (*top*) and the basic sequence of carbon nanotube growth (*bottom*). (**a**: Used with permission from Daraio C, Jin S. Synthesis and patterning methods for nanostructures useful for biological applications. In: Silva GA, Parpura V, editors. Nanotechnology for Biology and Medicine. New York: Springer Science+Business Media; 2012). (**b**) Photograph of a custom built plasma enhanced chemical vapor deposition reactor. (**b**: Courtesy of NASA Ames Center for Nanotechnology)

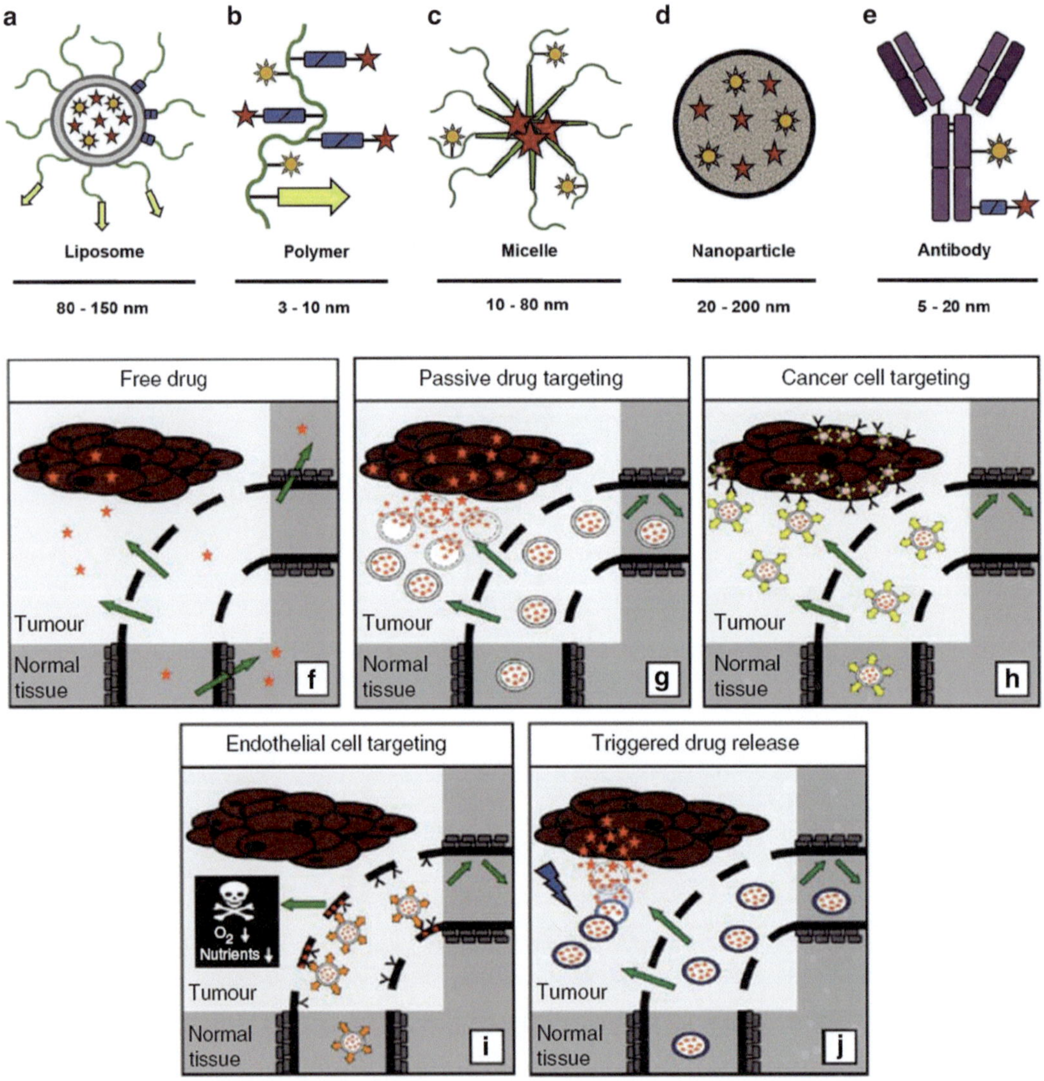

Fig. 4.3 (**a**–**j**) (**a**–**e**) Examples of nanomaterials, nanotechniques, and nanoparticles: liposomes and liposomal bilayers—*gray*; polymers and polymer coatings—*green*; linkers for drug release and "stealth" coatings—*blue*; targeting ligands—*yellow*; imaging agents—*orange*; conjugated or entrapped (chemo-) therapeutic agents—*red*. (**f**–**j**) Drug targeting strategies for tumors. Passive drug targeting with NPs (**g**) offers some benefit over free drug administration (**f**) (intravenous) but even more advantageous is active drug targeting of tumor cell surface receptors (**h**), local endothelial cell receptors (**i**), and triggered drug release (**j**) (by stimuli such as hyperthermia, pH change, or ultrasound). (**a**–**j**: Used with permission from Rizzo LY, Theek B, Storm G, Kiessling F, Lammers T. Recent progress in nanomedicine: therapeutic, diagnostic and theranostic applications. Curr Opin Biotechnol 2013;24(6):1–13; Lammers T, Kiessling F, Hennink WE, Storm G. Drug targeting to tumors: principles, pitfalls and (pre-) clinical progress. J Control Release. 2012 Jul 20;161(2):175–87; Lammers T, Aime S, Hennink WE, Storm G, Kiessling F. Theranostic nanomedicine. Acc Chem Res. 2011 Oct 18;44(10):1029–38)

(e.g., blood, cerebrospinal fluid). The impressive properties of NSs for both hemostasis and tissue repair are discussed below.

Carbon nanotubes (CNTs) and the closely related carbon nanofibers (CNFs)—see Figs. 4.2a, b and 4.6—have properties that allow novel interactions with tissues, from acting as carriers for antitumor drugs (Smalley's "nanoscale missiles") to tissue monitors and modulators with sensitivity orders of magnitude higher than non-nano techniques.

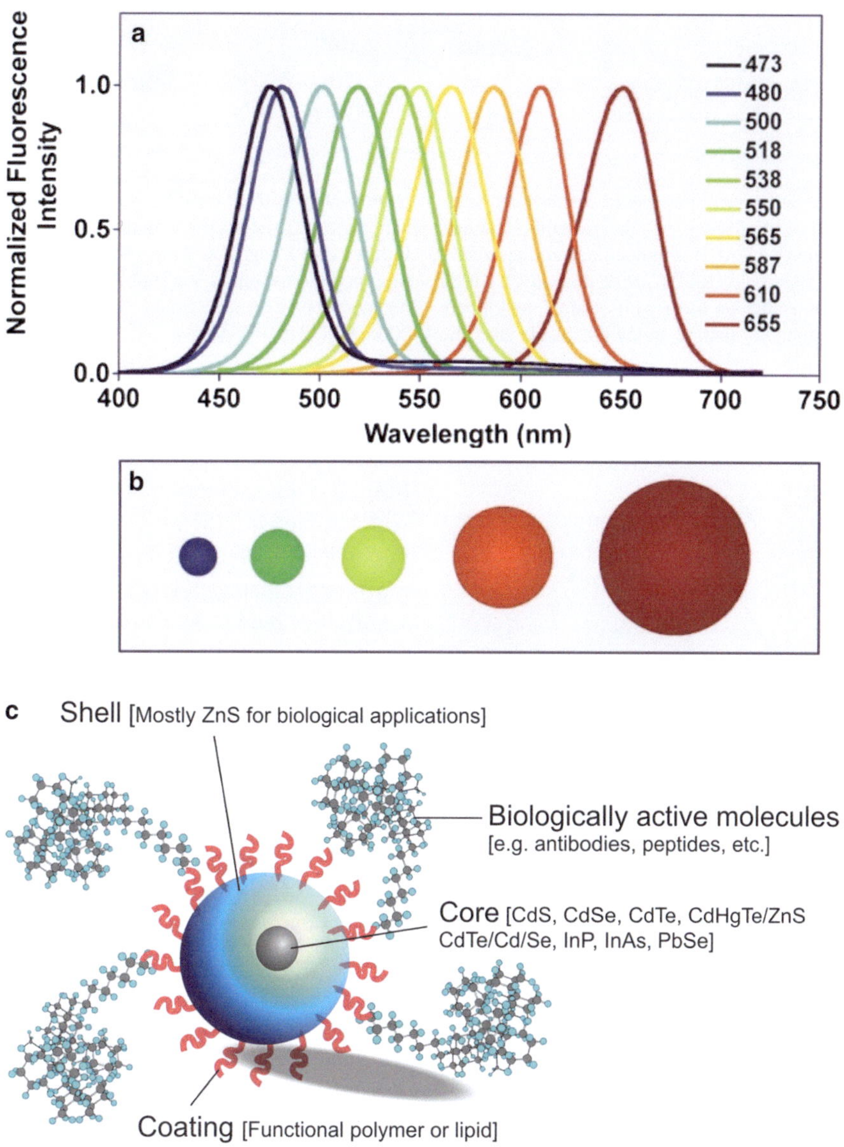

Fig. 4.4 (**a–c**) (**a**, **b**) Graph (**a**—*top*) showing that the wavelength of the light emitted by QDs varies with the diameter of the QD (**b**—*bottom*). (**a**, **b**: Used with permission from Smith AM, Nie S. Chemical analysis and cellular imaging with quantum dots. Analyst 2004;129:672–677.) (**c**) Structure of a semiconductor QD. The heavy metal core is responsible for the fluorescence properties of the QD. The shell stabilizes the core, while the coating provides anchor sites for organic and biological ligands such as antibodies, and peptides. (**c**: Used with permission from Pathak S, Cao E, Davidson MC, Jin S, Silva GA. Quantum dot applications to neuroscience: new tools for probing neurons and glia. J Neurosci 2006;26(7)1893–1895)

Figure 4.7 details some of the advantages of nanoelectrode arrays as biosensors based on size alone; other advantages—particularly important for recording and stimulating nervous system tissues (e.g., neuromodulation and deep brain stimulation)—include greatly reduced impedance and greatly increased capacitance with nanoarrays in comparison with traditional electrodes.

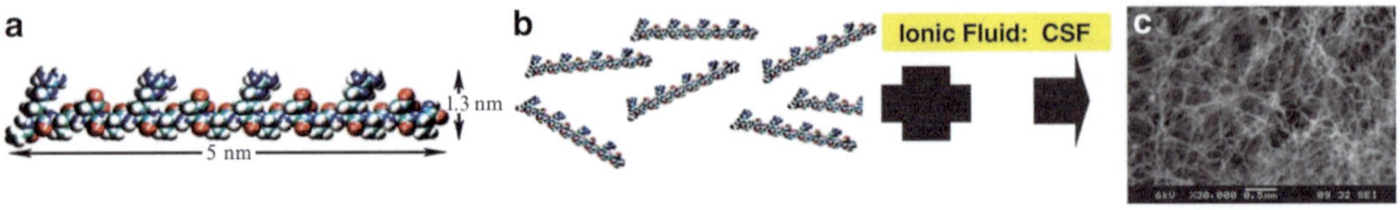

Fig. 4.5 (**a**–**c**) Self-assembling peptide nanofiber scaffold (SAPNS). (**a**) Model of the arginine-alanine-aspartate-alanine (RADA) 16-I molecular building block. (**b**) Model of numerous RADA 16-I molecules which undergo self-assembly to form well-ordered nanofibers with the hydrophobic alanine sandwich inside and the hydrophilic residues outside. (**c**) SEM of SAPNS (scale bar: 500 nm). (**a**–**c**: Used with permission from Ellis-Behnke RG, Liang YX, You SW, et al. Nano neuro knitting: peptide nanofiber scaffold for brain repair and axon regeneration with functional return of vision. PNAS 2006;103(13):5054–5059)

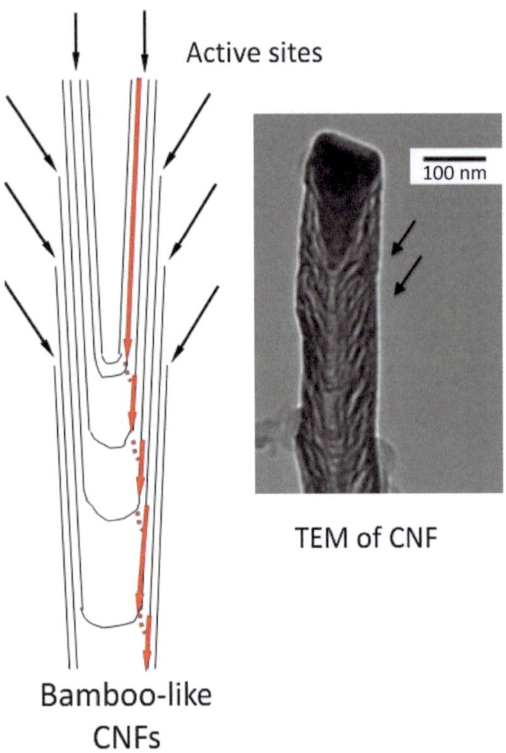

Fig. 4.6 Schematic of a carbon nanofiber showing the bamboo-like (or stacked dixie cup-like) structure of the multiple active sites (*left*) and TEM of a CNF (*right*). The multiple active sites result in very high electron transfer and very high capacitance. (Courtesy of NASA Ames Center for Nanotechnology)

Nanotechniques for Imaging, Targeting, and Healing

Superparamagnetic iron oxide NPs are being developed as improved MRI contrast agents for assessing the cerebral vasculature and malignant brain tumors [13]. Figure 4.8a presents MRI scans (7 T) of the human brain: (1) without contrast, (2) with gadoteridol (0.1 mmol/kg), and (3) with ferumoxytol (510 mg), a superparamagnetic iron oxide NP. Because ferumoxytol particles are much larger than gadoteridol particles (30 nm vs. 1 nm), they tend to leak out of the blood vessels into tumors more slowly (Fig. 4.8b). Gadoteridol enhancement peaks less than 30 min following injection; ferumoxytol enhancement peaks at about 24 h. This offers significant advantages: one can obtain an MRI of the brain immediately after ferumoxytol contrast injection and visualize the cerebral vasculature feeding the tumor, and repeated scans can be obtained over hours following contrast injection without repeating the contrast, especially important for intraoperative MRI scanning where several scans may be required during surgery.

Imaging of tumors with either gadoteridol or ferumoxytol relies on passive targeting, i.e., the tumor imaging or targeting depends on the tumor blood vessels being "leakier" than normal blood vessels. The leaky vessels adjacent to the tumor result in slow clearance of the contrast agent or QD-PEG (polyethylene glycol) NPs, causing an accumulation of NPs in the extracellular environment of the tumor. More effective imaging/targeting of tumors occurs with active techniques [8, 9, 14], Active targeting utilizes an antibody against the tumor cells conjugated to the QDs, by which the NPs accumulate on the tumor cell membrane and are incorporated within the tumor cells.

More sophisticated, multimodality NP techniques for tumor imaging and treatment are being developed, as illustrated in Figs. 4.3a–j and 4.9.

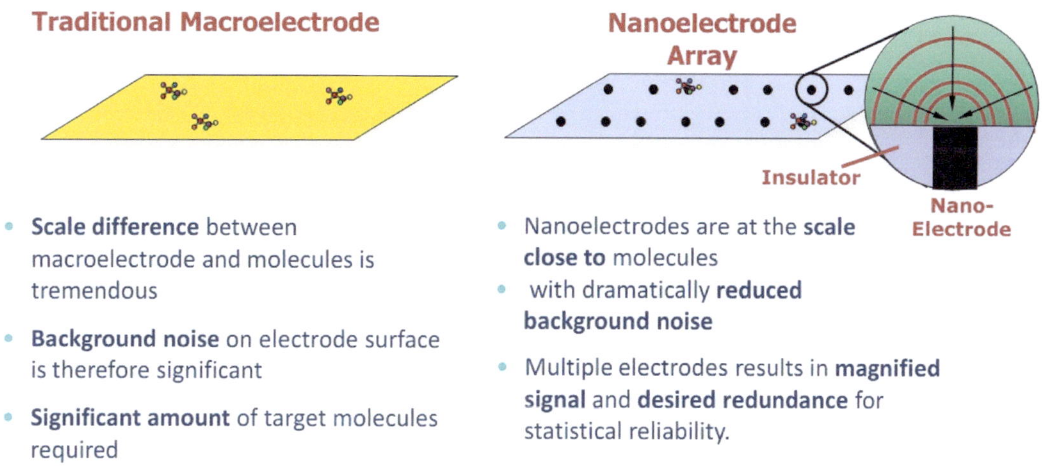

Fig. 4.7 Nanoscale electrodes offer dramatic improvement over traditional macro- or microelectrodes for detecting and quantifying small analytes in low concentrations. (Courtesy of NASA Ames Center for Nanotechnology)

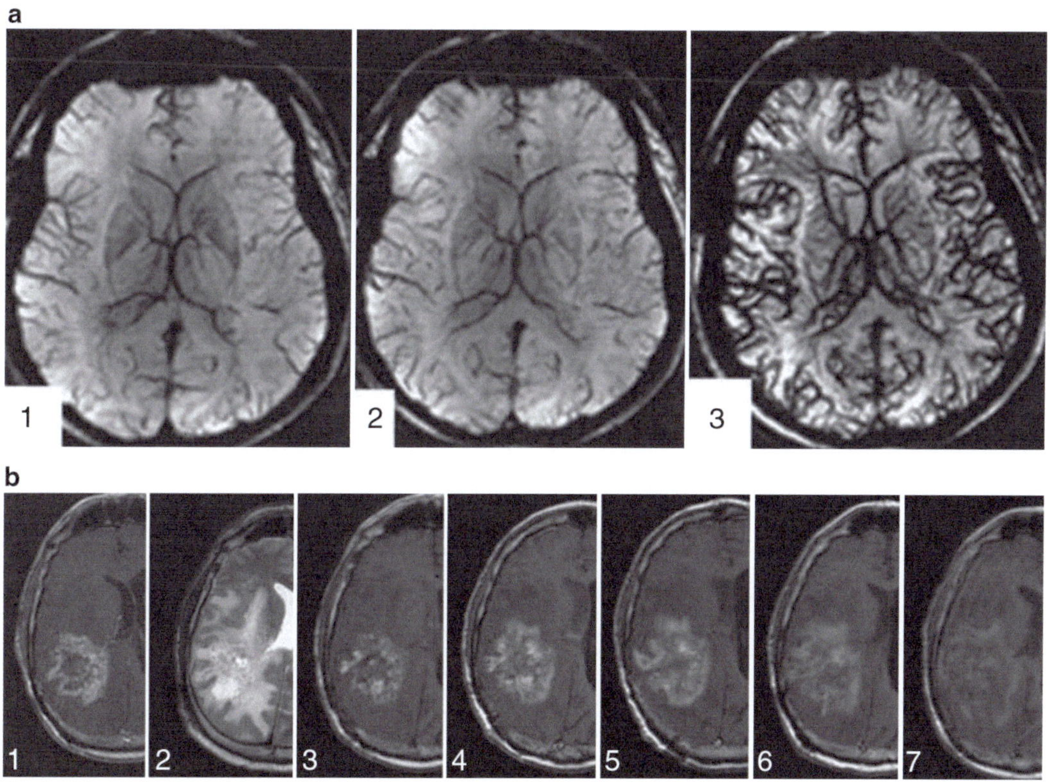

Fig. 4.8 (**a**, **b**) (**a**) Cerebral vasculature with 7T MRI. (1) Without contrast agent. (2) With gadoteridol 0.1 mmol/kg i.v. (3) With ferumoxytol 510 mg i.v. (**b**) Time course of ferumoxytol enhancement (1.5T MRI) in a patient with recurrent glioblastoma multiforme. (1) T1—gadoteridol. (2) T2. 3–7: T1—at the following five time points (hours post-injection of ferumoxytol): (3) 4–6 h; (4) 6–20 h; (5) 24–28 h; (6) 48–52 h; (7) ~72 h. Peak enhancement with ferumoxytol is at 24–28 h, much later than the ~30 min peak enhancement with gadoteridol. (**a**, **b**: Used with permission from Weinstein JS, Varallyay CG, Dosa E, et al. Superparamagnetic iron oxide nanoparticles: diagnostic magnetic resonance imaging and potential therapeutic applications in neurooncology and central nervous system inflammatory pathologies, a review. J Cereb Blood Flow Metab 2010;30:15–35)

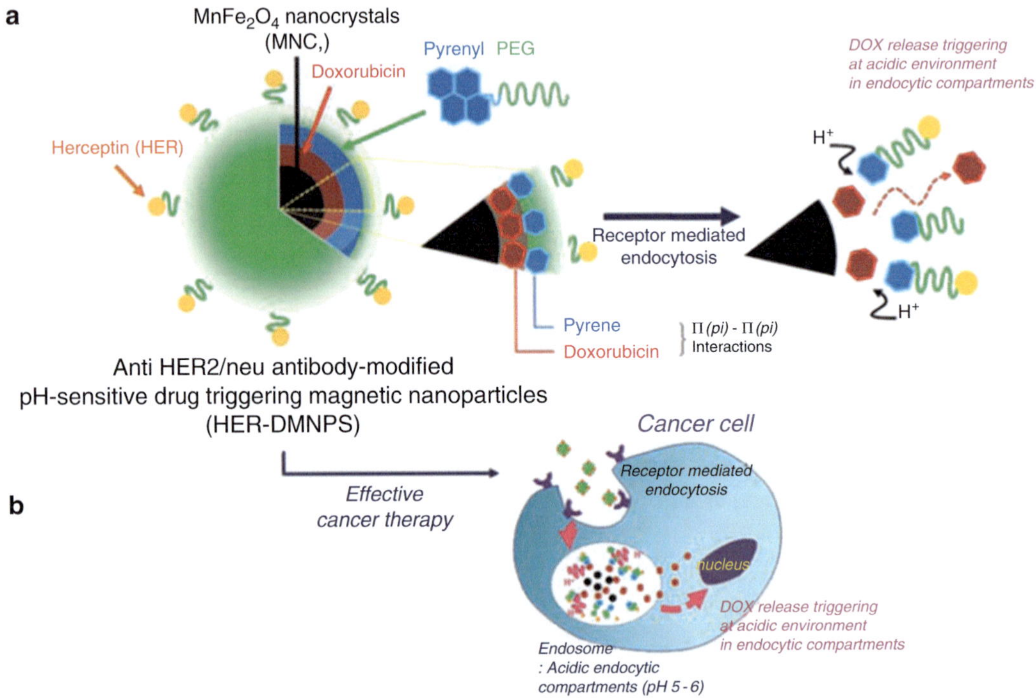

Fig. 4.9 Schematic illustration of anti-HER2/neu antibody-modified pH-sensitive drug-releasing magnetic NPs (HER-DMNPs) for cancer therapy followed by MRI. *DOX* doxorubicin, *HER* herceptin, *PEG* polyethylene glycol. (Used with permission from Wang LS, Chuang MC, Ho JA. Nanotheranostics—a review of recent publications. Int J Nanomed 2012;7:4679–4695)

In Fig. 4.9, a nanocrystal coated with polyethylene glycol (PEG) uses an antibody to target, pH sensitivity to release the chemotherapeutic agent, and magnetic properties for MRI detection [14]. Another technique by which NPs can improve cancer treatment is by thermotherapy (e.g., heating tumors using an MRI scanner once the tumor has been targeted with magnetic NPs) [15]. NPs can also enhance the efficacy of standard external beam radiation therapy for tumors. The radiation interacts with hafnium oxide NPs to generate a much larger number of electrons than radiation therapy alone, resulting in greatly increased treatment effect [16].

NPs are also being developed to reduce inflammation and improve healing in conditions ranging from arthritis to infection to endovascular stenting. The use of NPs incorporated into drug-eluting stents (to promote endothelial healing and minimize restenosis) for interventional cardiology has been reviewed [17]. NPs containing aspirin-triggered Resolvin D1 (a hexaenoic acid) have recently been shown to decrease inflammation in several conditions [18]. Examples of this nano-pro-resolving medicine (AT-RvD1 NPRM) are given in Fig. 4.10a, b, where a mouse model of (1) peritonitis (produced by intraperitoneal injection of zymosan) and (2) temporomandibular joint (TMJ) inflammation (produced by local injection of T Freund's adjuvant) were treated pre-insult by intravenous injection of AT-RvD1 NPRM. Figure 4.10a graphs the decrease in acute inflammation with the peritonitis model when AT-RvD1 NPRM was administered; Fig. 4.10b graphs the decrease in myeloperoxidase activity (MPO) by ELISA 12 h following injection of the TMJ.

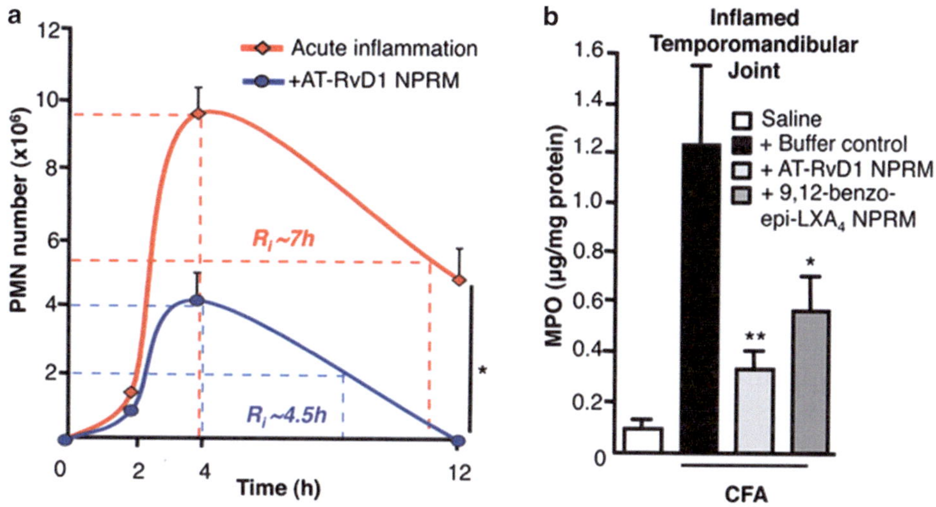

Fig. 4.10 (**a**, **b**) (**a**) Reduction in acute inflammation (PMN count) when AT-RvD1 NPRM was given i.v. prior to administration of inflammation-inciting zymosan i.p. in mice. PMN—polymorphonuclear cell. (**b**) Reduction in mouse temporomandibular joint (TMJ) inflammation (myeloperoxidase—MPO) induced by complete Freund's adjuvant (CFA) followed by i.v. NPRM (either AT-RvD1 or LXA_4). (**a**, **b**: Used with permission from Norling LV, Spite M, Yang R, Flower RJ, Perretti M, Serhan CN. Humanized nano-pro-resolving medicines mimic inflammation resolution and enhance wound healing. J Immunol 2011;186(10):5543–5547)

Nanotechniques for Hemostasis and Tissue Regeneration: Nanoscaffolds

Nanoscaffolds, being peptides composed of amino acids that self-assemble into nanofibers, are not recognized by the immune system as foreign, and thus do not incite an immune response. Moreover, peptidases remove the NS over time, an ideal intervention that performs its role and then disappears by natural means. The remarkable hemostatic properties of NSs—arresting bleeding even from small arteries within seconds—are well documented [19]. As illustrated in Fig. 4.11a–f, NPs form a clear gel through which one can operate in standard surgical fashion. NPs should be of significant utility in various surgical subspecialties, e.g., general, cardiovascular, cerebrovascular, urological.

NPs also possess remarkable properties to facilitate tissue regeneration. One example of central nervous system regeneration is documented in Fig. 4.12a–f [12]. Juvenile hamsters underwent superior colliculus (SC) sharp transection, as shown in Fig. 4.12a, b. Injecting 10 μl of a 1 % solution of the NP illustrated in Fig. 4.5a–c (arginine, alanine, aspartate, alanine—named RADA-1) into the region of SC transection, in contrast to 10 μl of saline control, resulted in the dark-field histological sections as shown: c and e are from 24 h and 30 days saline control animals, d and f are from 24 h and 30 days experimental (NP) animals. Impressively, 75 % of animals receiving NP treatment regained useful functional vision; recovery of vision was correlated with axonal reinnervation (up to 80 % of normal innervation), with no reinnervation (or visual return) being seen in the control animals.

Nanotechniques for the Tissue-Device Interface: Carbon Nanotubes and Nanofibers

Implanted medical devices such as cardiac pacemakers and deep brain stimulators depend on the electrical interaction of the device with tissues—

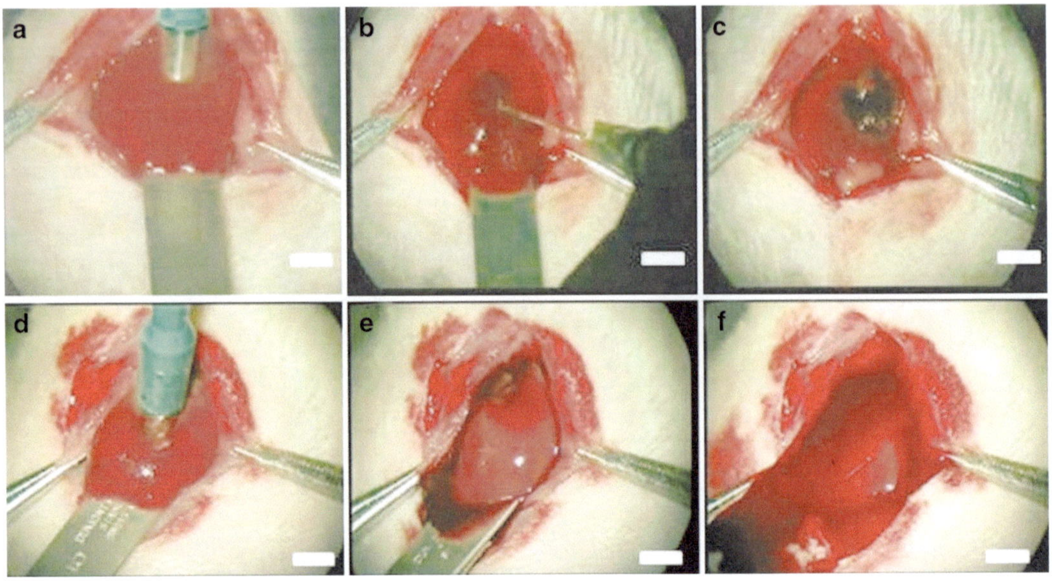

Fig. 4.11 (**a**–**f**) Rat liver punch biopsy (4 mm dia). (**a**–**c**) Topical treatment with a 3 % solution of the RADA SAPNS illustrated in Fig. 4.5. (**d**–**f**) Topical treatment with saline. (**a**, **d**) Time of punch biopsy, with profuse bleeding. (**b**) Treatment with RADA SAPNS, with complete hemostasis in approximately 10 s. (**e**) Treatment with iced saline and cautery, with continued bleeding. (**c**, **g**) 30 s after the punch biopsy—no bleeding with RADA SAPNS, continued bleeding with saline and cautery. (**a**–**f**: Used with permission from Ellis-Behnke R. At the nanoscale: nanohemostat, a new class of hemostatic agent. WIREs Nanomed Nanobiotechnol 2011;3:70–78)

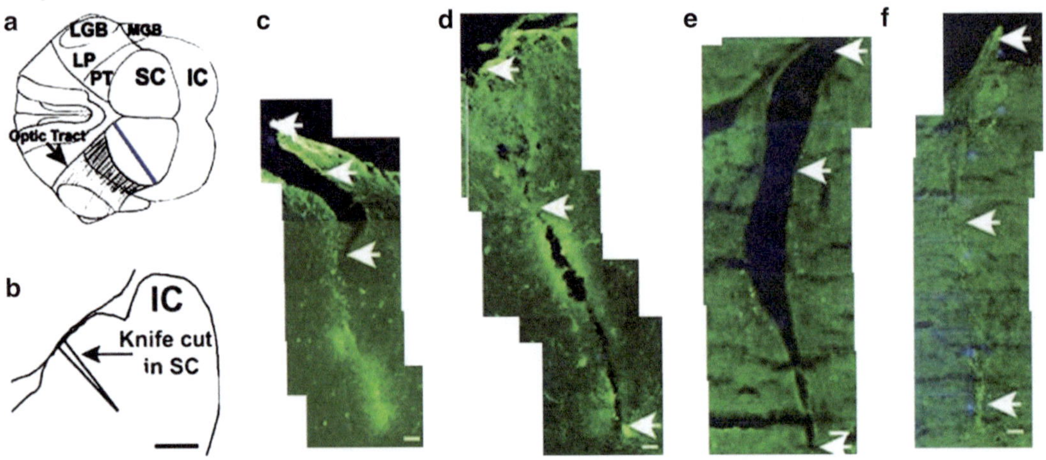

Fig. 4.12 (**a**–**f**) SAPNS for axonal regeneration in the hamster optic tract. Animals received saline 10 μl injection of 1 % SAPNS into the cut; controls received 10 μl saline injection. (**a**) Dorsal view of hamster brain with cortex removed; rostral to *left*, caudal to *right* in all figures. *Blue line*—optic tract transection at P2 in the SC of the midbrain. *IC* inferior colliculus, *LGB* lateral geniculate body, *LP* lateral posterior nucleus, *MGB* medial geniculate body, *PT* pretectal area, *SC* superior colliculus. (**b**) Parasagittal section of the hamster midbrain, indicating the optic tract transection in the SC. (**c**–**f**) Dark-field composite photos of parasagittal sections. (**c**, **d**) Animals sacrificed at 24 h after lesion and treatment, control (**c**) and treatment (**d**). (**e**, **f**) Animals sacrificed at 30 days after lesion and treatment, control (**e**) and treatment (**f**). Note the large gap in (**e**), not present in (**f**). (Used with permission from Ellis-Behnke RG, Liang YX, You SW, et al. Nano neuro knitting: peptide nanofiber scaffold for brain repair and axon regeneration with functional return of vision. PNAS 2006;103(13):5054–5059)

heart and brain, respectively. Improving the electrical charge transfer between the device and the tissue (by decreasing the impedance and/or increasing the capacitance) can markedly enhance clinical efficacy and battery life. CNTs and CNFs have been shown to improve charge transfer by orders of magnitude over electrodes not employing these nanotechniques. A simple but elegant example is the mere coating of standard electrodes for recording and stimulating the brain with CNTs; this provided a 20-fold decrease in impedance and a 40-fold increase in capacitance over uncoated electrodes [20]. By coating nanoarrays with conducting polymers, even more dramatic improvements in electrical charge transfer have been achieved [21].

Although the tissue-device interface has concentrated on electrical activity recording and stimulating, chemical activity (such as that of neurotransmitters in the brain) is clearly essential to understanding and correcting disorders of tissue function throughout the body. For example, Parkinson's disease (PD) occurs when there is a deficiency of dopamine in certain regions of the striatum of the brain. Drug treatment consists of replacing the dopamine deficiency with pills (orally); side effects such as dyskinesias often occur, which may—at least in part—be due to the replacement dopamine going to regions other than those deficient in dopamine (resulting in a relative excess). The most effective nondrug treatment for PD is deep brain stimulation of the subthalamic nucleus, which it is hypothesized tends to restore the electrical firing patterns in the brain to a more normal state. However, in a swine model, it has been shown that stimulation of the subthalamic nucleus (with parameters similar to those used in humans with PD) results in release of dopamine in the striatum [22]. The same group also showed that electrical stimulation (again similar to deep brain stimulation clinically) of astrocyte cell cultures results in release of another neurotransmitter, glutamate [23].

These data strongly suggest that monitoring neurotransmitters as well as electrical activity will greatly increase our understanding of many brain disorders and likely facilitate our treatment of those disorders. To that end, nanotechniques have been applied to our ability to monitor chemical activity in real time, in the brain (and potentially in other tissues such as the myocardium). Differential pulse voltammetry (DPV) is a well-established technique to monitor single neurotransmitters in the brain in near real time. However, DPV is unable to distinguish neurotransmitters such as dopamine and serotonin under in vivo conditions (e.g., when ascorbic acid is present) since dopamine and serotonin have oxidation potentials differing only by about 150 mV. It has recently been shown that CNF electrodes, unlike standard glassy carbon electrodes, can distinguish dopamine and serotonin in the presence of ascorbic acid (Fig. 4.13) [24].

Equally promising is the application of carbon nanotube techniques to myocardial disorders. Biomimetic extracellular matrices or scaffolds are a major thrust in myocardial tissue engineering. Problems with biocompatible scaffolds (polymers/gels) to date have included (1) mechanical weakness in comparison with myocardial tissues, (2) inability to match the conductive properties of myocardium, and (3) lack of submicron architectures that mimic myocardial tissues (architectures which are important in regulating cellular behavior) [25]. A recent publication demonstrates that gelatin methacrylate (GelMA) hydrogel (which has potential as a cardiac patch) demonstrates properties desirable in a cardiac patch when NT networks are embedded in the GelMA hydrogel [25]. The structure of the CNT-GelMA hydrogel is illustrated in Fig. 4.14a–d, the effect of various concentrations of CNTs on spontaneous beating and excitation threshold in Fig. 4.15, and proposed mechanisms for the cardioprotective effects of CNT-GelMA hydrogel against the reversible cardio-inhibitor heptanol and the cytotoxic agent doxorubicin in Fig. 4.16. CNT-GelMA hydrogel represents a significant advance in the search for a truly biomimetic cardiac patch, and the characteristics that CNTs (and other nanomaterials) add to tissue scaffolds are likely to prove effective for many tissue engineering challenges.

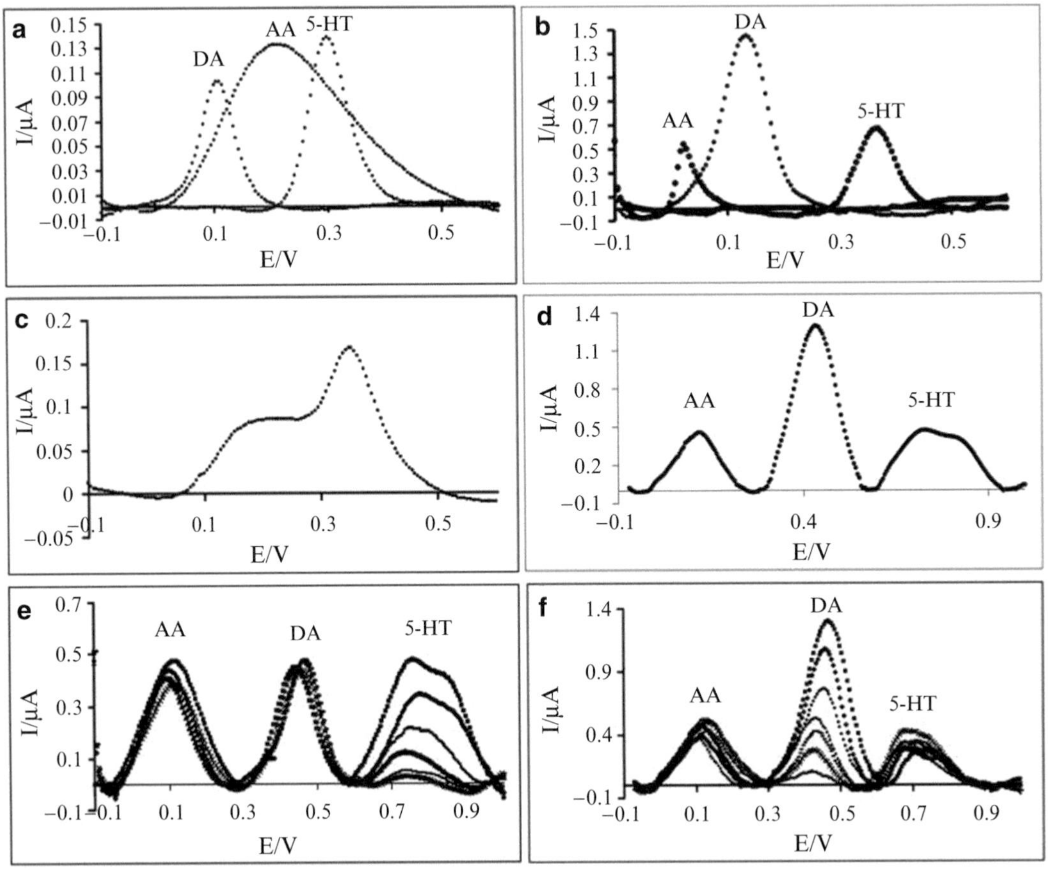

Fig. 4.13 Simultaneous detection of dopamine and serotonin in the presence of ascorbic acid. DPV plots of individual detection of 1 mM AA, 10 μM DA, 10 μM 5-HT (*left*), and a ternary mixture of 1 mM AA, 10 μM DA, 10 μM 5-HT (*right*) (glassy carbon electrode top row, carbon nanofiber electrode *middle row*). *Bottom row* (carbon nanofiber electrode): DPV plots of a ternary mixture of 1 mM AA, 10 μM DA, 5-HT (10, 5, 2.5, 1, 0.5, and 0.25 μM) (*left*), and a ternary mixture of 1 mM AA, DA (10, 5, 2.5, 1, 0.5, and 0.25 μM), 10 μM 5-HT (*right*). (Used with permission from Rand E, Eriyakaruppan A, Tanaka Z, et al. A carbon nanofiber based biosensor for simultaneous detection of dopamine and serotonin in the presence of ascorbic acid. Biosens Bioelectron 2013;42:434–438)

Conclusions

Richard Feynman did not address how the "swallowed surgeon" would get from the gastrointestinal tract to the blood vessels in order to operate on the faulty heart valve. Fortunately our endovascular colleagues have become adept at threading increasingly small catheters into increasingly small blood vessels. Indeed, the vascular "highway system"—from the aortic "interstate" to the capillary "alley"—can be employed to access all tissues in the body down to the cellular level. It has been demonstrated that electrical recordings and stimulations of the nervous system can be performed by an electrode in the blood vessel as effectively as by an electrode inserted into the brain parenchyma [26]. Furthermore, as suggested by Kendall Lee (personal communication, 2011), monitoring of chemicals in tissues (such as neurotransmitters in the brain) can be achieved by poking the electrode through the capillary wall. A nanoelectrode can be several hundred nanometers (or less) in diameter—only 1/10 the diameter of a red blood cell—so bleeding would not be a problem.

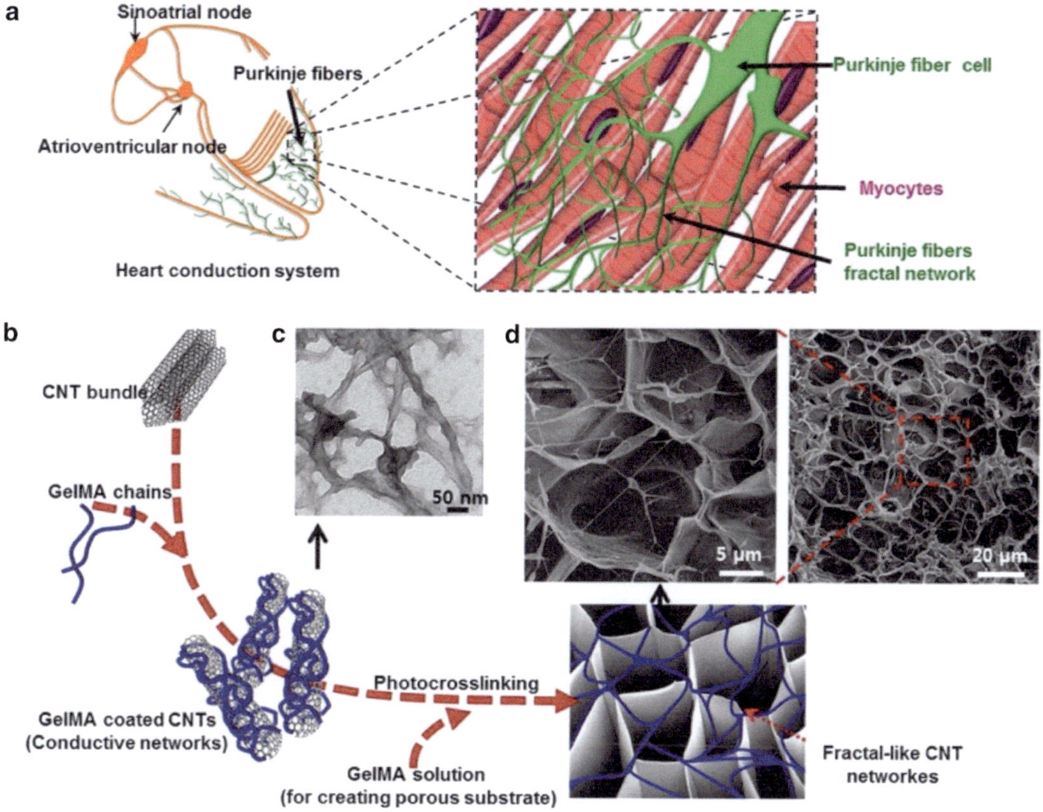

Fig. 4.14 (**a–d**) (**a**) Schematic of the isolated heart conducting systems. (**b**) Preparation procedure of fractal-like CNT networks embedded in GelMA hydrogel. (**c**) TEM of GelMA coated CNTs. (**d**) SEM of porous surfaces of 1 mg/ml CNT-GelMA thin film. Magnified image shows nanofibrous networks across and inside a porous structure. (**a–d**: Used with permission from Shin SR, Jung SM, Zalabany M, et al. Carbon-nanotube-embedded hydrogel sheets for engineering cardiac constructs and bioactuators. ACS Nano 2013;7(3):2369–2380)

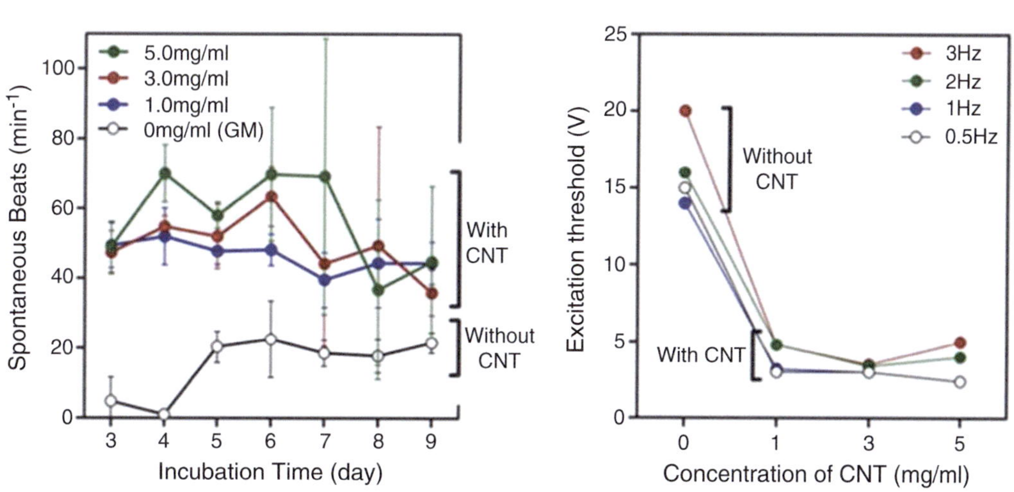

Fig. 4.15 *Left*. Spontaneous beating rates of cardiac tissues recorded from days 3 to 9. *Right*. Excitation threshold of cardiac tissues on CNT-GelMA was 85 % lower than on pristine GelMA. (Used with permission from Shin SR, Jung SM, Zalabany M, et al. Carbon-nanotube-embedded hydrogel sheets for engineering cardiac constructs and bioactuators. ACS Nano 2013;7(3): 2369–2380)

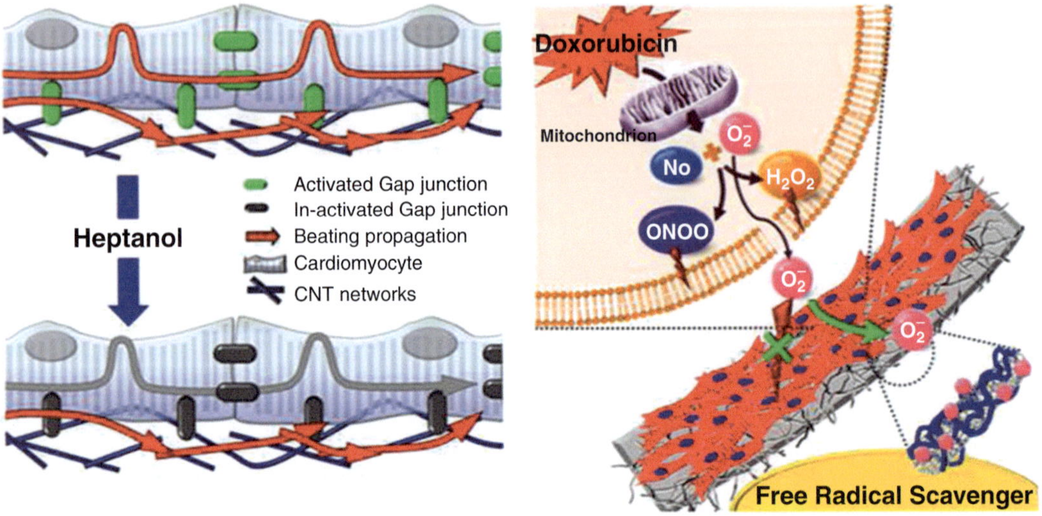

Fig. 4.16 *Left*. Schematic of alternative electric signal propagation through CNT networks after inhibition of direct intercellular gap junctions by heptanol. *Right*. Proposed mechanisms for CNTs to protect cardiac cells from oxygen free radical damage. (Used with permission from Shin SR, Jung SM, Zalabany M, et al. Carbon-nanotube-embedded hydrogel sheets for engineering cardiac constructs and bioactuators. ACS Nano 2013;7(3):2369–2380)

Feynman's vision is becoming a reality. In the present era of surgical technology, one must think small to make big advances!

References

1. Feynman RP. There's plenty of room at the bottom. Eng Sci. 1960;23(2):22–36.
2. Smalley RE. Testimony before the U.S. House of Representatives regarding the proposal to establish a National Nanotechnology Initiative. Available at www.rice.edu/media/smalleytestimony.htm. Accessed 22 June 1999.
3. Reibold M, Paufler P, Levin AA, Kochmann W, Pätzke N, Meyer DC. Carbon nanotubes in an ancient Damascus sabre. Nature. 2006;444:286.
4. Silva GA, Parpura V, editors. Nanotechnology for biology and medicine. New York: Springer Science + Business Media; 2012.
5. Kateb B, Heiss JD, editors. The textbook of nanoneuroscience and nanoneurosurgery. Boca Raton, FL: CRC Press; 2014.
6. Kateb B, Chiu K, Black KL, et al. Nanoplatforms for constructing new approaches to cancer treatment, imaging, and drug delivery: what should be the policy? Neuroimage. 2011;54:S106–24.
7. Daraio C, Jin S. Synthesis and patterning methods for nanostructures useful for biological applications. In: Silva GA, Parpura V, editors. Nanotechnology for biology and medicine. New York: Springer Science + Business Media; 2012.
8. Rizzo LY, Theek B, Storm G, Kiessling F, Lammers T. Recent progress in nanomedicine: therapeutic, diagnostic and theranostic applications. Curr Opin Biotechnol. 2013;24(6):1–13.
9. Provenzale JM, Silva GA. Uses of nanoparticles for central nervous system imaging and therapy. AJNR Am J Neuroradiol. 2009;30:1293–301.
10. Smith AM, Nie S. Chemical analysis and cellular imaging with quantum dots. Analyst. 2004;129:672–7.
11. Pathak S, Cao E, Davidson MC, Jin S, Silva GA. Quantum dot applications to neuroscience: new tools for probing neurons and glia. J Neurosci. 2006;26(7): 1893–5.
12. Ellis-Behnke RG, Liang YX, You SW, et al. Nano neuro knitting: peptide nanofiber scaffold for brain repair and axon regeneration with functional return of vision. PNAS. 2006;103(13):5054–9.
13. Weinstein JS, Varallyay CG, Dosa E, et al. Superparamagnetic iron oxide nanoparticles: diagnostic magnetic resonance imaging and potential therapeutic applications in neurooncology and central nervous system inflammatory pathologies, a review. J Cereb Blood Flow Metab. 2010;30:15–35.
14. Wang LS, Chuang MC, Ho JA. Nanotheranostics – a review of recent publications. Int J Nanomed. 2012; 7:4679–95.
15. Wankhede M, Bouras A, Kaluzova M, Hadjipanayis CG. Magnetic nanoparticles: an emerging technology

for malignant brain tumor imaging and therapy. Expert Rev Clin Pharmacol. 2012;5(2):173–86.
16. Nanobiotix website (www.nanobiotix.com). Accessed 27 Apr 2014.
17. Cyrus T, Wickline SA, Lanza GM. Nanotechnology in interventional cardiology. WIREs Nanomed Nanobiotechnol. 2012;4:82–95.
18. Norling LV, Spite M, Yang R, Flower RJ, Perretti M, Serhan CN. Humanized nano pro-resolving medicines mimic inflammation-resolution and enhance wound healing. J Immunol. 2011;186(10):5543–7.
19. Ellis-Behnke R. At the nanoscale: nanohemostat, a new class of hemostatic agent. WIREs Nanomed Nanobiotechnol. 2011;3:70–8.
20. Keefer EW, Botterman BR, Romero MI, Rossi AF, Gross GW. Carbon nanotube coating improves neuronal recordings. Nat Nanotechnol. 2008;3:434–9.
21. Nguyen-Vu TDB, Chen H, Cassell AM, Andrews R, Meyyappan M, Li J. Vertically aligned carbon nanofiber arrays: an advance toward electrical-neural interfaces. Small. 2006;2:89–94.
22. Shon YM, Lee KH, Goerss SJ, et al. High frequency stimulation of the subthalamic nucleus evokes striatal dopamine release in a large animal model of DBS neurosurgery. Neurosci Lett. 2010;475:136–40.
23. Tawfik VL, Chang SY, Hitti FL, et al. Deep brain stimulation results in local glutamate and adenosine release: investigation into the role of astrocytes. Neurosurgery. 2010;67:367–75.
24. Rand E, Periyakaruppan A, Tanaka Z, et al. A carbon nanofiber based biosensor for simultaneous detection of dopamine and serotonin in the presence of ascorbic acid. Biosens Bioelectron. 2013;42:434–8.
25. Shin SR, Jung SM, Zalabany M, et al. Carbon-nanotube-embedded hydrogel sheets for engineering cardiac constructs and bioactuators. ACS Nano. 2013;7(3):2369–80.
26. Llinas RR, Walton KD, Nakao M, Hunter I, Anquetil PA. Neuro-vascular nervous recording/stimulating system: using nanotechnology probes. J Nanopart Res. 2005;7:111–27.

Telemedicine for Trauma and Intensive Care: Changing the Paradigm of Telepresence

5

Rifat Latifi

Introduction

While principles of the surgical sciences and practice have remained the same over centuries, the way in which surgery is conducted has changed dramatically in the past 50 years. A key element of these changes is technological advances during this time period, with rapid advances in techniques such as laparoscopy, robotic surgery, and internet and remote presence introduction in the last two to three decades. Telemedicine and telepresence are not new phenomena and have been promoted and practiced by a number of surgeons over the last few decades. While few surgeons, such as Michael E. DeBakey and Ronald C. Merrell, were pioneers of telemedicine [1, 2], only in the last few years have telemedicine and telepresence been routinely accepted and practiced by a greater number of surgeons across multiple subspecialties. Yet, this number is very small compared to the overall number of surgeons worldwide and, in particular, in developed countries. Telemedicine offers great promise, specifically for people living in rural and remote areas because it reduces time and cost as well as provides specialists who are unavailable within those areas. It has also successfully been used from simple surgical consultations with low bandwidth [2] for a consulting second opinion, to intraoperative interventions, to transatlantic spectacular surgical interventions [3], to disaster response scenarios. Because of its potential uses with vulnerable populations, the World Health Organization (WHO) formulated the e-Health strategy in 2005. Within this e-Health strategy, several initiatives to foster development of telemedicine centers in member states began [4].

Recent technological advances have made possible telemedicine application in the management of trauma and emergency care and in the intensive care setting especially in remote areas and isolated communities. The biggest promise of teletrauma, teleresuscitation, and tele-ICU is the transformation of "Golden Hour" into "now care" and the stabilization of the patient and safe transport to trauma center when indicated. The initial experience with teletrauma in saving lives—managing critically ill and injured trauma patients at the rural site or safely transferring them when needed—reducing the overall cost of trauma care has been rewarding and very successful. The acceptance by trauma surgeons, referring physicians, nurses, and other providers, as well as patients, has been excellent. Other clinical specialties are making preparations and creating protocols to use the system as well. The telepresence of the trauma surgeon, through the teletrauma system, is being used to identify

R. Latifi (✉)
Department of Surgery, University of Arizona Medical Center, Tucson, AZ, USA
e-mail: latifi@surgery.arizona.edu

R. Latifi et al. (eds.), *Technological Advances in Surgery, Trauma and Critical Care*,
DOI 10.1007/978-1-4939-2671-8_5

knowledge gaps and the needs for instituting new outreach educational programs. As technology is becoming friendlier and cheaper, the concepts of teletrauma, telepresence, and teleresuscitation are evolving and will become an integral part of modern care of trauma and emergency care in rural settings, where there is a lack of specialists and other expertise.

Global advances in cellular telephony have made telemedicine even more readily available for poor and remote regions of the world. Agencies such as the National Institutes of Health are inviting proposals to facilitate the use of these technologies in low (LICs) and low middle income countries (LMICs) [5]; however, the use of these technologies for surgical practices still has been less than would be anticipated and is most likely reflective of being in the early phases of development.

Recent activities within the American College of Surgeons have increased the visibility of telemedicine for surgeons by having dedicated courses for surgeons as well as by creating a subcommittee on telemedicine within the Health Information Technology committee [6].

The primary benefit of telemedicine is the ability to provide medical care from and at the distance [7–14]. No other field of clinical telemedicine has proven more beneficial, has reduced mortality and morbidity, and has become more popular, in particular in organized major health systems, than telemedicine for intensive care. Variously known as "virtual e-ICU," "e-ICU," or "tele-ICU," all have the same meaning, however, and that means that an intensivist (surgeon, anesthesiologist, or an intensivist) manages a number of patients, often in a number of intensive care units in wide geographical areas, at the same time. Throughout this chapter, we will refer to telemedicine for intensive care units (ICU) as "tele-ICU," and to telemedicine for trauma and emergencies as "teletrauma."

Due to the growing demand of intensive care and the rising elderly population, it is expected that these numbers will continue to grow. On the other hand, there is a major shortage of intensivists caring for these patients, and telemedicine has been promoted as one solution to this major shortage of intensivists, in particular in a large healthcare system [7–15]. Patients are monitored live from a command and control center using audio and video connectivity, assisted with major set of evidence-based medicine guidelines and protocols.

While implementation of tele-ICU has expanded dramatically, there are a number of challenges to implement tele-ICU, both in developing countries and developed countries. These challenges include financial, economic, legislative, attitudinal, and cultural. Despite these barriers with the advancing of technological options, and as technology becomes cheaper, the use of tele-ICU will also grow. However, the benefits of tele-ICU programs outweigh the risks associated with them, and the barriers need to be overcome to allow for successful establishment and integration of tele-ICU services in the overall platform of healthcare system. For tele-ICU, geography and distance are meaningless, as is a case with any form of telemedicine. This chapter reviews the successful tele-ICU and teletrauma programs and discusses the challenges associated with implementing tele-ICU programs.

Prevalence of Tele-ICU and Models of Operations

Tele-ICU is becoming more and more prevalent. A recent review found that formal ICU telemedicine programs now support around 11 % of nonfederal hospital critically ill adult patients and have demonstrated lower ICU and hospital mortality and shorter ICU and hospital length of stay [14]. There is an expected annual growth rate of 1 % per year [11], indicating that critical care delivery models that include telemedicine will continue to grow [11, 15]. In addition to the continuous telemedicine care model, episodic care models continue to grow [15, 16]. In early 2013, there were 175 active robotic devices, 56 of which are known to be supporting ICU patients in 25 North American ICUs, that have been activated more than 10,000 times [15].

There are a couple of models of tele-ICU about which there have been reports. The most common one is Centralized Monitoring Model (CMM), usually applied in major healthcare systems, while the second one, Virtual Consultant Model (VCM), provides care to individual ICUs using a number of off-the-shelf technologies. This technology, especially for CMMs, is very expensive to set up and to maintain; in a most recent study [11], the capital cost of the tele-ICU was $1,186,220. The annual operational cost is $1,250,112, or $23,150 per monitored ICU bed [16].

A recent literature review of 91 studies on tele-ICU found that 46 of these studies assessed clinical outcomes, 36 assessed workload and staff acceptance, and nine assessed cost and financial indicators [17–19]. When these two models were studied side-by-side, it was found that CMMs showed better outcomes [19]. Of 46 studies reported, a reduced LOS and decrease in mortality were noted in all but six of the studies [18]. A review of 25 tele-ICU in the United States found that implementation of tele-ICU programs favorably affected morbidity rates and length of stay. Other studies also have shown decreased LOS and decrease in mortality when tele-ICU was applied [7, 11, 20, 21].

However, many argue against the cost-effectiveness of tele-ICU programs. Others [22] found that, while costs increased with the implementation of a tele-ICU, mortality rates decreased, but only among the sickest population. These authors reviewed the cost per bed for patients before and after the implementation of a tele-ICU in five hospitals within a large nonprofit group. The cost per bed for patients included software and hardware implementation. Costs per patient increased 28 %. Hospital cost per case increased 43 %. Because the sickest of the patients had lower mortality and length of stay, these authors suggest cautious implementation of tele-ICU programs [22] and possibly for the sickest of patients only. Additionally, a meta-analysis on studies that published results from tele-ICU implementation reported that mortality rates and LOS were reduced [23, 24], but the optimal tailoring of tele-ICU programs remains unclear [17]. Specifically, the best benefit to cost ratio has not been defined. Others have suggested further financial analysis [25]. Overall, however, the majority of studies do provide evidence for a reduction in mortality rates and a reduction in length of stay.

In addition, other important benefits come from using tele-ICU. It has been demonstrated that the experience of physicians in training with telemedicine intensivists is positive and that there is increased patient safety [14]. Numerous studies have been conducted on staff perception, usability, and satisfaction with tele-intensive care units. For example, physicians expressed that they were extremely satisfied [26]. Others found that there was an increase in satisfaction among nursing team members, particularly during nighttime hours [27]. Physicians felt they could manage critically ill patients better, were more equipped to communicate with bedside care teams, and were better able to provide reassurance to families [28]. Tele-ICU implementation was associated with improvement in nursing perceptions of working conditions and communications [29]. In one study, 93 % of clinicians felt that telemedicine was clinically useful in neonatal examinations [30]; others found that the use of telemedicine technology by nurses was affected by their perceived usefulness [31].

Overall, the majority of studies that included quantitative and qualitative data provide support for the use of telemedicine in intensive care settings, although in one study it was found that some nurses felt that the transition from bedside caregiver to information manager can be difficult [32]. Fewer studies that provide evidence for patient satisfaction are available. Evidence suggests that patients report higher satisfaction with tele-ICUs; however, vigilance of staff and nurses in the use of these services plays a role in patient satisfaction [33, 34]. Early studies suggest that implementation of ICU telemedicine programs has been associated with lower numbers of malpractice claims and costs. The requirements for Medicare reimbursement and states with legislation addressing providing professional services by telemedicine should be known by all providers involved in this exciting field [14]. A number of new directions and future uses of tele-ICU are being explored, including caring for the increasing geriatric population [35].

Tele-ICU protocols and procedures are based on the institutional policies and the setup. Most practices require 12–24 h telepresence of a critical care specialist. Providers such as physician assistants, nurse practitioners, or residents, in addition to bed site critical care nurses, are usually involved in the site where patients are present. Scheduled bedside rounds and rounds on demand are done. The main point is the fact that the critical care specialist has visual as well as audio access, and access to all the data and medical records as well. In addition, most of the tele-ICU models use guidelines, protocols, and algorithms to manage certain critical conditions.

Teletrauma and Emergency Management

Approximately 10 % of the world's deaths, or 5.8 million, are due to injuries each year. More than 90 % of deaths due to injuries occur in LICs and LMICs. It has been estimated that 40 % of deaths could be preventable in the United States if access to trauma care was uniform throughout the country. It has been postulated by a number of authors that adding telemedicine for trauma (teletrauma) will improve overall trauma care. To this end, a number of programs have been successfully designed and implemented [36].

The first attempt to simulate the use of telemedicine in trauma resuscitation in real time was recorded in 1978 by Dr. R. Adams Cowley, who staged a disaster exercise at Friendship Airport in an aged DC-6 aircraft, using old cumbersome satellite technology. Following the reports by Rogers et al. [37] on their use of a teletrauma, a number of other investigators established telemedicine services for trauma and emergencies, mostly for the management of injuries in rural settings. This certainly has major implications on the cost of transferring these patients to major medical centers, increased utilization of local healthcare facilities, and other social and financial issues of treating these patients away from their families. The clinical accuracy of telemedicine in evaluating other trauma patients also has been assessed and demonstrated. In order to fully implement remote trauma resuscitation, the remote trauma surgeons and referring healthcare providers must feel comfortable and confident in their ability to supervise and manage trauma resuscitation in the remote site from a central location.

While there are several studies that document the effectiveness of telemedicine in trauma, there were no reported randomized controlled trials. The benefits of teletrauma have been well documented and span from reduction of unneeded transfers, reduction in mortality, reduction of cost, to improvements in patients satisfaction. For example, a study comparing telemedicine consultations for a rural pediatric care facility found a high satisfaction rate among providers and patients [38]. Other studies evaluated 841 patients over a 5 years period in Mississippi and found that telemedicine significantly improved acute trauma management. Severely injured patients were more readily identified and transferred when necessary [39]. Several other studies have reported high clinical accuracy as well [40].

In a retrospective analysis of 59 teleconsults between five rural hospitals and a Level I trauma center, we reported the initial experience with 59 trauma and general surgery patients [41, 42]. Of those, 35 (59 %) were trauma patients, and 24 (41 %) were general surgery patients. Fifty patients (85 %) were from the first hospital at which teletrauma was established. For six patients, the teletrauma consults were considered potentially lifesaving; 17 patients (29 %) were kept in the rural hospitals (8 trauma and 9 general surgery patients). Treating patients in the rural hospitals avoided transfers, saving an average of $19,698 per air transport or $2,055 per ground transport. The authors concluded that the telepresence of a trauma surgeon aids in the initial evaluation, treatment, and care of patients, improving outcomes and reducing the costs of trauma care [42]. Others have recently published cumulative results for telemedicine in acute phase injury [43].

The use of telemedicine for wound and burn care has been extensive, and is one of the most common applications of telemedicine practices in surgeries. Burn centers in particular have documented the usefulness of telemedicine in burn and wound care [44–50].

Summary

There are numerous benefits and, as with anything, some limitations to the implementation and use of telemedicine for trauma and intensive care. The reduction in travel costs is significant; however, the initial capital costs for ICU and trauma units need to be balanced out by the benefits seen in the long term.

Successful telemedicine programs have been implemented and provide excellent examples for others, but the adoption of technology, programs, and systems has not happened as readily as expected. Of the successful programs that do exist, many have not spread to large-scale applications. These few successful programs typically have champions who facilitate program funding with government and private sector connections or who have successful grants. By continuing the mission of adopting technology and publishing results of the use of these technologies, empirical evidence supporting the effectiveness of these technologies will contribute to wider acceptance by patients and physicians, which will lead to the establishment of additional clinical telemedicine programs. This adoption will, in turn, contribute to saving lives. Despite the initial high cost of establishing tele-ICUs and teletrauma, the evidence for the effectiveness is unquestionable, and these services will continue to grow. While the technology is rapidly advancing and getting less expensive, the cost of setting it up may also eventually be reduced.

References

1. DeBakey ME. The living heart. New York: Charter Books; 1977.
2. Merrell RC. Changing the medical world order with technological advances: the future has only begun. In: Latifi R, editor. Establishing telemedicine in developing countries: from inception to implementation. Amsterdam: IOS Press; 2004.
3. Marescaux J, Leroy J, Rubino F, Smith M, Vix M, Simone M, et al. Transcontinental robot-assisted remote telesurgery; feasibility and potential applications. Am Surg. 2002;235:487–92.
4. World Health Organization National eHealth Strategy Toolkit. http://www.itu.int/pub/D-STR-E_HEALTH.05-2012. Accessed 24 Jan 2014.
5. National Institutes of Health, Fogarty Center. http://grants.nih.gov/grants/guide/pa-files/PAR-14-028.html. Accessed 8 Oct 2014.
6. American College of Surgeons. Health Information Technology Committee. https://www.facs.org/about-acs/governance/acs-committees/health-information-technology-committee. Accessed 8 Oct 2014.
7. Latifi R, Peck K, Satava R, Anvari M. Telepresence and telementoring in surgery. In: Latifi R, editor. Establishing telemedicine in developing countries: from inception to implementation. Amsterdam: IOS Press; 2004. p. 201–6.
8. Reynolds HN, Rogove H, Bander J, McCambridge M, Cowboy E, Niemeier M. A working lexicon for the tele-intensive care unit: We need to define teleintensive care unit to grow and understand it. Telemed J E Health. 2011;17:773–83.
9. Rosenfeld BA, Dorman T, Breslow MJ, et al. Intensive care unit telemedicine: alternate paradigm for providing continuous intensivist care. Crit Care Med. 2000;28:3925–31.
10. Thomas EJ, Lucke JF, Wueste L, et al. Association of telemedicine for remote monitoring of intensive care patients with mortality, complications, and length of stay. JAMA. 2009;302:2671–8.
11. Lilly CM, Thomas EJ. Tele-ICU: experience to date. J Intensive Care Med. 2010;25:16–22.
12. Zawada Jr ET, Herr P, Larson D, et al. Impact of an intensive care unit telemedicine program on a rural health care system. Postgrad Med. 2009;121:160–70.
13. Willmitch B, Golembeski S, Kim SS, et al. Clinical outcomes after telemedicine intensive care unit implementation. Crit Care Med. 2012;40:450–4.
14. Lilly CM, Zubrow MT, Kempner KM, Reynolds HN, Subramanian S, Eriksson EA, Jenkins CL, Rincon TA, Kohl BA, Groves Jr RH, Cowboy ER, Mbekeani KE, McDonald MJ, Rascona DA, Ries MH, Rogove HJ, Badr AE, Kopec IC, Society of Critical Care Medicine Tele-ICU Committee. Critical care telemedicine: evolution and state of the art. Crit Care Med. 2014;42(11):2429–36.
15. Reynolds EM, Grujovski A, Wright T, et al. Utilization of robotic "remote presence" technology within North American intensive care units. Telemed J E Health. 2012;18:507–15.
16. Fortis S, Weinert C, Bushinski R, Koehler AG, Beilman G. A health system-based critical care program with a novel tele-ICU: implementation, cost, and structure details. J Am Coll Surg. 2014;219(4):676–83.

17. Kumar S, Merchant S, Reynolds R. Tele-ICU: efficacy and cost-effectiveness approach of remotely managing the critical care. Open Med Inform J. 2013;7:24–9.
18. Ramnath VR, Ho L, Maggio LA, Khazeni N. Centralized monitoring and virtual consultant models of tele-ICU care: a systematic review. Telemed J E Health. 2014;20:936–61.
19. Ramnath VR, Khazeni N. Centralized monitoring and virtual consultant models of tele-ICU care: a side-by-side review. Telemed J E Health. 2014;20(10):962–71.
20. Kohl BA, Fortino-Mullen M, Praestgaard A, Hanson CW, Dimartino J, Ochroch EA. The effect of ICU telemedicine on mortality and length of stay. J Telemed Telecare. 2012;18(5):282–6.
21. Lilly CM, Cody S, Zhao H, et al. Hospital mortality, length of stay and preventable complications among critically ill patients before and after tele-ICU reengineering of critical care processes. JAMA. 2011; 305(21):2175–83.
22. Franzini L, Sail KR, Thomas EJ, Wueste L. Costs and cost-effectiveness of a tele-ICU program in six intensive care units in a large healthcare system. J Crit Care. 2011;26(3):329.e1–6.
23. Wilcox ME, Adhikari NKJ. The effect of telemedicine in critically ill patients: systematic review and meta-analysis. Crit Care. 2012;16(4):R127.
24. Sadaka F, Palagiri A, Trottier S, Deibert W, Gudmestad D, Sommer SE, Veremakis C. Telemedicine intervention improves ICU outcomes. Crit Care Res Pract. 2013;2013:456389.
25. Kumar G, Falk DM, Bonello RS, Kahn JM, Perencevich E, Cram P. The costs of critical care telemedicine programs: a systematic review and analysis. Chest. 2013;143(1):19–29.
26. Rogove H, Atkins C, Kramer J. Enhanced access to neurointensivists through a telemedicine program [abstract]. Crit Care Med. 2009;37(Suppl):A1.
27. Rincon T, Seiver A, Farrell W, Daly MA. Increased documentation of ICD-9-CM codes 995.92 and 785.52 with template-oriented monitoring and screening by a tele-ICU [abstract]. Crit Care Med. 2009;37(Suppl):A4.
28. Yager P, Whalen M, Cummings B, Noviski N. Use of telemedicine to provide enhanced communication between at-home attendings and bedside personnel in a pediatric intensive care unit [abstract]. Crit Care Med. 2010;38:U28.
29. Romig M, Latif A, Pronovost P, Gill R, Sapirstein A. Perceived benefit of a consultative telemedicine service in a highly staffed intensive care unit [abstract]. Crit Care Med. 2010;38:U27.
30. Armfield NR, Donovan T, Smith AC. Clinicians' perceptions of telemedicine for remote neonatal consultation. Stud Health Technol Inform. 2010;161:1–9.
31. Kowitlawakul Y. The technology acceptance model: predicting nurses' intention to use telemedicine technology (eICU). Comput Inform Nurs. 2011;29:411–8.
32. Hoonakker PLT, Carayon P, McGuire K, et al. Motivation and job satisfaction of tele-ICU nurses. J Crit Care. 2013;28:315.e13–21.
33. Goran SF. Measuring tele-ICU impact: does it optimize quality outcomes for the critically ill patient? J Nurs Manag. 2012;20(3):414–28.
34. Young LB, Chan PS, Cram P. Staff acceptance of tele-ICU coverage: a systematic review. Chest. 2011;139:279–88.
35. Hao JF, Cui HM, Han JM, Bai JX, Song X, Cao N. Tele-ICU: the way forward in geriatric care? Aging Clin Exp Res. 2014;26(6):575–82.
36. Latifi R, Peck K, Porter JM, Poropatich R, Geare III T, Nassi RB. Telepresence and telemedicine in trauma and emergency care management. In: Establishing telemedicine in developing countries: from inception to implementation. Amsterdam: IOS Press; 2004. p. 193–9.
37. Rogers F, Ricci M, Shackford S, Caputo L, Sartorelli K, Dwell J, Day S. The use of telemedicine for real-time video consultation between trauma center and community hospital in a rural setting improves early trauma care. Preliminary results. J Trauma. 2001; 51(6):1037–41.
38. Marcin JP, Schepps DE, Page KA, Struve SN, Nagrampa E, Dimand RJ. The use of telemedicine to provide pediatric critical care consultations to pediatric trauma patients admitted to a remote trauma intensive care unit: a preliminary report. Pediatr Crit Care Med. 2004;5:251–6.
39. Duchesne JC, Kyle A, Simmons J, Islam S, Schmieg Jr RE, Olivier J, et al. Impact of telemedicine upon rural trauma care. J Trauma. 2008;64:92–7. discussion: 97–98.
40. Lambrecht CJ. Telemedicine in trauma care: description of 100 trauma teleconsults. Telemed J. 1997;3(4):265–8.
41. Latifi R, Hadeed GJ, Rhee P, O'Keeffe T, Friese RS, Wynne JL, et al. Initial experiences and outcomes of telepresence in the management of trauma and emergency surgical patients. Am J Surg. 2009;198:905–10.
42. Latifi R, Weinstein RS, Porter JM, Ziemba M, Judkins D, Ridings D, et al. Telemedicine and telepresence for trauma and emergency care management. Scand J Surg. 2007;96:281–9.
43. Lewis ER, Thomas CA, Wilson ML, Mbarika VWA. Telemedicine in acute-phase injury management: a review of practice and advancements. Telemed J E Health. 2012;18(6):434–45.
44. Ong CA. Telemedicine and wound care. In: Latifi R, editor. Current principles and practices of telemedicine and e-health. Amsterdam: IOS Press; 2008. p. 211–25.
45. Massman NJ, Dodge JD, Fortman KK, Schwartz KJ, Solem LD. Burns follow-up: an innovative application of telemedicine. J Telemed Telecare. 1999;5 Suppl 1:52–4.

46. Saffle JR, et al. Telemedicine evaluation of acute burns is accurate and cost-effective. J Trauma. 2009;67:358–65.
47. Saffle JR. Telemedicine for acute burn treatment: the time has come. J Telemed Telecare. 2006;12:1–3.
48. Yoder LH, McFall DC, Cancio LC. Use of the videophone to collect quality of life data from burn patients. Int J Burns Trauma. 2012;2(3):135–44.
49. Knoblich K, Rennekampff HO, Vogt PM. Cell-phone based multimedia messaging service (MMS) and burn injuries. Burns. 2009;35:1191–3.
50. Smith AC, Kimble R, Mill J, Bailey D, O'Rourke P, Wootton R. Diagnostic accuracy of and patient satisfaction with telemedicine for the follow-up of paediatric burns patients. J Telemed Telecare. 2004;10:193–8.

6 Augmented Reality in Surgery

Timothy M. Rankin, Marvin J. Slepian, and David G. Armstrong

Introduction

Augmented reality involves the overlay of digital imagery onto the real world in real time [1, 2]. This has been used in a wide variety of applications and stems from virtual reality in which a user is able to interact with a virtual environment.

From a historic perspective, a "predictor" of the possibility of visually augmented reality may be seen in the work of Galileo Galilei in the sixteenth century. Early reports described a device of Galilei, referred to as a celatone, that was a face-mounted construct, which held a telescope while allowing basic vision, affording more precise visualization of celestial bodies to assist in navigation. Modern wearable technology began to take form in the 1970s when Steve Mann, a Canadian engineer, began wearing computers to improve his vision and was credited with being the first cyborg [3]. Subsequently there has been a surge in the number of manufacturers of devices as microchips have become smaller and "Heads Up" displays have become more delicate. At this time there are at least 45 companies, ranging from Sony (Minato, Japan) and Google (Mountain View, CA) to crowd funded start-ups such as Technical Illusions (Seattle, WA), with various forms of augmented reality devices in development and a handful with devices available for purchase. These range from $200 to $125,000 offering a range of capabilities with a wide variety of intended applications.

More recent augmented reality efforts began with smartphones, utilizing integrated cameras in order to merge app-based information and the real world. However, this hands-on approach is clearly not ideal for medical and certainly surgical applications. Over the past decade, physicians and surgeons have adopted this technology by way of heads-up displays both in training and to employ patient specific imaging in order to reference or guide intervention [4, 5].

While physicians, surgeons and other health care providers have identified potential applications for this technology, devices developed have suffered from high cost, uncomfortable form factors, suboptimal battery life, or lack of an app-based developer ecosystem [1]. The recent, limited release of wearable technologies using an eyeglass form-factor has begun to address these issues [6–8]. The advent of these wearable, consumer-based, augmented reality devices may provide economical, rapid communication, documentation, and consultation among clinicians.

T.M. Rankin, M.D., M.S. • M.J. Slepian, M.D.
D.G. Armstrong, D.P.M., M.D., Ph.D. (✉)
Department of Surgery, University of Arizona Medical Center, Tucson, AZ, USA
e-mail: Tmrankin.md@gmail.com; chairman.syns@gmail.com; Armstrong@usa.net

R. Latifi et al. (eds.), *Technological Advances in Surgery, Trauma and Critical Care*,
DOI 10.1007/978-1-4939-2671-8_6

Technology

The technology behind providing a heads-up display is based upon the use of a combiner. A combiner overlays a virtual image of an object with the actual object in order to provide a new augmented version of the object to the viewer. Combiners can be either curved mirror-based or waveguide-based (diffractive waveguide, holographic wave guide, polarized waveguide, etc.). Combiners vary in their thickness, weight as well as in the field of view provided. The Star™ 1200 manufactured by Vuzix (Rochester, NY) uses a curved mirror combiner (www.vuzix.com). Google® Glass by Google (Mountain View, CA), for example, uses a monocular Flat Combiner (45°) in order to provide a virtual image that is still translucent (Fig. 6.1). Though it is effective, this technology provides a medium field of view, has a medium eye box, and suffers from a relatively thick combiner. On the other end of the spectrum, Innovega (Bellevue, WA) has implemented a tapered opaque light guide that necessitates the use of a contact lens and glass in order to provide a thin, binocular glass, with a large eye box and a very large field of view (nearly 120°), and allows for true three-dimensional full augmented reality (innovega-inc.com).

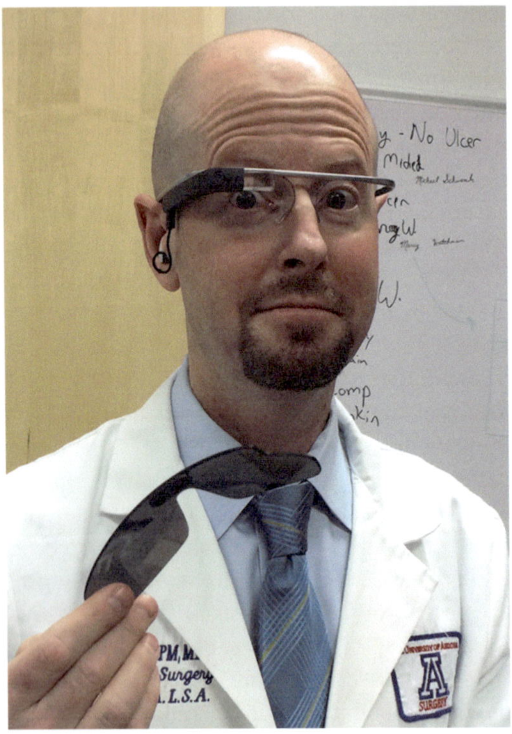

Fig. 6.1 Google Glass became available to the general public in May of 2014 and provides users with a natural language voice command user interface in order to provide a wearable hands-free computing experience

Devices

Augmented reality is the more modern term for mediated reality where our perception of the world is modified in some way. The simplest of these devices could be a rear-view mirror on a car; however, cutting edge augmented reality as we think of it today began in 1958 with Heads-up displays (HUD) for fighter pilots [9]. This overlay of computer-generated imagery has progressed since that time and has become infused into our vehicles, our smart phones and now our eyeglasses.

Smart Phones

Augmented reality for the smart phone became a reality with the integration of a camera. This allowed for the overlay of app-based information onto an image of the real world. Various apps used for locating restaurants and stores were the first to take advantage of this form of AR. Satellite AR (Analytical Graphics, Inc., Exton PA) even allows for the AR visualization of satellites as they orbit the earth (Fig. 6.2).

Head Mounted Displays

As previously stated, the original head mounted displays (HMD) were pioneered by the military for use by fighter pilots (Fig. 6.3). Though many companies have entered the race to engineer the ideal heads-up display, not all will be applicable for medical or surgical applications.

For example, Sony released the Glasstron™ in 1997, which did not have any transmissivity and was intended for viewing of multimedia such as movies. Since that time, Sony and most of its competitors have moved toward AR compatible eyewear with varying AR compatibility.

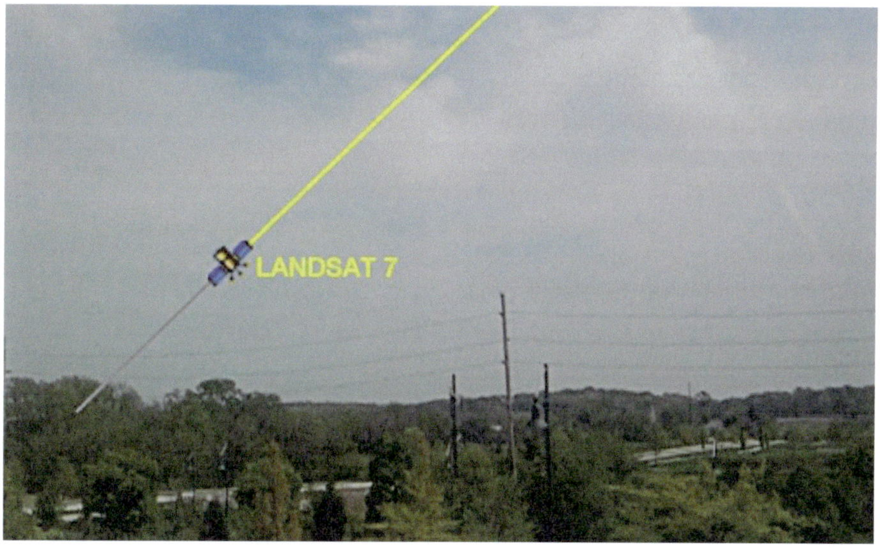

Fig. 6.2 A screen shot from Satellite AR (Analytical Graphics, Inc., Exton PA) shows the digital overlay of a satellite's current position and trajectory about the earth. (Source: https://play.google.com/store/apps/details?id=com.agi.android.augmentedreality. Permission granted under the terms of the GNU Free Documentation License, Version 1.2.)

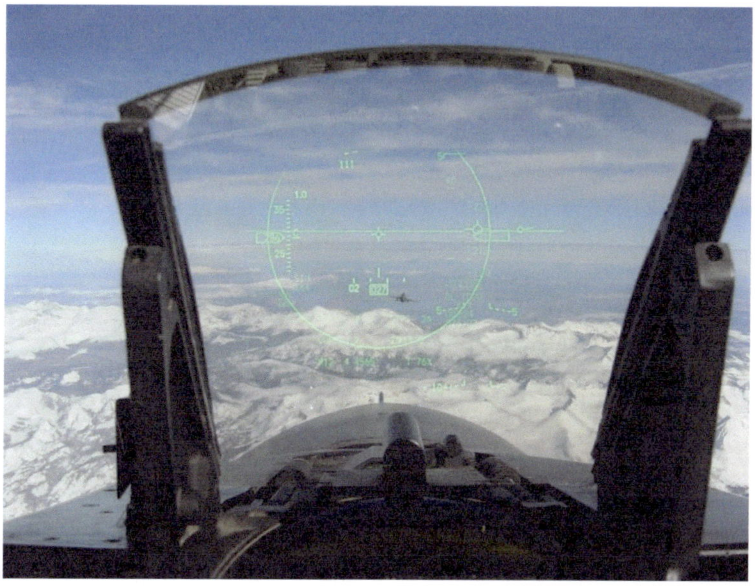

Fig. 6.3 The Heads-Up Display from the cockpit of an F-16 fighter plane displays altitude, artificial horizon, and magnetic heading along with other information to the pilot, without ever losing site of the external environment. (Source: http://www.defenseindustrydaily.com/39m-to-keep-f16-huds-aok-02131/. Permission granted under the terms of the GNU Free Documentation License, Version 1.2.)

Though many companies have thrown their hat into the head mounted display (HMD) arena, not all seek the same goal. Canon (Jamesburg, NJ) has developed their Mixed Reality eyewear with a price of $125,000, with the hope of providing a professional grade AR for use in multiple industries. Civil engineers would have the ability to visualize gas, water, and electrical lines as they exist or even as they are proposed prior to ever breaking ground.

Physicians and surgeons may be able to use the same device clinically and fully integrate the smart glass into the electronic medical record (EMR) of choice. This integration may allow for documentation, chart reviews, intraoperative communication, and information augmentation.

Not all groundbreaking work is being performed by tech based companies though. In 2007, the 3D Visualization and Imaging System Lab at the University of Arizona developed a unique polarized HMD and was subsequently awarded Army phase I and II Smart Business Innovation Research (SBIR) grants (www.sbir.gov) for its work in the field.

User Interface

As some authors have suggested, a HMD may cause information overload [10]. The user interface (UI) becomes important in order to tailor the content provided by the device. Google Glass uses a touchpad located on the side of the glass and voice commands in order to interact with the content of glass. Most of the newer devices have Bluetooth® (Bluetooth SIG, Kirkland, WA) connectivity and will allow for interface with a smartphone and computer, which can be used as the UI. The Technology Partnership (Melbourne, UK) has integrated electrodes capable of interpreting extraocular muscle activity as a proxy for eye tracking, which is implemented as the UI. Olympus Optical (Shinjuku, Japan) is one of the many users that have experimented with hand gesture recognition as the UI.

Google recently received recognition for their consumer smart glass (Google Glass) that did not require linkage to a device in order to display information. Google Glass is a computer with an optical head mounted display comparable to a 25″ HD television viewed from 8 ft. It uses bone conduction for audio, stores 16GB, possesses a 5MP camera, Wi-Fi, Bluetooth, voice recognition and has roughly 4 h of continuous, active battery life. It is incorporated into a familiar eyeglass form factor (Fig. 6.4).

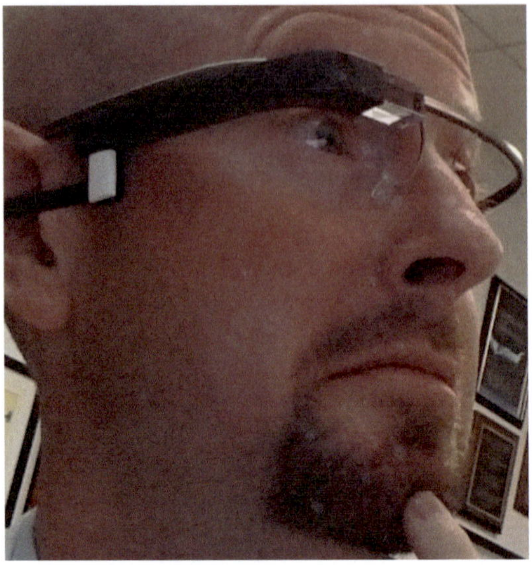

Fig. 6.4 Google Glass. One eye consists of a see-through monocle and integrated camera with bone-conducting or direct in-ear microphone. It connects to the Internet via Bluetooth and mobile phone or directly via WiFi

Inventors continue to push the envelope. Babak Parviz, an affiliate professor of electrical engineering at the University of Washington, has already created a contact lens with a single LED, and it is powered wirelessly with radio-frequency (RF) energy (Fig. 6.5) [11]. This is just the beginning. More recent works have shown the creation of contact lenses capable of sensing tear glucose concentrations [12].

Within our own group, the smart phone changed the way we performed telemedicine [6]. With the advent of Google Glass, we were able to further integrate telemedicine into our practice.

Intraoperative Case Example

As a surgical limb salvage group, we consulted with another surgical colleague and discussed requirements for resection and subsequent admixture of an antimicrobial bioactive implant to deliver into a previously infected bony defect following a combined vascular-soft tissue reconstructive limb salvage procedure (Fig. 6.6a–d). The Google Hangouts™ application was managed entirely by the operating surgeon using hands-free voice control. Additionally, real time diagrams and MRI measurements were developed

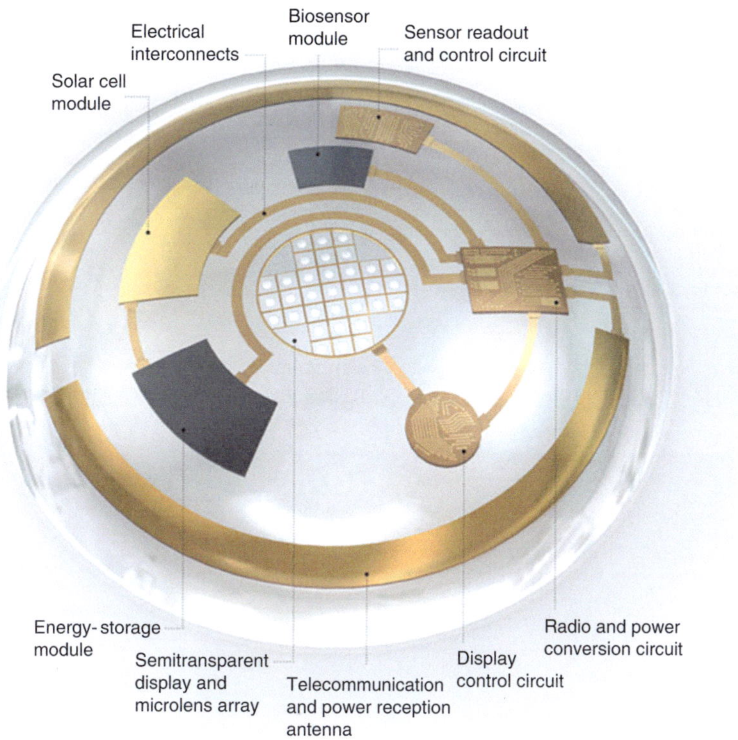

Fig. 6.5 A mock up of an augmented reality contact lens pioneered by Babak A. Parviz, PhD, a bionanotechnologist at the University of Washington. (Source: B. Parviz. 2009, September. Augmented Reality in a Contact Lens [Online]. Illustration by Emily Cooper. Available at: http://spectrum.ieee.org/biomedical/bionics/augmented-reality-in-a-contact-lens/eyesb1. Permission granted under the terms of the GNU Free Documentation License, Version 1.2.)

as a picture in picture, permitting two colleagues to effectively consult without the surgeon's eyes leaving the operative field to view intraoperative imaging along with surgical anatomy.

A consultation for the above patient was continued in clinic the next day. The clinician performed a dressing change along with the virtual consultant. The consultant was able to be virtually present for the first postoperative dressing change in the clinic, satisfactorily managing postoperative care.

Intraoperative Education

In a different patient at high risk for wound complications, we utilized Google Glass as an educational adjunct. A junior resident donned Google Glass during a scheduled delayed primary closure of a plantar defect and was engaged in an interactive "screen share" feature, which fed detailed descriptions on retention suture technique. This allowed for real-time, visual instruction in collaboration with a senior attending surgeon (Fig. 6.7a, b). This approach maximized hands on experience and autonomy for the resident. This was performed using bandwidth from a standard 3G CDMA connection using Glass-Bluetooth-Phone. A similar procedure followed demonstrating compartmental anatomy and assisting in planning a surgical decompression of a limb-threatening infection (Fig. 6.8a, b). Similarly, investigators have shown that AR education can shorten the learning curve during the acquisition of laparoscopic skills [13].

The above example is merely one of many ways that physicians are beginning to scratch the surface of what can be made possible.

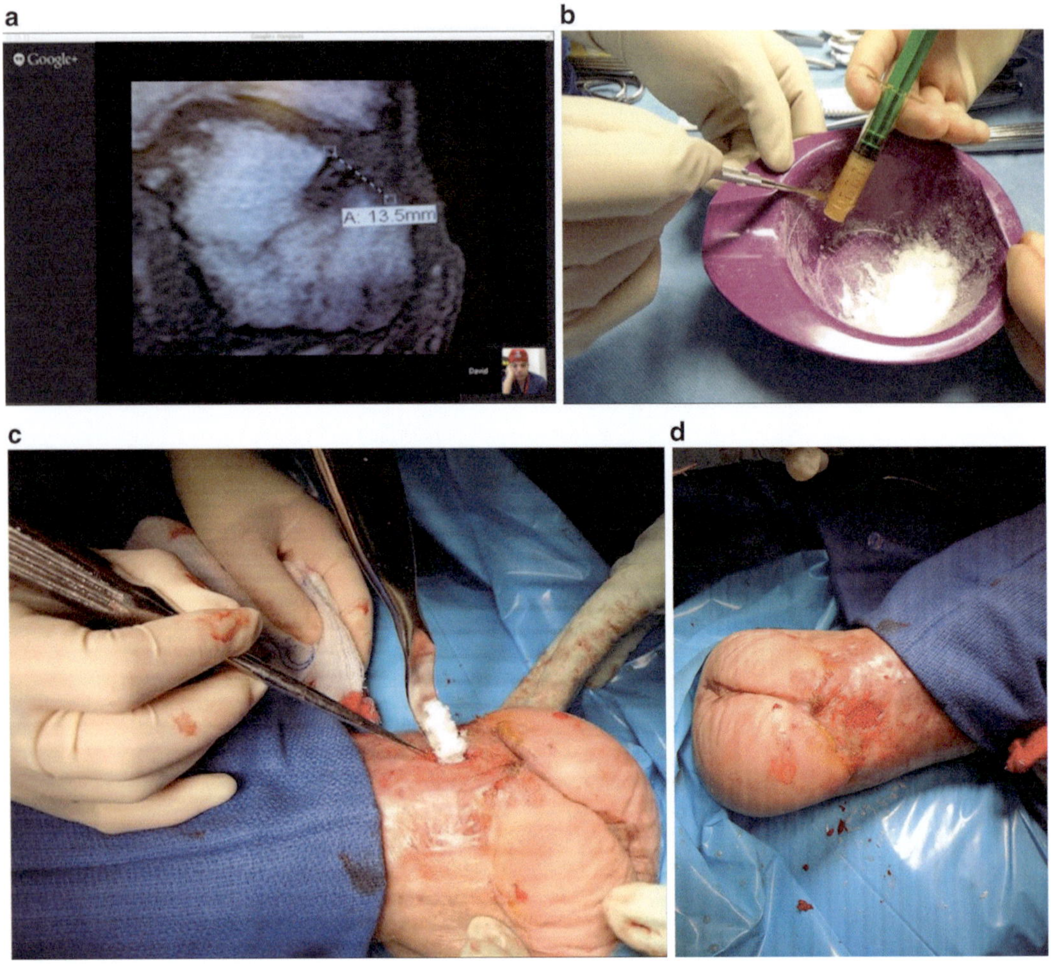

Fig. 6.6 (**a**–**d**) Visible defect on main screen with consultant clinician in lower right (**a**), real-time photograph of admixture of antibiotic-demineralized bone matrix (**b**) and measured delivery into defect (**c** and **d**). (**a**–**d**: Used with permission from Armstrong DG, Rankin TM, Giovinco NA, Mills JL, Matsuoka Y. A Heads-Up Display for Diabetic Limb Salvage Surgery: A View Through the Google Looking Glass. J Diabetes Sci Technol September 2014; 8: 951–956.)

Current Work

Surgeons are constantly faced with the task of mentally integrating two-dimensional radiographs and the three-dimensional surgical field, which is the very reason that augmented reality is so attractive. Researchers have been attempting to overcome this complexity for the last two decades [14].

Trauma

Trauma is the leading cause of mortality in patients aged 1–44 in the USA (CDC.gov). The ability to save lives is predicated upon a well-established system of responding to trauma patients and transporting them for definitive treatment. First responders are constantly faced with navigating unknown neighborhoods and homes

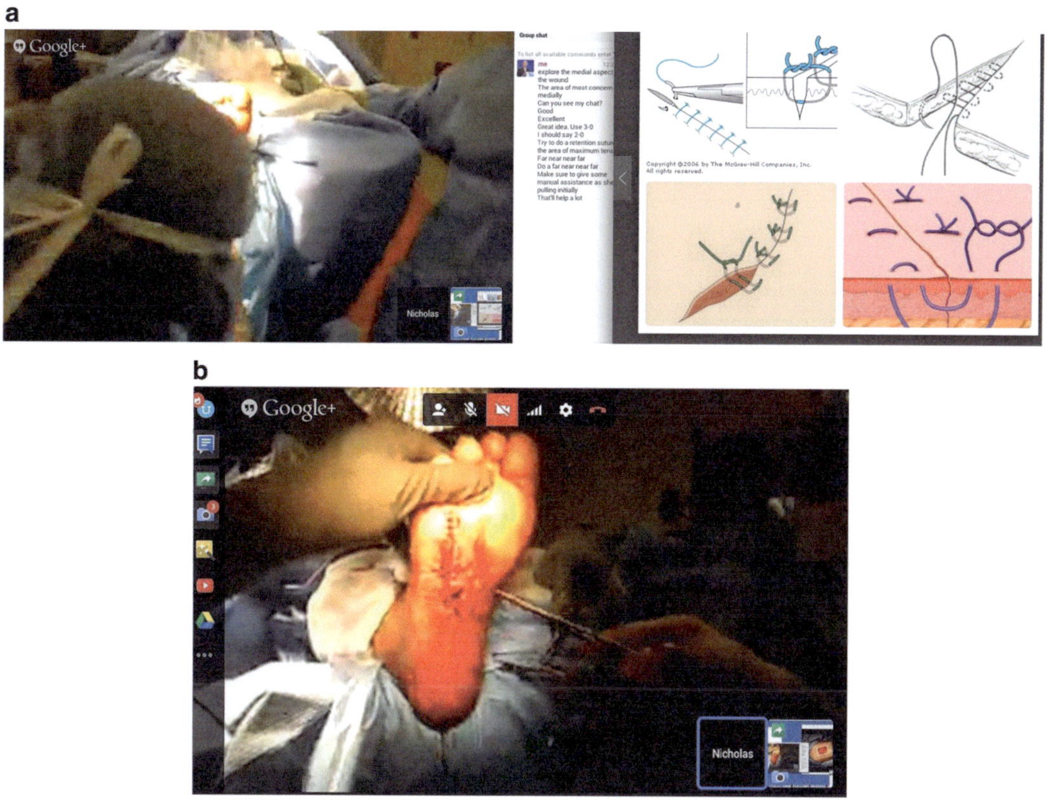

Fig. 6.7 (**a** and **b**) During a delayed primary closure of a high-risk plantar wound, real-time descriptions with instant “screen share” were fed through Glass to a junior resident during the surgical procedure to assist instruction by the senior attending surgeon. (**a** and **b**: Used with permission from Armstrong DG, Rankin TM, Giovinco NA, Mills JL, Matsuoka Y. A Heads-Up Display for Diabetic Limb Salvage Surgery: A View Through the Google Looking Glass. J Diabetes Sci Technol September 2014; 8: 951–956.)

in order to rescue injured patients. AR navigation could not only facilitate transportation to the distress call but also has been shown by researchers in France to make navigation within low-visibility environments, such as fires, safer [15]. This technology could be further modified to make the cellular signal of the 911 caller a beacon in order to accelerate the localization of the patient.

Orthopedic Surgery

Investigators have also been able to successfully apply AR to orthopedic trauma surgery by integrating the live feed/fluoroscopic radiographs onto the patient in a geometrically appropriate fashion so that the surgeon can visualize the underlying osseous structures during surgical intervention and manipulation (Fig. 6.9) [16]. Trauma surgeons have also utilized hybrid navigation [17].

Maxilofacial surgeons in Vienna, Austria, began applying this technology in the late 1990s in order to correct posttraumatic deformities of the zygomatic arch [18]. The use of patient specific CT imaging presented in a head mounted display allowed for accurate reconstruction of complex facial fractures, while minimizing the number of incisions typically required to do so.

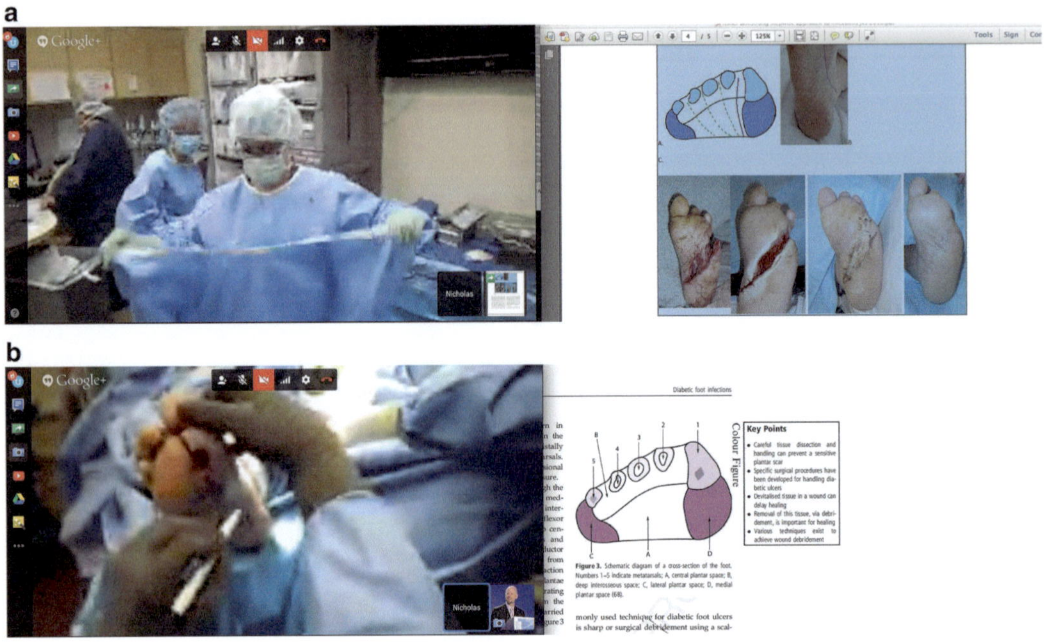

Fig. 6.8 (**a** and **b**) View during Intraoperative consultation for plantar deep space infection to assist in incision planning, exploration, and decompression using senior author's manuscript's figures as case example. (**a** and **b**: Used with permission from Armstrong DG, Rankin TM, Giovinco NA, Mills JL, Matsuoka Y. A Heads-Up Display for Diabetic Limb Salvage Surgery: A View Through the Google Looking Glass. J Diabetes Sci Technol September 2014; 8: 951–956.)

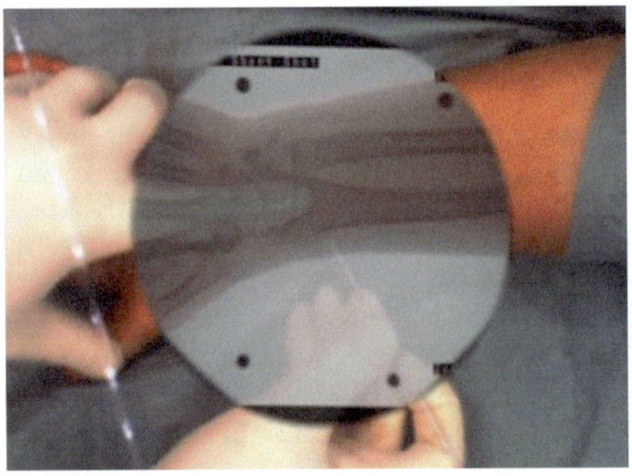

Fig. 6.9 The correctly oriented radiograph from a C-arm is displayed over the surgical field. (Used with permission from Weidert, S., L. Wang, A. von der Heide, et al., [Intraoperative augmented reality visualization. Current state of development and initial experiences with the CamC]. Unfallchirurg 2012; 115(3): 209–13.)

Otolaryngology

Otolaryngologists from the University of Toronto have evaluated the effect of AR on simulated intraoperative performance during an endoscopic approach to the skull base [19]. Though the AR was not based upon an HMD, the two experimental groups were provided either a full AR experience with critical structures visually highlighted or a standard display with an AR submonitor where the same information could be obtained but was not fully integrated into the primary display. Fifty otolaryngologists performed the task and they found that there was no significant difference in the speed or precision with which the task was completed. However, subjects were not informed that there would be a foreign body within the surgical field during the task. The group provided with full AR displayed inattentional blindness and did not identify the foreign body 68 % of the time vs. 40 % of standard display users.

Hepatobiliary Surgery

Trials have already been underway since 2009 investigating the utility of AR for liver resection. Seven hundred sixty nine patients have been

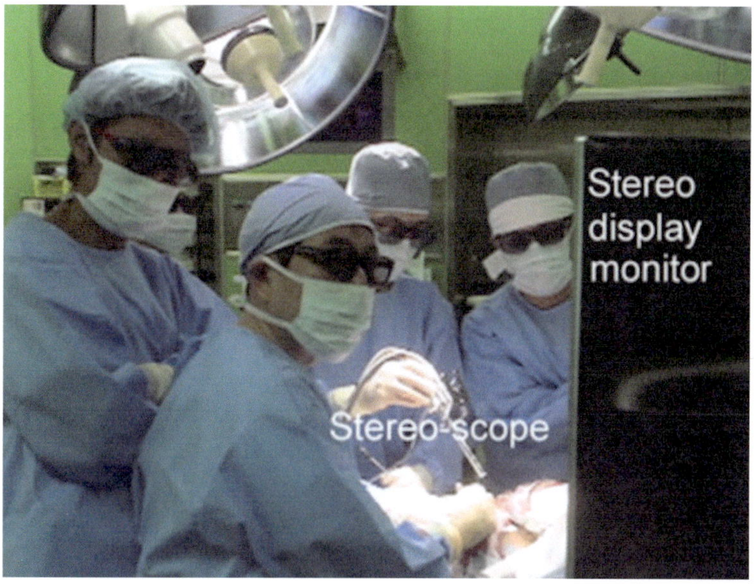

Fig. 6.10 Surgeons take advantage of the 3D, real time images captured by a stereoscope, which is then further augmented by the overlay of patient specific CT data upon the surgical field during a pancreatic dissection. (Used with permission from Onda, S., T. Okamoto, M. Kanehira, et al. Short rigid scope and stereo-scope designed specifically for open abdominal navigation surgery: clinical application for hepatobiliary and pancreatic surgery. J Hepatobiliary Pancreat Sci, 2013; 20(4): 448–53.)

modeled, leading to 50 operations. The authors believe that this technology may have increased the surgical eligibility of their patients. However, the authors comment that the issue in open surgery is deformation of organs. Other investigators have used a video see-through display whereby a short rigid stereoscope is used in to capture the operative field and then preoperative CT images are integrated on the 2D or 3D monitor (Fig. 6.10) [20]. The solution they found to organ deformation was the ability to quickly register defined points on the organ by using an infrared marker to co-register fiducial points. They used both soft tissue landmarks as well as blood vessels and found no significant difference in the accuracy of the two methods. These methods had a mean error of 6–10 mm, which is acceptable for open abdominal surgery, though it is not sensitive enough for neurosurgical applications (Fig. 6.11). The increasing availability of the hybrid OR may also be a solution to this problem as the patient could be reimaged once the surgical field was opened and retractors placed [21]. The surgical demands of a head mounted display are similar in some respects to those of the soldier, wherein the surgeon requires a simple design, with low head supported weight and low cost [22].

Neurosurgery

Neurosurgeons at the University of Florida have applied mixed reality or augmented reality in a slightly different way. Two hundred and sixty residents performed a ventriculostomy on a mixed reality model (real simulated skin/3D printed skull, but virtual brain) [23]. In this trial, augmented reality was not meant to guide the subject, but to evaluate the subject after the completion of the procedure. In this way, potential trainees have the advantage of very real physical feedback, and the detailed performance feedback typical of a virtual system. Junior and senior residents outperformed interns as would be expected, but, more importantly, this mixed simulation was able to distinguish levels of training. As a validated model, this reflects the potential of mixed reality simulators in order to educate our residents who

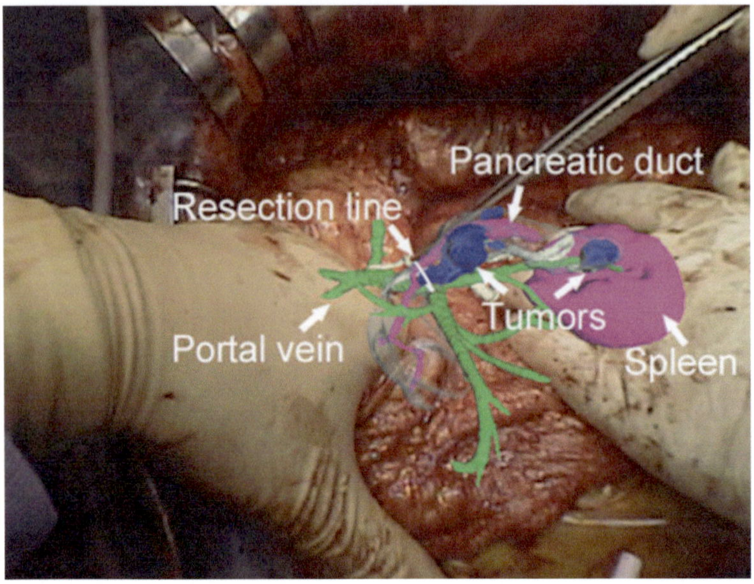

Fig. 6.11 Augmented reality created by the overlay of patient specific anatomy obtained from CT imaging and real-time, 3D imaging of the surgical field seen from a stereoscope. (Used with permission from Onda, S., T. Okamoto, M. Kanehira, et al. Short rigid scope and stereo-scope designed specifically for open abdominal navigation surgery: clinical application for hepatobiliary and pancreatic surgery. J Hepatobiliary Pancreat Sci 2013; 20(4):448–53.)

are faced with the responsibility of an ever-growing body of knowledge and fewer hours in which to master that knowledge.

The Future and Potential of AR

AR has the potential to increase surgical precision, increase patient safety, and facilitate physician education, but researchers have found limitations of the technology as it currently exists. During intracranial AVM surgery, AR was not as useful due to the complexity of AVMs; however, the authors felt that real-time information concerning hemodynamics would be more useful [24]. As investigators continue to push the envelope of this technology, its utility will become more defined.

Investigators have also looked at integrating other modalities separate from axial imaging. The use of an infrared camera allowed for the real-time visual display of cardiac ischemia in a pig model [25]. This could have direct implications during cardiac surgery or microvascular free tissue transfer. Depending on the sensitivity of the camera, this might even provide critical care specialists with real-time data concerning distribution of flow to myocardium or even pulmonary tissue. Theoretically, such technology could allow for the rapid diagnosis of pulmonary emboli or threatened limb ischemia. The military has also explored the use of ultra-wide band radars and stepped frequency continuous wave radars in order to detect the human heart beat at very long distances [26]. This is an additional technology that is being explored for noninvasive medical applications and could be used for evaluating real time, functional information.

While these procedures already are based largely on various imaging modalities—i.e., fluoroscopy, CT, or MRI—the ability to overlay for the operator additional information in the image field may allow for more meaningful interpretation of a given situation. For example, while focused on performing an interventional procedure and seeing a third dimension via an intraluminal ultrasound image that is now overlayed on hemodynamic data, ones clinical decision-making may be enhanced.

As outlined for surgical procedures, the ability to telemeter or broadcast this information to fellows, residents, students or other health care personnel may further enhance the efficacy of a given procedure and will serve as an augmented teaching modality.

The areas that AR appears to be most useful in are minimally invasive procedures where the tumor and or pathology are not palpable. This seems to be most obvious in the brain and skull base operations, arthroscopic procedures, and procedures within solid organs and the retroperitoneum.

A Word of Caution

It would be prudent to suggest caution in the use of the standard approach to research and development for AR technologies for medical applications, as we have seen high costs and slow progress with this approach. Though it may not integrate into our current systems readily, it will be of utmost importance to allow for a developer based ecosystem to drive the development of new software for these devices as this will result in lower costs and ultimately more rapid evolution.

Surgeons have been employing augmented reality in medicine and surgery for the last 20 years [27]. The key to successful introduction of new technologies is to seamlessly integrate them with existing technologies. The ability of oncologists to precisely eradicate a tumor using stereotactics, high-definition imaging, and focused radiation has had a significant impact on patient safety and survival [28]. Many new technologies suffer from high cost and size, and, therefore, widespread application is not possible. Until recently, augmented reality had neither the correct form factor to make intraoperative and in-clinic use practical, nor the efficacy to justify its application [29, 30].

In addition to size and cost, accessibility is key to the proliferation of a new technology. The cost of development for a commercially available technology is spread over an enormous consumer base. Most new medical technologies are slow to develop due to a relatively small consumer base—resulting in high costs—and proprietary restrictions. Google Glass, for example, is part of an app-based developer ecosystem, which greatly accelerates the maturation process as seen by mobile applications and the smart phone. Just as with smart phones a decade ago, the application ecosystem for Glass is rather small. However, the form factor and subsequent iterations of it allow for arguably enormous growth.

Summary

Although many of the issues concerning AR in surgery and medicine overall need further investigation, AR is here to stay, and surgeons should champion this technology in their quest to improve patient care. Despite these issues, it is clear this technology has the potential to enhance communication. Smart glasses and other forms of AR may increase individual physician efficiency, especially for surgeons, so that more efficient patient care can be provided. Surgeons now have the ability to provide or receive more meaningful consultation from their colleagues without having to leave the operating room, office, or clinic. Even intraoperative team communication could be improved. Each member of the operative team could be outfitted with smart glasses. The surgeon has heads-up real-time patient vitals, information and imaging. The anesthesiologist is able to administer critical medications, without ever losing sight of the operative field or communication with the surgeon. The surgical resident and medical students always have an ideal view of the operative field, which may help facilitate instruction. The operating room (OR) nurse knows exactly what tools the surgeon needs, even while outside of the OR: communication is never lost.

Concerning patient safety, many parallels might be drawn between the commercial airline industry and medicine. Surgical theaters have adopted checklists similar to pilots prior to take off, in order to make the journey safer. Smart glasses may even serve as an early "black box" in medicine. If every action of a physician, surgeon, and nurse is recorded, it could impact litigation, but it could also provide critical insight into surgical decision-making, technique and safety. Furthermore, anatomic "no fly zones" [31, 32] could be projected, like a road map, onto a head mounted display, which could reduce the risk of intraoperative complications. Immediate future works from our group include evaluating use of these "no fly zones" as well as merging with image overlay/anatomic registry to use techniques like indocyanine green angiography to identify tissue viability in real time [33, 34].

While the above points seem laudable, we must consider that the quest for increased efficiency could paradoxically result in decreased quality of care. While most people assume these devices are intended to increase the amount of information perceived, Steve Mann has also addressed the utility of degrading visual stimuli presented to the user. The low-tech version of this idea is sun glasses or a welding helmet that degrade the intensity of light presented in order to protect the user and improve visual acuity. This may be of utility to surgeons who use lasers in their practice.

Other industries have investigated the concept of cognitive blindness or in-attentional blindness [10]. Some authors concluded that, intraoperatively, similar objects seen during a challenging task are likely to not be differentiated. Given the difficulty or perceived difficulty of a surgical operation, particularly during surgical training, surgeons would be a high-risk population for this effect. Even early simulation conducted by NASA revealed a risk of in-attentional blindness during the use of head-up displays while landing aircraft [35].

We are ultimately now addressing the possibilities associated with implementing these systems. The application of AR is user- and application-specific [22]. It is unlikely that there will be one perfect system or technology that will suit every surgical specialty.

There are a number of issues that have not been addressed adequately. For example, we have not yet investigated how the additional stimulus of augmented reality impacts performance or whether it might prove too distracting [19]. We ultimately need to identify if AR positively impacts patients' outcomes. We look forward to further work in this area that might seek the requisite balance. We believe that the future in this area is promising. Enhancing communication, facilitating education, increasing safety and improving care are not virtual goals, but are rather virtuous and ultimately realistic.

Funding Sources: none

Acknowledgements: none

Disclosures: none

References

1. Mezzana P, Scarinci F, Marabottini N. Augmented reality in oculoplastic surgery: first iPhone application. Plast Reconstr Surg. 2011;127(3):57e–8.
2. Raposio E, DiSomma C, Fato M, et al. An "augmented-reality" aid for plastic and reconstructive surgeons. Stud Health Technol Inform. 1997;39:232–6.
3. Bilton N, Mann S. Wearable computing pioneer. The New York Times; 2012.
4. Yeniaras E, Navkar NV, Sonmez AE, et al. MR-based real time path planning for cardiac operations with transapical access. Med Image Comput Comput Assist Interv. 2011;14(Pt 1):25–32.
5. Tsutsumi N, Tomikawa M, Uemura M, et al. Image-guided laparoscopic surgery in an open MRI operating theater. Surg Endosc. 2013;27(6):2178–84.
6. Armstrong DG, Giovinco N, Mills JL, et al. FaceTime for physicians: using real time mobile phone-based videoconferencing to augment diagnosis and care in telemedicine. Eplasty. 2011;11, e23.
7. Mattos LS, Caldwell DG. Safe teleoperation based on flexible intraoperative planning for robot-assisted laser microsurgery. Conf Proc IEEE Eng Med Biol Soc. 2012;2012:174–8.
8. Lim TH, Choi HJ, Kang BS. Feasibility of dynamic cardiac ultrasound transmission via mobile phone for basic emergency teleconsultation. J Telemed Telecare. 2010;16(5):281–5.
9. Ercoline WR, DeVilbiss CA, Lyons TJ. Trends in U.S. Air Force spatial disorientation accidents: 1958–1992. In: Proceedings of the SPIE Conference (A95-12001-01-54 in Orlando, FL). Bellingham, WA: Society of Photo-Optical Instrumentation Engineers; 1994. p. 257–60.
10. Simons DJ, Chabris CF. Gorillas in our midst: sustained inattentional blindness for dynamic events. Perception. 1999;28(9):1059–74.
11. Parviz B. Augmented reality in a contact lens. IEEE: Spectrum; 2009.
12. Parviz BA. Of molecules, medicine, and Google Glass. ACS Nano. 2014;8(3):1956–7.

13. Vera AM, Russo M, Mohsin A, et al. Augmented reality telementoring (ART) platform: a randomized controlled trial to assess the efficacy of a new surgical education technology. Surg Endosc. 2014;28(12):3467–72.
14. Gleason PL, Kikinis R, Altobelli D, et al. Video registration virtual reality for nonlinkage stereotactic surgery. Stereotact Funct Neurosurg. 1994;63(1–4):139–43.
15. Klann M, Geissler M. Experience prototyping: a new approach to designing firefighter navigation support. IEEE Pervasive Computing. 2012;11:68–77.
16. Weidert S, Wang L, von der Heide A, et al. Intraoperative augmented reality visualization. Current state of development and initial experiences with the CamC. Unfallchirurg. 2012;115(3):209–13.
17. Traub J, Stefan P, Heining SM, et al. Hybrid navigation interface for orthopedic and trauma surgery. Med Image Comput Comput Assist Interv. 2006;9(Pt 1): 373–80.
18. Watzinger F, Wanschitz F, Wagner A, et al. Computer-aided navigation in secondary reconstruction of post-traumatic deformities of the zygoma. J Craniomaxillofac Surg. 1997;25(4):198–202.
19. Dixon BJ, Daly MJ, Chan HH, et al. Inattentional blindness increased with augmented reality surgical navigation. Am J Rhinol Allergy. 2014;28(5):433–7.
20. Onda S, Okamoto T, Kanehira M, et al. Short rigid scope and stereo-scope designed specifically for open abdominal navigation surgery: clinical application for hepatobiliary and pancreatic surgery. J Hepatobiliary Pancreat Sci. 2013;20(4):448–53.
21. Soler L, Nicolau S, Pessaux P, et al. Real-time 3D image reconstruction guidance in liver resection surgery. Hepatobiliary Surg Nutr. 2014;3(2):73–81.
22. Melzer J, Brozoski F, Letowski T, et al. Guidelines for HMD design. In: Helmet-mounted displays: sensation, perception, and cognition issues. Fort Rucker, AL: United States Army Aeromedical Research Laboratory; 2009. p. 805–84.
23. Hooten KG, Lister JR, Lombard G, et al. Mixed reality ventriculostomy simulation: experience in neurosurgical residency. Neurosurgery. 2014;10 Suppl 4:576–81. discussion 581.
24. Cabrilo I, Bijlenga P, Schaller K. Augmented reality in the surgery of cerebral arteriovenous malformations: technique assessment and considerations. Acta Neurochir (Wien). 2014;156(9):1769–74.
25. Szabo Z, Berg S, Sjokvist S, et al. Real-time intraoperative visualization of myocardial circulation using augmented reality temperature display. Int J Cardiovasc Imaging. 2013;29(2):521–8.
26. Shirodkar S, Barua P, Anuradha D, et al. Heart-beat detection and ranging through a wall using ultra wide band radar. International Conference on Communications and Signal Processing (ICCSP) 2011. IEEE, 10–12 Feb; 2011.
27. Giorgi C, Luzzara M, Casolino DS, et al. A computer controlled stereotactic arm: virtual reality in neurosurgical procedures. Acta Neurochir Suppl (Wien). 1993;58:75–6.
28. Senan S. Stereotactic body radiotherapy: do central lung tumors still represent a 'no-fly zone'? Onkologie. 2012;35(7-8):406–7.
29. Wiederhold M, Wiederhold B. Augmented reality: what is it and how is it enhancing healthcare today? Cyber Therapy and Rehabilitation 2012; Issue 1:10–12.
30. Sadda P, Azimi E, Jallo G, et al. Surgical navigation with a head-mounted tracking system and display. Stud Health Technol Inform. 2013;184:363–9.
31. Zoran A, Paradiso J. FreeD – a freehand digital sculpting tool. The 31th international conference extended abstracts on Human factors in computing systems (CHI '13). ACM, Paris; 2013.
32. Jaramaz B, Nikou C. Precision freehand sculpting for unicondylar knee replacement: design and experimental validation. Biomed Tech (Berl). 2012;57(4): 293–9.
33. Braun JD, Trinidad-Hernandez M, Perry D, et al. Early quantitative evaluation of indocyanine green angiography in patients with critical limb ischemia. J Vasc Surg. 2013;57(5):1213–8.
34. Perry D, Bharara M, Armstrong DG, et al. Intraoperative fluorescence vascular angiography: during tibial bypass. J Diabetes Sci Technol. 2012;6(1):204–8.
35. Fischer E, Haines R, Price T. Cognitive issues in head-up displays. NASA Technical Paper, 1980. 1711. NASA Ames Res Ctr, Moffett Field, CA.

The Lean Innovation Model for Academic Medical Discovery

7

Gabriel Gruionu and George C. Velmahos

Introduction

The goal of the present chapter is to provide a basic introduction to the innovation process in academia, based on our experience from four major US universities and a major US medical device company. Although there is a lot of information about industrial innovation, academic innovation—turning new scientific ideas into commercial products—is a very new endeavor for the academic scientist or clinician, and often diametrically opposed to the main goal of their career: basic scientific discovery, patient care, and education. To untangle the complicated process of academic innovation, we aim to offer some practical advice and exchange of information for academic scientists/clinicians about the steps they can take to turn their scientific ideas into innovative medical products. There could be differences among universities, but in general, the process described in this chapter applies to most US academic environments. For a more formal course in medical entrepreneurship, the reader can consult many specialized books and textbooks [1, 2]. Intentionally, the present approach is direct and personal, without the complicated lingo of business (text)books, in order to open the reader to the possibility that academic innovation is both fun and feasible for any scientist/ clinician with an entrepreneurial spirit and a useful idea.

G. Gruionu, M.S., Ph.D. (✉)
G.C. Velmahos, M.D., Ph.D., M.S.Ed., F.A.C.S.
Division of Trauma, Emergency Surgery, and Surgical Critical Care, Department of Surgery, Massachusetts General Hospital, Boston, MA, USA
e-mail: ggruionu@mgh.harvard.edu

The Medical Product

For illustration purposes, throughout this chapter we use a hypothetical new medical product, a classic Kelly hemostat locking forceps (in short the "forceps"). A forceps represents an example of a simple mechanical device defined as a "handheld, hinged instrument used for grasping and holding objects" (http://en.wikipedia.org/wiki/Forceps accessed on June 9th, 2014). Other surgical devices could contain electrical or electronic components (e.g., pacemakers), as well as biological or artificial biomaterials (e.g., biological surgical patches or vascular grafts). Although they are more complex, more expensive, and longer to develop, a similar methodology can be applied to develop these medical products.

R. Latifi et al. (eds.), *Technological Advances in Surgery, Trauma and Critical Care*,
DOI 10.1007/978-1-4939-2671-8_7

Industry vs. Academic Innovation

One of the first questions that come up about academic innovation is why we cannot just apply the industry innovation model in academia? Why do we need to reinvent the wheel? To answer those questions we first need to understand how the two innovation environments compare to each other:

1. Industry has a system in place where all functions (engineering, marketing, sales, management, legal, manufacturing) work in tandem to accomplish the same goal, which is the commercialization of new products. For a manufacturer of forceps, a new forceps design is a line extension and a matter of engaging the new development team, receiving approval from the leadership, and starting the production. The details of the process are the same: prototype design and execution, business plan, production, etc., but the execution is much faster, based on previous experience of the company.
2. Academic innovation at the level of the university works almost in complete isolation from the rest of the university. Among their peers, academic innovators work on their own and often in secrecy. Therefore, an innovator of a new forceps design has to first recreate and build the forceps prototype. The scientist has then to learn everything about writing a business plan and all other business aspects of the business. In particular, defining the market for the product, and sales and regulatory scenarios are very difficult for academic inventors and very easy for established medical device companies that already have a distribution network and an established market.

There are many other finer differences between industry and academia that mainly arise from academia having as its main mission, education and research. Once there is a common goal of commercializing innovation, an increase in communication and collaboration between industry and academia could solve many of these differences, and accelerate the academic innovation process.

The Lean Innovation Model in Academia

Medical innovation is becoming more of an integral part of academic research. In both clinical practice and laboratory research, there are many innovative solutions that could and need to be translated into practice. The present work exemplifies some of our work in medical device innovation at the Massachusetts General Hospital. At the time when this chapter was written, our work was still in progress, so for the purpose of maintaining confidentiality we have picked a hypothetical medical product to illustrate our experience and practices.

Lean innovation was initiated in lean manufacturing. *Lean Six Sigma* was developed by the Toyota car manufacturer [3], then applied to IT innovation [4]. Briefly, lean manufacturing or just-in-time production refers to producing only to customer demand. An example from the car industry would be producing a car with only the features that are requested by the customers and testing the car design as it is developed rather than waiting until all of the features of the car are in place and then tested by the customers. "One of the main fundamentals of the Toyota System is to make 'what you need, in the amount you need, by the time you need it', but to tell the truth there is another part to this and that is 'at lower cost.' But that part is not written down" [5].

Similarly, in the IT industry, when designing software, the features of such software can be tested early in the development process, often during the beta version of the software [4]. The early adopter customers then offer feedback early in the process such that the necessary changes can be made before too much time and money is spent on developing secondary and potentially unnecessary features.

For the first time, we are applying the concept of lean innovation to academia for medical product development. We believe that the academic environment is well suited for early customer feedback, particularly as it concerns medical products for which the customers are the doctors and hospitals affiliated with the university. Therefore, testing an early prototype could be as easy as contacting a clinician colleague while covered by the university confidentiality agreements. We have applied this concept at the Massachusetts General Hospital to accomplish both early feedback on our products as well as to keep the cost of the prototype production to a minimum. The remaining of the chapter describes how one can implement the lean innovation process in academia.

The Innovation Social Network

An innovation social network is crucial to the implementation of lean academic innovation. It contains all the people involved in developing the invention into a commercial product. It contains people from the university and also from the outside world: the innovation director who coordinates several innovation projects, the scientist/clinician inventor who came up with the idea, and the support system.

The Innovation Director

The central player of the academic innovation process is the innovation director (ID) rather than the inventor. The ID is a multidisciplinary scientist with experience in both academic research and industrial product development. The ID is responsible for integrating and coordinating the clinical, scientific, and industry aspects of the product development. The ID asks the right questions related to the medical device clinical need and finds the right answers that can generate hypotheses to be tested. For example, what is the strength of the forceps to hold but not crush the vessel? What is the best material for the forceps to be able to sustain steam sterilization? At the same time the ID acts as an early CEO for the start-up company and writes grant proposals for funding; in other words, the ID carries out the entire process. In industry, a similar function is performed by the product manager or specialist. The difference is that the product manager acts within the company infrastructure whereas the ID has to build the infrastructure for each medical product project in academia.

The Clinician Inventor

Usually, a single scientist/clinician—the inventor—initiates the medical innovation. This is partially due to the academic culture of "secrecy" vs. collaboration. An idea belonging to a clinician is perceived as the solution to a major medical need and therefore tends to be protected by the inventor who is the originator of idea. Although the academic environment is usually governed by the confidentiality agreements signed by every employee at the beginning of their employment, the clinicians and in general the inventors do not share their ideas with their peers. This approach has advantages and disadvantages. The advantage is that the inventor maintains a sense of ownership and leadership in the development process. Although by university rules all new ideas, even remotely related to the work being done at the university, belong to the university, inventors feel that they need to protect their idea within their own academic institution. At the same time, they are motivated to work diligently on developing their idea.

The disadvantage of the secrecy is that the entire process is developed in a silo, which makes the process of academic innovation very slow and individualized. Reinventing the wheel is almost the rule of the game, as every faculty has his/her own way of developing an idea and his/her own "connections" with the real world, inventors, developers, and so on. The disadvantage of working in silos greatly surpasses the advantage of secrecy at the level of the entire academic innovation environment and might be the single most important reason for the frustratingly slow academic innovation process.

The Engineering Team

The engineers could be from inside or outside the academic circle. Inside the academic circle, engineering students can be a useful resource. In particular, senior students are well prepared and willing to perform engineering design, especially if the project is designed to fulfill their senior design project requirements or a research internship. As tempting as it is to use free or low-cost engineering students for medical product development, one should resist this temptation unless the students are coordinated by someone with experience in medical product R&D, such as the ID. The danger is that the students can and will find all kinds of exciting and outside-the-box solutions to the clinical problems (the design output), but many of these solutions will not comply with necessary requirements, particularly as related to price or market value. For example, an atraumatic forceps could contain a pressure sensor at the tip of the forceps, which gives feedback to a small motor such that the grabbing force is continuously adjusted to the environment. Such a solution, although it could actually be a good engineering design project, is probably too complex and too expensive to ever be commercialized.

On the other hand, experienced engineers from outside the academic environment have the necessary market experience to design solutions that fit the design inputs and are at the same time practical and economically viable. However, such highly valuable engineers are very expensive. This is due to their experience, but also because they work for specialized companies who are certified to meet international standard for medical product development (i.e., ISO 13485). The ISO standards insure that the medical product is designed in a quality controlled environment and tested appropriately in bench-top, animal laboratory, and clinical settings [6].

A compromise could be reached between these two levels of expertise within the context of the lean innovation scenario in academia. For example, only the key feature of the forceps (atraumatic grabbing of the tissue) could be tested by the students while the esthetic and manufacturability aspects could be left for the later stages of the process to be done with experienced outside companies. Another long-term alternative is for universities to develop their own ISO 13485 certified laboratories, which could serve many inventors in the medical school. For a very large medical school, this solution could be a good long-term investment, considering that the prototype development services could run into ten of or even hundred of thousands of dollars, if done with external vendors.

The Business Expert(s)

A business expert (BE), preferably a person with a MBA degree, is desirable to assist with the development process. This person is initially the ID and later on the Chief Executive Officer (CEO) of the company. From setting up the start-up company to raising funds, the BE prepares the pathway to a start-up company. As much as the new product is novel and attractive, the investors will also look at how the company is organized. If there is no structure in place, it will be less likely they will invest in the company because they will have to organize the company themselves. They might have to bring in their own CEO to run the company. This strategy in itself could be a great alternative if the inventors/founders of the company do not have access to an experienced CEO as it is often the case in the academic environment. An experienced CEO is someone who not only has the business knowledge, but also a proven track record of commercializing the same category of medical products: it does not help us develop a forceps if the CEO has experience with medical IT, for example.

The University Support System

The Office of Technology Transfer (OTT) is usually the first line of support (and sometimes resistance!) for academic innovation. Essentially, OTT deals with patent search and filing and with licensing the technology to the outside world, i.e. either to large corporations, or another start-up or product development companies with the infrastructure to develop the product further.

The OTT can also license the technology (often under very attractive terms) to the original inventors if they decide to start they own company. The license rights means that the inventor start-up company can relicense the technology to another corporation. This could be a good strategy if the university OTT is not particularly fast in licensing the technology. We found that often the academic inventors assume that the OTT has their best interest in mind and they work diligently to license their technology. Although this is true in most cases, it is good to remember that the OTT serves the entire university. The OTT also serves its own interest because, at most universities, the OTT is organized as a nonprofit organization that is only affiliated to the university but is actually self-funded. Therefore, it will often focus its efforts on the technology that is most profitable to their office rather than the university or the individual inventor. It may often choose an area of innovation, for example, IT, that aligns with its own area of expertise and has a highly profitable profile. Other projects as, for example, the hemostat forceps, might not even be evaluated fairly in comparison to the area of emphasis of the OTT. Therefore, a higher responsibility should be assumed by the inventors in developing their own ideas rather that waiting for the OTT to do it.

Description of the Clinical Problem for the Medical Product

The very first step in the medical innovation process is defining the clinical problem to be solved. The clinical problem has to be defined in clinical terms and in as much detail as possible by a clinician who should be both familiar with the subject and preferably a key opinion leader (KOL) in the field. For our example, the hemostat forceps is used to stop the blood flow in an artery or a vein. Let us assume that the clinical problem with the existing hemostatic forceps is that it damages the blood vessel during normal use. So the clinical need is for an atraumatic hemostatic forceps (the medical product, MP to be developed). Most likely, the clinician inventor who realized this problem has already thought of a solution. Rarely or never in academia, the initial solution comes after the clinical need is referenced and researched in detail. So let us assume that the clinician, either by logical deduction, inspiration, or research experience, figured out that a different pattern of the forceps tip—a crisscross vs. straight lines—makes the forceps less traumatic. Regardless of the proposed solution, in order to define the clinical need, either the innovator director or the inventor has to document the clinical context: the conditions to be treated, the complications of the existing procedures, the number of patients that are affected have to be referenced. This information will define the solution and the market potential for the product. For the forceps, the clinical context is vascular repair. The complications could be: vascular wall damage, including thinning of the vessel wall, aneurysm, hemorrhage, luminal narrowing, and occlusion due to vascular stenosis. Such complications are encountered in the clinical practice of not only the clinician inventor but hopefully of many other clinicians (which makes for a serious problem without a solution). For a complete list of reportable complications (severe or less severe), the FDA website must be searched [7].

The clinical need is defined by the clinical problem created by the current solution, its adverse effects, and their incidence. Sometimes the clinical problem is very severe but the adverse effects have a very low incidence. For example the consequence of vessel trauma could be internal bleeding which can be fatal but this only happens in a very low percentage of the procedures. For the purpose of commercialization, such a clinical need will probably be ranked lower than a less severe clinical need but with a higher incidence.

Design Inputs

Once a clinical need is identified, the design inputs can be defined. The design inputs include physical but also commercial device attributes, and they all have to be described in as much detail as possible. Such device attributes for the forceps include the predominant goal of the device (manipulates the vessels atraumatically), how to do it (by grabbing or holding), how it should look and feel (like traditional forceps with a scissors-like shape), how much it should cost (inexpensive, comparable to the existing forceps), and what is the target market (similar to the traditional forceps). Once all the device attributes are captured (this might require several iterations of the process), it is recommended to rank the device inputs from the most critical, such as clinical function-related, to the least critical, such as cosmetic appearance (color, shape).

Based on the clinical need, the most important design input of the forceps is atraumatic manipulation of blood vessels. In addition, the forceps could be designed to be lighter, easier to handle, even a brighter color. Economically, the forceps has to be sold at an equal or lower price than the existing forceps. In addition, it has to be steam-sterilizable as existing medical instruments are, or disposable. The atraumatic feature is the highest-ranking feature (category 1). The next most important features are the smaller or equal price and sterilizable and disposable (category 2). The least important attributes are the lighter color and lighter weight assuming that the existing weight is not ideal but "it works" (category 3).

Design Outputs

Once the design inputs are formulated and ranked, the design outputs or the solution for each design input should be formulated keeping in mind all the design inputs. It is not advisable to generate design outputs for some of the design inputs but ignore the others. If, for example, a solution for the main function of the device (category 1) is found but requires very expensive components (such as electronics vs. mechanical, or biological vs. artificial), which disregards category 3 input, such a solution should be regarded only as a proof of principle solution rather than a final product solution. As before, a forceps with a mechanical pressure sensor and a motor, which senses and regulates the grasping force of the forceps such that the forceps does not cause vessel wall damage, might be scientifically solid. This solution might not make sense from an economic point of view as it will make the device much more expensive than existing devices. Unless the clinical need is very urgent, a drastic change in device design is probably not going to be received well by the market.

Testing Hypotheses

A R&D method that fits both the lean innovation model and the academic research is to formulate and test research hypotheses based on the design inputs. We should start with capturing the category 1 design input into a simple design that can be developed first and then tested. For example, we design a new configuration of the tip of the forceps to make it less traumatic for the blood vessels. The hypothesis is that the crisscross forceps tip design produces less vessel intima injury than the existing longitudinal design. This hypothesis can be tested by either performing a bench top study with either synthetic or animal blood vessel segment. A typical scientific study can then be designed and performed. The crisscross design could be easily implemented by modifying an existing forceps rather than designing a full new forceps. Once the category 1 outputs are tested, the other categories should also be formulated and tested as hypotheses for scientific studies. For the more advanced stages of the project, the preclinical animal and clinical studies could be designed.

Prior Art Search

When the clinical need and a draft of the design input are drafted, before moving to the design outputs, a thorough search of the literature has to be performed. In parallel with peer-reviewed journals that describe the procedure, a separate more extensive search should be performed for existing technologies in the field and patents. The key terms in the MP and CN should be used for the search. The search findings should be summarized in a table.

The findings of the prior art search could be surprising. For example, we could find that virtually all designs and configurations of the traditional forceps are already patented or publically disclosed and the only patentable solution is the pressure sensor and the motor complex. Then a decision has to be made between either securing a patent and developing a more complex device for a niche market or maybe making an improvement to an existing design and not worry about the IP protection (a less attractive option for investors).

Finding/Defining the Market for the New Technology

There is often a market for the MP but maybe not for the CN. The distinction should be carefully examined as only a subset of the MP market will also be the market for the CN. At the same time, additional markets for the CN might be possible. For example the market for surgical forceps is larger than the market for atraumatic vascular forceps. At the same time, an atraumatic forceps could be used in other medical applications such as soft tissue handling in plastic surgery.

The market can be defined in many ways:

1. The number of medical procedures in the USA, Europe, Japan, and the rest of the world (ROW) in which the device could be used.
2. The target patient population: for example, the number of patients suffering from vascular disease.
3. The number of medical units that perform this procedure: for example, all hospitals that perform vascular surgery.
4. Sales volume either in units or dollars: the number of vascular forceps sold annually or the money spent to buy vascular forceps.

A comprehensive business plan should include all the different aspects of the market, because the data complement each other. For example, it is not enough to know how many forceps units are sold but also who buys them and for how much in every region of the world. Also, the number of vascular repair procedures is not as important as how many units each hospital is purchasing and how often, because the forceps is a sterilizable medical device used in many vascular procedures.

From Concept to Object: Prototype Design and Execution

The ID will supervise the design execution. The prototype design is based on the design inputs and contains the design outputs or the engineering solutions to the clinical need. It can contain several variations of design to consider, such as a mechanical vs. electrical (motor-driven) solution. It can also contain variations of the exterior design of the device. It is recommended to run the design by the clinician to make sure it translates the critical design inputs.

The prototype execution can to be done in different stages. The critical design inputs have to be first incorporated in the design solution and the first generation of the prototype. Each of the device components will be subject to engineering optimization, then verification and validation. Therefore, the nonessential components (color and shape) could be reserved for the final versions of the prototype rather than the initial phase.

Big Money: Venture Funding and Licensing

Seed Money

Along with engineering design and preparation for commercialization, appropriate plans to secure the necessary funding have to be made. The seed money is the funds to design and build a prototype. The source for the money could be the proverbial FFF: friends, family and fools. Seed money is important because venture capital money (see below) usually requires a working prototype and a full business plan. The seed money and lean innovation concepts could take a project from an idea to a working prototype.

Venture Capital and Angel Investor Funding

The venture capital (VC) or angel investor funding is for commercializing the idea for a profit. Accepting venture capital money, although it is a complicated and sometime unorthodox process—a lawyer should be hired to represent the interest of the inventors during the entire process—it is probably the most efficient and fastest route to commercialization. This is due to the strict requirement of the venture fund administrator to make a profit within a certain period of time (typically up to 10 years). This means that, during this time, the VCs have to find a good product idea and a team, invest during the first 5 years, and make a profit during the remaining 5 years. From this perspective, it is easy to understand why the VCs seem driven and ruthless. On the other hand, it is almost guaranteed that if a VC is involved, the company will have an exit within 5–10 years of investment. This could be particularly beneficial for a serial entrepreneur who has several ideas that they want to develop. In that case, it is recommended to carefully pick the most profitable idea, run with it to commercialization, and then start another one. The second time around, things will go much smoother and faster due to the higher credibility of the entrepreneur.

If the inventors want to develop a company for themselves, a VC may not be the best option. Even if it takes longer, the inventors/entrepreneurs may prefer to do everything at their own pace with seed money coming from personal funds or sometimes bank loans such that they will maintain control of the company. To hope that the VCs will allow the inventors/entrepreneurs to keep their company at the end of the five years is unrealistic unless the company is so profitable that the VC will recuperate its money with a healthy profit and there is still enough equity left in the company that the inventor can keep control of the company. This is an unusual scenario, and it should be negotiated upfront.

Conclusions

Academic innovation is fit for lean innovation which is based on early customer feedback and testing hypotheses related to product function. The academic research environment is conducive for innovation and entrepreneurship, if there is adequate knowledge about the commercialization process especially during the early development stages. Only the early development steps are covered in the present chapter. The later aspects of commercialization related to launching the product on the market, selling and marketing it are probably implemented when a full business team is involved.

Related to the innovation social network, in addition to the inventor, an innovation director (ID) can coordinate several academic innovators through the entire R&D process to accelerate commercialization of academic innovation. The ID coordinates the design input and output process such that the clinical and commercial needs are fully met. Once there is a prototype and a business plan in place, there are several viable options for either licensing the technology or developing it further.

Although it might seem intimidatingly complex, the academic innovation fits with the existing academic scientist/clinician skills and environment and should be pursued as a part of the academic mission.

References

1. Hacker SM. The Medical Entrepreneur. Nano 2.0 Business Press; 2010.
2. Ireland BR, Ireland RD. Entrepreneurship: successfully launching new ventures. 4th ed. Pearson: Upper Saddle River, NJ; 2011.
3. Liker J. The Toyota Way: 14 management principles from the world's greatest manufacturer. New York: McGraw-Hill; 2003.
4. Ries E. The lean startup: how today's entrepreneurs use continuous innovation to create radically successful businesses. New York: Crown Business; 2011.
5. Ohno T. Workplace management. Milketo, WA: Gemba Press; 2007.
6. Standardization TIOf. ISO Catalogue: ISO 13485:2003 Medical devices—Quality management systems—Requirements for regulatory purposes. Available at: http://www.iso.org/iso/iso_catalogue/catalogue_tc/catalogue_detail.htm?csnumber=36786. Accessed 21 Jun 2014.
7. Administration USFaD. Medical Device Reporting (MDR). Available at: http://www.fda.gov/medicaldevices/safety/reportaproblem/default.htm. Accessed 21 Jun 2014.

8 Changing the Protocol: Is There Still Room for the Professor's Viewpoint?

Kenneth D. Boffard and Robert S. Boffard

I love my son, who is a 30-year-old writer living in Vancouver, but he has an unfortunate attraction to extreme sports. One of these is longboarding, which is essentially skateboarding on a type of elongated board designed for long, carving turns. It is very popular in Vancouver, where the city's hilly landscape and large parks provide ample opportunity to ride.

My son was travelling down a hill in the city, and decided he was going a little too fast for his comfort. Instead of stopping the board in the manner in which he had been taught (kicking out the back end to turn the board sideways, while simultaneously leaning back and dragging his hand across the ground using a specialised glove to reduce his speed), he thought it would be a good idea to jump off. It wasn't.

In the fall, he sustained an undisplaced fracture through the neck of the scaphoid bone. The wrist only became more painful a day or two later. He received excellent care through Canada's socialised medical system, including multiple X-rays and a CT scan to confirm the fracture. But at no point did the doctors—who, again, treated the injury extremely well—take a history, nor ever go into how and why, or how hard he fell. Did he blackout and then fall? Did he fall because he chose to jump off, or did he fall because something caused him to lose his balance? Does a scaphoid fracture point to something else, and would a machine (or a surgeon, who is increasingly becoming a technician) pick that something else up? (Throughout this chapter, I use the word machine to refer to any software or hardware system in a medical context, and the word professor to refer to not only the scholarly rank, but in this case, to any doctor of a sufficient age or experience to be considered senior.)

My son's case may be straightforward, but again, it shows the value of having the viewpoint of an experienced medical professional. The doctor says: "Here is a young man who has fallen onto his outstretched wrist. Now you can fall onto a wrist forwards—a young person's fall, where the impact is directly on the scaphoid bone—or you can fall backwards, which is an old person overbalancing, and most commonly causes a Colles' fracture. Young people generally don't fall backwards!" The protocol says: broken wrist, X-ray it, CT scan it, fix it. That is what a machine can do. The professor says: is the fracture compatible with what is supposed to have happened? Or is there a mismatch?

K.D. Boffard, M.B. F.R.C.S., F.A.C.S. (✉)
Department of Surgery, University of the Witwatersrand, Johannesburg, South Africa

Milpark Hospital, Johannesburg, South Africa
e-mail: kdboffard@pixie.co.za

R.S. Boffard, BJOURN(Rhodes)
Vancouver, BC, Canada
e-mail: robboffard@gmail.com

R. Latifi et al. (eds.), *Technological Advances in Surgery, Trauma and Critical Care*,
DOI 10.1007/978-1-4939-2671-8_8

One evening, about a year ago, a patient was admitted to our Trauma Center. The patient was a 65-year-old woman who had been in a car accident, but had no memory of the event. It was not certain whether she had lost consciousness and hit the car in front of her, or had lost consciousness afterwards. The CT scan was reported as normal, with neither injury to the brain nor any bony injury. By that stage, the woman was fully conscious, well oriented, and in accordance with protocol, was admitted for observation. She remained well overnight. Inevitably, by the following morning, there was pressure both from her family, and from the administration (there was the usual bed shortage) for an early discharge.

I looked at the scan. No breaks, nothing untoward, the patient was well. Something (a little voice in my ear?) told me it didn't look right. I went back and reviewed it. On one cut, there were a couple of small translucent areas in the skull itself. Myeloma changes the density of the skull. The bone of the skull table is usually homogenous, and there were minor areas of variable density in the scan. It turned out that she not only had a concussion, but had myeloma. That disease is fatal if untreated, and, as an added bonus, it usually presents late. But in this case, it was picked up early, because I looked at the scan and saw something that didn't look right.

I am a Trauma Surgeon, not a neurosurgeon, nor a radiologist. I wasn't sure what it was, but years ago, I had seen a similar picture in a patient I looked after as an intern, and my surgical radar started pinging. The irregularities were quite subtle, but shouldn't have been present in a normal skull. The Radiologist was senior, was asked to look at the brain for bleeding, and the skull for fractures, and came back with a normal report, reporting no pathology, because his brain programming did not consciously focus on bone density. Retrospective consensus was that the skull looked normal.

In many hospitals, the patient probably might not even have had a scan. She would have been observed, put in a ward overnight, then sent home. But because she was older, we had to exclude a bleed on the brain, and our thinking was that the scan would look at the contents of the skull rather than the skull itself. Had we stuck to that protocol—had we not had the experience to notice the irregular areas of the skull—she would have gone untreated until it was far too late to do anything. We did later confirm the diagnosis on blood tests and she was suitably referred, but the pathology was so subtle that we could have easily missed it. We wouldn't even have *done* the tests necessary to diagnose it, because it's so far from the realm of trauma surgery, or even *any* surgery.

My point here isn't to highlight my own particular skills as a diagnostician, but to highlight the value of experience. The question we're looking to answer here is whether there is room for professors' viewpoint; in this case, it was not only useful but necessary to have this view.

One might reasonably ask if all this—the possibilities, the mismatches, the peculiarities—can simply be reduced down to data, to a language that machine software can work with. After all, it's not difficult to teach a particular machine or piece of software about the differences between a straight scaphoid fracture and a Colles' fracture, and what they might mean, but that's not the problem.

The problem is not only single system pathology, but that you're talking about a *lot* of data that the machine has to sift through, looking for the bits that don't add up. That also results in a huge amount of choices for the person at the end. Unless the machine is performing the treatment as well (in which case we've created true artificial intelligence, capable of making clinical decisions on its own, and we have a much bigger problem!), then a human being must step in at some point to follow its recommendations. By offering so much choice, you risk making the wrong one.

Now, very obviously, these are all choices that a doctor has *anyway*, but very often their own intuition and experience can eliminate many of them. The less experience a doctor has, the fewer choices they will be able to eliminate, and greater risk to the patient:

Good judgement comes from experience
Experience comes from bad judgement!

The latter, we hope, primarily from somebody else's.

A human being can, very obviously, learn and gain experience, and to some extent a machine can as well. A machine can simply compare the outcome of a particular decision against the desired outcome, and adjust recommendations accordingly. Once again: it's just data. The issue isn't with the fact that machines can learn: it's how they learn. Automatic defibrillators (AEDs) work just fine. Every airport has them, and the chances of an experienced cardiologist being in precisely the right place at the right time are small.

There are significant distinctions between how machines operate and how humans operate. A human is capable of making errors of both commission and omission, but a machine can only make errors of omission. Machines can give you more possibilities, and a percentage of probability. The problem is that good judgement comes from experience, and experience comes from bad judgement. A machine cannot replicate that.

Another thing a machine cannot recognise is the limits of its own knowledge. It knows the limits of its own programming, and the parameters in which it operates, but there does not yet exist a machine which is aware of its own limitations in the way a human being is.

This is absolutely crucial to the argument here, and to the changing role of professors in a clinical environment. The role of a professor is twofold. Firstly: to educate enough to make the person he or she is teaching appreciate the need to ask for help, and, secondly, to leverage he or her own experience. And the definition of a good doctor is one who has the knowledge to deal with most situations and the humility to realise when that knowledge has gone beyond its capabilities. They know when to ask for help—ideally, early. At 3 am, I want what is often a junior, or inexperienced doctor to do the right things first, but if they're not working, I want that same doctor to phone for help.

All trauma, really, is protocol driven. Airway, Breathing, Circulation (ABC) is a protocol, or in the case of my son, Rest, Ice, Compression, Elevation. Damage Control Surgery is mandated if the core temperature is less than 34 °C. But is there a place where that isn't the correct or most appropriate treatment? Perhaps. And that's where the knowledge of the professor comes in. The dilemma is: *when* to break protocol and *who* is allowed to break protocol. A junior is allowed to break protocol only when instructed to do so, while as a professor, I can break protocol and be responsible for my actions (and be able to justify why I broke it, a statement my lawyers would prefer I note down).

Let's put this into context. Medicine across the entire Western world is suffering from a number of problems. One of these is that there is a reduction in the number of permitted working hours. You need to hire more people to cover the remaining hours, so what you have is the work spread across more people. The end result is that trainees end up with far less experience than they used to have. They have no choice but to focus on a much narrower sphere of knowledge and experience than their predecessors did. Fewer surgeons (and especially trauma surgeons) have had military exposure. The "darkness beyond the campfire" is drawing in and in many countries, the true General Surgeon is rare indeed. The expertise of many current surgeons is narrowed; they are better technically, but with less experience of patient care, especially the physiology and critical care of a patient, and this is why there is greater emphasis being placed on protocols. Trainees (and many super-specialists) do not have the experience necessary to work without them. Their results within their own disciplines may be far better than previously, but their ability to listen to hear the "little voice in their ear," is diminished, due to less access to a broader experience.

Should the professor just be there for when something goes wrong? Maybe, but then if the professor is not proactive, error will inevitably occur. You should never blame error: you should try and prevent it. Blame is at the centre of this question; breaking protocol allows you to blame somebody, which is very convenient. This is even more complex in litigation-friendly countries like the United States, although of course this is something that can happen anywhere. Everything has to be protocol-based: a rigid list of instructions which you have to follow. If you do not, you are deemed culpable, and it is more acceptable to follow them and get it wrong than to not follow them and get it right. What this means is that there is more *acceptance* for machines and protocol-based medicine than ever, and it is reducing the role for professors. Instead of their roles changing, they are being written out of the conversation altogether.

It is easy to straw-man this argument and accuse me of being a Luddite or a technophobe. That's not true. Every surgeon needs to have reliable diagnostic equipment, and equipment that is state of the art can only improve the chances of them getting it right. But consider this: Google is currently developing self-driving cars. If you get into an accident in a Google car, and you could see that crash coming but did not have the ability to tell the car to avoid it, because Google was working through a full set of protocols, wouldn't you be just a little bit angry?

That self-driving car needs a steering wheel that a human can take over and operate in case they disagree with the choices the machine is making. But what if the machine or protocol was right? However, if they no longer know how to drive, or there is no-one with them who knows how to drive, then if they crash, there is someone to blame. We not only need the option to take over, we need someone there who can advise and instruct if needed. But we also need to trust the machine.

If we believed entirely in technology, and protocols, then a patient with a scaphoid fracture or a change in cranium density that did not present on X-ray or CT would be sent home. And that is unacceptable. Experience should be preserved widely enough so that when something that ought to be right doesn't apply, there is still someone to ask!

Ethical Implications of Advanced Technologies in Surgical Care

9

Alberto R. Ferreres

"That any sane nation, having observed that you could provide for the supply of bread by giving bakers a pecuniary interest in baking for you, should go on to give a surgeon a pecuniary interest in cutting off your leg, is enough to make one despair of political humanity ... It is simply unscientific to allege or believe that doctors do not under existing circumstances perform unnecessary operations and manufacture and prolong lucrative illnesses."

GB Shaw
The Doctor's Dilemma: The Preface on Doctors
1911

Introduction and Framing the Issue

Without the contribution of innovative surgery to Medicine, there would not be organ transplantation, stapled gastrointestinal anastomosis, hip replacement, or substitute heart valves. Minimal invasive (laparoscopic, NOTES, single site and its variants) and robotic surgery belongs to this category and has revolutionized the treatment and approach of surgical conditions since the 1990s. Nonetheless surgical innovation also generates substantial ethical concerns with respect to surgeon's training, patient harm, patient autonomy and decision making, fair distribution of health resources, and conflicts of interest [1]. In that sense, the rate of biliary duct injuries was fairly increased after the wide adoption of standard 4-port laparoscopic cholecystectomy and similar data has been reported with single incision laparoscopic cholecystectomy [2, 3].

What is the meaning of advanced and novel technologies?

The Oxford Dictionary defines novel as "interestingly new or unusual," and innovation is a broad term defined as "the act of introducing something new or the use of a new idea or method." Surgical innovation includes a wide array of the necessary variations for usual practice and surgical research and development of new surgical procedures or improvement of existing ones. All definitions of innovation involve both ideas and an act of use or practice. New and innovative techniques have one thing in common: they are intended to lead to the renewal, refinement or betterment of the surgical technique offered for the treatment of human diseases.

Innovation in the surgical field tends to be more a process than an event, for example laparoscopic cholecystectomy, which was a huge innovation from 1990 on, should now be considered a standard procedure due to its rate of adoption. Other procedures cannot be termed exactly in the same way, and due to that fact, remain as innovative for longer periods and may never acquire the status of standard procedures.

A.R. Ferreres, MD, PhD, JD, MPH, FACS (Hon.) (✉)
Department of Surgery, Hospital Dr. Carlos A. Bocalandro, University of Buenos Aires, Vicente Lopez 1831 PB, Buenos Aires 1128, Argentina
e-mail: albertoferreres@gmail.com

R. Latifi et al. (eds.), *Technological Advances in Surgery, Trauma and Critical Care*,
DOI 10.1007/978-1-4939-2671-8_9

Ideally all surgical interventions should be controlled. When real hazard is involved in a new and unproven procedure, it may be urgent to determine the value of such intervention [4].

Due to its development and lack of wide acceptance, NOTES surgery may still be considered an innovation, though this approach may generate some discussion. Many times an early precursor does not gain wide acceptance and a couple of years later the same procedure presented by another physician gains widespread attention. For example Ortega proposed endoscopic myotomy for achalasia [5], which was very soon abandoned for the risks and 30 years later Inoue, amid the fashion of NOTES procedures, achieved POEM (Per Oral Endoscopic Myotomy) with worldwide impact [6].

The history of natural orifice surgery can be traced to three early developers such as N. Senn [7], Dimitri Oskarovich Von Ott [8], and Raoul Palmer [9].

Gynecologists were proficient in the culdoscopic approach and that may be the reason why Daniel Tsin performed the first transvaginal cholecystectomy and reported the case in 2003 [10], 4 years earlier than Zorron [11], Bessler [12], Marescaux [13], and Ramos [14].

The same can be said of single incision laparoscopic surgery, having reported Pelosi, the first single incision appendectomy years ago [15], and Navarra and Wg, the first single incision laparoscopic cholecystectomy [16, 17].

These procedures were not widely accepted. But after the first NOTES cases were reported and made clear the difficulties and necessary skills requested by this approach (flexible endoscopy, gynecologic approach, gastric closure), a bridge was inclined from NOTES to SILS, with the support of the industry.

Robotic surgery represents another field of innovation: this technology enables a surgeon to perform a procedure using laparoscopic instruments attached to robotic arms, which he or she manipulates from a console while viewing the cavity in three dimensions, very similar as if it were open surgery. First approved by the FDA in 2000, this approach was used in about 292,000 cases in 2011 and in about 367,000 the following year. The procedures performed with robotic technology include predominantly gynecologic, urologic and abdominal operations. Though this sounds like a wonderful addition to the surgeons' armamentarium, recent reports have raised concern regarding issues of safety, cost-effectiveness, and advertising by physicians and institutions [18]. Wu mentions "...The results show how direct-to-consumer marketing can lead to the explosion of an expensive new treatment—even when little evidence exists to support the therapy's superiority over standard care" [19]. More recently, a group from Johns Hopkins Institutions reported 245 adverse events due to the use of robotic surgery [20].

Nonetheless, in order to judge accordingly and to increase patients' knowledge and awareness, good science is mandatory for good ethics and may be considered a prerequisite. Which is the correct and adequate knowledge? From an epistemological point of view, three concepts must be considered: belief, truth, and justification. Belief is an individual faith and conviction regarding the truth of a proposition; truth is considered to be the reality and includes the meaning of veracity, and justification explains the basis or motives for believing [21].

Background

The Surgical Procedure and the Surgeon–Patient Relationship

Surgery has five unique characteristics that set it apart from any other kind of medical specialty:

1. Surgery harms before it heals.
2. It penetrates the patient's body and thus is highly invasive. According to the judgment of Judge Benjamin Cardozo in "Schloendorff v. Society of New York Hospitals" (1914): "A surgeon who performs an operation without patient's consent commits an assault."
3. It is fallible, which means that surgery is predisposed to human error. Increased awareness on this topic has developed since the Institute of Medicine's "To Err is Human" was published.

4. Surgeon's decision-making is performed under circumstances of uncertainty.
5. It is prone to risks and complications.

On the other hand, the surgeon–patient relationship is built around trust, so it is preferable to speak about fiduciarism and not about a contract. As John Gregory stated in the eighteenth century, the physician:

- Must be in a position to know reliably the patient's interest
- Should be concerned primarily with protecting and promoting the interests of the patient
- Should be concerned only secondarily with protecting and promoting his own interests

The concept of acting as a moral fiduciary of the patient is central to the core of surgical ethics. Being a fiduciary is legally understood to be "a person holding the character of a trustee, in respect of the trust and confidence involved in it and scrupulous good faith and candor which it requires" and also to be a "person having duty, created by his undertaking, to act primarily for another's benefit in matters connected with such undertaking."

The surgeon–patient relationship is attained and perfected throughout the process of the surgical informed process which includes the following elements:

1. Preconditions: competence and voluntariness of the patient
2. Information: disclosure and recommendations by the surgeon, and understanding by the patient
3. Consent: decision-making (acceptance or refusal), communication, registration, and authorization to proceed from the patient

Ethical Principles and Considerations

The principles of biomedical ethics as collated by Beauchamp and Childress and addressed by the Belmont Report (April 1979) have become one of the most widely used frameworks for considering bioethical issues. They are: respect for patient autonomy, beneficence, non-maleficence, and justice [22].

No concept overrides the other; there is no preeminence among them and all stand alike. Besides the four classical ethical principles, truthfulness, fairness, integrity, dignity and respect to people's rights, and honesty virtue should be added.

Respect for Patient Autonomy

The concept of autonomy examines individuals' decision-making in health care and research, as patients and as subjects in the surgical care process. In a properly structured theory, respect for autonomy is not excessively individualistic (thereby neglecting the social nature of individuals and the impact of individual choices and actions on others), not excessively focused on reason (thereby neglecting the emotions), and not unduly legalistic (thereby highlighting human rights and downplaying social practices and responsibilities).

The word autonomy is derived from the Greek "autos" (self) and "nomos" (rule, governance, law) and originally refers to the self-rule or self-governance of independent city states in Greece.

There are two conditions essential for autonomy: freedom (independence from external controlling influences) and agency (capacity for intentional action). Autonomous choice has to be obtained from the patient. The moral requirements of respect for autonomy include autonomous action in terms of normal choosers who act intentionally, with understanding and without controlling influences that determine their action.

The theories of two philosophers have powerfully influenced contemporary interpretations of respect for autonomy: Immanuel Kant and John Stuart Mill. Kant argued that respect for autonomy flows from the recognition that all persons have unconditional worth, each having the capacity to determine his or her own moral destiny. Mill concerned himself primarily with the individuality of autonomous agents, arguing that society should permit individuals to develop according to their own convictions, as long as they do not interfere with a like expression of freedom by others or unjustifiably harm others.

Kant's position entails a moral imperative of respectful treatment of persons as an end of itself.

The basic paradigm of autonomy in health care is represented by the informed consent process and entails a competent judgment. The conditions of a competent judgment must satisfy the standards for its determination in order to be valid.

Beneficence

Beneficence stands for acts of mercy, kindness, and charity and refers to the character trait or virtue of being disposed to act for the benefit of other persons. As opposed to utility, positive beneficence requires agents to provide benefit to others and is more an ideal than an obligation; according to the Good Samaritan's parable we cannot demand acts to exceed ordinary morality.

The principle of positive beneficence supports an array of moral rules of duty or obligations:

1. Protect and defend the rights of others
2. Prevent harm from occurring to others
3. Remove conditions that will cause harm to others
4. Help persons with disabilities
5. Rescue persons in danger

The rules of beneficence, in contrast to those of non-maleficence, include:

1. Positive requirements of action.
2. Need not always be followed impartially ("impartial adherence"). We are morally prohibited from causing harm to anyone. However, we are morally permitted to help or benefit those with whom we have special relationships, and we often are not required to help or benefit those with whom we have no such special relationships.
3. Generally do not provide reasons for legal punishment when agents fail to abide by them.

Physician obligations to patients represent philanthropic service, whereas obligations to their teachers represent debts incurred in the course of becoming physicians. However, today many physicians and health care professionals owe a large debt to society (for education and privileges) and to their patients, past and present (for research and practice). Because of this indebtedness the medical profession role of beneficent care of patients is misconstrued if modeled primarily on philanthropy, altruism, and personal commitment. This care is rooted in the reciprocity of giving after having received.

Non-maleficence

This principle imposes an obligation not to inflict harm on others. It is closely related to the aphorism "Primum non nocere." Often considered the fundamental principle in the Hippocratic tradition of medical ethics, it does not appear in the Hippocratic Corpus exception made of the translation of a single passage: "at least do no harm." Nonetheless the Hippocratic Oath expresses obligations of non-maleficence and of beneficence: "I will use treatment to help the sick according to my ability and judgment, but I will never use it to injure or wrong them."

The most important rule of this principle consists in not to inflict evil or harm; that means that this principle requires only intentionally refraining from actions that cause harm. When we refer to harm, we focus on physical harm, especially pain, suffering, disability, death, or loss of chance (survival) as well as mental harm. We can summarize as intending, causing, or permitting death or the risk of death.

The rules of non-maleficence are:

1. Negative prohibitions of actions
2. Must be followed impartially
3. Provide moral background for legal prohibitions of certain forms of conduct

The obligation of non-maleficence includes not only the duty not to inflict harm but also the duty not to impose risks of harm. In cases of risk imposition, both Law and Moral recognize a standard of due care that determines whether the agent who is causally responsible for the risk is legally or morally liable as well. This standard is a specification of the principle of non-maleficence.

On the other hand, negligence is the absence of due care, it involves a departure from the professional standards that determine due care in given circumstances. The term negligence covers two types of situations:

- Intentionally imposing unreasonable risks of harm (advertent negligence or recklessness)
- Unintentionally but carelessly imposing risks of harm (inadvertent negligence)

Justice

The concept of justice dates back to Aristotle, who conceptualized justice as "the rendering to each individual of what is due to him or her." Justice is interpreted as the fair, equitable and appropriate treatment of what is due or owed to persons. More recent influences in biomedical ethics originate from John Rawls' "A theory of justice," in which he argues that a social arrangement forming a political state is a communal effort to advance the good of all in society. Representing an egalitarian point of view, Rawls attempts to solve the problem of distributive justice (the socially just distribution of goods in a society) by using a variation of the familiar device of the "social contract." The resultant theory is known as "justice as fairness", from which the author derives his two principles of justice: the liberty principle and the difference principle.

In health care, justice primarily refers to the distribution of scarce resources in a fair way from a communitarian point of view, but includes the obligation to respect the patients' rights and morally acceptable laws from the patient's individual point of view. Hume considered that justice was a social virtue while benevolence was a principle of human nature.

The four ethical principles embrace more specific rules applicable to surgical care and innovative practice, providing a framework to consider systematically the ethics of surgical practice. In that sense the principles typology of surgical ethical issues includes the following:

- Respect for autonomy: surgical informed consent, truth telling, confidentiality, communication skills.
- Beneficence: surgical competence, sound judgment, continuing medical education, accountability, communication skills.
- Non Maleficence: surgical competence, sound judgment, recognizing one's limitations, disclosure and discussion of complications and surgical errors.
- Justice: allocation of scarce resources, legal issues, human rights.

Nonetheless, Sir David Ross (1877–1971) was the first one to achieve the prima facie ethical duties, originally in the number of five: fidelity, reparation, gratitude, promotion of a maximum of aggregate good and non maleficence [23]. Not all these duties bear the same importance. In his argumentation, the duty of non-maleficence overcomes the one to promote a maximum of aggregate good and the duties of fidelity, reparation, and gratitude are more preeminent than the one to promote the good. The four elements that are basically good include: virtue, knowledge, pleasure, and justice. He taught that moral decision-making sometimes requires us to think about the past and act according a sense of duty rather than focusing on the projected outcome, following the Kantian "moral imperative." His Duties-based (deontological) Ethics served as a foundation for the work of Beauchamp and Childress.

Ethical Considerations

The advancing technology and knowledge provide greater opportunities to save lives and relieve pain and suffering.

Many of the operations that are currently in use have never been formally tested by any rigorous scientific trial. They have been introduced into clinical practice as so many other procedures before them: as innovative therapies. As such, they were simply implemented without safeguards to protect patients. This has been, and largely still is, accepted, everyday surgical practice. Less high profile innovative surgeries, however, escape added scrutiny and eventually find their way into standard clinical care.

Some authors consider three minimal requirements that make a surgical innovation ethical: laboratory background, field strength and institutional stability, others include a fourth requirement, institutional review board (IRB) evaluation [24, 25]. Surgical innovation is an important driver of improvements in technique and technology, which ultimately translates into improvements in patients' outcomes. Nevertheless, patients may face new risks of morbidity and mortality when surgical innovation is used, and well-intentioned surgical "experimentation" on patients must be regulated and monitored. Besides, surgical innovation is not always a synonym of surgical evolution; patient safety must be the overriding ethical consideration.

Surgeons' responsibilities to individuals and to the society to which they belong cannot be disregarded in any sense. J.E. Dunphy stated them very clearly in his 1963 American College of Surgeons Presidential Address about "Responsibility and authority in American Surgery": "Surgeons have a collective responsibility to seek the benefit of humanity … the autonomy of the individual surgeon is only possible because society is in agreement with surgeons that they will act to benefit humanity and surgeons must have some form of central authority to ensure that certain standards of professionalism are met."

Some of the questions that need to be answered concerning the ethics of these new techniques include the following:

- Is this an experimental procedure?
- Is this frontline surgery?
- Who can perform this surgery?
- Requirements and training.

Probably we can consider NOTES as a combination of different approaches into a new one; more than a new surgical procedure of experimental nature, in the transvaginal approach we can find old historical landmarks of culdoscopic surgery, mostly in hands of gynecologists. Single site laparoscopy represents, on the other hand, a closer placement of the entry sites more than a radical new approach. Robotic surgery raises similar concerns, particularly regarding high cost, making it unavailable to many patients worldwide, cost/effectiveness, and the achievement of real benefits for the patient.

These procedures are not for every surgeon, not for every patient and not to be performed anywhere, but some talented surgeons should provide these approaches, under rigorous scrutiny and supervision and with a huge concern for patient safety.

Whenever a new technique is introduced, ideally a group of experts should encourage the critical evaluation giving answer to these crucial questions:

- Feasibility of the new procedure or technique, regarding its widespread acceptance, rate of adoption and efficacy for the condition to treat.
- Safety of the procedure, analyzing how easily this technique can be learned by the average surgeon, if there is an increased risk of complications and the requirements for training and education in this field.
- Clinical advantages, defining the real (and not the potential) benefits either to the patient or the health care system.

The four ethical challenges generated by innovative surgery can be grouped in the following categories:

1. Harm or disability to patients: Surgical innovative procedures have the ability to generate increased morbimortality in comparison to standard and/or conventional procedures. This is true and specially evident in the early stages of development, since the learning curve or curve of expertise needs a minimum number of cases to be attained. So the question posed is the following: How can the most obvious source of patient harm be minimized?
2. Compromise and threats to the surgical informed consent process: This addresses the concern regarding patient autonomy and the risk that patient freedom to decide may be compromised in different ways: Information may not be fully disclosed regarding the nature and type of the procedure, data about risks and dangers may be withhold to prevent patient's refusal to the procedure. An interesting point in informed consent for new proce-

dures is the general tendency among the public to equate newness with increased benefit or better quality. The role of IRB in supporting this process, as well as that of colleagues and faculty would sort any inconvenient in this sense.

3. Distribution of health-care resources: Innovative surgery presents—many times and particularly in developing countries—a challenge to the fair distribution of health-care resources. Common sense indicates limiting expenditure to interventions with proven safety and efficacy rather than "wasting" money on ineffective and/or unsafe and/or dangerous procedures. A fair distribution of resources revolves around notions of: liberty, associated with autonomy and the authority of individuals and institutions; equality, considered as the equity of surgical care and fraternity, targeted as the solidarity of the surgical profession within society.
4. Conflicts of interest: The last challenge is represented by the conflicts of interest, which may affect the individual surgeon, a faculty group, and sometimes their institutions. The most obvious is the economic one, usually associate with the willingness to attract more patients, to be considered a pioneer and its inherent prestige and with the development and use of new devices, provided by the manufacturing biomedical companies. This and other conflicts of interests can directly impact sound and appropriate decision making.

Some suggestions to aid in solving the above-mentioned issues include:

- Regulation by government agencies, in a similar way as in the pharmaceutical industry
- Control by scientific societies, which usually turns to be late and outdated
- Self-regulation by chairs, faculty, and colleagues
- Participation of the IRB or institutional Ethics Committee
- Mandatory collection in databases which allow a precise and prompt understanding of the innovation, facts and figures about outcomes, safety, and efficacy
- The implementation of randomized clinical trials, more challenging to run in surgery but not impossible

The Balliol Collaboration's IDEAL (innovation, development, exploration, assessment, and long-term study) model addresses some of the discussed topics and provides tools for the "surgical innovation ethics paradigm" [26]. It attempts to identify and describe stages of surgical innovation providing a basis for recommendations about regulation and assessment. They firmly propose the development of databases, which will provide the necessary collection of evidence:

- Innovation: the primary aims of this stage include safety and proof of the pursued concept. In this stage, the surgeons should inform hospitals and IRBs of their intention to perform innovative procedures.
- Development: regulation and evidence from well designed studies should be a requisite. Steps to be complied before patient recruitment include: mandatory monitoring, reporting of patient selection, detailed description of the procedure and modifications and outcomes of all cases.
- Early dispersion and exploration: with increasing adoption of the procedure, mentoring and learning assessment are pillars as is the collection of data for every patient.
- Assessment: the effectiveness of the innovation should be tested against current standards, including efficiency (economic assessment).
- Long term study: a registry should be established to monitor outcomes that are rare and those that only become apparent over time.

Conclusions

In conclusion, strict adherence to the following principles of the American College of Surgeons (The American College of Surgeons Statement of Principles, revised September 21, 2006) will provide a safe frame for innovation in surgical practice:

- *Performance of surgical procedures by those who are not properly trained to perform them should not be a frequent or continuing practice.*
- *Fellows are strongly encouraged to be actively involved as leaders of quality assessment and improvement activities in their own hospital.*
- *Acquisition of skills in new procedures should be fostered by attendance at courses with both didactic and hands-on sessions. The fellow should seek appropriate proctoring of cases as new procedures are added to his or her surgical portfolio. Continuous self- appraisal of surgical outcomes is strongly encouraged with the goal of improving patient outcomes.*

Besides, the Committee on Emerging Surgical Technologies of the American College of Surgeons published the following statement [27], which summarizes all the abovementioned issues:

"New surgical technologies are the combined product of basic and applied surgical research. The introduction and application of any new technology should proceed through a series of steps intended to ensure its safety, appropriateness, and cost-effectiveness.

1. The development of a new technology must be accompanied by a scientific assessment of safety, efficacy and need.
2. Diffusion into clinical practice requires appropriate education of surgeons and evaluation of their use of new technology. An in-depth knowledge of the relevant disease process and its management, gained through formal training and clinical experience, is a prerequisite. Acquisition of new technical skills and the development of appropriate support facilities must follow, and must be subject to initial assessment and periodic monitoring of outcomes.
3. Widespread application of new technologies must be continuously assessed and compared with alternative therapies to ensure appropriateness and cost-effectiveness through outcome studies."

Summary

This chapter surveys the foundations of the surgeon–patient relationship and the ethical principles of surgical care, providing a frame for those interested in achieving changes and/or innovations in surgical procedure. An analysis of the issues related to surgical innovation is also included as well as problem solving tools.

References

1. Angelos P. The ethical challenges of surgical innovation for patient care. Lancet. 2010;376:1046–7.
2. Goldfarb MA. Ethics and laparoscopy—concert or contest. In: Frezza EE, editor. Professionalism and ethics in a surgical practice, chapter 38. Woodbury: Cine-Med; 2008.
3. Joseph M, Phillips MR, Farrell TM, et al. Single incision laparoscopic cholecystectomy is associated with a higher incidence of bile duct injury rate. A review and a word of caution. Ann Surg. 2012;256:1–6.
4. Beecher HK. Surgery as placebo: a quantitative study of bias. JAMA. 1961;176:1354–60.
5. Ortega JA, Madureri V, Perez L. Endoscopic myotomy in the treatment of achalasia. Gastrointest Endosc. 1980;26:8–10.
6. Inoue H, Minami H, Kobayashi Y, et al. Peroral endoscopic myotomy (POEM) for esophageal achalasia. Endoscopy. 2010;42:265–71.
7. Senn N. The early history of vaginal hysterectomy. JAMA. 1895;XXV(12):476–82.
8. Von Ott DO. Die Beleuchtung der Bauchhohle als Methode bei. Vaginale Coeliotomie Abl Gynakol. 1902;231:817–23.
9. Palmer R. Instrumentation et technique de la coelioscopie gynecologique. Gynecol Obstet (Paris). 1947; 46:420–31.
10. Tsin DA, Sequeria RJ, Giannikas G. Culdolaparoscopic cholecystectomy during vaginal hysterectomy. JSLS. 2003;7:171–2.
11. Zorron R, Filgueiras M, Maggioni LC, et al. NOTES transvaginal cholecystectomy: report of the first case. Surg Innov. 2007;14:279–83.
12. Bessler M, Stevens PD, Milone L, et al. Transvaginal laparoscopically assisted endoscopic cholecystectomy: a hybrid approach to natural orifice surgery. Gastrointest Endosc. 2007;66:1243–5.
13. Marescaux J, Dallemagne B, Perretta S, et al. Surgery without scars: report of transluminal cholecystectomy in a human being. Arch Surg. 2007;142:823–7.

14. Ramos AC, Murakami A, Galvao Neto M, et al. NOTES transvaginal video-assisted cholecystectomy: first series. Endoscopy. 2008;40:572–5.
15. Pelosi MA, Pelosi III MA. Laparoscopic appendectomy using a single umbilical puncture (minilaparoscopy). J Reprod Med. 1992;37:588–94.
16. Navarra G, Pozza E, Occhionorelli S, et al. One-wound laparoscopic cholecystectomy. Br J Surg. 1997;84:695–7.
17. Wg WT, Kong CK, Wong YT. One wound laparoscopic cholecystectomy. Br J Surg. 1997;84:1627.
18. Satava RM. Laparoscopic surgery, robots and surgical simulation: moral and ethical issues. Semin Laparosc Surg. 2002;9:230–8.
19. Wu JC, Gu X, Lipsitz SR, et al. Comparative effectiveness of minimally invasive vs open radical prostatectomy. JAMA. 2009;302:1557–64.
20. Cooper MA, Ibrahim A, Lyu H et al. Underreporting of robotic surgery complications. J Healthcare Qual. doi:10.1111/jhq.12036. [Epub ahead of print].
21. Williams M. Problems of knowledge. A critical introduction to epistemology. Oxford: Oxford University Press; 2001.
22. Beauchamp TL, Childress JF. Principles of biomedical ethics. 4th ed. New York: Oxford University Press; 1994.
23. Ross WD. The right and the good. Oxford: Oxford University Press; 1930.
24. Johnson J, Rogers W. Innovative surgery: the ethical challenges. J Med Ethics. 2012;38:9–12.
25. McKneally MF. Ethical problems in surgery: innovation leading to unforeseen complications. World J Surg. 1999;23:786–8.
26. Barkun JS, Aronson JK, Feldman LS, For the Balliol collaboration, et al. Evaluation and stages of surgical innovation. Lancet. 2009;374:1089–96.
27. Statements on Emerging Surgical Technologies and the Evaluation of Credentials. American College of Surgeons. Bull Am Coll Surg. 1994; 79:40-1.

Part II

Trauma, Resuscitation, and Nutrition

Dedicated Resuscitation Operating Room for Trauma

10

Todd W. Costantini, Leslie Kobayashi, and Raul Coimbra

Concept of Operating Room Resuscitation: Introduction

Trauma is one of the most common causes of disability in the USA, and is the leading cause of death in patients age 1–45. The trimodal distribution of deaths describes the pattern of mortality in trauma patients. Nearly half of trauma deaths occur in the first hour after injury, and are generally caused by major vascular or severe head injury. The next peak in mortality occurs approximately 1–4 h post-injury and represents death caused by hemorrhage. It is this population that constitutes the majority of preventable deaths with outcomes potentially improved by developed trauma systems and prompt evaluation at a trauma center. The final peak occurs in the weeks following injury and is due to infection and multiple organ failure.

A major emphasis in the care of the injured patient has focused on the prompt identification and treatment of hemorrhage with the goal of minimizing deaths in the second peak of the trimodal distribution. Improvements in trauma systems and widespread application of advanced trauma life support (ATLS) protocols have led to prompt triage of injured patients to trauma centers and a common approach to identify and treat potentially life threatening injuries. With the goal of limiting the time to operative intervention for hemorrhage control, the concept of direct transport from the scene to the operating room was developed. A multicenter study by Hoyt et al. in 1990 demonstrated that delays to the operating room account for a significant portion of preventable deaths [1]. Operating room resuscitation has subsequently been utilized in several centers with the goal of minimizing the time to definitive treatment. The operating room resuscitation strategy also mobilizes significant resources at the time of initial evaluation including trauma physicians, trauma resuscitation nurses, anesthesiologists, radiology technicians, and operating room staff. Therefore, the concept of the operating room resuscitation theoretically offers the best of both worlds, providing a trauma resuscitation room for initial evaluation and diagnostic radiologic studies, with the potential for rapid conversion to open operative intervention and hemorrhage control. At the University of California San Diego (UCSD) level-1 Trauma Center we have had an operating room used exclusively for trauma resuscitations for more than 25 years. A detailed description of our OR resuscitation protocol is provided in this chapter.

T.W. Costantini, M.D., F.A.C.S. • L. Kobayashi, M.D., F.A.C.S. • R. Coimbra, M.D., Ph.D., F.A.C.S. (✉)
Division of Trauma, Surgical Critical Care, Burns and Acute Care Surgery, Department of Surgery, UC San Diego Health Sciences, San Diego, CA, USA
e-mail: tcostantini@ucsd.edu; lkobayashi@ucsd.edu; rcoimbra@ucsd.edu

R. Latifi et al. (eds.), *Technological Advances in Surgery, Trauma and Critical Care*,
DOI 10.1007/978-1-4939-2671-8_10

Prehospital Triage

In the field, patients can be categorized into three groups based on their injuries. The first group, which is comprised of approximately 5 % of all patients, is unlikely to benefit from prehospital care due to the severity of their injuries. The most common triage scenario, representing a vast majority of trauma patients, is patients with moderate injuries whose outcomes are unlikely to be significantly affected by delays in transport and evaluation. The final group, representing approximately 7–15 % of trauma patients, consists of those that have potentially fatal injuries. It is this group of patients that are most likely to benefit from prompt triage and transport to a trauma center. Due to the importance of hemorrhage control in this group of patients, triage for immediate evaluation, resuscitation, and treatment in the operating room may decrease the time to hemorrhage control and improve outcomes.

Since the operating room resuscitation is resource intensive it is clearly not appropriate for all trauma patients. Therefore, identifying the population of patients that would most benefit from initial evaluation in the operating room has been considered. Our current criteria for direct transportation from the field to the operating room (Table 10.1) include: (1) penetrating trauma with hypotension; (2) witnessed cardiac arrest; (3) hypotensive patients (systolic blood pressure <90 mmHg) who are unresponsive to fluid challenge in the field; (4) major, uncontrolled external hemorrhage (amputation); (5) direct injury to the neck with airway compromise. Physiologic changes may occur during transport to the trauma center. Therefore, patients can be upgraded to an operating room resuscitation while en route as long as this upgrade occurs at least 5 min prior to anticipated arrival. Patients meeting criteria for operating room resuscitation fewer than 5 min prior to arrival at the trauma center are evaluated in the trauma bay as this does not leave adequate time to mobilize personnel and resources to the operating room.

Table 10.1 Criteria for direct transport to the operating room

Penetrating trauma with hypotension (systolic blood pressure <90 mmHg)
Witnessed traumatic cardiac arrest
Hypotension unresponsive to prehospital fluid challenge
Major external hemorrhage/traumatic amputation of a limb
Direct injury to neck with airway compromise

Initial Assessment in an Operating Room Resuscitation

Once the decision is made for triage directly to the operating room, personnel are alerted to report to the designated trauma operating suite (Fig. 10.1). The trauma team responds and functions as the team leader, responsible for directing the activity and tasks of all other team members in the room (Fig. 10.2). During operating room resuscitation, the trauma team leader is positioned on the left side near the head of the bed in order to conduct the primary survey but allow anesthesia access to the airway. The team leader also directs the team members to prepare for any indicated procedures during the initial evaluation including control of external bleeding and the placement of central lines or chest tubes. While positioned at the head of the bed, the trauma team leader can also evaluate the need for a controlled airway, and can direct the anesthesia team to attempt orotracheal intubation when indicated. Trauma resuscitation nurses are present to record vital sign and exam findings, in addition to obtaining peripheral intravenous access, and administering medications under the direction of the trauma team leader. The anesthesia team reports to the head of the bed where they prepare for possible orotracheal intubation, if needed. The operating room nurses and technicians respond and prepare to open sterile laparotomy, thoracotomy, or major vascular trays when directed to do so by the trauma team leader. Radiology technicians also report to the operating room to obtain plain film radiographs during the initial evaluation.

The prehospital providers deliver the patient directly to the operating room and transfer the patient to the operating room table after giving a

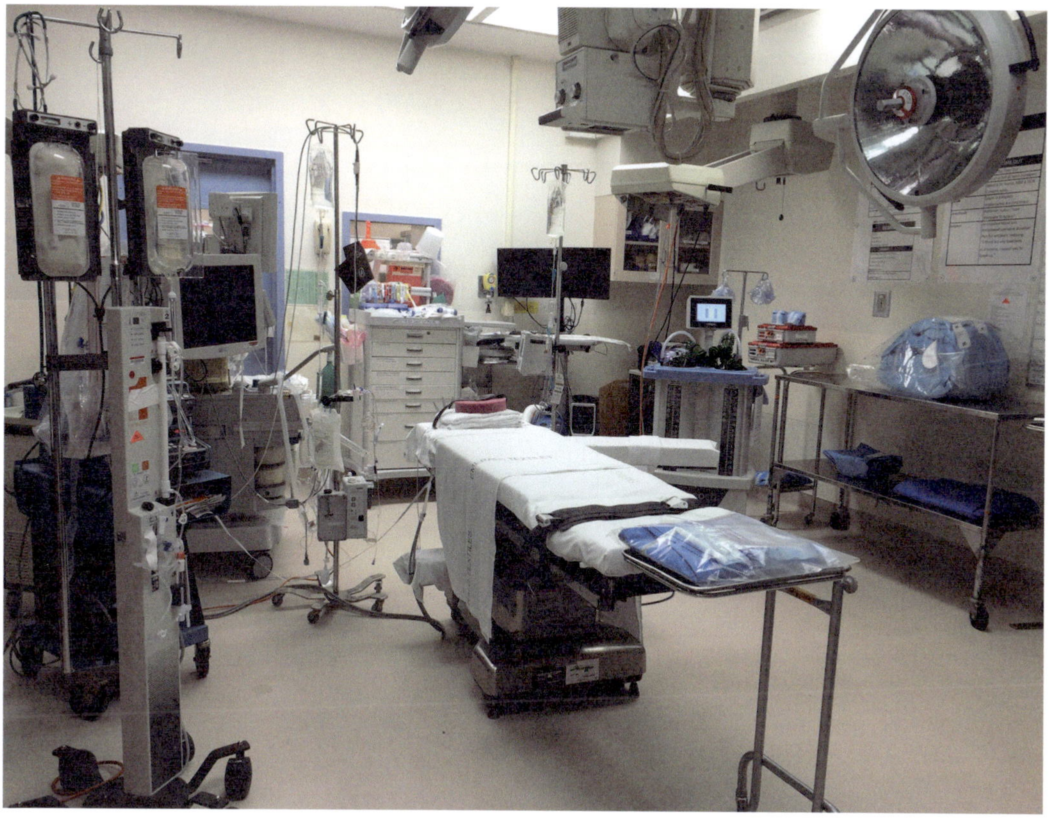

Fig. 10.1 Dedicated operating room resuscitation suite

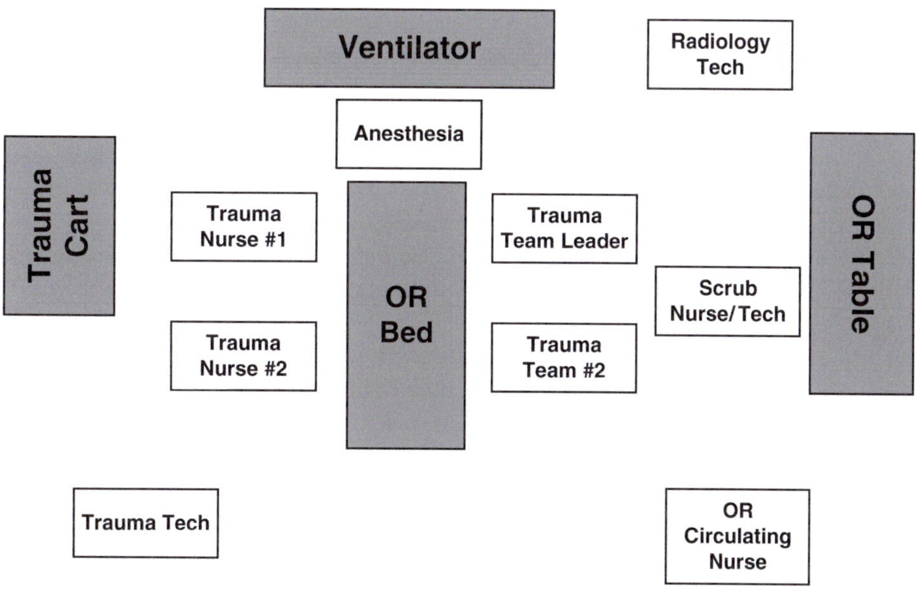

Fig. 10.2 Operating room resuscitation personnel

brief organized report detailing the *M*echanism of injury, obvious *I*njuries, the patient's *V*ital signs, and any *T*reatments provided (*MIVT*). The trauma team leader then begins the primary and secondary survey based on ATLS protocol.

Diagnosis and Treatment of Shock in the Operating Room

Hypovolemic shock due to hemorrhage is the most common cause of shock and can occur due to bleeding into the chest, abdomen, pelvis/retroperitoneum, into the extremities, or due to blood lost externally. Lack of response to fluid or blood product resuscitation indicates significant ongoing hemorrhage and necessitates immediate measures to identify and control the source of bleeding. Just as in the trauma bay, sources of external bleeding should be controlled with direct pressure or tourniquets prior to operative intervention aimed at proximal and distal control of any vascular injury. Bleeding into the chest can be diagnosed with a chest radiograph obtained in the operating suite and can be treated, and blood loss quantified, with chest tube placement. In-line or other types of devices should be arranged to collect shed blood after chest tube placement for autotransfusion (Fig. 10.3). Massive hemothorax can be addressed with immediate conversion to thoracotomy in the operating room. All patients with penetrating trauma to the chest, particularly those with injuries in the zone denoted by the clavicles superiorly, costal margin inferiorly, and bilateral mid-clavicular lines should be suspected of cardiac injury and evaluated with pericardial ultrasound and/or subxiphoid window. Findings of pericardial fluid or patients with hemodynamic instability and high index of suspicion for cardiac injury should undergo immediate midline sternotomy. Those *in extremis* or who undergo cardiac arrest should undergo immediate resuscitative thoracotomy if they are a victim of penetrating trauma with <15 min of prehospital CPR, or <10 min of prehospital CPR with a secured airway for a blunt mechanism of injury [2]. At UCSD most, if not all, resuscitative thoracotomies are performed in the Operating Room (OR),

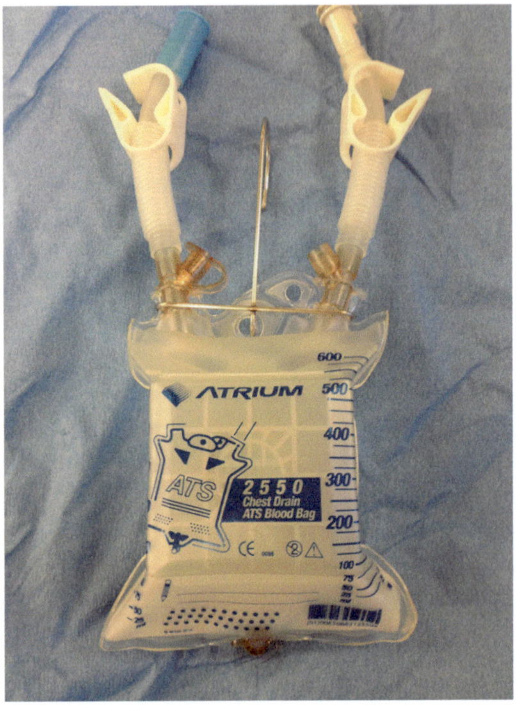

Fig. 10.3 Autotransfusion device (Chest Drain, ATS Blood Bag, Atrium, Merrimack, NH)

as those patients requiring the procedure do not stop in the trauma bay or in the Emergency Department (ED), and are transported from the scene directly to the OR. The advantages of performing the procedure in the OR compared to the ED are obvious, including but not limited to more available equipment options, better lighting, general anesthesia and airway control, absence of chaos and excessive noise, as well as improved sterility.

Patients with peritonitis should undergo laparotomy regardless of hemodynamic status which can occur promptly during an OR resuscitation as the OR staff is present and surgical instruments immediately available. Patients without peritonitis can be evaluated using a Focused Assessment with Sonography for Trauma (FAST) while in the OR, or diagnostic peritoneal aspiration/lavage (DPA/DPL). A positive FAST or DPA/DPL, in a hypotensive patient is another indication for immediate laparotomy which should be rapidly mobilized in the OR setting. Resuscitation in the

OR does not mandate operative intervention. Patients evaluated and resuscitated in the OR who do not require operative intervention can be transported to the computed tomography (CT) scanner for further imaging, or to the intensive care unit for further resuscitation based on the injuries diagnosed.

Outcomes Following Operating Room Resuscitation

The first report of immediate transport to the OR after major trauma was by Griswold and Drye in 1953 [3]. They reported their experience with 108 patients that were transported immediately to the OR based on history or physical findings suggestive of cardiac injury or other major thoracic trauma at the Louisville General Hospital. They reported an increase in the operability rate in this population with a decrease in total mortality. The notion of immediate evaluation in the OR was advanced by Noer, who applied the concept of bypassing the Emergency Department with early triage to the OR to a wider spectrum of injury patterns [4].

Fischer et al. reported their experience with direct transfer to the OR in a review of 4,000 patients over a 9-year period [5]. They utilized more liberal criteria to triage patients to the OR based on the presence of severe injury or obvious need for operative intervention. One-third of the patients reviewed required a major operative procedure while 57 % underwent a minor procedure. They found that direct transfer to the OR decreased the time to incision and improved blood transfusion rates in patients requiring splenectomy.

Rhodes et al. published a review of 240 trauma patients transported directly from the scene to the OR based on triage criteria that included penetrating torso trauma, systolic blood pressure <80 mmHg, major limb amputation, multiple long bone fractures, severe maxillofacial hemorrhage, and witnessed cardiac arrest [6]. They reported that 58.7 % of patients required major operative intervention. They also found that non-arrested, hypotensive patients requiring therapeutic laparotomy after blunt trauma had a higher than predicted survival based on TRISS methodology.

A previous study at our institution reviewed 323 patients that were taken directly to the OR for resuscitation during a 4-year period. This study demonstrated that patients who are hypotensive after sustaining penetrating wounds had observed survival that was greater than predicted when they were taken directly to the OR and underwent surgery within 20 min [7]. This study also found that no patients requiring thoracotomy after blunt cardiac arrest survived, consistent with prior studies demonstrating the limited utility of surgical intervention in this group regardless of time from presentation to operative intervention.

This study was followed by a retrospective review by Steele et al. of 879 patients admitted directly to the OR over an 11-year period [8]. This study found that the OR resuscitation triage criteria had a specificity of 98 % and sensitivity of 24 % for identifying patients needing immediate surgery. In this study, the average time to incision for all patients was 38.4 min compared to 99.4 min in the group resuscitated in the trauma bay. When further stratifying by injury mechanism, they demonstrated that 85.9 % of patients with penetrating injury admitted with a systolic blood pressure less than 90 mmHg required major operative intervention. The mean time to incision in this group was 21.7 min in the group resuscitated in the operating room, compared to 67.5 min in patients triaged to the trauma bay.

As part of a retrospective review of traumatic abdominal aortic injury in our institution over a 20-year period, we demonstrated that patients taken directly to the OR had a mortality rate of 40 % compared to a mortality rate of 78 % for those resuscitated in the trauma bay [9]. Resuscitation in the trauma bay remained a significant predictor of mortality on multivariate analysis in that study.

Martin et al. reviewed their experience with direct admission to the OR for resuscitation [10]. They studied 1,407 patients admitted directly to the OR from the scene over a 10-year period where they utilized more liberal triage criteria for initial evaluation in the operating room. In their study, the mean injury severity score of patients admitted directly to the OR was 19, with hypotension present in only 16 %. Forty-seven percent of their patients were admitted due to penetrating injury. They found that mortality was significantly lower than predicted for patients admitted directly to the OR (5 % observed vs. 10 % predicted). They identified penetrating truncal injury and hypotension as independent predictors of the need for surgical intervention, once again supporting the use of OR resuscitation for hypotensive patients with penetrating truncal trauma.

Future Directions

Endovascular techniques to achieve hemorrhage control have been the subject of increased preclinical and clinical study. Based on the success of endovascular balloon tamponade of bleeding in patients with ruptured abdominal aortic aneurysms and wider availability of endovascular devices, the use of resuscitative endovascular balloon occlusion of the aorta (REBOA) in trauma patients is increasing [11]. REBOA can be rapidly deployed using minimal imaging with the goal of achieving aortic control as a temporizing measure while resuscitation and open operative exposure are achieved. Studies are currently ongoing to identify patients that will most benefit from REBOA. The possibility of combining the features of the OR with the ability to perform fluoroscopic and angiographic evaluation has led to the evolution of the hybrid trauma OR [12]. In the future, severely injured patients may be directly triaged to a hybrid trauma OR that would provide the resources to evaluate and resuscitate patients and deploy either percutaneous or open techniques to achieve hemorrhage control.

Conclusion

Prompt identification of injuries and hemorrhage control is critical in the management of severe trauma patients. Triage directly to the OR speeds the time to incision and hemorrhage control. Ongoing research is needed to continue to define the ideal patients and injury patterns that will gain the most benefit from OR resuscitation. Advances in endovascular hemorrhage control techniques and the use of hybrid trauma operating rooms may further improve the benefit of OR resuscitation.

References

1. Hoyt DB, Bulger EM, Knudson MM, Morris J, Ierardi R, Sugerman HJ, et al. Death in the operating room: an analysis of a multi-center experience. J Trauma. 1994;37(3):426–32.
2. Burlew CC, Moore EE, Moore FA, Coimbra R, McIntyre Jr RC, Davis JW, et al. Western Trauma Association critical decisions in trauma: resuscitative thoracotomy. J Trauma Acute Care Surg. 2012;73(6):1359–63.
3. Griswold RA, Drye JC. Cardiac wounds. Ann Surg. 1954;139(6):783–5.
4. Noer RJ. Emergency care of critically injured. J Trauma. 1963;3:331–9.
5. Fischer RP, Jelense S, Perry Jr JF. Direct transfer to operating room improves care of trauma patients. A simple, economically feasible plan for large hospitals. JAMA. 1978;240(16):1731–2.
6. Rhodes M, Brader A, Lucke J, Gillott A. Direct transport to the operating room for resuscitation of trauma patients. J Trauma. 1989;29(7):907–13. discussion 13-5.
7. Hoyt DB, Shackford SR, McGill T, Mackersie R, Davis J, Hansbrough J. The impact of in-house surgeons and operating room resuscitation on outcome of traumatic injuries. Arch Surg. 1989;124(8):906–9. Discussion 9–10.
8. Steele JT, Hoyt DB, Simons RK, Winchell RJ, Garcia J, Fortlage D. Is operating room resuscitation a way to save time? Am J Surg. 1997;174(6):683–7.
9. Deree J, Shenvi E, Fortlage D, Stout P, Potenza B, Hoyt DB, et al. Patient factors and operating room resuscitation predict mortality in traumatic abdominal aortic injury: a 20-year analysis. J Vasc Surg. 2007;45(3):493–7.
10. Martin M, Izenberg S, Cole F, Bergstrom S, Long W. A decade of experience with a selective policy for direct to operating room trauma resuscitations. Am J Surg. 2012;204(2):187–92.
11. Brenner ML, Moore LJ, DuBose JJ, Tyson GH, McNutt MK, Albarado RP, et al. A clinical series of resuscitative endovascular balloon occlusion of the aorta for hemorrhage control and resuscitation. J Trauma Acute Care Surg. 2013;75(3):506–11.
12. Kirkpatrick AW, Vis C, Dube M, Biesbroek S, Ball CG, Laberge J, et al. The evolution of a purpose designed hybrid trauma operating room from the trauma service perspective: the RAPTOR (resuscitation with angiography percutaneous treatments and operative resuscitations). Injury. 2014;45(9):1413–21.

11 End Points of Resuscitation

T. Elizabeth Robertson, Shuntaye D. Batson, and John M. Porter

Introduction

Patients in shock have a lack of oxygen delivery to the mitochondria of vital organs. The goal of resuscitation is the perfusion of these cells with oxygenated hemoglobin. Earlier return to normal results in better outcomes [1]. Traditionally, tachycardia, oliguria, and hypotension have been used as markers, but this has been shown to leave more than half of patients without adequate oxygen delivery to mitochondria as evidenced by continued anaerobic metabolism [2, 3]. The ideal monitor of organ hypoperfusion is inexpensive, easy to perform and interpret, reliable, minimally invasive, and safe [1].

Macrocirculation

Indicators of global oxygen delivery have traditionally been used to identify underresuscitated shock. The problem with these types of indicators is that it does not evaluate regional ischemia and could miss focal ischemia. Physical exam is an initial indicator of shock, especially in the field, where the level of consciousness and radial pulse palpation are used as end points in combat [4]. In the intensive care unit, physical exam, especially cold extremities, is commented on, but rarely used as an end point for resuscitation. Heart rate and blood pressure are often used as targets, but patient specific factors make these targets unreliable in many cases. Beta blocker use and baseline hypertension cause otherwise normal numbers to be poor markers of cellular perfusion.

Laboratory findings are often used as markers of resuscitation as they are easy to obtain and seen as easy to interpret. Arterial lactate levels, base deficit levels, and serum bicarbonate levels provide information on the amount of anaerobic metabolism performed by cells, which is an indicator of inadequate oxygen delivery and unresolved shock. It has clearly been shown that the time to normalize the base deficit and lactate levels are predictive of survival [1]. In 2010, Dr. Jansen and colleagues showed that targeting lactate levels during the first 8 h of ICU admission using vasodilators, volume, inotropes, oxygen support, blood transfusions, and decreasing oxygen demand, decreased ICU and hospital mortality adjusted for predefined risk factors [4]. The lactate-targeted group had an increased amount of fluid and vasodilators administered, but had similar lactate measurements as compared to the control group [4]. This study excluded patients

T.E. Robertson, M.D., F.A.C.S. • S.D. Batson, M.D.
Department of Surgery, The University of Mississippi Medical Center, Jackson, MS, USA
e-mail: terobertson@umc.edu; sbatson@umc.edu

J.M. Porter, M.D., F.A.C.S. (✉)
Department of Surgery, Cooper University Hospital, Camden, NJ, USA
e-mail: jmporter@umc.edu; jpcut2cure@aol.com

R. Latifi et al. (eds.), *Technological Advances in Surgery, Trauma and Critical Care*,
DOI 10.1007/978-1-4939-2671-8_11

with known liver failure, as elevated lactate levels are seen in this group unrelated to organ hypoperfusion. Their conclusion was that lactate may be an early warning sign of hypoperfusion and therapy in response to an elevated lactate may attenuate mortality even though the indicator does not change in response to the therapy. There is no data on how frequently arterial lactates should be checked and therapy changes made.

Arterial lactate and base deficit levels do not always correspond and Martin evaluated this discordance concluding that when the base deficit is normal, elevated lactate can still be predictive of inadequate perfusion [5]. When lactate is normal, however, base deficit is not a reliable indicator [5]. Guidelines published by the Eastern Association for the Surgery of Trauma recommend rapid clinical reassessment of the patient for persistently high base deficit to determine if there was an underlying fixable pathology [1]. Serum bicarbonate is routinely measured on admission venous blood work and does not require an arterial sample as lactate and base deficit do. This has been found to provide equivalent mortality prediction and acid base evaluation in a trauma ICU [6].

Central venous oxygen saturation can be measured and demonstrates the amount of oxygen extraction by the cells. Low central venous oxygen saturation can indicate a high level of oxygen extraction, and thus presumed inadequate delivery and a shock state. Early goal directed therapy within the first 6 h of presentation with continuous central venous oxygen measurements was shown to decrease mortality as compared to standard care with central venous pressure, mean arterial pressure, and urine output goals [7]. The patients randomized to continuous central venous oxygen measurements received more fluid, transfusions, and inotropes early in their course and less fluid late in their course [7]. A recent study compared central venous oxygen saturation with lactate clearance and found a significant mortality benefit to lactate clearance of greater than 10 % within the first 6 h after presentation [8]. Lactates were measured every 2 h. This study showed that achieving central venous oxygen saturation goals but not lactate clearance is not good enough for prognostication and that the group targeting lactate clearance had similar therapies applied in terms of amount of volume and red blood cell resuscitation [8].

End tidal carbon dioxide measurements have also been shown to predict outcome during emergency trauma surgery [9]. Higher end-tidal CO_2 and greater differences between end-tidal CO_2 and arterial PaCO2 were both correlated with increased mortality [9]. In addition, baseline nasal cannula end tidal CO_2 measurements at presentation correlated with lactate as a predictor of requiring emergency trauma surgery [10]. Further research is needed to determine if this will be useful as a target of resuscitation.

Microcirculation

The classic work of Shoemaker led us to the understanding that maximizing oxygen delivery of systemic circulation should ensure adequate oxygen delivery to the organs and thereby decrease organ dysfunction and thus organ failure and mortality. However, we have come to realize that simply targeting parameters of systemic circulation does not automatically ensure adequate oxygen delivery to end organs. Inflammatory mediators and vascular autoregulatory mechanisms at the microcirculation level contribute to a mismatch of delivery and extraction of oxygen. It is this microcirculatory dysfunction that leads to organs dysfunction. Microcirculation monitoring has previously been limited to indirect measures such as lactate and tissue CO_2. With the advent of hand held microscopes, we may soon have a more direct look at the microvascular circulation.

Videomicroscopy

Videomicroscopy is a technique by which the microcirculation is visualized. Green light (530–550 nm), the isobestic point in the absorption spectrum on hemoglobin, is directed toward a superficial tissue layer. The light is absorbed by the hemoglobin in erythrocytes. The non-absorbed light is scattered around the tissue such that the red blood cells appear as gray or black against a white background. This video image is recorded and then analyzed for vascular density, capillary perfusion and flow. Multiple tissue sites have been used including eyes, brain, digestive tract, nail beds. However, the sublingual region is the most studied in humans. Numerous studies have reported impaired flow in critically ill pts. A study published in 2007 evaluated the use of videomicroscopy in septic patients upon presentation to the ER. They found that abnormalities in sublingual microcirculation correlated with outcomes [11]. A follow-up study by the same group found that improvement in microcirculation was associated with improved outcomes, specifically reduced organ failure [12]. One problem with this technique is that it cannot be performed continuously and is extremely operator dependent. Movement artifacts, secretions, and inadequate recordings, all impair the reliability of videomicroscopy. Additional criticisms include poor reproducibility and image quality. Videomicroscopy also requires time consuming off-line analysis of the acquired images. The use of videomicroscopy has added to our understanding of the significance of improving microcirculation however as a bedside tool for immediate assessment, more work is needed.

Near-Infrared Spectroscopy

Near-infrared resonance spectroscopy (NIRS) is a noninvasive technique based on the Beer–Lambert law which states that the absorption of light is proportional to the concentration of light-absorbing molecules present in a sample. This principle is applied with the use of tissue oxygen saturation (StO2) and pulse oximetry (SpO2). Tissue oxygen saturation differs from pulse oximetry in that it focuses on microcirculation or capillaries, the level at which gas exchange occurs. While SpO2 measures oxygenation in arterioles and thus is a reflection of the lungs' ability to oxygenate, the StO2 is calculated from the fractions of oxyhemoglobin and deoxyhemoglobin. The thenar eminence is the site most often used for monitoring. Changes in the tissue oxygen saturation reflect alterations in perfusion and metabolism. In 2005, Holcombe and colleagues found StO2 similar to base deficit in predicting mortality when assessed within the first hour of trauma [13]. Because StO2 is continuous, it allows for real-time assessment of the patients response to resuscitative efforts.

An extension of this modality is the dynamic vascular occlusion test (VOT). The test is performed by inflating a pneumatic cuff proximal to the StO2 sensor. The rate of deoxygenation is believed to reflect local metabolic rate. This may be more sensitive and specific in identifying shock than vitals alone [14, 15]. Here the rate of change in StO2 following arterial occlusion is calculated. This slope is decreased in patients in shock as compared to non-shock patients. Studies have demonstrated that StO2 is predictive of increased mortality when assessed early [16] and prehospital rate of deoxygenation can be predictive of need for life saving interventions [17]. The values derived can be affected by venous congestion, hypoalbuminemia, age, BMI, sex, race, and smoking.

Raman Spectroscopy

Raman spectroscopy is another tissue oxygenation monitor similar to near-infrared spectroscopy. "The spectroscopic basis for Raman spectroscopy of hemoglobin lies in the resonance vibrational enhancement of hemoglobin in the deep violet region, allowing simultaneous identification and monitoring of the proportion of oxy and deoxy species of hemoglobin in a concentration-dependent manner with a single wavelength of light." A recent study compared RRS-StO2 to NIRS-STO2 and found that in swine model, RRS was better at tracking central oxygenation during hemorrhage and predicting shock based on elevated lactate levels when compared to NIRS-StO2 [18].

CO_2 Tonometry

During times of anaerobic metabolism, the local increase in carbon dioxide is a reflection of the buffering of lactic acid by bicarbonate. The amount of CO_2 has been measured in various tissues, most notably the stomach. Originally, measuring gastric CO_2 was limited; it was time consuming and tedious. A semipermeable balloon filled with saline was placed in the stomach, the gases were allowed to equilibrate over 30 min, and then the saline from the balloon was then run thru a gas analyzer. Later an automated technique using infrared spectrophotometry was developed but did not show prognostic ability in clinical study. In recent years, there has been renewed interest in CO_2 tonometry. Clavijo-Alvarez et al. found that pCO2 in the bladder mucosa was comparable to changes seen in the GI tract [19]. They suggest the bladder mucosa as a potential site for continuous monitoring tissue perfusion during shock and resuscitation.

Noninvasive Hemodynamic Monitoring

Hemodynamic monitoring plays an important role in resuscitation in trauma and critically ill patients. Pulmonary artery catheter (PAC), once regarded as the gold standard of all hemodynamic monitors, has been used for years to direct resuscitation efforts and to aid in categorizing shock states. Information from PACs includes central venous pressure, pulmonary artery occlusion pressure, cardiac index, mixed venous saturation, oxygen delivery index, oxygen consumption index, and end diastolic volume index. These catheters can be cumbersome to use and place, are associated with complications and may damage the heart. They are invasive and there is no clear evidence of improved outcomes associated with their use. There are alternative technologies that provide the same information.

Echocardiography is an excellent way to evaluate the hemodynamic status in the ICU. One directly visualizes the cardiac chambers and valves, providing an aid in elucidating the etiology of hypotension. Transthoracic echo has its limitations. It requires significant training to accurately interpret the images obtained and this expertise is not always available for the intensivist. The image quality may also be impaired secondary to tubes, dressings, body habitus, etc. Transesophageal echo (TEE) is another option. The recent development of smaller and disposal probes has allowed for continuous monitoring (ClarTEE). There are only three views to master, 4 chamber mid esophagus view, transgastric short axis view, and superior vena cava (SVC) view.

The mid-esophageal 4 chamber view allows evaluation of biventricular size and function. The transgastric short axis view allows assessment preload by using left ventricle (LV) size and measuring the left ventricular end diastolic area (LVEDA) and left ventricular contractility by fractional area change (FAC). Fractional area change is a measure of LV function or grade of LV ejection. It is calculated as (LVEDA − LVESA)/LVEDA × 100. Fractional area change greater than 50 % is considered normal, 40–50 % is moderately decreased and less than 40 % is severely decrease. Finally, SVC view is used to assess volume responsiveness using SVC size and collapsibility. An index of greater than 35 % is predictive of hypovolemia and thus fluid responsiveness.

When only TTE is available, IVC diameter measurement can also be used to discriminate between patients who will be volume responsive and those who will not. The diameter of the IVC is used as an estimate of central venous pressure. The IVC is compliant and its size varies with changes in volume and throughout the respiratory cycle. During respiration, as negative intrapleural pressure develops, venous return to the heart increases. As flow increases through the IVC and intraluminal pressure decreases, the diameter of the IVC decreases. This difference in diameter at inspiration and expiration is referred to as the collapsibility index (CI). The CI has been shown to be higher in patients in shock and be used to estimate a patient's central venous pressures [20]. Yanagawa in his study of trauma patients found IVC diameter to be more sensitive than blood pressure alone for identifying hypovolemia [21]. Regardless of the hemodynamic monitoring system used, it is the interpretation of the information that alters patient outcome.

Waveform analysis has also been used in lieu of invasive PAC monitoring. Changes in pulse pressure and systolic pressure on invasive arterial line during mechanical ventilation have been shown to correlate with PAC findings and be predictive of fluid responsiveness [22]. These analyses are only valid with controlled mechanical ventilation in normal sinus rhythm. Intraoperatively, fluid management guided by pulse pressure has been shown to decrease length of stay in the hospital [23]. Pulse pressure variation and stroke volume variation has also been shown to predict volume responsiveness as compared to invasive pulmonary artery catheters in patients with acute respiratory distress syndrome on low tidal volumes and high positive end expiratory pressures [24].

Telemonitoring/Telepresence

Active resuscitation efforts are ideally led by medical professionals experienced in critical care as this has been associated with improved outcomes [25]. There is a known shortage of critical care experts [26] and many hospitals are using telemedicine resources to increase the number of patients managed by intensive care specialists. Advances in end points of resuscitation are only useful if they make it to the patient's bedside with a clinician available to correctly interpret and apply the data. Implementation of remote monitoring is associated with decreased ICU mortality and length of stay (LOS), but not hospital mortality or LOS [27]. Further investigation is needed to determine if telepresence of critical care specialists will improve outcomes and how to get health care providers experienced in critical care to the patient in a timely manner.

Summary

There is no inexpensive, easy-to-perform and -interpret, reliable, minimally invasive, and safe marker of adequate resuscitation that is easily applicable to all populations. Each target has to be interpreted considering the patient's underlying disease state and the length of time from the onset of physiologic insult. In addition, one must consider which tools are actually shown to improve clinical outcomes when targeted and which tools are useful for prognostication.

References

1. Tisherman SAM, et al. Clinical practice guideline: endpoints of resuscitation. J Trauma. 2004;57(4):898–912.
2. Abou-Khalil BM, et al. Hemodynamic responses to shock in young trauma patients: need for invasive monitoring. Crit Care Med. 1994;22(4):633–9.
3. Scale TMM, et al. Resuscitation of multiple trauma and head injury: role of crystalloid fluids and inotropes. Crit Care Med. 1994;22(10):1610–5.
4. Jansen TC, et al. Early lactate-guided therapy in intensive care unit patients: a multicenter, open-label, randomized controlled trial. Am J Respir Crit Care Med. 2010;182(6):752–61.
5. Martin MJ, et al. Discordance between lactate and base deficit in the surgical intensive care unit: which one do you trust? Am J Surg. 2006;191(5):625–30.
6. FitzSullivan E, et al. Serum bicarbonate may replace the arterial base deficit in the trauma intensive care unit. Am J Surg. 2005;190(6):961–7.
7. Rivers E, et al. Early goal-directed therapy in the treatment of severe sepsis and septic shock. N Engl J Med. 2001;345(19):1368–77.
8. Puskarich MA, et al. Prognostic value and agreement of achieving lactate clearance or central venous oxygen saturation goals during early sepsis resuscitation. Acad Emerg Med. 2012;19(3):252–8.
9. Tyburski JG, et al. End-tidal CO2-derived values during emergency trauma surgery correlated with outcome: a prospective study. J Trauma. 2002;53(4):738–43.
10. Caputo ND, et al. Nasal cannula end-tidal CO2 correlates with serum lactate levels and odds of operative intervention in penetrating trauma patients: a prospective cohort study. J Trauma. 2012;73(5):1202–7.
11. Trzeciak S, et al. Microcirculatory Alterations in Resuscitation and Shock Investigators: early microcirculatory perfusion derangements in patients with severe sepsis and septic shock: relationship to hemodynamics, oxygen transport, and survival. Ann Emerg Med. 2007;49(1):88–98.
12. Trzeciak S, et al. Microcirculatory Alterations in Resuscitation and Shock (MARS) investigators. Early increases in microcirculatory perfusion during protocol-directed resuscitation are associated with reduced multi-organ failure at 24 h in patients with sepsis. Intensive Care Med. 2008;34(12):2210–7.

13. Holcomb JB, et al. Prehospital physiologic data and lifesaving interventions in trauma patients. Mil Med. 2005;170(1):7–13.
14. Gómez H, et al. Use of non-invasive NIRS during a vascular occlusion test to assess dynamic tissue O2 saturation response. Intensive Care Med. 2008;34(9): 1600–7.
15. Creteur J, et al. The prognostic value of muscle StO2 in septic patients. Intensive Care Med. 2007;33(9):1549–56.
16. Cohn SM, et al. Tissue oxygen saturation predicts the development of organ dysfunction during traumatic shock resuscitation. J Trauma. 2007;62(1):44–55.
17. Guyette FX, et al. Prehospital dynamic tissue oxygen saturation response predicts in-hospital lifesaving interventions in trauma patients. J Trauma. 2012; 72(4):930.
18. Tiba MH, et al. Tissue oxygenation monitoring using resonance Raman spectroscopy during hemorrhage. J Trauma. 2014;76(2):402–8.
19. Clavijo-Alvarez JA, et al. Bladder mucosa pH and PCO2 as a minimally invasive monitor of hemorrhagic shock and resuscitation. J Trauma. 2004;57(6): 1199–210.
20. Wu TS. The CORE scan: concentrated overview of resuscitative efforts. Crit Care Clin. 2014;30(1): 151–75.
21. Yanagawa Y, Sakamoto T, Okada Y. Hypovolemic shock evaluated by sonographic measurement of the inferior vena cava during resuscitation in trauma patients. J Trauma. 2007;63(6):1245–8.
22. Michard F. Changes in arterial pressure during mechanical ventilation. Anesthesiology. 2005;103(2): 419–28.
23. Lopes MR, et al. Goal-directed fluid management based on pulse pressure variation monitoring during high-risk surgery: a pilot randomized controlled trial. Crit Care. 2007;11(5):R100.
24. Huang C-C, et al. Prediction of fluid responsiveness in acute respiratory distress syndrome patients ventilated with low tidal volume and high positive end-expiratory pressure. Crit Care Med. 2008;36(10):2810–6.
25. Pronovost PJ, et al. Physician staffing patterns and clinical outcomes in critically ill patients: a systematic review. JAMA. 2002;288(17):2151–62.
26. Angus DC, et al. Current and projected workforce requirements for care of the critically ill and patients with pulmonary disease: can we meet the requirements of an aging population? JAMA. 2000;284(21): 2762–70.
27. Young LB, et al. Impact of telemedicine intensive care unit coverage on patient outcomes: a systematic review and meta-analysis. Arch Intern Med. 2011;171(6):498–506.

12 Abdominal Trauma: Not Everything That Bleeds Needs an Operation

Marcie Feinman and David T. Efron

Introduction

Tradition has taught us that traumatic bleeding requires operative intervention. Without modern technology, an operation remains both diagnostic and therapeutic for trauma patients. From the time when ultrasound, CT scan, and angiography became mainstream, treatment options for patients have grown exponentially.

Physiology of a Trauma Patient

The lethal triad of trauma consists of hypotension, coagulopathy and acidosis. Bleeding leads to this downwards spiral, and extensive research has been done to determine the best way to prevent poor outcomes due to this physiology. Studies have shown that keeping patients warm can help minimize acidosis and coagulopathy. In addition, judicious use of intravenous fluids, focusing on early administration of packed red blood cells, fresh frozen plasma and platelets in a 1:1:1 ratio, can improve coagulopathy [1]. However, there is no substitute for rapidly controlling the bleeding. An operation remains the method of choice for unstable trauma patients, but alternatives now exist for the stable patient.

Blunt Intra-abdominal Injuries

Mechanism

Trauma is the leading cause of death in people between the ages of 1 and 44. Injuries to intra-abdominal organs are a huge source of morbidity and mortality among all age groups. There are three main mechanisms that lead to injuries during blunt trauma. The first mechanism is deceleration, which causes internal structures to stop moving from rapid speed. Some organs, such as the aorta, the liver and the kidneys, have fixed points of attachment and can have significant damage from the shear forces associated with rapid deceleration. Motor vehicle collisions, pedestrians' struck and falls from height are the most common mechanisms of injury associated with deceleration. The second mechanism involves crushing. Victims of this type of injury most often suffer damage to solid organs when they are crushed between the anterior abdominal wall and the vertebral column or posterior rib cage. Lastly there is external compression. This differs from the crush mechanism in that external compression causes a sudden,

M. Feinman, M.D.
Department of Surgery, Sinai Hospital of Baltimore, Baltimore, MD, USA
e-mail: mfeinman@jhmi.edu

D.T. Efron, M.D., F.A.C.S. (✉)
Division of Acute Care Surgery, Department of Surgery, Johns Hopkins Hospital, Baltimore, MD, USA
e-mail: defron1@jhmi.edu

R. Latifi et al. (eds.), *Technological Advances in Surgery, Trauma and Critical Care*,
DOI 10.1007/978-1-4939-2671-8_12

dramatic rise in the intra-abdominal pressure. This pressure change renders hollow organs the most susceptible to damage and is often suspected in bladder and bowel rupture.

Workup

While unrecognized bleeding in the abdomen may be rapidly fatal, the diagnosis of hollow viscus injury is equally important. The diagnostic workup is primarily geared towards these two types of potential injuries. Reliable physical exam remains essential. Hemodynamic lability suggests bleeding while peritonitis is suggestive of irritation from the spillage of a ruptured organ. Short of operative exploration and direct inspection, the remaining adjuncts to the physical exam include mainly imaging techniques including FAST and CT scanning. DPL continues to be an option in very few cases, but has largely been surplanted by the use of the FAST.

In 2002, the Eastern Association for the Surgery of Trauma (EAST) convened a work group to determine best practices for evaluation of patients with blunt abdominal trauma. The literature was reviewed and the following level 1 recommendations were made [2]:

1. Exploratory laparotomy is indicated for patients with grossly positive diagnostic peritoneal lavage (DPL).
2. CT is recommended for the evaluation of hemodynamically stable patients with equivocal findings on physical examination, associated neurologic injury, or multiple extra-abdominal injuries.
3. CT is the diagnostic modality of choice for nonoperative management of solid visceral injuries.
4. In hemodynamically stable patients, DPL and CT are complementary diagnostic modalities.

Of note, the following level 2 recommendations were made regarding focused abdominal sonography for trauma (FAST) [2]:

1. FAST may be considered as the initial diagnostic modality to exclude hemoperitoneum.
2. Exploratory laparotomy is indicated in hemodynamically unstable patients with a positive nonoperative management of select injuries.

These suggestions were based on the existing data that illustrated the strengths of FAST. Benefits included the ability to perform the test quickly in a noninvasive manner. The technology is portable and, therefore, the patient does not have to move from the trauma bay. In addition, the exam is repeatable. However, the reliability of the test is operator dependent, it does not give information regarding grade of injury and it is a poor determinant of hollow viscus injury. A positive FAST exam in a hemodynamically stable patient should lead to a CT scan for further diagnosis. CT has a sensitivity of ~95 % and a specificity of ~99 %, leading to reliable diagnosis of injuries. With a negative predictive value of over 99 %, providers can feel confident discharging patients from the emergency department if the abdominal CT scan is negative [3]. Figure 12.1 shows the suggested workup for a stable patient with blunt abdominal trauma [4].

Management

Successful nonoperative management of intra-abdominal injuries is predicated on the stability of the patient. Unstable patients or patients with diffuse peritonitis after blunt abdominal trauma require a laparotomy. Expectant management should only be attempted in a clinical setting capable of intensive monitoring, serial clinical examinations and where an operating room is available for urgent laparotomy at all times.

Liver

In the early 1900s, blunt hepatic injuries were treated primarily by observation alone. Due to poor outcomes, the pendulum then swung the complete opposite direction and laparotomy became the treatment of choice. For hemodynamically stable patients, several options exist for management [5].

The widespread use of CT scans for trauma patients has allowed for the development of a grading scale for solid organ injuries. Liver injuries range from mild (Grade I) to severely

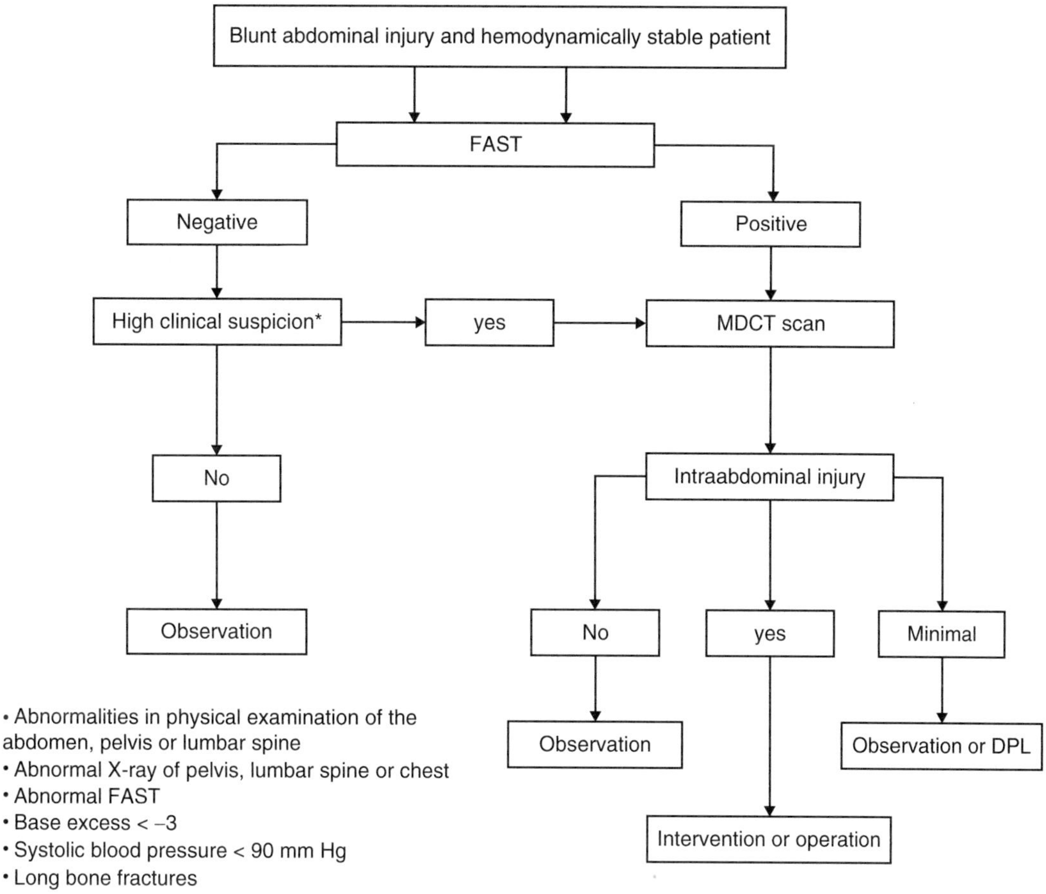

Fig. 12.1 Blunt abdominal trauma workup. (Used with permission from van der Vlies CH, Olthof DC, Gaakeer M, Ponsen KJ, van Delden OM, Goslings JC. Changing patterns in diagnostic strategies and the treatment of blunt injury to solid abdominal organs. Int J Emerg Med 2011 Jul 27;4:47-1380-4-47)

life-threatening (Grade VI) (Fig. 12.2a–c). Table 12.1 shows a representation of the AAST liver injury grading system.

In addition to allowing the injury to be graded, the newer multichannel detector CT scanners allow for more accurate visualization of vascular structures and active bleeding in the form of a "blush" (contrast extravasation). While certain CT findings, such as high grade injuries, active extravasation, periportal blood and large amount of hemoperitoneum, have previously been thought to preclude nonoperative management, recent literature suggests that these risk factors are not absolute contraindications to a trial of expectant management in a hemodynamically stable patient [6]. That said, more severe injuries and patients at with active bleeding are at high risk for needing intervention, and should be considered for early angiography with embolization.

While angioembolization of high-risk patients who suffer liver trauma is highly successful at controlling bleeding, it is not without its own morbidity. Contrast-induced nephropathy is a concern, especially since the vast majority of these patients have already undergone a CT scan with IV dye for diagnostic purposes. Embolization can lead to hepatic necrosis with the delayed complications of infection and abscess formation. Additionally, embolization only addresses vascular extravasation and cannot target bile ducts. Biliary leaks are especially prevalent in higher grade injuries, and can cause ongoing systemic inflammation, bilomas or biliary peritonitis.

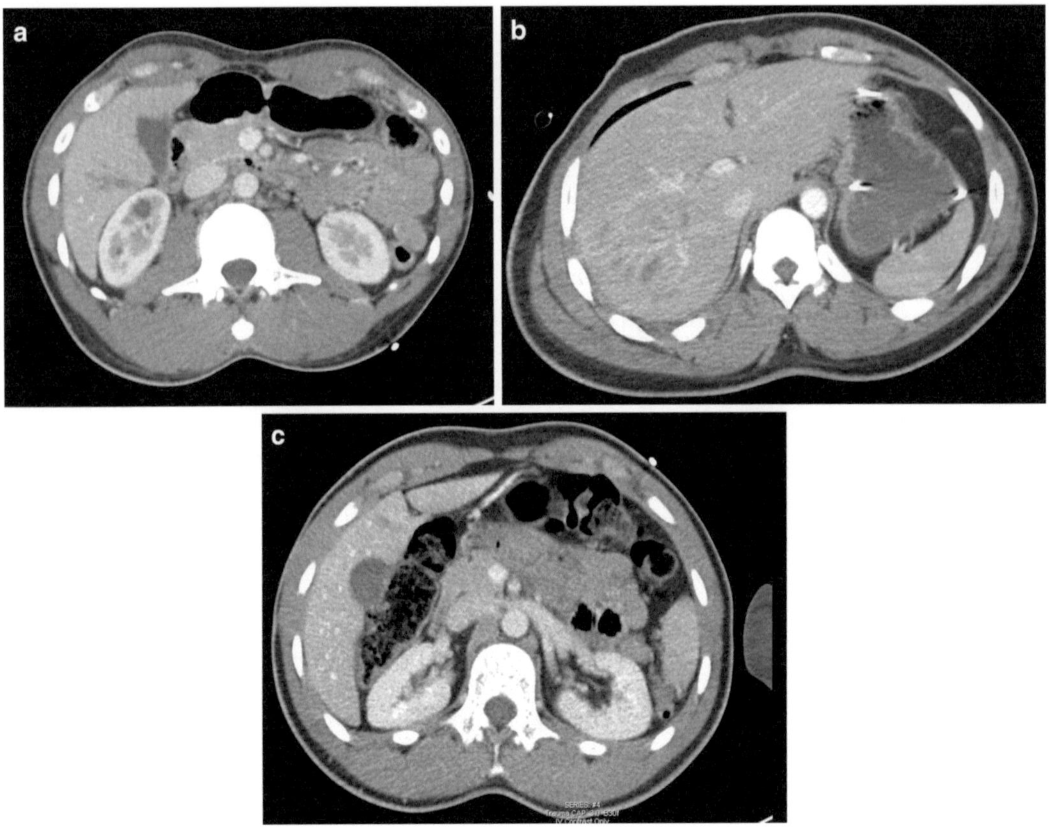

Fig. 12.2 (**a**–**c**) CT scan images of liver injuries following blunt trauma. (**a**) Grade II liver laceration. (**b**) Grade IV liver laceration. (**c**) Grade I liver laceration

Table 12.1 AAST hepatic injury grading scale

Grade	Injury type	Description
I	Hematoma	Subcapsular, <10 % surface area
I	Laceration	<1 cm parenchymal depth
II	Hematoma	Subcapsular, 10–50 % surface area
		Intraparenchymal, <10 cm diameter
II	Laceration	1-3 cm parenchymal depth, and <10 cm in length
III	Hematoma	Subcapsular, >50 % surface area or explanding/ruptured
		Intraparenchymal, >10 cm
III	Laceration	>3 cm parenchymal depth
IV	Laceration	Parenchymal disruption, 25–75 % of hepatic lobe
V	Laceration	Parenchymal disruption, >75 % of hepatic lobe
V	Vascular	Juxtavenous hepatic injuries (e.g., Major hepatic veins, retrocaval IVC)
VI	Vascular	Hepatic avulsion

Used with permission from Moore EE, Shackford SR, Pachter HL et al. Organ injury scaling: spleen, liver, and kidney. Journal of Trauma and Acute Care Surgery 1989; 29 (12): 1664–1666

Most of these patients can be treated without the need for laparotomy with percutaneous drainage and endoscopic retrograde cholangiopancreatography (ERCP) [7].

Spleen

Attempting splenic salvage after blunt trauma has become the norm in modern day trauma practice. While unstable patients still belong in the operating room, stable patients and transient responders have options for treatment that include expectant management and angiography with embolization. A CT scan with IV contrast should be performed in this patient population to define the severity of injury and guide the management [8] (Fig. 12.3). Much like with liver trauma, injuries to the spleen are graded based on severity. Table 12.2 shows the AAST grading scale for splenic injuries.

Common sense would dictate that patients with increased hemoperitoneum, higher grade injuries and active extravasation seen on CT would lead to higher failure rates of nonoperative management, and multiple studies proved this to be true [8]. However, there are no absolute contraindications to attempting splenic salvage based on age, severity of injury or presence of concomitant injuries as long as the infrastructure exists for appropriate monitoring [8]. The failure of nonoperative management can be significantly decreased by reevaluating patients with blunt splenic injury 48 h after their trauma with a repeat CT scan to look for pseudoaneurysms [9].

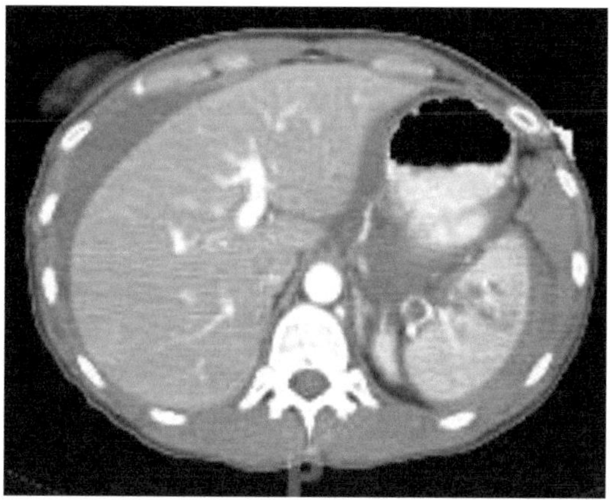

Fig. 12.3 CT scan image of grade III splenic laceration following blunt trauma to the abdomen

When embolization initially became popular, the main splenic artery was the most frequent target (Fig. 12.4a, b). As technology has improved, selective and superselective embolizations have become possible. One of the main reasons to attempt splenic salvage is to avoid overwhelming postsplenectomy sepsis (OPSI). There was concern that with main artery embolization, the immune function of the spleen would be compromised and patients could suffer the same fate as with splenectomy, hence the trend towards more selective targets. These fears have not been realized; small studies have shown that not only is immune function preserved in patients with main artery embolization [10] but there is no difference in complication rates between main artery and selective embolization [11].

Kidney

Historically, many blunt renal injuries were explored in the operating room with a resultant high nephrectomy rate. To attempt to increase the kidney salvage rate, nonoperative management of renal injuries became common. The proof that nonoperative management could be successfully carried out came in the form of retrospective

Table 12.2 AAST splenic injury grading scale

Grade	Injury type	Description
I	Hematoma	Subcapsular, <10 % surface area
I	Laceration	<1 cm parenchymal depth
II	Hematoma	Subcapsular, 10–50 % surface area
		Intraparenchymal, <5 cm diameter
II	Laceration	1–3 cm parenchymal depth that does not involve a trabecular vessel
III	Hematoma	Subcapsular, >50 % surface area or expanding/ruptured
		Intraparenchymal, >5 cm or expanding
III	Laceration	>3 cm parenchymal depth or involving trabecular vessels
IV	Laceration	Involves segmental or hilar vessels producing major devascularization (>25 % of spleen)
V	Laceration	Shattered spleen
V	Vascular	Hilar vascular injury with devascularized spleen

Used with permission from Moore EE, Shackford SR, Pachter HL et al. Organ injury scaling: spleen, liver, and kidney. journal of trauma and acute care surgery 1989; 29 (12): 1664–1666

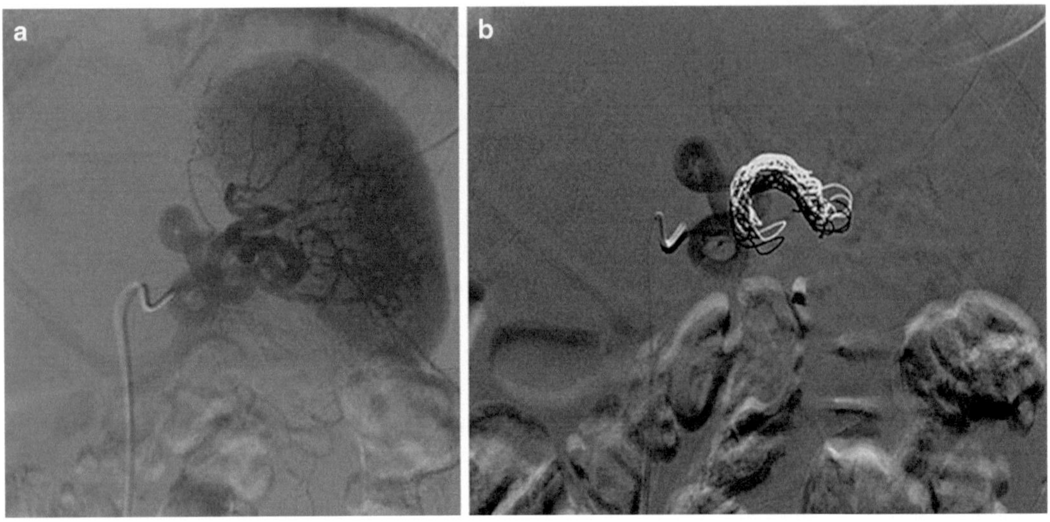

Fig. 12.4 (**a**, **b**) Angiographic management of a grade III splenic injury following blunt abdominal trauma. (**a**) Conventional angiography demonstrating injury and intra-parenchymal splenic blush. (**b**) Post-coil embolization of the main splenic artery

Table 12.3 AAST renal injury grading scale

Grade	Injury type	Description
I	Contusion	Microscopic or gross hematuria with normal urologic radiology
I	Hematoma	Subcapsular, nonexpanding, any size, without parenchymal laceration
II	Hematoma	Nonexpanding perirenal hematoma confined to renal retroperitoneum
II	Laceration	<1 cm parenchymal depth of renal cortex without urinary extravasation
III	Laceration	>1 cm, without extension into the renal pelvis or collecting system and with no evidence of urine extravasation
IV	Laceration	Extends through renal cortex, medulla, and collecting system
IV	Vascular	Main renal artery or vein injury with contained hemorrhage
V	Laceration	Shattered Kidney
V	Vascular	Devascularization of kidney due to avulsion of renal hilum

Used with permission from Moore EE, Shackford SR, Pachter HL et al. Organ injury scaling: spleen, liver, and kidney. Journal of Trauma and Acute Care Surgery 1989; 29 (12): 1664–1666

studies showing spontaneous healing of injured kidneys on CT imaging [12]. As with the other blunt solid organ injuries, age, severity of injury and presence of head trauma do not exclude non-operative management as a treatment option. The AAST recognizes five grades of injury for the kidney, as seen in Table 12.3.

High grade injuries (III–V) were specifically evaluated in the literature to determine if nonoperative management is safe and effective in this population. Not only did the patients managed without an operation have shorter ICU lengths of stay and lower transfusion requirements, they also had fewer complications [13]. Even if the kidney is shattered, as long as it is perfused non-operative management remains a viable option. Complications, though less than with operative intervention, may exist in the form of pseudoaneurysms, urinomas and unidentified uretural injuries. In the vast majority of cases, these can be addressed with angioembolization, percutaneous drainage or stenting as needed.

Hypertension secondary to renal parenchymal compression from a subcapsular hematoma (Page kidney) is rarely realized and even less frequently sustained.

Penetrating Abdominal Trauma

The dogma that all penetrating abdominal injuries require an operation has been challenged since the 1960s. While still uncommon, nonoperative management of this patient population is being attempted at several trauma centers around the country. Stab wounds are more commonly managed expectantly than gunshot wounds, though the evidence is strong enough to suggest that in stable patients without peritoneal signs, laparotomy is not indicated in either group [14]. Should nonoperative management be attempted, a CT scan to determine trajectory can be highly beneficial (Fig. 12.5). If the injury involves the flank, using oral, rectal, and IV contrast can increase the true negative value of the study to almost 100 % [15]. Tangential wounds are much more likely to be successfully managed without surgery than wounds that clearly penetrate the peritoneal cavity.

If injury should occur to a solid organ via a penetrating mechanism, nonoperative management remains a possibility. Angioembolization is a valuable adjunct for treatment (Fig. 12.6a–c). One prospective study by Demetriades and colleagues found that nonoperative management was feasible in patients with high grade (III–V) solid organ injuries with significantly shorter hospital length of stay than in patients managed operatively [16].

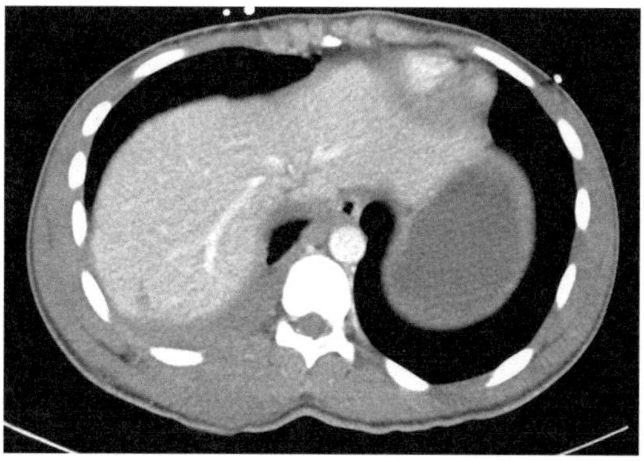

Fig. 12.5 CT scan image of a grade I liver laceration that resulted from a right flank stab wound which was successfully managed nonoperatively

Negative and nontherapeutic laparotomies are not without risk. Complications in general range from atelectasis and pneumonia to wound and urinary tract infections to prolonged ileus, and can occur in up to 40 % of patients. Significant complications have been documented in 8–12 % of patients [17, 18]. In addition, nontherapeutic laparotomies increase hospital length of stay and cost. Studies have shown that the vast majority of stable patients with stab wounds to the abdomen will develop an indication for surgery within 12 h of observation if they have a significant injury. The current recommendation is to observe stable patients with penetrating abdominal injuries of any mechanism for 24 h with serial clinical exams performed by the same individual or team of individuals. This includes patients with penetrating flank and buttock injuries. If they remain stable at 24 h, they can be safely discharged from the trauma service [14].

Pelvic Trauma

Pelvic injuries often exist in the setting of blunt trauma, and can be a major source of blood loss and remain highly mortal and morbid injuries. The majority of bleeding tends to be venous, but arterial sources do exist. The goal of managing pelvic fractures is to stabilize the pelvis and control the bleeding in an expeditious manner. In the trauma bay, a temporary pelvic binder or sheet wrap can be applied quickly and easily with a resultant decrease in pelvic volume by 10–20 %. Patients with pelvic fractures and hemodynamic instability or signs of ongoing bleeding after non-pelvic sources of blood loss have been ruled out should be considered for pelvic angiography/embolization [19]. In an unstable patient, it is essential to determine whether the bleeding is from the abdomen, pelvis or both. A positive fast exam in patients with significant pelvic and abdominal trauma mandates exploration in the operating room for damage control followed by

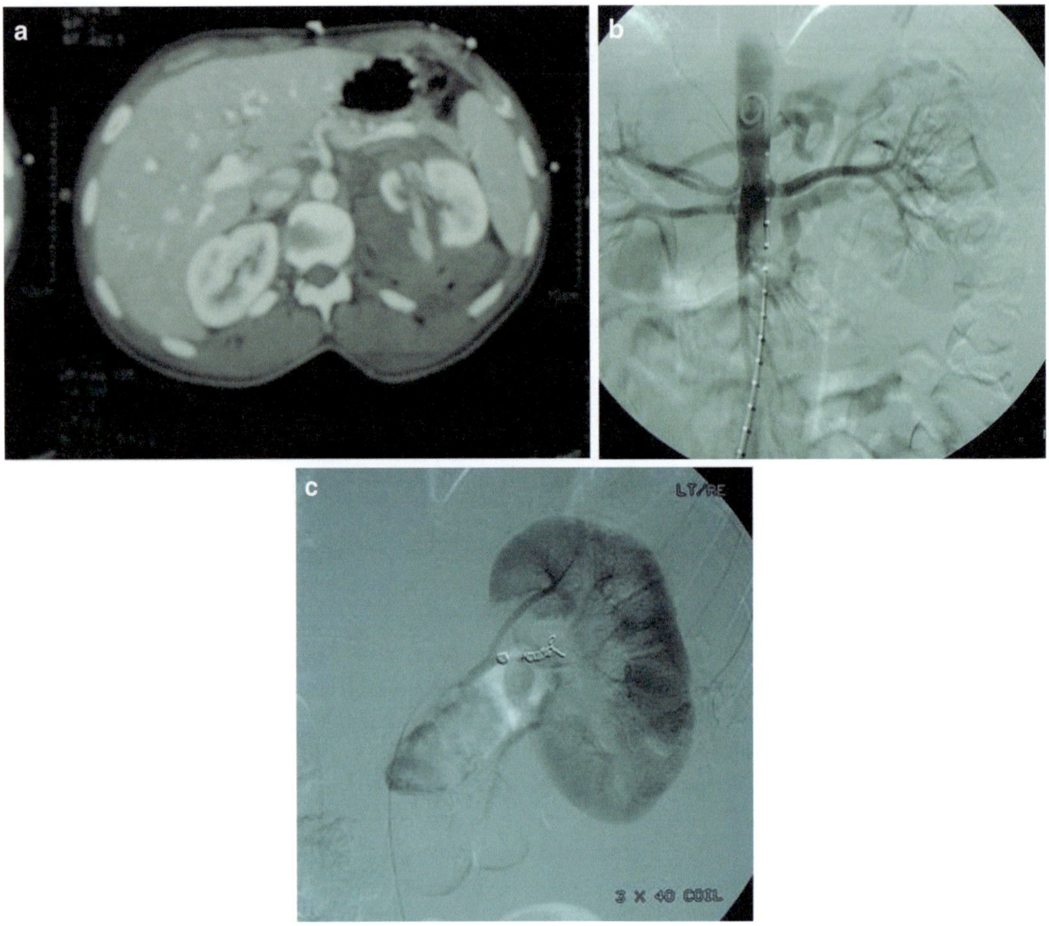

Fig. 12.6 (**a**–**c**) Stab wound to the left back demonstrating left renal hilar injury. (**a**) CT scan showing renal hilar injury and large perinephric hematoma and active contrast extravasation. (**b**) Diagnostic left renal artery angiogram showing intra-parenchymal blush and arterial–venous fistula. (**c**) Post-embolization angiography demonstrating successful control of bleeding and fistula, with minimal loss of perfused renal parenchyma

pelvic angiography. A negative FAST exam would lead to angiography first for definitive control of pelvic bleeding. If angio is not readily available, pelvic packing in the operating room remains a viable option for unstable patients. In a stable patient, a CT scan with IV contrast should be obtained to evaluate for abdominal injury. If the CT scan rules out intraperitoneal injury but shows active arterial extravasation in the pelvis, angiography should be strongly considered regardless of hemodynamic status as this is a significant risk factor for the need for embolization. Even without evidence of active bleeding on CT, there is an up to 18 % chance that patients with pelvic fractures may require embolization early in their hospital stay. Patients who are initially successfully embolized may require repeat embolization ~25 % of the time, and in the majority of those patients bleeding was found at a new site [19].

As with solid organ injuries, pelvic vessels can be embolized proximally or more selectively. There is concern that with proximal embolization, gluteal muscle ischemia and necrosis may ensue. Even though this phenomenon may be subclinical, there is concern in the orthopedic literature about increased complications after formal pelvic fixation in embolized patients [20]. The risks and benefits of pelvic embolization should be weighed, but this intervention remains a valuable option in the armamentarium of the trauma surgeon.

Major Vascular Injuries

Hemorrhage from major vascular injuries remains a substantial cause of morbidity and mortality in trauma patients. Regardless of mechanism, major vascular injuries require some type of intervention. In recent years, endovascular techniques have been employed with great success. Initially, blunt aortic injury was evaluated for feasibility of endovascular intervention. Outcomes were so promising that the Society for Vascular Surgery has recommended this approach preferentially over open surgery in their guidelines for traumatic thoracic aortic injury [21]. Endovascular techniques seem to be especially beneficial in areas of difficult exposure. One recent study evaluating carotid, subclavian and thoracic aortic injuries showed a significant increase in the use of endovascular repair with an associated 35 % decrease in mortality. Of note, 20 % of these patients were hypotensive on arrival but could still be successfully managed without an open operation [22].

Some patients are too unstable upon their arrival to the trauma bay to travel for intervention. These patients generally have severe ongoing blood loss that leads to decompensated shock. In such a population, resuscitative endovascular balloon occlusion of the aorta (REBOA) has been employed with some success. Similar to resuscitative thoracotomy with aortic cross-clamping, REBOA allows the trauma surgeon to occlude the aorta and prevent ongoing intra-abdominal blood loss while maintaining perfusion to the brain and heart. However, REBOA is much less invasive, and can be placed percutaneously or via cut down. Additional endovascular training for trauma surgeons may be beneficial prior to placing an intra-aortic balloon, though it is not necessary [23]. REBOA is a temporizing measure, and must be followed by either surgical exploration or interventional radiology techniques for definitive hemorrhage control.

Conclusion

Though there is a definite trend towards selective nonoperative management of trauma patients, operative intervention will always have a place in the care of the severely injured patient. Hemodynamically unstable patients and patients with diffuse peritonitis after blunt or penetrating abdominal wounds require an operation. Stable patients can be worked up with CT scan and managed nonoperatively regardless of severity of injury as long as the hospital has the capability of providing intensive monitoring and a staffed operating room should emergent intervention be required. As technology advances and imaging improves, we may be able to further delineate the best candidates for nonoperative management.

References

1. Feinman M, Cotton BA, Haut ER. Optimal fluid resuscitation in trauma: type, timing, and total. Curr Opin Crit Care. 2014;20(4):366–72.
2. Hoff WS, Holevar M, Nagy KK, Patterson L, Young JS, Arrillaga A, et al. Practice management guidelines for the evaluation of blunt abdominal trauma: the East practice management guidelines work group. J Trauma. 2002;53(3):602–15.
3. Livingston DH, Lavery RF, Passannante MR, Skurnick JH, Fabian TC, Fry DE, et al. Admission or observation is not necessary after a negative abdominal computed tomographic scan in patients with suspected blunt abdominal trauma: results of a prospective, multi-institutional trial. J Trauma. 1998;44(2):273–80. Discussion 280–2.
4. van der Vlies CH, Olthof DC, Gaakeer M, Ponsen KJ, van Delden OM, Goslings JC. Changing patterns in diagnostic strategies and the treatment of blunt injury to solid abdominal organs. Int J Emerg Med. 2011;4:47.
5. Stassen NA, Bhullar I, Cheng JD, Crandall M, Friese R, Guillamondegui O, et al. Nonoperative management of blunt hepatic injury: an Eastern Association for the Surgery of Trauma practice management guideline. J Trauma Acute Care Surg. 2012;73(5 Suppl 4):S288–93.
6. Sharma OP, Oswanski MF, Singer D, Raj SS, Daoud YA. Assessment of nonoperative management of blunt spleen and liver trauma. Am Surg. 2005;71(5):379–86.
7. Carrillo EH, Spain DA, Wohltmann CD, Schmieg RE, Boaz PW, Miller FB, et al. Interventional techniques are useful adjuncts in nonoperative management of hepatic injuries. J Trauma. 1999;46(4):619–22. Discussion 622–4.

8. Stassen NA, Bhullar I, Cheng JD, Crandall ML, Friese RS, Guillamondegui OD, et al. Selective nonoperative management of blunt splenic injury: an Eastern Association for the Surgery of Trauma practice management guideline. J Trauma Acute Care Surg. 2012;73(5 Suppl 4):S294–300.
9. Leeper WR, Leeper TJ, Ouellette D, Moffat B, Sivakumaran T, Charyk-Stewart T, et al. Delayed hemorrhagic complications in the nonoperative management of blunt splenic trauma: early screening leads to a decrease in failure rate. J Trauma Acute Care Surg. 2014;76(6):1349–53.
10. Malhotra AK, Carter RF, Lebman DA, Carter DS, Riaz OJ, Aboutanos MB, et al. Preservation of splenic immunocompetence after splenic artery angioembolization for blunt splenic injury. J Trauma. 2010;69(5):1126–30. Discussion 1130–1.
11. Ekeh AP, McCarthy MC, Woods RJ, Haley E. Complications arising from splenic embolization after blunt splenic trauma. Am J Surg. 2005;189(3): 335–9.
12. Matthews LA, Smith EM, Spirnak JP. Nonoperative treatment of major blunt renal lacerations with urinary extravasation. J Urol. 1997;157(6):2056–8.
13. Altman AL, Haas C, Dinchman KH, Spirnak JP. Selective nonoperative management of blunt grade 5 renal injury. J Urol. 2000;164(1):27–30. Discussion 30–1.
14. Como JJ, Bokhari F, Chiu WC, Duane TM, Holevar MR, Tandoh MA, et al. Practice management guidelines for selective nonoperative management of penetrating abdominal trauma. J Trauma. 2010;68(3): 721–33.
15. Ginzburg E, Carrillo EH, Kopelman T, McKenney MG, Kirton OC, Shatz DV, et al. The role of computed tomography in selective management of gunshot wounds to the abdomen and flank. J Trauma. 1998;45(6):1005–9.
16. Demetriades D, Hadjizacharia P, Constantinou C, Brown C, Inaba K, Rhee P, et al. Selective nonoperative management of penetrating abdominal solid organ injuries. Ann Surg. 2006;244(4):620–8.
17. Hasaniya N, Demetriades D, Stephens A, Dubrowskiz R, Berne T. Early morbidity and mortality of nontherapeutic operations for penetrating trauma. Am Surg. 1994;60(10):744–7.
18. Haan J, Kole K, Brunetti A, Kramer M, Scalea TM. Nontherapeutic laparotomies revisited. Am Surg. 2003;69(7):562–5.
19. Cullinane DC, Schiller HJ, Zielinski MD, Bilaniuk JW, Collier BR, Como J, et al. Eastern Association for the Surgery of Trauma practice management guidelines for hemorrhage in pelvic fracture—update and systematic review. J Trauma. 2011;71(6): 1850–68.
20. Matityahu A, Marmor M, Elson JK, Lieber C, Rogalski G, Lin C, et al. Acute complications of patients with pelvic fractures after pelvic angiographic embolization. Clin Orthop Relat Res. 2013;471(9):2906–11.
21. Lee WA, Matsumura JS, Mitchell RS, Farber MA, Greenberg RK, Azizzadeh A, et al. Endovascular repair of traumatic thoracic aortic injury: clinical practice guidelines of the Society for Vascular Surgery. J Vasc Surg. 2011;53(1):187–92.
22. Avery LE, Stahlfeld KR, Corcos AC, Scifres AM, Ziembicki JA, Varcelotti J, et al. Evolving role of endovascular techniques for traumatic vascular injury: a changing landscape? J Trauma Acute Care Surg. 2012;72(1):41–6. Discussion 46–7.
23. Brenner ML, Moore LJ, DuBose JJ, Tyson GH, McNutt MK, Albarado RP, et al. A clinical series of resuscitative endovascular balloon occlusion of the aorta for hemorrhage control and resuscitation. J Trauma Acute Care Surg. 2013;75(3):506–11.

13 Neurosurgical Advances in Trauma Management

ByoungJun Han and Uzma Samadani

Introduction

Traumatic brain injury (TBI) is the single greatest cause of death and disability in Americans younger than 35 years of age. The management of brain injury can be roughly divided into two modalities: surgical and nonsurgical. Surgical management has the general purpose of relieving mass effect, stopping active bleeding and securing the skull contents via repair of skull fractures. Nonsurgical management may include monitoring of the physical examination or for cerebral perfusion pressure, intracranial pressure or brain-tissue oxygenation and treatment with the goal of optimization of neurologic outcome. Purely traumatic injury will be discussed in this chapter, although many patients with TBI also have a concordant anoxic/ischemic injury. It should be noted that anoxic and ischemic injuries have a worse prognosis and fewer treatments than TBI. Advances in management of TBI include a tendency towards minimally invasive approaches to surgical management and experimentation with new diagnostics and therapeutics for nonsurgical management. Clinical trials for therapeutics for brain injury are limited by a lack of rigorous sensitive outcome measures. Recent increased media interest primarily driven by sports has stimulated grant applications in the field of TBI but not resulted in a proportionate increase in research funding.

B. Han, B.S.
Department of Neurosurgery, New York University School of Medicine, New York, NY, USA
e-mail: Byoungjun.han@med.nyu.edu

U. Samadani, M.D., Ph.D. (✉)
Department of Neurosurgery, Psychiatry, Physiology, and Neuroscience, NewYork Harbor Health Care System, New York University School of Medicine, New York, NY, USA
e-mail: uzma.samadani@nyumc.org

Acute Epidural Hematoma

Overview

Incidence

Epidural hematoma (EDH) occurs mainly in young adults with an incidence of 2.7–4 % of traumatic brain injury patients. The incidence is significantly lower before age 2 or after age 60 and the highest incidence occurs between the ages 20 and 30 [1, 2].

Pathogenesis

Traffic accidents, falls, and assaults comprise the majority of the reasons for EDH patient admissions representing 53 %, 30 %, and 8 % of total EDH cases respectively. In pediatric patients, 49 % of EDH cases result from falls, which is the most common cause of EDH in pediatric patient group [1]. The main source of bleeding from EDH is arterial bleeding (85 %) with the middle meningeal

R. Latifi et al. (eds.), *Technological Advances in Surgery, Trauma and Critical Care*,
DOI 10.1007/978-1-4939-2671-8_13

artery as the most common source in middle fossa EDH. Middle meningeal vein and dural sinus serve as the remaining source of bleeding in EDH [2].

Clinical Presentation

Patients with EDH present in comatose state on admission or prior to surgery in 22–56 % of the cases. About 10–27 % of patients have more classical presentation with loss of consciousness, followed by period of lucid interval that may last for several hours, and finally a rapid decline in state characterized by obtundation, contralateral hemiparesis, and ipsilateral pupillary dilatation. The lucid interval may be present in other scenarios, such as in patients with subdural hematoma; thus, a diagnosis of EDH cannot be made directly from observation of lucid interval. Other clinical symptoms of EDH include decerebrate posturing, seizures, elevated CSF pressure, hemi-hyperreflexia, and unilateral Babinski sign. In pediatric patients, a 10 % drop in hematocrit or early seizures should signal suspicion of EDH [1, 2].

Mortality

The mortality of all age groups with EDH undergoing surgery ranges from 7 to 12.5 %. Pediatric mortality lies around 5 %. Factors associated with increased mortality of patients undergoing surgery for EDH include poor Glasgow coma scale (GCS), age, pupillary abnormalities, associated intracranial lesions, increased time between neurological deterioration and surgery, and elevated intracranial pressure (ICP) [1].

Surgical Treatment

Indication

The indication for surgery of acute EDH relies on physical examination, GCS, pupillary exam, comorbidities, CT findings, age, and ICP. Often, EDH volume greater than 30 cm^3 is indicated for surgery regardless of the level of GCS. EDH with thickness >15 mm or midline shift (MLS) >5 mm may also suggest surgery is indicated. In a study of 74 patients with initial asymptomatic EDH managed nonoperatively but who required delayed surgery, 71 % of patients presented with EDH thickness >15 mm and 79 % presented with MLS >5 mm^2.

Standard of Care

Urgent craniotomy remains the gold standard for surgical treatment of EDH. Craniotomy is performed with the objectives of clot removal, hemostasis, and blood reaccumulation prevention. The removal of the clot lowers ICP and removes focal mass effect. Craniotomy allows greater access to the clot compared to burr hole procedures [2].

Latest Advances

The standard craniotomy procedure has the disadvantages of postoperative wound, increased blood loss, and longer operation time. Bone defects may also occur, leading to cosmetic and functional deficit problems [3]. Minimally invasive surgeries have been developed for patients who cannot tolerate general anesthesia required for craniotomy. Under local anesthesia, transfemoral endovascular embolization of the bleeding artery is performed to eliminate bleeding. Consequent hematoma evacuation through burr hole removes the hematoma with assist of endoscope to guide evacuation [4]. Experimental procedures for EDH may be difficult to justify in a deteriorating patient with an acute EDH for whom craniotomy is an option, so experimental procedures are, by necessity, reserved for rare, stable cases.

Nonsurgical Treatment

Indication

In patients with EDH volume <30 cm^3, thickness <15 mm, MLS <5 mm, GCS >8, and no focal neurologic deficit, nonsurgical treatment with close neurological observation can be performed [2].

Standard of Care

Nonsurgical treatment involves close observation and monitoring of level of consciousness, breathing pattern, hematocrit, headache, vomiting, and diplopia. CT scans may be performed at set intervals, with the first follow-up CT scan obtained within 6–8 h after TBI, to determine changes in size of the clot [1]. Hematomas usually are fully resorbed between 4 and 12 weeks after injury [5]. The critical component of non-surgical treatment is screening the right population of patients that do not require surgery.

Latest Advances

In patients with proven temporal EDH using CT but minimal symptoms, new endovascular techniques have been used to prevent continual bleeding. Angiography combined with embolization of the middle meningeal artery can be used in place of craniotomy to prevent further bleeding. Angiography can identify lucent areas inside EDH and determine patients who need immediate embolization. Lammy and Suzuki have applied endovascular therapy in EDH patients with encouraging results [6].

Acute Subdural Hematoma

Overview

Incidence

Acute Subdural hematoma (aSDH) is present in 12–29 % of patients admitted with severe TBI. The mean age for aSDH occurrence is between 31 and 47 years with male predominance, due to increased association of trauma with male gender [1].

Mechanism

Motor vehicle accidents (MVA) and falls comprise the majority of aSDH cases. In younger population (18–40 years), MVA presents as the major cause, resulting in 56 % and falls causing 12 % of aSDH within this population. In older population (>65 years) MVA causes 22 % and falls cause 56 % of aSDH cases. Patients on anticoagulants have increased risk of aSDH with a 7-fold rise in males and 26-fold rise in females [1].

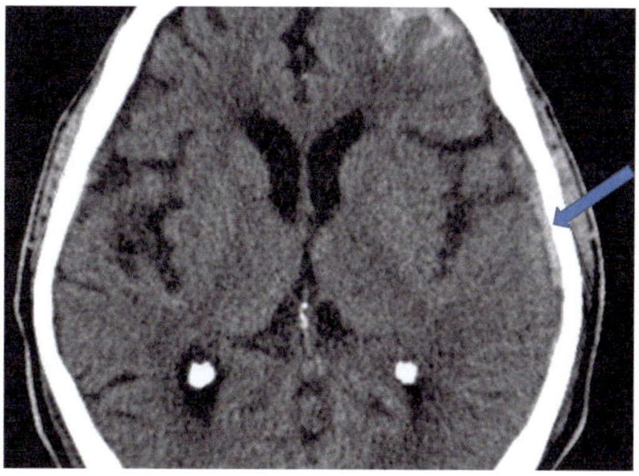

Fig. 13.1 Noncontrast CT scan of acute subdural hematoma

Clinical Presentation

37–80 % of aSDH patients presented with a GCS score 8 or less. A lucid interval is seen in traumatic aSDH caused by cerebral acceleration-deceleration events but not commonly seen in aSDH caused by accumulation around parenchymal laceration. 12–38 % of patients show a lucid interval pre-admission [1]. Figure 13.1 shows a CT scan of patient with acute SDH.

Mortality

Mortality in aSDH is high, ranging from 40 to 60 %. Underlying brain injury resulting from aSDH is the significant cause of the high mortality. Higher mortality is seen in older patients and patients on anticoagulants with mortality rates of 60 % and 90–100 % respectively. Factors influencing mortality include mechanism of injury, age, neurologic condition on admission, and post-operative ICP [2].

Surgical Treatment

Indication

Patients with aSDH thickness >10 mm or midline shift (MLS) >5 mm often receive surgery. If patients have aSDH thickness <10 mm and MLS <5 mm, surgery may be indicated if patients have GCS drop of two or more points from the time of injury to admission, asymmetric or fixed and dilated pupils, and/or intracranial pressure> 20 mmHg[2].

Standard of Care

Common surgical techniques used in treatment of aSDH are craniotomy, burr hole, twist drill, subtemporal decompressive craniectomy, and large decompressive hemicraniectomy. Choices of surgical techniques vary depending on situation and surgeon's training. One study comparing the efficacy of surgical techniques used for aSDH showed significantly increased mortality and reduced functional recovery rate for patients with GCS scores between 4 and 6 when burr hole trephination was used compared with craniotomy. Another study compared craniotomy, craniotomy with dural grafting, and decompressive craniectomy (DC) in 113 patients and found that all 17 patients undergoing DC died with no other significant differences found between treatment groups [1].

Latest Advances

The clinical cost-effectiveness of DC has been an important issue. The advantage of DC is that it allows more effective control of high ICP which is critical in determining outcome after traumatic brain injury. The disadvantage of DC is that it requires a cranioplasty procedure with its complications and that not all patients have brain swelling and do not benefit from the increased management of ICP provided by DC. Recent study showed that out of 91 patients, of whom 51 underwent DC and 40 underwent craniotomy, the overall mortalities of DC and craniotomy were 38 % and 32 % respectively. This showed that the unadjusted outcome of craniotomy and DC were not significantly different, even though there were higher proportion of major extracranial injury in patients undergoing DC. This suggests that DC may be more effective in selected patients as mortality rates did not significantly differ even with increased initial injury severity in patients who underwent DC [7].

Nonsurgical Treatment

Indication

Neurologically stable patients with aSDH <10 mm and MLS <5 mm with normal pupillary movements and no intracranial hypertension should be considered for nonsurgical management. Patients with a stable clinical condition and normal ICP are at lower risk than unstable patients with elevated ICP [8].

Standard of Care

Patients should be closely observed for neurological deterioration which may necessitate evacuation. Patients with traumatic brain injury often undergo serial follow-up head CT scans during the first 36 h post injury because of the high probability of clot expansion during this time [8].

Latest Advances

Hypertonic/hyperoncotic treatment (HHT) improves functional and histologic outcome after aSDH through decreasing ICP. HHT restores microcirculation through improved rheology. In addition, endothelial cell swelling is reduced, capillary diameters increased, and leukocyte endothelium interactions are reduced which all aid in reduction of ICP [9]. Recent study by Rahimi et al. has shown that recombinant human erythropoietin (EPO) applied locally as direct cortical application in rats can show similar neuroprotective events through potential mechanisms including anti-apoptosis, anti-inflammation, and anti-oxidation. EPO, in combination with hematoma evacuation, was shown to decrease post-ASDH lesion volume by 68 % [10].

Chronic Subdural Hematoma

Overview

Incidence

Chronic subdural hematoma (cSDH) mainly occurs in older patients. The incidence is 3.4 per 100,000 patients and 8.2 per 100,000 patients per year for adults younger than 65 and older than

65 years respectively [11]. Risk factors include atrophy, alcohol abuse, seizures, cerebrospinal fluid diverting shunts, coagulopathies, and patients at risk for falls [2].

Pathophysiology

Some cSDHs may start as acute subdurals triggering an inflammatory response. This results in fibroblast invasion into the clot and formation of neomembranes in both the cortical and dural surfaces. Ingrowth of neocapillaries, enzymatic fibrinolysis, and liquefaction of blood clot follow and the fibrin degradation products enter new clots to prevent hemostasis, resulting in cSDH [2].

Clinical Presentation

Common presenting symptoms include gait disturbance, hemiparesis, headaches, dementia, incontinence, and consciousness disturbance. In a study with 500 consecutive cases of cSDH patients, gait disturbance and hemiparesis were present in 63.0 and 58.6 % of the patients [2]. As many as half of patients may not recall significant traumatic events. Figure 13.2 shows a CT scan of patient with cSDH.

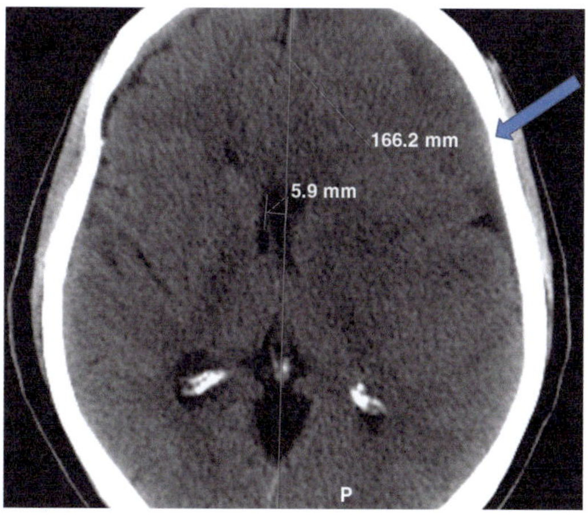

Fig. 13.2 Noncontrast CT scan of left frontoparietal chronic subdural hematoma with right midline shift

Mortality

Mortality of cSDH patients is high with perioperative mortality ranging from 1.2 to 11 % and the 1 year mortality of elderly patients treated with drainage intervention around 32 %. One study shows that out of 209 post-cSDH patients, the mean survival rate was 4.4 years which was significantly shorter than the mean survival of 6.0 years for an age matched non-cSDH group computed from actuarial life-tables [12].

Surgical Treatment

Indication

Surgical treatment is indicated in patients with symptomatic lesions including focal deficit and mental status changes. In addition, subdurals with maximum thickness >1 cm are often evacuated [2].

Standard of Care

Current surgical treatment options include craniotomy, burr holes, twist drill, and subdural evacuating port system (SEPS). No consensus exists as to which surgical method is the best to treat cSDH. Burr hole craniotomy is the most popular procedure for primary cSDH and can be done under general or local anesthesia [13]. Twist drill craniotomy decompresses the brain more slowly and avoids rapid pressure shifts which may be correlated with intracerebral hemorrhage complications. In addition, twist drill craniotomy can be performed at the bedside. SEPS is a variant of twist drill craniotomy with a hermetically sealed closed drainage which reduces infection rate [14].

Latest Advances

Twist drill craniostomy (TDC), although timesaving and cost-effective, has complications that include inadequate drainage, brain penetration, acute epidural hematoma and catheter folding. A modified technique of TDC has been developed to overcome these complications. From July

1992 to December 2011, 50 cSDH patients have been treated with modified TDC and no mortality related to the procedure was observed with 6 % mortality rate due to poor pre operative neurological status [15].

Nonsurgical Treatment

Indication

Patients without neurologic deficits are often managed without drainage.

Standard of Care

cSDH patients can be treated with seizure prophylactic anticonvulsants as seizure frequency in these patients range from 2 to 19 %. Conflicting viewpoints on risk and benefit of using anticonvulsants exist. Corticosteroids have also been used to treat cSDH with the rationale that anti inflammatory action will prevent hematoma and maintenance [16]. ACE inhibitors, which have antiangiogenic effects, have also been shown to reduce recurrence of cSDH. One study showed that out of 81 cSDH patients treated with ACE inhibitors, only 5 % showed recurrence of cSDH as compared to 18 % recurrence rate of patients who did not receive ACE inhibitors [17].

Latest Advances

Hyperfibrinolytic activity has been shown to be critical for liquefaction of hematoma and progression of cSDH. In addition, increased permeability of capillaries in hematoma leads to enlargement of cSDH. Plasmin acts on both fibrinolytic and kalikrein systems; thus targeting plasmin may ameliorate the progression of cSDH. Recently, tranexamic acid, an antifibrinolytic drug which inhibits plasminogen activation and plasmin activity, has been used to treat cSDH patients. Studies show that out of 18 cSDH patients treated with tranexamic acid only, clinical symptoms improved and hematomas were fully reduced in all patients. No recurrence or thromboembolic side effects have been observed. In addition, side effects of tranexamic acid are mild and uncommon with thromboembolic cerebrovascular events not occurring significantly more than control group. Tranexamic acid may be an effective medical therapy for cSDH [18].

Traumatic Parenchymal Lesions

Overview

Incidence

Traumatic parenchymal lesions comprise 8.2 % of all TBI, 13–35 % of severe TBI, and up to 20 % of operative intracranial lesions in representative series [1].

Classification

Traumatic parenchymal lesions are heterogeneous in nature, and these lesions have been divided into two broad classes: focal and nonfocal lesions. Focal lesions include intracerebral hematoma, delayed traumatic intracerebral hematoma, contusions and infarctions. Nonfocal lesions are comprised of cerebral edema, hemispheric swelling, and diffuse injury [1].

Clinical Presentation

Patients with traumatic parenchymal lesions may present with neurological deterioration, intracranial hypertension, and signs of mass effect on examination or imaging generally with CT [1].

Mortality

Mortality of the different classes of parenchymal lesions correlates with the prognostic variables of TBI in general. Age, postresuscitation GCS, cranial fracture presentation, pupillary response, respiratory insufficiency, ICP, and basal cistern status are factors affecting prognosis [1].

Surgical Treatment

Indication

Patients presenting with GCS between 6 and 8 with frontal or temporal contusions >20 cm^3 with MLS >5 mm and patients with lesion > 50 cm^3 in volume should be evacuated. Surgical indications, in addition to CT parameters, also need to take into account patients' clinical status and the occurrence of clinical deterioration [1].

Standard of Care

Current options for surgical treatment of focal parenchymal lesions include craniotomy with evacuation of the lesion. Surgical evacuation of the lesion aids in correcting cerebral shift and reduction of ICP. Study shows that craniotomy, when performed before neurological deterioration in patients, had significantly better outcomes when compared to delayed operation. Stereotactic evacuation of the lesions has also been used for treatment; however, stereotactic treatment is less effective if patient has a diffuse pathology and intracranial hypertension [1].

Latest Advances

Several studies show that decompressive procedures such as hemispheric DC may have a role in management of parenchymal injuries. One study shows that in 28 patients undergoing unilateral or bilateral DC for posttraumatic edema and intracranial hypertension, 57 % showed good outcome or moderate disability at 1 year. In 39 and 18 TBI patients with posttraumatic diffuse brain swelling who underwent primary decompression and secondary decompression respectively, 58 % of the first group and 65 % of the second group showed good outcome or moderate disability at 1 year [1].

In another recent, multicenter decompressive craniectomy (DECRA) trial, study showed that although DC decreased ICP, duration of mechanical ventilation, and time in ICU compared to standard, nonsurgical treatment, patients receiving the craniectomy had lower median score in Extended Glasgow Outcome Scale and resulted in higher risk of unfavorable outcome. This result may be associated with the possibility of the craniectomy allowing expansion of the swollen brain outside the skull, leading to axonal stretch and neural injury [19]. Critics of this trial noted that selection biases affecting randomization, nonstandard criteria for surgical indication and cross-over of subjects may have impacted outcomes.

Nonsurgical Treatment

Indication

Patients with stable ICP, no mass effect on CT scan, and no evidence of neurological deterioration are often managed nonsurgically [1].

Standard of Care

Medical treatment of traumatic parenchymal lesions include protocols involving head elevation, propofol sedation, mannitol and/or hypertonic saline, normocarbia, mild hypothermia to 33–35 °C, and electroencephalogram burst suppression. However, medical management alone shows 3.8 times increase in relative risk of unfavorable outcome compared to DC [1].

Latest Advances

Citicoline, also known as CDP-Choline, has been suggested to aid in both neuroprotection and neuro-restorative process. By increasing levels of glutathione, citicoline showed a reduction in oxidative stress, which reduces the risk of secondary injury in TBI. The Citicoline Brain Injury Treatment (COBRIT) trial tested the effects of 90 days of citicoline on functional outcomes of patients with TBI; however, the results showed that citicoline had no significant improvement compared to placebo as an acute/post acute therapy for TBI patients. 35.4 % of citicoline treated group showed improvement in Extended Glasgow Outcome Scale compared to 35.6 % improvement in the placebo group. The lack of improvement with citicoline treatment may be due to the heterogeneous pathophysiology of TBI and suggested that future drugs target specific subtypes of TBI [20].

Recent study also showed that the standard care of ICP monitoring in TBI patients does not have a significant increase in functional and cognitive status of patients when compared to treatment based on imaging and clinical examination. The 6 month mortality in ICP monitoring patients was 39 % and in imaging and clinical examination, 41 %. Length of stay in ICU in both groups was similar, with 12 days in ICP monitoring and 9 days in imaging-clinical examination. These results suggest that in the treatment of TBI patients, the role of current treatment protocol associated with ICP monitoring and manipulation should be reassessed [21].

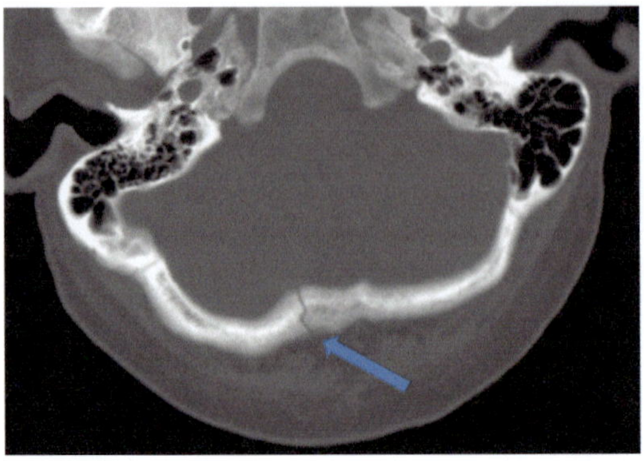

Fig. 13.3 Noncontrast CT scan of linear occipital skull fracture

Depressed Cranial Fractures

Overview

Incidence

Depressed cranial fracture (DCF) can be present and complicate up to 6 % of head injuries. 90 % of the depressed cranial fractures are comprised of compound cranial fractures [1].

Mortality

Compound cranial fractures have an infection rate of 1.9–10.6 % and an average neurological morbidity of 11 %, incidence of epilepsy of 15 %, and mortality rate of 14–19 % [1].

Clinical Presentation

Patients may present with head pain, swelling, overlying scalp disruption, or any symptoms typically associated with brain injury. Figure 13.3 shows a CT scan of patient with a linear occipital skull fracture.

Surgical Treatment

Indication

Surgery is indicated if fracture depression is greater than the thickness of cranium or as per the surgeon's judgment. Simple depressed fractures may be managed both surgically and nonsurgically [2].

Standard of Care

Although controversy exists in determination of appropriate surgical treatment of DCF, the conventional surgical treatment of compound DCF involves debridement and surgical elevation. Simple DCF requires surgical elevation only when depression is equal to or greater than the thickness of adjacent intact bone. Reasons for aggressive treatment of DCF involve potential occurrence of infection, epilepsy, and for cosmetic deformity. Study shows that compound cranial fracture patients show 10.6 % incidence of infection and 15 % incidence of late epilepsy [1].

Latest Advances

Traditional treatment of DCF removes bone fragments in order to reduce danger of infection, unstable fixation and intracranial pressure. Recent studies have shown that replacement of the bone fragments did not show a significant increase in risk of infection compared to the removal of bone fragments. By replacing bone fragments in the first operation, second cranioplasty may be obviated. Dissociate bone flap cranioplasty has been shown to provide additional benefits in comparison to lever-up cranioplasty. The advantages of this method is that it avoids epidural hematoma which may form during lever-up craniplasty procedures, can repair dura rupture, treat complicated fractures comminuting across superior sagittal sinus, allow direct vision for surgeons, and avoid secondary operation [22].

Nonsurgical Treatment

Indication

Nonsurgical treatment may be considered if all of the following criteria are met:

No evidence of dural penetration
No significant intracranial hematoma
No frontal sinus involvement
No wound infection or gross contamination
No gross cosmetic deformity [1]

Standard of Care

Antibiotics are used for all compound depressed fractures to prevent infection. Nonsurgical therapy is often reserved for nondisplaced closed fractures. Continuous monitoring of the wound should be done. If significant hematoma does not resolve within 2–3 days, surgery should be performed [1].

Penetrating Intracranial Injury

Overview

Incidence

Penetrating intracranial injury comprises all traumatic brain injuries not resulting from blunt trauma. Of the penetrating injuries, gunshot wound to the head (GSWH) is most common and occurs in 35 % of deaths in brain injury patients and is the proximal cause of the death in greater than 90 % of the victims [2].

Mechanism

Primary injury from GSWH results from injury to soft tissue, comminuted fracture of bone, cerebral injuries from missile, and coup/contrecoup injury from missile impact. Extent of primary injury is correlated to impact velocity. Secondary injury consists of cerebral edema with rapid rise in ICP. Intracranial hemorrhage from lacerated blood vessels may also occur [2].

Prognosis

Factors that worsen prognosis include the following:

Increase in age
Bilateral involvement/trajectory
Intraventricular trajectory
Brainstem injury
Suicide attempts
Coagulopathy
GCS <3 with bilaterally fixed and dilated pupils
High initial intracranial pressure [22]

Surgical Treatment

Indication

Patients with little CNS function will not likely benefit from craniotomy and supportive measures are indicated [2].

Standard of Care

Surgical operation should be made within 12 h to minimize opportunities for infection and abscesses. Small entrance wounds should be treated with local wound care and closure in patients with no significant intracranial pathologic findings on CT scan. If significant mass effect is present, necrotic brain tissue and safely accessible bone fragments should be debrided. Deeply seated bone fragments in sensitive areas should not be debrided as it is correlated with worse outcomes. Watertight closure of the dura may decrease risk of abscess formation and CSF fistulas [23].

Latest Advances

Angiographic and endovascular techniques may be used to assess and treat vessel injuries associated with penetrating trauma.

Nonsurgical Treatment

Indication

Patients with superficial trajectories and reassuring prognoses, or deep trajectories with poor prognoses may not require surgery.

Standard of Care

Antibiotic prophylaxis should be used to prevent infections complications which can occur in up to 15 % of all PBI cases. CSF fistulas and air sinus wounds place the patient at an even greater increased risk of infection with an incidence of 49.5 %. Cephalosporin is a preferred broad spectrum antibiotic for use in penetrating intracranial injuries.

Antiepileptic prophylaxis should also be administered to reduce mortality and morbidity of patients. Seizures during the first week post injury may increase intracranial pressures and metabolic demands which can cause morbidity and mortality. Prophylactic anticonvulsant treatment beyond 1 week post injury has not been shown to prevent development of new seizures [2].

Diffuse Axonal Injury

Overview

Incidence

Diffuse axonal injury (DAI) is found in patients with trauma ranging in severity from sever to concussive. Studies show that the mean age of occurrence was 28 ± 15.8 years and was caused mainly by traffic injury (92 %) followed by fall (3.2 %), assault (2.4 %), and work injury (1.6 %) [24].

Mechanism

In contrast to focal brain injury, diffuse axonal injuries after TBI are found scattered throughout subcortical white matter in corpus callosum, thalamus, and brain stem. The acceleration and deceleration phenomena creates rotational shear forces that lead to progressive changes that interfere with axonal transport, which results in local swelling of the axon prior to detachment from its downstream segment. Studies have suggested that inflammatory responses also participate in the neural injury of DAI that differ from the inflammatory mechanism following focal brain injury [25–27].

Clinical Presentation

Average GCS of DAI patients was 6.80 ± 2.37. Anisocoria was seen in 29.5 % of the patients and the remaining patients presented with bilateral myosis [24].

Mortality

Mortality of DAI patients was correlated to the absence of consciousness recovery. 51 % of DAI patients had poor outcome, which was related to initial hypotension, anisocoria, hyperglycemia at admission, disseminated intravascular coagulation, and transfusion [24].

Surgical Treatment

Surgery is not generally indicated for isolated diffuse axonal injury. If a patient has elevated ICP in addition to DAI, the ICP elevation is treated, and may even potentially require hemicraniectomy.

Nonsurgical Treatment

Latest Advances

The neuroprotective effect of progesterone on ischemia has been shown in various animal models with its reductive effect on cerebral edema and secondary neuronal death due to decreased free radicals. In patients with diffuse axonal injury, progesterone administration in patients with severe brain injury ($5 < GCS < 8$) showed significantly higher GOS score than the control group. However, in patients with critical brain injury ($GCS < 5$), progesterone administration did not show significant GOS improvement [26].

Recent study has also suggested that the formation of membrane pores caused by mechanical deformation may result in axon degeneration and disconnection. Treatment aimed at sealing the porous membrane has been tried with monomethoxy poly ethylene glycol poly D,L-lactic acid di-block copolymer micelles (mPEG-PDLLA) which have been shown to restore compound action potentials in injured spinal cord in rat model. mPEG-PDLLA administration in controlled cortical impact (CCI) mice showed improved function of both myelinated and unmyelinated axons of corpus callosum in the CCI mice model; however, the improvement was shown independent of membrane resealing mechanism [28].

Stem cell transplantation is another potential treatment that can provide functional recovery following DAI. Recent study has shown that embryonic stem cell transplantation significantly improved functional outcomes of behavioral tasks after fluid-percussion injury, which produced DAI in an animal model. The tumorigenic potential of introducing stem cells can be mitigated by in vitro pre differentiation before transplantation [29]. Stem cell transplantation for DAI has not yet been performed in humans.

Carotid and Vertebral Artery Dissection

Overview

Incidence

Cerebral arterial dissections usually occur in middle aged patients with a mean age of 45 years, occurring more frequently in men. Vertebral artery (VA) dissection is the most common occurrence followed by internal carotid artery (ICA) dissection [2]. Approximately 2.6 per 100,000 people in the United States have an incidence of spontaneous ICA dissection, which is the leading cause of strokes in young people [30, 31].

Mechanism

Traumatic ICA dissection is caused by neck hyperextension with lateral rotation causing ischemic symptoms. Motor vehicle accidents are the most common cause of ICA. Spinal manipulation therapy can also result in both ICA and VA dissections. Spontaneous ICA dissection is associated with trivial trauma from coughing, nose blowing, and neck turning. Spontaneous VA dissection is associated with fibromucular dysplasia, migraine, and oral contraceptives [2].

Clinical Presentation

In spontaneous ICA dissection, ipsilateral headache is the most common initial symptom. Pain is mostly orbital/periorbital and can produce sudden onset of carotidynia. Incomplete Horner's syndrome sparing the external carotid artery plexus can occur. ICA dissection may also cause hemiplegia and hemiparesis in children.

In VA dissection, neck pain is the most prominent early finding with severe headache. Additionally, altered consciousness may be seen in VA dissection patients and subarachnoid hemorrhage (SAH) may also be seen [2].

Mortality

Overall mortality of cerebral arterial dissection is 26 % with ICA dissection mortality of 49 % and vertebrobasilar artery dissection mortality of 22 % [2].

Surgical Treatment

Indication

Presence of SAH requires surgery or endovascular techniques. Persistent symptoms in spite of medical therapy and progression of dissection also indicate surgical treatment.

Standard of Care

Endovascular stent angioplasty is used to treat carotid dissections. This procedure has shown to improve symptoms, resolve cerebral ischemia and cause return of neurological functions. However, such procedures have 12 % incidence of stroke and death, and a 58 % incidence of cranial neuropathy. As such, they are reserved for patients whose status does not improve with medical treatment [32].

Endovascular techniques are also used to treat VA; however, if endovascular techniques are not available, alternative surgical procedures may be performed, including Hunterian occlusion of the VA, VA clipping combined with vascular bypass, resection accompanied by autogenous interposition vein graft, and non-occlusive surgical techniques [2].

Latest Advances

Flow diverter stents, which are a new generation of self-expanding, stent-like devices with high metal surface area, have been used in management of vertebral dissections. Flow diverters have been designed to occlude aneurysms through endoluminal reconstruction of the dysplastic segment of the parent artery. The increased surface area of the flow diverter also provides tighter clot containment and allows post-stenting angioplasty [33].

Nonsurgical Treatment

Indication

In cases without hemorrhage or large ischemic stroke, medical therapy should be started emergently.

Standard of Care

Anticoagulation medication starting with acute administration of heparin followed by oral agents, such as Coumadin, for total of 6 months is recommended. Antithrombotic therapy has been suggested to retard thrombosis in the false lumen, which can delay the healing of the dissection. In addition, the risk of bleeding from anticoagulation therapy may outweigh the benefits provided by the therapy [2, 34, 35].

Blast Injury

Overview

Incidence

The wars in Iraq and Afghanistan have increased the incidence of TBI significantly, with 267,000 US soldiers sustaining TBI since 2000. Of these soldiers, 69 % of the TBI were caused by blast injury with the principal source of blast from improvised explosive devices [36, 37].

Pathophysiology

Explosion creates an instantaneous expansion of gas, causing blast wave that can travel at a velocity between 3,000 and 8,000 m/s. Primary blast injury results when the blast wave contacts the body and creates both stress waves and shear waves leading to microvascular damage, tissue disruption, and disruption of tissue attachments. Organs most commonly affected from primary blast waves are ears, lungs, and colon. Secondary blast injury results from solid matter expulsed from the blast leading to penetrating wounds. Tertiary injury is due to collapse of surrounding structures or from propulsion of the victim due to the blast wave, causing injury. Quaternary injury is from chemical and thermal factors and quinary injury results from radiation and bacteria [36, 38, 39].

Clinical Presentation

Traumatic brain injury due to blast injury can cause cranial fractures and focal neurologic deficits due to air embolism. In addition, diffuse or focal axonal injury can also occur. Blast induced TBI can also result in concussive syndrome with mild TBI, leading to symptoms of posttraumatic stress disorder, which includes depression, anxiety, memory and attention deficits, sleep problems, and emotional disturbances [36, 38, 39]. Severe TBI due to blast injury is characterized by cerebral edema, intracranial hemorrhage, delayed vasospasm, and pseudoaneurysm formation with GCS between 3 and 8 [40].

Mortality

Casualties with head injuries is similar to previous wars, but mortality has reduced significantly due to increased effectiveness of body armor and Kevlar helmets that provides improved shielding from bullets and fragmentation [39]. However, patient temperature control post blast injury may be a challenge, as hyperthermia due to TBI is the most common secondary insult [40].

Surgical Treatment

Indication

Altered level of consciousness following blast exposure, or rapidly increasing refractory ICP in a monitored patient are both indications for DC.

Standard of Care

Current surgical treatment of choice for blast injury induced TBI is large DC. DC allows ICP to be maintained under control and prevent secondary damage resulting from ICP. However, the use of DC raises controversy due to its high invasiveness. Although DC is highly effective in reducing ICP and improving cerebral perfusion pressure, GOS outcome is low, with only 29 % of patients with DC having favorable outcome [39].

Nonsurgical Treatment

Indication

All penetrating head injury requires administration of antibiotics. ICP monitoring is advised for patients who cannot be awoken hourly for neurologic evaluation and/or those who have ongoing intracranial lesion with potential for cerebral edema development [41]. Patients with blast injury are also at risk for vasopasm, which may require endovascular management.

Standard of Care

Cefazolin is recommended for 5 days after all penetrating head injuries. ICP monitoring can include ventriculostomy or intracranial bolt. Hyperthermia should be avoided in patients as temperatures above 99 °F may increase risk of vasopasm. In patients without evidence of ongoing hemorrhage, deep vein thrombosis prophylaxis should be administered with enoxaparin or subcutaneous heparin [41].

Latest Advances

Blast injury TBI is associated with early complement activation and inflammatory response. One study showed a potential efficacy of recombinant human decay-accelerating factor (rhDAF) within 30 min of moderate blast exposure in rats showed protective effect on brain histological damage, blood–brain barrier breakdown, and formation of brain edema. rhDAF was also shown to attenuate blast triggered systemic complement activation, reduce complement interaction and decrease tau phosphorylation during first 24 h post blast exposure. These effects suggest a potential use of rhDAF as an effective therapeutic treatment for blast-induced neurotrauma and neuroinflammation [42].

Abbreviations

aSDH	Acute subdural hematoma
CCI	Controlled cortical impact
CNS	Central nervous system
COBRIT	Citicoline brain injury treatment
cSDH	Chronic subdural hematoma
CSF	Cerebrospinal fluid
CT	Computed tomography
DAI	Diffuse axonal injury
DC	Decompressive craniectomy
DCF	Depressed cranial fracture
EDH	Epidural hematoma
EPO	Erythropoietin
GCS	Glasgow coma scale
GSWH	Gunshot wound to the head
HHT	Hypertonic/hyperoncotic treatment
ICA	Internal carotid artery
ICP	Intracranial pressure
MLS	Midline shift
MVA	Motor vehicle accidents
PBI	Penetrating brain injury
rhDAF	Recombinant human decay-accelerating factor
SAH	Subarachnoid hemorrhage
SEPS	Subdural evacuating port system
TBI	Traumatic brain injury
TDC	Twist drill craniostomy
VA	Vertebral artery

References

1. Bullock M, Chesnut R, Ghajar J, Gordon D, Hartl R, Newell D, et al. Guidelines for the surgical management of traumatic brain injury author group: acknowledgments. Neurosurgery. 2006;58(3):2.
2. Greenberg M. Handbook of neurosurgery. 1st ed. Tampa, FL: Greenberg Graphics; 2010.
3. Xiaoyu W, Guoping L. Surgical treatment of supra-and infratentorial epidural hematoma. Turk Neurosurg. 2012;23(3):299–303.
4. Ohshima T, Tajima H, Fujii K, Nagakura M, Nishizawa T, Kato K, et al. Combined endovascular and endoscopic surgery for acute epidural hematoma in a patient with poor health. Neurol Med Chir. 2012;52(11):829–31.
5. Cucciniello B, Martellotta N, Nigro D, Citro E. Conservative management of extradural haematomas. Acta Neurochir. 1993;120(1-2):47–52.
6. Lammy S, McConnell R, Kamel M, Rennie I, Al-Haddad S. Extradural haemorrhage: is there a role for endovascular treatment? Br J Neurosurg. 2013;27(3):383–5.
7. Li L, Kolias A, Guilfoyle M, Timofeev I, Corteen E, Pickard J, et al. Outcome following evacuation of acute subdural haematomas: a comparison of craniotomy with decompressive craniectomy. Acta Neurochir. 2012;154(9):1555–61.
8. Gerard C, Busl K. Treatment of acute subdural hematoma. Curr Treat Options Neurol. 2014;16(1):1–15.
9. Jussen D, Papaioannou C, Heimann A, Kempski O, Alessandri B. Effects of hypertonic/hyperoncotic treatment and surgical evacuation after acute subdural hematoma in rats. Crit Care Med. 2008;36(2):543–9.
10. Rahimi Nedjat M, Wähmann M, Bächli H, et al. Erythropoietin neuroprotection is enhanced by direct cortical application following subdural blood evacuation in a rat model of acute subdural hematoma. Neuroscience. 2013;238:125–34.
11. Asghar M, Adhiyaman V, Greenway M, Bhowmick B, Bates A. Chronic subdural haematoma in the elderly—a North Wales experience. J R Soc Med. 2002;95(6):290–2.
12. Miranda L, Braxton E, Hobbs J, Quigley M. Chronic subdural hematoma in the elderly: not a benign disease: clinical article. J Neurosurg. 2011;114(1):72–6.
13. Cenic A, Bhandari M, Reddy K. Management of chronic subdural hematoma: a national survey and literature review. Can J Neurol Sci. 2005;32(4):501–6.
14. Asfora W, Schwebach L. A modified technique to treat chronic and subacute subdural hematoma: technical note. Surg Neurol. 2003;59(4):329–32.
15. Helezon K, Tekniugi M. Modified twist drill technique in the management of chronic subdural hematoma. Turk Neurosurg. 2013;23(1):50–4.
16. Santarius T, Lawton R, Kirkpatrick P, Hutchinson P. The management of primary chronic subdural haematoma: a questionnaire survey of practice in the United Kingdom and the Republic of Ireland. Br J Neurosurg. 2008;22(4):529–34.
17. Weigel R, Hohenstein A, Schlickum L, Weiss C, Schilling L. Angiotensin converting enzyme inhibition for arterial hypertension reduces the risk of recurrence in patients with chronic subdural hematoma possibly by an antiangiogenic mechanism. Neurosurgery. 2007;61(4):788–93.
18. Kageyama H, Toyooka T, Tsuzuki N, Oka K. Nonsurgical treatment of chronic subdural hematoma with tranexamic acid: clinical article. J Neurosurg. 2013;119(2):332–7.
19. Cooper D, Rosenfeld J, Murray L, Arabi Y, Davies A, D'Urso P, et al. Decompressive craniectomy in diffuse traumatic brain injury. N Engl J Med. 2011; 364(16):1493–502.
20. Zafonte R, Bagiella E, Ansel B, Novack T, Friedewald W, Hesdorffer D, et al. Effect of citicoline on functional and cognitive status among patients with traumatic brain injuryciticoline brain injury treatment trial (COBRIT) use of citicoline in traumatic brain injury. JAMA. 2012;308(19):1993–2000.
21. Chesnut R, Temkin N, Carney N, Dikmen S, Rondina C, Videtta W, et al. A trial of intracranial-pressure monitoring in traumatic brain injury. N Engl J Med. 2012;367(26):2471–81.
22. Wan Y, Li X, Qian C, Xue Z, Yang S, Wang Y. The comparison between dissociate bone flap cranioplasty and traditional cranioplasty in the treatment of depressed skull fractures. J Craniofac Surg. 2013; 24(2):589–91.
23. Van Den Heever C, van der Merwe D. Management of depressed skull fractures: selective conservative management of nonmissile injuries. J Neurosurg. 1989;71(2):186–90.
24. Chelly H, Chaari A, Daoud E, Dammak H, Medhioub F, Mnif J, et al. Diffuse axonal injury in patients with head injuries: an epidemiologic and prognosis study of 124 cases. J Trauma. 2011;71(4):838–46.
25. Skandsen T, Kvistad K, Solheim O, Strand I, Folvik M, Vik A. Prevalence and impact of diffuse axonal injury in patients with moderate and severe head injury: a cohort study of early magnetic resonance imaging findings and 1-year outcome: Clinical article. J Neurosurg. 2010;113(3):556–63.
26. Shakeri M, Boustani M, Pak N, Panahi F, Salehpour F, Lotfinia I, et al. Effect of progesterone administration on prognosis of patients with diffuse axonal injury due to severe head trauma. Clin Neurol Neurosurg. 2013;115(10):2019–22.
27. Lin Y, Wen L. Inflammatory response following diffuse axonal injury. Int J Med Sci. 2013;10(5):515.
28. Ping X, Jiang K, Lee S, Cheng J, Jin X. PEG-PDLLA micelle treatment improves axonal function of the corpus callosum following traumatic brain injury. J Neurotrauma. 2014;31(13):1172–9.
29. Li X, Feng D. Diffuse axonal injury: novel insights into detection and treatment. J Clin Neurosci. 2009;16(5):614–9.

30. Schievink W, Mokri B, Whisnant J. Internal carotid artery dissection in a community. Rochester, Minnesota, 1987–1992. Stroke. 1993;24(11):1678–80.
31. Bogousslavsky J, Regli F. Ischemic stroke in adults younger than 30 years of age: cause and prognosis. Arch Neurol. 1987;44(5):479–82.
32. Edgell R, Abou-Chebl A, Yadav J. Endovascular management of spontaneous carotid artery dissection. J Vasc Surg. 2005;42(5):854–60.
33. Cohen J, Gomori J, Moscovici S, Bala M, Itshayek E. The use of flow diverter stents in the management of traumatic vertebral artery dissections. J Clin Neurosci. 2013;20(5):731–4.
34. Touz'e E, Randoux B, M'eary E, Arquizan C, Meder J, Mas J. Aneurysmal forms of cervical artery dissection associated factors and outcome. Stroke. 2001;32(2):418–23.
35. Lyrer P. Extracranial arterial dissection snticoagulation is the treatment of choice: against. Stroke. 2005;36(9):2042–3.
36. Ritenour A, Baskin T. Primary blast injury: update on diagnosis and treatment. Crit Care Med. 2008; 36(7):311–7.
37. Taylor P, Ludwigsen J, Ford C. Investigation of blast-induced traumatic brain injury. Brain Inj. 2014;28(7): 879–95.
38. Chen Y, Huang W, Constantini S. Concepts and strategies for clinical management of blast-induced traumatic brain injury and posttraumatic stress disorder. J Neuropsychiatry Clin Neurosci. 2013;25(2): 103–10.
39. Wang E, Huang J. Understanding and treating blast traumatic brain injury in the combat theater. Neurol Res. 2013;35(3):285–9.
40. Rosenfeld J, McFarlane A, Bragge P, Armonda R, Grimes J, Ling G. Blast-related traumatic brain injury. Lancet Neurol. 2013;12(9):882–93.
41. United States Army Institute of Surgical Research. Joint theater trauma system clinical practice guideline [online]. http://www.usaisr.amedd.army.mil/assets/cpgs/Neurosurgical_Management_7_Mar_12.pdf. Accessed 16 June 2014.
42. Li Y, Chavko M, Slack J, Liu B, McCarron R, Ross J, et al. Protective effects of decay-accelerating factor on blast-induced neurotrauma in rats. Acta Neuropathol Commun. 2013;1(1):52.

14 Damage Control and Organ Injury Priority Management of Trauma Patients

Riaan Pretorius, Frank Plani, and Elias Degiannis

Introduction

During damage control surgery, physiological recovery is prioritized above anatomical reconstruction by doing an abbreviated procedure and minimizing the insult [1–3]. It has undergone significant changes (Table 14.1). The insult with the initial injury together with prolonged surgery causes an increased release of histones and cytokines that contribute to multiorgan failure. Histones have been proven to cause damage to endothelial cells, stimulate cytokine release, and induce neutrophil extracellular trap formation [4]. With prolonged surgery there is an increased risk of the "vicious cycle of the lethal triad" described by Kashuk in 1982 of hypothermia, acidosis, and coagulopathy with an increased mortality [5]. Hypothermia in the polytrauma patient is usually multifactorial with external heat loss, cold IV fluids, anaerobic metabolism and theatre multiple cavity exposure as some of the most important causes. When the patient's temperature drops below 35 °C, the patient becomes coagulopathic due to decreased platelet count and function, while when body temperature gets below 33 °C the synthesis of clotting factors drops. Hypothermia worsens acidosis by peripheral vasoconstriction, increased oxygen consumption with shivering and the oxygen dissociation curve shift to left. Acidosis in the severely injured patients is caused due to poor tissue perfusion and anaerobic metabolism. Most enzyme activity is dependant on the pH, as is clotting enzymes. Furthermore, with a drop of the pH to 7.0 the activity of Factor VIIa decreases by 90 % and that of Factor Xa/Va complex by 70 % [5–8]. The response to inotropes is also compromised in the acidotic patient.

Coagulopathy in polytrauma is complex and has multiple components. It is divided into dilutional coagulopathy and non-dilutional coagulopathy. Dilutional coagulopathy is due to diluting the clotting factors with crystalloids, colloids, and blood administration and is directly related to the amount of fluids that was received. To avoid dilutional coagulopathy during a massive transfusion, fresh frozen plasma and platelets are transfused as part of a transfusion protocol.

R. Pretorius, MBChB, FCS (✉)
Department of Surgery/Trauma, Chris Hani Baragwanath Academic Hospital, University of the Witswatersrand, Johannesburg, South Africa
e-mail: drriaanp@yahoo.com

F. Plani, MD, PhD, FRCS, FCS
Department of Surgery, Chris Hani Baragwanath Academic Hospital, Johannesburg, South Africa
e-mail: frankplani@icloud.com

E. Degiannis, MD, PhD, FRACS, FCS
Department of Surgery, Chris Hani Baragwanath Academic Hospital, University of the Witwatersrand, Johannesburg, South Africa
e-mail: degiannis@yebo.co.za

R. Latifi et al. (eds.), *Technological Advances in Surgery, Trauma and Critical Care*,
DOI 10.1007/978-1-4939-2671-8_14

Table 14.1 Three historical stages of surgery for trauma

	Past	Current	Future
Surgery	Aggressive definitive surgery	Damage control surgery	Prehospital control of bleeding
			Improvement of haemostatic agents.
		Haemostatic agents	Improvement of interventional radiology with hybrid theatre
Coagulopathy	"Catch up" correction in coagulopathic patients	Massive transfusion protocols	Genetic guidance to treatment.
		TEG return	Early treatment (prehospital)
Perfusion/ BP	Aggressive resuscitation with clear fluids	Early blood and blood products	Development of the optimal oxygen carrier
		Restriction of clear fluids	
Inflammation	None	Decrease fluids that stimulate an immune response	Targeting genetic targets
			Early treatment

Non-dilutional coagulopathy is the initial type of coagulopathy that develop in the poly trauma patient due to the systemic factors and hypoperfusion. This lead to acidosis and the activation of protein C. Activation of protein C causes coagulopathy by inhibiting plasminogen activators and Factors V and VIII.

"Truncated laparotomy" was first described by Stone and colleagues in 1983 for patients with clinical coagulopathy. Rotondo and Schwab used the term "damage control laparotomy" in 1992 mainly referring to an abbreviated procedure for patients with massive hemorrhage [9]. It created the concept of a limited initial operation to stop the hemorrhage and control the contamination rather than definitive repair. The aim is not only to take the patient alive out of the operating theatre but also to limit the possibility of postoperative multiorgan failure. Initially Rotondo et al. described damage control for abdominal trauma in three stages (initial laparotomy, resuscitation in ICU, and definitive surgery) [9, 10]. Johnson and Swab later on added a fourth phase which include the pre-theatre phase. Currently it has been expanded into five stages: Stage 1: Patient selection and resuscitation in Emergency Department; Stage 2: Initial operation; Stage 3: Resuscitation in ICU; Stage 4: Definitive surgery; and Stage 5: Abdominal wall reconstruction. Currently the principles of damage control applies not only to abdominal but also to thoracic, vascular, orthopedic, and neurosurgical trauma.

Patient Selection

Early and appropriate identification of patients who can potentially benefit from damage control is critical and should be made early, best if it is done in the emergency department. There is no isolated "physiological threshold" that should trigger damage control, but a combination of injuries, physiological parameters, expected hemorrhage and response to treatment, as well as the surgeon's clinical decision should be the key factors. Patients with indications for damage control surgery that would undergo definitive surgery inevitably would have a poor outcome or lead to unplanned damage control. On the other hand, overzealous use of damage control deny patients a single definitive procedure, increase ICU and hospital stay and cost, increase morbidity (intra-abdominal infections, fistulas, hernias) and mortality. Our current emergency department indications for damage control are: injury severity score >25; persistent hypotension with systolic blood pressure of less than 70 mmHg; temperature of <34 °C; pH<7.2; lactate of >5 and worsening; INR and PTT >50 % of normal. On occasion, damage control is applied as part of disaster management aiming to free up overwhelmed resources. Patients that were not initially triaged for damage control in the emergency department might undergo damage control in theatre due to the following: Worsening of physiology (decreased temperature, decreased pH, increased lactate); Increasing inotropic requirements; continuous of massive transfusion protocol (ten or more packed red blood cells in less than 24 h or replace half of the blood volume in less than 3 h); inability to control hemorrhage that force packing; and operative time greater than 90 min. Overall it is estimate that 10 % of major trauma patients might benefit from damage control surgery.

Damage control resuscitation includes ATLS resuscitation with the ABCs. In military resuscitation where a large source of bleeding is visible they adopted the <C>ABC resuscitation approach with immediate control of the hemorrhage. Damage control resuscitation classically consists of permissive hypotension, hemostatic resuscitation, and damage control surgery for control of bleeding and contamination.

Recently two other components have been added to damage control resuscitation, namely rewarming and correction of acidosis. The goal is to minimize the physiological insult on the patient and to improve outcome by decreasing the volume of blood loss. If all three components are adhered to, the amount of blood and blood products used will be reduced, with an improvement in 24 h mortality and a 2.5-fold improvement in 30-day mortality [11].

Permissive Hypotension

The aim of permissive hypotension is to maintain a lower systolic BP than normal until surgical control of the hemorrhage can be obtained. It was initially described in 1918 by Cannon et al. [12] and later reinforced by Bickell et al. in 1994, who showed an 8 % absolute reduction in mortality in hypotensive patients with penetrating torso trauma and delayed resuscitation until surgical control of the hemorrhage was obtained [13]. With hypotensive resuscitation only a limited amount of fluids are given to the patient. Aggressive resuscitation with saline-based fluids is associated with increased blood loss due to coagulopathy and the displacement of established clots. It is also associated with acidosis, cardiac dysfunction, increased abdominal compartment syndrome, severe inflammation and ARDS, multiple-organ failure, and increased mortality [14]. On the other hand restricting fluids contributes to systemic ischemia due to hypoperfusion. This ischemic stress can also cause coagulopathy and a systemic inflammatory response. An attempt to bridge this hypoperfusion with the use of vasopressors worsens outcome. The theory is that it causes capillary vasoconstriction, which worsens cellular ischemia [15, 16]. Some studies suggest that permissive hypotension should only be practiced for 90–120 min to avoid organ damage. The role for permissive hypotension is well described in penetrating trauma but the evidence is not clear on blunt trauma. It is yet to be established what would be safe in patients with head injuries and known cardiac patients. Morrison et all looked at 90 patients where the intraoperative mean arterial pressures were kept at 50 instead of 65 and found that less clear fluid and blood products were administered, and improved early postoperative survival and a trend to improved 30 day survival [17]. The ideal fluid for resuscitation should be a fluid that has oxygen-carrying capabilities, is able to reduce tissue ischemia and will not cause coagulopathy or inflammation. Unfortunately despite many pharmaceutical trails there is no perfect fluid at this stage. The overall current consensus among trauma surgeons is that crystalloids and colloids must be limited as much as possible. In the prehospital environment according the EAST and other guidelines, IV access should only be obtained in transit to hospital if the patient is not entrapped, and radial pulses should be used as indication for 250 ml fluid boluses. However, the controversy with crystalloids vs. colloids is an ongoing debate. Some studies suggest that colloids are better than crystalloids [18]; other studies suggest that colloids—especially the starches—cause coagulopathy and acute renal failure. A meta-analysis done to look at all fluids used for resuscitation in patients in hemorrhagic shock found there was no fluid that was better than another in mortality endpoints [19]. Initial studies suggested hypertonic saline to be the ideal resuscitation fluid in patients with traumatic brain injury and hypotension, but studies that were conducted by the Resuscitation Outcomes Consortium

(ROC) were stopped due to safety concerns. Currently hypertonic saline is not recommended for hypotensive resuscitation [20, 21].

Hemorrhagic Resuscitation

Early resuscitation with blood and blood products has been shown to reduce coagulopathy and mortality. Whole blood makes up the best resuscitation fluid and is being used by the US military. Due to limited availability and short shelf life of whole blood it is not readily used and components of blood are transfused separately. Military studies have shown a 46 % reduction in mortality in patients that required massive transfusion and were resuscitated with FFP–Blood in a 1:1 ratio. Platelets are added on to the ratio FFP–Blood–Platelets at 1:1:1 although there is very limited evidence to support this practice at the time of this writings. Part of the controversy is that the ratio does not constitute whole blood and only makes up a half to two-thirds of the active elements in blood. Currently, the first prospective study looking at the optimal ratio of blood, FFP, platelets, and other products is PROPPR (Pragmatic, randomized optimal platelet and plasma ratios) study. The thrombo-elastogram should still be used to guide component therapy [22]. Massive blood transfusion is defined as ten or more units of red blood cells in 24 h or more than 50 % of the blood volume in 3 h. Early activation of the massive transfusion protocol is essential in patients with ongoing bleeding; usually after the second unit is administered, the practitioner should activate the protocol if it is anticipated that the patient will need a massive transfusion. Early activation decreases the amount of blood products required as coagulopathy is better controlled due to early component transfusion. The recognition of the impact of coagulopathy in trauma developed an interest in pharmaceutical agents that could help with clotting:

- Factor VII a: Factor VII a plays a major role in the initiation phase of clot formation. Several studies confirmed it decreased transfusion requirements in blunt trauma but not in penetrating trauma. However, it has shown no effect on mortality [23, 24] and is very expensive.
- Fibrinogen: Fibrinogen is depleted earlier than other clotting factors and can be given as fibrinogen concentrate or as part of cryoprecipitate (Fibrinogen, factor VIII, and Factor XIII and von Willebrand factor). Current evidence shows no benefit unless thromboelastography has shown a deficiency, and the large number of required donors increases the risk for infections.
- Tranexamic Acid: Tranexamic acid inhibits plasmin, which plays a vital role in coagulation and inflammation. A large randomized control study (Crash-2) showed a reduction in mortality when administered early in bleeding patients [25]; however, further high powered studies are required to confirm its role. Similar antifibrinolytics include aprotinin and aminocaproic.
- Calcium: Calcium plays a vital role in coagulation and is an important cofactor for various enzymes. Levels must be continuously monitored during massive transfusion and should be replaced when depleted. Component resuscitation in a coagulopathic patient should only be done using thromboelastogram or ROTEG.

Early control of hemorrhage is also part of hemorrhagic resuscitation. Tourniquet has recently been extensively used to control extremity bleeding. Local hemostatic agents have been developed and form a large part of hemorrhage control.

It is a very commercially driven part and there are numerous products that can be used and include amongst others:

- Factor concentrators [26]: These products concentrate the clotting factors by rapidly absorbing the water in the blood.
- Mucoadhesives: These products adhere to the adjacent tissues to form a plug to bleeding wounds.
- Pro-coagulant supplementors: These products contain clotting factors that are delivered into

a bleeding wound and promote clotting. Local hemostatic agents, while they do not replace surgical techniques and should not be used with active arterial bleeds as the sole treatment method, can be helpful. The development of cellulose minisponges that can be placed into cavities with severe incompressible hemorrhage have proven to have a significant reduction of hemorrhage and have reduced transfusion requirements and improved outcome [23]. High-frequency argon beams can be also used on raw surfaces.

The Development of Hemorrhagic Shock Management

Rewarming the Patient

Preventing or reversing hypothermia is part of resuscitation. Rewarming the patient should be started at the torso rather than the extremities to prevent acidosis and hypotension due to peripheral vasodilatation. The following three methods of rewarming are most frequently used:

1. Passive external warming (blankets and ambient temperature)
2. Active external warming (warm air devices)
3. Active internal warming (warm fluids and blood, irrigation via an intercostal drain, warm fluid gastric lavage, or washing of the abdomen with warm fluids)

Correcting Acidosis

The best way to correct acidosis is stopping the bleeding and ensuring optimal resuscitation and restoration of end-organ perfusion. Currently, base excess and lactate are used most commonly to monitor end points of resuscitation. The initial levels and the level of clearance of lactate correlate with the mortality of the patient. There is no convincing data to support the use of bicarbonate in patients with a pH less than 7.2.

Damage Control Surgery as a Team Approach

Damage control surgery is a team approach where the main goal is to limit surgery time, to control the bleeding and contamination and minimize the physiological insult.

Each team member plays a vital role in ensuring the best possible outcome. The following steps must be adhered to:

1. The operating theatre is warmer than usual.
2. The *nursing staff* must ensure that all possible equipment that may be required is readily available (this includes, but is not limited to gastrointestinal staplers, nasogastric tubes for shunts, suture materials, vacuum dressings, vascular sets, etc.). Patients with torso injuries must be prepped and draped from the chin to the knees (Fig. 14.1), and areas not being

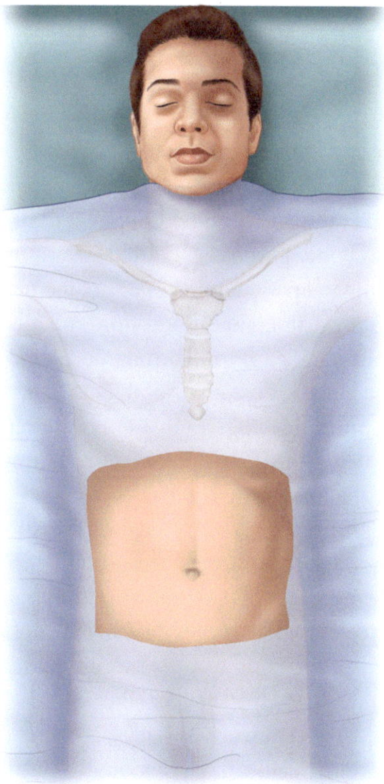

Fig. 14.1 Draping of the patient should allow access to all potential cavities. Areas not used should be covered to prevent hypothermia

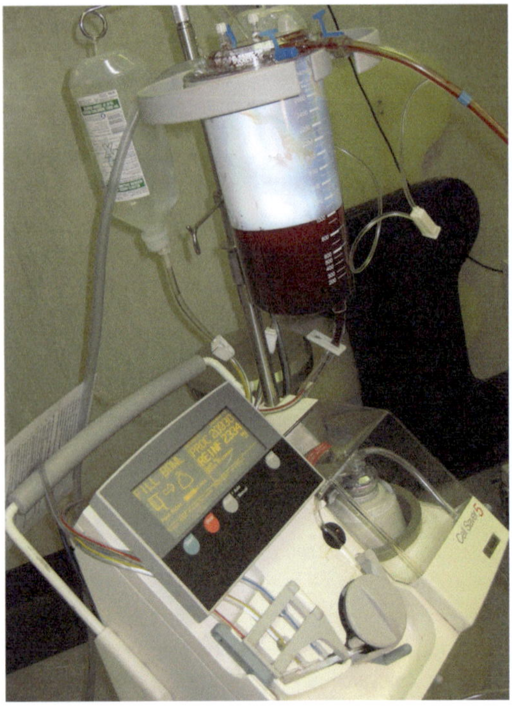

Fig. 14.2 Cell saver (Cell Saver® 5, Harmonetics, Braintree, MA)

operated on must be covered. The nursing staff must ensure that accurate records are kept of swab count and all blood must be removed for cell saving purposes. Folded swabs must be kept on the patient upon opening the peritoneal cavity, warm blankets and fluid must be available to prevent hypothermia, and local hemostatic agents must be available as required.

3. The *anesthesiologist* must continue resuscitation using the damage control principles, prepare the autologous blood recovery system for cell saving (Fig. 14.2), ensure the surgeon is completely ready prior to administering any muscle relaxants or putting the patient to sleep, and give prophylactic antibiotics and repeat if the patient loses more than his blood volume. Perhaps the anesthesiologist's team most important role is that of keeping the surgeon informed of the physiologic status of the patient (i.e., inotropic requirements, blood gases, and vital signs) as the surgeon may need to change to damage control if the surgical findings and response to treatment do not correlate. Is the surgeon missing something or is in the wrong cavity?
4. The *surgeon* must keep everyone in theatre informed about the injuries found and the future management plan, as well as have the ability to change to damage control if the injuries are more severe than initially anticipated or if the patient deteriorated.
5. The *blood bank* needs to have an established massive transfusion protocol that can be activated immediately.

The intensive care unit personnel must be able to continue with resuscitation and ensure the coagulopathy, acidosis and hypothermia is reversed. The most difficult part of ICU management is to differentiate between coagulopathy that requires ongoing resuscitation versus a surgical bleed that needs to go back to operating theatre. With surgical bleed, it will be nearly impossible to correct the patient's physiological parameters without surgical control; however, it is ill advised to send an unstable patient to theatre unnecessarily and compromise the resuscitation. Embolization should be considered before transfer to ICU or at any point thereafter.

Damage Control Laparotomy for Solid Organ Injuries

Liver

One of the most common organs when damage control has been applied is liver. When the liver is identified as the source of bleeding the principles of "Ps" is used to control the bleeding and perform damage control:

- "Push"—Pushing the edges of the liver together and restoring the anatomy as much as possible can cease the bleeding. This will allow time to plan the next steps and provide an impression of what might be needed to stop the bleeding.
- "Pringle"—If pushing does not work, the Pringle maneuver is used to stop the inflow of blood. With a Pringle maneuver, the Foramen

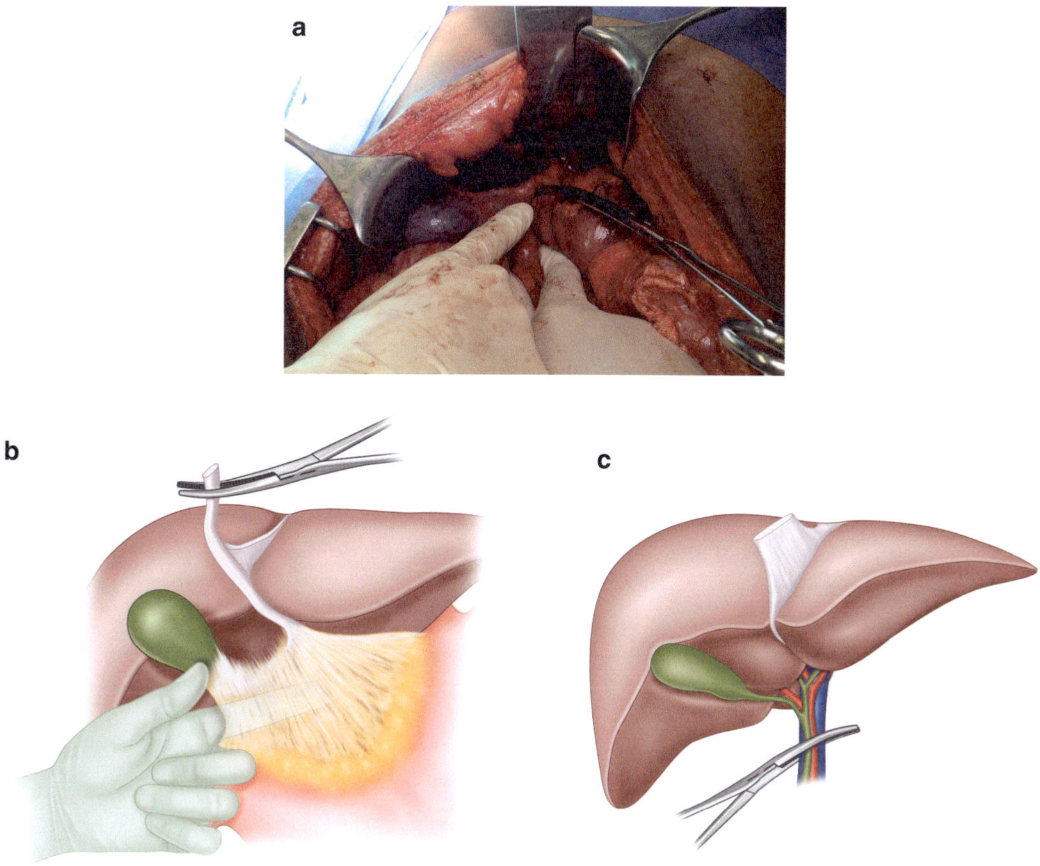

Fig. 14.3 (**a**) Pringle maneuver being applied. (**b**) With a Pringle, the hand gets inserted into the Foramen of Winslow to help to identify the area to apply the clamp and see the efficiency of a Pringle. (**c**) Schematic diagram of a soft noncrushing clamp (can also use a Foley's) to do a Pringle cutting of the inflow (common bile duct, hepatic artery, and portal vein)

of Winslow must be located at the free edge of the lesser omentum, where the common bile duct, hepatic artery, and portal vein are found. The inflow can be controlled by putting a soft bowel clamp, direct finger pressure or by making a hole through the lesser omentum and putting a Foley's catheter around the bundle (Fig. 14.3a–c). If the Pringle does not control the bleeding it may indicate that some of the bleeding is coming from the hepatic veins. With the Pringle the bleeding will slow down enough to allow suture ligation of individual vessels or the use a LIGACLIP. After hemostasis is obtained the Pringle must be removed to determine if the bleeding has stopped.

- "Plug"—In patients with a gunshot wound of the liver the tract has small entrance and exit wounds, making it very difficult to control individual vessels without opening a large incision into the liver. For this injury a Caltostat plug or a Sengstaken Blakemore tube for balloon tamponade can be used (Fig. 14.4a, b).
- "Packing"—In packing of the liver vectors are created with the pack that will restore normal anatomy and tamponade the bleed. Packs between the liver and the diaphragm should be put in gently, as they may compromise ventilation, and potentially compromise vena cava. When packing, the liver is pushed up and

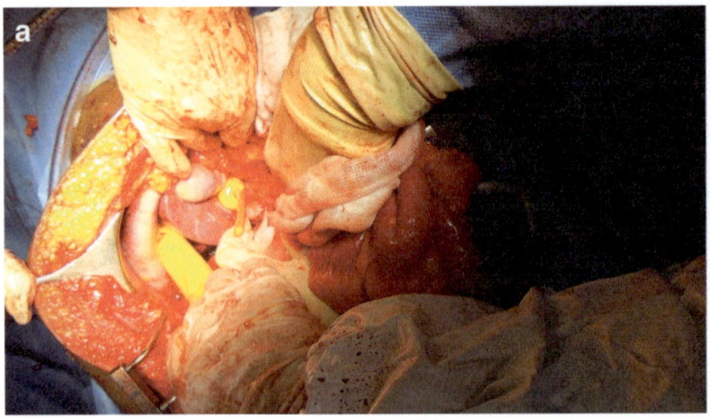

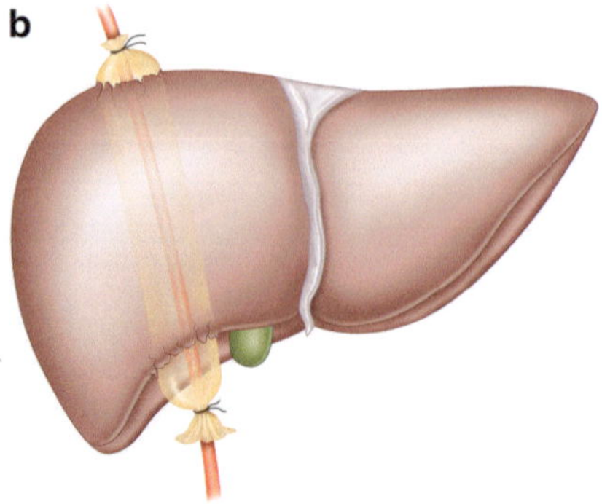

Fig. 14.4 (**a**) Sengstaken Blakemore tube inserted for GSW liver. (**b**) Schematic diagram of the Sengstaken in this GSW liver

laterally with folded swabs. If there was a major arterial bleed the patient can go for angio-embolization of selective branches before the relook is done. On occasion, surgical selective vascular isolations should be used.

With retro-hepatic IVC injuries the liver should not be mobilized and should be packed. Atrio-caval shunts are very ambitious, perhaps even desperate, with an almost 100 % mortality. Two major pitfalls of packing the liver is over-packing or under-packing. Over-packing compromises venous return to the heart by compressing the IVC and causes hypotension. Under-packing is when the packing is not effective enough to control the bleed and the packs are quickly soaked with blood. Wrapping the liver in a Vicryl mesh requires extensive mobilization and takes time, does not offer any more benefit than packing, and should not be used during damage control. Resection of a segment of the liver should be avoided during damage control unless the trauma has done most of the resection and it is the only way to get control of the hemorrhage. Drains are always left in the right upper quadrant after closure of the abdomen for severe liver injuries to prevent bile collections. The incidence of biliary complications post damage control is 15 %. Most of these complications can be treated with ERCP and stenting or a pigtail to drain biliary collections [27].

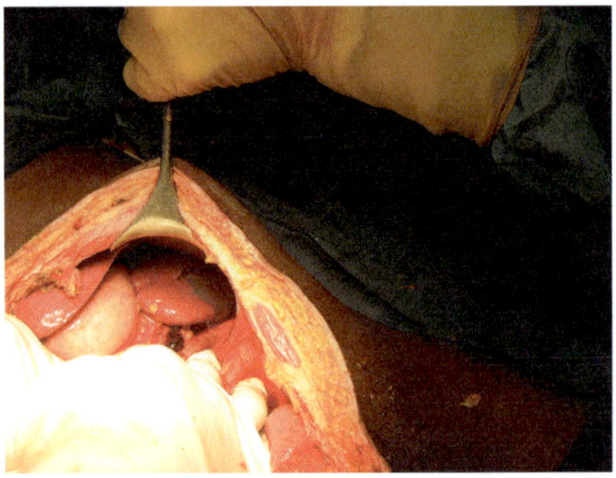

Fig. 14.5 Splenic laceration

Spleen

Several splenic preserving maneuvers are described including partial splenectomy or wrapping the spleen in a Vicryl mesh. In damage control, however, there is no place for spleen salvage since the simplest laceration (Fig. 14.5) might bleed later when the patient is coagulopathic. Splenectomy is a far safer option. Post-splenectomy oozing from the splenic bed is possible and may require packing. Placement of drains post splenectomy is still controversial, with some surgeons leaving the drains in situ in order to monitor bleeding and leaks from the pancreas.

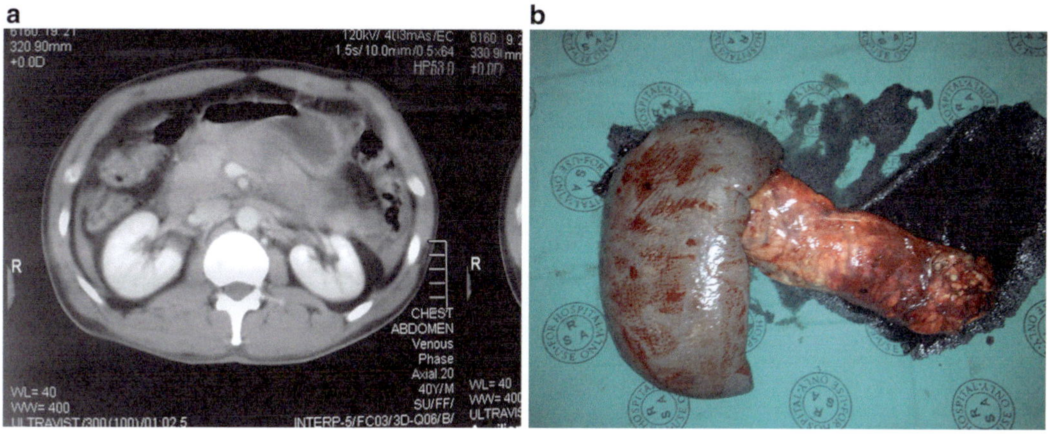

Fig. 14.6 CT scan (**a**) and distal pancreatectomy and splenectomy (**b**)

Kidney

All zone II penetrating retroperitoneal hematoma or those that are rapidly expanding must be explored. In blunt trauma, on the other hand, if the hematoma is not expanding, try to avoid opening Gerota's fascia since it is associated with a high nephrectomy rate. In Grade IV and Grade V renal injuries a nephrectomy must be done as part of damage control. If there is mild ooze the kidney can be packed. Selective renal artery embolization can be done in areas of small blush if the patient is stable.

Pancreas

Small pancreatic lacerations that bleed can be controlled with hemostatic sutures and packing. Large lacerations with ductal disruptions to the left of the superior mesenteric vessels are usually treated with a distal pancreatectomy. In damage control situations a splenectomy with a distal pancreatectomy is done to save time (Fig. 14.6a, b). With large lacerations to the right of the superior mesenteric vessels the hemorrhage is controlled with hemostatic sutures and packing. Pancreatic leaks are managed with large drains. Delayed collections can be drained by percutaneous pigtail or with an Endoscopic Retrograde Cholangiopancreatography (ERCP).

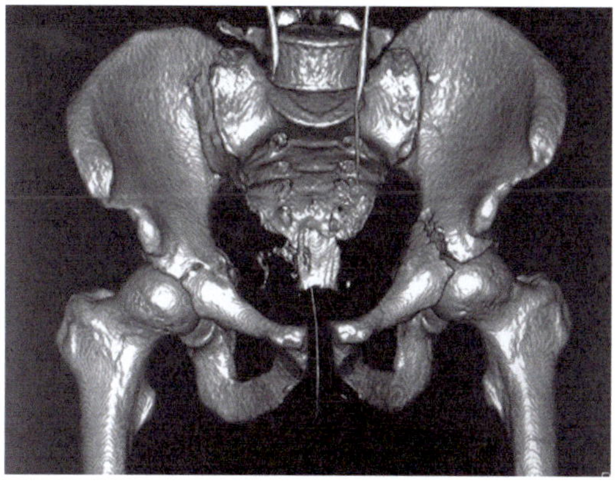

Fig. 14.7 Pelvic fracture with right SI joint disruption, bilateral acetabulum fractures. Had a sheath applied for hemodynamic instability

Pelvis

In a hemodynamically unstable patient, part of the initial resuscitation is tying down of the pelvis with a wrapping sheath or a pelvic binder (Fig. 14.7). The sheath must be positioned over the greater trochanters. If angiography is immediately available, angio-embolization of the bleeding vessels is recommended. Both internal iliac arteries can be embolized. Unlike selective embolization, injecting gelatin sponge particle is much faster, promotes clotting, and allows for some distal organ perfusion.

In most centers, angio-embolization is not easily accessible, and embolization itself takes a long time. In this case, if the patient remains unstable after tying the pelvis they must be taken to operating theatre for a laparotomy and extraperitoneal packing of the pelvis [28]. In the case of extraperitoneal packing a space is created anterior to the bladder, blunt dissected downwards, the peritoneum is mobilized medially, and packing is started posterior from the sacrum. If obvious bleeding arterial vessels are visible a LIGACLIP can be used to stop the bleeding. Abdominal laps are packed into this space and the lower sheath closed.

The use of intra-aortic balloons to occlude the aorta has been described in severe hemorrhagic shock due to unstable pelvic fractures [29]. Early open reduction and internal fixation (ORIF) of the pelvic bones was always thought to be associated with increased hemorrhage and mortality. For this reason the pelvic binder or sheath is left on until relook and removal of the packs. The orthopedic surgeons will then do a staged ORIF of the pelvis. Some studies suggest that it might be beneficial to do the ORIF in the acute setting, which has shown similar results [30]. At this stage it is dependent on the expertise available.

Damage Control for Hollow Organ Injuries

After liver packing, hollow organ injuries are most common organs treated with damage control. This is usually done quickly using stapler or ligation, which basically controls the contamination and bleeding from mesentery. In the following section, we will address briefly each organ injured. It is up to the surgeon and patient's physiology to dictate what operation is usually done.

Stomach

The majority of stomach injuries will be repaired as part of damage control due to good blood supply and proximity. When a quick repair is done, the stitches are left long so that on relook the quality of the repair can be reviewed.

Duodenum

Primary repair is the best damage control for the duodenum due to the position and poor results with delayed repair. Pyloric exclusion is becoming less popular due to a high rate of complications [31] and pancreatico-doudenectomy as part of damage control surgery has an exceptionally high mortality.

Small Bowel

Complete occlusion of bowel lumen used to be the standard for bowel injuries or mesenteric tears. Current practice, however, allows the preservation of some gut lumen by either staple or ties to reduce the risk of bacterial translocation [32].

Special care should be taken to suture ligate mesenteric bleeders since they tend to present with delayed bleeds when the blood pressure has been restored and the patient is coagulopathic (Fig. 14.8a, b).

Colon

Colon injuries are also tied or stapled off as part of damage control. In the past all colonic injuries were brought out as a stoma as definitive management but Miller, Chang et al. showed that delayed colonic anastomosis is safe [33].

Rectum

For intraperitoneal rectal injuries primary repair is adequate. For extraperitoneal injury a colostomy should be done as a definitive and delayed procedure. Washing out the distal rectal stump was standard protocol previously but is no longer done as it is thought that the feces are pushed into the tissue. Patients should be monitored for potential pre-sacral abscess.

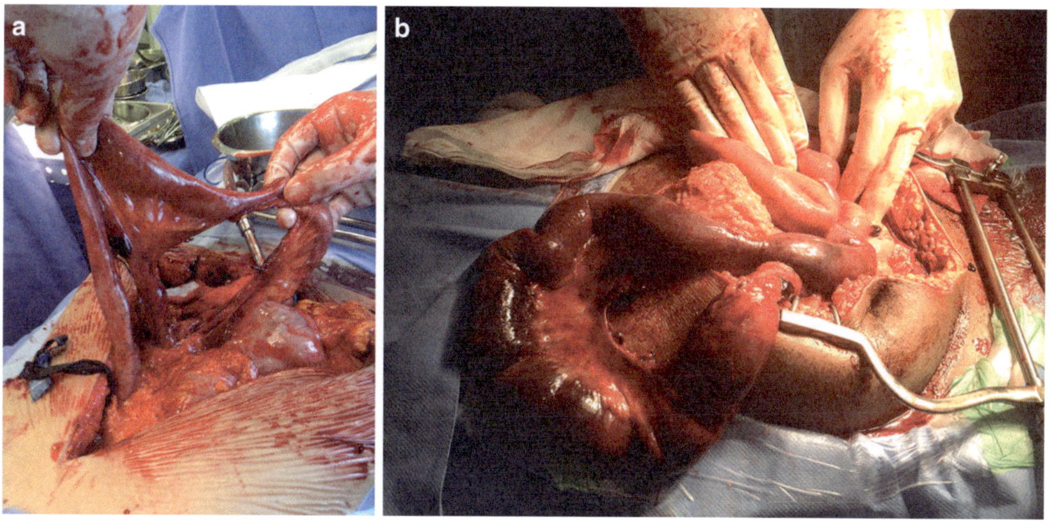

Fig. 14.8 (**a**) MVC with free fluid and no solid organ injury on CT scan. Multiple mesenteric tears. (**b**) Dead bowel due to mesenteric tear

Biliary Tract Injuries

Any injury to the gallbladder requires a cholecystectomy.

Minor damage to the bile ducts can be controlled with a T-tube whilst with severe injuries the bile duct should be ligated. On relook with a stable patient a hepatico-jejunostomy can be done, if the patient remains unstable, a drain can be inserted to drain the bile.

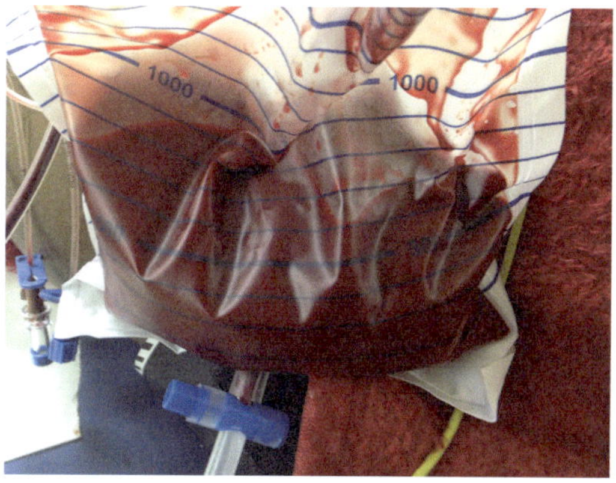

Fig. 14.9 Hematuria with a bladder rupture

Ureter and Bladder Injuries

Ureters can be drained and repaired over via a double J stent. Alternatively, external drainage can be obtained with a small nasogastric tube. In extreme situations the ureters may be ligated and a nephrostomy done later.

All intraperitoneal bladder ruptures must be repaired whilst an extraperitoneal bladder rupture can be treated with a Foley's catheter decompressing the bladder for 10 days. Extraperitoneal bladder injury repairs must be considered if the patient requires a laparotomy for any other indication, if there are bone fragments in the bladder wall that might compromise healing and any associated intraperitoneal injuries. In the past all bladder repairs used to have suprapubic and transurethral catheters placed in order to decompress the bladder. Current evidence shows that placement of a transurethral catheter on its own is sufficient (Fig. 14.9).

Abdominal Vascular Injuries

Aorta

All suprarenal aortas should be repaired and infrarenal aortic injuries can be either repaired or shunted. Depending on the level of the lesion,

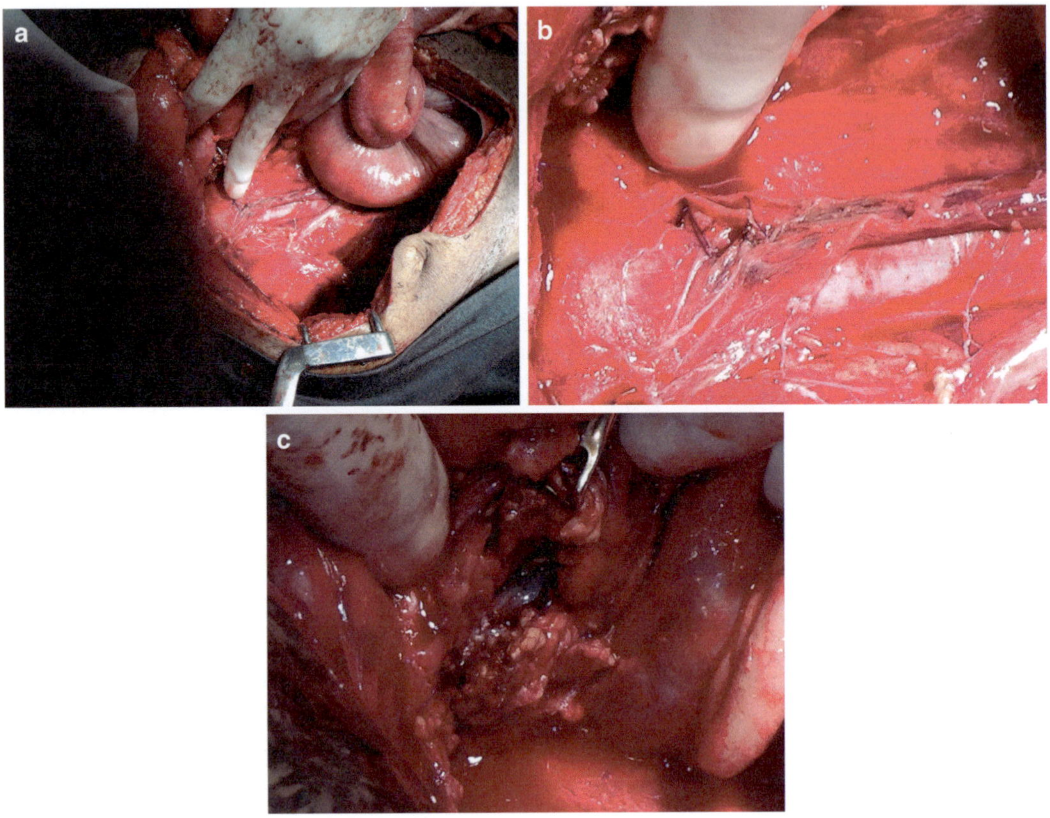

Fig. 14.10 (**a–c**) Stab abdomen through the head of the pancreas with right visceral rotation for IVC and portal vein repair

the size of the hematoma and the patients stability, proximal control can either obtained via the intrathoracic, supra-celiac, or infrarenal route. If the patient is stable an intra-aortic balloon can be used to get proximal control.

A left anterolateral thoracotomy is used to get intrathoracic control. The lung is mobilized anteriorly, the mediastinal pleura is opened, and a vascular clamp is applied to the aorta. For supra-celiac control the left lobe of the liver must be mobilized and the lesser omentum opened. For infrarenal control a left visceral rotation is done. If the possibility of tamponade release prior to proximal control exists, the left mesocolon can be divided to get control prior to visceral rotation.

The *celiac artery* and inferior *mesenteric artery* can be ligated. The superior mesenteric artery must be repaired or shunted.

Inferior Vena Cava

A right visceral rotation and Kocherization of the duodenum can obtain exposure of the IVC (Fig. 14.10a–c). Control of the bleeding can then be obtained with proximal and distal compression with swabs. The IVC should not be mobilized, as this will cause tears of the posterior lumbar vessels and bleeding.

The IVC is usually repaired with PROLENE. If a posterior laceration needs to be sutured, the anterior wound is extended and the posterior wound is sutured from inside the vessel. There tends to be ooze from the suture line that will usually stop bleeding with mild pressure or with a hemostatic agent. The infrarenal vena cava can be ligated. Ligation of the suprarenal vena cava however is associated with a high morbidity and mortality and should thus be avoided. Adequate packing of the

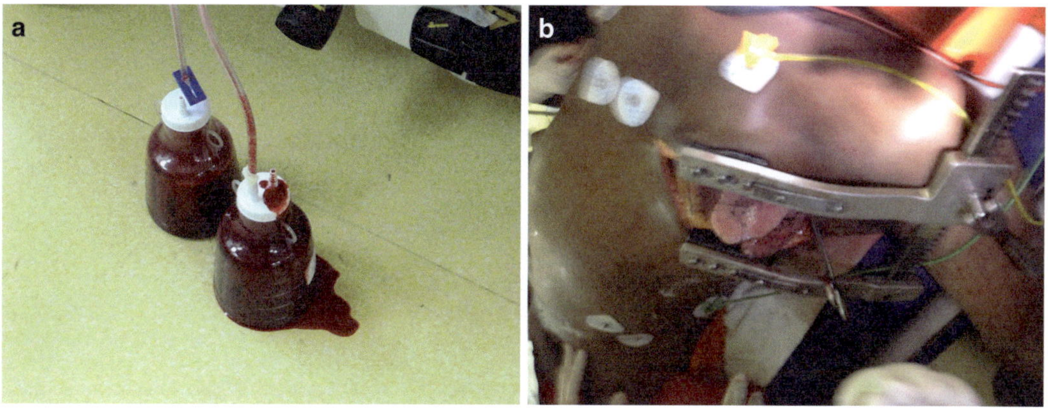

Fig. 14.11 (**a**, **b**) Massive hemothorax and emergency room thoracotomy

IVC, due to low-pressure system, can control the hemorrhage and is the treatment of choice for retro-hepatic IVC injuries.

The *hepatic artery* can be ligated. Ligation of the *portal vein* can be cautiously done but is associated with a high mortality. If both are injured at least one must be repaired or shunted.

Thoracic Damage Control

Thoracic damage control is often definitive repair due to the extent of the injuries but with the emphasis on simpler and quicker procedures. Emergency room thoracotomy is part of damage control surgery in the chest (Fig. 14.11a, b).

The choice of incision will often determine how successful the operation will be. The suspected injuries and the stability of the patient should guide you as to the best and most appropriate incision. A number of incision used currently have not changed over time. These include median sternotomy, anterolateral thoracotomy, and posterolateral thoracotomies. In emergency trauma setting, the most common incision is emergency anterolateral thoracotomy for cardiac injuries.

Packing in the abdomen is well described, but packing in the chest is much more complex due to cardiopulmonary physiology and dynamic movement of thoracic structures. Thoracic cavity packing is usually applied as a last resort in patients who have defuse oozing from the thoracic wall secondary to multiple fractures of the ribs. Packing the thoracic cavity after blunt trauma can cause cardiac dysrhythmias when next to the heart. Packing of the upper mediastinum and the apex of the pleural cavities is better tolerated [34, 35].

Conclusion

Damage control most certainly improves mortality but at the cost of a higher morbidity, longer hospital and ICU stay and increased theatre procedures. Hence, choosing the patient that will benefit most from damage control, and avoidance of overuse, is vitally important [36]. It can be used just about in any of the cavities and organs.

References

1. Steward RM, Myers JG, Dent DL, et al. Seven hundred fifty-three consecutive deaths in a level one trauma center: the argument for injury prevention. J Trauma. 2003;54:66–70.
2. Pringle JH. Notes on the arrest of hepatic hemorrhage due to trauma. Ann Surg. 1908;48:541–9.
3. Holcomb JB. The 2004 Fitts. Lecture: current perspective on combat casualty care. J Trauma. 2005; 59:990–1002.

4. Abrams ST, Zhang N, Manson J. Circulating histones are mediators of trauma-associated lung injury. Am J Respir Crit care Med. 2013;187(2):160–9.
5. Kashuk JL, Moore EE, Millikan JS, Moore JB. The bloody vicious cycle. J Trauma. 1982;22:672–9.
6. Kaafarani HM, Velmahos GC. Damage control resuscitation in Trauma. Scand J Surg 2014 Apr 28:103 (2):81–88
7. Meng ZH, Wolberg AS, Monroe III DM, et al. The effect of temperature and pH on the activity of Factor VIIa: implications for the efficacy of high-dose factor VIIa in hypothermic and acidotic patients. J Trauma. 2003;55(5):886–91.
8. Martini WZ, Pusateri AE, Uscilowicz JM, et al. Independent contributions of hypothermia and acidosis to coagulopathy in swine. J Trauma. 2005;58(5): 1002–9.
9. Rotondo MF, Schwab CW, McGonigal MD, Phillips 3rd GR, Fruchterman TM, Kauder DR, et al. "Damage control": an approach for improved survival in exsanguinating penetrating abdominal injury. J Trauma. 1993;35:375–82.
10. Holcomb JB, Jenkins D, Rhee P, Johannigman J, Mahoney P, Mehta S, et al. Damage control resuscitation: directly addressing the early coagulopathy of trauma. J Trauma. 2007;62:307–10.
11. Cotton BA, Reddy NBS, Hatch QM. Damage control resuscitation is associated with a reduction in resuscitation volumes and improvement in survival in 390 damage control laparotomies. Ann Surg. 2011; 254(4):598–605.
12. Cannon W, Fraser J, Cowell E. The preventative treatment of wound shock. JAMA. 1918;70:618.
13. Bickell WH, Wall Jr MJ, Pepe PE, Martin RR, Ginger VF, Allen MK, et al. Immediate versus delayed fluid resuscitation for hypotensive patients with penetrating torso injuries. N Engl J Med. 1994;331:1105–9.
14. Cotton BA, Guys JS, Morris Jr JA, Abumrad NN. The cellular, metabolic and systemic consequences of aggressive fluid resuscitation strategies. Shock. 2006;26:115–21.
15. Sperry JL, Menei JP, Frankel HL, et al. Early use of vasopressors after injury: caution before vasoconstriction. J Trauma. 2008;64:9–14.
16. Plurad DS, Talving P, Lam L, Inaba K, Green D, Demetriades D. Early vasopressor use in critical injury is associated with mortality independent from volume status. J Trauma Injury Infect Crit Care. 2011;71:656–72.
17. Morrison CA, Carrick MM, Norman MA, et al. Hypotensive resuscitation strategy reduces transfusion requirements and severe postoperative coagulopathy in trauma patients with hemorrhagic shock: preliminary results of a randomized controlled trial. J Trauma. 2011;70(3):652–63.
18. Guidry C, Gleeson E, Simms E. Initial assessment on the impact of crystalloids versus colloids during damage control resuscitation. J Surg Res. 2013;185:294–9.
19. Gruen RL, Brohi K, Schreiber M, Balogh ZJ, Pitt V, NArayan M, Maier RV. Hemorrhage control in severely injured patients. Lancet. 2012;380:1099–108.
20. Bulger EM, May S, Brasel KJ, et al. Out-of-hospital hypertonic resuscitation following severe traumatic brain injury: a randomized controlled trial. JAMA. 2010;304(13):1455–64.
21. Bulger EM, May S, Kerby KJ, et al. Out-of-hospital hypertonic resuscitation after traumatic hypovolemic shock: a randomized, placebo controlled trial. Ann Surg. 2011;253(3):431–41.
22. Jansen JO, Thomas R, Loudon MA, Brooks A. Damage control resuscitation for patients with major trauma. BMJ. 2009;338:1436–40.
23. Boffard KD, Riou B, Warren B. Recombinant factor VIIa as a adjunctive therapy for bleeding control in severely injured trauma patients: two parallel randomized, placebo-controlled, double-blind clinical trails. J Trauma Injury Infect Crit Care. 2005;59:8–18.
24. Hauser CJ, Boffard K, Dutton R, et al. Results of the CONTROL trial: efficacy and safety of recombinant activated Factor VII in the management of refractory traumatic hemorrhage. J Trauma Injury Infect Crit Care. 2010;69:489–500.
25. CRASH-2 Collaborators. Effects of tranexamic acid on death, vascular occlusive events, and blood transfusions in patients with significant hemorrhage: a randomized placebo-controlled trail. Lancet. 2010;376:23–32.
26. Mueller GR, Pineda TJ, Xie HX, Teach JS. A novel sponge-based wound stasis dressing to treat lethal non-compressible hemorrhage. J Trauma Acute Care Surg. 2012;73:134–9.
27. Hommes M, Kazemier G, Schep NWL. Management of biliary complications following damage control surgery for liver trauma. Eur J Trauma Emerg Surg. 2013;39:511–6.
28. White CE, Hsu JR, Holcomb JB. Haemodynamically unstable pelvic fracture. Injury. 2008;40:1023–30.
29. Martinelli T, Thony F, Declety P. Intra-aortic balloon occlusion to salvage patients with life-threatening hemorrhagic shock from pelvic fractures. J Trauma. 2010;68:942–8.
30. Enninhorst N, Toth L, King KL. Acute definitive Internal Fixation of pelvic ring fractures in polytrauma patients: A feasible option. J Trauma. 2010;68(4):935–41.
31. Mayberry J, Fabricant L, Anton A. Am Surg. 2011;77:681–4.
32. Wang P, Wei X, et al. Influences of intestinal ligation on bacterial translocation and inflammatory response in rats with hemorrhagic shock: implication for damage control surgery. J Invest Surg. 2008;21(5):244.
33. Miller PR, Chang MC, Hoth JJ, Holmes 4th JH, Meredith JW. Colonic resection in the setting of damage control laparotomy: is delayed anastomosis safe. Ann Surg. 2007;73(6):606–9.
34. Rotondo MF, Bard MR. Damage control surgery for thoracic injuries. Injury Int JCare Injured. 2004;35: 649–54.
35. Wall Jr MJ, Soltero E. Damage control for thoracic injuries. Surg Clin North Am. 1997;77(4):863–78.
36. Higa G, Friese R, O'Keeffe T, Wynne J, Bowlby P, Ziemba M, Latifi R, Kulvatunyou N, Rhee P. Damage control Laparotomy: a vital tool once overused. J Trauma. 2010;69:53–9.

Multiorgan Dysfunction in Trauma and Surgical Intensive Care Units

15

Ayman Ahmed El-Menyar, Mohammad Asim, and Hassan Al-Thani

Introduction

Multiple organ dysfunction syndrome (MODS) is a systemic, dysfunctional inflammatory response that requires longer intensive care unit (ICU) stay and is associated with higher rate of mortality (27–100 %) depending upon the number of organs involved [1–3]. MODS is the leading cause of mortality in those patients who survived the initial hours after trauma [2] and is a major driver of high hospital cost. Generally, the cause of post-injury MODS involves a mixed layering of patient, injury, and treatment factors. However, a deregulated immunological response is the key factor that governs the pathophysiology of post-injury MODS [3].

Irrespective of injury mechanism, all trauma patients could develop a resuscitated clinical state of systemic hyperinflammation known as "systemic inflammatory response syndrome" (SIRS). A mild to moderate SIRS response might be both beneficial and compensatory in the early stage and resolves in the majority of patients as they recover. However, organ failure occurs if this inflammatory response is exaggerated or sustained, leading to MODS. The initial magnitude of post-injury inflammatory response is dependent on the amount of tissue injury, the degree of shock, and host factors [4].

Initially, MODS is thought to be an overwhelming, uncontrolled sepsis response. However, this concept has been modified after the introduction of "Bimodal model" of MODS and recognition that early MODS is unrelated to sepsis. The one-event model corresponds to massive SIRS response that has the potential to cause early multiple organ failure. While, in two-event model, patient who was initially resuscitated to a mild or moderate systemic inflammation (primed) are vulnerable to a second (activating) event that leads to dysfunctional hyper-inflammation and organ dysfunction [1, 5]. Lung dysfunction is the primary indicator of early MODS development which may occur in the majority of post-injury MODS patients. On an average, lung dysfunction

A.A. El-Menyar, M.D., F.R.C.P(Glasg). (✉)
Department of Surgery, Clinical Research, Hamad General Hospital & Clinical Medicine,Weill Cornell Medical College, Trauma Main Office, Quality Management Building, PO Box 3050, Doha, Qatar
e-mail: elmenyar@yahoo.com

M. Asim, Ph.D.
Department of Surgery, Clinical Research, Hamad General Hospital, Trauma Main Office, Quality Management Building, PO Box 3050, Doha, Qatar
e-mail: Asim.jmi@gmail.com

H. Al-Thani, M.D.
Department of Surgery, Trauma Surgery Section, Hamad General Hospital, Trauma Main Office, Quality Management Building, PO Box 3050, Doha, Qatar
e-mail: althanih@hotmail.com

R. Latifi et al. (eds.), *Technological Advances in Surgery, Trauma and Critical Care*,
DOI 10.1007/978-1-4939-2671-8_15

precedes cardiac dysfunction by 0.6 days, hepatic dysfunction by 4.8 days, and renal dysfunction by 5.5 days [1, 5]. The failures of other organ systems can be associated with or without sepsis, and usually occurs after 72 h (late MODS). Such patients require a second insult to progress to MODS, and this is often caused by sepsis due to compensatory anti-inflammatory syndrome. Nosocomial pneumonia, a common ICU complication, is the major infection associated with late MODS [1, 6].

Epidemiology of MODS

Interestingly, the overall incidence, morbidity, and mortality of MODS have been reduced during the past few decades. It is noteworthy that the advancement of prehospital care and resuscitation attributed to such reduction, which eventually improved the early survival rate in severe trauma patients. However, still there is an increased risk of late MODS (developed 4–10 days post injury) in trauma patients mainly due to development of sepsis which leads to extended ICU stay and deaths in vast majority of cases [7, 8]. Particularly, the reported incidence of post-injury MODS varies from 7 to 66 % and the MODS-related mortality ranges from 31 to 80 % in severe trauma patients [9]. An earlier prospective study from United States observed 25 % incidence of MODS among high-risk severe trauma patients [10]. Similarly, a multicenter prospective cohort study reported the overall incidence of MODS to be 29 % in blunt trauma patients [11]. However, during the past few years, investigators have observed either a marginal reduction [10, 12] or no overall change in MODS incidence among trauma patients [13].

A retrospective analysis of 31,154 severely injured trauma patients (mean age: 45 years, 73 % males, mean ISS: 28, blunt trauma: 96 %) over 10-years identified 33 % incidence of MODS from the nationwide prospective database in Germany [14]. Though, the incidence of MODS has significantly increased (24.6–31.5 %), but the mortality rate among MODS patients has declined (42.6 % vs. 33.3 %) during the study period (2002–2011). Moreover, the MODS patients were older in age, sustained severe injuries and require longer ICU stay as compared to non-MODS patients. Frohlich and colleagues [14] also observed an increasing trend of age in MODS patients, which reflects the general demographic changes among aging German population. However, a recent study from Australia reported a lesser incidence (15 %) and mortality (24 %) among post-injury MODS patients [8]. In addition, MODS patients showed three-fold higher ICU stay and require 4 times greater ventilatory days in comparison to non-MODS patients. Sauaia et al. [15] presented the temporal trend of MODS in post-injury patients enrolled from four institutions during 2003–2010. The study included 1,643 trauma patients, of which 13.6 % developed MODS. Though, the incidence of MODS declined from 17 to 9.8 % over the years but, the rate of mortality, ICU stay, and duration of mechanical ventilation in MODS patients remains unchanged.

Furthermore, the incidence and mortality of MODS patients also depend upon the mechanism of injury. Patients who sustained blunt trauma developed MODS more frequently and had higher mortality rate in comparison to patients with penetrating injuries [7, 16]. It has also been observed that greater proportion of trauma patients developed late MODS (60 %) which mainly depends on the length of resuscitation, need of blood transfusion, development of pneumonia and sepsis [17, 18]. On the other hand, the incidence of early MODS is relatively lower (40 %) which usually reflects the host response to injury [19].

Understanding the Pathophysiology and Mechanisms of MODS

To date various hypotheses have proposed possible pathophysiology and underlying mechanisms of MODS. Some investigators have suggested uncontrolled, occult sepsis as the initiator of MODS [20, 21]. However, others have reported lesser association with infectious complications and suggested that MODS is primarily triggered by a SIRS caused by host immune response to tissue injury [22, 23]. Of note, unusual SIRS plays a central role in the pathogenesis of MODS [23]. It has been established that various mechanisms of MODS have overlapping events and multiple sequential insults are involved in the pathogenesis of MODS as suggested by the two-hit model [24]. According to this model an initial insult leads to priming of host immune cells followed by an excessive SIRS on the second insult which eventually evolves into overt MODS. Studies focusing on the mechanism and pathogenesis of end-organ injury and MODS in trauma patients have observed a cause-effect relationship [25]. Specifically, in such patients three possible pathophysiologic events have been proposed which are based on time and extent of tissue injury. First of all ischemia is considered as the primary event in pathophysiology of MODS that results from persistent and progressive splanchnic vasoconstriction and hypoperfusion [26]. The second hypothesis is *the gut-derived systemic inflammatory response,* which is caused by the ischemic gut [27]. It describes that injury causes decline in gut barrier which facilitates translocation of gut microorganisms to distant organs that activates SIRS and ultimately culminates in MODS. The third possible mechanism is the *development of ionic-disequilibrium* that leads to fluid shifts at the cellular and capillary level after injury [28].

Moreover, it has been established that various host immune cells and pro- and anti-inflammatory cytokines play an important role in the pathophysiology of MODS. Innate immune cells release pro-inflammatory mediators such as interleukins, tumor necrosis factor, and platelet activation factor (PAF) in response to local inflammation [9]. Particularly, predominance of pro-inflammatory cytokines leads to SIRS, whereas exaggeration of anti-inflammatory cytokines is responsible for immunosuppression which results in infection, sepsis, and MODS [29]. Further, interaction of these mediators and bacterial components leads to priming (pre-activation) of polymorphonuclear granulocytes (PMNs). Particularly, during early inflammatory phase in trauma cases, PMNs facilitate recognition and elimination of pathogens. In trauma patients, hemorrhagic shock leads to hypoperfusion, which is managed by aggressive resuscitation. This reperfusion of ischemic gut results in the release of cytokines and proinflammatory cells which facilitate PMNs prime and causes excessive neutrophilia within the first few hours of injury and during this period a second hit might lead to MODS [17, 25]. Therefore, the exponential increase in PMNs within the initial hours post injury is associated with an increased risk of MODS and mortality [30].

Major Risk Factors of MODS

The rates of morbidity and mortality remain higher among MODS patients, and in case of post-organ dysfunction, there are not many treatment options available and such patients could only be managed by supportive treatment [9]. Also, various studies have proposed potential risk factors of MODS development in trauma and surgical ICU patients. The risk factors could be classified on the basis of early or late onset of MODS. The major contributors of early MODS include the severity of tissue injury, shock-ischemia or reperfusion, and the severity of systemic inflammatory response. On the other hand, late MODS is mainly associated with blood transfusion, development of infection, secondary operative procedures, and host factors (age and preexisting disease) [31]. In case of severe tissue injury, improper distribution of blood flow affects delivery of oxygen, nutrients, and other substrates that are crucial for normal functioning of vital organs and eventually leads to organ failure [31]. Moreover, microaggregation by various blood components can affect the microcirculatory flow causing tissue ischemia. In trauma patients, resuscitation allows reperfusion of previously ischemic tissue which induces pro-inflammatory cytokines that causes impaired systemic inflammatory response [3]. Also, toxic oxygen metabolites (free radicals), cytokines, and other mediators can initiate apoptotic process, leading to reperfusion injury. Together these factors result in endothelial damage which might contribute to the development of early MODS

[32]. Furthermore, the severity of SIRS has been proposed as a contributing factor in the pathogenesis of MODS. An earlier study observed SIRS in more than 90 % of surgical ICU patients but it was not found effective in predicting severe sepsis and septic shock in these patients [33]. Gando et al. [34] demonstrated coagulation and sustained SIRS to be the strong determinants of post-injury MODS. Among critically ill patients admitted in ICU, nosocomial pneumonia is the most frequent cause of infection and is mainly associated with the development of MODS [35]. Due to extensive screening of blood for infectious agents, the risk of transfusion related diseases has been substantially reduced. However, investigators have identified an association between liberal blood transfusion with an increased risk of nosocomial infection, MODS, and mortality [36, 37]. Shorr et al. [38] observed a positive dose–response relationship among the amount of transfused blood units and the chances of acquiring ventilator-associated pneumonia. Similarly, Johnson et al. [39] reported a higher risk of MODS in post-injury patients who received fresh frozen plasma during early resuscitation. The stored blood components could contain proinflammatory mediators that may act as a second inflammatory stimulus and promote MODS [38].

Operative procedures also pose surgical trauma to the patients which activates host immune response in similar fashion to that of traumatic injuries. Hence, such operative interventions might be involved in a second insult resulting in the development of MODS in patients who survived the first hit of inflammatory response [40]. Particularly, surgical trauma induces the activation of pro- as well as anti-inflammatory cytokines which create an immunological imbalance, leading to postoperative complications such as multiorgan failure [41]. An earlier study analyzed the association between secondary operations and the development of late MODS [42]. The authors suggested that an increased inflammatory response might be useful for prediction of postoperative organ failure with 79 % accuracy. Moreover, the secondary operations pose a subsequent inflammatory response hit which probably leads to late MODS in severe trauma patients. Though it is difficult to determine the appropriate timing of secondary operations in severe trauma patients, many studies have tried to investigate this important issue. Pape et al. [43] reported a greater incidence of MODS in severe injury patients who underwent early surgery within 2–4 days of trauma compared to those subjected to late surgical intervention after the sixth day post injury. Consistently, an earlier prospective trial of severely injured patients demonstrated higher rate of postoperative organ failure among early secondary surgery group (within 2–4 days of injury) than that of late secondary surgery group (5–8 days post trauma) [44]. The authors reported that on-admission increased IL-6 levels had a predictive value for the development of postoperative MODS among the early secondary surgery group.

Advanced age is also a contributing factor of increased morbidity (ARDS, MODS) [45, 46] and mortality in ICU and trauma patients [47, 48]. Morris et al. [48] identified comorbidities such as liver cirrhosis, preexisting blood coagulopathy, ischemic heart disease, chronic obstructive pulmonary disease, and diabetes mellitus to be the significant predictors of mortality in these patients. A Brazilian study involving 587 non-cardiac surgery patients admitted to ICU identified that older age, unplanned surgery, peritonitis, and presence of diabetes are the primary factors associated with increased risk of mortality due to MODS [49].

Therefore, identification of major risk factors involved in the development of MODS is crucial for developing effective preventive strategies as evidenced by various predictive models of MODS.

Genetic Predisposition and MODS

Most studies focusing on the development of MODS have included both medical as well as surgical patients who developed organ failure [50]. It is now recognized that organ failure does not occur as an all-or-none phenomenon, but rather a range of organ dysfunction exists that leads to clinical organ failure [50]. It has been suggested that this continuous process of varying degree of organ dysfunction could be designated as MODS [51]. It is not well-understood, under similar circumstances of trauma, why certain and not all patients may develop MODS. There is an ample evidence in the literature that gene-host and gene-environment interactions may play a major role in the morbidity and mortality associated with these complications [52].

Since trauma is sporadic, genetic association studies are more useful for investigating the possible relationships between MODS and genetic predisposition. Therefore, identification of candidate susceptibility genes associated with the development of MODS are of great clinical and research interest in patients of trauma as well as surgery. Genetic variants, particularly single-nucleotide polymorphisms (SNPs), are critical determinants of inter-individual differences in both inflammatory responses and clinical outcome in trauma patients [53]. MODS is a systemic process which involves inflammatory as well as coagulation pathways. Particularly, a complex range of humoral substances, cellular effectors, and bacterial products act as potential mediators in MODS process [31, 54–56].

The proinflammatory cytokine; Tumor necrosis factor-alpha (TNF-α) and its SNP (-308G/A) is an important humeral mediator that has been studied in the development of sepsis and its severity [57, 58]. The other relevant polymorphic cytokines include interleukin (IL)-1 (isoforms α and β) IL-6, IL-10, TNF-β, and IFN-γ [52].

Gu and Jiang [52] found that polymorphisms of (8 SNPs) IL-1*β*/-1470, IL-1*β*/-511, IL-1*β*/-31, IL-4/-589, IL-6/-572, IL-8/-251, IL-10/-819, and TNF*α*/-308 are susceptibility loci for the development of sepsis and organ dysfunction in major trauma patients. Moreover, patients with greater than four risk alleles showed increased risk of sepsis and organ dysfunction by more than 50% [59]. A recent study showed that cytokine expression in patients with septic shock may enable earlier identification of patients at risk for development of MODS [60].

Various studies have been performed to link receptor gene polymorphism with disease phenotypes, including sepsis. Toll-like receptor (TLR) signaling plays an important role in the innate immune response and has been associated with the activation of inflammatory immune responses after blunt trauma [61, 62]. Because of their importance in both the innate immune response and the induction of adaptive immunity, TLRs are currently at the center of the current research. TLR9 expression is upregulated following severe trauma and sepsis. Macrophages and lymphocytes produce greater numbers of proinflammatory cytokines after trauma in response to microbial CpG-DNA stimulation [62].

In addition to microbial infection, cellular disruption by injury could release mitochondrial DNA with evolutionarily conserved similarities to bacterial DNA into the circulation, inducing a systemic inflammatory response, also via TLR9 [62]. Although TLR9 signaling may play an important role in the innate immune response inducing sepsis and organ dysfunction, little is known about the clinical relevance of *TLR9* gene polymorphisms in trauma patients [19]. There are few prospective studies that focus on incidence, early detection and prevention of MODS in the literature [7, 63].

Table 15.1 shows the effect of genetic polymorphism on sepsis or MODs in trauma and surgical ICU patients [62, 64–71]. Patients who developed MODS had higher levels of systemic proinflammatory cytokines such as, IL-6, IL-8, and IL-10. Biomarkers such as procalcitonin (PCT) may predict the occurrence of sepsis in its early stages and discriminate sepsis from an intense inflammatory response in sick patients. Moreover, organ-specific biomarkers like pentraxin-3 and IL-18 (Lung), NT-pro BNP, and Adrenomedullin (Heart), Neutrophil gelatinase-associated lipocalin (NGAL) (kidney), and Glutamate/Glutamine ratio (liver) are useful for better understanding of early organ failure. Therefore, early detection of specific biomarkers have clinical implications in the decision-making for selection of patients and the optimal time points of surgery to limit second hit inflammatory response. To date, therapeutic strategies to combat the post-injury MODS have focused on control of the post-injury inflammatory response [7].

Table 15.1 Effect of genetic polymorphism on sepsis or MODs in trauma and surgical ICU patients

Gene	Function	Study origin	Sample size	Criteria	Polymorphic sites	Clinical implications on the development of sepsis or MODS
TLR9	Pathogen recognition and activation of innate immunity	China [62]	557	Severe blunt trauma (ISS > 16); presence of at least one life-threatening injury	TLR9 polymorphisms rs187084 and rs352162	It has a trend of association with MOD score. There is significant association with TNF-α production and higher rates of sepsis morbidity
		Netherlands [64]	219	Polytrauma patients with ISS ≥ 16 and age between 18 and 80 years	-1486T/C	This SNP has a trend toward reduced prevalence of gram + ve bacteria/ fungi but no significant association with SIRS, or septic shock
TNFα	Regulation immune cells and respond to sepsis via IL1, IL6 producing cells	United States [65]	152	Severe trauma, ISS ≥ 16; admitted to the ICU for more than 24 h	-308G/A	TNF-α promoter increases the risk for severe sepsis and possibly for death after trauma
		Germany [66]	159	Multiple trauma, age 18–65 years, ISS ≥ 12, time of admission to the ICU within 12 h of accident, >3 days of survival	rs1800629A or rs909253G	TNF gene variants are associated with sepsis syndrome and death after severe injury
		United States [67]	68	Blunt and penetrating trauma with ISS ≥ 15	-308G/A	Lack of association between the TNF-α G/A or A/A high producer genotypes and sepsis
		Netherlands [68]	70	Severe blunt trauma; age 18–65 years; admission <8 h after trauma or secondary admission	-308G/A	Significantly associated with development of sepsis
		Latvia [69]	103	ICU patients with severe sepsis	-308G/A	TNF-α -308 A allele is not associated with a higher mortality rate in septicemic patients without shock
IL-6	To stimulate immune response, e.g., after trauma	Germany [70]	112	Critically ill patients admitted to the surgical ICU; age ≥ 18	-174G/C	IL-6 -174G/C promoter genotype is associated with shock in patients with sepsis
		Germany [71]	326	Severe sepsis and/or shock	-174G/C	IL-6 promoter polymorphism (-174G/C) does not affect the incidence of sepsis
		Latvia [69]	103	Severe sepsis	-174G/C	An increased association of IL-6 -174 observed with mortality

Therefore, methods for early detection of MODS must be developed by prospective studies.

Prediction Models of MODS

Till date several prediction models have been proposed for early detection of high-risk patients susceptible for the development of MODS. These models are crucial for the development of early interventional strategies, planning intensive care resource allocation and risk-stratification of vulnerable patient population to prevent second hit. An initial prediction model of MODS was proposed in 1998, which demonstrated shock parameters, age, ISS and platelet count as the predictor of MODS [18]. Since then efforts have been put to minimize the effect of shock through improved resuscitation strategies. Currently, early hemostatic resuscitation helped in reducing the impact of shock and now it is not considered as a predictor of MODS. A recent study [8] demonstrated age and on-admission platelet count to be independent predictors of MODS. Dewar and colleagues reported that the prediction power could be further enhanced by considering creatinine and bilirubin levels within first 24 h of admission [8]. Ciesla et al. [7] observed that ISS is ineffective in predicting MODS, as there is an injury threshold level above which MODS is likely to occur. Moreover, several investigators have identified advanced age as a marker of comorbidity and consider it as an independent predictor of the development of post-injury MODS in severe trauma patients [7, 63, 72]. An earlier study observed male gender to be an independent predictor of the development of severe infection in surgical patients [73]. Nydam et al. [74] reported thrombocytopenia (<80,000) at 12 h post admission to be an independent predictor of MODS. Consistently, Dewar et al. [8] also observed a similar association showing on-admission thrombocytopenia ($<150\times10^9$/L) to be a significant predictor of MODS. Also, base deficit has been considered as a surrogate marker of hypovolemic shock and is used to identify patients who need early hemostatic resuscitation [75]. Regardless of MODS occurrence, base excess is a strong predictor of mortality in severely injured patients [76]. In addition, base deficit along with other significant predictors of MODS has the potential to stratify high-risk MODS patients initially during admission. A recent prospective cohort study from the USA identified male gender, preexisting liver disease, severe ISS, use of early vasopressors, higher volumes of FFP and crystalloid resuscitation, duration of shock, and more severe depth of shock (lactate values <12 h) to be the independent predictors of MODS [10].

Groeneveld et al. [77] analyzed the utility of immunomodulating interventions for the management of posttraumatic complications. The authors [77] found little significance of immune markers (cytokines) for prognosis of MODS due to lower sensitivity and specificity. Another recent promising approach to predict MODS is the assessment of immune cell functionality. It has been shown that phenotyping of blood Polymorphonuclear granulocytes (PMNs) in post-injury patients help to estimate the kinetics and extent of initial SIRS [78]. Furthermore, it has been observed that prior to sepsis development the PMNs functionality reaches its minimum level, so this approach could be used for determining the high-risk patients at earlier stage [79]. Recently, Anne Morrison et al. [80] demonstrated that trauma patients with hemorrhagic shock who had higher PMN apoptosis are at reduced risk of tissue injury and susceptibility to infection which might lead to MODS.

Based on the available predictors, to some extent MODS can be predicted at early stage after injury and so early prevention and treatment could be initiated at this point [18]. Particularly, a reliable prediction model might be supportive for patient recruitment and inclusion in trauma studies, in which MODS marks the primary end point. Finally, identification of major risk factors and predictors helps to stratify and enroll patients for clinical trials during the initial phase of trauma care and surgery. It also supports the assessment of quantifiable outcome of trials in critical ill patients. Although, numerous studies have focused on MODS, majority of prediction models have restricted applicability which may be attributed to the genetic variation among the individual trauma and surgery patients. Therefore, current studies based on genetic predisposition of multiple trauma and surgery patients will favorably improve these prediction models and will enhance their applicability in the near future [81].

Management of MODS Patients

Over the years extensive clinical and experimental studies have been performed for early detection and treatment of post-injury MODS, however it remains a challenging issue for the emergency physicians and trauma surgeons. The current management strategies of high-risk MODS patients are mainly based on preventive and therapeutic interventions.

Preventive Strategies

In trauma patients, preventive strategies usually focus on pre-injury (such as controlling severity of injuries, and limiting the intensity and duration of prehospital shock) and post-injury (to prevent secondary insults) phases, whereas the management strategies in surgical ICU patients mainly depend upon the postoperative course. The rate of post-injury and postoperative MODS could be minimized through improvement in metabolic defects and early hemostatic resuscitation among high-risk population [54]. Moreover, proper mechanical ventilation, antibiotic use, early nutritional support, detection of missed injuries and continuous monitoring for septic complications could be useful for reducing the risk of MODS [54]. O'Brien [82] showed that the risk of developing acute respiratory distress syndrome (ARDS) and MODS could also be minimized by early fixation of major orthopedic injuries in multiple trauma patients. During early phase of injury, the triad of hypothermia, coagulopathy, and acidosis is harmful for severe trauma patients, and such patients are at increased risk of MODS [3]. Therefore, early posttraumatic complications could be mitigated or prevented through rapid hemorrhage control, proper resuscitation, and correction of coagulopathy. Moreover, rapid prehospital transport, early hemostatic resuscitation, and minimal use of blood products might help in reducing the duration and severity of shock which controls PMN priming and decrease the risk of developing MODS post-injury [7]. Johnson et al. [83] investigated the association between red cell substitute and hyperinflammatory response in post-injury patients. The authors found that patients treated with red cell substitutes had lower immunological response (IL6, IL8, and IL10) than those treated with packed red blood cells [83]. The approach of damage control surgery particularly in orthopedics have been recognized in reducing the delayed initial surgery (act as second hits in primed patients) and the risk of developing MODS [1]. A number of factors are found to reduce the development of MOF and or improve the outcomes of MODS patients. These include improvement in critical care medicine facilities, modernization of ICUs, timely recognition of missed injuries, lung protective ventilation strategies, optimal timing of surgery, early enteral nutrition, and renal replacement therapies [1]. Therefore, the primary objective of these therapies is to prevent MODS in critically ill patients.

Therapeutic Strategies

For better prognosis of MODS patients, several therapeutic strategies have been developed to modulate the inflammatory response. The current therapeutic options are mainly focused on modulating the detrimental effects of the exaggerated immune system and at the same time maintaining favorable host immune response. Particularly, timing of intervention is a crucial factor for appropriate modulation of immune response in high-risk sepsis and MODS patients [84]. A variety of targets has been identified to develop therapeutic interventions which range from exogenous trigger (endotoxin or bacterial infection), systemic mediators (such as IL-1, TNF-α), effector cell (e.g., the neutrophil), to specific target cell (the endothelium) [54]. Despite current therapeutic advancement, MODS remains a deadly syndrome. So, in order to limit secondary damage and degeneration in severely injured patients, damage control surgery has been implemented as a preferred therapeutic intervention [9].

Administration of C1-esterase inhibitor (acute-phase protein) is another promising approach to reduce the levels of circulating pro-inflammatory cytokines. Recently, CAESAR study identified C1-esterase inhibitor to be a safe and strong anti-inflammatory agent which is capable of controlling systemic inflammation among trauma patients [85].

It has been observed that immunomodulation strategies are often useful for modulating the favorable changes in the inflammatory response. A recent systematic review analyzed the implications of various immunomodulative strategies on the outcomes of severe trauma patients [86]. Even though the authors found reduction of immune response by many interventions, effective decline in infectious complications and mortality was only observed by the use of immunoglobulin, IFN-γ, or glucan. Moreover, it has been observed that the levels of circulating IgG are reduced in trauma patients. Douzinas et al. [87] demonstrated that the administration of exogenous immunoglobulins improves IgG-mediated antigen presentation which in turn modulates favorable immune response. Earlier studies reported that the administration IgG (0.25–1.0 g/kg) together with antibiotics is effective in lowering the infection in trauma patients [87, 88]. Similarly, IFN-γ induces antigen presentation to lymphocytes and two studies have reported a positive response of administrating exogenous IFN-γ (100 μg daily) on reducing rate of infection [89] and mortality [90].

Glucan, (a component of the inner cell wall of yeast), reduces prostaglandin discharge by macrophages and triggers bone marrow proliferation which improves immune response during late immune paralysis [91]. Earlier studies have suggested that the administration of Glucan (50 mg/m^2 daily [91] or 30 mg every 12 h [92]) demonstrated significant reduction in the rates of infectious complications and mortality in severe trauma patients.

Interestingly, many novel therapeutic modalities have been investigated in clinical trials, but most of them failed to demonstrate efficacy in large-scale, randomized clinical trials. Therefore, use of combination therapy appears to be effective approach in minimizing infectious complications and improving survival rate among severely ill patients.

Conclusions

Although, there is a considerable improvement in the understanding of the underlying mechanism, MODS remains the main cause of resource utilization in surgical and trauma ICUs and had greater burden of morbidity and late mortality. It has been speculated that several predictors of MODS development among surgery and trauma patients might remain unidentified which mandate further exploration based on clinical and experimental studies. Moreover, further understanding of MODS mechanisms will provide better management option which will improve trauma care. Understanding the pathophysiology of early MODS will discriminate the signs of intense inflammatory response from early signs of sepsis. This will reduce the inappropriate use of antibiotics and guide the judicious therapy at the early stages of sepsis and subsequently reduce hospital stay and mortality. Furthermore, there is a need for newer therapeutic strategies for early detection of MODS and risk-stratification of trauma and surgical ICU patients using biomarker based prospective studies. Till date, implications of the efficacy of immune modulating therapies in trauma patients are not well explored. Therefore, advanced research focusing on the implications of novel immunomodulation strategies based on steroid therapy might be useful for minimizing the risk of MODS in multiple trauma and surgery patients.

References

1. Dewar D, Moore FA, Moore EE, Balogh Z. Postinjury multiple organ failure. Injury. 2009;40:912–8.
2. Maier B, Lefering R, Lehnert M, Laurer HL, Steudel WI, Neugebauer EA, Marzi I. Early versus late onset of multiple organ failure is associated with differing patterns of plasma cytokine biomarker expression and outcome after severe trauma. Shock. 2007;28:668–74.
3. Dewar D, Butcher N, King K, Balogh Z. Post injury multiple organ failure. Trauma. 2011;13:81–91.
4. Ciesla DJ, Moore EE, Johnson JL, Sauaia A, Cothren CC, Moore JB, Burch JM. Multiple organ dysfunction during resuscitation is not postinjury multiple organ failure. Arch Surg. 2004;139:590–4.
5. Ciesla DJ, Moore EE, Johnson JL, Burch JM, Cothren CC, Sauaia A. The role of the lung in postinjury multiple organ failure. Surgery. 2005;138:749–57.
6. Moore FA, Sauaia A, Moore EE, Haenel JB, Burch JM, Lezotte DC. Postinjury multiple organ failure: a bimodal phenomenon. J Trauma. 1996;40:501–2.
7. Ciesla DJ, Moore EE, Johnson JL, Burch JM, Cothren CC, Sauaia A. A 12-year prospective study of postinjury multiple organ failure: has anything changed? Arch Surg. 2005;140:432–8.
8. Dewar DC, Tarrant SM, King KL, Balogh ZJ. Changes in the epidemiology and prediction of multiple-organ failure after injury. J Trauma Acute Care Surg. 2013;74(3):774–9.
9. van Wessem KJP, Leenen LPH. The effect of evolving trauma care on the development of multiple organ dysfunction syndrome. Eur J Trauma Emerg Surg. 2014;40:127–34.
10. Minei JP, Cuschieri J, Sperry J, Moore EE, West MA, Harbrecht BG, O'Keefe GE, Cohen MJ, Moldawer LL, Tompkins RG, et al. The changing pattern and implications of multiple organ failure after blunt injury with hemorrhagic shock. Crit Care Med. 2012;40:1129–35.
11. Aldrian S, Koenig F, Weninger P, Vecsei V, Nau T. Characteristics of polytrauma patients between 1992 and 2002: what is changing? Injury. 2007;38:1059–64.
12. Kahl JE, Calvo RY, Sise MJ, Sise CB, Thorndike JF, Shackford SR. The changing nature of death on the trauma service. J Trauma Acute Care Surg. 2013;75:195–201.
13. Nast-Kolb D, Aufmkolk M, Rucholtz S, Obertacke U, Waydhas C. Multiple organ failure still a major cause of morbidity but not mortality in blunt multiple trauma. J Trauma. 2001;51:835–41.
14. Fröhlich M, Lefering R, Probst C, Paffrath T, Schneider MM, Maegele M, Sakka SG, Bouillon B, Wafaisade A, Committee on Emergency Medicine, Intensive Care and Trauma Management of the German Trauma Society Sektion NIS. Epidemiology and risk factors of multiple-organ failure after multiple trauma: an analysis of 31,154 patients from the TraumaRegister DGU. J Trauma Acute Care Surg. 2014;76:921–7.
15. Sauaia A, Moore EE, Johnson JL, Chin TL, Banerjee A, Sperry JL, Maier RV, Burlew CC. Temporal trends of postinjury multiple-organ failure: still resource intensive, morbid, and lethal. J Trauma Acute Care Surg. 2014;76:582–92.
16. Sauaia A, Moore FA, Moore EE, et al. Epidemiology of trauma deaths: a reassessment. J Trauma. 1995;38:185–93.
17. Moore EE, Moore FA, Harken AH, et al. The two-event construct of post-injury multiple organ failure. Shock. 2005;24 Suppl 1:71–4.
18. Sauaia A, Moore FA, Moore EE, Norris JM, Lezotte DC, Hamman RF. Multiple organ failure can be predicted as early as 12 h after injury. J Trauma. 1998;45:291–301.
19. Antonelli M, Caricato A. Post-injury multiple organ failure and late outcome. Is it just an association? Crit Care. 2007;11:166.
20. Peitzman AB, Udekwu AO, Ochoa J, et al. Bacterial translocation in trauma patients. J Trauma. 1991;31:629–38.
21. Sprung CL. Definitions of sepsis: have we reached a consensus? Crit Care Med. 1991;19:849–51.
22. Rotstein OD. Modeling the two-hit hypothesis for evaluating strategies to prevent organ injury after shock/resuscitation. J Trauma. 2003;54 Suppl 5:203–6.
23. Keel M, Trentz O. Pathophysiology of polytrauma. Injury. 2005;36:691–709.
24. Moore FA, Moore EE. Evolving concepts in the pathogenesis of post injury multiple organ failure. Surg Clin North Am. 1995;75:257–77.
25. El-Menyar A, Al-Thani H, Zakaria E, Zarour A, Tuma M, AbdulRahman H, Parchani A, Peralta R, Latifi R. Multiple organ dysfunction syndrome (mods): is it preventable or inevitable? Int J Clin Med. 2012;3:722–30.
26. Zakaria ER, Garrison RN, Spain DA, Matheson PJ, Harris PD, Richardson DJ. Intraperitoneal resuscitation improves intestinal blood flow following hemorrhagic shock. Ann Surg. 2003;237:704–13.
27. el Zakaria R, Campbell JE, Peyton JC, Garrison RN. Postresuscitation tissue neutrophil infiltration is time-dependent and organ-specific. J Surg Res. 2007;143:119–25.
28. el Zakaria R, Li N, Matheson PJ, Garrison RN. Cellular edema regulates tissue capillary perfusion after hemorrhage resuscitation. Surgery. 2007;142:487–96.
29. Tsukamoto T, Chanthaphavong RS, Pape HC. Current theories on the pathophysiology of multiple organ failure after trauma. Injury. 2010;41:21–6.
30. Botha AJ, Moore FA, Moore EE, et al. Early neutrophil sequestration after injury: a pathogenic mechanism for multiple organ failure. J Trauma. 1995;39:411–7.
31. Balk RA. Pathogenesis and management of multiple organ dysfunction or failure in severe sepsis and septic shock. Crit Care Clin. 2000;16(2):337–52.

32. Dunham CM, Damiano AM, Wiles CE, Cushing BM. Post-traumatic multiple organ dysfunction syndrome-infection is an uncommon antecedent risk factor. Injury. 1995;26:373–8.
33. Pittet D, Rangel-Frausto S, Li N, Tarara D, Costigan M, Rempe L, Jebson P, Wenzel RP. Systemic inflammatory response syndrome, sepsis, severe sepsis and septic shock: incidence, morbidities and outcomes in surgical ICU patients. Intensive Care Med. 1995;21: 302–9.
34. Gando S, Nanzaki S, Kemmotsu O. Disseminated intravascular coagulation and sustained systemic inflammatory response syndrome predict organ dysfunctions after trauma: application of clinical decision analysis. Ann Surg. 1999;229:121–7.
35. Baue AE, Faist E, Fry DE, editors. Multiple organ failure: pathophysiology, prevention, and therapy. New York: Springer Science; 2000.
36. Moore FA, Moore EE, Sauaia A. Blood transfusion. An independent risk factor for postinjury multiple organ failure. Arch Surg. 1997;132:620–4.
37. Malone DL, Dunne J, Tracy JK, Putnam AT, Scalea TM, Napolitano LM. Blood transfusion, independent of shock severity, is associated with worse outcome in trauma. J Trauma. 2003;54:898–905.
38. Shorr AF, Duh MS, Kelly KM, Kollef MH, CRIT Study Group. Red blood cell transfusion and ventilator-associated pneumonia: a potential link? Crit Care Med. 2004;32:666–74.
39. Johnson JL, Moore EE, Kashuk JL, Banerjee A, Cothren CC, Biffl WL, Sauaia A. Effect of blood products transfusion on the development of post injury multiple organ failure. Arch Surg. 2010;145: 973–7.
40. Roumen RM, Hendriks T, van der Ven-Jongekrijg J, Nieuwenhuijzen GA, Sauerwein RW, van der Meer JW, Goris RJ. Cytokine patterns in patients after major vascular surgery, hemorrhagic shock, and severe blunt trauma. Relation with subsequent adult respiratory distress syndrome and multiple organ failure. Ann Surg. 1993;218:769–76.
41. Ni Choileain N, Redmond HP. Cell response to surgery. Arch Surg. 2006;141:1132–40.
42. Waydhas C, Nast-Kolb D, Trupka A, Zettl R, Kick M, Wiesholler J, Schweiberer L, Jochum M. Posttraumatic inflammatory response, secondary operations, and late multiple organ failure. J Trauma. 1996;40:624–30.
43. Pape H, Stalp M, v Griensven M, Weinberg A, Dahlweit M, Tscherne H. Optimal timing for secondary surgery in polytrauma patients: an evaluation of 4,314 serious-injury cases. Chirurg. 1999;70:1287–93.
44. Pape HC. Major secondary surgery in blunt trauma patients and perioperative cytokine liberation: determination of the clinical relevance of biochemical markers. J Trauma. 2001;50:989–1000.
45. Sauaia A, Moore FA, Moore EE, Haenel JB, Read RA, Lezotte DC. Early predictors of postinjury multiple organ failure. Arch Surg. 1994;129:39–45.
46. Tran DD, Cuesta MA, van Leeuwen PA, Nauta JJ, Wesdorp RI. Risk factors for multiple organ system failure and death in critically injured patients. Surgery. 1993;114:21–30.
47. Grossman MD, Ofurum U, Stehly CD, Stoltzfus J. Long-term survival after major trauma in geriatric trauma patients: the glass is half full. J Trauma Acute Care Surg. 2012;72:1181–5.
48. Morris Jr JA, MacKenzie EJ, Edelstein SL. The effect of preexisting conditions on mortality in trauma patients. JAMA. 1990;263:1942–6.
49. Lobo SM, Rezende E, Knibel MF, Silva NB, Páramo JA, Nácul FE, Mendes CL, Assunção M, Costa RC, Grion CC, Pinto SF, Mello PM, Maia MO, Duarte PA, Gutierrez F, Silva Jr JM, Lopes MR, Cordeiro JA, Mellot C. Early determinants of death due to multiple organ failure after noncardiac surgery in high-risk patients. Anesth Analg. 2011;112:877–83.
50. Durham RM, Moran JJ, Mazuski JE, Shapiro MJ, Baue AE, Flint LM. Multiple organ failure in trauma patients. J Trauma. 2003;55:608–16.
51. Bone R, Balk R, Cerra F, et al. Definitions for sepsis and organ failure and guidelines for the use of innovative therapies in sepsis:the ACCP/SCCM Consensus Conference Committee—American College of Chest Physicians/Society of Critical Care Medicine. Chest. 1992;101:1644–55.
52. Gu W, Jiang J. Genetic polymorphisms and posttraumatic complications. Comp Funct Genomics. 2010;2010:814086. Article ID 814086, 7 pages.
53. Jiang JX. Genomic polymorphisms and sepsis. Chin J Traumatol. 2005;21:45–9.
54. Deitch EA, Goodman ER. Prevention of multiple organ failure. Surg Clin North Am. 1999;79: 1471–88.
55. Casey LC. Immunologic response to infection and its role in septic shock. Crit Care Clin. 2000;16:193–213.
56. de Bel EE, Goris RJA. Systemic inflammation after trauma, infection, and cardiopulmonary bypass: is autodestruction a necessary evil? In: Bruce AE, Faist E, Fry DE, editors. Multiorgan failure: pathogenesis, prevention and therapy. New York: Springer-Verlag; 2000. p. 71–81.
57. Read RC, Teare DM, Pridmore AC, et al. The tumor necrosis factor polymorphism TNF (-308) is associated with susceptibility to meningococcal sepsis, but not with lethality. Crit Care Med. 2009;37:1237–43.
58. Barber RC, Aragaki CC, Rivera-Chavez FA, Purdue GF, Hunt JL, Horton JW. TLR4 and TNF-α polymorphisms are associated with an increased risk for severe sepsis following burn injury. J Med Genet. 2004;41:808–13.
59. Gu W, Zeng L, Zhou J, et al. Clinical relevance of 13 cytokine gene polymorphisms in Chinese major trauma patients. Intensive Care Med. 2010;36:1261–5.
60. Pettila V, Pettila M, Sarna S, Voutilainen P, Takkunen O. Comparison of multiple organ dysfunction scores in the prediction of hospital mortality in the critically ill. Crit Care Med. 2002;30:1705–11.
61. Takeda K, Akira S. Regulation of innate immune responses by toll-like receptors. Jpn J Infect Dis. 2001;54:209–19.

62. Chen KH, Zeng L, Gu W, Zhou J, Du DY, Jiang JX. Polymorphisms in the toll-like receptor gene associated with sepsis and multiple organ dysfunction after major blunt trauma. Br J Surg. 2011;98: 1252–9.
63. Dewar DC, Mackay P, Balogh Z. Epidemiology of post-injury multiple organ failure in an Australian trauma system. ANZ J Surg. 2009;79:431–6.
64. Bronkhorst MW, Boyé ND, Lomax MA, et al. Single-nucleotide polymorphisms in the toll-like receptor pathway increase susceptibility to infections in severely injured trauma patients. J Trauma Acute Care Surg. 2013;74:862–70.
65. O'Keefe GE, Hybki DL, Munford RS. The G→A single nucleotide polymorphism at the -308 position in the tumor necrosis factor-alpha promoter increases the risk for severe sepsis after trauma. J Trauma. 2002;52:817–25.
66. Menges T, König IR, Hossain H, et al. Sepsis syndrome and death in trauma patients are associated with variation in the gene encoding tumor necrosis factor. Crit Care Med. 2008;36:1456–62.
67. McDaniel DO, Hamilton J, Brock M, et al. Molecular analysis of inflammatory markers in trauma patients at risk of postinjury complications. J Trauma. 2007;63:147–57.
68. Majetschak M, Obertacke U, Schade FU, et al. Tumor necrosis factor gene polymorphisms, leukocyte function, and sepsis susceptibility in blunt trauma patients. Clin Diagn Lab Immunol. 2002;9:1205–11.
69. Sabelnikovs O, Nikitina-Zake L, Krumina A, et al. Associations between TNF-α, IL-6 and IL-10 promoter polymorphisms and mortality in severe sepsis. J Sci Res Rep. 2012;1:17–28. Article no. JSRR.2012.002.
70. Tischendorf JJ, Yagmur E, Scholten D, et al. The interleukin-6 (IL6)-174 G/C promoter genotype is associated with the presence of septic shock and the ex vivo secretion of IL6. Int J Immunogenet. 2007;34:413–8.
71. Schlüter B, Raufhake C, Erren M, et al. Effect of the interleukin-6 promoter polymorphism (-174 G/C) on the incidence and outcome of sepsis. Crit Care Med. 2002;30:32–7.
72. Brattstrom O, Granath F, Rossi P, Oldner A. Early predictors of morbidity and mortality in trauma patients treated in the intensive care unit. Acta Anaesthesiol Scand. 2010;54:1007–17.
73. Offner PJ, Moore EE, Biffl WL. Male gender is a risk factor for major infections after surgery. Arch Surg. 1999;134:935–40.
74. Nydam TL, Kashuk JL, Moore EE, et al. Refractory postinjury thrombocytopenia is associated with multiple organ failure and adverse outcomes. J Trauma. 2011;70:401–6.
75. Mutschler M, Nienaber U, Brockamp T, Wafaisade A, Fabian T, Paffrath T, Bouillon B, Maegele M. Renaissance of base deficit for the initial assessment of trauma patients: a base deficit-based classification for hypovolemic shock developed on data from 16,305 patients derived from the TraumaRegister DGU. Crit Care. 2013;17:R42.
76. Rixen D, Raum M, Bouillon B, Neugebauer E. Base excess as prognostic indicator in patients with polytrauma [in German]. Anasthesiol Intensivmed Notfallmed Schmerzther. 2002;37:347–9.
77. Groeneveld KM, Leenen LP, Koenderman L, Kesecioglu J. Immunotherapy after trauma: timing is essential. Curr Opin Anaesthesiol. 2011;24:219–23.
78. Hietbrink F, Koenderman L, Althuizen M, Pillay J, Kamp V, Leenen LP. Kinetics of the innate immune response after trauma: implications for the development of late onset sepsis. Shock. 2013;40:21–7.
79. Hietbrink F, Oudijk EJ, Braams R, Koenderman L, Leenen L. Aberrant regulation of polymorphonuclear phagocyte responsiveness in multitrauma patients. Shock. 2006;26:558–64.
80. Anne Morrison C, Moran A, Patel S, Vidaurre Mdel P, Carrick MM, Tweardy DJ. Increased apoptosis of peripheral blood neutrophils is associated with reduced incidence of infection in trauma patients with hemorrhagic shock. J Infect. 2013;66:87–94.
81. Warren HS, Elson CM, Hayden DL, et al. A genomic score prognostic of outcome in trauma patients. Mol Med. 2009;15:220–7.
82. O'Brien PJ. Fracture fixation in patients having multiple injuries. Can J Surg. 2003;46:124–8.
83. Johnson JL, Moore EE, Gonzalez RJ, et al. Alteration of the postinjury hyperinflammatory response by means of resuscitation with a red cell substitute. J Trauma. 2003;54:133–9.
84. Ronco C, Kellum JA, Bellomo R, House AA. Potential interventions in sepsis-related acute kidney injury. Clin J Am Soc Nephrol. 2008;3:531–44.
85. Heeres M, Visser T, van Wessem KJ, Koenderman AH, Strengers PF, Koenderman L, Leenen LP. The effect of C1-esterase inhibitor on systemic inflammation in trauma patients with a femur fracture—the CAESAR study: study protocol for a randomized controlled trial. Trials. 2011;12:223.
86. Spruijt NE, Visser T, Leenen LPH. A systematic review of randomized controlled trials exploring the effect of immunomodulative interventions on infection, organ failure, and mortality in trauma patients. Crit Care. 2010;14:R150.
87. Douzinas EE, Pitaridis MT, Louris G, Andrianakis I, Katsouyanni K, Karmpaliotis D, Economidou J, Sfyras D, Roussos C. Prevention of infection in multiple trauma patients by high-dose intravenous immunoglobulins. Crit Care Med. 2000;28:8–15.
88. Glinz W, Grob PJ, Nydegger UE, Ricklin T, Stamm F, Stoffel D, Lasance A. Polyvalent immunoglobulins for prophylaxis of bacterial infections in patients following multiple trauma. A randomized, placebo-controlled study. Intensive Care Med. 1985;11:288–94.
89. Nakos G, Malamou-Mitsi VD, Lachana A, Karassavoglou A, Kitsiouli E, Agnandi N, Lekka ME. Immunoparalysis in patients with severe trauma and the effect of inhaled interferon-gamma. Crit Care Med. 2002;30:1488–94.

90. Dries DJ, Walenga JM, Hoppensteadt D, Fareed J. Molecular markers of hemostatic activation and inflammation following major injury: effect of therapy with IFN-gamma. J Interferon Cytokine Res. 1998;18:327–35.
91. Browder W, Williams D, Pretus H, Olivero G, Enrichens F, Mao P, Franchello A. Beneficial effect of enhanced macrophage function in the trauma patient. Ann Surg. 1990;211:605–12.
92. de Felippe Júnior J, da Rocha e Silva Júnior M, Maciel FM, Soares Ade M, Mendes NF. Infection prevention in patients with severe multiple trauma with the immunomodulator beta 1-3 polyglucose (glucan). Surg Gynecol Obstet. 1993;177:383–8.

Advances in Burn Care

16

Kareem R. AbdelFattah and Steven E. Wolf

Introduction

Thermal injury became a problem in human existence simultaneously with the discovery of fire, and descriptions of burns and burn treatment have been documented since the introduction of the written word. Egyptian, Chinese, and Ayurvedic records indicate that a myriad of salves and procedures were used in combination to alleviate the suffering associated with burns. While management of burns has been ongoing thousands of years, it has been the last half-century in which significant strides have changed the outcome of patients suffering from this most devastating of injuries. Improved knowledge of fluid resuscitation, burn wound excision, and wound coverage has vastly changed the mission of practitioners caring for these patients from simply trying to improve survival to trying to improve rehabilitation, recovery, and reinsertion into society. This chapter covers advances in the treatment of the burned patient, from prehospital care and trauma systems that have improved delivery and triage of these patients, through advancements in the acute care of these patients during their hospital course, including advances in resuscitation and burn wound management.

K.R. AbdelFattah, M.D.
Department of Surgery, Parkland Memorial Hospital, University of Texas—Southwestern Medical Center, Dallas, TX, USA
e-mail: Kareem.abdelfattah@utsouthwestern.edu

S.E. Wolf, M.D., F.A.C.S. (✉)
Department of Surgery, University of Texas—Southwestern Medical Center, Dallas, TX, USA
e-mail: Steven.wolf@utsouthwestern.edu

Prehospital Care of the Thermally Injured Patient

The first patient transport system was created by Dominique Jean Larrey, Napoleon's surgeon-in-chief from 1797 to 1815. His "Flying Ambulances" would provide rapid transport from the front lines of battle to field hospitals. Since that time, the transport of patients from the site of injury to definitive care has been one of the keystone features of a mature trauma system, whether that be military or civilian. The rapid delivery of these patients to centralized clinical expertise has been cited as one of the major determinants in survival not only following severe injury, but in a myriad of other conditions as well.

The American Burn Association (ABA) has suggested guidelines for the transfer of burn injuries [1] (Table 16.1). These are now used through much of the world.

Thermal injuries represent a special problem in terms of transporting patients to major burn centers. Thermal injuries, however, tend to occur away from centralized burn centers, most often in

R. Latifi et al. (eds.), *Technological Advances in Surgery, Trauma and Critical Care*,
DOI 10.1007/978-1-4939-2671-8_16

Table 16.1 Guidelines for the transfer of burn injuries

Partial thickness burns greater than 10 % TBSA.
Burns involving the face, hands, feet, genitalia, perineum, or major joints.
Third degree burns in any age group.
Electrical burns including lightning injuries.
Chemical burns.
Inhalational injuries.
Burn injuries in patients with preexisting medical disorders which could complicate management.
Combined burns and trauma.
Burned children in facilities that are not equipped to handle the care of children.
Burn injuries in those who will require social, emotional, or rehabilitative interventions.

the rural setting. The first point of care for these patients then becomes smaller hospitals and clinics, in which practitioners may have limited experience in treating burned patients, and the estimation of the severity of burns is one of the key components of burn care, and determines the proper triage of patients. The combination of the relative rarity of encountering these injuries for the rural practitioner along with the development of centralized expertise results in a tendency towards both over- and under-triage of burned patients. At least one study demonstrated that 48 % of patients treated at a non-burn center meet criteria for transfer but were never transferred. The same study demonstrated that 12 % of patients treated at burn centers did not meet criteria for transfer [2]. Other studies have shown upwards of 30 % of transfers to burn centers not meeting criteria [3]. In an effort to optimize triage of burn patients to centralized centers from rural areas, several groups have looked to telemedicine as an initial tool in evaluation, prior to transfer.

Telemedicine and Triage of the Burned Patient

Telemedicine has been proposed as a solution to providing limited availability of clinical expertise in areas where it is not feasible to routinely have those clinicians on-site. The use is currently being explored in rural and international medicine, along with the possibility of aiding in disaster management [4–7]. Telemedicine technology is already being used in many burn centers in the USA. A survey submitted to directors of 126 burn center directors showed that 84 % of the 50 respondents were already using telemedicine in some form, with the majority using it routinely. While the majority of current telemedicine involves the use of remote patient data via home computer or personal devices, several reported the remote evaluation of acute burns for consultation, help in determining the need for transfer, and for follow-up visits [8].

While telemedicine has been thought of as an expensive solution to the problem of a lack of specialized clinical expertise in rural areas, the modern situation is such that most healthcare practitioners own or have access to common technology such as cellular phones and desktop computers which have free and user-friendly technology to be able to consult experts easily and quickly. The challenge for the current generation of practitioners will be ensuring the security of these interactions when utilizing this technology and compliance with the Health Insurance Portability and Accountability Act [9].

Initial Care of the Burned Patient

Acute care of the severely burned patient follows ATLS guidelines, ensuring that the patient has suffered no other significant traumatic injury, determination of the size of the patient's burn, with potential transfer to a designated burn center. Burn injuries that are large enough to cause pathophysiologic responses such as hypotension and tachycardia warrant admission to the Intensive Care Unit. This response is secondary to intravascular fluid deficit within the first 24–48 h, and can lead to hypovolemic shock coupled with significant edema secondary to capillary leak. Early fluid administration in this group of patients has been shown to improve survival and decrease morbidity. While several formulas have been developed to estimate the fluid requirements to abate the associate morbidity and mortality, most centers utilize urine output as a measure of end-organ perfusion during this resuscitation, with a target output for most adults of 0.5 cc/kg/h.

Burn Resuscitation: Development of Closed-Loop and Decision-Assist Technologies

The logistics of how burn resuscitation actually occurs at most major burn centers involves practitioners using one of several available formulas (e.g., Parkland, Brooke Army) to determine a starting point for fluid volumes to be given to a severely burned patient. From that point on, most decisions are made either by institutional protocols driven by historical data, or clinical gestalt of the practitioners at the bedside. This frequently results in either fluid rates being reduced too quickly, or in the phenomenon of "fluid creep" whereby too much fluid is given in patients whose resuscitations are difficult. Studies have demonstrated that a vast majority of patients, in fact, are given more fluid than formulas estimate. The end product of either issue is a worse outcome for the patient. The need for automated systems has arisen out of these concerns, and allows for the skills and knowledge of expert practitioners to be utilized when they themselves are not available.

Personnel trained in burn care must provide prompt initialization of fluid therapy coupled with continuous attentive care at admission to the ICU, as described above. Appropriate fluid titration during this resuscitation has been one of the cornerstones of effective burn care; however, it is labor- and experience-dependent. Some groups have utilized computerized decision-support systems as early as 2007 [10]. These systems capture urine output volumes from a digital urimeter throughout the resuscitation, and have infused fluid volumes recorded and entered by bedside practitioners.

Computerized decision support system use has been shown to lower infused crystalloid volumes while maintaining urine output at goal a higher percentage of the time compared with traditional fluid resuscitation strategies. Furthermore, the use of this technology may also reduce ventilator free days and mortality in severely burned patients. While these tools have been developed to make the resuscitation of severely burned patients more standardized and hopefully safer, they are likely not a solution for a lack of expertise.

Determination of Burn Depth

Practitioners with expertise in burn wound management understand that the depth of a burn can be difficult to ascertain at its initial presentation. Determining which wounds would benefit most from excision and grafting versus a strategy of waiting for healing within 3 weeks remains one of the most important components of surgical planning for burned patients, and yet remains one of the most subjective. One of the developing technologies in the field of burns relates to being able to determine the precise depth of injury such as to preserve areas of skin that are still viable and/or to prevent unnecessary full-thickness excisions. The gold standard for assessing depth is a biopsy with histologic analysis. While it has been well studied as a reliable method for depth assessment, it is not always readily available, depending on local resources. Furthermore, it is largely impacted by sampling error, and as most burn wounds are not completely homogenous could lead to the need for multiple biopsies, increasing cost and possibly worsening the cosmetic outcome if the burn is not full-thickness.

As histologic analysis proves to be difficult to use in the clinical setting, the most commonly used method of determining burn depth currently is clinical evaluation. It is the least expensive method available, and relies on a subjective evaluation of the features of the burn wound, such as its appearance, sensitivity to touch, and pain [11–13]. However, none of the features of clinical appraisal of a burn have been shown to be reliable, and the accuracy has been called into question [14]. Studies have demonstrated, however, that this assessment is accurate in only 60–75 % of cases and that the clinical observation between examiners is not always consistent. Most frequently, the error is in depth overestimation [15].

Measurement of tissue perfusion has become an area of interest for groups examining technology to measure burn wound depths. Experimental data has demonstrated that the preservation of microvascular blood flow is related to the severity of a burn wound [16–18]. Technologies such as thermal imaging, vital dye use, and laser Doppler imaging are being considered for commercial use in determining burn depth.

Thermal imaging, or thermography, is a promising technology in that it is fast and noninvasive. It is based on temperature measurements of the wound to determine depth with the assumption that deep wounds are cooler by virtue of less or nonexistent vascular perfusion. Thermography has been criticized for falsely reporting deeper wounds secondary to ambient heat losses to the environment, and has been shown to have poor accuracy as wounds age [11].

Several variations of vital dyes have been utilized in research to differentiate between superficial and deep burns. The majority of these proved to have little clinical utility; however, some of these dyes have made a resurgence in many areas of medicine. Fluorescein fluorescence involves IV injection of fluorescein dye, followed by illumination via ultraviolet light over the area of interest. This has been utilized in burn wounds, however could not differentiate between deep and superficial burns, and had difficulty penetrating eschar [19, 20]. Another dye, Indocyanine green (ICG), is also administered intravenously, and has a peak spectral absorption at 800 nm. ICG binds to plasma proteins, becoming trapped in the vascular system, and is cleared with a half-life of 180 s via biliary excretion. This technology has been adapted to a videography image allowing practitioners to view this indicator of tissue perfusion on a monitor. Studies have confirmed that this allows for determining dermal viability from a structural and functional standpoint [21]. This technique is in use in several other fields of medicine via the SPY Elite® (LifeCell Corp, Branchburg, NJ) device and other similar technologies. Currently, the technology is being used in colorectal surgery, breast oncology, abdominal wall reconstruction, and vascular surgery/wound care. The most useful aspect of the SPY Elite is that it can be used in real-time, in an operating room, and can allow for sequential measurements in burned areas that are in question. While indocyanine green technologies appear promising, they are currently limited by availability and expense.

Laser Doppler imaging is the technology that has received the most attention thus far, and has a long list of studies supporting its use in burn wound assessment and treatment [14, 22, 23]. It has been used since the 1970s to evaluate cutaneous circulation. Doppler signals are produced when waves are reflected moving objects, and measured by the change in frequency based on the space between the object and the transducer. Such techniques have been examined in burns and demonstrated the highest positive predictive values of any of the technologies available currently [24]. As such, it is the only technology which has been FDA approved for burn wound assessment. It has consistently been shown to be better than clinical assessment at multiple time points following injury [23].

Management of the Burn Wound

Burn Eschar Excision

Debridement of burn eschar typically involves sharp dissection using instruments such as Bovie electrocautery, scalpels, and Humby knives. These methods of debridement are swift and effective; however, healthy collateral tissue around the wound may be removed as well. Furthermore, while experienced burn surgeons can typically perform this easily for full-thickness burns, superficial and partial-thickness burns do not need such deep excision, and sharp dissection may result in a much deeper excision than is necessary. Blood loss can also be an issue when very large surface areas are involved. To reduce unnecessary excision depth and size, more sophisticated technology is being developed for excision of burn eschar, especially for the case of partial-thickness burns. One example, the Versajet™

(Smith & Nephew, London, UK) system, uses pressurized sterile saline which is forced into a specialized nozzle which focuses the liquid into a jet. This jet is passed along tissue and takes with it ablated tissue and debris, moving the mixture into an evacuator port. This system has been shown to reduce bacterial burden and reduces the volume of normal tissue excised. Further examination of this and similar excision technologies will delineate the patients that most benefit from this form of debridement.

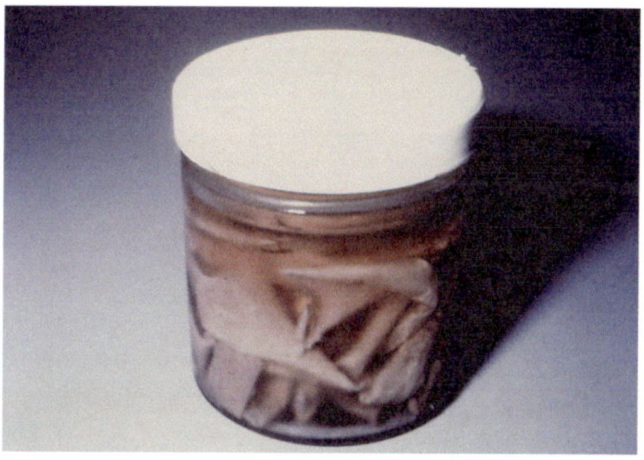

Fig. 16.1 Fresh allograft skin prior to freezing. Fresh skin can be used without freezing which many claim to have better results through better graft take

The Skin Bank

One of the most important and advanced technologies stemming from the care of thermally injured patients is the development of the Skin Bank. While skin grafting techniques developed in the 1800s, it was not until the early 1900s that the storage of human skin began. Early on, skin could be stored for up to 2 weeks prior to use. By the 1940s, the use of allograft skin in burn wound coverage had been described in children with extensive burns [25]. Finally, in 1949, the United States Navy Tissue Bank was established, heralding the era of the modern Skin Bank. Soon after, the American Association of Tissue Banks and the Food and Drug Association set policies and standards for tissue harvesting, processing, and banking of human tissues.

The technical aspects of skin banking include a rigorous donor screening process, followed by skin recovery within 24 h of the death of the donor. The skin is then processed in a laminar flow clean room. This processing involves microbiologic testing for bacteria, yeast, and fungi. These tests are performed on multiple samples of skin from each 10 % of the body surface area from which the skin was removed. Fresh allograft skin is then stored at 4 °C in tissue culture medium. This typically allows for storage for up to 7–10 days, after which the skin is cryopreserved (Fig. 16.1).

Cryopreserved skin can be maintained in a mechanical freezer for up to 6 months, or in liquid nitrogen for up to 10 years with maintained viability. Rewarming of cryopreserved skin is done in such a fashion as to preserve the structural integrity of the skin, and is done at rates of 50 °C/min, resulting in 90 % graft survival [25].

Burn Wound Coverage

In all vertebrates, skin has multiple critical functions for survival, including protection from the environment, a surface area for interaction with the environment, temperature control, control of evaporation, and a membrane to prevent the loss of essential nutrients. Thermal injury represents a disruption of this system and at least a partial loss of these functions, resulting in a higher risk of infection, evaporative losses, and dysfunction in thermoregulation. For these reasons, coverage of the burn wound as quickly as possible in order to restore an intact barrier is another key element of advanced burn care.

The ideal wound coverage is easily available, inexpensive, provide a mechanical barrier to the environment, offer antibacterial protection, maintain moisture within the wound, remain non-adherent, and be a comfortable non-restrictive option for the patient. Unfortunately, no single available dressing meets all of these criteria. Similar to the development of the skin bank, the technology involved in the development of new types of wound coverage materials has been paramount to the long-term care of the burned patient.

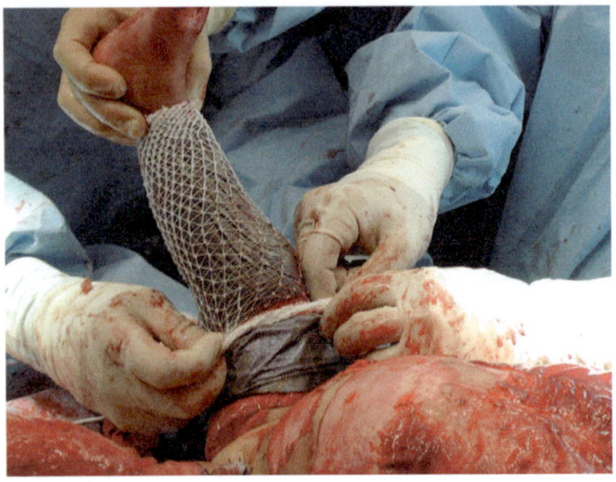

Fig. 16.2 Silver dressing applied to a partial thickness wound

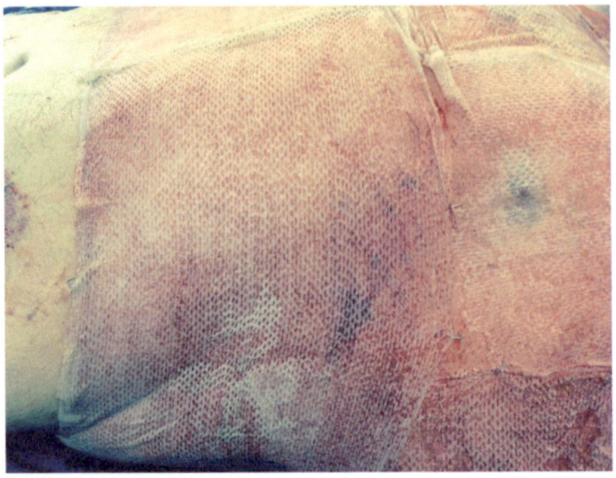

Fig. 16.3 Xenograft skin applied to a deep partial thickness burn

Until the 1980s, readily available wound coverage options were sorely limited, consisting of gauze-based products and paste-based bandages. Modern development has focused on the ability to have all of the properties of prior dressings as well as conformability to parts of the body which are difficult to cover (e.g., hands, feet) as well as patient comfort, with some options allowing for as little as once-weekly dressing changes (Fig. 16.2).

Burn wound management and coverage depends on the thickness of the wound. Excisions can involve only removal of damaged epidermis, allowing for reepithelialization over time, typically with one of several available wound coverings protecting the underlying dermis until healing occurs. Conversely, a full-thickness burn and excision may benefit from autograft, when available; however, these excisions often require the use of a dermal substitute.

Superficial/Partial-Thickness Wound Coverage Materials

Synthetic Dressings

Synthetic dressings include silicone, barrier films, foams, tissue adhesives, hydrogels, and silver-impregnated dressings. The most commonly used variety in the acutely burned patient are the silver-based dressings, such as Acticoat™ (Smith & Nephew, London, UK), Aquacel® (Convatec, Skillman, NJ) , and Mepilex® (Mölnlycke, Gothenburg, Sweden). These dressings are generally soft and conformable, can remove excess exudate without causing desiccation of the wound. These dressings have advanced to become less painful and can be left in place for several days to minimize painful dressing changes while also reducing skin irritation. They are often used for coverage of split-thickness skin graft donor sites.

Xenogenic Graft Coverage

Tissues derived from animal origins have been used for wound coverage much longer than any other tissue-type coverage. While they only provide temporary wound coverage, they are readily available and relatively inexpensive options, making them useful in many situations. Pigskin, or porcine skin, is the most commonly used xenograft because of similar properties to human skin. Bovine xenograft has been used when cultural beliefs prohibit the use of porcine skin. Similar to other tissue-derived skin substitutes, the processing of the skin following harvest involves an irradiating and freeze-drying cycle to ensure sterility (Fig. 16.3). Glycerin has alternatively been used as a sterile wash to reduce processing costs.

Acellular Matrices and Combination Products: Biobrane®, Promogran®, AWBAT®, Suprathel®

The synthetic and biosynthetic materials which have been developed for wound coverage have been in use since initial efforts at engineering a

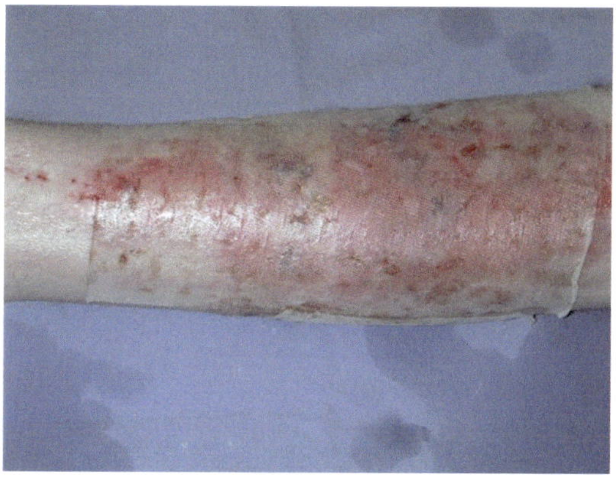

Fig. 16.4 Biobrane® (Smith & Nephew, London, UK) applied to a partial thickness wound. The dressing is transparent allowing for direct inspection of the wound. Epithelialization occurs under the dressing

dermal component to substitute the volume of missing tissue occurred in the mid-1970s. The first used in burn care was Biobrane® (Smith & Nephew, London, UK), which is a temporary biosynthetic skin dressing used on superficial and partial-thickness wounds or donor sites (Fig. 16.4). It is composed of a silicone membrane bonded to a nylon mesh to which peptides from a porcine dermal collagen source have been bonded to the nylon membrane to form a conformable composite dressing. The product has been beneficial in that it has been safe to use, controls evaporative losses, is flexible, has some hemostatic properties, and is relatively inexpensive. It has also been demonstrated to reduce local wound pain and to have some antibacterial properties. AWBAT® (Advanced Wound Bioengineered Alternative Tissue, Aubrey Inc., Carlsbad, CA) is a similar silicone-based membrane that is more porous with the advantage of allowing more exudate out of the wound, resulting in better adherence. Suprathel® (PolyMedics Innovations, Denkendorf, Germany) is a synthetic copolymer with similar porous properties, and is applied with an overlay of paraffin or gauze. The material begins to peel off within 2 weeks, when reepithelialization begins to occur beneath the dressing. The main benefit to this technique has been in decreasing pain associated with dressing changes.

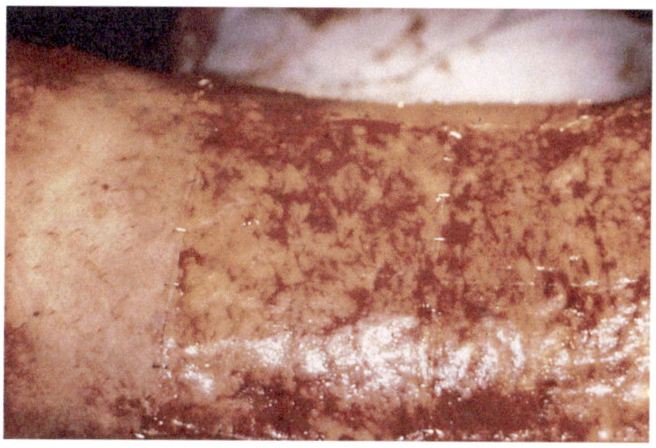

Fig. 16.5 Transcyte® (Shire Regenerative Medicine, La Jolla, CA) applied as a skin substitute to a full thickness excised wound. This is only a temporary coverage which should be closed with autografting at a later date

Single-Element Biologic Dressings

Amnion as a biologic material in medicine has been increasingly used in a variety of applications. While the use of amnion has been described since at least the early 1900s, its use as a burn dressing has only been popularized over the last three decades. This development coincides with the improvement in all of human tissue banking as previously described. Currently, amnion is supplied in either a fresh-frozen form or a glycerol-preserved form, although they are not readily available in all burn centers. Amniotic membrane has many of the characteristics of an ideal skin substitute in that it is thin and pliable, can easily be removed while having excellent adherence to the wound, has very low immunogenicity, decreases pain, has some bacterial control, and allows for some promotion of wound healing. Some practitioners also prefer its translucency to other dressings as it allows visual inspection of the wound.

Cellular Allogeneic Analogs

Biologic wound coverage options such as TransCyte® (Shire Regenerative Medicine, La Jolla, CA), Apligraf® (Organogensis, Canton, MA), and Dermagraft® (Organogensis, Canton, MA) all use human keratinocytes and/or fibroblasts to seed a synthetic matrix and create a biologic dermal dressing (Fig. 16.5). While Apligraf and Dermagraf are approved for stasis ulcers and diabetic foot ulcers, respectively, their use is being explored in burn care. TransCyte uses human newborn fibroblasts cultured on the nylon mesh of Biobrane, and has been used to cover wounds in a single application until wound healing occurs.

Full-Thickness Burn Wound Coverage

Full-thickness wounds involve loss of the epidermis and dermis, often resulting in the loss of epidermal appendages that supply the epithelial cells that allow regeneration in partial thickness burns. The elements providing these cells include sweat glands, apocrine glands, and hair follicles, and often penetrate deep into the dermis, and even into the subcutaneous fat. This allows skin to reepithelialize in most wounds; however, the length of time for this to occur may be dangerous to survival if depth and surface area is large enough. The best option for wound coverage is the patient's own skin; however, in tertiary care burn centers, some wounds are large enough that autografting is not an option.

Autograft

Autograft is skin taken from the patient for transplantation onto the same patient. Autografting has been described since the late 1800s, and the utility of autologous skin as a coverage for wounds became clearer soon after. The work of Dr. Thiersch in the 1870s describing the use of partial-thickness grafts also advanced the field of wound coverage. As the field of skin grafting grew, it became apparent that partial thickness grafts left a wound that would regenerate from deep islands of hair follicles and sebaceous gland epithelium allowing for deeper partial-thickness grafting [25]. One of the major differences between full- and partial-thickness grafts is the amount of contraction that occurs after placement, with contraction degree being dependent on the amount of dermis in the graft. Full-thickness grafts contracts initially after harvest, but have less contraction in the long-term and are used in areas where such contracture would be detrimental. Conversely, split-thickness grafts have much more contraction but can be used to cover larger surface areas.

Donor site selection is typically based on skin color, thickness needed, vascularity, and the cosmetic effects of the donor site itself. Full-thickness grafts are often small, and can be taken from the supraclavicular skin to match coloring of the face. Partial-thickness grafts are taken from locations that can be covered by clothing, such as back, buttocks, and most typically the thigh. These grafts are taken using either a Weck blade or a powered instrument such as the Zimmer Dermatome. These instruments can be adjusted to variable depths in order to achieve either a partial or full thickness graft.

Key points for the operative technique of placing these grafts includes ensuring a hemostatic wound bed such that a hematoma does not prevent application of the graft, meshing the graft for seromas and blood to escape through, and providing gentle pressure on the graft to ensure contact with the wound bed. Grafts survive based on their ability to take up nutrition from the wound bed, first through the process of imbibition, which is a form of capillary action. The graft then undergoes inosculation (alignment of capillary beds) and finally revascularization of the graft through the growth of new blood vessels. While autograft has been used with great success, there exist several skin substitutes when autografting is not possible.

Acellular Dermal Analogs

AlloDerm® (LifeCell Corp, Branchburg, NJ), an acellular human dermis substitute, is healthy human dermis with all cellular materials removed. The tissue is screened for viruses, and is freeze-dried for preservation and later use. They are prepared from cadaver skin by a process involving purification by washing and radiation treatment, followed by freezing (Fig. 16.6). The harvest and purification process leads to an increased expense associated with these products.

Keratinocyte Coverage

CEA (cultured epithelial autograft) is a novel material that is indicated for the coverage of deep and extensive wounds (Fig. 16.7). The major drawback of this technique is the time required for growth of cells in vitro and the associated cost.

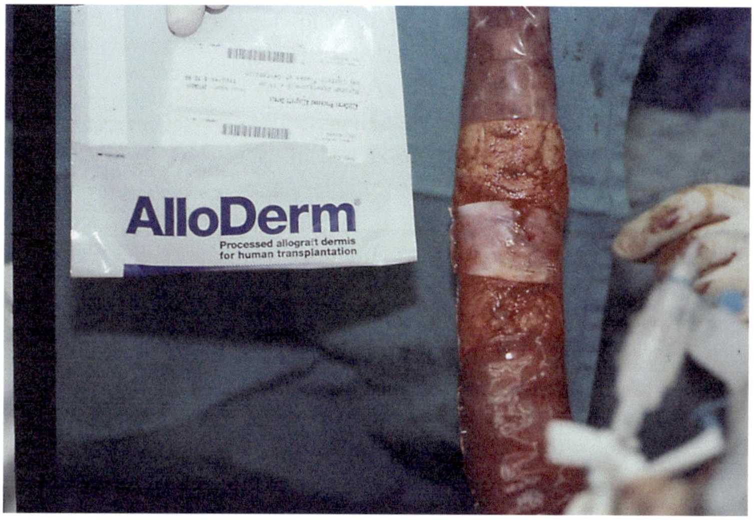

Fig. 16.6 AlloDerm® (LifeCell Corp, Branchburg, NJ) applied across the elbow joint as a dermal substitute. Autograft can be immediately applied with equivalent graft take to autograft alone

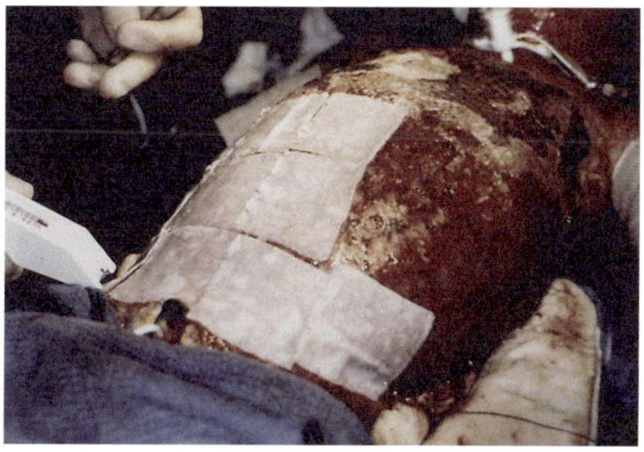

Fig. 16.7 CEA grafts applied to an excised and prepared wound on the anterior torso

Some evidence suggests that allogeneic cultured epithelial sheet grafts do not actually survive, being rejected within 2 weeks in mice. Instead, the allograft may actually induce faster healing of the wound via the residual keratinocytes already in the wound.

Another form of keratinocyte coverage comes in the form of "spray-on skin." This technology was an advancement when compared to the cultured epithelial autograft sheets previously described and was an effort to reduce wound contraction and healing times. The technique involves obtaining split-thickness skin from unburned areas and shaking the skin in a 2 % dispase (neutral protease) solution to separate the epidermal layer. The cells are then cultured and aerosolized for application onto the wound. This process takes over 3 weeks to complete, however, which may result in significant treatment delays in cases where other options exist.

Tissue regeneration through the use of stem cell therapy is an evolving technique in burn care, and is purported to improve the quality of burn wound healing, minimize scarring, and reestablish the protective barrier of skin. Adult stem cells have been an area of interest in burn treatment, with cells being isolated from bone marrow, adipose tissue, and skin. Stem cells are self-renewing and multipotent, allowing for differentiation into different skin cell lineages such as epidermis, hair follicles, and dermis. Researchers are determining the optimal environment in which these stem cells will appropriately differentiate into these cell types. Stem cell therapy has also been shown to accelerate the wound healing process via blood vessel and collagen synthesis, all while diminishing some of the inflammatory response to the burn wound. While the promise of stem cell technology is extremely promising, there remain many challenges to overcome before it can become part of standard practice.

Rehabilitation of the Severely Burned Patient

While the vast field of rehabilitation after burn injury is well beyond the scope of this chapter, there are some notable uses of existing technology that have assisted patients in regaining function after severe burns. Initially thought to be a fad in rehabilitation of burned children and adolescents, the use of video games, and more specifically, interactive video games, have now been in use for several years. Commercially available video game systems have been shown to enhance recovery of active limb motion. Video games were noted to improve compliance with physical therapy by encouraging movement while acting as a distraction from pain [26]. These systems have been found useful in both the inpatient and outpatient rehabilitation arenas. Similarly, virtual reality has been explored as an assistive device in lessening pain in burned patients, however is currently not as accessible or available as commercially produced video game systems. While not examined for physical rehabilitative possibilities, the upcoming merge of virtual reality into currently available video game technology promises interesting ways of aiding patients both psychologically and physically.

Conclusion

While burn injuries are relatively rare occurrences, they represent one of the most devastating events that can occur in trauma. Technological advancements over the last 50 years have rapidly changed the way that burned patients are cared for. The next half-century will likely see an expansion of these technologies to minimize costs, morbidity, and time to return of function for severely burned individuals.

References

1. American Burn Association/American College of Surgeons. Guidelines for the operation of burn centers. J Burn Care Res. 2007;28(1):134–41.
2. Carter JE, Neff LP, Holmes JHT. Adherence to burn center referral criteria: are patients appropriately being referred? J Burn Care Res. 2010;31(1):26–30.
3. Reiband HK, et al. Optimization of burn referrals. Burns. 2014;40(3):397–401.
4. Latifi R, Tilley EH. Telemedicine for disaster management: can it transform chaos into an organized, structured care from the distance? Am J Disaster Med. 2014;9(1):25–37.
5. Latifi R, et al. Preoperative telemedicine evaluation of surgical mission patients: should we use it routinely? Bull Am Coll Surg. 2014;99(1):17–23.
6. Latifi R. Using telemedicine to strengthen medical systems in limited-resource countries. Bull Am Coll Surg. 2012;97(10):15–21.
7. Latifi R. Telepresence and telemedicine in trauma and emergency. Stud Health Technol Inform. 2008; 131:275–80.
8. Holt B, et al. Telemedicine use among burn centers in the United States: a survey. J Burn Care Res. 2012; 33(1):157–62.
9. Zangbar B, et al. Smartphone surgery: how technology can transform practice. Telemed J E Health. 2014; 20(6):590–2.
10. Salinas J, et al. Computerized decision support system improves fluid resuscitation following severe burns: an original study. Crit Care Med. 2011;39(9): 2031–8.
11. Devgan L, et al. Modalities for the assessment of burn wound depth. J Burns Wounds. 2006;5, e2.
12. Heimbach D, et al. Burn depth: a review. World J Surg. 1992;16(1):10–5.
13. Watts AM, et al. Burn depth and its histological measurement. Burns. 2001;27(2):154–60.
14. Pape SA, Skouras CA, Byrne PO. An audit of the use of laser Doppler imaging (LDI) in the assessment of burns of intermediate depth. Burns. 2001;27(3):233–9.
15. Droog EJ, Steenbergen W, Sjoberg F. Measurement of depth of burns by laser Doppler perfusion imaging. Burns. 2001;27(6):561–8.
16. Jackson DM. The diagnosis of the depth of burning. Br J Surg. 1953;40(164):588–96.
17. Boykin JV, Eriksson E, Pittman RN. In vivo microcirculation of a scald burn and the progression of postburn dermal ischemia. Plast Reconstr Surg. 1980; 66(2):191–8.
18. Zawacki BE. Reversal of capillary stasis and prevention of necrosis in burns. Ann Surg. 1974;180(1):98–102.
19. Still JM, et al. Diagnosis of burn depth using laser-induced indocyanine green fluorescence: a preliminary clinical trial. Burns. 2001;27(4):364–71.
20. Gatti JE, et al. Evaluation of the burn wound with perfusion fluorometry. J Trauma. 1983;23(3):202–6.
21. Sheridan RL, et al. Burn depth estimation by use of indocyanine green fluorescence: initial human trial. J Burn Care Rehabil. 1995;16(6):602–4.
22. Pape SA, Byrne PO. Safety and efficacy of TransCyte for the treatment of partial-thickness burns. J Burn Care Rehabil. 2000;21(4):390.
23. Holland AJ, Martin HC, Cass DT. Laser Doppler imaging prediction of burn wound outcome in children. Burns. 2002;28(1):11–7.
24. O'Reilly TJ, et al. Laser Doppler flowmetry evaluation of burn wound depth. J Burn Care Rehabil. 1989; 10(1):1–6.
25. Kagan RJ, Robb EC, Plessinger TR. Human skin banking. Clin Lab Med. 2005;25(3):587–605.
26. Haik J, et al. The use of video capture virtual reality in burn rehabilitation: the possibilities. J Burn Care Res. 2006;27(2):195–7.

17 Biology of Nutrition Support and Gut Access in Critically Ill Patients

Norio Sato and Rifat Latifi

Background

Nutrition support for critically ill and injured patients has undergone significant advances in recent decades as the direct result of scientific progress and our increased knowledge of the biology and biochemistry of key nutrient changes induced by injury, sepsis, and other critical illnesses, both in adults and in children. The science of nutrition support (or, more accurately, of nutrition therapy) has become more disease-based. Also called "specialized" or "artificial" nutrition support, nutrition therapy refers to the provision of either enteral nutrition (EN) via tube feeding or total parenteral nutrition (TPN). In contrast, "standard therapy" refers to a patient's own volitional intake, without the provision of nutrition therapy [1].

Of all the advances in nutritional support, the development of Total Parenteral Nutrition by Dr. Stanley J. Dudrick and his team is the most significant event to have clearly changed the way we think about nutrition, the way we feed the critically ill and the way we support these patients who cannot, should not, or will not be fed orally [2]. Furthermore, in the past three to four decades, the understanding of the molecular and biological effects of nutrients in maintaining homeostasis in the critically ill population has made exponential advances. Traditionally, nutrition support in the critically ill population was regarded as adjunctive care designed to provide exogenous fuels to support the patient during the stress response. This support had three main objectives: to preserve lean body mass, to maintain immune function, and to avert metabolic complications. Recently, these goals have become more focused on nutrition therapy; specifically attempting to attenuate the metabolic response to stress, prevent oxidative cellular injury, and favorably modulate the immune response.

Depending on the individual patient's metabolic needs, nutrition therapy helps ensure that key nutrient substrates are replenished, or added in larger amounts, to supplement specific deficiencies or to simply prevent further deterioration and clinical consequences. The benefit of early institution of either EN or TPN in the overall care of critically ill and injured patients has now been well-established. After a critical illness or injury, the patient's energy and overall metabolic requirements greatly increase in order to sustain increased metabolism and the process of wound repair. Given current evidence derived from

N. Sato, M.D., Ph.D.
Department of Primary Care and Emergency Medicine, Kyoto University Hospital, Kyoto City, Japan
e-mail: drnori@kuhp.kyoto-u.ac.jp

R. Latifi, M.D., F.A.C.S. (✉)
Department of Surgery, University of Arizona Medical Center, Tucson, AZ, USA
e-mail: latifi@surgery.arizona.edu

R. Latifi et al. (eds.), *Technological Advances in Surgery, Trauma and Critical Care*,
DOI 10.1007/978-1-4939-2671-8_17

randomized controlled trials (RCTs), early provision of nutrition for critically ill and injured patients is now a level I recommendation [3].

Critical illness and tissue injury initiate a complex series of rapidly responding homeostatic events in an attempt to prevent ongoing tissue damage and to activate the repair process. Classically, inflammation has been recognized as the hallmark of the homeostatic response. But more recently, attention has been focused on defining the complexities of response at the cellular, metabolic, and molecular levels. There is mounting evidence regarding the multiple specific metabolic changes in critically ill and injured patients and their need for fundamental nutrients and special substrates.

The benefit of the early institution of adequate enteral or parenteral nutrition in the overall management of critically ill patients has been well-established. Early nutritional support has the potential to reduce disease severity, diminish complications, and decrease the intensive care unit (ICU) length of stay and favorably impact patient outcome. Recognizing the importance of the appropriate nutritional support of trauma and critically ill patients with severe and/or multiple injuries, we have implemented a standard nutritional assessment and support program that aligns with guidelines set by the SCCM, ASPEN, ESPEN, and EAST. Despite all of this, it is very difficult to extrapolate nutritional support alone as the major factor impacting the patient's outcome. Sophisticated delivery tubing systems for enteral feeding, complex pharmacological mixtures of various nutrients in the form of parenteral nutrition, and recognition of various nutrients as pharmaco-nutrients have exploded in recent years. Gut access for provision of nutrition support has undergone major changes as well. Advanced laparoscopic approaches, percutaneous endoscopic access, and fine technology of these tubing systems have been refined continuously for the last few decades. In the following pages we describe some of the key nutrients and their effect on the biology of the disease.

n-3 Fatty Acids

Pharmacological Effects of n-3 Fatty Acids

Fatty acids are categorized as either saturated or unsaturated fatty acids. Monounsaturated fatty acids have one double bond while polyunsaturated fatty acids have two or more double bonds. Depending on the number of carbon atoms, fatty acids are also referred to as "short chain" (<8 carbons), "medium chain" (8–14 carbons), or "long chain" (≥15 carbons) fatty acids. Unsaturated fatty acids are also distinguished by where the first double bond occurs, counting from the carbon atom at the very end. These are typically designated ω3 (n-3), ω6 (n-6), and ω9 (n-9). The role of fatty acids include important aspects such as (1) sources of energy, (2) components of cell membranes, and (3) conversion into lipid metabolites that take part in physiological activities (e.g., prostagladins). Fatty acid administration leads to their incorporation into cell membranes. Arachidonic acid, which is an n-6 series fatty acid, plays a role in the formation of cell membranes, along with the n-3 series fatty acids eicosapentaenoic acid (EPA) and docosahexanoic acid (DHA). These fatty acids are discharged from cell membranes if cell injury or phospholipase activation occurs in association with a cellular insult. Although n-3 and n-6 fatty acids are metabolized by the same enzymes (cyclooxygenase and 5-lipoxygenase), the final metabolic products are different. When inflammatory mediators such as prostaglandin (PG) E_2, thromboxane (TX) A_2, or leukotriene (LT) B_4 are produced from n-6 fatty acids in excessive amounts, neutrophil activation is triggered which leads to systemic inflammatory response syndrome (SIRS). PGE_3, TXA_3, LTB_5, and other similar factors are produced from n-3 fatty acids; they are known to compete with metabolites of n-6 fatty acids and bring about anti-inflammatory activity. Reports indicate that n-3 fatty acids inhibit the production of the inflammatory cytokines interleukin (IL)-1 and tumor necrosis factor (TNF) by neutrophils and reduce the production of inducible nitric oxide synthase (iNOS) by macrophages. Furthermore, it has been demonstrated that n-3 fatty acids metabolize into resolvins and protectins, which promote convergence of inflammation, and have gained particular attention for their anti-inflammatory effects. The anti-inflammatory effect of n-3 fatty acids has been corroborated by many fundamental studies.

Clinical Studies Involving n-3 Fatty Acids

n-3 fatty acids is commonly found in a number of IEN or IMN, but one formula that has received particular attention is known that Oxepa® (Abbott Labs, Abbott Park, IL), which contains EPA, DHA, γ-linoleric acid (GLA), and antioxidants, is recommended for Acute lung injury (ALI) and Adult respiratory distress syndrome (ARDS) by guidelines in Europe, the USA, Canada, and other countries [3–5].

Pontes-Aruda et al. [6] studied 165 patients with severe septicemia involving acute lung injury (ALI) and acute respiratory distress syndrome who received Oxepa® and Pulmocare® (Abbott Labs, Abbott Park, IL). They reported that Oxepa® significantly improved the survival rate (67.3 % vs. 47.9 %) and decreased the number of days under artificial respiration control (14.6 days vs. 22.2 days) and the number of days patients remained in the intensive care unit (ICU) (17.2 days vs. 23.4 days). Furthermore, significant improvements were seen in oxygenating function and there was a significant reduction in the occurrence of new organ dysfunction. The fact that the control group in this study received a nutritional supplement that contained 55 % n-6 polysaturated fatty acid became an issue. In a study of the effectiveness of Oxepa® that included 106 patients with early-stage septicemia, the control group was given an ordinary nutritional supplement that contained 29 % fatty ingredients [7]. In that study, Oxepa® significantly decreased the incidence of septicemia (26.2 % vs. 51.0 %), the incidence of new organ dysfunction such as cardiovascular failure (21.0 % vs. 36.2 %) or respiratory failure (24.6 % vs. 39.6 %), the number of days patients remained in the ICU (7 days vs. 13 days), and the number of days patients remained in the hospital (9 days vs. 19 days). However, there was no significant change in mortality rates. Grau-Carmona et al. [8] compared Oxepa® to an ordinary nutritional supplement that contained 30 % fatty acids in 133 patients with septicemia. In that study, Oxepa® did not lead to any significant differences in mortality, oxygenation function, infection outbreak rate, or organ dysfunction incidence rate. However, Oxepa® was associated with significantly fewer days in the ICU (16 days vs. 18 days). Investigators also conducted a randomized controlled trial to examine the effectiveness of enteral bolus administration of EPA and DHA to patients with ALI. Stapleton et al. performed bolus administration of EPA and DHA to 90 patients with ALI and compared them to a group that did not receive this treatment. The group treated with bolus administration experienced a significant rise in the concentrations of EPA and DHA in the blood, but no significant differences were found in proinflammatory cytokine levels in the bronchoalveolar lavage fluid. Furthermore, there were no significant differences in mortality, number of days in the hospital, number of days in the ICU, or organ dysfunction incidence. Rice et al. [9] performed bolus administration of EPA, DHA, GLA, and antioxidants in 272 patients with ALI and compared them to a group that did not receive this treatment. The group that received the bolus administration had a significantly increased concentration of EPA in the blood but no significant differences were found in proinflammatory cytokines in the blood or in LTB4 concentration. Furthermore, a significant rise in the rate of death was observed in the group that received the bolus administration. It is necessary to consider the rise in death rate observed after bolus administration of EPA, DHA, and GLA separately from the anti-inflammatory effects of Oxepa® that support the guidelines.

Fat emulsions containing fish oil (EPA and DHA) have been widely administered intravenously, primarily in Europe, and clinical studies of their effectiveness have been conducted [10]. A recent meta-analysis of critically ill patients conducted by Manzanares et al. [11] confirmed a tendency toward decreased mortality and shortened period of mechanical ventilation; however, no effect was found on the infection rate or number of days in the ICU. Pradelli et al. [12] conducted a meta-analysis of patients who underwent elective surgery and critically ill patients, and they found significant decreases in infection rates, the number of days in the ICU, and the number of days in the hospital. When Palmer et al. [13] conducted a meta-analysis of critically ill patients in a similar manner, the conclusions were somewhat different; they reported no improvements in mortality, infection rate, or number of days in the ICU in patients who used fish oil. Currently, clinical studies have not yielded consistent conclusions. Although the issue of the sale of fish oil in the USA and Japan has not yet been available, there are physicians who are awaiting the permission of usage fat emulsions containing fish oil.

Glutamine

Pharmacological Effects of Glutamine

Glutamine is synthesized from other amino acids. Therefore, it is not necessary to ingest it as a nutrient when cells are not subject to insult. However, when the body is experiencing an insult such as trauma and sepsis the demand for glutamine increases, and the amount that can be synthesized by the body cannot keep up with demand. For this reason, it is considered a conditionally essential amino acid. Supplementation with glutamine to make up for relative shortages is considered beneficial for the body. Glutamine plays a diverse range of roles and can be converted into metabolites such as ammonia, nucleic acids, glutathione, arginine, and glucosamine. When the body is experiencing an insult, glutamine acts as an energy substrate in the intestinal mucosa, lymphocytes, macrophages, and neutrophils, and administration of glutamine to the intestinal tract is considered effective for sustaining the intestinal tract barrier function and preventing bacterial translocation. Many reports have demonstrated that glutamine increases levels of heat shock proteins (HSPs) as an anti-inflammatory mechanism. Intravenous administration of glutamine after the onset of septicemia activates the transcription factor heat shock factor-1, causing expression of HSP-70 and HSP-25 and thereby reducing the occurrence of acute lung disorders. Similarly, HSP-32 (heme oxygenase-1) is also expressed to reduce apoptosis and decrease tissue damage in the intestinal tract [14]. A report indicated that administration of glutamine inhibits apoptosis following stress or injury, and depletion of glutamine triggers apoptosis, which then activates caspase-3 and -9. Intravenous administration of glutamine inhibits the activation of nuclear factor-κB in the septicemia model [15]. It also inhibits activation of the stress-related p38 mitogen-activated protein kinase and extracellular signal-related kinase, resulting in reduced TNFα, IL-6, and IL-18. Similarly, enteral administration of glutamine has been shown to reduce serum IL-6 levels, increase IL-4 production by lymphocytes, and reduce interferon-γ production [16]. In an ischemia reperfusion model where a jenunal pouch was prepared and glutamine was administered, researchers confirmed inhibited activation of activator protein-1 and enhanced activation of peroxisome proliferator-activated receptor (PPAR). PPAR has drawn attention as a transcription factor with anti-inflammatory functions that is associated with reduced iNOS, reduced accumulation of neutrophils in the jejunum, retention of adenosine triphosphate levels in the jejunum, inhibition of intestinal tract permeability, and reduced tissue damage. Another study found that syndecan 1 was involved in reducing the action of glutamine in intestinal tract ischemia reperfusion damage [17]. It has also been noted that there is potential for arginine conversion through metabolism of glutamine to produce nitric oxide (NO), which can be harmful.

Clinical Studies Related to Glutamine

Many clinical trials have supported the usefulness of glutamine administration for reducing the infection rate during insult to the body. The results of large-scale clinical studies for determining the effectiveness of glutamine administration (enteral administration or intravenous administration) have been debatable, as some papers have cast doubt on the effectiveness of glutamine. Wernerman et al. [18] conducted a clinical study involving intravenous administration of glutamine (0.28 g/kg/day). The targeted number of cases was 1,000 over a 4-year period at 9 facilities in Sweden, 1 facility in Norway, and 1 facility in Finland (11 facilities in total). However, the study did not reach the target number of subjects; instead, the study included only 413 cases. Intravenous administration of glutamine in targeted patients with Acute Physiology and Chronic Health Evaluation II scores of 10 or higher, as well as in some mild cases, confirmed differences in the ICU death rate and the 28-day death rate; however, no difference was found in the mortality over a longer period. Andrews et al. [19] conducted a clinical study involving intravenous administration of glutamine (20.2 g/day) and intravenous administration of selenium (500 μg/day); this was known as the SIGNET trial. Analysis of 502 cases from ten ICU facilities in Scotland could not confirm that glutamine effectively reduced the infectious disease occurrence rate, number of days in the ICU, or the death rate. Heyland et al. [20] found astounding results when they conducted a large-scale clinical study of glutamine administration (intravenous administration of 0.35 g/kg/day and enteral administration of 30 g/day) along with selenium and antioxidant administration. They analyzed 1,223 critically ill patients with dysfunction of two or more organs from 40 facilities in Canada, the USA, and Europe, and found that the death rate increased with glutamine. The results of this study, known as the REDOX study, indicate that excessive amounts of glutamine must not be administered to patients with highly critical illnesses. It is important to note that this study did not completely refute the benefits of glutamine yet. Additionally SIGNET Trial [19] and REDOX Trial [20] tested the antioxidant nutrient using selenium. There was a reduction in the infection rate after intravenous administration of selenium (500 μg/day) for 5 days or more during the SIGNET Trial. However, in the REDOX study, when intravenous selenium administration (500 g/day) and enteral administration of selenium (300 μg), zinc (2 mg), β-carotene (10 mg), Vitamin E (500 mg), and Vitamin C (1,500 mg) was compared to groups without them, there were no differences in outcomes between the two groups.

Arginine

Pharmacological Effects Related to Arginine

Similar to glutamine, arginine is a conditionally essential amino acid. Arginine is metabolized in the body primarily through two routes [21]. One route leads to ornithine and urea owing to the action of arginase, while the other route leads to NO and citrulline because of the action of nitric oxide synthase (NOS). Arginase I is found primarily in the liver, and ornithine is metabolized further into polyamine and proline to improve collagen synthesis and wound healing. Alternatively, arginase II occurs primarily outside the liver and produces creatine in the small intestine mucous membrane to store muscle energy. Arginine increases the secretion of hormones such as growth hormones, glucagon, prolactin, and somatostatin, raising immune function when insults occur. Although appropriate concentrations of ornithine are essential for sustaining immune function, a report found that the differentiation of B-cells and the number of intestinal Peyer patch cells deceased in mice with a large amount of arginase, inhibiting production of T-cells and the T-cell receptor CD3. An appropriate amount of NO is essential for bactericidal action, and the vasodilation action of NO improves microcirculation, making oxygen transport to the periphery possible. However, excessive NO production leads to peroxynitrite production and tissue damage and can cause septic shock owing to vasodilation. The three arginase I and II enzymes as well as iNOS are all induced when inflammation occurs, and arginase and NOS compete in immune cells. There is a rise in the demand for arginine and because the metabolic behavior of arginine changes according to its concentration, it is difficult to confirm or repudiate the benefits of arginine.

Trends of Clinical Studies Related to Arginine

There have not been any clinical studies of arginine administration alone; clinical studies have used arginine-containing nutritional supplements that are commercially available. Galban et al. [22] studied 176 septicemia patients and reported that the group that received a nutritional supplement with enhanced arginine had a significantly reduced death rate compared to the control nutritional supplement group (19 % vs. 32 %). Kieft et al. [23] studied 597 ICU patients and compared a group that received a nutritional supplement containing enhanced arginine to a control group. They found that there were no differences between the groups in death rate, infection rate, or the number of days in the ICU. A meta-analysis of septicemia patients and critically ill patients except those with external injuries or burns, who received arginine found no differences in mortality or infection rate [24]. However, arginine administration in patients undergoing elective surgery has been found to reduce the infection rate and shorten the number of days in the hospital. It is also economically beneficial. Arginine administration in patients with critical septicemia for whom the hemodynamics may deteriorate is considered a situation to be avoided from a theoretical perspective [25].

Pharmacological Nutrients and Clinical Studies Related to Leucine

Reducing lean body mass index is known to be associated to mortality; therefore, avoiding reduction of skeletal muscles is essential. Among the amino acids, some have functions that contribute to important aspects of body function such as signal transmission, phosphorylation, and gene expression. Leucine is a branched amino acid (BCAA), along with valine and isoleucine. Unlike other amino acids, leucine is directly metabolized in skeletal muscles. Leucine has cell growth promoting action and has been shown to stimulate the mammalian target of rapamycin (mTOR) to promote protein synthesis in skeletal muscles, cardiac muscles, and other tissues. Protein synthesis declines with septicemia, but administration of leucine is known to affect mTOR and increase protein synthesis. Studies on BCAAs have been conducted for more than 30 years, including a clinical study conducted in the 1990s investigating the administration of BCAAs for septic patients [26]. Jimenes et al. [27] conducted a study of 80 peritonitis patients in which they compared a group treated with 22.5 % BCAAs to another group treated with 45 % BCAAs at a nitrogen quantity of 12 g/day. While there was no difference in the death rate, there was an improvement in nitrogen balance and a reduction in 3-methylhistidine levels in the urine. Garcia-de-Lorenzo et al. [28] compared three groups of septic patients for whom enteral administration of nutrients was not possible. One group received 1.5 kg/kg of protein included 23 % BCAA, one group was given 1.5 g/kg of protein included 23 % BCAAs, and the last group was given 1.1 g/kg protein included 45 % BCAAs. While there were no improvements in nitrogen balance or similar outcomes, the two groups that received higher concentration of BCAA of 45 % had reduced mortality rates. The BCAAs included a combination of isoleucine, leucine, and valine in a 0.8:1.4:1 ratio. Many studies with high quantities of leucine have indicated the effectiveness of BCAAs in patients who are experiencing an injury. With the focus on early rehabilitation of ICU patients, the expectations for leucine increase in relation to the effectiveness of hydroxymethylbutyrate (HMB), a metabolite of leucine, as adjustment of skeletal muscle metabolism (suppression of protein catabolism and promotion of protein synthesis) and sustaining and increasing muscle mass lead to patient recovery and enhanced quality of life. Although there are metabolic behaviors in which functional amino acids are important, it is important to remember that administering amino acids in a proper balance is important for maintenance of homeostasis of the entire body.

Pharmacological Nutrients and Clinical Studies Related to Whey Protein

Protein in milk is made up of 20 % whey protein and 80 % casein. The protein component that remains in milk when coagulated is referred to as whey protein (milk whey). Milk whey consists of α-lactalbumin, β-lactalbumin, glycomacropeptide, lactoferrin, and albumin. Reports have highlighted the capabilities of whey protein, including promotion of protein synthesis, anti-inflammatory action, and antioxidative action, among others. Suppression of phospholipase A2 and cyclooxygenase 2 by α-lactalbumin has an anti-inflammatory effect. While whey protein suppresses production of cytokines such as TNF and IL-6 in a rodent liver injury model, it also increases production of cytokines via neutrophils and epithelial cells to improve immune function. Lactoferrin is an important factor for natural immunity related to biophylaxis in the digestive tract and mucous membranes. Discharge of lactoferrin included in the granules of neutrophils from activated neutrophils is known to raise the lactoferrin concentration in blood, from normal levels of 0.5–1 μg/mL to 200 g/mL. Lactoferrin has antioxidant properties, suppresses cytokine production, and functions in immunoregulation. Lactoferrin is known to bond with lactoferrin-lipopolysaccharide (LPS), alleviate toll-like receptor signal transmission, stabilize circulatory behavior for administration of LPS, and suppress TNF-α and IL-6 production.

Manzoni et al. studied 472 newborns weighing 1,500 g or less in neonatal ICUs at 11 facilities [29]. They compared a group that received lactoferrin to a placebo control group and found that administration of lactoferrin significantly suppressed the occurrence of tardive septicemia, significantly reduced fungal infection, and reduced mortality. A group in the USA conducted a double-blinded randomized comparison in adults with severe sepsis at 24 facilities in a phase 2 study of talactoferrin, which is a recombinant form of human lactoferrin [30]. In this study of 194 targeted patients, the 28-day death rate of the group treated with human lactoferrin was 14.4 %, which was significantly lower than the 26.9 % death rate in the control group. The death rate was also significantly lower after 6 months. This clinical study indicated the effectiveness of lactoferrin in adults.

Gut Access

The indications for EN are fairly straightforward and well established. All resuscitated critically ill and trauma patients who cannot, will not, or should not receive nutrition orally and who have a functional GI tract should receive nutrition support via GI access as early as possible. EN delivery can be via temporary nasoenteric tube placement (orogastric, nasogastric, nasoduodenal, or nasojejunal) or via more long-term techniques (gastrostomy or gastrojejunostomy, which can each be done either surgically or endoscopically). Factors to consider in terms of the individual patient include the anticipated duration of EN, aspiration risk, GI tract function, ability to tolerate the given EN technique, degree of critical illness or injury, and specific goal of EN.

As stated above, gut access has undergone major technological changes. A recent study by Tuma et al. [31] that reviewed all articles on gut access found that the most common gut access techniques included nasoenteric tube placement (nasogastric, nasoduodenal, or nasojejunal) as well as a percutaneous endoscopic gastrostomy (PEG). Other open or laparoscopic techniques such as a jejunostomy or a gastrojejunostomy are also used. Early EN continues to be preferred whenever feasible. In addition, evidence is mounting that, during the early phase of critical illness or trauma, trophic feeding has an outcome comparable to that of full-strength formulas. Most patients tolerate EN through the stomach, so post pyloric tube feeding is not needed initially. In critically ill and trauma patients early EN through the stomach should be instituted whenever feasible. Other approaches can be used according to patient needs, available expertise, and institutional guidelines. Nonetheless, more research is needed to ensure the safe use of surgical tubes in the open abdomen.

Indications for Gut Access

The indications for EN are fairly straightforward and well-established. All critically ill and trauma patients who cannot, will not, or should not receive nutrition orally and who have a functional GI tract need gastrointestinal access, as early as possible after they are fully resuscitated for nutritional support [32–36].

Techniques for Gut Access

Various techniques to obtain gut access and deliver EN exist. These include short-term options (nasogastric, nasoduodenal, or nasojejunal tube placement) or more long-term or even permanent options (gastrostomy or gastrojejunostomy). All of these techniques can be done either surgically or endoscopically. The decision which technique to use depends on the individual patient and on anticipated duration of nutrition support, aspiration risk, GI tract function, ability to tolerate the given placement technique, degree of critical illness or injury, and the goals of EN [37–39].

Whichever technique for gut access is used, the tube placement must be confirmed by the presence of aspirating gastric fluid or by radiologic or other techniques of verification (for example, intraoperative view). The position of the feeding tube should be confirmed at the time of insertion before intermittent feedings, and during continuous feedings; a chest or abdominal radiograph may confirm placement, and the mark on the tube at the exit site indicates that the exposed tube length has not changed [40].

Post-pyloric Versus Gastric Tubes

The debate over post-pyloric tube feeding versus gastric feeding continues to this date [41–44]. Many critically ill and trauma patients can be started with orogastric or nasogastric tube feeding; if they continue to be intubated and require prolonged tube feeding, they may be switched to post pyloric feeding. However, if patients do not tolerate gastric feeding, switching them to nasojejunal nutrition was not associated with better outcomes [45].

While nasogastric tubes or orogastric tubes (for intubated patients) constitute the initial short-term access for many patients, this is not ideal access for long-term access. Potential complications, although they are rare, include erosion of the nasal cartilage, sinusitis, and gastroesophageal reflux which in turn can lead to aspiration, pneumonitis, or pneumonia. Furthermore, dislodgment and blocking of these tubes is not uncommon.

Percutaneous Endoscopic Gastrostomy (PEG)

Ever since Ponsky and Gauderer [46] first reported a technique for percutaneous endoscopic gastrostomy (PEG) in the early 1980s, countless patients have been provided with EN through PEG. PEG is relatively safe and it is minimally invasive when compared with open surgical procedures. The indications and contraindications for PEG placement have been reported and are established [23]. The technique, however, has been standardized and does need further elaborations except to note that there are two ways of advancing the wire: the push and the pull technique. Two methods are possible for advancing the guidewire. If the pull method is used, the tapered gastrostomy tube is attached to the guidewire outside the patient's mouth; gentle tension is applied to the guidewire from the abdominal side to introduce the gastrostomy tube and guidewire unit into the esophagus and then into the stomach [47]. If the push method is used, the gastrostomy tube is passed over the guidewire, and the endoscope is used to grasp and stabilize the end of the wire beyond the gastrostomy tube; the gastrostomy tube is then pushed, by the endoscope, through the abdominal wall into the stomach, while tension is applied to both ends of the guide wire. With both methods, the endoscope may be reintroduced to confirm optimal placement (but without undue tension) of the internal bumper against the gastric mucosa. An external bumper is then used to secure PEG placement, with care taken to avoid undue pressure on the skin. A distance of 1–2 mm between the bolster and the skin is advisable, in order to decrease ischemic necrosis and subsequent infection.

PEG Gastrojejunostomy

Another technique for patients who cannot tolerate stomach feeding is the percutaneous gastrojejunostomy (PEGJ). The J-tube is passed through the existing PEG; the suture on the distal end of the J-tube is grasped with an endoscopic clip applicator passed through the working channel of the endoscope. The gastroscope and jejunal tube are then passed, under direct visualization, through the pylorus and into the small bowel. By firing the endoscopic clip, the surgeon secures the suture loop to the small-bowel mucosa. This technique allows for easier removal of the endoscope from the small bowel and minimizes the risk for inadvertent dislodgement of the jejunal feeding tube back to the stomach.

Surgical Gastrostomy

If PEG placement is contraindicated (see above), a surgically placed gastrostomy is an option, either via open technique or laparoscopy [48]. The Stamm open technique begins with the surgeon placing inner and outer purse string sutures on the mid-anterior gastric wall then an incision is made in the central portion of the purse string.

Laparoscopic approaches can be used as a modification of the Stamm procedure [49]. With two ports, one at the umbilicus for a 30° camera and the other in the right upper quadrant for use as a working port, the surgeon grasps the stomach and elevates it to the anterior abdominal wall, then selects an appropriate location for gastrostomy tube placement. The use of T-fasteners through the anterior abdominal wall and the gastric wall ensures the stomach is secured well and reduces overall morbidity if dislodgement occurs [50]. Through a small incision, a 14-gauge needle is introduced into the stomach and a guide wire is passed into the gastric lumen. The tract is serially dilated until the gastrostomy tube can be introduced.

Laparoscopically Assisted PEG

Laparoscopically assisted PEG is a preferred procedure in obese patients, in patients that have undergone previously laparotomies, and in those when we "do not see the light" as this ensures the gastrostomy-tube placement is checked by both the endoscopist and the surgeon [51]. The peritoneal cavity is accessed in the usual fashion. We use an open technique to insert a 30-degree laparoscope. A one or two 5 mm port is inserted also under direct vision. The stomach is inflated with a gastroscope and the needle from the anterior abdominal wall is inserted into the stomach under direct vision. The rest of the procedure is similar to PEG described above. One has to remember to lower the intraperitoneal pressure to 8–10 cm of H20 in order to allow the approximation of the stomach to the posterior abdominal wall.

Surgical Jejunostomy

Surgical jejunal access for feeding is another option. Both open and laparoscopic approaches are acceptable. Which technique the surgeon selects depends on experience and the clinical situation. When the patient is undergoing laparotomy and is in need of long-term nutrition support, an open Witzel jejunostomy is the preferred technique. Although in good hands, this procedure is safe and easy to perform, numerous technical and mechanical complications have been described [52].

Summary

This chapter outlined clinical studies of representative nutrients that are relevant to anti-inflammation and some of the basic techniques for gut access. Nutritional studies performed in ICUs have historically been conducted using guidelines based on relatively small-scale clinical studies or opinions based on experience and there have been clear differences and unspecified aspects in the guidelines set by various nations and societies. Large-scale clinical studies have been conducted to clarify recommendations but their results and predictions are sometimes contradictory, which adds to the confusion. While it is important to pay attention to the outcomes of clinical studies, the studies conducted in different nations at numerous facilities have provided results that were not obtained consistently with regard to the treatment details, leading to a detrimental reduction in accuracy. Clinical studies with higher accuracy are believed to have more significance even if the number of targeted patients is smaller. Cases involving distress of critically ill patients require medical treatment over longer periods so anti-inflammatory action against persistent and recurring inflammation as well as immune-enhancing action is extremely important. Therefore, we should consider administration of nutrients with renewed focus on the actions of the nutrients in the living body. While nutrition support has changed dramatically in the recent two to three decades, it is imperative that, in order to improve our practice of nutritional support for trauma and critically ill patients, we should continue to pursue further understanding of their metabolism, energy requirements and specific requirements of each nutrient, and not rely on old dogma and guidelines established by experts' opinions and semi-quasi data [32, 33].

Specifically, we need to continue to challenge the current understanding of nutritional science, the biology of nutrients and the interaction of these nutrients with trauma, injury and critical illness, and how to further advance timely and disease-directed nutritional support. In the meantime, we need to provide nutritional support to critically ill or injured patients early and we should tailor nutritional formulas based on the content of the nutrient compositions [34].

References

1. Latifi R. Nutritional therapy in critically ill and injured patients. Surg Clin North Am. 2011;91(3):579–93.
2. Dudrick SJ, Wilmore DW, Vars HM, Rhoads JE. Long-term total parenteral nutrition with growth, development, and positive nitrogen balance. Surgery. 1968;64(1):134–42.
3. McClave SA, Martindale RG, Vanek VW, et al. Guidelines for the provision and assessment of nutrition support therapy in the adult critically ill patient: Society of Critical Care Medicine (SCCM) and American Society for Parenteral and Enteral Nutrition (A.S.P.E.N.). JPEN. 2009;33:277–315.
4. Kreymanna KG, Bergerb MM, Deutz NEP, et al. ESPEN guidelines on enteral nutrition: intensive care. Clin Nutr. 2006;25:210–23.
5. Canadian Clinical Practice Guidelines 2014. Summary of topics and recommendations. (http://www.criticalcarenutrition.com/)
6. Pontes-Arruda A, Aragao AM, Albuquerque JD. Effects of enteral feeding with eicosapentaenoic acid, gamma-linolenic acid, and antioxidants in mechanically ventilated patients with severe sepsis and septic shock. Crit Care Med. 2006;34:2325–33.
7. Pontes-Arruda A, Martins LF, de Lima SM, et al. Enteral nutrition with eicosapentaenoic acid, gamma-linolenic acid and antioxidants in the early treatment of sepsis: results from a multicenter, prospective, randomized, double-blinded, controlled study: the INTERSEPT study. Crit Care (London, England). 2011;15:R144.
8. Grau-Carmona T, Moran-Garcia V, Garcia-de-Lorenzo A, et al. Effect of an enteral diet enriched with eicosapentaenoic acid, gamma-linolenic acid and anti-oxidants on the outcome of mechanically ventilated, critically ill, septic patients. Clin Nutr (Edinburgh, Scotland). 2011;30:578–84.
9. Rice TW, Wheeler AP, Thompson BT, deBoisblan BP, Steingrub J, Rock P. Enteral omega-3 fatty acid, gamma-linolenic acid, and antioxidant supplementation in acute lung injury. JAMA. 2011;306:1574–81.
10. Singer P, Berger MM, Van den Berghe G, et al. ESPEN guidelines on parenteral nutrition: intensive care. Clin Nutr. 2009;28:387–400.
11. Manzanares W, Dhaliwal R, Jurewitsch B, Stapleton RD, Jeejeebhoy KN, Heyland DK. Parenteral fish oil lipid emulsions in the critically ill: a systematic review and meta-analysis. JPEN. 2014;38(1):20–8.
12. Pradelli L, Mayer K, Muscaritoli M, Heller AR. n-3 fatty acid-enriched parenteral nutrition regimens in elective surgical and ICU patients: a meta-analysis. Crit Care (London, England). 2012;16:R184.
13. Palmer AJ, Ho CK, Ajibola O, Avenell A. The role of omega-3 fatty acid supplemented parenteral nutrition in critical illness in adults: a systematic review and meta-analysis. Crit Care Med. 2013;41:307–16.
14. Uehara K, Takahashi T, Fujii H, et al. The lower intestinal tract-specific induction of heme oxygenase-1 by

glutamine protects against endotoxemic intestinal injury. Crit Care Med. 2005;33:381–90.
15. Singleton KD, Beckey VE, Wischmeyer PE. Glutamine prevents activation of Nf-kappab and stress kinase pathways, attenuates inflammatory cytokine release, and prevents acute respiratory distress syndrome (ARDS) following sepsis. Shock (Augusta, Ga). 2005;24:583–9.
16. Yeh CL, Hsu CS, Yeh SL, Chen WJ. Dietary glutamine supplementation modulates Th1/Th2 cytokine and interleukin-6 expressions in septic mice. Cytokine. 2005;31:329–34.
17. Peng Z, Ban K, Sen A, et al. Syndecan-1 plays a novel role in enteral glutamine's gut protective effects of the post ischemic gut: role of syndecan-1 in gut protection by glutamine. Shock. 2012;38(1):57–62.
18. Wernerman J, Kirketeig T, Andersson B, et al. Scandinavian glutamine trial: a pragmatic multicentre randomised clinical trial of intensive care unit patients. Acta Anaesthesiol Scand. 2011;55:812–8.
19. Andrews PJ, Avenell A, Noble DW, et al. Randomised trial of glutamine, selenium, or both, to supplement parenteral nutrition for critically ill patients. BMJ (Clin Res ed). 2011;342:d1542.
20. Heyland D, Muscedere J, Wischmeyer PE, et al. A randomized trial of glutamine and antioxidants in critically ill patients. N Engl J Med. 2013;368:1489–97.
21. Wu G. Amino acids: metabolism, functions, and nutrition. Amino Acids. 2009;37:1–17.
22. Galban C, Montejo JC, Mesejo A, et al. An immune-enhancing enteral diet reduces mortality rate and episodes of bacteremia in septic intensive care unit patients. Crit Care Med. 2000;28:643–8.
23. Kieft H, Roos AN, van Drunen JD, Bindels AJ, Bindels JG, Hofman Z. Clinical outcome of immunonutrition in a heterogeneous intensive care population. Intensive Care Med. 2005;31:524–32.
24. Waitzberg DL, Saito H, Plank LD, et al. Postsurgical infections are reduced with specialized nutrition support. World J Surg. 2006;30:1592–604.
25. Zaloga GP, Roberts PR, Marik P. Feeding the hemodynamically unstable patient: a critical evaluation of the evidence. Nutr Clin Pract. 2003;18:285–93.
26. Kazi AA, Pruznak AM, Frost RA, Lang CH. Sepsis-induced alterations in protein-protein interactions within mTOR complex 1 and the modulating effect of leucine on muscle protein synthesis. Shock (Augusta, Ga). 2011;35:117–25.
27. Jimenez Jimenez FJ, Ortiz Leyba C, Morales Menedez S, Barros Perez M, Munoz Garcia J. Prospective study on the efficacy of branched-chain amino acids in septic patients. JPEN. 1991;15:252–61.
28. Garcia-de-Lorenzo A, Ortiz-Leyba C, Planas M, et al. Parenteral administration of different amounts of branch-chain amino acids in septic patients: clinical and metabolic aspects. Crit Care Med. 1997;25:418–24.
29. Manzoni P, Stolfi I, Messner H, et al. Bovine lactoferrin prevents invasive fungal infections in very low birth weight infants: a randomized controlled trial. Pediatrics. 2012;129:116–23.
30. Manzoni P, Rinaldi M, Cattani S, et al. Bovine lactoferrin supplementation for prevention of late-onset sepsis in very low-birth-weight neonates: a randomized trial. JAMA. 2009;302:1421–8.
31. Tuma M, Latifi R, El-Menyar A, Al-Thani H. Gastrointestinal tract access for enteral nutrition in critically ill and trauma patients: indications, techniques, and complications. Eur J Trauma Emerg Surg. 2013;39:235–42.
32. Joseph B, Wynne JL, Dudrick SJ, Latifi R. Nutrition in trauma and critically ill patients. Eur J Emerg Surg. 2010;36(1):25–30.
33. Latifi R. Editorial: nutritional support of critically injured patients: do it early and do it right. Eur Surg. 2011;43(1):5–6.
34. Latifi R, Uranues S. Feed the gut, feed early and with the right stuff, but do not forget total parenteral nutrition. Eur J Trauma Emerg Surg. 2013;39:201–2.
35. DeLegge M. Enteral access—the foundation of feeding. JPEN. 2001;25:58.
36. Burlew CC, Moore EE, Cuschieri J, Jurkovich GJ, Codner P, Nirula R, Millar D, Cohen MJ, Kutcher ME, Haan J, Macnew HG, Ochsner MG, Rowell SE, Truitt MS, Moore FO, Pieracci FM, Kaups KL, the WTA Study Group. Who should we feed? A Western Trauma Association multi-institutional study of enteral nutrition in the open abdomen after injury. J Trauma Acute Care Surg. 2012;73(6):1380–7. Discussion 1387–8.
37. Gopalan A, Khanna S. Enteral nutrition delivery technique. Curr Opin Clin Nutr Metab Care. 2003;6(3):313–7.
38. Huang HH, Chang SJ, Hsu CW, et al. Severity of illness influences the efficacy of enteral feeding route on clinical outcomes in patients with critical illness. Acad Nutr Diet. 2012;112(8):1138–46.
39. Rice TW. Can we stomach gastric feeding in critically ill patients with gastrointestinal intolerance? Crit Care Med. 2012;40(8):2508–9.
40. Metheny NA, Titler MG. Assessing placement of feeding tubes. Am J Nurs. 2001;101:36–46.
41. Montecalvo MA, Steger KA, Farber HW, et al. Nutritional outcome and pneumonia in critical care patients randomized to gastric versus jejunal tube feedings. Crit Care Med. 1992;20:1377–87.
42. Kearns PJ, Chin D, Mueller L, et al. The incidence of ventilator-associated pneumonia and success in nutrient delivery with gastric versus small intestinal feeding: a randomized clinical trial. Crit Care Med. 2000;28(6):1742–6.
43. ChienWei H, ShuFen S, Shoa L, et al. Duodenal versus gastric feeding in medical intensive care unit patients: a prospective, randomized, clinical study. Crit Care Med. 2009;37:1866–72.
44. Kulvatunyou N, Joseph B, Tang A, et al. Gut access in critically ill patients: where have we gone thus far? Eur Surg. 2011;43(1):24–9.
45. Davies AR, Morrison SS, Bailey MJ, et al. Multicenter, randomized controlled trial comparing early nasojejunal with nasogastric nutrition in critical illness. Crit Care Med. 2012;40(8):2342–8.

46. Ponsky JL, Gauderer MW. Percutaneous endoscopic gastrostomy: a nonoperative technique for feeding gastrostomy. Gastrointest Endosc. 1981;27:9–11.
47. Jane P. Technique of upper gastrointestinal endoscopy. Gastrointest Endosc Clin N Am. 1994;4:501–52.
48. Zollinger Jr RM, Zollinger Sr RM. Plate 10. Percutaneous endoscopic gastrostomy—PEG. In: Zollinger Jr RM, Zollinger Sr RM, editors. Zollinger's atlas of surgical operations. 9th ed. New York: McGraw-Hill; 2011.
49. Zollinger Jr RM, Zollinger Sr RM. Plate 9. Gastrostomy. In: Zollinger Jr RM, Zollinger Sr RM, editors. Zollinger's atlas of surgical operations. 9th ed. New York: McGraw-Hill; 2011.
50. Duh Q, Way L. Laparoscopic gastrostomy using T-fasteners as retractors and anchors. Surg Endosc. 1993;7:60–3.
51. Charlesworth P, Hallows M, van der Avoirt A. Single-center experience of laparoscopically assisted percutaneous endoscopic gastrostomy placement. J Laparoendosc Adv Surg Tech A. 2010;20(1):73–5.
52. Tapia J, Murguia R, Garcia G. Jejunostomy: techniques, indications, and complications. World J Surg. 1999;23(6):596–602.

Part III

System-Oriented Technological Advances: Section A—Head and Neck

Advances in Head and Neck Surgery

18

Michael E. Stadler, Mihir R. Patel, and Marion E. Couch

Introduction

Head and neck cancers (HNC) encompass a diverse group of tumors in terms of clinical behavior and involved subsites. However, roughly 90 % are diagnosed as squamous cell carcinoma of the head and neck (SCCHN). In 2014, there were an estimated 55,070 new cases of HNC in the USA, with an estimated 12,000 deaths, representing roughly 4 % of all cancer deaths in the USA that year [1]. Worldwide, HNC is the sixth most common cancer, with roughly 650,000 new cases reported annually. Historically, the traditional risk factors for the development of SCCHN were tobacco and alcohol abuse, synergistically working together as potent risk factors for the disease.

M.E. Stadler, M.D. (✉)
Department of Otolaryngology and Communication Sciences, Medical College of Wisconsin, Milwaukee, WI, USA
e-mail: mstadler@mcw.edu

M.R. Patel, M.D.
Department of Otolaryngology—Head and Neck Surgery, Winship Cancer Institute of Emory University, Atlanta, GA, USA
e-mail: mihir.r.patel@emory.edu

M.E. Couch, M.D., Ph.D., M.B.A.
Department of Otolaryngology—Head and Neck Surgery, Indiana University School of Medicine, Indianapolis, IN, USA
e-mail: couchma@iupui.edu

The treatment for SCCHN has become quite complex, now importantly involving multidisciplinary teams and multimodality therapy. Yet tumors of the head and neck have historically been treated primarily with open surgical approaches. The utilization of postoperative adjuvant radiation therapy (RT) became much more commonly administered in the 1970s, although its use in SCCHN dated back decades earlier. Mounting data subsequently followed, showing that adjuvant treatment with radiotherapy after surgical resection improved locoregional control rates, thus improving overall survival. Further investigations have also led to the use of RT alone for the primary treatment of certain early stage SCCHNs with excellent outcomes. However, for most advanced stage disease of the head and neck, multimodality therapy is required.

Along with surgery and radiation therapy, a third efficacious modality to treat HNC is chemotherapy. Investigated most thoroughly in the last few decades of the twentieth century, chemotherapeutic regimens, combined with radiation therapy in the preoperative and postoperative setting, have shown great promise as adjuvant therapy in further improving oncologic outcomes. And in the mid to late-1990s, concomitant chemoradiation therapy (CRT) became a viable primary treatment option for certain patients with advanced stage SCCHN. Yet, despite the continued advances in the therapeutic options available for SCCHN

R. Latifi et al. (eds.), *Technological Advances in Surgery, Trauma and Critical Care*,
DOI 10.1007/978-1-4939-2671-8_18

patients over the past 20+ years, overall survival (OS), disease-free survival (DFS), functional outcomes, and toxicity profiles from therapy, have remained relatively poor. To date, patients with SCCHN continue to have some of the lowest survival rates of all major cancer types.

These historically suboptimal results have helped drive continued progress and innovation, including improved minimally invasive surgical procedures, advanced technological developments in radiation therapy, and expanded research and development of targeted chemotherapeutics and biologic therapies. These efforts have coincided with a new era for SCCHN, in which an increasing number of patients are presenting with a unique disease process that is biologically distinct from the more traditional HNC previously seen. This distinct disease process has demanded a thorough reevaluation of current practices, further promoting innovative efforts to improve patient care.

Table 18.1 Epidemiologic and clinical differences between HPV-positive and HPV-negative SCCHN

HPV-negative tumors	HPV-positive tumors
Decreasing incidence	Increasing incidence
Tobacco abuse common	Tobacco abuse less common
Alcohol abuse common	Alcohol abuse less common
Low oral sex exposure	High oral sex exposure
Marajuana use less common	Marajuana use more common
More advanced age	Less advanced age
Lower socioeconomic status	Higher socioeconomic status
All head and neck subsites	Predominantly oropharynx subsite
Relatively poor locoregional control	Excellent locoregional control
Poor disease-free and overall survival	Good disease-free and overall survival
Comorbid disease common	Comorbid disease less common

Transoral Surgery (TOS) of the Head and Neck

The incidence of oropharyngeal squamous cell cancer (OPSCC) is estimated to be increasing at a rate of 5 %/year in the USA, rising to epidemic levels. This is in clear contradistinction to other head and neck subsites, whose rates have been in decline due to decreased tobacco use. Extensive epidemiologic and clinical data has shown that these rising rates of OPSCC are related to the causative role of the human papilloma virus (HPV). HPV-related OPSCC (HPV-OPSCC) has been shown to have unique risk factors, patient demographics, and an improved prognosis compared to traditional, tobacco-related OPSCC (Table 18.1). The improved survival has also been shown to be treatment-modality independent, with excellent outcomes in patients treated with either primary surgical or radiation therapy [2]. This HPV-OPSCC patient population is usually younger and healthier than the more "traditional" SCCHN patient. This, along with the fact that these patients have improved outcomes, translates to the HPV-OPSCC patient living longer with the side effects that are caused by their treatment(s). It has therefore become clear that HPV-OPSCC demands tailored therapy that focuses on maintaining excellent oncologic outcomes, while also reducing unnecessary acute and late treatment-related toxicities, and providing efficient, cost-effective care.

Improved technical precision, access, and visualization with minimally invasive surgical approaches have allowed for a reemergence of primary surgical therapy for many head and neck tumors, including that of OPSCC. Minimally invasive surgery of the head and neck consists of techniques that reduce the extent of surgery through the use of natural orifices, small incisions, and tools that enhance visualization. The proposed benefits of these approaches are to maintain or improve oncologic outcomes, reduce operative morbidity, improve patient function and quality of life, and decrease hospital stay and overall cost of care.

While these techniques have long been used for accessible oral cavity tumors, transoral surgery (TOS) has increasingly been utilized as a primary treatment modality for both early and late-stage OPSCC as well. The two most popular and proven techniques, transoral laser microsur-

Table 18.2 Differences between TLM and TORS for minimally invasive approaches to SCCHN

	TLM	TORS
Advantages	Precise tissue differentiation with laser use	No line of sight limitations
	High resolution binocular visualization of tumor	High resolution 3D visualization of tumor
	Relative ease in addressing larynx and hypopharynx tumors	Tremor-filtration and motion scaling
	Tactile feedback	Instrument range of motion
Disadvantages	Laser safety considerations/risks	Cost of robotic system use
	Relative steep learning curve	Lack of tactile feedback
	Line of site limitations	Credentialing and training requirements
	Requirement for skilled pathologist to accurately assess piecemeal resection margins	Access: need to share with other services
		Need for skilled surgical assistant at head of bed

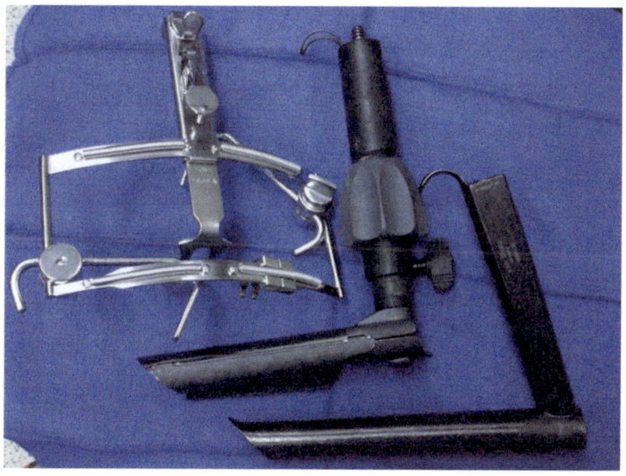

Fig. 18.1 In TLM, surgical exposure of the tumor within the upper aerodigestive tract is achieved with use of various oropharyngeal retractors, pharyngoscopes, and laryngoscopes

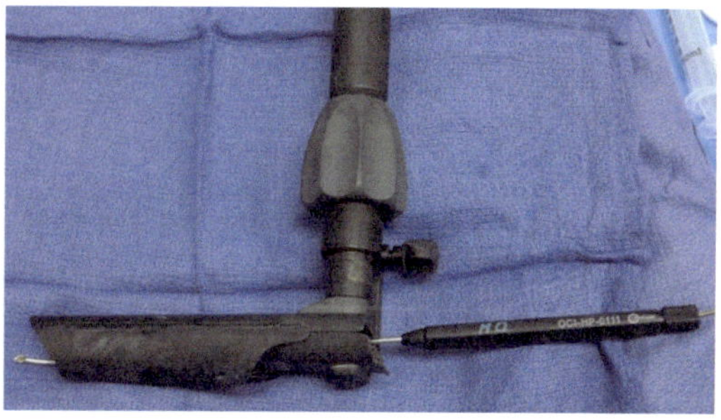

Fig. 18.2 Handpieces designed to transmit a flexible laser fiber can be then passed through the device used for surgical exposure. Pictured here is a bivalved expandable pharyngoscope with a laser handpiece

gery (TLM) and transoral robotic surgery (TORS), are also sometimes utilized to treat oral cavity and laryngeal tumors of the head and neck (Table 18.2). There has been growing interest in these minimally invasive TOS techniques that avoid the morbidity associated with traditional open en bloc resections, which often included a mandibulotomy and extensive dissection of non-cancerous, normal tissues to gain access to the tumor.

With the TLM technique, a modified mouth gag and/or expandable distending bivalved laryngoscope is used to expose the primary tumor (Figs. 18.1 and 18.2). As tumors extend more proximally into the upper aerodigestive tract, this process becomes more challenging, with tumors of the base of tongue (BOT) and vallecula requiring precise placement of these instruments for adequate tumor exposure and resection. A rigid telescope, or more commonly, high-magnification operating microscope, is then used to magnify and illuminate the exposed operative field (Figs. 18.3 and 18.4). This improved visualization of the tumor then provides the surgeon the ability to utilize either the line-of-site carbon dioxide (CO_2) laser or handheld CO_2 laser fiber for tumor resection. With the TLM technique, tumors are usually transected through the midportion to gain valuable and accurate information on depth of invasion and of the critical neurovascular structures adjacent to these tissues. Tumors are excised segmentally and ultimately removed piecemeal, mapping margins and paying close attention to both the peripheral and deep extension of the tumor as the procedure proceeds. This utilization of trans-tumoral cuts goes against the classic dogma within the surgical world of en bloc resection. However, long-term follow-up

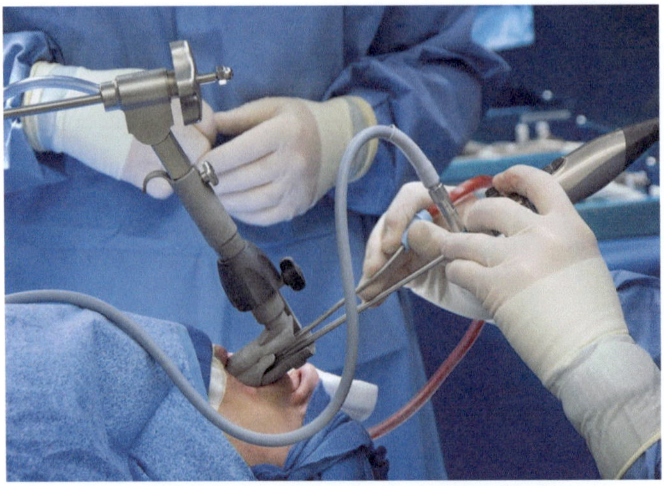

Fig. 18.3 Surgical exposure of the base of tongue tumor is obtained with use of a bivalved expandable pharyngoscope and patient is placed in suspension. Use of a rigid telescope or microscope allows for high magnification view of the tumor

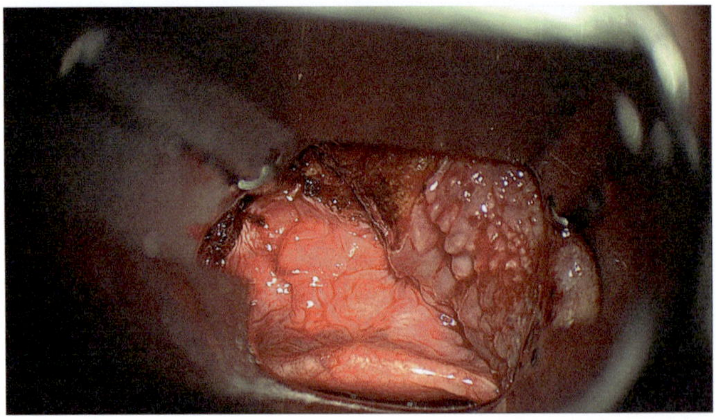

Fig. 18.4 High magnification view of right base of tongue tumor resection bed through a bivalved expandable pharyngoscope. Epiglottis is noted posteriorly with residual base of tongue tissue noted superiorly and laterally on the *right*. Evidence of tumor resection seen laterally on the *left* and superiorly

data from both Europe and the USA has shown that this method of tumor extirpation does not negatively impact local control.

With the high-magnification operative view that the microscope provides, along with the distinct tissue characteristics that are seen when the laser cuts through cancerous and normal tissues, margin control has been shown to be excellent with this technique. A reasonable margin of normal-appearing tissue (usually 1 cm) is then excised beyond the invading front of the tumor. The resected tissues are then inked in the operating room by the surgeon, as the three-dimensional complexity of the tissues removed can lead to processing issues if precise orientation is not maintained. Intraoperative frozen section margins can be assessed from the tissues removed and/or additional margins can be sent for analysis as well.

The role of TLM has been expanding since the early 1980s, when Wolfgang Steiner in Goettingen, Germany described line-of-site laser ablation of upper aerodigestive tract tumors. The excellent oncologic and functional results from the TLM approach in Europe were reinforced in the USA with multi-institutional data showing excellent outcomes with primary TLM resections of advanced stage oropharyngeal malignancies [3, 4]. With TLM, oncologically sound tumor ablation can be accomplished with minimal collateral damage to adjacent soft tissues and neurovascular structures. This has ultimately led to excellent locoregional tumor control rates, with improved recovery of swallowing function, low rates of tracheotomy dependence, and decreased length of hospital stay [4]. TLM has been widely accepted for treatment of early-stage T1 and T2 tumors of the upper aerodigestive tract, and there is evidence to support its effectiveness for select advanced-stage T3 and T4 lesions of the oral cavity, larynx, and oropharynx as well.

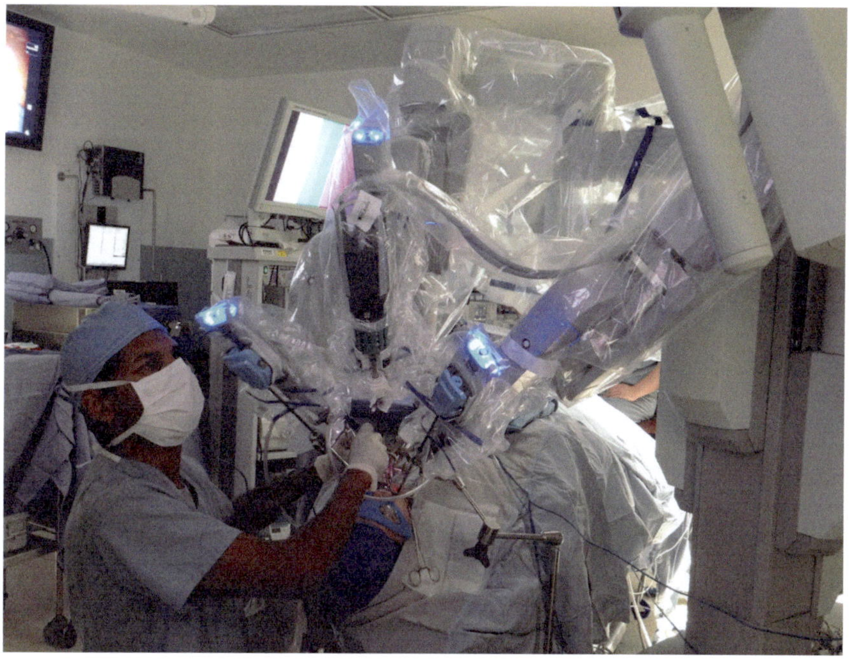

Fig. 18.5 Surgical assistant seated at the head of the patient during Transoral Robotic Surgery (TORS) while viewing primary surgeon's view on monitor

TLM for BOT tumors can be quite challenging, however, and the technique requires specific training, patience, and experience to successfully gain access and remove many of these tumors. More recently, TORS has rapidly gained recognition as an effective minimally invasive modality for the surgical resection of upper aerodigestive tract cancers, with particular benefits in the treatment of BOT tumors. In 2009, the US Food and Drug Administration (FDA) approved the da Vinci® Surgical System (Intuitive Surgical, Inc, Sunnyvale, CA) for transoral surgical procedures restricted to early stage malignant and benign lesions.

The da Vinci® Surgical System was not the first robotic system developed for the use in the operative theater. While both the military and the National Aeronautics and Space Administration (NASA) were interested in developing a surgical robotic system, the first surgical application was in 1985 when the PUMA 560 performed a needle-guided biopsy of a brain tumor with CT guidance. In 1993, the FDA approved the first robotic system, known as Automated Endoscopic System for Optimal Positioning (AESOP), to assist with laparoscopic surgery, providing a robotic-controlled arm to "drive" the endoscope during these procedures. The FDA then approved the Da Vinci robotic system in 2000 for laparoscopic surgery, culminating in its eventual approval for head and neck surgery in 2009. Leading up to this approval, the safety and feasibility of TORS using the da Vinci® robotic system was reported in both preclinical and clinical work, mainly from the University of Pennsylvania [5, 6].

The surgical robotic system consists of a surgeon console, the surgical robotic device with associated specialized instrumentation, and a monitoring system for the remainder of the surgical team to view (Figs. 18.5 and 18.6). The main operative surgeon sits remotely from the patient at the surgeon console, while the surgical assistant sits at the head of the patient's bed. The console provides the surgeon with three-dimensional (3D) images of spectacular high-definition quality, which is obtained through the use of either straight or angled endoscopes placed transorally. From this console, this endoscope is controlled, along with two transorally positioned robotic arms. The robotic arms hold a variety of specialized,

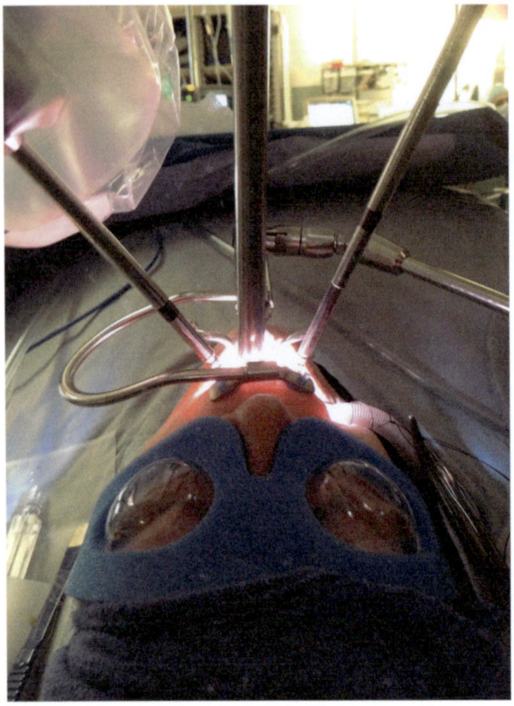

Fig. 18.6 Two robotic arms with midline robotic endoscope placed through the mouth to gain access to the oropharynx for Transoral Robotic Surgery (TOS)

wristed instruments with tremor filtration and seven degrees of freedom. This articulating freedom of motion within tight spaces, along with the visualization "around corners," is what sets TORS apart from any other surgical approach to the BOT. The operative assistant typically utilizes a suction in hand to function as a retractor and suction the surgical smoke. The assistance role is critical for providing hemostasis as well with the use of surgical clips that must be exchanged with the suction as needed. Therefore, four instruments and an endoscope are transorally operating through the mouth of the patient at any given time. The CO_2 laser fibers can be utilized with TORS as well, but more commonly, a Bovie cautery robotic handpiece is utilizes for resection of the tumor. Resection is usually performed en bloc with an appropriate margin of normal surrounding tissues. Intraoperative frozen section margins are then sent to ensure oncologically sound resections.

Regardless of technique utilized, TOS for the oropharynx, as well as for other subsites within the head and neck, has been thoroughly studied and oncologic results are comparable to nonsurgical modalities of therapy. Compared to open resections, TOS provides improved functional outcomes for patients, including swallowing and speech outcomes. Gastrostomy and tracheostomy tube dependency rates are lower as well, allowing for improved quality of life. Hospital stays have been shown to be lower, leading to an overall decreased cost of treatment [7]. If negative margin resections are obtained on final pathology, depending on tumor biology and stage, adjuvant radiation therapy can sometime be avoided, or at the very least, its dose can be decreased. In advanced stage disease, a primary surgical approach may also allow for the ability to omit chemotherapy from the multi-modality treatment regimen, thus eliminating its associated side effects and accompanying cost.

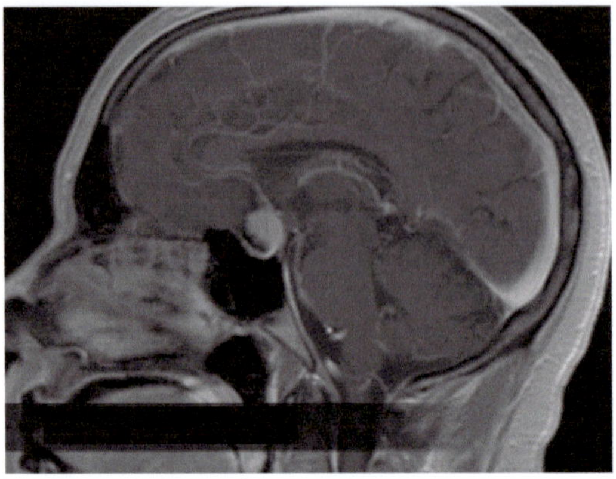

Fig. 18.7 Coronal MRI showing craniopharyngioma of the anterior skull base. (Used with permission of Dr. Adam Zanation)

Minimally Invasive Approaches to the Skull Base

Advances in transnasal endoscopic techniques have dramatically changed the way in which skull base tumors have been approached over the last two decades. These techniques, initially developed for the treatment of benign paranasal sinus disease, have matured to become known as expanded endonasal approaches (EEA) to the skull base (Figs. 18.7 and 18.8). Open craniofacial

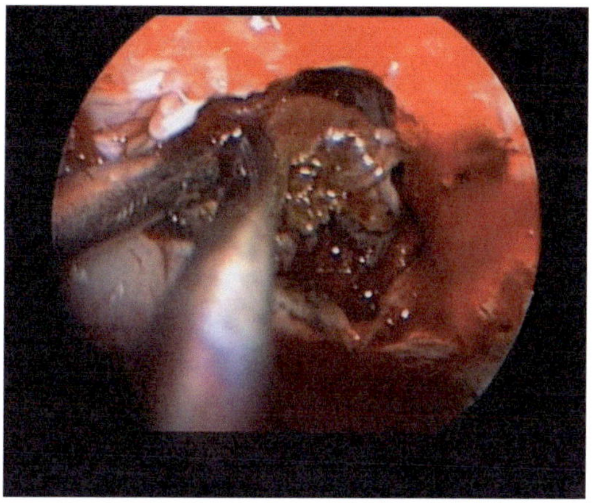

Fig. 18.8 Intraoperative view of transnasal endoscopic resection of craniopharyngioma. Total resection was carried out without external incisions or craniotomy. (Used with permission of Dr. Adam Zanation)

resection (CFR) approaches to the skull base have traditionally been used to resect tumors of the anterior and anterolateral skull base. However, these approaches, while providing excellent surgical exposure, require large facial and/or cranial incisions, entail dissection through extensive "normal" soft tissues of the face, head, and neck, and often require sacrifice of important neurovascular anatomy. While at times necessary, these complex and highly technical approaches have the potential of leaving patients with long-term functional and cosmetic deficits.

The endoscopic approach to the skull base has its roots in the neurosurgical arena with the surgical management of pituitary tumors. The purely endoscopic transsphenoidal approach to pituitary tumors was popularized in the 1990s by Jho and Carrau. Compared to the transseptal, transsphenoidal approach using the operative microscope, the purely endoscopic approach has been shown to offer improved operative visualization, shorter operative times, less blood loss, reduced hospital stay, and decreased need for nasal packing [8]. This endoscopic approach has also reigned in an era in which collaboration between the neurosurgical and otolaryngologic fields for the management of skull base tumors has greatly expanded.

With the safety and effectiveness of the endoscopic transsphenoidal approach to the sella well-established, further work was undertaken to expand this approach beyond the sella and pituitary gland. Expanded endonasal approaches (EEA) to the skull base can be divided into six main sagittal plane corridors: transfrontal, transcribiform, transplanum, transsellar, transclival, and transodontoid. Major progress has been made over recent years, as extensive cadaveric and anatomic studies have shown the safety and feasibility of these various approaches and creative exposure techniques. Clinical work has substantiated these claims and has also shown that these EEAs to the skull base provide equivalent, if not improved, oncologic outcomes. Similarly, studies have shown that reconstruction of the skull base, one of the biggest issues initially appreciated with these EEA to the skull base, can also be carried out safely and effectively with an endonasal approach, thus decreasing cerebrospinal fluid (CSF) leak rates [9].

This clinical work has paralleled the constant progress and innovation seen in diagnostic and intraoperative imaging, surgical instrumentation, and image-guided navigation systems. These various factors have culminated in an increased interest and utilization of EEA to the skull base. Indications have therefore gradually expanded to include lesions of the clivus, olfactory cleft, petrous apex, infratemporal fossa, and planum sphenoidale to name a few.

As mentioned, the major advantages of the EEA is that it can provide direct anatomical access to the anterior and anterolateral skull base, while avoiding skin incisions, facial and/or cranial bone flaps, and brain retraction, all of which are involved with conventional open craniofacial surgical approaches. These advantages lead to patient benefits, with decreased morbidity and functional deficits, and subsequent improved quality of life. These EEA have also been shown to decreased recovery time, therefore decreasing length of hospital stay and overall cost of treatment [10]. One of the major criticisms of the EEA to the skull base is the technique's inability to perform en bloc resections. Yet, with better visualization of tumors and the ability to use angled endoscopes to see around corners, excellent negative-margin oncologic resections can to be carried out. Similar to what has been shown in

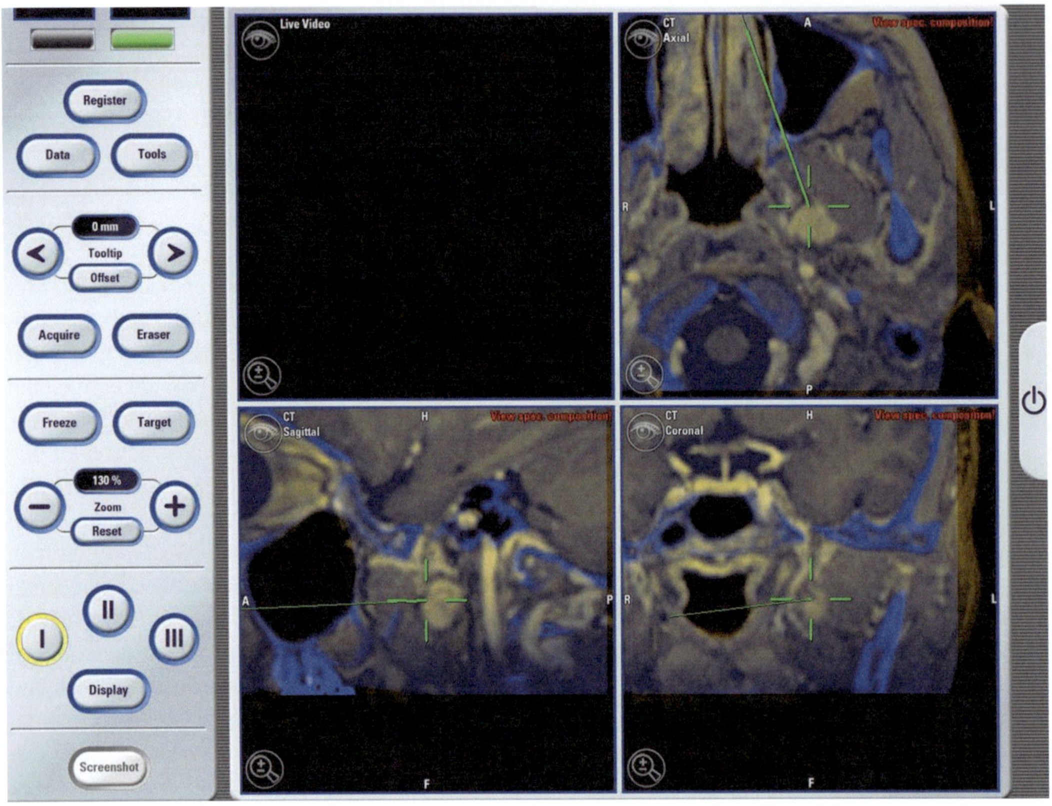

Fig. 18.9 Intraoperative view of surgical monitor with use of image guidance. Pictured here is a lesion of the masticator space being accessed through an endonasal, minimally invasive approach

the oropharyngeal literature with TLM techniques, local control of tumors and overall oncologic results are equivalent with piecemeal resections [11].

Image-guided surgery (IGS) (also referred to as image-guided navigation systems) is nearly uniformly utilized with EEA and the resection of skull base tumors (Fig. 18.9). IGS is the use of preoperative imaging data in the operating room for real-time correlation of the surgical field with precise radiographic localization of anatomy and surgical instrumentation. Along with the excellent endoscopic visualization that these approaches provide, IGS images are utilized to help confirm precise surgical localization within the complex skull base anatomy. Navigation systems, while initially developed for neurosurgical use, have expanded and are now commonly utilized in endoscopic sinus surgery (ESS) for benign inflammatory sinus disease. While CT scans are most often utilized, MRI scans can also be "fused" along with CT scan images, to assist in improved IGS applications such as tumor removal. Similarly, preoperative angiography studies can also be "fused" with these images to be used intraoperatively with IGS, further expanding the anatomical delineations of important vascular structures of the skull base and intracranial cavity. The navigational capabilities that this technology provides for skull base surgery teams are tremendous.

Next-generation IGS systems will likely incorporate intraoperative imaging techniques so that real-time IGS can be carried out, adapting the procedure to the intraoperative changes of the surgical bed anatomy. Currently, intraoperative MRI scanning is most commonly being utilized in the EEAs to the pituitary gland, allowing for real-time information on the extent of pituitary tumor resection. This provides valuable information to the skull base surgery teams on their intraoperative progress, so that additional surgical resection can take place immediately if deemed to be beneficial for the patient.

Advances in surgical instrumentation are also ongoing. Multidirectional rigid endoscopes, combined with three-dimensional visualization screens, will likely further advance the visualization of the skull base with endoscopic endonasal techniques. Articulating instrumentation, similar to that of current surgical robotic systems, will likely be developed and brought to market for utilization within the paranasal and skull base regions as well. Regardless of the improvements in technology and instrumentation, the combined skull base teams of otolaryngologists and neurosurgeons will most certainly continue to revolutionize skull base surgery with expanded indications, safe and effective procedures, and improved patient outcomes.

Optical Imaging

The advancements in optical imaging have clearly served a role in improved visualization and surgical navigation. However, optical imaging devices and technology have also been developed to allow surgeons to better visualize subclinical foci of disease that otherwise would be impossible to assess with even current high-magnification visualization methods. Optical imaging refers to a number of different technologies that utilize light reflectivity and absorption changes to identify tissue changes that may be associated with malignancy [12]. These technologies include use of autofluorescence to detect differential absorbance of mucosal surface tissues to better delineate normal and abnormal tissues, as well as use of exogenous fluorescent contrast agents that are preferentially absorbed by tumor cells. Fluorescence angiography technology is currently being investigated in surgical oncology. Through the use of targeted fluorophores, such as fluorescently labeled antibodies, cancer-specific optical contrast agents can accumulate with high specificity within tumor tissues, and subsequently utilized to delineate tumor margins with tremendous accuracy. This technology can be combined with specialized optical imaging technologies built in to the latest generation microscopes to allow for improved intraoperative tumor clearance and margin control [12].

While these techniques and technologies are still in their infancy in terms of clinical utilization, they have the potential to provide a tremendous advancement in intraoperative, real-time, surgical margin assessment. With the known prognostic importance of negative surgical margins, these technologies can allow the surgeon to be less dependent on subjective assessment of subtle, and sometimes imperceptible, tissue characteristics that have historically driven margin assessment.

Improved Precision of Head and Neck Radiation Therapy

The utilization of radiation therapy has long been a part of the treatment armamentarium for HNC. Since the early 1960s, when linear accelerator development was refined, extensive developments have been made in both technologies and treatment protocols. Since the 1990s, External beam radiotherapy (EBRT) techniques have given way to Intensity-modulated radiotherapy (IMRT) techniques. With IMRT, multiple specifically shaped radiation beams are modulated to produce improved dose conformity, subsequently allowing for the delivery of high doses to targeted tissues with sharp dose gradients. These improved conformal dose distributions lead to improved protection and preservation of adjacent normal structures, thus decreasing the severity of untoward side effects of radiation therapy (Fig. 18.10).

Imaged-guided radiotherapy (IGRT) is a broad term that conveys the incorporation of multidimensional imaging into treatment planning and execution. While the concept is nothing new, the improvements in the three-dimensional imaging, including magnetic resonance imaging (MRI) and positron emission tomography/computed tomography (PET/CT), have helped improve accuracy of treatments provided to patients. Similarly, the utilization of day-of-treatment cone-beam computed tomography (CBCT) scans has allowed

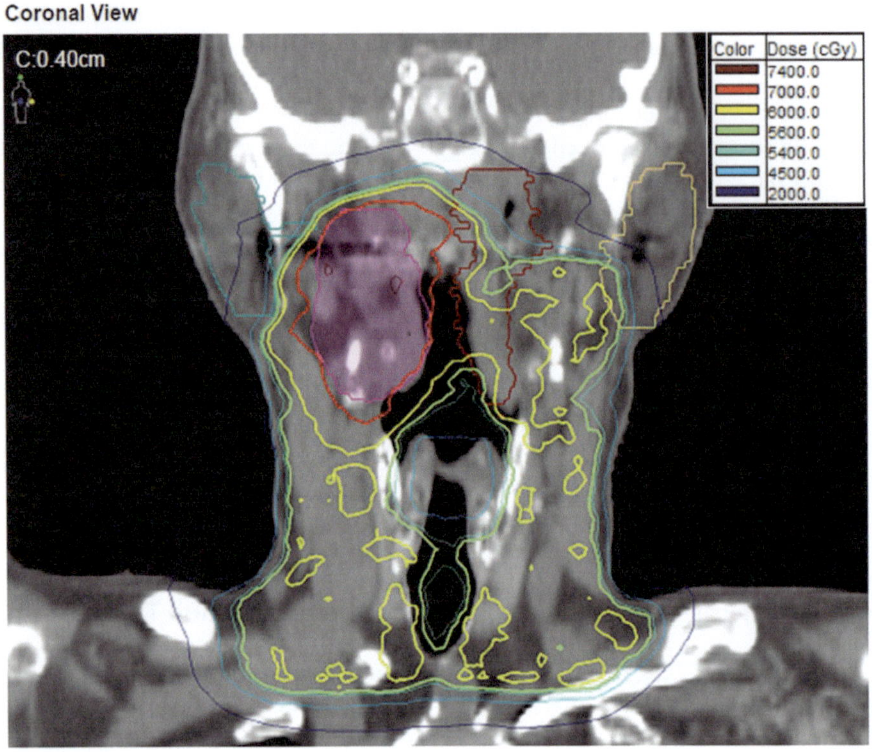

Fig. 18.10 IMRT dose distribution overlayed on a coronal CT scan of a patient with a T2N0M0 squamous cell carcinoma of the right tonsil

for improved treatment precision through correction of daily set-up variables [13].

The concept of maximizing the therapeutic ratio (TR), or enhancing the antitumor effects while minimizing the toxicity to critical adjacent normal structures, has been the ultimate goal in any advancement in radiation oncology made over the last many decades. "Particle therapy" utilizes protons, heavy ions (i.e., carbon ions), or neutrons, instead of standard photons (electrons) to help improve this TR. In standard photon-based therapy, most of the radiation energy is deposited along the entrance and exit portions of the beam path, which usually lie outside of the cancer target. In contrast, protons travel in tissue only a finite distance and release most of their energy at the end of their range, immediately before they come to rest. This characteristic radiation dose-deposition peak is called the "Bragg Peak." This energy peak can be modified and controlled by varying the acceleration of the particles, thus allowing for precise delivery of ionizing radiation with limited damage to surrounding tissues. This may allow for an opportunity to increase the TR of radiotherapy treatments to the head and neck while also being able to carry out dose escalation and/or intensification, thus improving local control.

Despite these proposed benefits, the emerging technology committee of the American Society for Radiation Oncology (ASTRO) currently reports that there are insufficient data to recommend proton beam therapy for routine head and neck radiation therapy outside of clinical trials [14]. Particle therapy is theoretically well-suited for targets near critical structures such as the optic chiasm, spinal cord, and skull base, yet these tumors are quite rare and therefore only minimal data is available on treatment outcomes. Many of the studies currently published for head and neck tumors involve combinations of photons and protons, further complicating analysis of the potential beneficial effects of particle therapy. However, emerging data has shown the beneficial effects of utilizing proton or carbon ion therapy in a variety of skull base tumors, including esthesioneuroblastomas, chondrosarcomas, chordomas, meningiomas, and pituitary adenomas. Further clinical studies are needed to delineate the exact clinical indications for the use of particle therapy in the head and neck, as the cost of this therapy is currently not insignificant.

Stereotactic radiosurgery (SRS) refers to the delivery of radiation dose in a single fraction with precise stereotactic targeting, whereas stereotactic radiotherapy (SRT) refers to this same process delivered with multiple fractions. To date, the majority of clinical experience and data with SRS deals with treatment of benign tumors of the skull base, such as meningiomas and vestibular schwannomas. However, emerging evidence has shown benefits with SRS and SRT in the treatment of recurrent, unresectable nasopharyngeal carcinomas, and non-nasopharyngeal carcinomas of the skull base (often from metastases). With these methods of treatment, local disease control rates have been shown to be comparable to that of salvage surgery, albeit with much less morbidity to the patient [15].

The Genomic and Molecular Landscape of Head and Neck Cancer

HNCs possess a large degree of heterogeneity with very few consistent mutations that are seen across various patient cohorts. This poses a tremendous challenge in establishing effective molecular targeting strategies, for both diagnosis and treatment, for the greater population of HNC patients. In addition to this issue, there has also an epidemic rise in a unique, biologically distinct, virally induced type of HNC. HPV-positive oropharyngeal squamous cell carcinoma (HPV+ OPSCC) is a distinct epidemiologic, molecular, and clinical disease and is increasing at epidemic rates here in the USA and in other westernized countries [16]. Data has shown that virally associated HPV+ OPSCC carries an improved prognosis when compared to HPV negative disease of the oropharynx. HPV+ OPSCC is associated with the expression of E6 and E7 oncoproteins, as well as with expression of p16, the most commonly utilized surrogate marker for HPV positivity within tumor cells. While the ability to diagnose HPV+ OPSCC is tremendously important for prognostic purposes and patient counseling, it currently is not recommended that this information be used to drive treatment decisions. However, ongoing clinical studies will likely provide data that will be used to modify the staging of this distinct disease process, and guide treatment recommendations in the future.

The epidermal growth factor receptor (EGFR) is a member of the human epidermal receptor (HER)/ERb-B family, a group of tyrosine kinases. Binding of ligands to EGFR results in activation of tyrosine kinase activity, subsequently initiating a host of downstream signaling pathways involved in angiogenesis, invasion, and metastasis of SCCHN [17]. Overexpression of EGFR has been found to occur in SCCHN in roughly 90 % of cases, and it is for this reason that many of the targeted therapeutic efforts to date have focused on this receptor. Strategies have included targeting EGFR ligand binding within the extracellular domain as well as inhibiting the intrinsic receptor tyrosine kinase activity within the intracellular domain. However, a mutated version of EGFR (EGFRvIII) is the most common variant of EGFR and has been reported in over 40 % cases of SCCHN. To help predict which patients might benefit most from these anti-EGFR therapies, EGFR-related biomarkers have been extensively studied, including protein expression measured by immunohistochemistry, *EGFR* gene copy number by fluorescence in-situ hybridization (FISH), and EGFR mutations in the tyrosine kinase domain. While initial evidence has shown that EGFR overexpression and/or increased gene copy number may be related to a worse prognosis in SCCHN, use as predictive biomarkers for therapeutic response has been disappointing to date.

Other biomarkers have included the excision repair cross-complementation group 1 (ERCC1) protein, which plays a key role in repairing DNA damage caused by platinum chemotherapy agents. ERCC1 has been shown in preliminary studies to have a role in predicting patient response to cisplatin-based therapy for SCCHN, with low levels correlating with improved response to cisplatin and improved survival in certain subsites [18]. Messenger RNA, mitochondrial DNA, DNA hypermethylation, DNA microsatellite instability, and specifically, HPV DNA have all been targets of biomarker detection within salivary secretions to assist in early detection of SCCHN as well. Despite correlations found on limited initial studies, these methods remain in the investigative phase and further study is warranted. Even the most commonly mutated genes in SCCHN, such as *PIK3CA*, *FAT1*, *EGFR*, *SOX2*, *TP53*, *CCND1*, *E2F1*, and *NOTCH1*, occur in only 10–15 % of head and neck malignancies. This has precluded the widespread application of genomic medicine in SCCHN.

Table 18.3 Anti-EGFR and anti-VEGF targeted therapeutic agents being studied for use in SCCHN

Category	Agent	Delivery
Anti-EGFR monoclonal antibodies		
	Cetuximab	Intravenous
	Panitumumab	Intravenous
	Zalutumumab	Intravenous
	Nimotuzumab	Intravenous
EGFR tyrosine kinase inhibitors		
	Gefitinib	Oral
	Erlotinib	Oral
	Lapatinib	Oral
	Afatinib	Oral
	Dacomitinib	Oral
Anti-VEGF monoclonal antibodies		
	Bevacizumab	Intravenous
VEGF tyrosine kinase inhibitors		
	Vandetanib	Oral
	Sorafenib	Oral
	Sunitinib	Oral

Targeted Chemotherapeutics

Chemotherapy has increasingly been utilized in the multi-modality treatment for locoregionally advanced HNC. Cisplatin is considered the "gold standard" chemotherapeutic agent for concomitant chemoradiation treatments. However, these platinum-based regimens carry significant acute and long-term toxicities. Therefore, new approaches to the treatment of patients with advanced HNCs have been investigated in efforts to limit the significant toxicities associated with systemic therapy (Table 18.3).

As previously mentioned, EGFT and its downstream pathways, are of particular importance in HNC, as aberrant levels of expression of EGFR are associated with decreased survival, radiotherapy resistance, increased risk of locoregional failure, and higher rates of distant metastases [19]. Anti-EGFR agents have been the primary focus of targeted therapy development for HNCs. Cetuximab, a recombinant human-murine chimeric anti-EGFR immunoglobulin G (IgG) monoclonal antibody (mAb), is currently approved by the US FDA to be used in combination with radiotherapy for locally advanced HNC. It is also approved for use as a single-agent, or in combination with platinum-based chemotherapy, for recurrent and/or metastatic SCCHN. Cetuximab has a much more desirable side effect profile compared to platinum-based agents, with diarrhea and acneiform rashes being the most common potential negative effects. Infusion reactions also occur and usually are mild, but can rarely be life-threatening. With this overall favorable side effect profile, it is therefore not surprising that investigators are studying this drug aggressively in ongoing clinical trials in hopes of expanding the drug's indications in the treatment of SCCHN.

Other anti-EGFR agents have been developed as well, including three other mAb drugs: Panitumumab, Zalutumumab, and Nimotuzumab. However, to date, these agents have shown limited improvements in patient outcomes with SCCHN. Of note, Nimotuzumab has been of particular interest however, as initial phase II studies have shown that this specific humanized anti-EGFR mAb does not cause the sometimes severe skin, renal and GI side effects seen with Cetuximab.

EGFR tyrosine kinase inhibitors (TKIs) block the phosphorylation and activation of EGFR, thus inhibiting the pathway through a different mechanism compared to Cetuximab. These agents, which include Gefitinib, Erlotinib, Lapatinib, Afatinib, and Dacomitinib, are all orally administered, making them convenient to administer. Similar to anti-EGFR mAb, common side effects include acneiform rash and diarrhea. Gefitinib and Erlotinib are currently approved for treatment of locally advanced and/or metastatic non-small-cell lung cancer, while Lapatinib is FDA approved for the treatment of metastatic breast cancer. These agents have all undergone at least phase II study for the treatment of SCCHN, and initial results have been mixed. Currently, none of these agents are FDA approved for the treatment of SCCHN, but additional clinical studies are ongoing.

Other targeted therapies currently under investigation include agents that target the vascular endothelial growth factor (VEGF) pathway, the MET pathway and its downstream P13K/AKT/mTOR pathways, and Type I Insulin-like Growth Factor receptors (IGF-1R). With VEGF being one of the most essential cytokines involved in tumor angiogenesis, it is of no surprise that targeted agents blocking this pathway are being developed and heavily studied. Bevacizumab is a mAb directed against VEGF and is currently approved for a number of cancers outside of HNC, but is currently being studied in combination with more traditional chemotherapy regimens for the treatment of SCCHN. Up-regulation of VEGF has been associated with resistance to anti-EGFR agents, thus leading to additional studies exploring the utilization of both anti-EGFR and anti-VEGF targeted therapies to address this resistance. A VEGF receptor TKI, Vandetanib, has already been approved for the use in medullary thyroid cancer and has also been shown to have some anti-SCC tumor activity that is currently being studied as well.

References

1. Siegel R, Ma J, Zou Z, Jemal A. Cancer statistics, 2014. CA Cancer J Clin. 2014;64(1):9–29.
2. de Almeida JR, Byrd JK, Wu R, Stucken CL, Duvvuri U, Goldstein DP, Miles BA, Teng MS, Gupta V, Genden EM. A systematic review of transoral robotic surgery and radiotherapy for early oropharynx cancer: a systematic review. Laryngoscope. 2014;124(9):2096–102.
3. Steiner W, Fierek O, Ambrosch P, Hommerich CP, Kron M. Transoral laser microsurgery for squamous cell carcinoma of the base of the tongue. Arch Otolaryngol Head Neck Surg. 2003;129(1):36–43.
4. Haughey BH, Hinni ML, Salassa JR, Hayden RE, Grant DG, Rich JT, Milov S, Lewis Jr JS, Krishna M. Transoral laser microsurgery as primary treatment for advanced-stage oropharyngeal cancer: a United States multicenter study. Head Neck. 2011;33(12):1683–94.
5. Hockstein NG, Malley O, Jr BW, Weinstein GS. Assessment of intraoperative safety in transoral robotic surgery. Laryngoscope. 2006;116(2):165–8.
6. O'Malley BW, Weinstein GS. Robotic skull base surgery: preclinical investigations to human clinical application. Arch Otolaryngol Head Neck Surg. 2007;133(12):1215–9.
7. Li RJ, Richmon JD. Transoral endoscopic surgery: new surgical techniques for oropharyngeal cancer. Otolaryngol Clin North Am. 2012;45(4):823–44.
8. Senior BA, Ebert CS, Bednarski KK, Bassim MK, Younes M, Sigounas D, Ewend MG. Minimally invasive pituitary surgery. Laryngoscope. 2008;118(10):1842–55.
9. Patel M, Stadler M, Snyderman C, Carrau R, Kassam A, Germanwala A, Gardner P, Zanation A. How to choose? Endoscopic skull base reconstructive options and limitations. Skull Base. 2010;20(06):397–404.
10. Nicolai P, Battaglia P, Bignami M, Bolzoni Villaret A, Delù G, Khrais T, Lombardi D, Castelnuovo P. Endoscopic surgery for malignant tumors of the sinonasal tract and adjacent skull base: a 10-year experience. Am J Rhinol. 2008;22(3):308–16.
11. Snyderman CH, Carrau RL, Kassam AB, Zanation A, Prevedello D, Gardner P, Mintz A. Endoscopic skull base surgery: principles of endonasal oncological surgery. J Surg Oncol. 2008;97(8):658–64.
12. Rosenthal EL. Optical imaging of head and neck cancer. JAMA Otolaryngol Head Neck Surg. 2014;140(2):93.
13. Kubicek GJ, Machtay M. New advances in high-technology radiotherapy for head and neck cancer. Hematol Oncol Clin North Am. 2008;22(6):1165–80.
14. Allen AM, Pawlicki T, Dong L, et al. An evidence based review of proton beam therapy: the report of ASTRO's emerging technology committee. Radiother Oncol. 2012;103(1):8–11.

15. Gardner E, Linskey ME, Peñagarícano JA, Hanna EY. Stereotactic radiosurgery for patients with cancer of the head and neck. Curr Oncol Rep. 2003;5(2):164–9.
16. Chaturvedi AK, Engels EA, Anderson WF, Gillison ML. Incidence trends for human papillomavirus-related and -unrelated oral squamous cell carcinomas in the United States. J Clin Oncol. 2008;26(4):612–9.
17. Stadler ME, Patel MR, Couch ME, Hayes DN. Molecular biology of head and neck cancer: risks and pathways. Hematol Oncol Clin North Am. 2008;22(6):1099–124.
18. Patel MR, Zhao N, Ang MK, et al. ERCC1 protein expression is associated with differential survival in oropharyngeal head and neck squamous cell carcinoma. Otolaryngol Head Neck Surg. 2013;149(4):587–95.
19. Dorsey K, Agulnik M. Promising new molecular targeted therapies in head and neck cancer. Drugs. 2013;73(4):315–25.

Neck Cancer: Imaging Techniques and Progress on the Operative Approach

19

Diego Sinagra and Fernando Dip

Imaging Techniques

When cancers of the head and neck are suspected by physical examination, biopsies are performed to determine and confirm this suspicion. A confirmed biopsy may warrant a positron emission tomography (PET) scan to determine the spread of cancer. Imaging studies have proved to be useful in evaluating primary lesions and cervical metastases. Ultrasonography demonstrates to be the least sensitive for assessing metastases of the head and neck. Magnetic resonance imaging (MRI) is comparable in sensitivity to computed tomography (CT) but CT is considerably more cost effective in the detection of metastases when compared to MRI.

CT is able to assess the amount of tumor infiltration in surrounding tissue including bones. Malignancy in the cervical lymph node could be detected by CT scans (Fig. 19.1a, b). Publications have reported 1.2–1.5 cm in cervical lymph node size to be indicative of malignancy. However, necrosis remains to be a superior and more reliable indicator. The CT DentaScan is performed on a conventional CT scanner but this specialized exam is equipped with a special software platform that enhances the extent of bony involvement.

Compared to CT, PET is more accurate in staging or re-staging cancer of the head and neck. After surgery and/or medical treatments, PET is used to monitor the return of cancer cells which could determine the restart of treatment. In many patients with head and neck cancers, a mass may remain after surgery, chemotherapy, and/or radiation. This mass could be visible on CT, however, it cannot determine the presence of residual cancer or if this mass was successfully treated. Consequently a PET scan could image responses from therapy and detect recurrence of treated lesions/masses.

Modern PET/CT scanners combine both imaging techniques increasing their functionality. This combination offers several gains. While the PET component illustrates the spatial circulation of biochemical activity, the CT component depicts anatomic structures. Imaging from PET is more precisely correlated with CT images in this manner. The significance of PET for the diagnosis of cervical lymph node metastases have been discussed controversially as a meta-analysis have shown that PET examination may achieve a sensitivity of up to 80 % and a specificity of 86 %, however, only half of the patients with clinical N0 neck and histologically identified metastasis could be identified by means of PET (Fig. 19.2). Nevertheless, PET/CT scanning

D. Sinagra, M.D. • F. Dip, M.D. (✉)
Department of Surgical Oncology, Hospital de Clinicas Jose de San Martin, Buenos Aires, Argentina
e-mail: diegosinagra@hotmail.com; fernandodip@gmail.com

R. Latifi et al. (eds.), *Technological Advances in Surgery, Trauma and Critical Care*,
DOI 10.1007/978-1-4939-2671-8_19

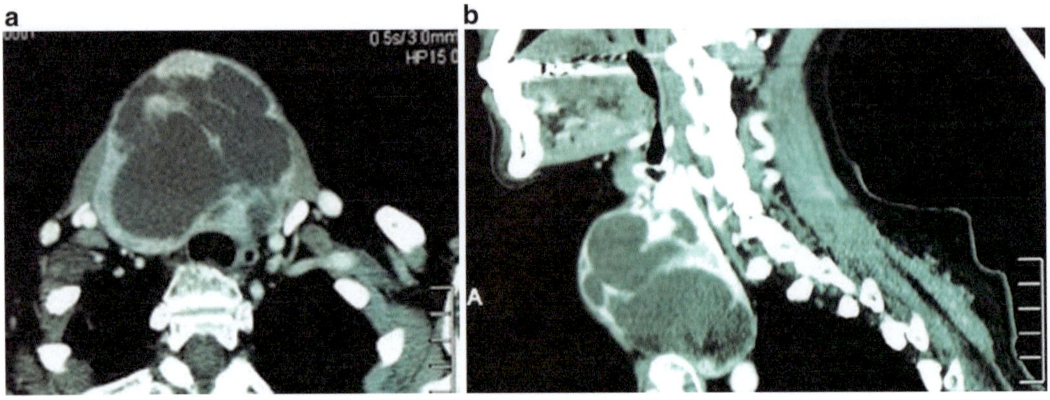

Fig. 19.1 (**a**, **b**) CT scan. Tumor extension evaluation

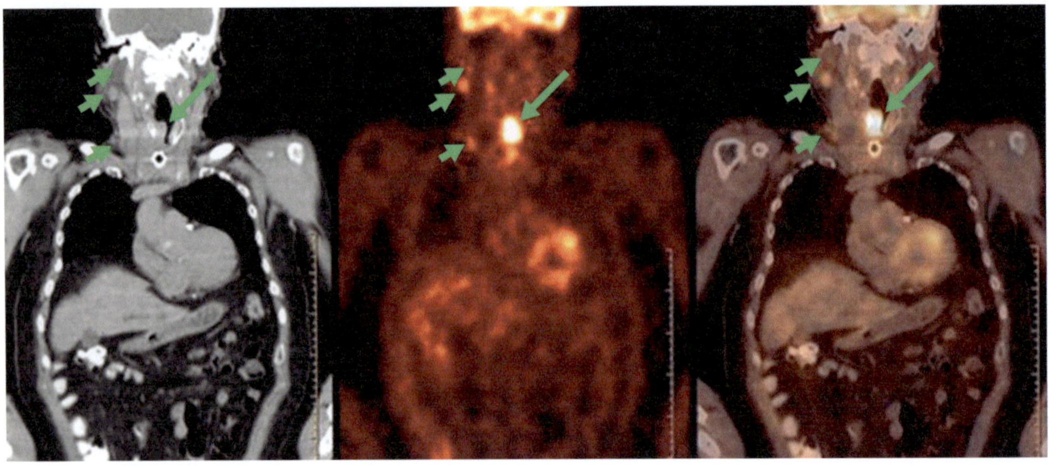

Fig. 19.2 PET CT tumor identification

in the post-treatment stage for assessing response and residual disease is increasingly performed and is proving to be vital in cancer treatment [1].

Head and Neck Cancer Targeted Gene Therapy

Gene therapy in head and neck squamous cell carcinoma (HNSCC) involves delivering therapeutic genes into target tissues. Though it is still confined to trials, this evolving field is likely to progress to clinical use in combination with surgery, radiotherapy, and/or chemotherapy. HNSCC tumors serve as an ideal model for gene therapy research due to abilities of directly injecting tumors intramurally and obtaining biopsies for biomarkers evaluations.

The epidermal growth factor receptor (EGFR) is a transmembrane tyrosine kinase receptor consisting of mainly four members: ErbB1/EGFR, ErbB2/HER2, ErbB3, and ErbB4. Activation of EGFR leads to cell cycle progression that stimulates numerous antiapoptotic signals. Ninety percent of squamous cell cancers of the head and neck express high levels of EGFRs. Poor prognosis with locoregional failure and radioresistance is associated with higher levels of EGFRs via increased EGFR gene amplification.

The first gene therapy protocol for cancer was submitted in 1993. Since then, over 1,000 gene therapy and 12 HNSCC clinical protocols have been registered on Clinicals.gov. INGN 201, a promoter to encode the wild-type p53 gene, is a treatment that increases programmed cell death in tumors of HNSCC. A clinical phase III trial comparing survival to methotrexate is currently underway. Augmenting p53 in HNSCC tumors does appear to have antitumor effects. Another approach is to inhibit oncogenes as the epidermal growth factor receptor (EGFR) is greatly upregulated in 90 % of HNSCC. Inhibiting or blocking ligand binding to this receptor may prevent downstream signaling that mediate HNSCC growth. An EGFR-specific antibody, cetuximab, in combination with radiation was reported to improve survival. Although it is approved by the FDA for HNSCC, the response rate is less than 10 % as a monotherapy.

Cetuximab blocks EGFRs from the outside of cancer cells. Research has shown that cancer cells can turn proliferation and antiapoptotic signals back on by the EGFR joining with a related receptor called ErbB2, also known as HER2. Lapatinib blocks both EGFR and HER2 from the inside of cancer cells. Combining drugs that target both EGFR and HER2 may improve response in turning this signal off. An irreversible inhibitor of EGFR and HER2, the oral agent lapatinib is a recent approach in clinical studies. Current phase II studies investigate the use of lapatinib in combination with cisplatin-based chemoradiation for HPV-negative tumors. Prior to transoral surgery, lapatinib as induction therapy with carboplatin and paclitaxel is demonstrating promising results. Another such trial is assessing the progression-free survival of lapatinib and capecitabine for recurrent or metastatic disease. However, early data suggest a marginal benefit as monotherapy or in combination with platinum-based chemoradiation therapy [2].

Efficient and stable transgene expression remains a challenge in gene transfer, although several methods have been developed. Encapsulating DNA in liposomes is one such method. Genes encoding HLA-B7, interleukin (IL)-2, and E1A have demonstrated transferability by cationic liposomes. However, liposomes do not facilitate DNA integration into the genome, requiring retreatment. Conversely, viral vectors allow permanent gene integration into genomic DNA, particularly retroviruses and adenoviruses. Though transfection of DNA into tumor tissue has low efficiency, preclinical studies using naked DNA have shown moderate effects in HNSCC xenograft tumors. These injections are known to be technically challenging and usually performed by a surgeon. Ultrasound-guided injections of DNA are advantageous in identifying and avoiding blood vessels and necrotic regions.

MHC-I expression has been reported to reject leukemic cells after their gene transfer and reverse oncogenesis of transformed cells. Allovectin-7 is a plasmid DNA that expresses MHC class I molecules required for HLA-B7. In an initial phase I and phase II studies, gradual reduction in tumor size was demonstrated. Although oncolytic viruses itself do not modulate gene expression, they serve as gene delivery vectors. COX-2, which is responsible for prostaglandin production, is undetectable in normal tissue but is overexpressed in HNSCC. A COX-2 promoter-driven replication-selective adenoviral vector, Ad-COX2-E1a, demonstrated antitumor effects against COX-2-expressing HNSCC in vitro and in vivo. The most widely tested oncolytic virus in HNSCC is ONYX-015. In a phase II trial, tumor regression was observed with some demonstrating stable disease. ONYX-015 mouthwash was evaluated in the treatment of premalignant dysplasia. Histologic resolution of dysplasia was reported, however, the responses were transient. Further studies with larger sample sizes are needed to determine the effectiveness of ONYX-015 mouthwash in the treatment of premalignant oral dysplasia. A modified version of ONYX-015, called H101 was approved by the Chinese State Food and Drug Administration for cancer treatment.

A meta-analysis published in 2005 has demonstrated an increased prevalence of HPV in oropharyngeal compared to oral or laryngeal carcinoma, with HPV16 accounting for the majority of oncogenic infections. However, this systematic review only included studies on PCR-based analysis that were not combined with p16 immunohistochemistry to identify integrated HPV. HPV positive and negative tumors are reported to have different clinical and molecular presentations. HPV-positive oropharyngeal cancer patients are younger with less consumption of alcohol and tobacco. They are also inclined to have more sexual partners. The primary tumor is frequently smaller. HPV positive tumors are characterized by the inactivation of the p53 tumor suppressor gene by the oncoprotein E6, and overexpression of the p16 cell cycle protein due to the loss of negative feedback caused by the oncoprotein E7 on the retinoblastoma suppressor gene.

Studies have shown that patients with HPV positive, p16 positive, or p53 wild type tumors have better overall survival and disease free survival rates than patients with HPV negative, p16 negative, and p53 altered SCCHN. Exome sequencing revealed more mutations in HPV negative tumors. Furthermore, TP53 mutations are generally not identified in HPV positive tumors but were found in 78 % of HPV negative tumors. Therapeutic vaccines and immunotherapy targeting HPV specific epitopes are investigated in cervical cancer patients where tumor regressions are observed. Currently, a phase I trial in SCCHN is ongoing which investigates a HPV DNA vaccine using electroporation devices associated to an immunomodulatory agent, cyclophosphamide, in HPV-16 SCCHN [3].

Preclinical studies have reported enhanced antitumor effects when combining gene therapy with radiation or chemotherapy. Docetaxel in combination with EGFR antisense gene therapy resulted in reduction of HNSCC xenograft growth in vivo. Another such study resulted in significant antitumor efficacy when partial resection of HNSCC xenograft tumors was followed by a human IL-2 plasmid formulation. In radiotherapy, toxicity to adjacent structures has posed significant problems. To increase the radiosensitivity of HNSCC tumors, adenoviral particles encoding the Nijmegen breakage syndrome (NBS1) protein were used to transduce HNSCC cells. Expression of this protein resulted in enhanced sensitivity of HNSCC xenograft tumors to ionizing radiation. Combing all three modalities of transducing HNSCC xenografts to encode a tissue inhibitor of matrix metalloproteinase-2 (TIMP-2), cisplatin treatment, and radiotherapy have showed an additive antitumor effect compared to any single agent alone. Further research will improve efficacies of gene delivery and discover other potential molecular targets in HNSCC.

Minimally Invasive Approach

Robotics

While open surgery remains the gold standard for skull base, sinonasal, oral, salivary gland, sarcoma, and thyroid cancer, head and neck surgeons must embrace the advancement of endoscopic, laser, robotics, and image-guided surgery. Research in laryngeal transplantation is progressing and evolving, with a bio-engineered larynx becoming a reality. Nonetheless, open surgery has progressed and now includes more salvage surgery and organ-preservation with complex reconstruction and free flaps.

Compared to 20 years ago, the rate of open surgery as the primary initial treatment for head and neck cancer is decreasing, particularly with pharyngeal and laryngeal squamous cell carcinoma. Concurrently, the rate of primary chemotherapy and irradiation is increasing. Suboptimal functional outcomes from any treatment approach still exist and present significant issues. A 30 % risk of long-term gastrostomy tube feeding, mucositis, and tracheostomy tubes after primary chemoradiation or open surgery with postoperative chemoradiation is present in current practice today. Furthermore, pharyngectomy with concurrent neck dissection and subsequent radiation may lead to pharyngocutaneous fistulas. Thus, this presents opportunities for surgeons to participate in the development of new approaches in treatment. Oncologic surgical technology is shifting toward reducing morbidity and mortality without compromising oncologic outcomes.

In 2009, transoral robotic surgery (TORS) was approved by the Food and Drug Administration for the treatment of oropharynx and larynx benign and malignant disease. TORS with postoperative adjuvant treatment is a valid option that has produced excellent functional results. Robotics offer a reduced invasive approach with potentially fewer complications, reduced operative times, and shorter intensive care unit stays for select patients compared to extensive incisions of open surgery. Many patients are able to eat within days after TORS. For head and neck cancer patients, quicker return of speech and swallowing functions may be experienced following robotic surgery compared to split-lip mandibulotomy and pharyngectomy of open surgery. Lacking the need for skin incision, TORS does not create through-and-through defects [4].

The robotic technique allows high resolution three-dimensional visualization of mucosal surfaces by an endoscope. The da Vinci system is equipped with at least two instrument arms that allow manipulation through the mouth of the patient. Adequate mouth opening is verified in TORS candidates. Inadequate neck extension, micrognathia, non-resectable cervical lymph node metastases are contraindications of TORS. A retropharyngeal internal carotid artery or lack of normal tissue between the carotid and tumor presents concerns which TORS would not be considered. Neck dissections are generally performed before or after TORS in primary tumor treatment to decrease the risk of pharyngocutaneous fistulas. Currently, application of TORS includes resection of most T1 and T2 tumors in the oropharynx, supraglottis, and piriform sinus.

TORS have extended to resections below the base of the skull in prestyloid parapharyngeal spaces, salivary glands, and retropharyngeal lymph nodes. Open surgery at the skull base often requires split-lip mandibulotomy with large cervical incisions.

Robotic-assisted thyroidectomy with the gasless axillary approach is a further advancement of robotic surgery in thyroid glands. Studies have shown shorter lengths of hospitalization and improved cosmetic outcomes. Robotic total thyroidectomies (TT) with modified radical neck dissection (MRND) have been performed in N1b papillary thyroid carcinoma patients with improved swallowing functions postoperatively and decreased neck sensory changes. Increased operating times, temporary hyperparathyroidism, brachial plexus neuropathy, and tracheal injury have limited its widespread application.

Robotic-assisted neck dissections using a transaxillary and retroauricular (TARA) approach and modified facelift and retroauricular approaches are also current robotic developments for HNSCC. Patients with clinical negative nodes or lateral regional metastases have undergone this technique with increased satisfaction of cosmesis. Further studies on functional outcomes and safety in robotic head and neck surgery are needed to determine and evaluate long-term effects [5].

Endoscopy

Natural orifice transluminal endoscopic surgery (NOTES) was presented a decade ago to be the next generation of surgery in various fields. Although abdominal organs have been successfully resected and explored transorificially, NOTES has demonstrated to be not as cost effective when compared to laparoscopic approaches. However, valuable experiences have been gained and produced improvements in this field.

Newer generations of endoscopes with small instruments have allowed unique tactics in benign and malignant tumor resections of the head and neck. Endoscopes are coupled with high resolution cameras and powerful light sources that illuminate and magnify surgical fields. The evolution of smaller endoscopes with video capabilities enables visualization of small and narrow areas that may be difficult to examine with open surgery. This permits greater accuracy in identification of anomalous tissue and improve margin visualization.

Creating huge flaps are often associated with open surgery. The risk of bleeding, infections, and elevated postoperative pain are increased compared to minimally invasive approaches. Endoscopic application on sinusonasal regions is gaining acceptance from surgeons. Although a learning curve exists, the endoscopic approach has demonstrated to achieve results comparable with open surgery as small malignant tumors can be resected with safe pathological margins. Endoscopic tumor resections in the sinus and skull base are proven feasible while improving significantly the quality of life of patients.

Endoscopic techniques can be performed on endocrine tumors. The transaxillary or substernal approaches are common for thyroidectomies, avoiding incisions of the neck. The technique starts by dissecting one or two subcutaneous tunnels in the axilla and ligating the pectoral pedicle. Magnification of structures by the endoscope can potentially reduce the complications. With detection of parathyroid glands by endoscopes, hypocalcemia could be avoided postoperatively as well as lesions to recurrent laryngeal nerves. Advantages of endoscopy include satisfactory cosmetic outcomes by avoiding neck incisions and decreased risk of hematoma. Endoscopic approaches, even though they are feasible, are not easy to perform as technical skills and training are necessary [6].

Fluorescence Technology

In the last decade, improvements in minimally invasive instruments have impacted the surgical approaches of head and neck tumors. However, poor margins and indiscernible microscopic tumors are responsible for poor outcomes. In the last years, a novel technology has developed to evaluate and visualize tumor margins, lymph vessels, and sentinel lymph nodes by a fluorescent dye.

This fluorescent dye is indocyanine green (ICG), approved by the FDA in 1959. It has a low rate of toxicity of 0.003 % per dose in 0.5 mg/ml. Fluorescence image-guided surgery (Figs. 19.3 and 19.4) is gaining grounds for liver function evaluation, determination of cardiac output, and extrahepatic biliary recognition. ICG is intravenously administered at the moment of the surgery. The ICG dye travels through vessels and is captured by tumors with ICG receptors. Nerves of vascularized tumors and their margins are then illuminated and visualized by near infrared light. Parapharyngeal tumors can be easily detected with margins, avoiding the need of multiple resections after frozen section (Figs. 19.3 and 19.4). The same concept is applied to sentinel lymph node detection. The dye is administered at the tumor site with fluorescence light use to detect the node, avoiding any need of Tc99m. This method allows the surgeon real time evaluation of the head and neck cancer [7].

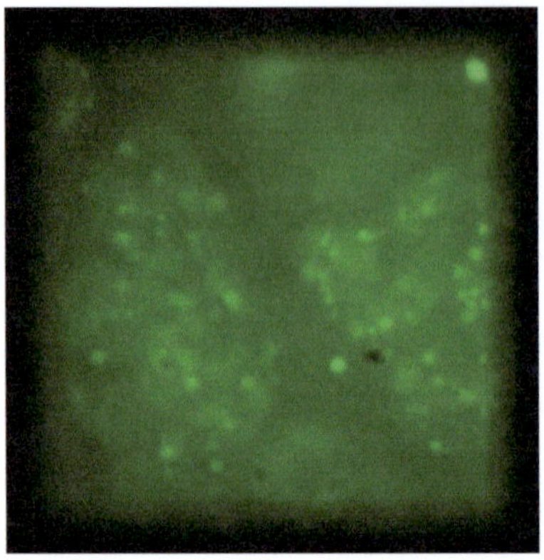

Fig. 19.3 Autofluorescence of parathyroid adenoma

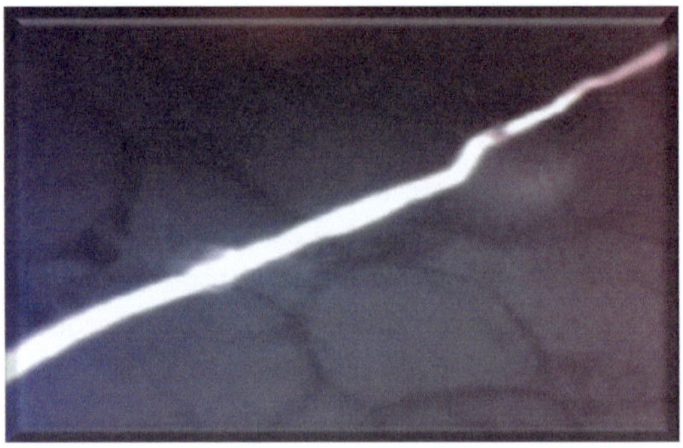

Fig. 19.4 Fluorescence of recurrent laryngeal nerve

Laser Applications

One of the advantages of this type of energy is that it stays narrow along the path. The concept of laser technology in surgery is not new. It was described in the 1960s and has evolved over the years. Today, laser has an important role in the diagnosis and treatment of head and neck cancer. In has demonstrated to be precise as the light is concentrated to a specific area potentially decreasing the risk of infection. Laser applications are generally superficial as their properties results in prompt tissue healing with reduced bleeding, swelling, and scarring [8].

Historically different types of laser were developed such as diode, yellow light, and ruby. Argon and CO_2 lasers are most frequently used with major clinical impact. Laser treatment of tumors was first described for benign lesions, particularly for laryngeal papillomatosis. Gradually it has been introduced as part of the microsurgical armamentarium for carcinomas. Promising results of this technology opened the spectrum to others areas in the ear, nose, and throat. The main objective of lasers is organ preservation, specifically in advanced cases.

The decision to perform laser treatment has to be based on TNM staging. Achieving good oncological results require microsurgical resection of areas outside the margins not compromised by the tumor. High level of expertise is needed similar to the open surgical approach. A longer learning curve is required for endoscopic laser resections. Laser microsurgical techniques on the tongue, floor of mouth, buccal mucosa, oral surface of the soft palate, and posterior wall of oropharynx are being assessed presently. Prospective randomized studies are needed to evaluate laser therapy as standard of care for head and neck cancer.

References

1. Omami G, Tamimi D, Branstetter BF. Basic principles and applications of (18)F-FDG-PET/CT in oral and maxillofacial imaging: a pictorial essay. Imaging Sci Dent. 2014;44(4):325–32.
2. Schmitz S, Ang KK, Vermorken J, Haddad R, Suarez C, Wolf GT, Hamoir M, Machiels JP. Targeted therapies for squamous cell carcinoma of the head and neck: current knowledge and future directions. Cancer Treat Rev. 2014;40(3):390–404.
3. Zandberg DP, Rollins S, Goloubeva O, Morales RE, Tan M, Taylor R, Wolf JS, Schumaker LM, Cullen KJ, Zimrin A, Ord R, Lubek JE, Suntharalingam M, Papadimitriou JC, Mann D, Strome SE, Edelman MJ. A phase I dose escalation trial of MAGE-A3- and HPV16-specific peptide immunomodulatory vaccines in patients with recurrent/metastatic (RM) squamous cell carcinoma of the head and neck (SCCHN). Cancer Immunol Immunother. 2015; 64(3):367–79.
4. de Almeida JR, Moskowitz AJ, Miles BA, Goldstein DP, Teng MS, Sikora A, Gupta V, Posner M, Genden EM. Transoral robotic surgery is cost-effective compared to (Chemo) radiotherapy for early t-classification oropharyngeal carcinoma: a cost-utility analysis. Head Neck. 2014. doi:10.1002/hed.23930.
5. Loevner LA, Learned KO, Mohan S, O'Malley Jr BW, Scanlon MH, Rassekh CH, Weinstein GS. Transoral robotic surgery in head and neck cancer: what radiologists need to know about the cutting edge. Radiographics. 2013;33(6):1759–79.
6. Meining A, Spaun G, Fernández-Esparrach G, Arezzo A, Wilhelm D, Martinek J, Spicak J, Feussner H, Fuchs KH, Hucl T, Meisner S, Neuhaus H. NOTES in Europe: summary of the working group reports of the 2012 EURO-NOTES meeting. Endoscopy. 2013; 45(3):214–7.
7. van der Vorst JR, Schaafsma BE, Verbeek FP, Keereweer S, et al. Near-infrared fluorescence sentinel lymph node mapping of the oral cavity in head and neck cancer patients. Oral Oncol. 2013; 49(1):15–9.
8. Cömert E, Tunçel Ü, Dizman A, Güney YY. Comparison of early oncological results of diode laser surgery with radiotherapy for early glottic carcinoma. Otolaryngol Head Neck Surg. 2014;150(5): 818–23.

Advances in Thyroid and Parathyroid Care

20

Randall P. Scheri, Julie A. Sosa, and Sanziana A. Roman

Introduction

Over the last several years, new techniques and technologies have changed the surgical approach to patients with thyroid and parathyroid disease. The preoperative evaluation of patients includes sophisticated radiological imaging, molecular testing and other adjuncts which allow the surgeon to better select and tailor surgery for patients. While meticulous surgical technique and attention to detail remain the hallmarks of endocrine surgery, several intraoperative adjuncts have been developed along with minimally invasive techniques to permit safe and efficient surgery with reduced morbidity, excellent cosmetic outcomes, and quick recovery. Some new technologies have been enthusiastically endorsed and incorporated by many surgeons while others have fallen out of favor due to lack of proven benefit or replacement by better technology. This chapter reviews new technology and surgical techniques that are available for the surgical management of thyroid and parathyroid disease.

R.P. Scheri, M.D. • J.A. Sosa, M.D., M.A.
S.A. Roman, M.D., F.A.C.S. (✉)
Department of Surgery, Duke University, Durham, NC, USA
e-mail: r.scheri@duke.edu; Julie.sosa@duke.edu; Sanziana.roman@duke.edu

Thyroid

Molecular Testing

Thyroid nodules are common in the USA; they are present in over 50 % of thyroid ultrasounds, 16 % of computed tomography scans, and 2–3 % of positron emission tomography scans (PET) [1]. Ultrasound-guided fine needle aspiration biopsy (FNA) with cytological assessment has become the gold standard for evaluation of nodules, enabling a diagnosis of benign or malignant disease in the majority of cases. The addition of ultrasound to the FNA has allowed for better diagnostic evaluation of the nodule in question by reducing false negative and insufficient aspirations. FNA cytology results in an indeterminate diagnosis in 15–30 % of cases [2], which often leads to diagnostic thyroid lobectomy. However, the majority of these lesions are ultimately benign [3].

Molecular analysis of thyroid tissue has been evaluated as an adjunct to cytology to improve diagnostic accuracy. Nearly 70 % of thyroid cancers [4] harbor a known genetic mutation; therefore, testing for specific genes can improve the diagnostic accuracy of cytology in indeterminate cases. Several molecular tests have been developed and tested, and they can be broadly categorized as either "rule in" or "rule out" malignancy tests. The "rule in" test assesses for single gene

R. Latifi et al. (eds.), *Technological Advances in Surgery, Trauma and Critical Care*,
DOI 10.1007/978-1-4939-2671-8_20

mutations or gene rearrangements to predict cancer probability in an indeterminate nodule, thus avoiding a diagnostic lobectomy and allowing definitive treatment for thyroid cancer. The "rule out" test uses a proprietary gene expression classifier designed to reclassify an indeterminate nodule as benign, and thus potentially helps to avoid surgery altogether.

"Rule In" Testing

Individual point mutations in BRAF, RAS genes and rearrangements of RET/PTC and PAX/PPARG genes have been evaluated to assess for thyroid cancer, but are of relatively limited utility individually because of low sensitivity. A collective panel of 17 mutations among these four oncogenes has been developed and is available at several academic medical centers and commercially. The results of validation studies for the commercially available tests have not been reported. However, in a single center prospective study by Nikiforov et al. [4], a panel of the same genes was analyzed for 1,056 consecutive cytologically indeterminate nodes. Cytology was classified as atypia of undetermined significance (AUS)/follicular lesion of undetermined significance (FLUS) (Bethesda Category 3), follicular or Hurthle cell neoplasm (FN) (Bethesda Category 4), or suspicious for malignancy (SM) (Bethesda Category 5). Molecular testing and definitive histopathological assessment was performed for 513 nodules. A total of 83 mutations, including 17 BRAF, 61 RAS, one RET/PTC, and four PAX8/PPARG rearrangements were identified. The risk of malignancy based on cytology alone for nodules categorized as AUS/FLUS, FN, and SM was 14 %, 27 %, and 54 %, respectively. However, when a mutation was identified, the risk of malignancy increased to 88 %, 87 %, and 95 % for AUS/FLUS, FN, and SM, respectively. The BRAF, RET/PTC and PAX8/PPARG were associated with 100 % risk of malignancy, while the RAS mutation carried an 85 % risk of cancer. The non-malignant RAS-positive nodules were all follicular adenomas. Based on the high likelihood of malignancy, the authors suggested that patients with a positive BRAF, RET/PTC, and/or PAX8/PPARG mutation should undergo definitive thyroid cancer treatment (i.e., total thyroidectomy), and could avoid a diagnostic lobectomy first. For patients with a RAS mutation, there should be an informed discussion of the cancer risk and consideration of a diagnostic lobectomy; however, definitive surgical treatment may be warranted, given the high cancer risk.

However, the overall sensitivity for this "rule in" test is only 60 %, leading to a negative predictive value (NPV) of 94 %, 86 %, and 72 % for AUS/FLUS, FN, and SM, respectively. Importantly, the NPV decreases as the prevalence of malignancy increases, such that for a 24 % risk of malignancy in the AUS/FLUS group, the NPV falls to 89 %, demonstrating the importance of knowing the prevalence of malignancy at each individual institution. Using this "rule in" test, diagnostic lobectomy may still be indicated for mutation-negative, cytologically indeterminate nodules; however, patients with mutation-positive nodules could undergo definitive thyroidectomy for cancer.

A cost analysis by Yip et al. [5] revealed that the molecular panel indeed appeared to be cost-effective. Molecular testing resulted in fewer diagnostic lobectomies than standard cytological evaluation (9.7 % vs. 11.6 %) and more frequent upfront total thyroidectomies (18.2 % vs. 16.1 %). While the added diagnostic cost for molecular testing for each total thyroidectomy was $5,031, leading to a total cost of $16,414 per case, it was less than the cost of diagnostic lobectomy ($7,684) followed by completion thyroidectomy ($11,954). A sensitivity analysis revealed that molecular testing remained cost effective if the cost of the test was less than $870.

Another molecular test available through the Cleveland Clinic Foundation measures serum thyrotropin receptor mRNA (TSHR mRNA) levels in order to identify thyroid cancer. In a study of 368 patients, TSHR mRNA measurement alone had 61 % sensitivity and 83 % specificity for the presence of thyroid cancer [6]. In a subset analysis of nodules with a cytological diagnosis of FN, TSHR mRNA had a sensitivity of 76 % and specificity of 96 %. When ultrasound characteristics were considered for FN, the sensitivity increased to 97 %, but specificity fell to 84 %. In addition to diagnosing thyroid cancer in an indeterminate nodule, the same study evaluated TSHR mRNA as a marker for thyroid cancer recurrence. For 134 thyroid cancer patients in active surveillance without thyroglobulin antibodies in long term follow up, TSHR mRNA only identified 10 of 25 patients with recurrent cancer (sensitivity 40 %) but identified 107 of 109 patients without recurrence (specificity 98 %). TSHR mRNA did not detect recurrences for radiologically occult disease with elevated thyroglobulin levels ($n=8$), recurrences only identified on PET ($n=3$), and cervical recurrences ($n=4$). The performance was much better for 60 patients with thyroglobulin antibodies in long term follow up; TSHR mRNA identified four of six patients with recurrent cancer (sensitivity 67 %) and all 54 patients without recurrence (specificity 100 %). These results are compelling but have not been validated at other institutions.

"Rule Out" Testing

This molecular test is comprised of a gene expression classifier (GEC) that analyzes 167 genes from the FNA of an indeterminate nodule, and compares them to gene signatures of benign and malignant lesions using a proprietary algorithm to classify the nodule as either benign or suspicious. The test was designed to confirm the high likelihood of a benign nodule and "rule out" malignancy for indeterminate nodules. The GEC test was validated against surgical histopathology in a large, prospective, blinded multicenter trial enrolling 3,789 patients [7]. The performance of the test was evaluated for 265 nodules with indeterminate cytology with adequate material for evaluation. The sensitivity and specificity was 92 % and 52 %, respectively, for the entire group of indeterminate nodules. Many nodules categorized as suspicious ultimately were benign (48 %) on final histopathology. The NPV for AUS/FLUS and FN was 95 % and 94 %, respectively, which is on par with a diagnosis of benign cytology; therefore, many argue that it is sufficient to "rule out" malignancy. On the other hand, the NPV for SM was only 85 %, which is inadequate to exclude malignancy. The authors concluded that a benign result could rule out malignancy for nodules characterized by cytology as AUS/FLUS and FN and reclassify them as benign. For nodules with cytology SM, the GEC testing provided little benefit, as it could not adequately exclude malignancy and avoid diagnostic surgery. In the setting of SM, it is therefore not indicated.

A cost-effective analysis by Li et al. [8] revealed that GEC testing appeared to be cost effective. The analysis assumed a cost of $3,200 for the test and a sensitivity of 91 %. The cost of care without molecular testing was $12,172 per patient compared to $10,719 when GEC testing was used, leading to a potential cost savings of $1,453 per patient compared to current standard of care; this was due to the reduction in the number of unnecessary diagnostic thyroid lobectomies when a nodule was classified as benign on the GEC.

In addition to diagnostic evaluation, molecular markers have been evaluated for prognostic value to identify patients at risk for persistent or recurrent thyroid cancer. BRAF mutations are common in papillary thyroid cancer and are thought to confer more aggressive disease and a worse prognosis. Tufano et al. [9] conducted a meta-analysis of 14 studies and 1,470 patients to determine the prevalence and prognostic value of BRAF mutation for thyroid cancer. The mean prevalence of the BRAF mutation was 45 %, and it ranged from 32 to 73 %. The presence of the BRAF mutation was significantly associated with recurrence (odds ratio (OR) of 1.93 (1.61–2.32), $p<0.0001$), lymph node metastases (OR 1.32 (1.20–1.45), $p<0.0001$), extrathyroidal extension (OR 1.71 (1.50–1.94), $p<0.0001$), and advanced stage of disease (OR 1.70 (1.45–1.99), $p<0.0001$). Accordingly, preoperative knowledge of BRAF mutation status may facilitate treatment strategy so that a tailored approach may be used to minimize risk of recurrence.

Molecular testing holds great promise as an adjunct to cytopathology to help discriminate benign from malignant nodules, as well as possibly predicting biological behavior of thyroid cancer. Data evaluating the performance of the available molecular tests are limited to relatively few studies, and long-term outcomes are not yet available. This is reflected in the American

Thyroid Association guidelines [10], where currently there is no recommendation for or against the use of molecular diagnostic testing for indeterminate nodules.

Intraoperative Nerve Monitoring

Intraoperative nerve monitoring (IONM) was developed as an adjunct to the "gold standard" of recurrent laryngeal nerve (RLN) visualization to minimize the risk of nerve injury. In the USA, IONM has gained popularity; based on recent surveys, it is used by 53 % of general surgeons [11] and 65 % of otolaryngologists [12]. Despite its widespread use, there is considerable debate regarding the benefit of IONM for improving outcomes for thyroid or parathyroid surgery.

Multiple studies have evaluated the efficacy of IONM. A systematic review of the literature by Dralle et al. [13] identified six observational studies with more than 100 nerves at risk that compared IONM to standard nerve visualization alone and found that the incidence of RLN injury was not significantly different in any of the studies. Another study by Chan et al. [14] evaluated 1,000 nerves at risk and found no difference in the frequency of RLN injury with IONM in primary surgery. However, it did show a significant benefit for remedial surgery (19 % vs. 7.8 %, $p=0.017$). There was also a trend towards lower RLN injury rates for patients with cancer and retrosternal goiters. The only randomized controlled trial evaluating IONM of the RLN [15] randomized 1,000 patients to nerve visualization alone or IONM. Transient nerve injury was significantly more frequent in the visualization group than the IONM group (3.8 % vs. 1.9 %, respectively, $p=0.011$). The frequency of permanent nerve injury was similar for both groups (1.2 % vs. 0.8 %, $p=0.368$). A subgroup analysis of patients stratified by surgical risk revealed that for high risk patients, the frequency of transient injury to the RLN was higher with nerve visualization alone compared to IONM (4.9 % vs. 2.0 %, $p=0.011$), but there was no difference in frequency of transient RLN injury for low risk patients (2.8 % vs. 1.8 %). There was no difference in permanent RLN injury rates based on risk stratification.

Proponents of IONM have advocated that its use facilitates nerve identification and dissection. In a study by Snyder et al. [16], IONM assisted in nerve identification for 3 % of nerves at risk with aberrant anatomy (extralaryngeal bifurcation, medial displacement, and non-RLNs) and 7 % of nerves at risk with difficult dissections (large thyroid lobes, scar tissue, and morbid obesity). Another perceived benefit of IONM is the ability to prognosticate nerve function at the conclusion of surgery. This is most important for bilateral surgery, where injury to both RLNs may lead to tracheostomy. Blunt injuries from crush or stretch to the RLN are difficult to identify and are only detected visually 10–15 % of the time [17]. On the other hand, IONM is highly specific for nerve injury and has a NPV of 92–100 % [13]. A study by Goretzki et al. [18] revealed that when loss of nerve signal on the first side led to a change in surgical strategy, no bilateral RLN injuries occurred. However, when loss of signal was ignored, 17 % of patients sustained bilateral RLN injury.

Recently, novel real time IONM with continuous vagal stimulation has been developed to potentially identify impending nerve injuries so that the surgeon can alter the surgical approach or technique in order to avoid injury [19]. Although the studies evaluating this new technology are small, there do appear to be changes in nerve signal prior to loss of nerve function, particularly for traction and stretch injuries. Furthermore, modification in surgical technique allowed nerve recovery in many patients at the time of surgery, thus avoiding loss of nerve function. Additional studies are needed to determine if this technology may reduce the rate of RLN injury.

Several guidelines regarding the implementation and use of IONM have been published. The International Neural Monitoring Study Group guidelines [20] state that neural monitoring should be used routinely, since technically difficult surgeries cannot always be predicted preoperatively. Although IONM provides the greatest benefit in difficult surgeries, routine use enhances familiarity and intricate knowledge of the device, and improves interpretation of signals and troubleshooting of the system. The American Academy of Otolaryngology and Head and Neck Surgery (AAOHNS) has recently published guidelines [21] for improving voice outcomes after thyroid surgery. The guidelines state that IONM may be considered for patients having thyroid surgery due to the proven benefit in shortening RLN identification time in complex and remedial cases, and avoidance of bilateral RLN paralysis. The guidelines recommend that surgeons may consider IONM for bilateral thyroid surgery, remedial thyroid surgery, and surgery in the setting of existing RLN paralysis.

Hemostatic Devices

Over the last 10 years, innovative hemostatic devices have been developed to facilitate surgery by permitting effective hemostasis and reducing operative times. The most commonly used devices are the ultrasonic coagulators, which use high frequency ultrasound to coagulate and cut tissue simultaneously, and the tissue sealers, which use a modified computer-controlled bipolar dissecting and sealing technology. Both devices have been used for thyroidectomy and have been evaluated in multiple studies. A meta-analysis by Melck et al. [22] comparing the ultrasonic device to conventional techniques for thyroidectomy included nine randomized controlled trials and 822 patients. The mean operative time for thyroidectomy with the device was significantly shorter by 23 min ($p<0.001$). The frequency of transient hypoparathyroidism was significantly less using the ultrasonic device than conventional techniques (14.5 % vs. 21.5 %, respectively; $p=0.01$). The frequency of permanent hypoparathyroidism, RLN injury, and postoperative hematoma were the similar using the device and conventional technique. A meta-analysis comparing the tissue sealer to conventional techniques for thyroidectomy by Yao et al. [23] included nine trials and 927 patients. Similar to the results for the ultrasonic device, thyroidectomy with the tissue sealer was significantly shorter than conventional technique by 20 min ($p<0.05$). The frequency of transient or permanent hypoparathyroidism, RLN injury, and postoperative hematoma were the same for both groups. Cost was not evaluated in these studies, but has been assessed in smaller single institutional studies which found that these devices were cost-effective, given the shorter operative time [24].

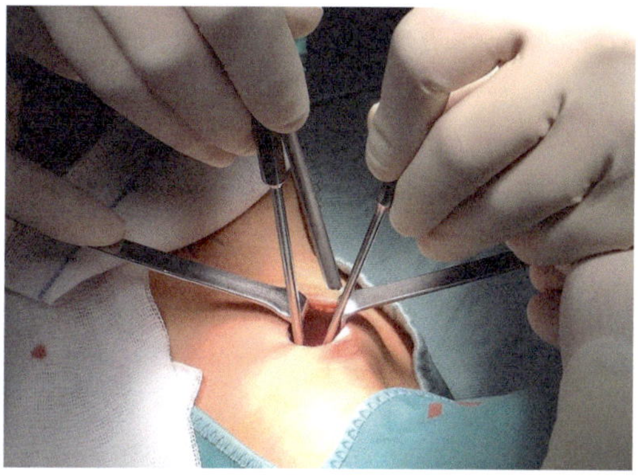

Fig. 20.1 Intraoperative image of incision and instrumentation used for MIVAT

Minimally Invasive Thyroidectomy

Minimally invasive techniques were late to be adopted in thyroid surgery because open thyroidectomy already has very low morbidity, little postoperative pain, and excellent cosmetic results. The perceived benefit of these techniques for thyroid surgery is primarily cosmetic by avoiding or minimizing the cervical incision. Miccoli developed a minimally invasive video-assisted thyroidectomy (MIVAT) gasless technique through a cervical incision < 2 cm in length with the assistance of a 3–5 mm endoscope (Fig. 20.1) [25]. The technique is limited to the removal of thyroid nodules <3 cm in diameter, thyroid gland volume < 20 mL as estimated by ultrasound, no history of thyroiditis, no previous surgery or radiation, presence of a benign nodule or low risk thyroid cancer, and absence of lymph nodes suspicious for malignancy. These requirements limit the general applicability of the technique. A meta-analysis by Pisano et al. [26] comparing MIVAT to conventional thyroidectomy

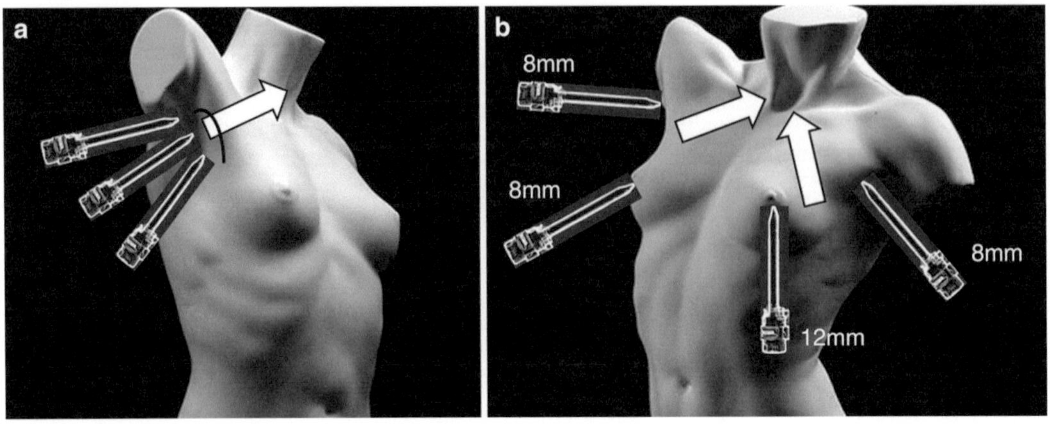

Fig. 20.2 (**a**) Port site location for robotic thyroidectomy: transaxillary approach. (**b**) Port site location for robotic thyroidectomy: axillo-breast approach

included nine prospective randomized studies with 581 patients. There was no significant difference between the groups in the frequency of transient or permanent RLN injury, transient hypoparathyroidism, postoperative hematoma, or wound infection. The mean operative time was significantly longer for MIVAT than conventional thyroidectomy (75 vs. 59 min, respectively, $p<0.0001$). Patients treated with MIVAT had better patient satisfaction, although no validated questionnaires were used, and the follow-up was short. Cost–effectiveness was not evaluated in the study, but would be expected to be lower for MIVAT, given the longer operative times and similar complication rates.

Robotic assisted thyroid surgery through either a transaxillary or axillo-breast approach avoids a cervical incision altogether (Fig. 20.2a, b). The ideal patients for this approach have a small body habitus, low body mass index (BMI), and a normal-sized thyroid with small tumors. The vast majority of studies evaluating these techniques are from South Korea. The largest study to date [27] included 3,000 patients with thyroid cancer (99.3 % papillary, 0.4 % follicular, and 0.3 % medullary) who had robotic assisted thyroidectomy through an axillary approach. The average patient BMI was 22.2±3.1, and the average tumor size was 0.7 cm±0.6 cm. A total thyroidectomy was performed on 1,090 patients (36 %) and less than total thyroidectomy on 1,910 patients (64 %). The mean operative time was 125±33 min. The most common complications observed were transient hypoparathyroidism (37.4 %), permanent hypoparathyroidism (1.1 %), transient RLN injury (1.2 %), and permanent RLN injury (0.3 %). The technique-specific complications were axillary skin flap perforation in three patients and brachial plexus traction injuries in four patients. Post-operative chest wall numbness was also reported. Other studies have reported additional complications, such as esophageal perforation and higher risks of hematoma formation. A meta-analysis by Sun et al. [28] comparing robotically assisted to conventional thyroidectomy included 11 studies with 726 patients undergoing robotic surgery, and 1,205 undergoing conventional thyroidectomy for either thyroid cancer or thyroid nodules. The robotic group was younger (40.5 vs. 49.2 years, respectively), had a lower BMI (23.1 vs. 24.2), and was less likely to undergo total thyroidectomy (58.1 % vs. 75.1 %). The tumors were small, with a mean size of 8 mm. None of the studies evaluated cost. The mean operative time was 77 min longer for the robotic group ($p<0.001$). There was no significant difference between the groups in the frequency of RLN injury, hypoparathyroidism, postoperative hematoma, or seroma. The robotic group had higher cosmetic satisfaction scores, but follow up was only 3 months, and validated patient questionnaires were not used.

Although there was initial enthusiasm for minimally invasive techniques for thyroidectomy in the USA, the technology has not been embraced except in select centers. Critics of MIVAT and the robotically assisted thyroidectomy have identified the limited applicability of these techniques to a select group of patients [29]. Furthermore, these techniques are associated with longer operative times, novel possible complications, and increased resource utilization without long-term oncological follow-up, and a small cosmetic benefit.

Outpatient Thyroidectomy

In recent years, outpatient thyroidectomy has become increasingly frequent. Several studies, comprised of more than 4,500 patients, have reported the safe implementation of ambulatory thyroidectomy [30]. The frequency of postoperative hematoma in these studies ranged from 0 to 2 %, with no fatalities. Hypocalcemia occurred in 0–10 % of patients, and hospital readmission was required in 0–3.9 % of patients. In 2013, the American Thyroid Association published a statement on outpatient thyroidectomy to identify eligibility criteria and factors that should be considered in order to safely and efficiently perform thyroidectomy in an ambulatory setting. The statement stressed the importance of careful preoperative patient selection, postoperative evaluation prior to discharge, patient education regarding the early identification and treatment of postoperative complications, and communication between patient and the care team. Suggested eligibility criteria for outpatient thyroidectomy included: no major comorbidities, an understanding of preoperative education, a social setting conducive to safe postoperative care, an available primary care giver, and proximity to a skilled facility. Factors identified that were felt to be relative contraindications to outpatient thyroidectomy included massive goiter, extensive substernal goiter, locally advanced cancer, challenging hemostasis, Graves' disease, severe thyroiditis, significant medical comorbidities, and social barriers to care. After outpatient thyroid surgery, patients should be observed for at least 2 h and should meet discharge criteria. These included: ability to take liquids, adequate pain control, ability to void, adequate oxygenation and blood pressure, and satisfactory postoperative evaluation without concern for hematoma, dysphonia, dysphagia, or dyspnea. While experienced surgeons can safely perform outpatient thyroidectomy, it is essential that patients are carefully selected and a mechanism is set in place to rapidly and safely identify and treat postoperative complications. This requires an experienced, multidisciplinary care team as well as an experienced surgeon.

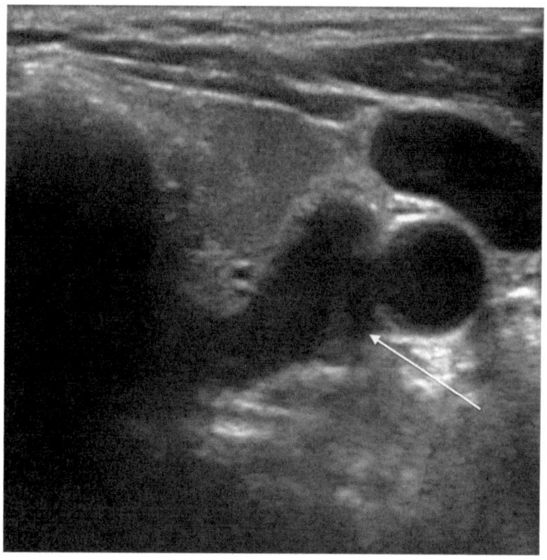

Fig. 20.3 Ultrasound of left superior parathyroid adenoma (*arrow*) with typical hypoechoic appearance

Parathyroid

Preoperative Imaging

Traditionally, parathyroidectomy was performed with a bilateral neck exploration and excision of the abnormal parathyroid gland(s). Advances in radiological imaging have allowed improved preoperative localization of the hyperfunctioning parathyroid gland(s), thus permitting a focused minimally invasive parathyroidectomy. The most well established imaging modalities are ultrasound (US) and sestamibi imaging. US is widely available (Fig. 20.3), inexpensive, evaluates the

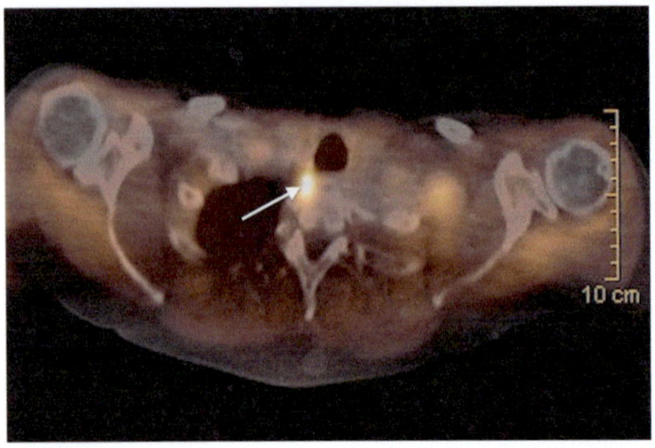

Fig. 20.4 Sestamibi SPECT-CT demonstrating a right superior parathyroid adenoma (*arrow*) in the tracheoesophageal groove

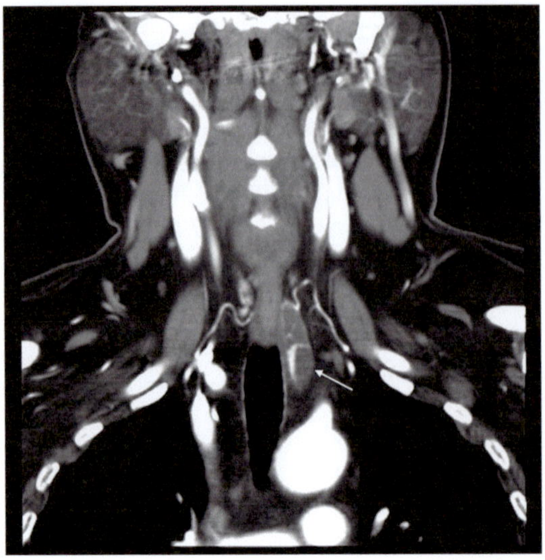

Fig. 20.5 4-Dimensional CT scan of cystic parathyroid (*arrow*) with internal septations located in the upper mediastinum

thyroid for concomitant pathology, and does not expose patients to ionizing radiation. However, it is user dependent, cannot evaluate ectopic locations, and performs poorly for patients with enlarged nodular goiters or challenging body habitus. Sestamibi is a radiocolloid that is retained in parathyroid adenomas, but not in the thyroid gland or other surrounding tissue. Sestamibi scanning with the addition of single photon emission computed tomography (SPECT) has been used to allow for more precise localization of the abnormal parathyroid gland(s) in a three-dimensional approach (Fig. 20.4). Sestamibi/SPECT imaging is widely available, operator independent, and can evaluate for ectopic locations. Nonetheless, expert radiologists are needed to accurately read the scans, and the technique is expensive, time consuming, and exposes patients to ionizing radiation.

Historically, standard computed tomography (CT) has played little role in localization of hyperfunctioning parathyroid glands because of low sensitivity for parathyroid adenomas. Recent modifications of the conventional 3-dimensional anatomic protocol, termed four-dimensional computed tomography (4D-CT), have been developed. The term 4D-CT originates from the added "dimension" of timing of the scanning protocol based on the intravenous contrast phases. Hyperfunctioning parathyroid glands rapidly take up and wash out contrast in comparison to the surrounding thyroid tissue and lymph nodes, thus enabling accurate localization (Fig. 20.5). The images obtained can precisely locate hyperfunctioning glands. In a study by Rodgers et al. [31], 75 patients with primary hyperparathyroidism underwent US, Sestamibi/SPECT, and 4D-CT. The sensitivity for localization of the abnormal parathyroid glands for 4D-CT (88 %) was superior to SPECT (65 %) and US (57 %). Also, 4D-CT identified 45 % of patients who ultimately had multigland disease in contrast to US or SPECT, which identified none of these patients. Advantages of 4D-CT are that it is operator independent, intermediate in cost, and evaluates ectopic locations. However, it is not widely available, requires expert radiologist interpretation, should not be used in patients with renal insufficiency due to the intravenous contrast load, and exposes patients to relatively higher doses of ionizing radiation.

There is considerable debate among surgeons regarding which of these imaging modalities is the best for preoperative localization for patients with primary hyperparathyroidism. A meta-analysis by Cheung et al. [32] of 43 studies evaluated preoperative localization techniques for primary hyperparathyroidism comparing US, SPECT, and 4D-CT. US and SPECT had similar pooled sensitivities of 76 % and 79 %, respectively. Although there was an insufficient number of 4D-CT studies (only 2), the weighted sensitivity was 89 %. The authors cautiously concluded that 4D-CT shows great promise and may allow better localization, but more studies need to be performed to confirm these results. Cost-effectiveness studies have also been done to determine which preoperative imaging techniques or combination of techniques is most effective. A study by Wang et al. [33] determined that US + SPECT, and, if discordant, followed by 4D-CT was the most cost-effective algorithm because it reduced the need for bilateral neck exploration and increased the possibility of undergoing minimally invasive parathyroidectomy, which was always associated with lower costs. However, the results were dependent on the sensitivity of each imaging technique, and this varies among institutions. Accordingly, each institution should evaluate their own data to determine the optimal imaging algorithm at that institution for patients with primary hyperparathyroidism.

Minimally Invasive Parathyroidectomy

The advent of preoperative imaging techniques and intraoperative parathyroid hormone (ioPTH) monitoring has permitted experienced surgeons to perform focused minimally invasive parathyroidectomy (MIP) for the majority of their patients. Patients with preoperative localization identifying a hyperfunctioning parathyroid gland are candidates for a focused, minimally invasive procedure. The surgery is performed using regional anesthesia with a surgeon-performed superficial cervical plexus block and mild sedation, using rapid, intraoperative PTH monitoring to assure adequate parathyroidectomy in an ambulatory setting. If needed or based on patient preference, general anesthesia can be used.

This technique involves the following general protocol: prior to the surgical incision, a baseline rapid, intraoperative PTH level is obtained. A 2–4 cm cervical incision is created, and the abnormal parathyroid gland identified and excised. Intraoperative PTH levels are obtained at the time of gland excision and at 5, 10, and 15 min post-excision. Intraoperative criteria for a successful parathyroidectomy are a drop of the intra-operative PTH level by greater than 50–65 % of baseline (typically at 10 min, but this can vary based on a number of factors, including the starting level, amount of gland manipulation during the dissection, and renal clearance), and in to the normal range. If the criteria are met, the procedure is terminated. If the 15 min sample fails to decrease sufficiently, additional cervical exploration is performed to evaluate for multigland disease. In circumstances where PTH may be metabolized more slowly (such as elderly patients or those with renal or hepatic insufficiency), additional intraoperative PTH levels can be obtained after 10–15 min prior to undertaking additional exploration. The success of the minimally invasive parathyroidectomy has been confirmed by several studies, with cure and recurrence rates that are similar to standard bilateral neck exploration [34]. In a study by Udelsman et al. [35], 1,650 patients underwent parathyroidectomy by a single surgeon. Bilateral neck exploration was performed in 613 patients and minimally invasive parathyroidectomy in 1,037 cases. The cure rate for the minimally invasive technique was superior to bilateral neck exploration (99.4 % vs. 97.1 %, respectively; $p<0.001$), and the complication rate was lower (1.5 % vs. 3.1 %, $p=0.02$). In addition, minimally invasive parathyroidectomy was associated with a shorter mean hospital length of stay compared to bilateral neck dissection patients (0.2 vs. 1.3 days, $p<0.0001$), and the total hospital charges were less by $1,471 per case.

Parathyroid Imaging with Magnetic Resonance Imaging (MRI)

Due to its ability to evaluate soft tissue, MRI was initially thought to be a good imaging modality to localize hyperfunctioning parathyroid glands. However, variability in signal intensity and long imaging times leading to poor spatial resolution have hampered the ability of MRI to localize abnormal parathyroid glands [36]. MRI has been largely replaced by other imaging modalities due to its high cost and inferior sensitivity.

Radioguided Parathyroidectomy

Radioguided parathyroidectomy is another surgical adjunct to identify hyperfunctioning parathyroid glands. Patients are injected with sestamibi approximately 2 h prior to surgery, and then a gamma probe is used to direct the incision and help identify the hyperfunctioning parathyroid gland(s). After the abnormal gland is removed, the gamma probe is used to measure its activity compared to the surgical bed; radiation counts greater than 20 % of background are considered to be definitive for representing parathyroid tissue. Early reports for radioguided parathyroidectomy revealed a sensitivity of 93 %, positive predictive value of 88 %, and an overall accuracy of 83 % for parathyroid localization [37]. However, another study [38] reported that radioguidance was felt to be unhelpful because of confusing or inaccurate counts, increased counts only after the parathyroid gland was fully exposed, or equipment failure. Use of radioguided parathyroidectomy has not expanded widely among parathyroid surgeons because many feel that it offers little overall benefit in the setting of higher cost. One potential use may be in patients who have recurrent or persistent hyperparathyroidism and have had prior explorations, as this technique may facilitate identification of the overactive parathyroid gland amidst scar.

Conclusion

There have been numerous technological advances in the treatments for thyroid and parathyroid disease, and overall these have helped to improve patient outcomes and reduce surgical morbidity. This remains an area of dynamic change and ongoing technological and scientific development; however, long-term examination of the benefit of some of these novel approaches still needs to be undertaken. In particular, cost-effectiveness analysis should be performed as part of this evaluation, especially given the challenges of our current resource-constrained health care environment. It will be important that practice guidelines remain contemporary, helping surgeons to evaluate the evidence underlying these developments, such that adoption is appropriate and driven by compelling data. Professional societies and associations might need to play a role.

References

1. Jin J, McHenry CR. Thyroid incidentaloma. Best Pract Res Clin Endocrinol Metab. 2012;26(1):83–96.
2. Cooper DS, Doherty GM, Haugen BR, Kloos RT, Lee SL, Mandel SJ, et al. Revised American Thyroid Association management guidelines for patients with thyroid nodules and differentiated thyroid cancer. Thyroid. 2009;19(11):1167–214.
3. Cibas ES, Ali SZ. The Bethesda System for reporting thyroid cytopathology. Am J Clin Pathol. 2009; 132(5):658–65.
4. Nikiforov YE, Ohori NP, Hodak SP, Carty SE, LeBeau SO, Ferris RL, et al. Impact of mutational testing on the diagnosis and management of patients with cytologically indeterminate thyroid nodules: a prospective analysis of 1056 FNA samples. J Clin Endocrinol Metab. 2011;96(11):3390–7.
5. Yip L, Farris C, Kabaker AS, Hodak SP, Nikiforova MN, McCoy KL, et al. Cost impact of molecular testing for indeterminate thyroid nodule fine-needle aspiration biopsies. J Clin Endocrinol Metab. 2012;97(6): 1905–12.
6. Milas M, Shin J, Gupta M, Novosel T, Nasr C, Brainard J, et al. Circulating thyrotropin receptor mRNA as a novel marker of thyroid cancer: clinical applications learned from 1758 samples. Ann Surg. 2010;252(4):643–51.
7. Alexander EK, Kennedy GC, Baloch ZW, Cibas ES, Chudova D, Diggans J, et al. Preoperative diagnosis of benign thyroid nodules with indeterminate cytology. N Engl J Med. 2012;367(8):705–15.
8. Li H, Robinson KA, Anton B, Saldanha IJ, Ladenson PW. Cost-effectiveness of a novel molecular test for cytologically indeterminate thyroid nodules. J Clin Endocrinol Metab. 2011;96(11):E1719–26.
9. Tufano RP, Teixeira GV, Bishop J, Carson KA, Xing M. BRAF mutation in papillary thyroid cancer and its value in tailoring initial treatment: a systematic review and meta-analysis. Medicine. 2012;91(5):274–86.
10. Hodak SP, Rosenthal DS. Information for clinicians: commercially available molecular diagnosis testing in the evaluation of thyroid nodule fine-needle aspiration specimens. Thyroid. 2013;23(2):131–4.
11. Sturgeon C, Sturgeon T, Angelos P. Neuromonitoring in thyroid surgery: attitudes, usage patterns, and

predictors of use among endocrine surgeons. World J Surg. 2009;33(3):417–25.
12. Singer MC, Rosenfeld RM, Sundaram K. Laryngeal nerve monitoring: current utilization among head and neck surgeons. Otolaryngol Head Neck Surg. 2012; 146(6):895–9.
13. Dralle H, Sekulla C, Lorenz K, Brauckhoff M, Machens A. Intraoperative monitoring of the recurrent laryngeal nerve in thyroid surgery. World J Surg. 2008;32(7):1358–66.
14. Chan WF, Lang BH, Lo CY. The role of intraoperative neuromonitoring of recurrent laryngeal nerve during thyroidectomy: a comparative study on 1000 nerves at risk. Surgery. 2006;140(6):866–72. discussion 72–3.
15. Barczynski M, Konturek A, Cichon S. Randomized clinical trial of visualization versus neuromonitoring of recurrent laryngeal nerves during thyroidectomy. Br J Surg. 2009;96(3):240–6.
16. Snyder SK, Sigmond BR, Lairmore TC, Govednik-Horny CM, Janicek AK, Jupiter DC. The long-term impact of routine intraoperative nerve monitoring during thyroid and parathyroid surgery. Surgery. 2013;154(4):704–11. discussion 11–3.
17. Lo CY, Kwok KF, Yuen PW. A prospective evaluation of recurrent laryngeal nerve paralysis during thyroidectomy. Arch Surg. 2000;135(2):204–7.
18. Goretzki PE, Schwarz K, Brinkmann J, Wirowski D, Lammers BJ. The impact of intraoperative neuromonitoring (IONM) on surgical strategy in bilateral thyroid diseases: is it worth the effort? World J Surg. 2010;34(6):1274–84.
19. Phelan E, Schneider R, Lorenz K, Dralle H, Kamani D, Potenza A, et al. Continuous vagal IONM prevents recurrent laryngeal nerve paralysis by revealing initial EMG changes of impending neuropraxic injury: a prospective, multicenter study. Laryngoscope. 2014;124(6):1498–505.
20. Randolph GW, Dralle H, Abdullah H, Barczynski M, Bellantone R, Brauckhoff M, et al. Electrophysiologic recurrent laryngeal nerve monitoring during thyroid and parathyroid surgery: international standards guideline statement. Laryngoscope. 2011;121 Suppl 1: 1–16.
21. Chandrasekhar SS, Randolph GW, Seidman MD, Rosenfeld RM, Angelos P, Barkmeier-Kraemer J, et al. Clinical practice guideline: improving voice outcomes after thyroid surgery. Otolaryngol Head Neck Surg. 2013;148(6 Suppl):S1–37.
22. Melck AL, Wiseman SM. Harmonic scalpel compared to conventional hemostasis in thyroid surgery: a meta-analysis of randomized clinical trials. Int J Surg Oncol. 2010;2010:396079.
23. Yao HS, Wang Q, Wang WJ, Ruan CP. Prospective clinical trials of thyroidectomy with LigaSure vs conventional vessel ligation: a systematic review and meta-analysis. Arch Surg. 2009;144(12):1167–74.
24. Ortega J, Sala C, Flor B, Lledo S. Efficacy and cost-effectiveness of the UltraCision harmonic scalpel in thyroid surgery: an analysis of 200 cases in a randomized trial. J Laparoendosc Adv Surg Tech A. 2004;14(1):9–12.
25. Miccoli P, Berti P, Materazzi G, Minuto M, Barellini L. Minimally invasive video-assisted thyroidectomy: five years of experience. J Am Coll Surg. 2004; 199(2):243–8.
26. Pisanu A, Podda M, Reccia I, Porceddu G, Uccheddu A. Systematic review with meta-analysis of prospective randomized trials comparing minimally invasive video-assisted thyroidectomy (MIVAT) and conventional thyroidectomy (CT). Langenbecks Arch Surg. 2013;398(8):1057–68.
27. Ban EJ, Yoo JY, Kim WW, Son HY, Park S, Lee SH, et al. Surgical complications after robotic thyroidectomy for thyroid carcinoma: a single center experience with 3,000 patients. Surg Endosc. 2014;28(9): 2555–63.
28. Sun GH, Peress L, Pynnonen MA. Systematic review and meta-analysis of robotic vs conventional thyroidectomy approaches for thyroid disease. Otolaryngol Head Neck Surg. 2014;150(4):520–32.
29. Perrier ND. Why I, have abandoned robot-assisted transaxillary thyroid surgery. Surgery. 2012;152(6): 1025–6.
30. Terris DJ, Snyder S, Carneiro-Pla D, Inabnet 3rd WB, Kandil E, Orloff L, et al. American Thyroid Association statement on outpatient thyroidectomy. Thyroid. 2013;23(10):1193–202.
31. Rodgers SE, Hunter GJ, Hamberg LM, Schellingerhout D, Doherty DB, Ayers GD, et al. Improved preoperative planning for directed parathyroidectomy with 4-dimensional computed tomography. Surgery. 2006; 140(6):932–40. discussion 40–1.
32. Cheung K, Wang TS, Farrokhyar F, Roman SA, Sosa JA. A meta-analysis of preoperative localization techniques for patients with primary hyperparathyroidism. Ann Surg Oncol. 2012;19(2):577–83.
33. Wang TS, Cheung K, Farrokhyar F, Roman SA, Sosa JA. Would scan, but which scan? A cost-utility analysis to optimize preoperative imaging for primary hyperparathyroidism. Surgery. 2011;150(6):1286–94.
34. Lew JI, Solorzano CC. Surgical management of primary hyperparathyroidism: state of the art. Surg Clin North Am. 2009;89(5):1205–25.
35. Udelsman R, Lin Z, Donovan P. The superiority of minimally invasive parathyroidectomy based on 1650 consecutive patients with primary hyperparathyroidism. Ann Surg. 2011;253(3):585–91.
36. Udelsman R, Pasieka JL, Sturgeon C, Young JE, Clark OH. Surgery for asymptomatic primary hyperparathyroidism: proceedings of the third international workshop. J Clin Endocrinol Metab. 2009;94(2): 366–72.
37. Chen H, Mack E, Starling JR. Radioguided parathyroidectomy is equally effective for both adenomatous and hyperplastic glands. Ann Surg. 2003;238(3):332–7. discussion 7–8.
38. Inabnet 3rd WB, Kim CK, Haber RS, Lopchinsky RA. Radioguidance is not necessary during parathyroidectomy. Arch Surg. 2002;137(8):967–70.

Neuron Based Surgery: Are We There Yet? Technical Developments in the Surgical Treatment of Brain Injury and Disease

21

Whitney Sheen James and G. Michael Lemole Jr.

Introduction

Over the past 25 centuries, technical developments in the surgical treatment of brain injury have both persisted and progressed. From early trephination of the skull in prehistoric Europe and pre-Columbian Peru [1], to syntheses of boutique nanoscale agents targeting specific cells in an individual's brain, patients suffering from disease of the central nervous system now have treatment options ranging from primitive to postmodern. Indeed, over the ages, the progression of therapeutic technologies for the treatment of neurological diseases has been cumulative. While neurosurgeons continue to employ techniques that mimic those of ancient trephination, such as drilling burr holes in the skull and creating "cookie cutter" craniotomies for evacuation of subdural and epidural brain hemorrhages, they now also employ twenty-first century neuronavigation-guided approaches for the treatment of highly focal brain pathologies. With the advancement of our understanding of neuroanatomy and neurophysiology, scientists and surgeons have been able to continually refine primitive practices while developing novel ones in an ongoing effort to improve clinical outcomes and patients' quality of life and drive down rates of morbidity and mortality. A noteworthy paradigm shift, beginning in the late 20th century and growing in popularity today, is a holistic, multidisciplinary approach to the neurosurgical patient. We now recognize that to achieve best outcomes in the treatment of a traumatic brain injury, we must incorporate not only surgical but also environmental, mechanical, biochemical, and genetic based treatments for cure and optimum outcomes.

Origins of Surgical Treatment for Brain Trauma and Disease

Written historical evidence of neurosurgical treatment for brain injury and disease dates back to 3,000 years B.C. The Edwin Smith Surgical Papyrus, thought to originate from ancient Egypt or Asia in 1700 B.C., is one of the oldest known medical papyri describing cases of brain trauma and proposed treatments. In the papyrus, there are descriptions of surface features of the brain, cerebral spinal fluid, and certain bodily functions that can be impaired by injury to the brain and spinal cord [2]. The papyrus is the first known

W.S. James, M.D., M.H.S.
Division of Neurosurgery, Department of Surgery, University of Arizona Medical Center, Tucson, AZ, USA
e-mail: wsheen@surgery.arizona.edu

G.M. Lemole Jr., M.D. (✉)
Division of Neurosurgery, Department of Surgery, University of Arizona, Tucson, AZ, USA
e-mail: mlemole@surgery.arizona.edu

R. Latifi et al. (eds.), *Technological Advances in Surgery, Trauma and Critical Care*, DOI 10.1007/978-1-4939-2671-8_21

written description of the cranial sutures, the meninges, the external surface of the brain, and the cerebral vasculature. It includes the first description of surgical suturing as well as various types of surgical dressings. Localization of areas of brain damage according to physical symptoms, such as damage to the temporal lobe with presentation of aphasia, is also described. The document recommends active treatment of simple skull fractures, while it advises against treatment of head injuries with "protruding or swollen brain." Such advice can be viewed as an accurate prediction of the difficulties neurological surgeons of the future would face in treating severe cases of traumatic brain injury.

The Advent of Modern American Neurosurgery

In the first half of the twentieth century, Harvey Williams Cushing, commonly referred to as the father of American neurosurgery, developed myriad operating procedures and techniques that are now the foundation of neurosurgical practice in the twenty-first century. It was in large part due to his techniques that the high mortality rates previously associated with brain injury were more than halved. Some of his important contributions to the field included continuous monitoring of blood and intracerebral pressures, application of local anesthesia, the use of X-ray technology to diagnose brain tumors, the use of electrical stimuli to study the human sensory cortex, and the development of the Bovie electrocautery tool.

The Advent of Neuron Based Surgery

Prompted by Cushing and his colleagues, the field of neurosurgery experienced an accelerated evolution in the twentieth century. The advent of neuron-based surgery can be traced to multiple origins, including that of Richard Feynman, an American theoretical physicist and Nobel laureate [3], who in 1959 delivered a famous talk "There's Plenty of Room at the Bottom." In this talk, he discussed the possibility of small-scale surgical treatments, stating:

> ...A friend of mine (Albert R. Hibbs) suggests a very interesting possibility for relatively small machines. He says that, although it is a very wild idea, it would be interesting in surgery if you could swallow the surgeon. You put the mechanical surgeon inside the blood vessel and it goes into the heart and 'looks' around. (Of course the information has to be fed out.) It finds out which valve is the faulty one and takes a little knife and slices it out. Other small machines might be permanently incorporated in the body to assist some inadequately-functioning organ... [3]

In 1974, a Japanese professor, Norio Taniguchi, coined the term "nanotechnology" in a paper entitled "On the Basic Concept of Nanotechnology" [4], and in 1986, Eric Drexler at the Massachusetts Institute of Technology published the book *Engines of Creation: The Coming Era of Nanotechnology* [5] in which he described his idea that one day, "molecular assemblers" would be able to manipulate individual atoms and discussed the technological significance of nanoscale technologies. The idea of neuron-based surgery with nanoscale therapies had been planted. With President William J. Clinton's Presidential Proclamation, the 1990s were proclaimed "The Decade of the Brain" and scientists went to work turning nanoscale neuron-based therapies from an idea into a reality. The momentum continued into the 21st century with President Barak Obama's Brain Initiative (NIH: http://www.nih.gov/science/brain/). With the development of nanoscale therapies on the horizon, scientists now face the challenge of identifying neurophysiological mechanisms and markers of traumatic brain injury and injury severity. As knowledge regarding mechanisms and markers of traumatic brain injury advances, researchers will be able to develop neuron-based therapeutics to intercept processes that lead to exacerbation of morbidity and increased rates of mortality and promote processes that lead to neuronal preservation.

Advancements in Treatment of Neurotrauma

Advancement in Development of Serum Biomarkers for Detection of Trauma Severity

Systemic autoimmunity is now a recognized phenomenon in traumatic brain injury. Detailed mechanisms for the role of immunoexcitotoxicity in traumatic encephalopathy have been described [6]. Several groups have begun investigating the role of serum autoantibody markers in the quantification of traumatic brain injury severity [7, 8]. Glial fibrillary acidic protein (GFAP), an intermediate filament protein in the cytoskeleton of astroglia, is highly correlated with brain injury. Elevated serum levels of GFAP on post brain injury day 2 have been shown to increase odds of mortality (odds ratio 1.45, p value 0.028) [8], and autoantibodies to glial fibrillary acidic protein (GFAP) and GFAP breakdown products have been shown to increase 7 days after traumatic brain injury [7]. Additionally, anti-GFAP autoantibody has been shown to enter living astroglia cells in culture where it acts to compromise glial cell viability. In a study by Zhang et al. from 2014, TBI patients showed an average 3.77 fold increase in anti-GFAP autoantibody levels from early (0–1 days) to late (7–10 days) times post injury. Changes in autoantibody levels were negatively correlated with outcomes as measured by extended Glasgow Coma Outcomes Scale score at 6 months [7], suggesting that TBI patients with greater anti-GFAP immune-responses have worse outcomes, and making anti-GFAP antibodies a potential target for nanotherapeutics in traumatic brain injury.

Several groups have developed technologies that use serum biomarkers to distinguish TBI symptoms from those of other traumatic injuries outside the brain, allowing physicians to distinguish acute brain injury from other organ damage [9]. For example, choice of treatment in stroke patients depends on whether the stroke is hemorrhagic or ischemic. A serum biomarker distinguishing the two that could be measured in the field has the potential of providing patients with much faster, and potentially lifesaving, interventions. Indeed, research points to GFAP as a valuable marker for the diagnosis and determination of prognosis in stroke and TBI [9].

Amyloid-beta peptides and tau protein have been used as biomarkers in cerebrospinal fluid (CSF) and interstitial fluid following TBI [10]. Amyloid precursor protein (APP) accumulates with the shearing of axons and as a result of diffuse axonal injury in patients with TBI. It is the post-injury enzymes, such as caspases, that cleave APP to yield amyloid-beta (Aβ) peptides, commonly associated with Alzheimer's disease. Indeed, brains of a subset of TBI victims look histologically similar to those of patients with Alzheimer's disease on autopsy, with accumulations of Aβ peptides and neurofibrillary tangles of phosphorylated tau proteins [10]. Epidemiological evidence suggests a direct link between TBI and the development of Alzheimer's disease, and researchers are presently looking into the use of Aβ and tau proteins as serum and CSF biomarkers for establishment of prognosis after TBI. Furthermore, it has also been noted that high levels of Aβ peptide may be neurotoxic in and of themselves [10]. Finally, because traumatic brain injury involves degradation of brain tissues, including axonal damage, necrotic cell death, and both delayed and acute products of neuronal apoptosis, a process activated by caspases, other groups have looked at caspase inhibition therapy as a means of decreasing TBI increases in Aβ peptide [11].

Post-injury lack of oxygen delivery to the brain results in prolonged neuroinflammation with an increase in cerebral cytokine production and extravasation, lending serum and cerebral spinal fluid cytokines as additional markers of TBI [12]. Serum cytokines that can be measured to diagnose and determine prognosis for hypoxic TBI include albumin, S100, myelin basic protein (MBP), neuronal specific enolase (NSE), ubiquitin C-terminal hydrolase (UCH-L1), granulocyte macrophage-colony stimulating factor (GM-CSF), interferon-gamma (IFN-gamma), tumor necrosis factor (TNF), interleukin (IL)-2, IL-4, IL-6, and IL-10, and increases of these serum biomarkers following TBI correlate with poorer outcomes [13]. Proposals have been suggested to use serum markers, such as S100 and MBP, to track the occurrence of post-TBI hypoxia and prompt expedited and adequate treatments [14]. Additionally, research has shown that serum levels of S100B protein correlate with IL-6 levels, hypoperfusion indices and outcomes in patients requiring surgical control of traumatic brain hemorrhages [14]. In sum, with sensitive and specific biomarkers that reflect brain injury, physicians are able to gather important information regarding TBI pathophysiology and severity while formulating more accurate prognoses for outcomes [15].

Advancements in Understanding of Environmental Factors Affecting Patient Outcomes in Neurotrauma

In the twenty-first century we continue to learn about the important influence of environment in neuronal injury, death and survival. By controlling or influencing the environment of neurons and glial cells immediately after injury, physicians and surgeons can attempt to limit secondary insults and injury to the brain. Hemodynamic instability must be immediately addressed. Likewise, secondary insults, such as hypoxia, hypotension and hypoglycemia, must be treated before an accurate neurological assessment can be obtained. Finally, monitoring and management of intracerebral pressures is paramount for maintaining adequate blood supply to neuron and glial cells in the severely injured brain.

Ischemia, or lack of oxygen delivery, is an ongoing threat to cell viability in the injured brain. There exist three described phases of ischemic brain injury: an immediate no-flow state, in which there is an absence of blood flow and oxygen delivery to the brain, a secondary reperfusion injury, in which resumed oxidative phosphorylation results in formation of reactive oxygen species and subsequent cell damage, and a tertiary delayed postreperfusion injury, marked by neuronal calcium overload, activation of pathologic proteases, alteration of gene expression and activation of the inflammatory cascade [16]. Each of theses three phases is a potential target for cell saving therapeutic interventions.

Much research has looked into the effects of cooling the body and brain as a means of protecting neuron and glial cells from ischemic injury. Though targeted temperature management has been shown to be of benefit for adult patients with post cardiac arrest syndrome and neonates with hypoxic-ischemic encephalopathy [16], the vast body of the scientific literature points toward a detrimental effect of hypothermia and a beneficial effect of normothermia after brain injury [17–19]. Randomized control trials looking at the effects of cooling the brain after traumatic brain injury are still lacking [20].

Sex hormones, such as estrogen and progesterone, play neuroprotective and neuron-sparing roles in brain trauma [21]. Premenopausal women have better survival than men after intracerebral hemorrhage, a phenomenon postulated to be associated with the ability of estrogen to inhibit iron-induced autophagy of injured cells [22], leading researchers to look at estrogen as a potential drug for inhibiting autophagy in patients suffering TBI. Similarly, progesterone is being utilized as a therapeutic means to ward off neuron death and cognitive dysfunction following brain injury [23]. Evidence suggests that progesterone inhibits "several physiological processes that are detrimental to neuron function and survival including inflammation, edema, demyelination and excitotoxicity," the mechanism of which is thought to be related to the blockage of voltage-gated calcium channels [23].

Glycemic control has historically been an issue of debate in the management of patients with TBI. Elevated glucose levels with prolonged hyperglycemia are associated with increased rates of mortality and worse outcomes in TBI patients [24–26]. Vespa et al. [27] published a study in 2012 demonstrating that TBI patients tend to have increased glucose metabolism followed by increased cellular distress with elevations in lactate/pyruvate ratios and glutamate levels when cerebral glucose levels are tightly controlled and maintained between 80 and 110 mg/dL. Following traumatic brain injury, the brain loses its ability to maintain cerebral autoregulation and is unable to compensate for low glucose levels. Hence, subsequent fluctuations in cerebral blood flow after TBI may cause increased susceptibility to the effects of hypoglycemia [28]. Additionally, it is now believed that glucose delivery to the brain is limited when oxidative metabolism is impaired, such as in settings of TBI, and therefore, loose glycemic control (90–150 mg/dL) is not only permissible, but actually preferable in the immediate post injury period.

Monitoring and management of intracerebral pressures is of critical importance in maintaining adequate blood supply to the injured brain. Management of intracranial pressures has long been a mainstay treatment of patients with TBI. Well-maintained ICPs are essential for ensuring adequate cerebral perfusion for oxygen and substrate delivery as well as metabolite waste removal. Advances in neuroimaging and neuromonitoring technologies have the potential to significantly improve the detection of neural compromise and our understanding of the pathophysiology of TBI, including the nature of the perihematomal penumbra and role of mitochondrial dysfunction [29]. Osmotherapy with hypertonic saline and mannitol continues to be a mainstay of treatment of elevated ICPs [30].

Advancements in Surgical Therapies and Techniques for Treatment of Neurotrauma

Nanotherapeutics

Most neurosurgeons are familiar with the adage, "Time is brain." The speed with which a patient is transported to the hospital and into the operating room is still considered to be one of the greatest determining factors of outcome and survival in cases of severe TBI. Diagnostic and therapeutic interventions for patients with severe TBI continue to be refined and developed. With the introduction of diagnostic and therapeutic nanoparticles, the field of neurosurgery is embarking upon a new revolution of neuron-based surgery.

Nanoparticles are defined as "... solid colloidal particles ranging in size from 10 to 1,000 nm (1 μm). They consist of macromolecular materials in which the active principle (drug or biologically active material) is dissolved, entrapped, encapsulated and/or to which the active principle is adsorbed or attached" [31]. Nanoparticles can be categorized into polymeric nanoparticles, polymeric nanoconjugates, micelles, peptides, metal complexes, carbon nanoplatforms, and dendrimers [30]. They are often made of biodegradable synthetic polymers, such as polylactic acid (PLA), polylactic-*co*-glycolic acid (PLGA) and poly-L-caprolactone (PCL). They can also be constructed with the use of natural polymers such as albumin, collagen, gliaden, gelatin, chitosan, pullulan and curdlan [32]. The nanoparticle surface can be conjugated with various ligands, such as polyethelene glycol, monoclonal antibodies, antisense oligonucleotides, endosomal escape units, gadolinium and fluorescent molecules for desired diagnostic and therapeutic properties. Such ligands can also be used to selectively target certain cell types for nanoparticle drug delivery.

Nanoparticle conjugates that target molecules of specific cell types make it possible to treat specific neuronal or diseased tissues for imaging, drug delivery, radiation, surgical excision and chemotherapies [33]. For example, the chemotherapeutic agent paclitaxel (Abraxane®, Abraxis BioScience, LLC, Bridgewater, NJ) can be loaded into protein-bound nanoparticles conjugated with protein ligands that allow the nanoparticles to selectively target and treat cancer cells in the brain. Other applications currently under investigation include nanoparticle delivery of doxorubicin, 5-fluorouracil and dexamethasone. Targeted nanoparticle drug delivery has been shown to increase therapeutic effects, decrease systemic side effects and improve patient outcomes as compared to delivery of unbound, systemically delivered drugs [34]. Similarly, Paunesku et al. [35] demonstrated that nanoparticles loaded with titanium dioxide, DNA oligonucleotides, and gadolinium contrast have increased intracellular accumulation in central nervous system tissues as compared to systemically delivered gadolinium dye, the current standard of care. Such technology allows for diseased tissue to be injected with greater sensitivity. With cell specific drug delivery, it is now possible to selectively deliver antiepileptic drugs, calcium channel blockers, and agents potentiating the dopaminergic response, such as amantadine, to specific areas of disease in the nervous system. Additionally, these technologies now allow clinicians, surgeons and scientists to directly visualize cells of interest via immunofluorescence, which occurs when ligands bind to markers of a specific disease [36].

Delivery methods of nanoparticles are myriad and include both local and systemic methods. Though the specific methods by which nanoparticles cross the blood brain barrier are unknown, two primary pathways are described in the literature and include: (1) axonal translocation from peripheral sensory nerves; and (2) uptake from the systemic circulation via passive diffusion, opening of tight junctions, receptor-mediated transport and inhibition of efflux systems by coating agents at the blood-brain-barrier [31, 32, 37, 38]. Particles can be effectively delivered by intravenous or intra-arterial injection. Alternatively, the blood brain barrier may be bypassed altogether via local infusion of nanoparticles or placement of polymeric implants. Pressurized catheters can be introduced into brain regions of interest and nanoparticles delivered via convection-enhanced delivery. Intrathecal, intranasal, oral and transdermal methods of nanoparticle delivery are currently under investigation as well [32]. Finally, gadolinium-diethylenetriamine pentaacetate (DTPA) can be co-infused with targeted nanoparticles and monitored using real-time magnetic resonance imaging to accurately adjust the volume of distribution of delivered therapeutic agents [32, 39, 40].

At the time of this publication, the FDA had not yet approved a nanomedicine for neurological or neurosurgical application. Numerous nanotechnologies are undergoing clinical trials. For instance, carbon nanotubes are being investigated for their ability to selectively deliver drugs and genes to treat malignant cells in the central nervous system [32, 41]. Gold nanoparticles are being used in thermal ablation applications for targeted treatment of diseased central nervous system cells [42–44]. Holding much promise, the delivery of nanoparticles in the diagnosis and treatment of neurological diseases requires more research to establish safety and efficacy of this treatment modality.

Nano Neurosurgery, Robotics, and Bioelectronics

Scientists are presently working on the development of nanoparticle scaffolds in the treatment of acute and chronic neuronal injury. One such nanoscale scaffold is made from (RADA)4, a synthetic biological material formed through self-assembly of ionic complementary peptides using alternating positively and negatively charged amino acids that form highly hydrated β-sheet nanoscaffolds in the presence of physiological-concentration salts, such as saline, tissue culture media, cerebrospinal fluid, and other body fluids. Researchers are investigating potential uses of the (RADA)4 nanoparticle scaffold, including the establishment of frameworks for partial reinnervation of axons in patients with trauma to peripheral nerves, the inhibition of scar formation in neural tissues, the promotion of de novo central nervous system tissues from stem cell precursors, and the improvement of intraoperative and postoperative hemostasis [32, 45].

In addition to nanoscale tissue scaffolding, researchers are working to develop nanoscale surgical instruments. Leary et al. [46] showed that femtosecond laser pulses, lasting only one quadrillionth of a second, can manipulate molecular structures of single cells with exquisite precision and spatial resolution in the nanometer range. Femtosecond laser pulses can be used to transfect cells with DNA, RNA and other genetic code, dissect away subcellular organelles without affecting cellular viability, and incise individual neuronal fibers. Nanoneedles, microscopy tips sharpened to diameters of 200–300 nm, are used to penetrate cellular and nuclear membranes for the insertion of various molecular constructs while preserving cell viability, and nanotweezers, made from carbon nanotubes attached to electrodes, are applied to manipulate subcellular structures within living cells [46].

In addition to the development of nanoscale surgical instruments, researchers are working on engineering synthetic and biological nanorobots to manipulate and treat neuronal diseases and tissues [32]. Tumor-targeting peptides can be incorporated into the coats of viruses and contrast-enhancing agents or chemotherapies can be loaded into viral capsules for targeted nanoscale contrast and drug delivery [47]. Peptides, designed to release diagnostic and therapeutic agents in specified environments, are being synthesized to selectively target and treat certain diseased cell types [48]. Nanomotors, naturally occurring enzymes or bacteria conjugated to metal-binding amino acid residues controlled by certain environmental electrochemical reactions [47], can be used to propel nanoscale instruments to the appropriate targets.

Finally, scientists are currently working on the development of nanoscale bioelectronics for non-invasive treatments of neuronal disease. Neural electrotherapy, or the use of electrical energy for purposes of treatment of neural tissues, has been a topic of conversation in the scientific and medical communities since 1980 when Cohen et al. discovered stronger magnetic fields in brain and nervous system tissues as compared to other tissues in the body [49]. Electrically active polymers can be incorporated into nanoscale scaffolds that guide and promote nerve regeneration in patients with peripheral nerve injury [50]. Nanofibers can be applied in damaged tissues to magnetically align collagen fibers to direct new nerve growth [51]. Carbon nanotubes are being used to replace bulkier implant electrodes in deep brain stimulation for patients with Parkinson's disease [52]. Finally, glioblastoma multiforme brain tumor cells can be selectively targeted and destroyed by low-intensity, intermediate frequency electrical pulses [53].

Conclusion

Neuron-based surgery is the twenty-first century frontier in neurosurgery. With the advent of nanoneurosurgery, the subcellular, nanoscale manipulation of nervous system tissues using nanotechnology combined with molecular biology, electrochemistry and electrophysics [32] is opening doors in neurodiagnostics and neurotherapeutics that were previously considered in the realm of science fiction. Nanoparticles can be surgically infused via direct inoculation, convection enhanced delivery, and implantation using nanosurgical instruments and techniques. Nanoparticles themselves are being constructed to deliver DNA, RNA, siRNA, shRNA, pharmaceuticals, labeling markers, electrical impulses, and other therapeutics that are able to selectively target neurons, glial cells, tumor cells, necrotic cells, and other tissues directly responsible for diseases of the nervous system. While not yet clinically implemented, the science has proven feasible. We stand on the brink of a brave new world of neuron based neurosurgical treatments.

References

1. Laws ER, Udvarhelyi GB, editors. The genesis of neuroscience by A. E. Walker. Park Ridge, IL: American Association of Neurological Surgeons; 1998.
2. Wilkins RH. Neurosurgical classic–XVII: Edwin Smith Surgical Papyrus. J Neurosurg. 1964;240–4.
3. Feynman RP. There's plenty of room at the bottom. Eng Sci. 1960;23:22–36.
4. Nano.gov. 2014. United States Nanotechnology Initiative.
5. Drexler KE. Engines of creation: the coming era of nanotechnology. New York: Anchor Books; 1986.
6. Blaylock RL, Maroon J. Immunoexcitotoxicity as a central mechanism in chronic encephalopathy—a unifying hypothesis. Surg Neurol Int. 2011;2(1):107.
7. Zhang Z, Zoltewicz JS, Mondello S, Newsom KJ, Yang Z, Kobeissy F, et al. Human traumatic brain injury induces autoantibody response against glial fibrillary acidic protein and its breakdown products. PLoS One. 2014;9(3), e92698.
8. Lumpkins KM, Bochicchio GV, Keledjian K, Simard JM, McCunn M, Scalea T. Glial fibriallary acidic protein is highly correlated with brain injury. J Trauma. 2008;65(4):778–82.
9. Schiff L, Hadker N, Weiser S, Rausch C. A literature review of the feasibility of glial fibrillary acidic protein as a biomarker for stroke and traumatic brain injury. Mol Diagn Ther. 2012;16(2):79–92.
10. Tsitsopoulos PP, Marklund N. Amyloid-beta peptides and tau protein as biomarkers in cerebrospinal and interstitial fluid following traumatic brain injury: a review of experimental and clinical studies. Front Neurol. 2013;4:79.

11. Abrahamson EE, Ikonomovic MD, Ciallella JR, Hope CE, Paljug WR, Isanski BA, et al. Caspase inhibition therapy abolishes brain trauma-induced increases in Abeta peptide: implications for clinical outcome. Exp Neurol. 2006;197(2):437–50.
12. Yan EB, Satgunaseelan L, Paul E, Bye N, Nguyen P, Agyapomaa D, et al. Post-traumatic hypoxia is associated with prolonged cerebral cytokine production, higher serum biomarker levels and poor outcome in patients with severe traumatic brain injury. J Neurotrauma. 2014;31(7):618–29.
13. Hayakata T, Shiozaki T, Tasaki O, Ikegawa H, Inoue Y, Toshiyuki F, et al. Changes in CSF S100B and cytokine concentrations in early-phase severe traumatic brain injury. Shock. 2004;22(2):102–7.
14. Stamataki E, Stathopoulos A, Garini E, Kokkoris S, Glynos C, Psachoulia C, et al. Serum S100B protein is increased and correlates with interleukin 6, hypoperfusion indices, and outcome in patients admitted for surgical control of hemorrhage. Shock. 2013;40(4): 274–80.
15. Mondello S, Schmid K, Berger RP, Kobeissy F, Italiano D, Jeromin A, et al. The challenge of mild traumatic brain injury: role of biochemical markers in diagnosis of brain damage. Med Res Rev. 2014;34(3): 503–31.
16. Perman SM, Goyal M, Neumar RW, Topjian AA, Gaieski DF. Clinical applications of targeted temperature management. Chest. 2014;145(2):386–93.
17. Hutchinson JS, Guerguerian AM. Cooling of children with severe traumatic brain injury. Lancet Neurol. 2013;12(6):527–9.
18. Biswas AK, Bruce DA, Sklar FH, Bokovoy JL, Sommerauer JF. Treatment of acute traumatic brain injury in children with moderate hypothermia improves intracranial hypertension. Crit Care Med. 2002;30:2742–51.
19. Adelson PD, Wisniewski SR, Beca J, Brown SD, Bell M, Muizelaar JP, et al. Comparison of hypothermia and normothermia after severe traumatic brain injury in children (Cool Kids): a phase 3, randomized controlled trial. Lancet Neurol. 2013;12(6):546–53.
20. Harris B, Andrews PJ, Murray GD, Forbes J, Moseley O. Systematic review of head cooling in adults after traumatic brain injury and stroke. Health Technol Assess. 2012;16(45):1–175.
21. Johann S, Beyer C. Neuroprotection by gonadal steroid hormones in acute brain damage requires cooperation with astroglia and microglia. J Steroid Biochem Mol Biol. 2013;137:71–81.
22. Chen CW, Chen TY, Tsai KL, Lin CL, Yokoyama KK, Lee WS, et al. Inhibition of autophagy as a therapeutic strategy of iron-induced brain injury after hemorrhage. Autophagy. 2012;8(10):1510–20.
23. Luoma JI, Stern CM, Mermelstein PG. Progesterone inhibition of neuronal calcium signaling underlies aspects of progesterone-mediated neuroprotection. J Steroid Biochem Mol Biol. 2012;131(1-2):30–6.
24. Whitcomb BW, Pradhan EK, Pittas AG, Roghmann MC, Perencevich EN. Impact of admission hyperglycemia on hospital mortality in various intensive care unit populations. Crit Care Med. 2005;33:2772–7.
25. Jeremitsky E, Omert LA, Dunham CM, Wilberger J, Rodriguez A. The impact of hyperglycemia on patients with severe brain injury. J Trauma. 2005;58:47–50.
26. Oddo M, Schmidt JM, Carrera E, Badjatia N, Connolly ES, Presciutti M, et al. Impact of tight glycemic control on cerebral glucose metabolism after severe brain injury: a microdialysis study. Crit Care Med. 2008;36:3233–8.
27. Vespa P, McArthur DL, Stein N, Huang SC, Shao W, Filippou M, et al. Tight glycemic control increases metabolic distress in traumatic brain injury: a randomized controlled within-subjects trial. Crit Care Med. 2012;40:1923–9.
28. Itoh Y, Suzuki N. Control of brain capillary blood flow. J Cereb Blood Flow Metab. 2012;32(7): 1167–76.
29. Kirkman MA, Smith M. Supratentorial intracerebral hemorrhage: a review of the underlying pathophysiology and its relevance for multimodality neuromonitoring in neurointensive care. J Neurosurg Anesthesiol. 2013;25(3):228–39.
30. Grape S, Ravussin P. PRO: osmotherapy for the treatment of acute intracranial hypertension. J Neurosurg Anesthesiol. 2012;24(4):402–6.
31. Kreuter J. Nanoparticluate systems for brain delivery of drugs. Adv Drug Deliv Rev. 2001;47:65–81.
32. Kateb B, Heiss J. The textbook of nanoneuroscience and nanoneurosurgery. New York: Taylor and Francis Group; 2014.
33. Hu G, Lijowski M, Zhang H, Partlow KC, Caruthers SD, Kiefer G, et al. Imaging of Vx-2 rabbit tumors with alpha(nu)beta3-integrin-targeted 111In nanoparticles. Int J Cancer. 2007;120:1951–7.
34. Robidoux A, Buzdar AU, Quinaux E, Jacobs S, Rastogi P, Fourchotte V, et al. A phase II neoadjuvant trial of sequential nanoparticle albumin-bound paclitaxel followed by 5-fluorouracil/epirubicin/cyclophosphamide in locally advanced breast cancer. Clin Breast Cancer. 2010;10:81–6.
35. Paunesku T, Ke T, Dharmakumar R, Mascheri N, Wu A, Lai B, et al. Gadolinium-conjugated TiO2-DNA oligonucleotide nanoconjugates show prolonged intracellular retention period and T1-weighted contrast enhancement in magnetic resonance images. Nanomedicine. 2008;4:201–7.
36. Khurana R, Coleman C, Ionescu-Zanetti C, Carter SA, Krishna V, Grover RK, et al. Mechanism of thioflavin T binding to amyloid fibrils. J Struct Biol. 2005;151:229–38.
37. Agarwal A, Lariya N, Saraogi G, Dubey N, Agrawal H, Agrawal GP. Nanoparticles as novel carrier for brain delivery: a review. Curr Pharm Des. 2009;15: 917–25.
38. Lockmann PR, Mumper RJ, Khan MA, Allen DD. Nanoparticle technology for drug delivery across the blood-brain barrier. Drug Dev Ind Pharm. 2002;28: 1–13.

39. Croteau D, Walbridge S, Morrison PF, Butman JA, Vortmeyer AO, Johnson D, et al. Real-time in vivo imaging of the convective distribution of a low-molecular weight tracer. J Neurosurg. 2005;102:90–7.
40. Heiss JD, Walbridge S, Asthagiri AR, Lonser RR. Image-guided convection-enhanced delivery of muscimol to the primate brain. J Neurosurg. 2010;112:790–5.
41. VanHandel M, Alizadeh D, Zhang L, Kateb B, Bronikowski M, Manohara H, et al. Selective uptake of multi-walled carbon nanotubes by tumor macrophages in a murine glioma model. J Neuroimmunol. 2009;208:3–9.
42. Etame AB, Diaz RJ, O'Reilly MA, Smith CA, Mainprize TG, Hynynen K, et al. Enhanced delivery of gold nanoparticles with therapeutic potential into the brain using MRI-guided focused ultrasound. Nanomedicine. 2012;8:1133–42.
43. O'Neal DP, Hirsch LR, Halas NJ, Payne JD, West JL. Photo-thermal tumor ablation in mice using near infrared-absorbing nanoparticles. Cancer Lett. 2004;209:171–6.
44. Sperling RA, Rivera Gil P, Zhang F, Zanella M, Parak WJ. Biological applications of gold nanoparticles. Chem Soc Rev. 2008;37:1896–908.
45. Ellis-Behnke RG, Liang YX, Tay DK, Kau PW, Schneider GE, Zhang S, et al. Nano hemostat solution: immediate hemostasis at the nanoscale. Nanomedicine. 2006;2:207–15.
46. Leary SP, Liu CY, Apuzzo ML. Toward the emergence of nanoneurosurgery: part III. Nanomedicine: targeted nanotherapy, nanosurgery, and progress toward the realization of nanoneurosurgery. Neurosurgery. 2006;58:1009–26.
47. Freitas RA. Current status of nanomedicine and medical robotics. J Comput Theor Nanosci. 2005;2:1–25.
48. Douglas SM, Bachelet I, Church GM. A logic-gated nanorobot for targeted transport of molecular payloads. Science. 2012;335:831–4.
49. Cohen D, Palti Y, Cuffin N, Schmid SJ. Magnetic fields produced by steady currents in the body. Proc Natl Acad Sci U S A. 1980;77(3):1447–51.
50. Ghasemi-Mobarakeh L, Prabhakaran MP, Morshed M, Nasr-Esfahani MH, Ramakrishna S. Electrospun poly (ε-caprolactone)/gelatin nanofibrous scaffolds for nerve tissue engineering. Biomaterials. 2009;29:4532.
51. Biazar E, Khorasani MT, Zaeifi D. Nanotechnology for peripheral nerve regeneration. Int J Nanomed. 2010;1(1):1–23.
52. Kabanov AV, Gendelman HE. Nanomedicine in the diagnosis and therapy of neurodegenerative disorders. Prog Polym Sci. 2007;32:1054–82.
53. Kirson ED, Dbaly V, Tovarys F, Vymazal J, Soustiel JF, Itzhaki A, et al. Alternating electric fields arrest cell proliferation in animal tumor models and human brain tumors. Proc Natl Acad Sci. 2007;104(24):10152–7.

22 Brain Cancer: The New Frontiers

Brian J. Scott and Santosh Kesari

Introduction

There have been numerous exciting advances in cancer care, and specifically to the field of neuro-oncology. Basic science research has dramatically increased the understanding of tumor biology, and better defined the role of cancer stem cells in maintaining tumor growth and resistance to therapy. The result of this work has been the identification of numerous potential targets for therapy, making neuro-oncology a prime area for translational research. Clinically, a coordinated team approach among surgical, medical, neuroimaging, and radiation oncology and pathology ensures a timely and accurate diagnosis, and that the most up-to-date and effective treatment options are available to the patient for their specific cancer. This chapter reviews some of the promising areas in diagnostic testing, neuroimaging, and therapies that are impacting the understanding of brain tumors and brain tumor care.

B.J. Scott, M.D.
Tufts University School of Medicine,
Boston, MA, USA

Lahey Hospital and Medical Center,
Burlington, MA, USA
e-mail: Brian.j.scott@lahey.org

S. Kesari, M.D., Ph.D. (✉)
Department of Neurosciences, UC San Diego,
Moores Cancer Center, La Jolla, CA, USA
e-mail: skesari@ucsd.edu

Background/Epidemiology

Metastasis

The most common malignant intracranial tumors are metastases, which spread hematogenously from systemic solid tumors or hematologic malignancies (Fig. 22.1a, b). Less frequently, systemic cancer may spread to the central nervous system (CNS) as dural (Fig. 22.2) or leptomeningeal metastasis (Fig. 22.3a, b). CNS metastases are often a manifestation of advanced and progressive systemic cancer, but rarely may be the presenting feature of an occult malignancy. The likelihood of developing brain metastasis varies greatly depending on the primary cancer site. Individuals with lung cancer develop brain metastasis at an estimated incidence of 19.9 %, breast cancer 5.1 %, and GU malignancies 1 % or less [1].

Brain metastases characteristically present with focal neurologic dysfunction related to the site of involvement, or progressively worsening headache. Typical radiographic features are a peripherally enhancing lesion or lesions occurring at the cortical/subcortical junction. Posterior fossa lesions, cystic lesions, and tumors with an imaging appearance similar to primary brain tumors may also occur. Headache, confusion/depressed level of consciousness, and cranial neuropathies are the most common presenting signs and symptoms of meningeal carcinomatosis, with

R. Latifi et al. (eds.), *Technological Advances in Surgery, Trauma and Critical Care*,
DOI 10.1007/978-1-4939-2671-8_22

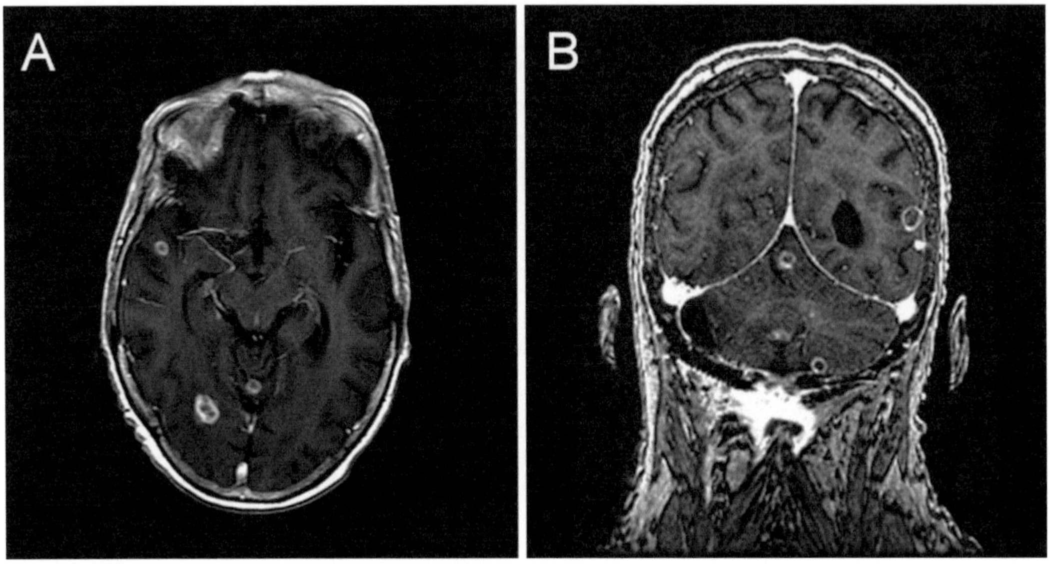

Fig. 22.1 T1 axial (**a**) and coronal (**b**) post-gadolinium-enhanced MRI showing multiple peripherally enhancing metastatic lesions in an individual with known metastatic breast cancer

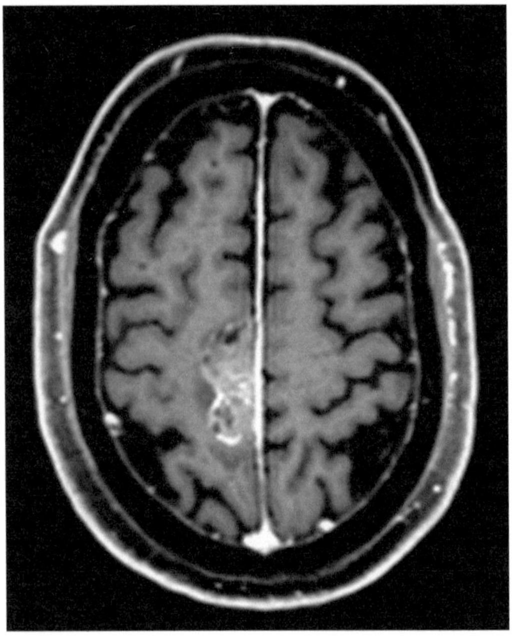

Fig. 22.2 T1 axial post-gadolinium-enhanced MRI showing a dural-based mass lesion along the right side of the falx, histologically confirmed to be a brain metastasis from prostate cancer

imaging showing leptomeningeal or subependymal enhancement. The diagnosis of leptomeningeal cancer is made when cerebrospinal fluid cytology shows malignant cells, and/or characteristic neuroimaging features are present in the appropriate clinical context.

Primary Brain Tumors

Unlike brain metastasis, primary brain tumors arise from cells normally found in the brain (Fig. 22.4a). The overall incidence of primary brain tumors in adults is 21.03/100,000 [2]. Benign tumors are more common (10.5/100,000). Meningioma occurs more commonly in women, with an estimated incidence of 8.36/100,000 person-years in women compared to 3.61/100,000 in men [2]. The incidence increases with age and with estrogen supplementation. Additional risk factors include elevated body mass index, low self-rated physical activity levels, and a history of uterine fibroids [3]. Meningiomas are extra-axial, dural-based mass lesions that characteristically demonstrate avid homogeneous contrast enhancement (Fig. 22.4b), and are graded on a World Health Organization (WHO) scale from I to III depending on their histologic characteristics. Complete surgical removal, when possible, provides the greatest chance of cure.

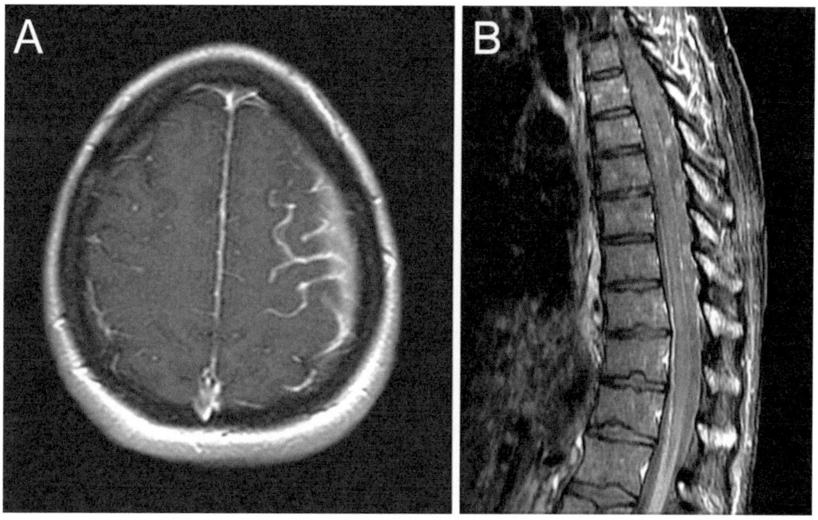

Fig. 22.3 Axial T1 post-contrast brain MRI (**a**) and sagittal post-contrast spine MRI (**b**) demonstrating abnormal leptomeningeal enhancement due to leptomeningeal metastasis

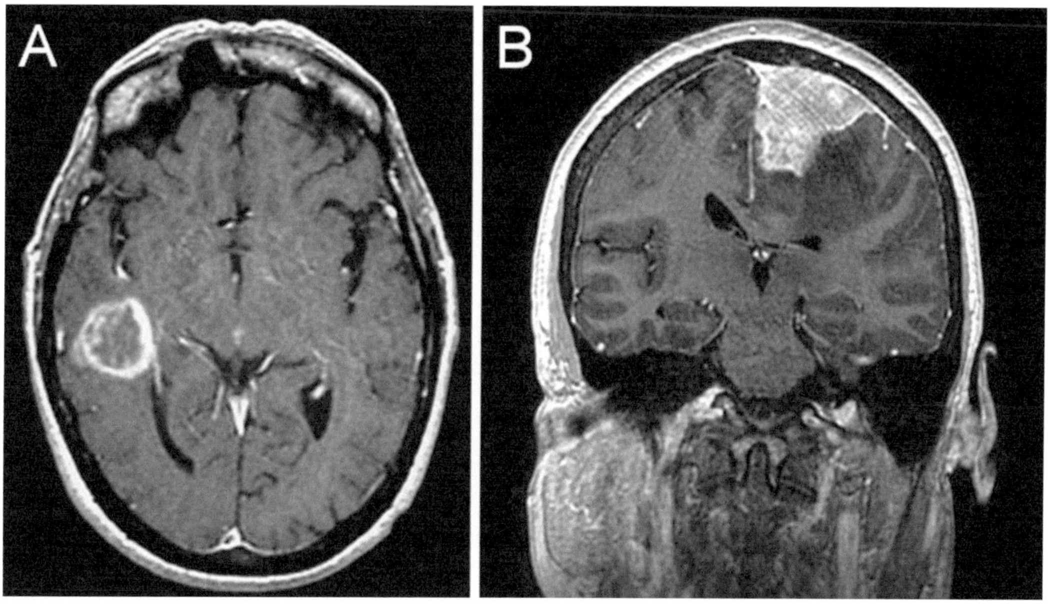

Fig. 22.4 T1 coronal post-gadolinium-enhanced MRI showing an intraaxial enhancing lesion, histologically confirmed to be a glioblastoma (**a**). T1 coronal post-gadolinium-enhanced MRI showing a dural-based homogeneously enhancing lesion, histologically confirmed to be a meningioma (**b**)

Radiation therapy is an effective treatment for residual or recurrent disease, and is also important in the treatment of grade II and III tumors as these carry a higher risk of recurrence.

Gliomas are the most common malignant brain tumor in both adults and children, and represent 1.4 % of all new cancer cases diagnosed in the USA. They comprise 36 % of all brain and

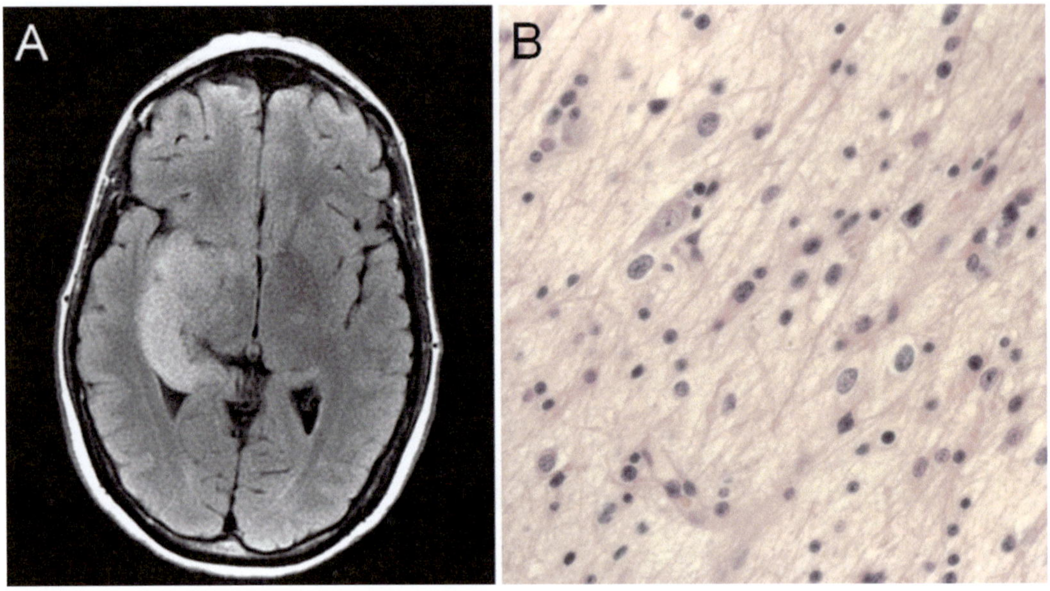

Fig. 22.5 T2 fluid-attenuated inversion recovery (FLAIR) MRI showing a T2 hyperintense, expansile abnormality in the right temporal lobe (**a**). Histologic analysis revealed a grade II astrocytoma that showed increased cellularity, pleomorphism, and infiltration (**b**)

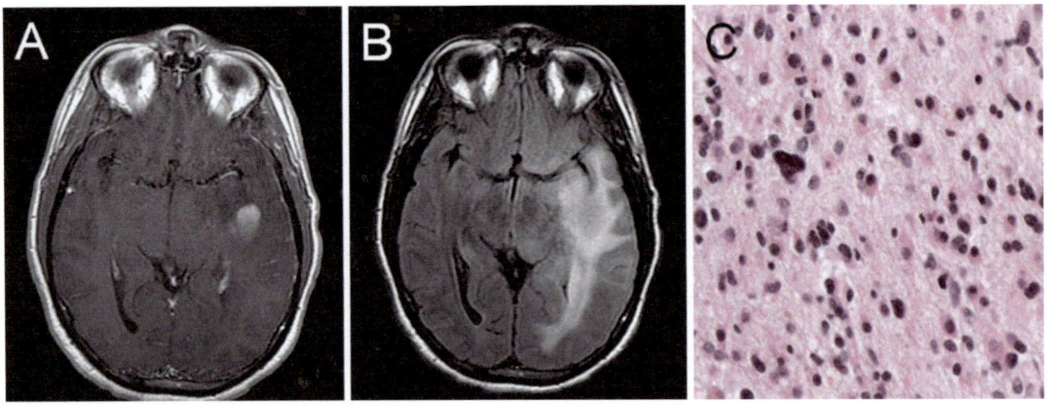

Fig. 22.6 T1 axial post-gadolinium-enhanced MRI (**a**) and T2 axial fluid-attenuated inversion recovery (**b**) images showing a left temporal anaplastic astrocytoma with a central focus of homogeneous enhancement. Histologic analysis revealed a grade III astrocytoma that showed high cellularity, pleomorphism, and mitotic figures (**c**)

CNS tumors, and 81 % of all malignant brain tumors [2]. Gliomas are graded from WHO grades I to IV, with grades II (Fig. 22.5a, b) and III (Fig. 22.6a–c) characterized by increasing cellular atypia and anaplasia respectively, and WHO grade IV (Fig. 22.7a–e) demonstrating vascular proliferation and necrosis. Medulloblastoma (Fig. 22.8a, b), ependymoma (WHO grades II–III) (Fig. 22.8c), pilocytic astrocytoma (WHO grade I) (Fig. 22.8d), and diffuse infiltrative pontine glioma (WHO grade II) (Fig. 22.8e) are more often seen in children, while glioblastoma (WHO grade IV) is the most common malignant brain tumor in adults.

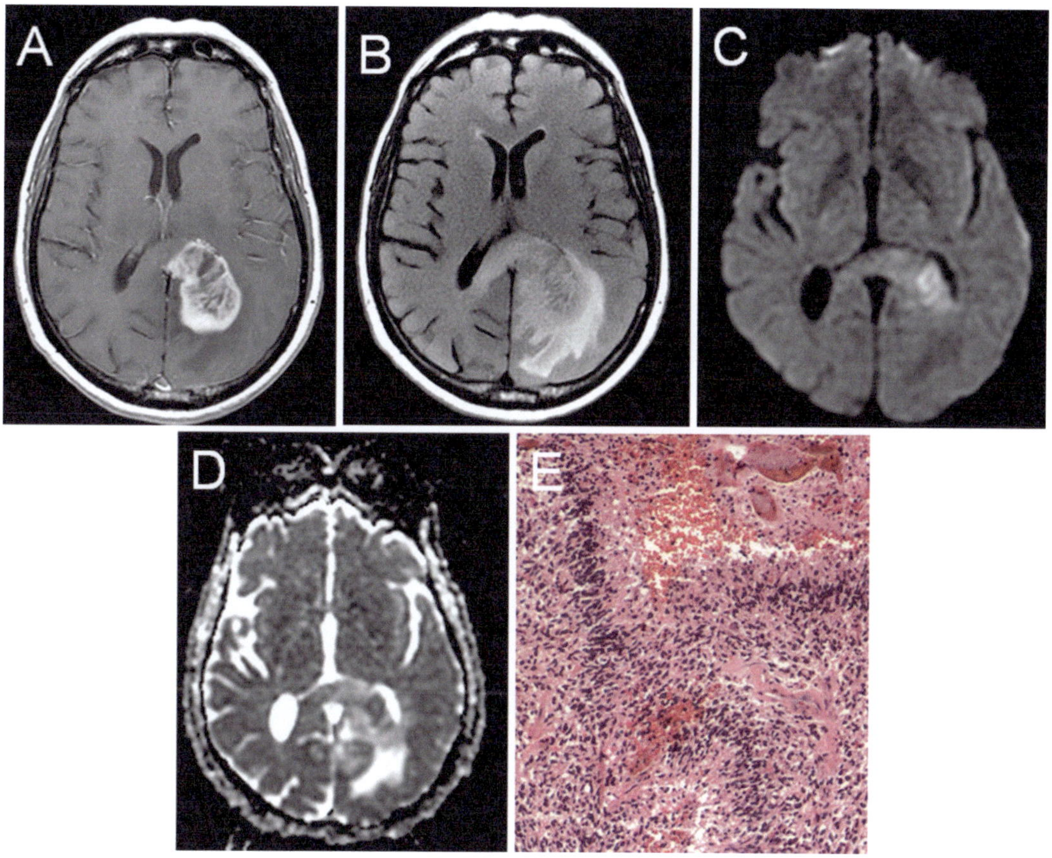

Fig. 22.7 T1 axial post-gadolinium (**a**), T2 FLAIR (**b**), diffusion-weighted imaging (**c**), and apparent diffusion coefficient (**d**) imaging of a left-hemisphere glioblastoma. The peripheral enhancing pattern and nonenhancing expansile changes crossing the midline via the corpus callosum are characteristic. DWI (**c**) and ADC (**d**) imaging reveal an area of diffusion restriction consistent with increased cellular density in the region. Histologic analysis revealed a grade IV glioblastoma that showed high cellularity, pleomorphism, microvascular proliferation, and necrosis (**e**)

Classification and Grading

Unlike systemic cancer, staging is not undertaken for primary brain tumors, and spread of systemic malignancy to the CNS would qualify as stage IV disease. However, an extent of disease evaluation in known or suspected CNS malignancies such as CNS lymphoma or brain metastasis presenting when the status of systemic disease is unknown is important. Spine imaging in known or suspected leptomeningeal cancer, especially if there are signs or symptoms of nerve root involvement, is also appropriate.

CNS tumors are traditionally graded upon acquisition of tumor tissue based on histologic appearance. The World Health Organization (WHO) Classification of Central Nervous System Tumors is the most widely accepted histologic grading system [4]. It classifies tumors based on histopathologic and immunohistochemical features, and is revised periodically to reflect advances in the field based on expert consensus. In the WHO classification, grade I and II tumors are designated as low grade, and grade I tumors are considered potentially curable with surgery. Grade III and IV tumors are high grade, with more aggressive growth potential. They often require radiation and/or chemotherapy in addition to surgical resection.

In some tumors, better understanding of the genetic abnormalities in the tumor has led to advances in molecular phenotyping. The Cancer Genome Atlas (TCGA) project, for example, completed genomic sequencing of 206 glioblastomas [5]. TCGA provided new insights into the

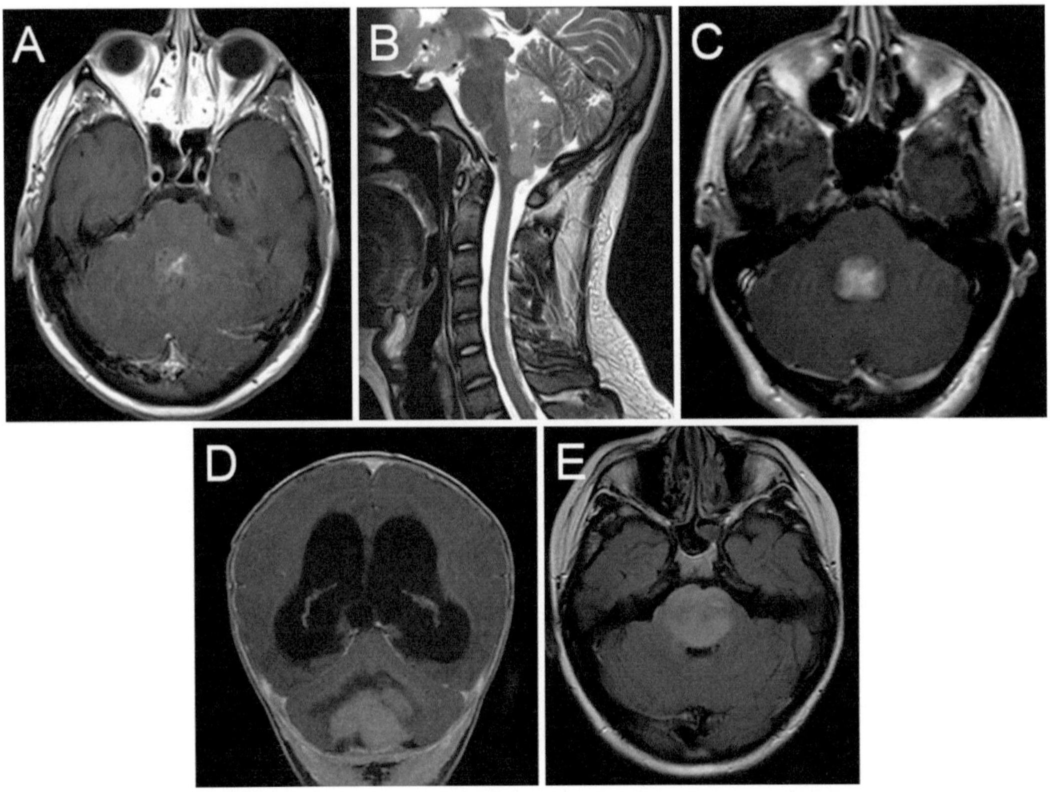

Fig. 22.8 Axial T1 post-gadolinium (**a**), and sagittal T2 (**b**) MRI showing a posterior fossa mass lesion with an enhancing component. Surgical resection revealed a medulloblastoma. Axial T1 post-gadolinium (**c**) shows a fourth ventricular ependymoma. Coronal T1 post-gadolinium (**d**) shows a cerebellar pilocytic astrocytoma with obstructive hydrocephalus. Axial FLAIR (**e**) shows a diffuse infiltrative pontine glioma

frequency of specific genetic abnormalities in glioblastoma. The information from TCGA led to a proposed classification scheme in which four distinct molecular phenotypes in glioblastoma were derived by consensus clustering based on abnormalities in platelet-derived growth factor receptor (PDGFR)-A, isocitrate dehydrogenase (IDH)-1, epidermal growth factor receptor (EGFR), and neurofibromatosis (NF)-1 [6].

The four molecular phenotypes are designated classical, mesenchymal, neural, and proneural. The classical glioblastoma subtype is characterized by chromosome 7 amplification paired with chromosome 10 loss. There was also a higher frequency of EGFR amplification, and less frequent TP53 mutation than other GBM subtypes. The mesenchymal subtype was characterized by focal deletions of a region of chromosome 17 that contains the NF1 gene, and high expression of genes in the tumor necrosis factor and NF-kappa B pathways. The neural subtype showed prominent expression of neural markers.

The proneural subtype demonstrated amplification and increased gene expression of PDFGRA and a higher frequency of point mutation in IDH-1 than other subtypes. Proneural classification was somewhat less common, associated with younger age at onset and a tendency toward better overall survival than other GBM subtypes. When the molecular phenotyping was expanded to include analysis of histologic grade II and III gliomas, a number of lower grade gliomas were found to have a proneural molecular signature. These were characterized by the coexistence of IDH1 mutation and CpG island methylator phenotype (CIMP). Codeletion of chromosomes 1p and 19q, long identified as a favorable prognostic feature in oligodendroglial tumors, was found in many grade II and III tumors as well. The combination of IDH-1 mutation/CIMP+ and 1p;19q codeleted molecular signature predicted longer survival when compared to IDH-1 wild-type/ CIMP– and 1p;19q non-deleted tumors independent of tumor histology [7].

DNA repair is one mechanism of resistance to chemoradiation in high-grade gliomas. The most common chemotherapeutic agent for glioblastoma, temozolomide, is an alkylating agent with good CNS penetration that acts by methylation of guanine at the O-6 position. Methylation disrupts DNA replication and ultimately leads to apoptosis. The DNA repair enzyme methylguanine methyltransferase, or MGMT, reverses the methylation activity of temozolomide. High-grade gliomas that have a methylated (inactive) MGMT promoter show prolonged median overall survival and improved 2-year survival with concurrent radiation and temozolomide chemotherapy plus adjuvant monthly temozolomide. Tumors with an unmethylated (active) MGMT promoter region have no significant benefit from treatment with alkylating chemotherapy [8]. MGMT promoter methylation is associated with the CIMP phenotype found most commonly in the proneural glioma subtype. Strategies to inactivate the DNA repair activity of MGMT or administer a chemotherapy that is not dependent on DNA methylation are potential strategies to improve outcomes in individuals with MGMT unmethylated tumors.

A more detailed understanding of molecular phenotyping will continue to provide insight into differences in the biologic behavior among malignant glioma subtypes, as well as differences in survival and response to treatment with chemotherapy. Identifying important molecular pathways also provides potential targets for future therapies.

Advances in Diagnosis

Molecular Diagnostic Tools

As the field of cancer genomics provides new insight into specific genetic alterations that characterize CNS cancers, better tests are being devised that achieve less invasive and potentially earlier detection, improve diagnostic certainty, and will give information about prognosis, or one or more specific therapeutic targets.

Cerebrospinal fluid (CSF) analysis is a diagnostic test that, if successful, may provide information to guide treatment without requiring craniotomy. This approach would be especially important for mass lesions that are in areas that are high risk to biopsy. Historically, the main CSF diagnostic tools are CSF cytology, flow cytometry, and a handful of molecular tests including CSF lactate dehydrogenase, beta-2-microglobulin, and Epstein-Barr virus DNA by polymerase chain reaction (PCR). Unfortunately, all of these tests are limited by low sensitivity or specificity.

More recently, proteomics and micro-RNA analysis of cerebrospinal fluid has emerged with the potential to differentiate lymphoma from other CNS inflammatory disorders, and potentially improve the detection of solid tumor CSF spread as well (Fig. 22.9a–c). Compared to conventional cytology, which had a sensitivity of 17 %, elevated levels of proteins associated with B-cell proliferation and migration (interleukin-10 and chemokine CXCL-13) in combination were shown to be 54 % sensitive and 99 % specific in the detection of CNS lymphoma [9]. Elevations in a combination of three specific micro-RNA levels from CSF in individuals with primary CNS lymphoma were 95.7 % sensitive and 96.7 % specific compared to controls [10]. CSF micro-RNAs in the diagnosis of glioma have a 90 % sensitivity and 100 % specificity to identify glioma compared to controls [11]. Micro-RNA levels in CSF have been used to successfully differentiate cancer from nonneoplastic brain lesions, and in some cases to distinguish metastasis from lung cancer versus breast cancer [12]. In solid tumors, elevated levels of CSF vascular endothelial growth factor (VEGF) had 75 % sensitivity, 97 % specificity, and 94 % negative predictive value in the diagnosis of breast cancer leptomeningeal metastasis compared to CSF cytology [13].

Circulating Tumor Cell Detection

Over the past 5–10 years, it has become possible to isolate circulating tumor cells (CTCs) in whole blood. Cells are obtained by using markers to

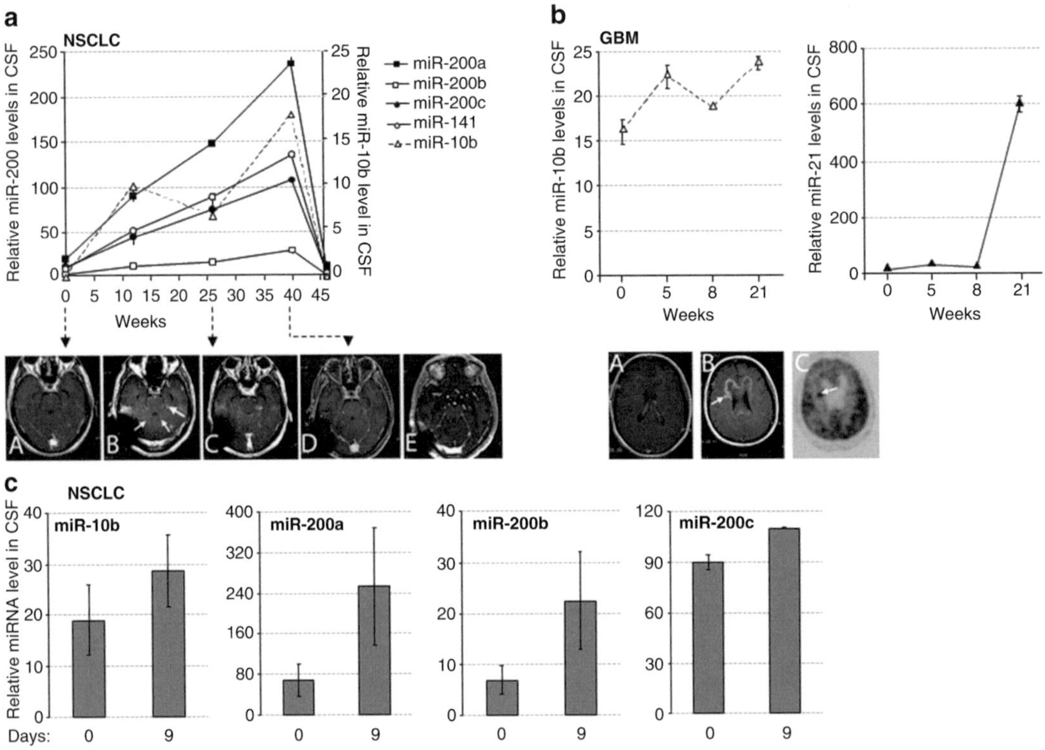

Fig. 22.9 The CSF levels of miRNA markers in metastatic lung cancer and GBM patients during treatment with erlotinib. miRNA levels were examined by qRT-PCR in CSF samples of lung cancer patients (**a**, **c**) and GBM patient (**b**) during the time course of erlotinib treatment. The disease progression and the drug response were concomitantly monitored by MRI, as follows. For Patient A: serial axial post-gadolinium MRIs of lung cancer patient's brain during course of progression of disease and stability and improvement on MRI with escalating doses of erlotinib. (A) Time 0 weeks while patient on erlotinib, there is no leptomeningeal and parenchymal enhancement and CSF cytology was negative; (B) 3 weeks progression on erlotinib 150 mg daily dosing with new cerebellar leptomeningeal enhancement (*small arrows*) and nodule (*large arrow*), erlotinib increased to 600 mg every 4 days at 9 weeks; (C) 29 weeks on showing stable leptomeningeal enhancement and nodule; (D) 40 weeks showing reduction in leptomeningeal enhancement and nodule, erlotinib increased to 900 mg every 4 days at 41 weeks; (E) 64 weeks after six cycles of chemotherapy with carboplatinum and pemetrexed due to lung cancer progression showing further reduction in leptomeningeal enhancement and nodule has disappeared. For Patient B: (A) time 2 weeks for patient with recurrent GBM with prominent mass effect and enhancement felt to be radiation changes rather than tumor based on MRI spectroscopy and FDG-PET scan on erlotinib at 600 mg every 4 days; (B) 26 weeks on treatment showing progression on MRI with new lesion (*arrow*) concerning for tumor; (C) 27 weeks on treatment showing hypermetabolic area (*arrow*) on PET consistent with tumor and biopsy confirmed. For Patient C: Had inadequate treatment due to functional status and rapidly progressed over a few weeks, which was reflected by an increase in levels of miR-200 family members in a short interval. (All: Reproduced with permission from Teplyuk NM, Mollenhauer B, Gabriely G, Giese A, Kim E, Smolsky M et al. MicroRNAs in cerebrospinal fluid identify glioblastoma and metastatic brain cancers and reflect disease activity. Neuro-oncology 2012;14(6):689–700)

detect epithelial cell adhesion molecules that are present on tumor cells, but not expressed on normal blood cells. The same technology used in whole blood may be used with CSF, and live tumor cells can be isolated this way [14, 15]. The clinical significance of asymptomatic CTCs in cerebrospinal fluid, and the reliability of following CTC counts as a marker of response to therapy as an adjunct or in lieu of cytology, remains to be determined. It is possible that CTC technology will allow considerably earlier detection of CNS involvement. Earlier detection and initiation of CNS-directed therapies may positively impact survival outcomes in brain and leptomeningeal metastasis.

Neuroimaging

Contrast-enhanced magnetic resonance imaging (MRI) is the diagnostic test of choice for identification and characterization of brain tumors (Fig. 22.1a, b through 22.8a–e, Figs. 22.10a–c, 22.11, 22.12a, b). Among other advantages, increases in field strength from 1.5 to 3 T scanners for clinical use have resulted in greater distinction between contrast-enhancing and nonenhancing regions, improved spatial resolution, and more clear differentiation of tissue types (spectral resolution). Perfusion-weighted imaging and assessment of relative cerebral blood volume to identify areas of hyperperfusion make it possible to more accurately discriminate between neoplastic and inflammatory brain lesions or subacute infarction (Fig. 22.12a, b).

Imaging assessment following radiation therapy for brain tumors presents a potential challenge. Increases in the volume of abnormal enhancement and surrounding T2 hyperintensity may be seen with tumor progression or treatment effect from radiation. Distinguishing between the two based on neuroimaging can be difficult or sometimes impossible. Radiographic assessment of tumor progression or response to treatment was traditionally performed using MacDonald criteria [16]. More recently, the Response Assessment in Neuro-Oncology (RANO) working group created modified criteria that account for the confounding effects of radiation therapy and anti-angiogenic treatments (Table 22.1) [17]. The RANO criteria provide a standardized approach to response assessment in brain tumors, which is useful for clinical trials and to avoid inaccuracies in imaging interpretation. To account for the potential confounding effects of radiation therapy on imaging, RANO criteria specify that increased volume of enhancing abnormality within the first 12 weeks following radiation therapy will not qualify as progression without tissue confirmation of active tumor or evidence of growth outside the radiation field. Additionally, RANO differs from MacDonald criteria in that progression of disease may occur with an increase in the volume of the nonenhancing T2 abnormality, or with clinical worsening that occurs without an alternate explanation.

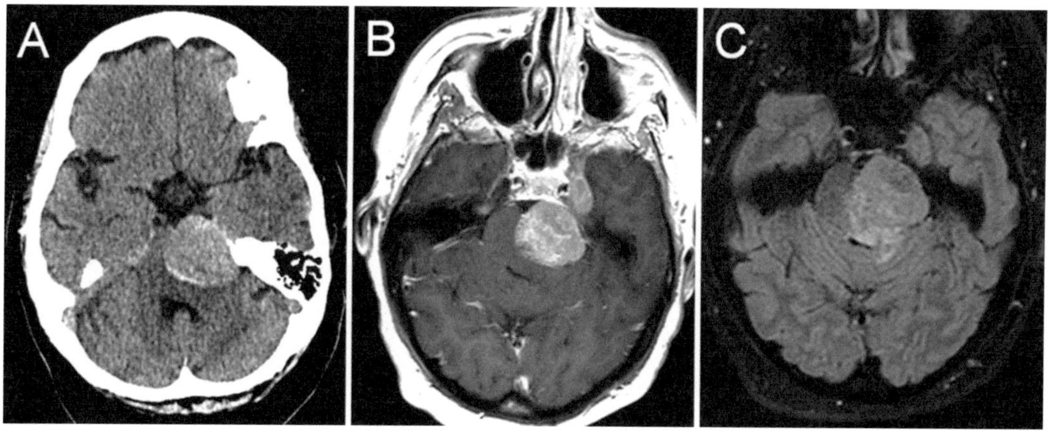

Fig. 22.10 Radiographic features of CNS melanoma. Axial non-contrast head CT shows a hyperdense mass lesion on the left displacing the pons (**a**). Axial T1-weighted MRI with contrast demonstrates homogeneous contrast enhancement (**b**), and axial T2 FLAIR (**c**) at the same level demonstrates an expansile T2 hyperintense lesion

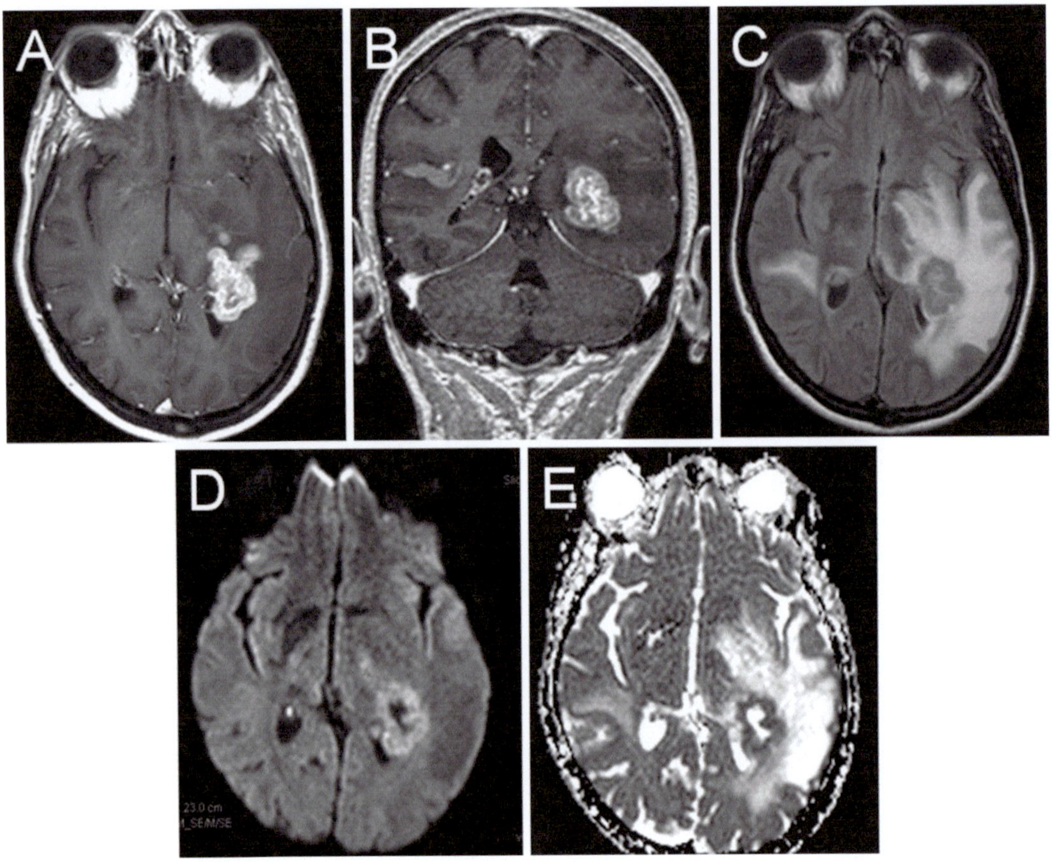

Fig. 22.11 MRI characteristics of diffuse large B-cell lymphoma. T1-weighted axial (**a**) and coronal (**b**) post-contrast imaging reveals an avidly contrast-enhancing mass lesion in the deep white matter with extension into the lateral ventricle on the *left*. There is a substantial amount of vasogenic edema surrounding the lesion (**c**), and restricted diffusion of water seen on DWI (**d**) and ADC (**e**)

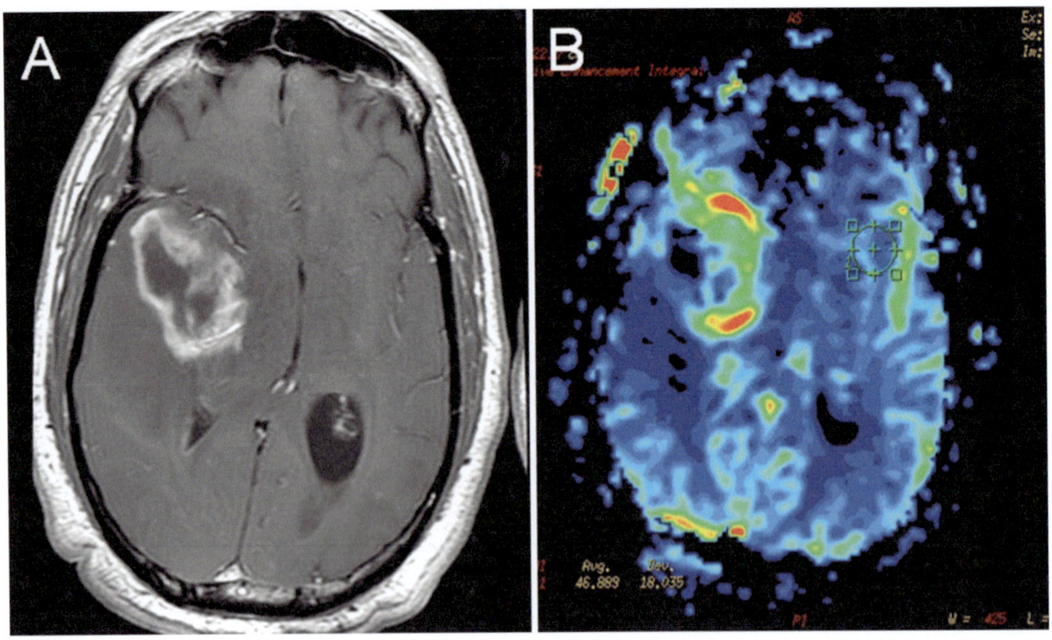

Fig. 22.12 Axial T1 post-gadolinium (**a**) and perfusion (**b**) MRI showing areas of increased cerebral blood volume corresponding to areas of contrast enhancement within a right frontal lobe glioblastoma

Table 22.1 A comparison of the MacDonald versus RANO criteria for the radiographic assessment of response to therapy in malignant glioma

	MacDonald criteria [16]	Response Assessment in Neuro-Oncology (RANO) criteria [17]	
Complete response (CR)	*All* of the following:	*All* of the following:	
MRI T1-post-Gd	Disappearance of all enhancing tumor on consecutive CT or MRI scans at least 1 month apart	Complete disappearance of all enhancing measurable and nonmeasurable disease sustained for at least 4 weeks; no new lesions	
MRI T2/FLAIR	–	Stable or improved nonenhancing (T2/FLAIR) lesions	
Corticosteroid	Off steroids	Off corticosteroids (or on physiologic replacement only)	
Clinical	Neurologically stable or improved	Stable or improved clinically	
Partial response (PR)	*All* of the following:	*All* of the following:	
MRI T1-post-Gd	≥50 % reduction in size of enhancing tumor on consecutive CT or MRI scans at least 1 month apart	≥50 % decrease compared with baseline in the sum products of perpendicular diameters of all measurable enhancing lesions sustained for at least 4 weeks; no progression of nonmeasurable disease; no new lesions	
MRI T2/FLAIR	–	Stable or improved nonenhancing (T2/FLAIR) lesions on same or lower dose of corticosteroids compared with baseline scan	
Corticosteroid	Steroids stable or reduced	Steroid dose no greater than the baseline scan dose	
Clinical	Neurologically stable or improved	Stable or improved clinically	
Progressive disease (PD)	*Any* of the following:	≥12 weeks after completion of chemoradiotherapy, *any* of the following:	<12 weeks after completion of chemoradiotherapy
MRI T1-post-Gd	≥25 % increase in size of enhancing tumor or any new tumor on CT or MRI scans	≥25 % increase in sum of the products of perpendicular diameters of enhancing lesions compared with the smallest tumor measurement obtained either at baseline (if no decrease) or best response. Any new lesion or clear progression of nonmeasurable disease	Only if there is new enhancement outside of the radiation field (beyond the high-dose region or 80 % isodense line) or if there is unequivocal evidence of viable tumor on histopathologic sampling

(continued)

Table 22.1 (continued)

	MacDonald criteria [16]	Response Assessment in Neuro-Oncology (RANO) criteria [17]	
MRI T2/FLAIR	–	Significant increase in T2/FLAIR nonenhancing lesion	
Corticosteroid	Steroids stable or increased	Stable or increasing doses of corticosteroids	
Clinical	*Or* neurological worsening	Clear clinical deterioration not attributable to other causes apart from the tumor (e.g., seizures, medication adverse events, complications of therapy, cerebrovascular events, infection) or changes in corticosteroid dose; failure to return for evaluation as a result of death or deteriorating condition	Insufficient to determine progression in the period < 12 weeks after completion of chemoradiotherapy given the potential impact of radiation treatment effect
Stable disease (SD)	"All other situations"	*All* of the following:	
MRI T1-post-Gd		Does not qualify for complete response, partial response, or progression	
MRI T2/FLAIR		Stable nonenhancing (T2/FLAIR) lesions on same or lower dose of corticosteroid compared with baseline scan	
Corticosteroid		In the event that the corticosteroid dose was increased for new symptoms and signs without confirmation of disease progression on neuroimaging, and subsequent follow-up imaging shows that this increase in corticosteroids was required because of disease progression, the last scan considered to show that stable disease will be the scan obtained when the corticosteroid dose was equivalent to the baseline dose	
Clinical		Stable or improved clinically	

Advances in Therapy

Surgery

Cytoreduction via maximal safe surgical resection is an extremely important part of treatment for gliomas. The extent of resection has been shown to impact survival, especially in low-grade glioma [18], but also in retrospective series of grade III and IV gliomas [19]. Advances such as intraoperative MRI and fluorescence-guided resection have been investigated as potential ways to achieve more complete resection.

Intraoperative imaging has been employed by brain tumor surgeons in tertiary care centers (Fig. 22.13a–c). In some series, the real-time assessment of extent of resection has impacted surgical planning, and has made it possible to achieve more complete surgical resection of brain tumors compared to preoperative MRI and direct visualization during surgery. Some have combined intraoperative MRI with awake craniotomy and functional brain mapping. Further evaluation is needed to determine whether the added resources, surgical time, and demand on the patient result in an impact on survival or functional outcomes.

In gliomas, the extent of infiltrating (nonenhancing) tumor can be difficult to determine on preoperative imaging, and so techniques that employ fluorescent labeling of tumor cells are of potential utility. Improved visualization of residual tumor and less residual tumor following surgery were achieved with presurgical administration of 5-aminolevulinic acid-induced porphyrins and intraoperative fluorescence compared to conventional neuronavigation [20]. Prolonged survival was also observed in those who had no residual fluorescence following surgery. More recently, other tumor markers have been employed such as chlorotoxin conjugated with indocyanine green for visualization in the near-infrared spectrum [21]. For high-grade gliomas, additional treatment with chemotherapy and/or radiation is required to prolong survival and delay growth of the tumor.

Angiogenesis Inhibition

Vascular proliferation has long been identified as a hallmark of cancer, and is especially prominent in high-grade gliomas. Bevacizumab, a humanized monoclonal antibody to circulating vascular endothelial growth factor (VEGF), was approved by the US Food and Drug Administration for treatment of recurrent high-grade glioma in 2010. Bevacizumab treatment at recurrence resulted in a 6-month overall survival of 77 %, and 57 % with at least a partial radiographic response on imaging [22].

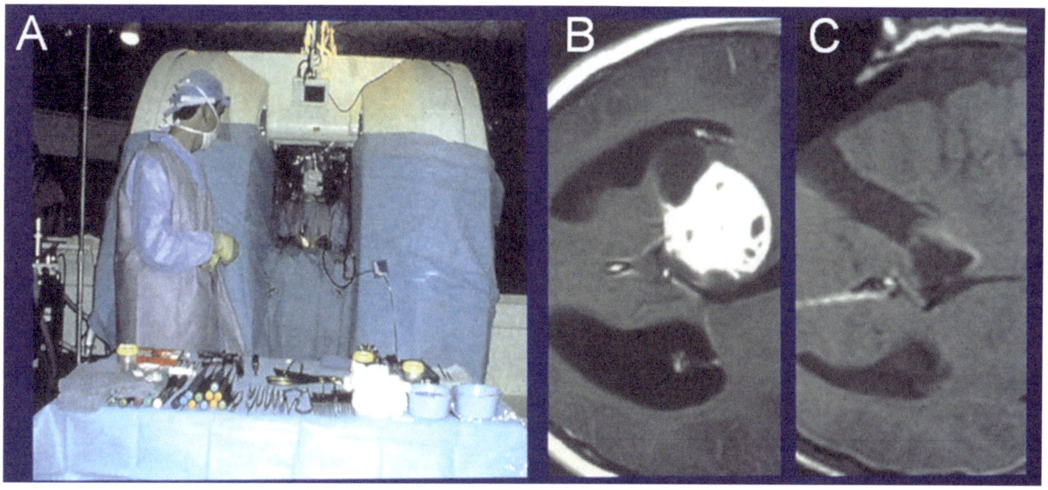

Fig. 22.13 Intraoperative MRI (**a**) can be used to obtain better extent of resection safely. Preoperative axial T1 post-gadolinium MRI shows a large deep thalamic tumor (**b**), which was totally resected under guidance of intraoperative MRI (**c**)

Phase III studies of bevacizumab in addition to standard chemoradiation with temozolomide for treatment of glioblastoma in the up-front setting are ongoing. In addition to monoclonal antibody therapy, receptor tyrosine kinase inhibitors targeting multiple receptors involved in angiogenesis and cellular growth and proliferation have been studied with limited impact on survival.

Vaccine-Based Therapies

The interplay between the immune system and cancer is an area of ongoing interest in glioma biology. As more is understood, vaccine-based therapies have been created that show T-cell responses to tumor antigens, and in some instances have resulted in increased overall survival compared to matched controls. The epidermal growth factor receptor (EGFR) vIII mutation is not found in normal tissue, but is present in approximately 1/3 of glioblastomas. A vaccine to EGFR vIII administered to 18 glioblastoma patients showed that among those who showed evidence of mounting an antibody response, the median overall survival was 47.7 months, compared to 22.8 months who did not mount a response and 15 months for the control group [23]. Another approach to vaccine therapy is the development of dendritic cell vaccines using the patient's own serum and cell lines cultured from their own tumor tissue to create vaccines to tumor-associated antigens. This approach allows for targeting of multiple patient-specific tumor antigens, including those expressed on glioma stem cells, with the goal of inciting an immune response against the tumor [24].

Virus-Based Therapies

Viruses have been of interest in brain tumor therapy because of their ability to transfect tumor cells. Most virus therapies are injected directly into the tumor bed at the time of surgery. Delivery may also be accomplished with stereotactic guidance or convection-enhanced delivery. Intravenous administration of virus is being studied. There are a number of mechanisms by which viruses may be used therapeutically. Oncolytic viruses infect tumor cells, and cause direct damage or apoptosis. Enzyme/prodrug therapy is a mechanism by which a virus delivers a prodrug to the tumor that is subsequently activated. Viral gene transfer is a third mechanism in which normal genes are delivered to the tumor using viral vectors with the goal of restoring normal function of specific genetic pathways such as TP53 [25]. Ongoing early clinical trials and combining virus therapies with immunotherapy or radiation hold promise to provide better treatment options in glioma as well as brain metastasis.

Tumor Treating Fields

Regional therapy with a device that delivers alternating electrical fields (200 kHz) to disrupt cell division has been studied in recurrent glioblastoma, and is currently under investigation for up-front therapy and in brain metastasis. The Tumor Treating Fields (TTFields) (Optune™, Novocure, Ltd, Haifa, Israel) device is an electrode array that is configured based on the tumor location, and delivers alternating electrical fields to the tumor bed intended to selectively disrupt the process of cell division (Fig. 22.14). In the recurrent setting, TTFields demonstrated non-inferiority to chemotherapy, without hematologic side effects or interactions with other chemotherapies [26]. More recently, a planned

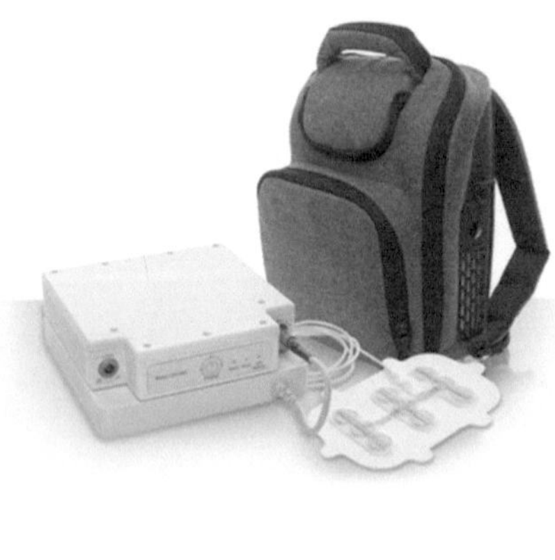

Fig. 22.14 Novo-TTF portable device with battery pack and scalp electrodes (Copyright © 2014 Novocure. All Rights Reserved)

interim analyses from a randomized phase 3 trial of TTFields plus temozolomide in patients with newly diagnosed glioblastoma showed significantly increased progression-free survival and overall survival compared with standard therapy (temozolomide) alone. Systemic toxicity did not increase with addition of TTFields therapy to temozolomide [27].

Radiosurgery

Advances in radiosurgical technique and image guidance have led to the ability to deliver high-dose radiation to areas that would previously be treated with conventional fractionated radiotherapy. As more is learned about the detrimental long-term neurocognitive effects of whole-brain irradiation, stereotactic radiosurgery is often considered as an alternative to whole-brain irradiation in the treatment of brain metastasis [28].

Conclusions

The future of neuro-oncology is promising on a number of new frontiers. More sensitive diagnostic modalities will improve accuracy and provide a less invasive means to establish a diagnosis. Better classification and characterization of tumors based on genetic features will more accurately predict prognosis and response to treatment. A better understanding of tumor stem cells and immunology has provided new therapeutic targets and modes of treatment delivery, many of which are being studied in clinical trials. In virtually all aspects, advances in the basic and clinical sciences have impacted care and contributed to new therapies for individuals with brain tumors.

References

1. Davis FG, Dolecek TA, McCarthy BJ, Villano JL. Toward determining the lifetime occurrence of metastatic brain tumors estimated from 2007 United States cancer incidence data. Neuro Oncol. 2012; 14(9):1171–7.
2. CBTRUS. CBTRUS statistical report: primary brain and central nervous system tumors diagnosed in eighteen states in 2002–2006. Hinsdale, IL: Central Brain Tumor Registry of the United States; 2009–2010.
3. Johnson DR, Olson JE, Vierkant RA, Hammack JE, Wang AH, Folsom AR, et al. Risk factors for meningioma in postmenopausal women: results from the Iowa Women's Health Study. Neuro Oncol. 2011; 13(9):1011–9.
4. Louis DN, Ohgaki H, Wiestler OD, Cavenee WK, editors. World Health Organization classification of tumors of the central nervous system. Lyon, France: IARC Press; 2007.
5. McLendon R, Friedman A, Bigner D, Van Meir EG, Brat DJ, Mastrogianakis GM, et al. Comprehensive genomic characterization defines human glioblastoma genes and core pathways. Nature. 2008;455(7216): 1061–8.
6. Verhaak RG, Hoadley KA, Purdom E, Wang V, Qi Y, Wilkerson MD, et al. Integrated genomic analysis identifies clinically relevant subtypes of glioblastoma characterized by abnormalities in PDGFRA, IDH1, EGFR, and NF1. Cancer Cell. 2010;17(1):98–110.
7. Guan X, Vengoechea J, Zheng S, Sloan AE, Chen Y, Brat DJ, et al. Molecular subtypes of glioblastoma are relevant to lower grade glioma. PLoS One. 2014;9(3), e91216.
8. Hegi ME, Diserens AC, Gorlia T, Hamou MF, de Tribolet N, Weller M, et al. MGMT gene silencing and benefit from temozolomide in glioblastoma. N Engl J Med. 2005;352(10):997–1003.
9. Rubenstein JL, Wong VS, Kadoch C, Gao HX, Barajas R, Chen L, et al. CXCL13 plus interleukin 10 is highly specific for the diagnosis of CNS lymphoma. Blood. 2013;121(23):4740–8.
10. Baraniskin A, Kuhnhenn J, Schlegel U, Chan A, Deckert M, Gold R, et al. Identification of microRNAs in the cerebrospinal fluid as marker for primary diffuse large B-cell lymphoma of the central nervous system. Blood. 2011;117(11):3140–6.
11. Baraniskin A, Kuhnhenn J, Schlegel U, Maghnouj A, Zöllner H, Schmiegel W, et al. Identification of microRNAs in the cerebrospinal fluid as biomarker for the diagnosis of glioma. Neuro Oncol. 2012;14(1):29–33.
12. Teplyuk NM, Mollenhauer B, Gabriely G, Giese A, Kim E, Smolsky M, et al. MicroRNAs in cerebrospinal fluid identify glioblastoma and metastatic brain cancers and reflect disease activity. Neuro Oncol. 2012;14(6):689–700.
13. Groves MD, Hess KR, Puduvalli VK, Colman H, Conrad CA, Gilbert MR, et al. Biomarkers of disease: cerebrospinal fluid vascular endothelial growth factor (VEGF) and stromal cell derived factor (SDF)-1 levels in patients with neoplastic meningitis (NM) due to breast cancer, lung cancer and melanoma. J Neurooncol. 2009;94(2):229–34.
14. Patel AS, Allen JE, Dicker DT, Peters KL, Sheehan JM, Glantz MJ, El-Deiry WS. Identification and enumeration of circulating tumor cells in the cerebrospinal fluid of breast cancer patients with central nervous system metastases. Oncotarget. 2011;2(10):752.

15. Muller C, Holtschmidt J, Auer M, Heitzer E, Lamszus K, Schulte A, Matschke J, Langer-Freitag S, Gasch C, Stoupiec M, Mauermann O, Peine S, Glatzel M, Speicher MR, Geigl JB, Westphal M, Pantel K, Reithdorf S. Hematogenous dissemination of glioblastoma multiforme. Sci Transl Med. 2014; 6(247):101.
16. Macdonald DR, Cascino TL, Schold SC, Cairncross JG. Response criteria for phase II studies of supratentorial malignant glioma. J Clin Oncol. 1990;8(7): 1277–80.
17. Wen PY, Macdonald DR, Reardon DA, Cloughesy TF, Sorensen AG, Galanis E, et al. Updated response assessment criteria for high-grade gliomas: response assessment in neuro-oncology working group. J Clin Oncol. 2010;28(11):1963–72.
18. Smith JS, Chang EF, Lamborn KR, Chang SM, Prados MD, Cha S, et al. Role of extent of resection in the long-term outcome of low-grade hemispheric gliomas. J Clin Oncol. 2008;26(8):1338–45.
19. Sanai N, Polley MY, McDermott MW, Parsa AT, Berger MS. An extent of resection threshold for newly diagnosed glioblastomas: clinical article. J Neurosurg. 2011;115(1):3–8.
20. Zhao S, Wu J, Wang C, Liu H, Dong X, Shi C, et al. Intraoperative fluorescence-guided resection of high-grade malignant gliomas using 5-aminolevulinic acid-induced porphyrins: a systematic review and meta-analysis of prospective studies. PLoS One. 2013;8(5), e63682.
21. Butte PV, Mamelak A, Parrish-Novak J, Drazin D, Shweikeh F, Gangalum PR, et al. Near-infrared imaging of brain tumors using the Tumor Paint BLZ-100 to achieve near-complete resection of brain tumors. Neurosurg Focus. 2014;36(2), E1.
22. Vredenburgh JJ, Desjardins A, Herndon JE, Marcello J, Reardon DA, Quinn JA, et al. Bevacizumab plus irinotecan in recurrent glioblastoma multiforme. J Clin Oncol. 2007;25(30):4722–9.
23. Sampson JH, Heimberger AB, Archer GE, Aldape KD, Friedman AH, Friedman HS, et al. Immunologic escape after prolonged progression-free survival with epidermal growth factor receptor variant III peptide vaccination in patients with newly diagnosed glioblastoma. J Clin Oncol. 2010;28(31):4722–9.
24. Phuphanich S, Wheeler CJ, Rudnick JD, Mazer M, Wang H, Nuno MA, et al. Phase I trial of a multi-epitope-pulsed dendritic cell vaccine for patients with newly diagnosed glioblastoma. Cancer Immunol Immunother. 2013;62(1):125–35.
25. Piccione DE, Kesari S. Clinical trials of viral therapy for malignant gliomas. Expert Rev Anticancer Ther. 2013;13(11):1297–305.
26. Stupp R, Wong ET, Kanner AA, Steinberg D, Engelhard H, Heidecke V, et al. NovoTTF-100A versus physician's choice chemotherapy in recurrent glioblastoma: a randomised phase III trial of a novel treatment modality. Eur J Cancer. 2012;48(14): 2192–202.
27. Stupp R, Wong E, Scott C, for the EF-14 Trial Investigators, et al. Interim analysis of the EF-14 trial: a prospective, multi-center trial of NovoTTF-100A together with temozolomide compared to temozolomide alone in patients with newly diagnosed GBM. Neuro Oncol. 2014;16 suppl 5:167.
28. Chang EL, Wefel JS, Hess KR, Allen PK, Lang FF, Kornguth DG, et al. Neurocognition in patients with brain metastases treated with radiosurgery or radiosurgery plus whole-brain irradiation: a randomised controlled trial. Lancet Oncol. 2009;10(11):1037–44.

Part IV

System-Oriented Technological Advances: Section B—Chest, Lungs, and Heart

Advanced Thoracoscopic Surgery to Modern Pulmonary Disease: The Japanese Approach

23

Masato Kanzaki

Introduction

Thoracoscopy has become an important procedure in thoracic surgery. Recently in Japan, thoracoscopic surgery has been performed in about 60 % of operations for primary lung cancer and more than 90 % of operations for spontaneous pneumothorax [1]. The rapid aging of the Japanese population has increased the importance of relatively noninvasive patient-tailored treatment. In thoracic surgery, thoracoscopy has contributed to reducing the physical stress of patients while maintaining the quality of surgery. As compared with open lobectomy, thoracoscopic lobectomy has been reported to decrease the incidence of complications, with no significant change in the overall survival rate at 5 years in patients with early-stage, non-small-cell lung cancer. Many studies have thus reported that thoracoscopic lobectomy is a safe and an effective procedure [2, 3].

The standard treatment for resectable, non-small-cell lung cancer is parenchymal resection of at least one lobe with systematic hilar and mediastinal lymph-node dissection. However, a study assessing the outcomes of segmentectomy in patients who had small peripheral lung cancers with tumors 2 cm or less in diameter that could be treated by lobectomy reported similar survival rates for segmentectomy and lobectomy. If surgical N0 disease is confirmed on strictly performed preoperative imaging studies and intraoperative frozen section diagnosis of lymph nodes, segmentectomy with resection of adjacent segments and subsegments as required by tumor location may be established to be a standard procedure for curative surgery [4].

Thoracoscopic surgery performed while monitoring two-dimensional images has the drawback of a limited field of view. In lung resection, the pulmonary arteries and veins have many diverse branches, and bleeding caused by intraoperative vascular damage can further limit the field of vision. On the other hand, remarkable progress has been made in imaging technology, allowing three-dimensional (3D) processing of computed tomographic (CT) images. 3D image processing is now used to perform navigation surgery in the fields of brain surgery and head and neck surgery. However, navigation surgery of the lung is difficult to perform because the surgical site may be displaced considerably; however, reconstructed 3D images can be used for preoperative simulation. In addition, 3D endoscopy is now available, and endoscopic surgery can be performed with the use of a 3D monitor [5].

M. Kanzaki, M.D., Ph.D. (✉)
Department of Surgery I, Tokyo Women's Medical University, Tokyo, Japan
e-mail: kanzaki@twmu.ac.jp

R. Latifi et al. (eds.), *Technological Advances in Surgery, Trauma and Critical Care*,
DOI 10.1007/978-1-4939-2671-8_23

Surgical robots enable more complex and delicate surgical procedures to be done. The availability of more accurate 3D imaging data may also allow safer, minimally invasive surgery to be performed.

Preoperative Simulation and Intraoperative Navigation Performed Using a 3D Pulmonary Model Reconstructed Using a Homemade Software Program

Enhanced processing power of the central processing units of personal computers and a marked increase in memory capacity have enabled 3D images to be analyzed by anyone on a desktop personal computer. Previously, 3D image analysis could only be done on a large computer system.

In open surgery, thoracic surgeons have intraoperatively evaluated the anatomic relations of the pulmonary arteries and veins from various perspectives during dissection of the pulmonary hilum, even though they did not completely understand the branches of the pulmonary arteries and veins before surgery. As the number of patients increased, they learned that various branching patterns exist. Owing to the current increase in thoracoscopic surgery with its restricted field of view, it is difficult to understand the anatomic relations of the pulmonary vasculature during surgery. Vascular injury is an important intraoperative complication of thoracoscopic surgery, occurring in about 60 % of Japanese patients. To avoid vascular injury and to perform surgery safely and quickly, we have preoperatively reconstructed 3D lung images with the use of a homemade software package, designated as CTTRY (Tokyo Women's Medical University, Tokyo, Japan) and have used these images to select the surgical procedure [6–8]. In the operating room, a 3D reconstructed model of the lung is used for intraoperative navigation. Next, we describe our method for preparing 3D reconstructed images of the lung.

Methods

CT scanning is performed at 1-mm intervals for at least 12 cm from the pulmonary hilum to the tumor, without using contrast media. In patients with enlarged hilar lymph nodes, however, contrast medium is used. Imaging data are viewed in the DICOM format. A thoracic surgeon manually traces the bronchi, pulmonary arteries and veins, tumor, and pulmonary lobes on all generated CT scans with the use of CTTRY (Fig. 23.1) [5–8].

The cylindrical numeric data on the three-dimensional images of the bronchi, pulmonary vessels, tumor, and pulmonary lobes are reconstructed as 3D graphic images with the use of a freeware version of Metasequoia LE (http://metaseq.net/; Tetraface Inc, Tokyo, Japan), a free software package (Fig. 23.2). This software allows 3D images of the lung to be modified, and 3D images of the pulmonary vessels and bronchi to be transected and moved, thereby simulating surgery.

The pulmonary blood vessels and the bronchi are depicted as cylinders, which is adequate for understanding the anatomic spatial relations at the time of surgery. Because the data are simple, images of the pulmonary blood vessels, bronchi, and lung can be modified, transected, and moved, even on a notebook personal computer. Because CT scanning is performed during inhalation, the resulting 3D images are also in the inhalation phase. However, the 3D images can be modified to prepare 3D images of the collapsed lung during differential lung ventilation. On the other hand, when 3D images are reconstructed from conventional contrast-enhanced CT scans, it is difficult to separately depict arteries and veins. Two-stage images obtained in different phases have been reported to be useful, but exposure to radiation increases. Separate imaging of arteries and veins in different phases is generally performed to distinguish arteries from veins in the lung. However, this also requires an increased dose of contrast agents. In this respect, CTTRY allows 3D images to be reconstructed without using contrast media and produces very accurate

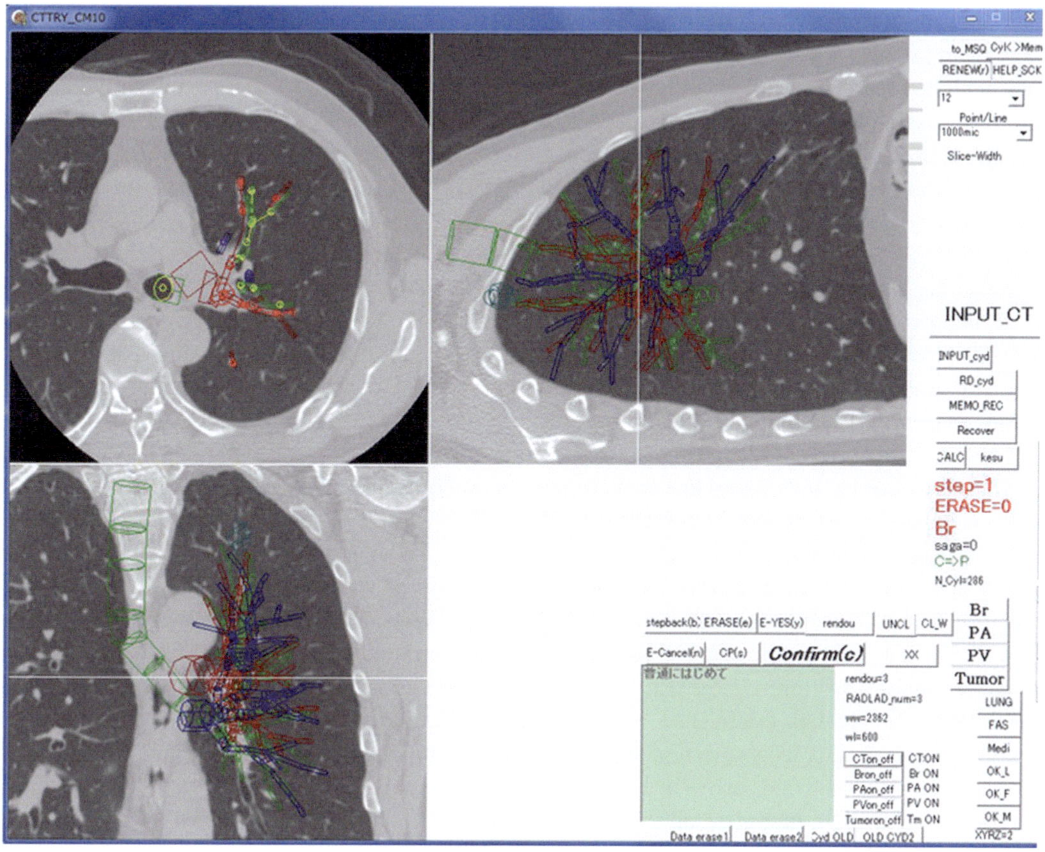

Fig. 23.1 CTTRY. Procedural images of CTTRY picture are shown. A thoracic surgeon carefully manually traces the bronchi, pulmonary vessels, and tumor on CT images. The pulmonary arteries are shown in *red*, the pulmonary veins in *blue*, the bronchi in *yellowish green*, and the tumors in *green*

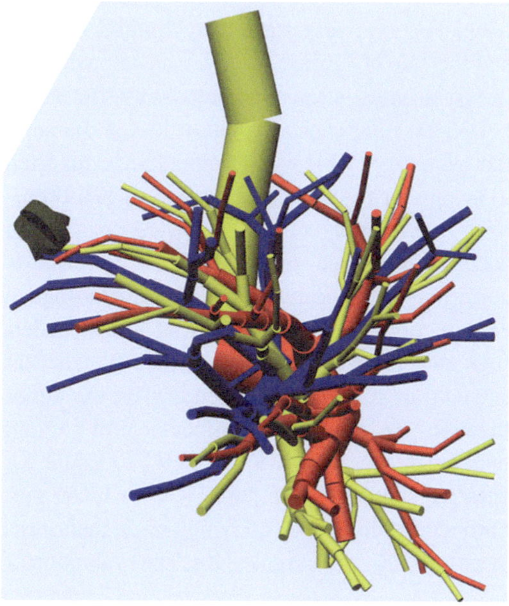

images because reconstructed images are manually confirmed by comparing the images with CT scans [5–8].

Thoracoscopic Lung Segmentectomy

Surgery, radiotherapy, and chemotherapy are the mainstays of treatment for lung cancer. The therapeutic effectiveness of radiotherapy and chemotherapy remains unsatisfactory, and surgery is the standard treatment for clinical early-stage lung cancer.

Fig. 23.2 Reconstructed 3D images of the lung using a freeware version of Metasequoia LE (http://metaseq.net/), a free software package

Improved performance of diagnostic imaging devices and routine use of CT have dramatically increased the detection rate of small lung cancers. However, even small tumors can be associated with advanced disease. Therefore, parenchymal resection of at least one lobe with extensive hilar and mediastinal lymph-node dissection has become the standard surgical treatment throughout the world.

Since the later half of the 1970s, segmentectomy and partial resection have been indicated as limited surgery for compromised hosts with lung cancer. However, a randomized clinical trial comparing lobectomy with limited surgery in patients with clinical stage T1N0M0 lung cancer, reported by Ginsberg et al. in 1995, found that limited surgery, segmentectomy, or wedge resection were associated with higher rates of local recurrence and poorer outcomes as compared with lobectomy [9]. They concluded that lobectomy should be performed in patients who can tolerate the procedure, even for small lung cancers.

In Japan, which has established a national health checkup system, the proportion of patients who present with small and early-stage lung cancer associated with ground-glass opacity (GGO) on CT is higher than that in the USA. Consequently, many Japanese investigators reported that there is no distinct difference in outcomes between lobectomy and limited surgery. The surgical procedure of choice for early-stage, small lung cancers is thus shifting from lobectomy to segmentectomy, and techniques for limited surgery have received considerable attention.

As for the surgical approach, studies comparing open surgery with thoracoscopic surgery have yet to adequately demonstrate the superiority of thoracoscopic surgery in terms of invasiveness, safety, or curability. However, there is apparently no difference between these procedures in complications, local recurrence rate, length of hospital stay, or 5-year survival rate. Many studies thus reported that thoracoscopic surgery is a viable option [2, 3, 6].

Because lung resection can directly cause functional disorders, minimally invasive surgery should be performed while maintaining good outcomes. Thoracoscopic surgery can decrease postoperative pain and hasten recovery. Thoracoscopic surgery requires a small incision and is associated with less postoperative pain if no rib or muscle is transected. It is therefore considered minimally invasive surgery.

Recently, thoracoscopic segmentectomy with a small thoracic incision and minimal resection of lung volume has been increasingly performed as limited surgery in patients with small peripheral lung cancers, metastatic lung tumors located in the central portion of the lung, and impaired pulmonary function. Partial resection of lung has the smallest range of resection and can be performed thoracoscopically. However, partial resection of lung has limited indications and is not suited for resection of lesions located near the hilum. Another drawback of partial resection is the inability to evaluate lymph-node metastasis. Lung segmentectomy is associated with a smaller resection volume than lobectomy and allows resected tissue to be easily removed through a small incision, retaining the advantages of thoracoscopic surgery. Segmentectomy was initially used to manage benign lung tumors, infections, and inflammatory diseases, but was then performed as limited surgery in some poor-risk patients with lung cancer [2, 3]. The increased detection of early-stage small lung cancers and of peripheral lung cancer with a high air content then led to an increased number of patients who could be curatively treated by limited surgery, and the role of limited surgery was reconsidered. Survival rates after segmentectomy for small peripheral lung cancers 2 cm or less in diameter that were resectable by lobectomy were reported to be similar to those after lobectomy [2]. If preoperative imaging studies are strictly performed and the presence of surgical N0 disease is confirmed on the intraoperative histopathological examination of frozen sections of lymph nodes, segmentectomy including resection of an adjacent segment or subsegment depending on the tumor location (i.e., extended segmentectomy) might thus be established as a standard procedure for curative surgery. Some pure GGO or GGO predominant lesions have no lymph-node metastasis or postoperative recurrence [10]. The evaluation of

GGO on high-resolution CT is thus useful for deciding whether limited surgery is indicated. Positron emission tomography (PET) also has an important role in deciding the treatment policy. A larger tumor size and a higher standardized uptake value (SUV) are directly related to the risks of metastasis and invasion. For example, tumors 2 cm or less in diameter with an SUV of ≤1.5 have low risks of metastasis and invasion. Small lung cancers range from low-grade bronchoalveolar cancers presenting with GGO to locally advanced lung cancers consisting primarily of solid components that are accompanied by lymph-node metastasis. Segmentectomy can be indicated for GGO-predominant lesions and predominantly solid lesions 1.5 cm or less in diameter. However, lobectomy is indicated for solid lesions exceeding 1 cm in diameter and should be indicated with caution even for tumors measuring 1 cm or less.

In our department, thoracoscopic limited surgery was intentionally performed in 131 patients with clinical stage IA peripheral lung cancers 2 cm or less in diameter from July 2001 through September 2013 [6–8]. Intentional limited surgery is a procedure designed to reduce the range of resection in patients able to undergo lobectomy. The details of the surgical procedures are shown in Tables 23.1 and 23.2. Single segmentectomy was performed in 63 patients, upper division resection in 15, lingulectomy in 9, extended segmentectomy in 21, single subsegmentectomy in 7, and multiple subsegmentectomy in 16. In segmentectomy with dissection of the pulmonary arteries, veins, and bronchi at the hilum up to the level of the divisions of the segments, the hilar lymph nodes can be evaluated. If lymph-node metastasis is diagnosed on intraoperative histopathological examination of frozen sections of lymph nodes, the surgical procedure is switched to lobectomy. The pros and cons of systematic lymph-node dissection or sampling remain controversial. Systematic lymph-node dissection is recommended for an accurate diagnosis of disease stage. However, the therapeutic effectiveness of this procedure remains a matter of debate. There are certain trends in the most common sites of lymph-node metastasis according to lobe. If no metastasis is found at the most common sites, it has been proposed that selective (rational) lymph-node dissection with omission of more extensive dissection can be performed.

Table 23.1 Segmentectomy

Single segmentectomy	($n=63$)	Extended segmentectomy	($n=21$)
Right		Right	
S^1	8	S^1+S^2a	1
S^2	8	S^1+S^3	1
S^3	8	S^1+S^3a	1
S^6	10	S^2+S^1a	1
S^8	3	S^6+S^8a	1
Left		S^8+S^9	2
S^{1+2}	7	S^9+S^{10}	3
S^3	3	Left	
S^4	1	$S^{1+2}+S^3a+S^3b$	1
S^6	10	$S^6+S^9a+S^{10}a$	1
S^8	2	S^8+S^9	3
S^9	1	S^9+S^{10}	5
S^{10}	2	$S^9+S^{10}b$	1
Upper division resection	15		
Lingulectomy	9		

Abbreviations: *S* denotes segment, S^1 apical, S^2 posterior, S^{1+2} apical posterior, S^3 anterior, S^6 superior, S^8 anterior basal, S^9 lateral basal, S^{10} posterior basal, *a* posterior subsegment, *b* anterior subsegment

Table 23.2 Subsegmentectomy

Single subsegmentectomy	($n=7$)	Multiple subsegmentectomy	($n=16$)
Right		Right	
S^3a	3	S^1a+S^3a	1
S^3b	1	S^1a+S^2a	1
S^4a	1	S^1b+S^3a	1
		S^2b+S^3a	5
Left		Left	
$S^{1+2}c$	1	$S^{1+2}a+S^{1+2}b$	3
S^6a	1	$S^{1+2}a+S^3c$	1
		$S^{1+2}b+S^3a$	1
		$S^{1+2}c+S^3a$	2
		$S^{1+2}c+S^3a+S^4a$	1

Abbreviations: *S* denotes segment, S^1 apical, S^2 posterior, S^{1+2} apical posterior, S^3 anterior, S^4 right; lateral, left; superior lingular, S^6 superior, *a* posterior subsegment, *b* anterior subsegment, *c* horizontal subsegment

A preoperative understanding of the branches of the pulmonary vasculature allows lung segmentectomy to be performed safely and smoothly. An understanding of the pulmonary arteries and veins is particularly important for performing anatomic segmentectomy, and it is thus useful to prepare reconstructed 3D images on the basis of CT data. A 3D understanding of the intersegmental veins allows segments to be defined without relying on tactile perception.

We have actively performed segmentectomy of the anterior basal, lateral basal, and posterior basal segments of the lower lobes of the lung, which are relatively rare procedures. Reconstruction of 3D images by CTTRY, the homemade software described above, allowed these procedures to be performed.

Next, we describe the technique for segmentectomy (anterior basal segment, lateral basal segment, posterior basal segment) and extended segmentectomy of the lower lobes. Our technique for segmentectomy of the lower lobes of the lung utilizes the anatomic characteristics of the pulmonary ligament. In contrast to other ligaments, the pulmonary ligament comprises a double-serous layer of visceral pleura, which forms the intersegmental septum. The intersegmental septum can easily be used to divide the right lung into the medial basal segment and posterior basal segment and the left lung into the anterior basal segment and the posterior basal segment. Division of the intersegmental septum formed by the pulmonary ligament exposes the lower pulmonary veins. The 3D reconstructed lung images prepared before surgery are compared with the surgical field displayed on a monitor to confirm the courses of the pulmonary veins, and then surgery is continued. Branches of segmental pulmonary veins that should be resected and those that should be preserved are identified, and intersegmental dissection is performed. The bronchi of the segment are dissected, confirmed on bronchoscopy, and transected. Then, the pulmonary arteries are transected (Fig. 23.3a–f). To visualize the intersegmental border, the affected lung is inflated and then deflated. The inflation-deflation line is used to define the intersegmental border. Division at the intersegmental border is performed while applying traction to the transected bronchus. Dissection is done with an electrocautery and ultrasonic activated device to identify the intersegmental veins. Dissection proceeds from the hilum towards the periphery. Small branches entering the resected segment are appropriately divided. The peripheral part of the lung is divided with an automatic stapler. Thoracoscopic lung segmentectomy is challenging because it is difficult to identify and divide the intersegmental border. However, 3D images reconstructed from CT data are useful for understanding the 3D branching pattern of the intersegmental pulmonary veins, allowing the intersegmental plane to be identified, without the use of tactile perception. To maintain an adequate distance from the tumor, multiple segments, subsegments, or adjacent segments of the lung should be resected, without hesitation. In patients suspected to have lung cancer, a margin exceeding the tumor diameter, which is at least 1 cm even for small tumors, should be secured [6]. In accordance with this basic concept, if it is difficult to secure an adequate margin by resection of the affected segment, extended partial resection of

Fig. 23.3 (continued) along the lower pulmonary veins. (**d**) On transection of the intersegmental veins in the left lateral basal segment and the posterior basal segment, the bronchi (*black arrow*) can be confirmed. (**e**) On transection of B9–10, the pulmonary artery A10 is exposed (*black arrow*). (**f**) On transection of the pulmonary artery A10, the pulmonary artery A9 appears. The pulmonary artery A9 (*black arrow*) is transected. The affected lung is inflated and then deflated. The segments are divided along the intersegmental plane, using the inflation-deflation line as a guide. While applying traction to the transected bronchus, dissection proceeds from the hilum towards the periphery. The dissected bronchus is pulled and dissected towards the distal part of the pulmonary hilum. The peripheral part of the lung is divided with an automatic stapler, and the segmentectomy is completed. *Abbreviations*: *PV* denotes inferior pulmonary vein, *PC* pericardium, *Ao* aorta, *S* segment, *S8* anterior basal, *S10* posterior basal, *B9–10* lateral basal and posterior basal bronchi, *A9* lateral basal segmental artery, *A10* posterior basal segmental artery

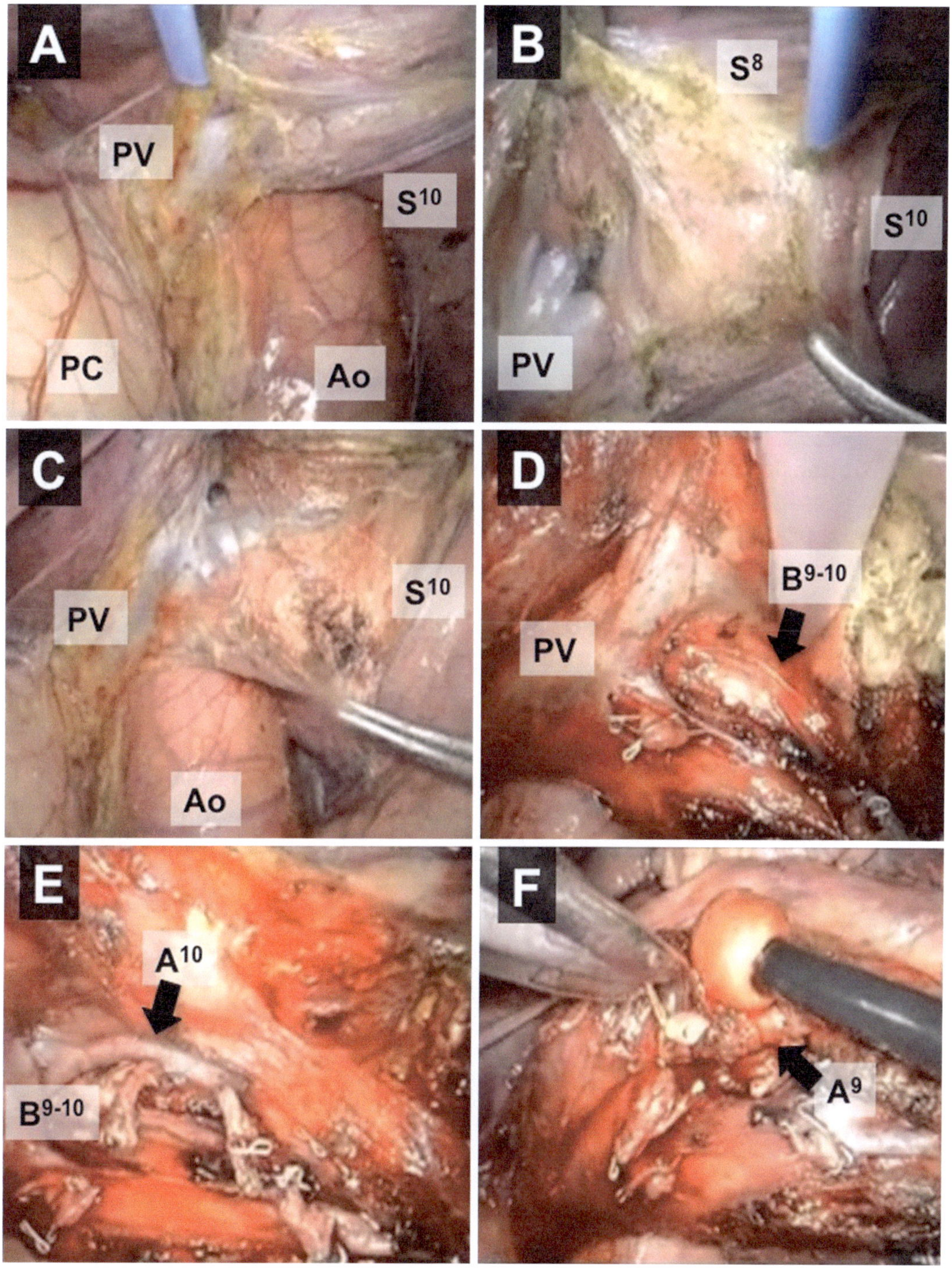

Fig. 23.3 Thoracoscopic extended segmentectomy. Thoracoscopic resection of the left lateral basal segment and the posterior basal segment is shown. (**a**) The lower pulmonary ligament is divided in a cranial direction to reach the inferior margin of the left lower pulmonary veins. (**b**) In contrast to other ligaments, the pulmonary ligament consists of a double-serous layer of visceral pleura, which forms the intersegmental septum. The intersegmental septum can easily be used to divide the left lung into the anterior basal segment and the posterior basal segment. (**c**) The anterior basal segment and the posterior basal segment are divided towards the periphery

adjacent segments or resection of the adjoining subsegment should be performed.

In patients in whom radical limited surgery is performed, the advantages of lung segmentectomy include the significant preservation of postoperative lung function, maintenance of the postoperative quality of life, and prevention of the development of second and third asynchronous lung cancers [2, 3, 6]. The functional preservation of segmentectomy combined with the minimal invasiveness of thoracoscopic surgery allows the advantages of each of these procedures to be effectively maintained.

Three-Dimensional Video-Assisted Thoracoscopic Surgery

We perform thoracoscopic surgery with a 3D stereo endoscope to obtain a visual field approximating that of open surgery. In conventional thoracoscopic surgery, operative procedures are performed while viewing a two-dimensional display monitor. In contrast, when a 3D stereo endoscope is used, the operator, assistants, and nurses wear polarized glasses and perform surgical procedures while watching a 3D monitor.

Data on 3D images prepared by CTTRY as described above are converted into interactive 3D contents by Autodesk 3DS Max® (Autodesk, San Rafael, CA), a commercially available software package, and are displayed on a 3D monitor with the use of a Remo Viewer (3D Incorporated, Kanagawa, Japan) [5]. These images are used for preoperative simulation and intraoperative navigation (Fig. 23.4).

As compared with conventional thoracoscopic surgery, the senses of depth and distance are more easily perceived intraoperatively for procedures assisted by 3D stereo endoscopy. From January 2012 through February 2014, the following procedures were performed in patients with primary lung cancer or metastatic lung tumors: lobectomy in 7 patients, segmentectomy in 13, and other procedures such as wedge resection in 7. To date, vascular damage has not occurred during operation.

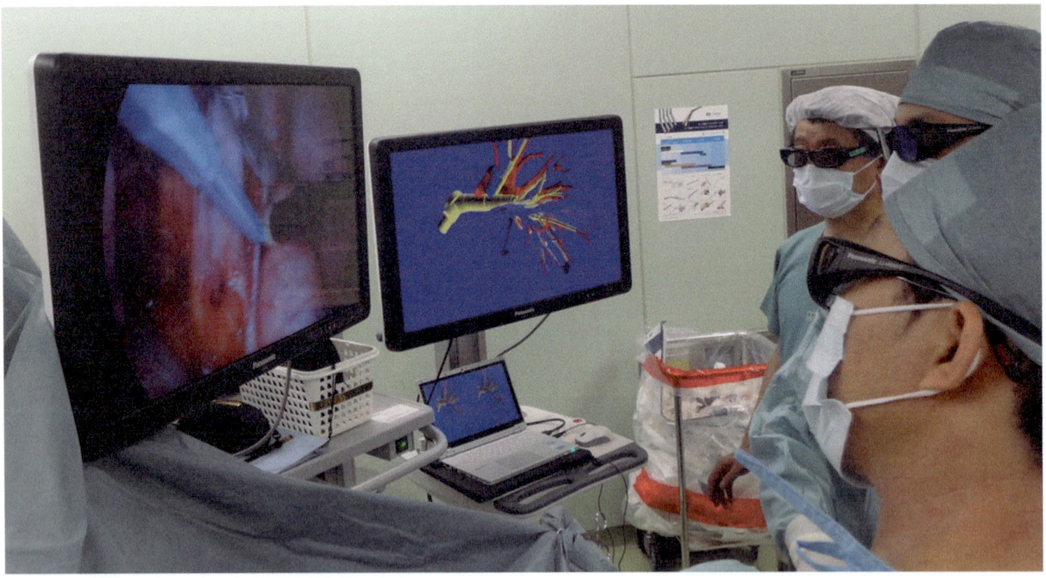

Fig. 23.4 3D stereo endoscopy. The operator, assistants, and nurses wear polarized glasses and perform surgical procedures while viewing a 3D monitor. Static images appear to be double on the 3D monitor. The 3D reconstructed images of the lung on *right side* 3D monitor, generated by the personal computer at the *lower right side* of the screen

Thoracoscopic Surgery Using Bioabsorbable Polymers

In spontaneous pneumothorax, in addition to closing the air leak intraoperatively or postoperatively, the prevention of recurrence is important. In Japan, many studies have reported that applying polyglycolic acid (PGA) felt or regenerated oxidized cellulose to the surface of the pleura reduces the recurrence rate of pneumothorax [11]. We focus on reinforcement of the pleura and apply a sheet of regenerated oxidized cellulose to the resection stump and the surrounding region. This is done because experimental studies have shown that application of regenerated oxidized cellulose thickens the underlying surface of the pleura, suggesting that this step may effectively prevent recurrence of pneumothorax. Our experience has indicated that adhesion between the lung and chest wall was very mild when regenerated oxidized cellulose was used, as compared with PGA felt. In secondary pneumothorax, we sometimes cover the entire surface of the pleura with a sheet of regenerated oxidized cellulose (Fig. 23.5).

When bullectomy is performed in patients with pneumothorax, the air leak in the lung is closed during surgery, and a sheet of regenerated oxidized cellulose is applied to the resection stump and the portion of the pleura showing emphysematous changes, without the use of fibrin glue, to prevent the recurrence of pneumothorax.

In lung segmentectomy and subsegmentectomy, the intersegmental pulmonary veins are exposed peripherally to prepare a plane between segments or subsegments, creating a pleural defect. Because an air leak was found in the pleural defect, the defect was covered with a sheet of PGA felt and fibrin glue, thereby closing the air leak in the lung (Fig. 23.6).

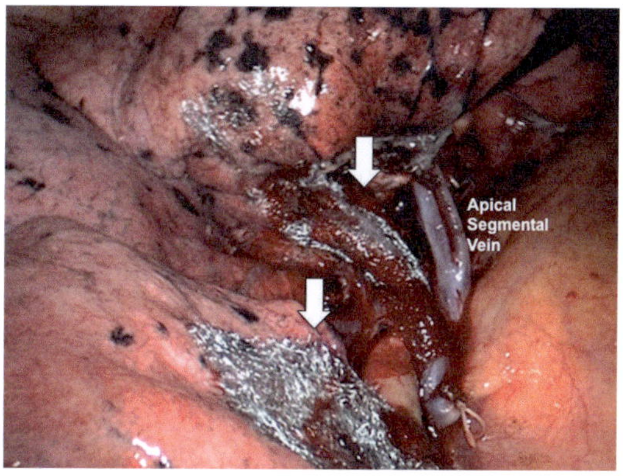

Fig. 23.6 Thoracoscopic lung subsegmentectomy. During thoracoscopic anatomic subsegmental resection (resection of the right anterior subsegment of the anterior segment), an air leak is seen in the pleural defect between the subsegments. A sheet of polyglycolic acid felt (*white arrow*) and fibrin glue are applied to the pleural defect to close the air leak in the lung

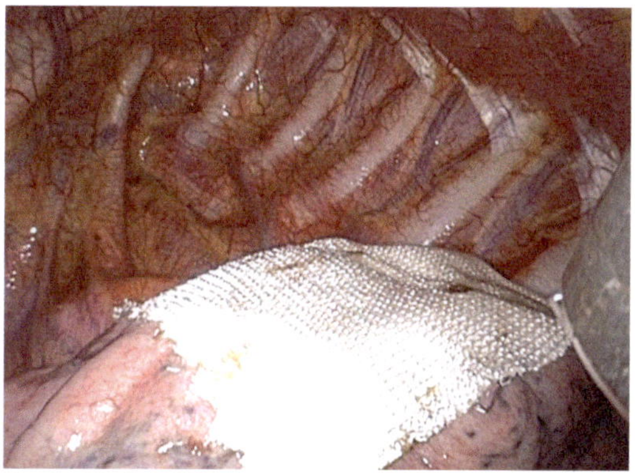

Fig. 23.5 Thoracoscopic surgical findings of pneumothorax

In refractory pneumothorax associated with conditions such as secondary pneumothorax or empyema with bronchopleural fistula are sutured to close pulmonary air leaks. The use of muscle flaps such as the latissimus dorsi or intercostal muscles, pericardial adipose tissue, or omentum can lead to suture failure and the recurrence of pulmonary air leaks. The recurrence of air leaks in the lung is a technical problem, and we use sheets of PGA felt to prevent recurrence. PGA undergoes hydrolysis and is absorbed. During this process, inflammatory reactions are known to be induced by oxidation [12]. To take advantage of these inflammatory reactions, rather than simply suturing the fistula and muscle flap, PGA felt is first inserted between the fistula and muscle flap to promote adhesion between the fistula and muscle flap. The local inflammatory reactions at the site applied PGA promote tight adhesion between the fistula and muscle flap, resulting in tighter suture closure (Fig. 23.7a–f).

To treat a giant pulmonary bulla, the wall of the bulla is incised, and PGA felt is applied to the lung parenchyma. The pulmonary bulla is

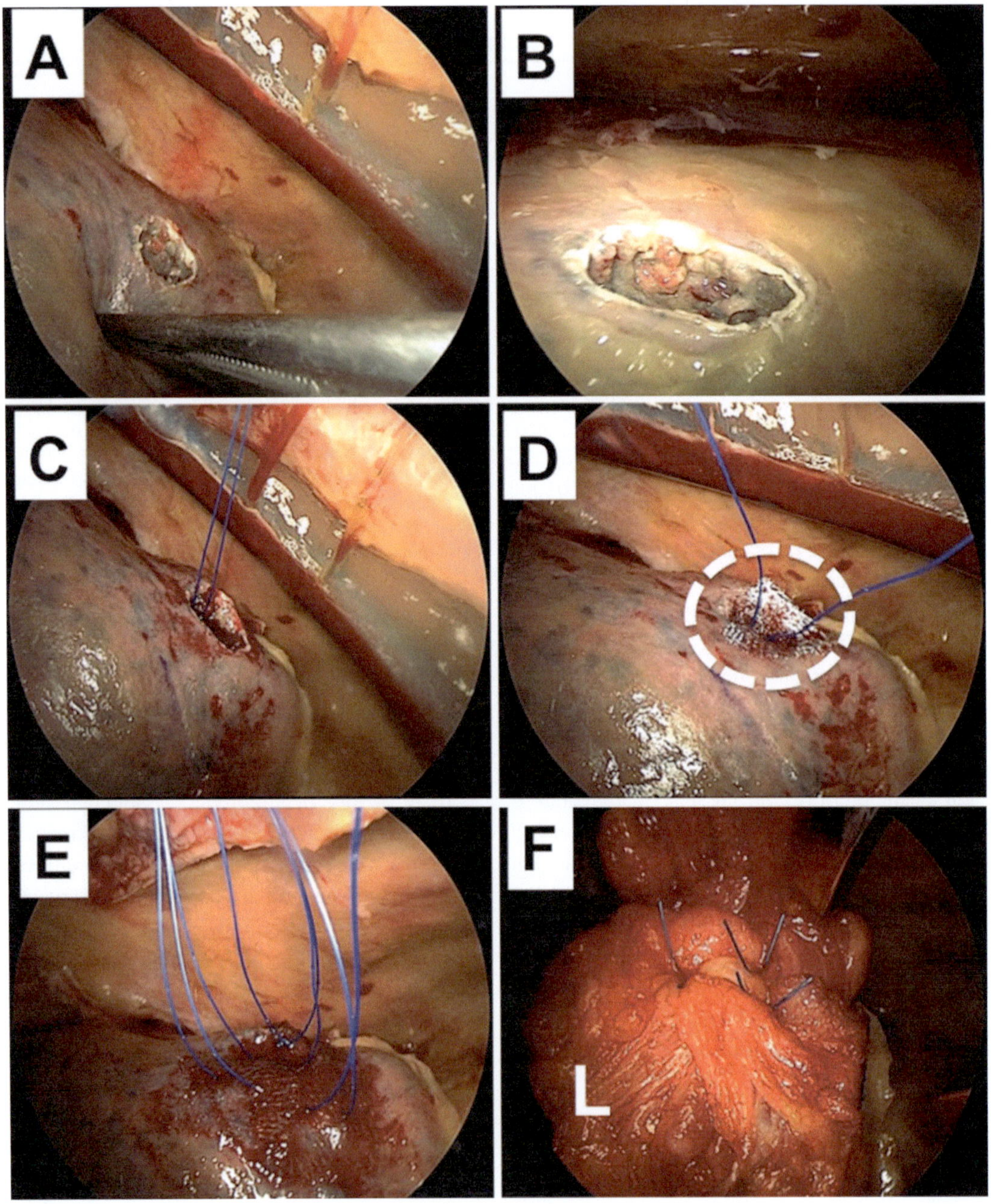

Fig. 23.7 Thoracoscopic surgical findings of refractory pneumothorax. (**a**) An air leak is seen in the ruptured visceral pleura. (**b**) A magnified view of the pulmonary air leak. (**c**) A nonabsorbable suture is used to support the parenchyma in a pulmonary bulla. (**d**) A sheet of polyglycolic acid felt is passed through the support suture (within the *dotted circle*) and applied to the lung parenchyma. (**e**) A muscle flap is sutured to the outer perimeter of the ruptured visceral pleura with nonabsorbable suture. (**f**) The latissimus dorsi muscle (L) is sutured to the lung parenchyma, using the nonabsorbable suture shown in (**e**)

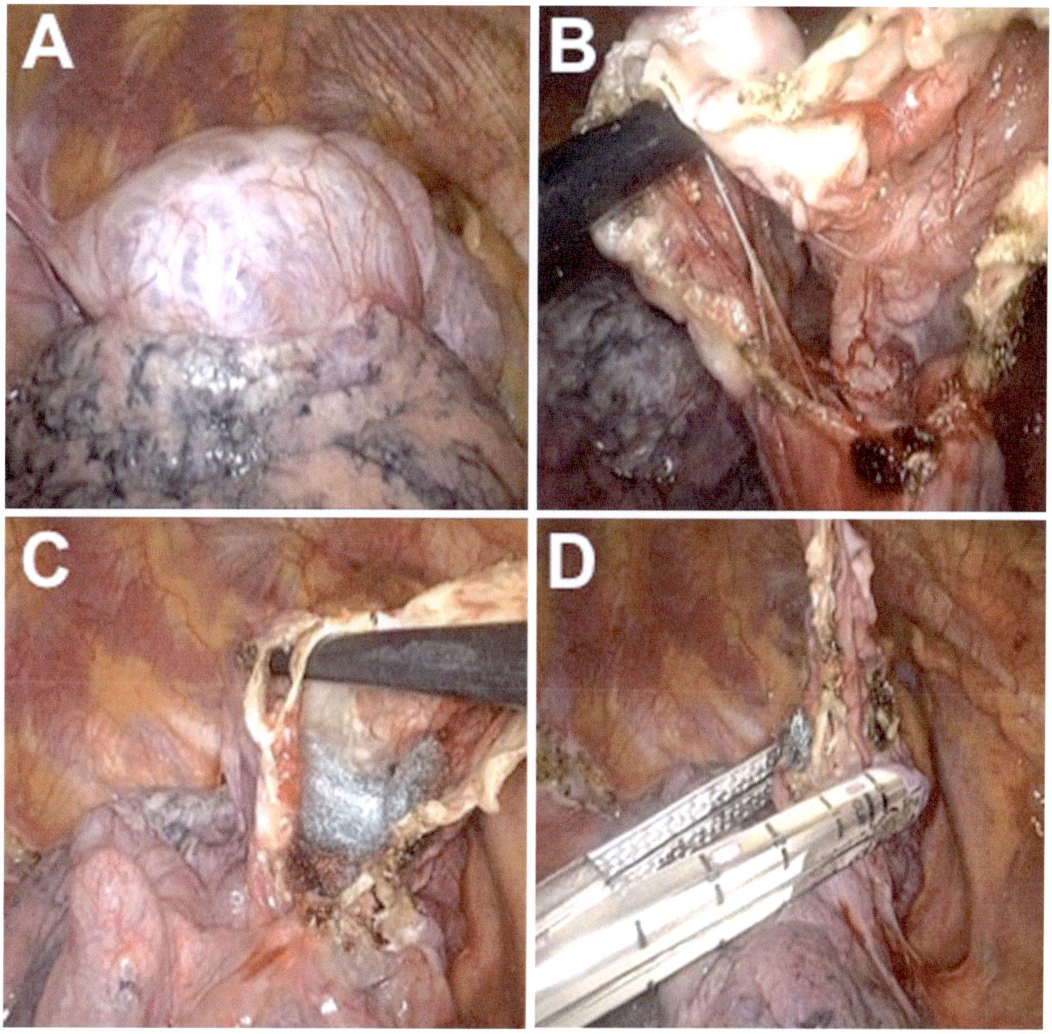

Fig. 23.8 Thoracoscopic surgical findings of a giant pulmonary bulla. (**a**) Thoracoscopy shows a giant pulmonary bulla. (**b**) The wall of the bulla is incised with an ultrasonic scalpel. (**c**) The lung parenchyma is confirmed through the incision in the resected bulla, and a sheet of polyglycolic acid felt (*light blue*) is applied to the lung parenchyma. (**d**) Traction is applied to the pulmonary bulla, and the wall of the bulla is resected using an automatic stapler, without resecting the lung parenchyma

resected without resecting the parenchyma. The residual pulmonary bulla contained air at the time of surgery. However, after 2–3 months the PGA is absorbed, and the inflammatory reactions induced by oxidation promote adhesion between the wall of the residual pulmonary bulla and the lung parenchyma. Consequently, the retained air disappears (Fig. 23.8a–d).

References

1. Kawano H, Amano J, Yokomise H. Erratum: thoracic and cardiovascular surgery in Japan during 2010. Gen Thorac Cardiovasc Surg. 2013;61:57–9.
2. Okada M, Koike T, Higashiyama M, Yamato Y, Tsubota N. Radical sublober resection for small-sized non-small cell lung cancer: a multicenter study. J Thorac Cardiovasc Surg. 2006;132:769–75.

3. Nomori H, Mori T, Ikeda K, Yoshimoto K, Iyama K, Suzuki M. Segmentectomy for selected cT1N0M0 non-small cell lung cancer: a prospective study at a single institute. J Thorac Cardiovasc Surg. 2012; 144:87–93.
4. Naruke T, Tsuchiya R, Kondo H, Nakayama H, Asamura H. Lymph node sampling in lung cancer: how should it be done? Eur J Cardiothorac Surg. 1999;16 Suppl 1:S17–24.
5. Kanzaki M, Kikkawa T, Sakamoto K, Maeda H, Wachi N, Komine H, Oyama K, Murasugi M, Onuki T. Three-dimensional simulation, surgical navigation and thoracoscopic lung resection. J Surg Case Rep. 2013;3. pii: rjt015.
6. Kanzaki M, Kikkawa T, Shimizu T, Maeda H, Wachi N, Isaka T, Murasugi M, Onuki T. Presurgical planning using a three-dimensional pulmonary model of the actual anatomy of patient with primary lung cancer. Thorac Cardiovasc Surg. 2013;61:144–50.
7. Kanzaki M, Wachi N, Onuki T. Simulating video-assisted thoraoscopic lung resection using a virtual 3-dimensional pulmonary model on a personal computer. J Thorac Cardiovasc Surg. 2011;142:243–4.
8. Kanzaki M, Maeda H, Wachi N, Kikkawa T, Komine H, Isaka T, Oyama K, Murasugi M, Onuki T. Complete video-assisted thoracoscopic multi-subsegmentectomy based on patients' specific virtual 3-D pulmonary models. Asian J Endosc Surg. 2013;6:110–5.
9. Ginsberg RJ, Rubinstein LV, Lung Cancer Study Group. Randomized trial of lobectomy versus limited resection for T1 N0 non-small cell lung cancer. Ann Thorac Surg. 1995;60:615–23.
10. Noguchi M, Morikawa A, Kawasaki M, et al. Small adenocarcinoma of the lung. Histologic characteristics and prognosis. Cancer. 1995;75:2844–52.
11. Kurihara M, Kataoka H, Ishikawa A, Endo R. Latest treatment for spontaneous pneumothorax. Gen Thorac Cardiovasc Surg. 2010;58:113–9.
12. Ceonzo K, Gaynor A, Shaffer L, Kojima K, Vacanti CA, Stahl GL. Polyglycolic acid induced inflammation: role of hydrolysis and resulting complement activation. Tissue Eng. 2006;12:301–8.

The Role of Robotics in Selective Thoracic Surgical Problems: Technical Considerations

24

Farid Gharagozloo

Introduction

The daVinci® system (Intuitive Surgical, Mountain View, CA) consists of three main components: (1) the surgical console with two master controls and an integrated 3D display stereo viewer; (2) the surgical cart with a camera arm and up to three instrument arms (Fig. 24.1); and (3) the vision cart, which contains camera and image-processing equipment. While seated at the surgical console, the surgeon operates by placing his fingers in the masters and moving the masters within the console. The instruments within the surgical field are aligned with the masters. There is natural and predictable instrument movement within the operative field. The relationship of the masters to the instruments within the surgical field coupled with 3D visualization ensures hand/eye coordination and orientation as well as natural operative feel found in open surgery. The 3D visualization is provided by a stereo viewer which is provided for the surgeon's head. Open surgery techniques which are employed by the surgeon's hands are instantly converted into minimally invasive surgical movements at the surgical site. Furthermore the system electronically scales the surgeon's hand movements to correspondingly smaller movements at the instrument tips located in the surgical field. The instrument tips have six degrees of freedom plus grip and the tip articulations mimic the movements of the human wrist. The daVinci Surgical Robotic system has been upgraded four times and the most recent model, daVinci Xi, represents the pinnacle of robotic surgical technology.

Although the daVinci surgical robot was originally marketed for cardiac surgical applications, it has found widespread use in urologic surgery. In addition to urology, the daVinci Robot is used in cardiac, thoracic, general surgical, and gynecologic surgical applications.

The enhanced dexterity of the daVinci Robot has enabled the application of video-assisted thoracic surgery to complex procedures such as (1) totally endoscopic lobectomy for lung cancer; (2) endoscopic esophagectomy for esophageal cancer; (3) endoscopic resection of mediastinal masses; (4) endoscopic thymectomy for myasthenia gravis; and (5) endoscopic transthoracic esophageal myotomy for achalasia.

Totally Endoscopic Robotic Pulmonary Lobectomy for Lung Cancer

Lobectomy remains the standard of care for the treatment of early-stage non-small-cell lung cancer. Until recently, thoracotomy has been the standard

F. Gharagozloo, M.D., F.A.C.S. (✉)
Department of Surgery, University of Arizona, Arizona Cancer Center, Tucson, AZ, USA
e-mail: gharagozloof@aol.com

R. Latifi et al. (eds.), *Technological Advances in Surgery, Trauma and Critical Care*,
DOI 10.1007/978-1-4939-2671-8_24

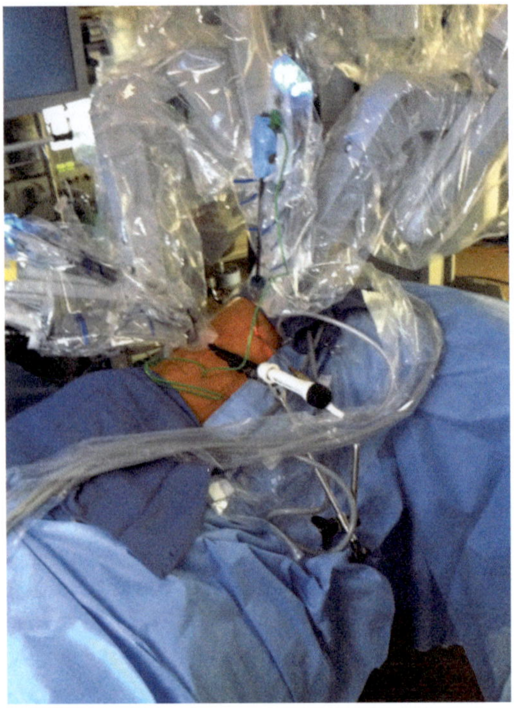

Fig. 24.1 The daVinci® surgical cart (Intuitive Surgical, Mountain View, CA) during a procedure

approach to lobectomy. However, the standard posterolateral thoracotomy and even a muscle-sparing thoracotomy are associated with significant acute and chronic pain as well as a lengthy recovery. It has been reasoned that a less invasive approach to lobectomy by the use of VATS techniques may be advantageous. It is hypothesized that the advantages of the VATS approach would stem from small incisions without transection or spreading of ribs, less postoperative pain, and a shorter hospital stay [1–7]. However, no uniform definition for VATS lobectomy has been accepted [8–11]. VATS lobectomy techniques can be describes as [1] mini-thoracotomy with video assistance; [2] simultaneously stapled lobectomy; [3] individual ligation lobectomy with a utility thoracotomy; and [4] a hybrid VATS lobectomy technique with features of isolation ligation and simultaneously stapled lobectomy [11].

One of the shortcomings of the VATS technique stems from the fact that the instruments are introduced through ports or small incisions which amount to holes in the chest wall. The instruments pivot at the entry hole and can be moved in four directions. The limited mobility of conventional endoscopic instruments, whether in the abdomen or the chest, has been referred to by some investigators as "chopstick surgery." The chopstick nature and the limited maneuverability of the effector instruments stem from the rigid shaft axis fixed to the thorax by the entry hole. This technical shortcoming limits the surgeon in performing fine dissection and complex three-dimensional maneuvers. Pivoting instruments on the chest wall results in a large radius of curvature for the tip of the instrument and makes fine dissection in deep spaces such as the mediastinum very difficult and even dangerous. Indeed, it is this fact which has necessitated the need for a utility thoracotomy. Using the utility thoracotomy, the surgeon is able to utilize conventional instruments and his own wrist in order to provide additional degrees of freedom.

Another shortcoming of the VATS technique is in the lack of the three-dimensional visualization. The surgeon has to use two-dimensional information from the video monitor in order to create a three-dimensional mental image. This fact requires significant experience and can prove to be a source of fatigue for the surgeon. Most importantly, using such indirect means of judging depth perception is rarely equivalent to binocular vision. In the thoracic hilum, binocular vision is paramount for lymphadenectomy and individual vascular and bronchial dissection.

The use of the robotic technology obviates these difficulties. As has been pointed out in other chapters in this book, our view is that the daVinci Robot represents an ideal tool for dissection of the hilum and can be combined with VATS techniques to reach our ultimate goal of completely endoscopic lobectomy. In our view, the indispensable features of the daVinci Robot in performing VATS lobectomy are the following:

1. The EndoWrist® (Intuitive Surgical, Mountain View, CA), or the cable-driven wrist at the end of the robotic arm: The placement of the robotic arm through the VATS hole is comparable to and accomplishes the chopstick maneuvers performed by conventional VATS

instruments. However, the EndoWrist at the distal end of the robotic arm is positioned in the confined spaces within the chest and brings four more degrees of freedom and six additional directions of movement compared to normal VATS techniques. The EndoWrist provides the surgeon with fine instrument maneuverability in a very confined space.
2. The daVinci Robotic system is designed to provide downscaling from the motion of the surgeon's hand to that of the robotic instrument. This is invaluable in dissecting fine and fragile intrathoracic structures. Furthermore, a 6 Hz motion filter is used to filter out any tremor in the surgeon's hand.
3. The binocular robotic camera provides superb three-dimensional visualization, and by nature of being mounted on the central robotic arm, it can be manipulated by the surgeon. The surgeon's ability to manipulate the camera and the arms recreates the natural biologic motion of the surgeon's head, eyes, and hands in providing optimal hand-eye coordination.

Operative Technique

Anesthesia

Patients undergoing robotic-assisted VATS lobectomy require single-lung ventilation. We prefer a left-sided double-lumen endotracheal tube to a bronchial blocker. With a double-lumen tube, lung collapse is superior and hilar manipulation does not result in movement of the blocker and compromise in patient ventilation and surgical visualization. Longer tubing is required as the robot is brought in over the patient's head and the anesthesiologist will occupy a more remote position than in usual video-assisted thoracic surgical procedures.

Patient Positioning

The patient is placed in a full lateral decubitus position. The table is flexed to open the intercostal spaces. The position of the double-lumen tube is reconfirmed after final patient positioning. The patient is then prepared and draped as in routine VATS procedures. The superior portion of the drape is allowed to cover the patient's head. The table is unlocked and rotated 30° from its normal position in order to facilitate the positioning of the robot over the patient's head.

Stage I: Routine VATS

The procedure is started using standard VATS instrumentation and incisions. The surgeon stands facing the patient's back (Figs. 24.2 and 24.3). A 2 cm incision (camera incision) is made in the eighth intercostal space in the midaxillary line. A 10 mm metal trocar is introduced, and the Olympus EndoEYE (Center Valley, PA) video endoscope which is used in the VATS portion of the operation is positioned over the dome of the diaphragm.

The oblique fissure is identified and an incision is made anteriorly on the chest wall overlying the oblique fissure in the anterior axillary line at least five fingerbreadths from the camera incision.

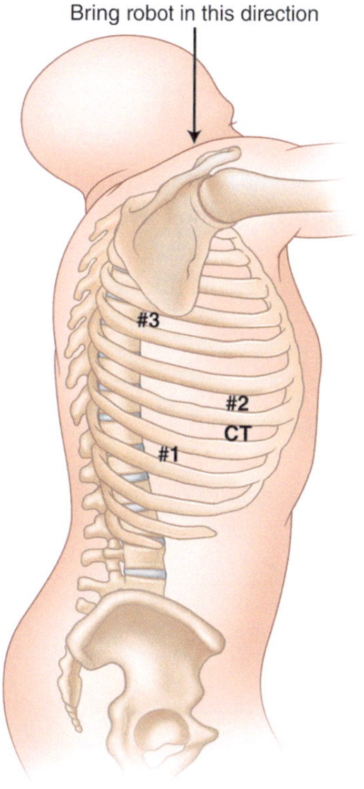

Fig. 24.2 Port placement for robotic lobectomy in the right chest

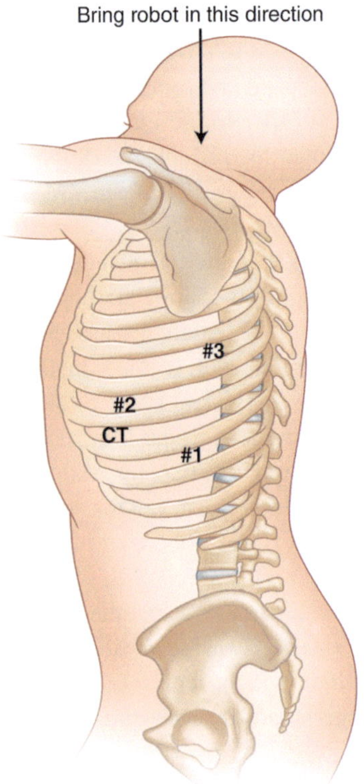

Fig. 24.3 Port placement for robotic lobectomy in the left chest

This incision will be used for the left robotic arm during the robotic portion of the operation. A third 2 cm incision is made one interspace below the interspace for the anterior incision in the posterior axillary line at least five fingerbreadths from the camera incision. This incision will be used by the right robotic arm. It is important to note that as different pulmonary pathology results in changes in relationships between the fissures and the overlying intercostal spaces, the planning of our incisions is based on the initial view of the oblique fissure rather than an arbitrary predetermined positioning over certain intercostal spaces. This technique allows us to have the optimal visualization and access to the hilum in all patients. Furthermore, it is important to note that the anterior and posterior incisions need to be separated at least by the width of the surgeon's hand in order to ensure optimal movement of the robotic arms. A fourth 1 cm incision is made in the same interspace and three fingerbreadths anterior to the camera incision. An atraumatic paddle retractor (Covidien, Inc. Minneapolis, MN) is introduced through this incision for retraction of the lung in an anterior and medial direction during robotic mediastinal dissection.

At the end of the procedure, a 28 Fr straight chest tube is introduced through this incision and positioned in the posterior aspect of the pleural space. The paddle retractor is used to sweep the lung medially and enhances the exposure of the mediastinum. Once the optimal positioning of the retractor is attained, it is held in place by a mechanical holder and fixed to the operating room table. For lobectomy procedures, the robot is positioned and repositioned two to three times depending on the lobe being resected.

Stage II: Robotic Dissection

1. Mediastinal dissection: At this point, the robot is brought into the operating field over the patient's head. The camera arm is introduced through the camera incision. In the right pleural space, the right robotic arm with the robotic hook cautery is positioned through the anterior incision and the EndoWrist is positioned over the mediastinum. The left robotic arm with a robotic DeBakey forceps is positioned through the posterior incision over the paddle retractor and its EndoWrist is also positioned over the mediastinum. A metal suction is introduced by the first assistant through the posterior incision below the robotic arm and is used to evacuate smoke, provide occasional retraction, and remove blood from the field. In the left pleural space, the hook cautery is introduced through the posterior incision and the forceps through the anterior incision. At all times the robotic arms are oriented such that the hook is manipulated by the surgeon's right hand and the forceps by the surgeon's left hand. At this juncture, the surgeon assumes his position at the robotic console. It is our preference for the surgeon to remain gowned and gloved such that he can rapidly attend to any unanticipated events without the need to rescrub. In the event of complication, the surgeon can remove the contaminated

gown and glove, quickly change into a sterile gown and gloves, and attend to the patient in an expeditious manner. The pleura overlying the mediastinum is opened and all visible nodal tissue from the subcarinal and paraesophageal spaces as well as the pulmonary ligament area are removed at this portion of the operation. It is paramount to perform a complete mediastinal lymphadenectomy at this point of the lobectomy procedure. Nodes are placed in a small endobag and removed by the assistant at the table. Following the mediastinal dissection, the robotic camera and the robotic arms are repositioned by the surgeon to view the paratracheal region and a complete nodal dissection of the paratracheal region is completed. We find that the daVinci robot affords a deeper and more complete mediastinal lymphadenectomy as compared to the VATS technique and is comparable to an open procedure. Following the lymphadenectomy, the robotic arm and the camera are moved back to the posterior aspect of the hilum and used to dissect the proximal portion of the pulmonary artery, the anterior branch of the pulmonary artery, the bronchus, and the inferior pulmonary vein in cases which require a lower lobectomy.

2. Anterior hilar dissection (upper lobectomy patients only): At this point, the surgeon changes his gown and gloves and the robotic arms are moved out of the chest. In patients undergoing upper lobectomy, paddle retractor is repositioned to retract the lung posteriorly and to expose the anterior aspect of the hilum. Once again, once optimal visualization is obtained, the paddle retractor is affixed to the table. The robotic camera is repositioned, this time to view the anterior hilum, and the right and the left arms are repositioned as described previously with similar instruments. However, this time, the EndoWrists are positioned over the anterior mediastinum. The robotic arms are then used to dissect the superior pulmonary vein and the anterior hilum.
3. Pulmonary artery and dissection of the oblique fissure: As a third robotic maneuver in patients undergoing upper lobectomies or as a second robotic maneuver in patients undergoing middle or lower lobectomies, the robot is repositioned over the fissure. During this phase of the procedure, the N_1 nodes are dissected and the pulmonary artery over its entire length is dissected and skeletonized.

A few principles are strictly adhered to in the robotic phase of the VATS lobectomy:

1. A much wider dissection of the vascular and bronchial structures is performed. This allows for more mobility of the fragile structures and decreases the risk of catastrophic events.
2. The robot is an excellent tool for dissection. The robotic platform is used for dissection of the fragile thoracic structures. Once the dissection is complete, we feel that manipulation and division of the vascular and bronchial structures are better accomplished using VATS instruments and stapling devices.
3. In the event of bleeding, the assistant places pressure over the bleeding site with the metal suction. At this point, the robotic arms and camera are withdrawn and the control of bleeding is obtained using VATS techniques as have been described earlier in this chapter. After the bleeding is brought under control, the robot is repositioned and surgery continues. We have found the robotic platform to be unsuitable for control of bleeding or other catastrophic events. Once dissection is completed, the robot is withdrawn and lobectomy is completed by VATS. The vessels and bronchus are divided using conventional endoscopic staplers.

Following the completion of the lobectomy, the specimen is retrieved in the manner which was described earlier in this chapter through the anterior incision. The pulmonary vein stump is inspected for hemostasis and repaired with endoscopic suturing techniques using 4-0 Prolene® (Ethicon Endo-Surgery, Blue Ash, OH) if necessary. Sealant (Evicel®, Johnson and Johnson, New Brunswick, NJ) is applied to the staple lines as described earlier. The bronchial stump is tested with 30 cm airway pressure and the remaining lung is inflated under direct vision. A 28 French chest tube is positioned through the retraction incision as described earlier. The incisions are closed in two layers. The deeper muscle layer is closed with three separate simple sutures of 3-0 PDS. The skin and subcutaneous tissues are closed en bloc with three vertical mattress sutures of 2-0 Prolene. All patients undergo videobronchoscopy with inspection of the bronchial stump and removal of any obstructing secretions. All patients are extubated in the operating theater.

Robotic technology has the potential of greatly improving the accuracy and oncologic efficacy of video-assisted lobectomy for patients with early-stage lung cancer [12, 13].

Endoscopic Robotic Esophagectomy

> The history of esophageal surgery is a tale of men repeatedly losing to a stronger adversary yet persisting in this unequal struggle until the nature of the problems became apparent and the war was won. [14]

Although surgery has been the mainstay of treatment of esophageal carcinoma, the high morbidity and mortality rates associated with surgery have necessitated more palliative procedures as well as the search for nonsurgical therapies. Results of surgical resection have improved. In the 1960s and 1970s, the operability rate of esophageal carcinoma was 58 %, the resectability rate was 39 %, and the mortality associated with resection was 29 %, with an overall 5-year survival of 4 % [15]. In the 1980s, the resectability rate was 56 %, the mortality rate with resection was 13 %, and the 5-year survival was 10 % [16]. Presently in specialized centers which perform greater than 50 procedures per year, the mortality rate is reported at 4.5 % with a 5-year survival of 50.4 % overall [17]. Clearly this dramatic change in the overall survival and operative risk is due to the earlier diagnosis of esophageal carcinoma, refinement of surgical technique and perioperative care, and greater use of multimodality therapy.

Over the past decade, our program for esophageal carcinoma has followed the concept of en bloc resection of the tumor with extensive periesophageal lymphadenectomy. The en bloc resection of esophageal cancer has been accomplished using the Ivor-Lewis approach. In 2004, based on the Society of Thoracic Surgeons database, for patients undergoing esophageal resection using this technique at our institution, the mortality rate was 2 %, pneumonia was seen in 11 % of patients, and there were no anastomotic leaks.

This experience has formed the basis for robotic esophagectomy program at our institution [18]. At the outset of the robotic esophagectomy program, a number of parameters were identified:

1. Our experience with VATS and laparoscopy had clearly demonstrated the feasibility of esophagectomy using minimally invasive techniques. However, in our experience the thoracoscopic approach impaired the ability to perform mediastinal nodal exoneration which has been a requirement of our conventional approach. The thoracoscopic approach was more akin to the lymphadenectomy that was achieved by the transhiatal esophagectomy.
2. Posterior gastric dissection and celiac as well as mediastinal nodal exoneration were far less satisfactory with laparoscopy.
3. The significant morbidity of conventional esophagectomy is due to the cervical esophagogastrostomy during the THE and the morbidity associated with a thoracotomy during the TTE. In order for the robotic program to obviate these difficulties, the thoracic portion of the procedure would need to be performed by minimally invasive techniques and the esophagogastric anastomosis needed to be positioned in the chest.
4. The ideal robotic procedure would be one where a combined robotic video-assisted thoracoscopic and laparoscopic procedure would be accomplished with the placement of an esophagogastrostomy in the chest.

With the advent of the daVinci Robot, robotic surgical techniques have been applied to robotic laparoscopic mobilization of the stomach, transhiatal resection of the esophagus, and an open cervical esophagogastrostomy and robotic transthoracic mobilization of the esophagus combined with transhiatal esophagectomy and a cervical esophagogastrostomy. To the best of our knowledge, our program has been one of few centers which have emphasized video-assisted approach to esophagogastrostomy in the chest. It has been our contention that the addition of new robotic technology to the technique of transhiatal esophagectomy suffers from the shortcomings of the conventional THE.

Based on our experience with conventional esophagectomy, we determined that a robotic esophagectomy program should be designed based on the following parameters: (1) Oncologic efficacy of conventional procedures should be retained; (2) the complications associated with thoracotomy should be obviated; and (3) an intrathoracic esophagogastrostomy should be performed.

At the present time, the patients undergoing robotic esophagectomy at our institution undergo a transabdominal robotic laparoscopic mobilization of the stomach followed by a transthoracic robotic thoracoscopic esophagectomy and an intrathoracic video-assisted esophagogastrostomy.

Part I: Laparoscopic Gastric Dissection

The patient is placed in a supine position. Five abdominal ports are placed on the anterior abdominal wall, an approach similar to laparoscopic antireflux procedures. We prefer a 10–12 VersaPort™ (Covidien Autosuture™, Minneapolis, MN) for each of the trocar sites and Visiport™ (Covidien Autosuture™, Minneapolis, MN) instrument for entry into the peritoneum. The peritoneum is entered below the umbilicus using the Visiport instrument. The abdomen is inflated, and ports #2 and #3 are placed at the level of the umbilicus at the right and left mammary lines. A Diamond-Flex® (Snowden Penser®, Tucker, GA) liver retractor is introduced through port number two and placed under the left lateral segment of the liver. The retractor is fixed by a self-retaining system (Mediflex, Velmed, Wexford, PA) to the operating table. This maneuver exposes the esophageal hiatus. An endoscopic Babcock is introduced through port #3 and used to retract the stomach inferiorly. Ports #4 and #5 are placed in the subcostal region and are positioned to "line up" with the left and right sides of the esophageal hiatus. The phreno-esophageal ligament is opened using Endoshears and the esophagogastric junction is exposed. The Harmonic® Scalpel (Ethicon Endo-Surgery, Blue Ash, OH) is used to divide the gastrocolic omentum and the short gastric vessels. The gastroepiploic artery is preserved. The endoscopic Babcock is removed and a fan retractor (Auto Suture, U.S. Surgical Inc) is positioned through incision #3 and the stomach is retracted superiorly. The left gastric pedicle is divided using an endoscopic reticulating 45 mm vascular stapler (Ethicon Endo-Surgery, Blue Ash, OH). We generally do not perform a pyloromyotomy or pyloroplasty during the laparoscopic procedure. The occasional postoperative pyloric obstruction has been shown to be easily amenable to balloon dilatation. The gastric tube is constructed by dividing the stomach using an EZ 45 stapler (Ethicon Endo-Surgery, Blue Ash, OH) starting just proximal to the right gastric artery on the lesser curve of the stomach and proceeding to the apex of the greater curve. Due to the greater ease of suturing in the chest, the gastric suture line is oversewn using 000 polypropylene suture during the robotic video-assisted portion of the procedure. The esophagus is divided using the EZ-45 stapler at just above the gastroesophageal junction. Using an endostitch with 0 Ethibond (Ethicon Endo-Surgery, Blue Ash, OH) suture, the proximal gastric tube is attached to the transected distal esophagus. The jejunostomy is fashioned by suturing a loop of proximal jejunum onto the anterior abdominal wall with an endostitch instrument and 00 Ethibond suture. A needle catheter jejunostomy kit (Compact Biosystems, Minneapolis, MN) is used to percutaneously place a jejunostomy catheter into the jejunum. The jejunal entry site is further fixed to the anterior abdominal wall in order to prevent spillage and torsion. At the conclusion of the procedure, the right and left sides of the right crural arch are sutured using an endostitch instrument with 0 Ethibond suture. This maneuver facilitates the suture ligation of the phrenic vein which overlies the crural arch. The crural arch is opened with Endoshears™ (Covidien, Minneapolis, MN) and the distal esophagus is further mobilized. This maneuver invariably results in loss of pneumoperitoneum and should be reserved for the conclusion of the procedure. The trocar sites are closed using an EXIT instrument and 0 Vicryl (Ethicon Endo-Surgery, Blue Ash, OH). Subcutaneous tissues are closed with 00 Vicryl® and the skin is closed with staples. In these patients esophagectomy and an intrathoracic esophagogastrostomy are accomplished using robotic right video-assisted thoracic surgical techniques.

Part II: Robotic Right Video-Assisted Thoracic Surgical Esophagectomy with an Intrathoracic Esophagogastrostomy

This portion of the procedure is similar for Groups 1 and 2. The room setup on preparation of the robot has been covered in a separate chapter in this book.

Anesthesia

Patients undergoing robotic esophagectomy require single-lung ventilation. We prefer a left-sided double-lumen endotracheal tube to a bronchial block. With a double-lumen tube, lung collapse is superior and hilar manipulation does not result in movement of the blocker and compromise in patient ventilation and surgical visualization. It is imperative for the lungs to remain deflated during the robotic procedure. Longer tubing is required as during the robotic procedure the anesthesiologist occupies a more remote position than in the usual video-assisted thoracic surgical procedures.

Patient Positioning

The patient is placed in a full lateral decubitus position. The table is flexed to open the intercostal spaces. The position of the double-lumen tube is reconfirmed after final patient positioning. The patient is then prepared and draped in a routine manner as with all video-assisted thoracic surgical procedures. The superior portion of the drape is allowed to cover the patient's head. The robot is brought in perpendicular to the patient's back. Final fine docking maneuvers are performed by unlocking the table and positioning the patient into the robotic arms.

Stage I: Routine Vats for Division of the Azygous Vein

The procedure starts using standard video-assisted thoracic surgical instrumentation and incisions. The surgeons stand facing the patient's back. A 2 cm incision is made in the sixth intercostal space in the midaxillary line (incision # 1) (Fig. 24.4). A 10 mm metal trocar is introduced, and a zero degree Olympus EndoEYE video endoscope is used for this portion of the procedure. Three other 2 cm incisions are made. Incision # 2 is made in the third intercostal space in the anterior axillary line. Incision # 3 is made in the fifth intercostal space in the posterior axillary line. Incision # 4 is made in the eighth intercostal space in the anterior axillary line. Incisions # 1, # 2, and #3 are used during the VATS portion of the procedure. Incisions # 1, #2, and #4 are used during the robotic portion of the procedure. An atraumatic paddle retractor (Auto Suture, Covidien, Minneapolis, MN) is introduced through a 10 mm port in the seventh intercostal space in the anterior axillary line. At the end of the procedure a 28-French straight chest tube is introduced through this port and positioned in the posterior aspect of the pleural space. The paddle retractor is used to sweep the lung medially and enhances exposure of the posterior mediastinum. Once the optimal position of the retractor is attained, it is held in place by a mechanical holder (Mediflex, Velmed, Wexford, PA) and fixed to the operating room table. At this point a 30° Olympus EndoEYE video endoscope is introduced through incision # 1. Incisions # 2 and #3 are used to dissect the azygous vein. An endoscopic reticulating 45 mm vascular stapler (Ethicon Endo-Surgery, Blue Ash, OH) is used to divide the azygous vein.

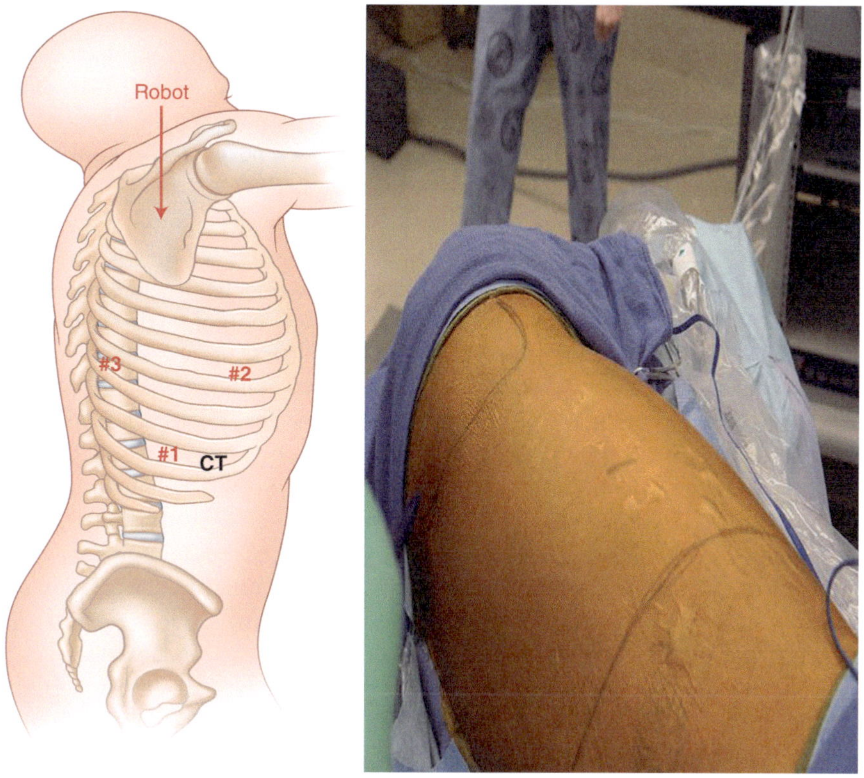

Fig. 24.4 Port placement for robotic esophagectomy through the right chest

Stage II: Robotic Esophagectomy

Following the division of the azygous vein, esophagectomy is accomplished using the robot. A paddle retractor is introduced through incision #4 and the lung is retracted medially. The robot is brought over the head of the patient. The camera port is positioned in incision #1. The right robotic arm with the hook cautery is positioned through incision # 2. The left robotic arm with a robotic DeBakey forceps is positioned through incision # 3. A metal suction is introduced by the first assistant under the robotic arms in incisions # 2 and 3 and used to evacuate smoke, provide retraction, and remove blood from the field. Dissection is started just posterior to the right mainstem bronchus and the subcarinal nodes are dissected away from the carina and towards the esophagus. Next dissection is continued in a caudad direction just posterior to the lung down to the level of the esophageal hiatus. Tissue is removed from back of the pericardium and the inferior pulmonary vein and all tissues are swept towards the esophagus. Next a posterior dissection is begun in a line parallel to the anterior border of the azygous vein. All periesophageal tissue is dissected from the esophageal hiatus to above the azygous vein. At the conclusion of the dissection, the left pleura should be seen at the depth of the field of dissection. Furthermore, the posterior pericardium should be seen anteriorly, the aorta should be seen posteriorly, and the left mainstem bronchus and distal trachea should be clearly visible superiorly. Following the en bloc dissection of the esophagus, the right robotic arm is used to place Hemoclips on the thoracic duct which is invariably damaged as the result of the extensive mediastinal exoneration. The nasogastric tube is withdrawn and the esophagus is transected above the azygous vein.

Stage III: Intrathoracic Stapled Esophagogastrostomy or Robotic Hand-Sewn Robotic Esophagogastrostomy

We have used two anastomotic techniques. Both techniques will be presented. Presently, our preference is a robotic hand-sewn end to side esophagogastrostomy.

After the extensive esophageal dissection, which is enabled by the robot, conventional video-assisted thoracic surgical techniques are used for the creation of the esophagogastric anastomosis. A 30° Olympus EndoEYE video endoscope is placed in incision # 4 and provides a panoramic view of the pleural space. The esophagus specimen is placed in an Endopouch and withdrawn through incision # 2. The pathologist is instructed to examine the proximal and distal resection margins. Using atraumatic pediatric lung clamps, the stomach tube is delivered into the right chest. Great care is exercised to avoid excessive tension on the gastric wall in order to avoid disruption of the intraluminal vessels. Furthermore, just enough stomach is pulled to the level of the thoracic inlet in order to prevent kinking at the level of the hiatus. Finally the greater curve is positioned in the mediastinum and care is taken not to twist the stomach tube. For the creation of an intrathoracic esophagogastric anastomosis, we prefer a circular 25 mm End-to-End Anastomosis Stapler (EEA, Ethicon Endo-Surgery Inc, Blue Ash, OH). In order to ensure incorporation of the esophageal mucosa, into this staple line, the esophageal mucosa and muscle are sutured together at 3, 6, 9, and 12 o'clock positions. Long 000 silk sutures are used and two dots are placed using extracorporeal knot-tying techniques and a knot pusher. A purse string suture of 000 polypropylene is placed on the esophagus using "Lewis" thoracoscopic needle drivers introduced through incisions # 2 and #3 and used to drive and retrieve the needle. The anvil of the stapling device is introduced into the esophagus and the purse string suture is tightened using a knot pusher. At this point the anvil is held in place using a kidney pedicle clamp which is introduced through incision # 2. The placement of the clamp on the distal aspect of the anvil prevents migration into the proximal esophagus. The anterior wall of the stomach tube is opened using electrocautery and two full-thickness sutures of 00 polypropylene are placed at the 3 and 9 o'clock positions and brought out through incision #1. These sutures will provide appropriate traction on the stomach wall during the stapling maneuvers. A disposal suction is used to clear the stomach tube of all contents. This allows manipulation of the stomach without spillage into the pleural space. The shaft of the EEA instrument is introduced through incision #1 into the pleural space. The EEA is then passed through the gastrostomy towards the apex of the stomach tube. After exiting through the apex of the stomach, the EEA instrument is used to engage the anvil and closed, thus creating an esophagogastrostomy. Following the creation of the anastomosis, the instrument is withdrawn from the gastrostomy, placed in an Endopouch® (Ethicon Endo-Surgery Inc, Blue Ash, OH), and withdrawn out of the pleural space. The doughnuts of tissue are examined in order to determine the need for further reinforcement of a specific location on the circular anastomosis. The internal aspect of the anastomosis is further inspected by visualization through the gastrostomy. We routinely place 000 silk horizontal mattress seromuscular sutures at the anastomosis. These sutures are tied using extracorporeal knot-tying techniques and a knot pusher. The gastrostomy is closed using a roticulating 45 mm endoscopic stapler (Ethicon Endo-Surgery, Blue Ash, OH) with a thick tissue insert. The staple line is further reinforced with a running 000 polypropylene suture. The nasogastric tube is passed by the anesthesiologist through the esophagogastric anastomosis and positioned at the distal portion of the stomach tube. All suture lines are covered with Evicel® (Ethicon Endo-Surgery, Blue Ash, OH) fibrin sealant. The gastric tube is tacked to the posterior pleural using 000 silk sutures. A small flat Jackson-Pratt drain is introduced through incision # 4 and positioned in the mediastinum adjacent to the esophagogastric anastomosis. As stated earlier, the retractor is removed and replaced with a 28 French straight chest tube which is positioned in the posterior aspect of the pleural space. The lung is reinflated. The four incisions are closed with en bloc musculosubcutaneous sutures of 0 PDS (Ethicon Endo-Surgery, Blue Ash, OH). Skin is closed with interrupted mattress sutures of 00 polypropylene.

In order to accomplish the robotic hand-sewn anastomosis, the robot is positioned with camera through incision #1, and the right and left robotic arms each carrying a needle driver through incisions #2 and 3. A two-layer running anastomosis in fashioned. The esophagus is placed onto the superior aspect of the stomach tube. A running barbed nonabsorbable suture (V-Loc™ PBT, Covidien, Minneapolis, MN) is used to approximate the posterior layer of the esophagus to the serosa of the stomach. This suture is left in the chest and used to complete the anterior nonabsorbable layer. The stomach is opened, and, using a running barbed absorbable suture (V-Loc™ 180, Covidien, Minneapolis, MN), the inner posterior and anterior layer of the anastomosis is completed. Following the inner layer the nonabsorbable suture is picked up and used to complete the anterior second layer of the anastomosis. Patients routinely undergo bronchoscopy with removal of secretions and tracheobronchial toilet prior to extubation. An upper gastrointestinal study with water-soluble contrast is obtained on postoperative day 7.

Robotic Resection of Mediastinal Masses

In the era of VATS and robotic surgery the approach to the diagnosis and treatment of anterior mediastinal masses (in the anterosuperior compartment) has undergone a significant change. Traditionally, image-guided transthoracic needle biopsy (TTNA) and anterior mediastinotomy (Chamberlain Procedure) have been used for the diagnosis of lesions in this anatomic region. In this particular application, the technique of TTNA has a number of shortcomings: (1) the inability to provide adequate tissue for a meaningful diagnosis and appropriate subtyping of lymphoma; (2) the inability to differentiate lymphoma from thymoma; and (3) the inability to differentiate a benign from an invasive thymic epithelial neoplasm (thymoma). On the other hand, aside from the inherent risks of surgery, the anterior mediastinotomy approach suffers from (1) the inability to adequately visualize the surgical field due to a small "keyhole" incision; (2) the risk of surgical complications resulting from inadequate exposure and visualization; (3) the delay in the application of radiotherapy following tissue diagnosis due to the need for wound healing prior to application of radiation; (4) occasional incisional wound breakdown following the application of radiation to the area encompassing the mediastinotomy; and (5) the need for a second definitive surgical procedure for certain types of anterior mediastinal masses.

With the advent of VATS and robotic thoracic surgery the algorithm for the diagnosis and therapy of anterior mediastinal masses has changed. The advantages of these approaches are as follows: (1) The incisions are placed in the lateral chest wall away from the field of radiation which typically encompasses the entire anterior chest wall. Using the laterally placed incisions, in patients with lymphoma there is no need to delay radiation therapy while awaiting wound healing. (2) The minimally invasive video endoscopic techniques yield adequate tissue for appropriate differentiation of thymic epithelial neoplasms from lymphoma. (3) In patients with resectable lesions surgical resection can be accomplished in the same setting [19, 20].

Robotic Transthoracic Heller Myotomy

The emergence of video endoscopic techniques changed the approach to the surgical therapy of achalasia. Laparoscopic techniques allowed for better transabdominal visualization and manipulation of the gastroesophageal junction. Until the advent of laparoscopy, visualization of the GE junction by virtue of its location deep under the costal arch required extensive retraction. Even with the use of self-retaining retractors, visualization of the GE junction remained suboptimal.

As the direct result of the inability to see, open transabdominal myotomy was associated with poor results. The extensive use of laparoscopy for fundoplication in patients with gastroesophageal reflux disease provided greater facility and familiarization with the anatomy of the gastroesophageal junction. It was not difficult to extrapolate the techniques used for fundoplasty to the procedure of esophageal myotomy which, if performed transabdominally, required an antireflux procedure at any rate. Unlike conventional surgery, video endoscopic techniques were associated with lower morbidity and pain, as well as shorter hospital stays. Therefore, these minimally invasive techniques with the promise of better long-term results were more favorable to nonsurgical approaches and found acceptance among patients and medical practitioners.

In 1991, Shimi et al. reported the first laparoscopic experience for Heller myotomy, and Pellegrini et al. reported a series of patients who had undergone esophageal myotomy using the thoracoscopic approach [21, 22].

Laparoscopic Approach

The object of the laparoscopic esophageal myotomy and anterior fundoplication is to perform myotomy of the lower 6 cm of the esophagus and the proximal 2 cm of the stomach. In order to access the intrathoracic esophagus, this procedure requires full dissection of the right crus of the diaphragm and the entire esophageal hiatus. Consequently, following myotomy, a partial anterior gastric fundoplication is performed as an antireflux procedure. Invariably, all series reporting the laparoscopic approach to Heller myotomy have shown excellent relief of dysphagia. In one series of 133 patients who had undergone laparoscopic myotomy with a partial fundoplication, Patti et al. reported 11 % persistent dysphagia, 17 % new gastroesophageal reflux, and 5 % mucosal perforations which were amenable to laparoscopic closure [23, 24]. The majority of difficulties with the laparoscopic approach were related to reflux and the technical aspects of the fundoplication. In a series of 69 patients undergoing laparoscopic myotomy and fundoplication for achalasia, Finley et al. reported a median operative time of 1.9 h, one mucosal perforation which was amenable to laparoscopic repair, 96 % patient satisfaction for relief of dysphagia, and a 9 % rate of new postoperative gastroesophageal reflux [25].

Thoracoscopic Approach

During the thoracoscopic approach, the esophagus is approached through the left chest. The myotomy is carried down to the gastroesophageal junction. During this approach, either the gastroesophageal junction is left intact or the left rim of the right crus is opened and subsequently reapproximated following the myotomy. With the thoracoscopic approach, an antireflux procedure has not been necessary. Whereas the complications of the laparoscopic approach have been related to reflux and the antireflux procedures, the thoracoscopic approach has suffered from the difficulty of residual achalasia and the steep learning curve associated with obtaining a complete myotomy. The most important complication following the thoracoscopic approach has been incomplete myotomy and persistent dysphagia [26]. Pellegrini et al. have reported that after thoracoscopic myotomy, dysphagia was relieved in 70 % of patients, 12 % of patients had residual achalasia, and mild reflux was seen in 20 % of patients. Stewart et al. reported esophageal perforation in 12 % of patients undergoing the thoracoscopic esophageal myotomy and conversion to thoracotomy in 21 % of patients. The mean hospitalization for this group of patients was 6 days. In the same group at 42 months, 31 % of patients had relief of dysphagia and 23 % of patients had new gastroesophageal reflux. Patti et al. reported a 6 % conversion to a thoracotomy, a 73 % rate of relief of dysphagia, and a 25 % rate of incomplete myotomy. The data have shown the laparoscopic procedure to have a lower conversion rate to an open procedure and to be associated with lower morbidity and shorter hospitalization. Most importantly, the laparoscopic Heller myotomy with an anterior fundoplasty has shown excellent relief of dysphagia at the expense of the higher rate of new gastroesophageal reflux.

Due to these results at the present time, the laparoscopic approach has become the initial approach of choice for patients undergoing the surgical palliation for achalasia [27, 28].

Operative Technique

Anesthesia

Patients undergoing video-assisted thoracic surgical Heller myotomy require single-lung ventilation. We prefer a left-sided double-lumen endotracheal tube to a bronchial blocker. With a double-lumen tube, lung collapse is superior and hilar manipulation does not result in movement of the blocker and inadvertent expansion of the lung. As is addressed in a separate chapter in this book, the facility of the anesthesiologist with the robotic techniques is crucial to the conduct of the operation. Following the induction of anesthesia, with the patient in the supine position, upper GI endoscopy is performed. The gastroesophageal junction is identified and a nasogastric tube is positioned under direct vision into the stomach. Decompression of the stomach facilitates retraction of the diaphragm and enhances visualization of the gastroesophageal junction. While the patient is in the supine position, the gastroscope is pulled back to the distal esophagus and secured for patient positioning. As has been described by Pellegrini et al., the gastroscope plays a significant role during the myotomy procedure. First, it allows for identification of the left lateral wall of the esophagus without the need for extensive mobilization of a circumferential dissection of the esophagus. Second, it transilluminates the esophageal mucosa and helps in identification of the area of incomplete myotomy. Third, by application of intraluminal suction to the mucosa during the myotomy procedure, the mucosa is pulled towards the lumen of the esophagus, thereby exposing the anterior plane between the esophageal mucosa and the muscle of the esophagus.

Patient Positioning

The patient is placed in an extended right lateral decubitus position. The table is fully flexed to enlarge the space between the ribs. The surgeon

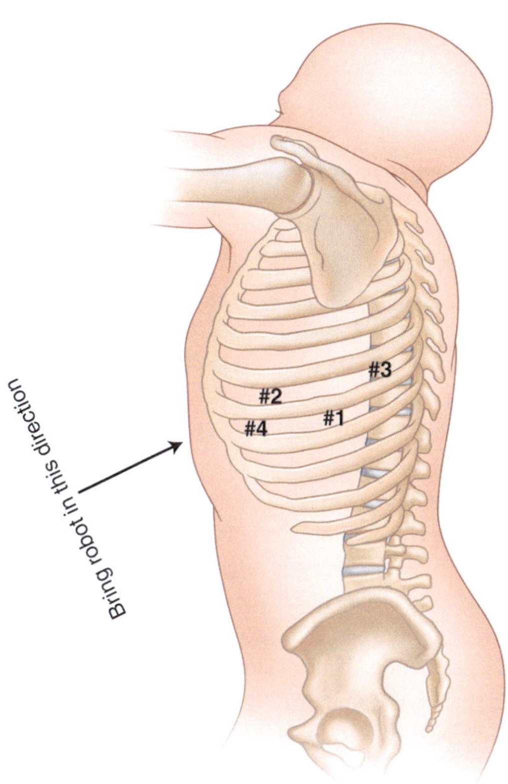

Fig. 24.5 Port placement for robotic Heller myotomy through the left chest

stands behind the patient. A monitor is positioned at the patient's feet and a second monitor is positioned in front of the patient facing the surgeon. The robot is positioned in front of the patient (Fig. 24.5). During the robotic portion of the procedure, the robot is brought into the operative field from an anterior to posterior direction facing cephalad at a 30° angle to the axis of the patient.

Myotomy

After the patient is prepped and draped, a 2 cm incision (# 1) is made in the seventh intercostal space in the midaxillary line. This incision will serve as a camera port during the VATS and robotic portion of the operation. A second 2 cm incision (# 2) is made in the sixth intercostal space anteriorly at the anterior axillary line. A third 2 cm incision (# 3) is made in the sixth intercostal space posteriorly at the midscapular line. A fourth 1 cm incision is made one interspace below the anterior incision and as far inferiorly as possible. This incision will be used for placement of the diaphragmatic retractor, and, at the conclusion of the procedure, it will be used for the placement of the drainage chest tubes. It is paramount that this incision be positioned as far anteriorly from incision # 2 in order to decrease interference with the robotic arm. We prefer the Olympus EndoEye Video Endoscopic System. A 10 mm 0° end-viewing scope is positioned initially viewing cephalad over the diaphragm using conventional video-assisted thoracic surgical techniques and viewing the monitor located in front of the patient and facing the surgeon, the inferior pulmonary ligament is divided and the lung is retracted superiorly. The table is positioned in Trendelenburg in order to allow the lung to fall into the apex of the chest. The camera is then rotated 180° in order to view the distal esophagus at the diaphragm. The surgeon and the surgical team then rotate their field of vision and use the video monitor at the patient's feet for the next phase of the procedure. In order to retain intuitive spatial relationships, it is imperative that the surgical team view the surgical site in the same direction and axis as the video endoscope. The gastroscope is rotated to the patient's left, and its tip is flexed, thus allowing the surgeon to visualize the distal esophagus without the need for further dissection (Fig. 24.5). Using conventional Endoshears (Ethicon Endo-Surgery, Blue Ash, OH) with cautery attachment, the pleura overlying the esophagus is divided. An endostitch instrument (Autosuture, Covidien, Minneapolis, MN) with a 2-0 Ethibond suture is used to place retraction sutures on the two edges of the pleura. The sutures are then brought out through the anterior and posterior incisions (incisions # 2 and #4) and fixed to the drapes. This maneuver creates a pleural sling and elevates the esophagus from its normal mediastinal location into the left pleural space. A fan retractor (Ethicon Endo-Surgery, Blue Ash, OH) is introduced through the anterior (#4) incision and positioned on the posteromedial aspect of the diaphragm and used to retract the diaphragm inferiorly. This retractor is fixed to the table by the use of a mechanical holder (Mediflex, Velmed, Inc., Wexford, PA). The esophageal hiatus is identified and the left lateral limb of the right crus of the diaphragm is divided using the Endoshears with cautery. The dissection is discontinued with the visualization of the phreno-esophageal ligament on the underside of the diaphragm. Using the endostitch instrument with a 0 Ethibond suture, full-thickness retraction sutures are placed on the cut edges of the diaphragm and brought out through the anterior and posterior incisions, respectively (#2 and #4). The sutures are fixed to the drapes. This maneuver allows for the full visualization of the esophagogastric junction. At the end of the procedure, the cut edges of the right limb of the right crus of the diaphragm are re-approximated using an endostitch instrument with 0 Ethibond suture. Usually, three such sutures are necessary. By avoiding disruption of the anterior crural arch and by restoring the integrity of the right limb of the right crus of the diaphragm, the crural sling is preserved and the antireflux barrier remains intact. At this point, the VATS camera is removed and the robot is positioned. The robot is brought in from the anterior aspect of the patient. It is positioned caudad to cephalad with 30° rotation in the cephalad direction on the patient's axis. The camera port is positioned in the camera incision (# 1) and a 30° down-viewing scope is positioned viewing caudally onto the distal esophagus. The right robotic arm with a hook end-effector instrument connected to a cautery is placed through the anterior incision (#2) and its EndoWrist is positioned directly over the distal esophagus. A left robotic arm with a DeBakey forceps as its distal end-effector instrument is positioned through the posterior incision (#3) and its EndoWrist is positioned directly over the distal esophagus. A metal suction with a blunt tip is positioned through the anterior incision below the entry point of the right robotic arm. The suction is used by the assistant to evacuate cautery smoke, control bleeding, and provide downward force on the esophageal mucosa during the myotomy, should this become necessary. With binocular view and depth perception and the facility of the EndoWrist movements, the performance of esophageal myotomy is quite accurate and uncomplicated. The muscular wall of the esophagus is exposed and the muscle is divided with a hook cautery at the midpoint of the exposed esophagus. The anatomic plane between the mucosa and the muscle is identified. The blunt metal suction is positioned on the mucosa; endoluminal suction is also applied using the video gastroscope. The robotic forceps are used to elevate the muscle layers. The culmination of these maneuvers allows for the hook cautery (blended coagulation current set at 30 W) to be used to divide the muscle of the esophagus. At the distal aspect of the esophagus and the intussuscepted portion of the esophagus into the proximal stomach is approached, the robotic forceps are used to reduce the intussusception by pulling the esophagus in a cephalad direction. The hook cautery then completes the myotomy approximately 1 cm onto the cardia of the stomach. Myotomy is discontinued when the submucosal vascular plexus of the stomach wall is visualized. At this point, the gastroscope is advanced past the GE junction into the stomach. The ease of movement of the gastroscope into the stomach and the lack of resistance confirm the complete division of the esophageal muscles at the GE junction. Furthermore, the gastroscope is retroflexed to view the GE junction from a caudad-to-cephalad direction. Observation of the transilluminated mucosa of the proximal portion of the stomach cardia from the light of the robotic camera serves as the final confirmation for the completion of the esophageal myotomy. Following the completion of the myotomy, the chest is filled with saline and the gastroscope is used to insufflate air into the stomach and esophagus in order to rule out any mucosal perforation. Any mucosal perforations are easily repaired by the endoscopic techniques and the use of 4-0 Prolene® (Ethicon Endo-Surgery, Blue Ash, OH) sutures. The robotic arms are retracted and the robot is moved away from the table. At this juncture, the conventional VATS EndoEYE camera is inserted through the camera port and the left limb of the right crus of the diaphragm is re-approximated as described earlier. At this point, a 2 cm square piece of Vicryl® mesh (Ethicon Endo-Surgery, Blue Ash, OH) is positioned at the distal aspect of the mediastinum. This absorbable mesh was attached to the edges of the mediastinal pleura using the endostitch with 2-0 Ethibond sutures. We have found that the Vicryl mesh which is absorbed and replaced by scar tissue approximately 8 weeks following implantation reestablished the integrity of the pleura on the left lateral aspect of the esophagus and repositions the distal esophagus into the mediastinum. Furthermore, this maneuver with the resultant scarring of the pleura prevents the formation of a mucosal diverticulum at the distal portion of the esophagus. It has been hypothesized that the mucosal diverticulum may be one of the causes of chronic dysphagia even with an adequate myotomy when a fundoplasty is not performed. In fact, some authors have proposed that one of the benefits of the fundoplasty is the prevention of a mucosal diverticulum by placing external pressure on the mucosa. Prior to the employment of this technique, we had observed mucosal outpouching at the distal esophagus and the level of the gastroesophageal junction in a number of patients. This technique seems to have addressed that issue without any negative sequelae. Following the pleural closure, the diaphragmatic retractor is removed. The lung is reinflated under direct vision. A 28-French straight chest tube is inserted through incision No. 4 and positioned posteriorly in the pleural space. ON-Q® PainBuster® (Halyard Health, Alpharetta, GA) catheters are positioned in a subpleural tunnel extending from the second to the eighth intercostal spaces, and the incisions are closed as done in video-assisted surgery. The gastroscope is used to confirm the appropriate position of the nasogastric tube. The patient is extubated in the operating room. Postoperatively, we routinely obtain an upper GI contrast study with water-soluble contrast in order to rule out mucosal perforation and to confirm completeness of the distal esophageal myotomy. With a satisfactory study, a soft diet is started, the chest tube is removed, and most patients are discharged on the second postoperative day.

References

1. American Cancer Society. Cancer facts and figures-2001. Atlanta: American Cancer Society; 2001.
2. Jacobeus HC. Possibility of the use of the cystoscope for investigation of serous cavities. Munch Med Wochenschr. 1910;57:2090.
3. Kaiser LR. Diagnostic and therapeutic uses of pleuroscopy (thoracoscopy) in lung cancer. Surg Clin North Am. 1987;67:1081.
4. Kirby TJ. Invited commentary. Ann Thorac Surg. 1997;63:1421–2.
5. Braimbridge MV. Thoracoscopy—a historical perspective. In: Yim APC, Hazelrrig SR, Izzat MB, et al., editors. Minimal access cardiothoracic surgery. Philadelphia: WB Saunders; 2000.
6. McKenna RJ, Wolf RK, Brenner M, et al. Is lobectomy by video-assisted thoracic surgery an adequate cancer operation? Ann Thorac Surg. 1998;66:1903–7.
7. Mack MJ, Scruggs GR, Kelly KM, et al. Video-assisted thoracic surgery: has technology found its placed? Ann Thorac Surg. 1997;64:111.
8. Yim APC, Landreneau RJ, Izzat MB, Fung ALK. Is video-assisted thoracoscopic lobectomy a unified approach? Ann Thorac Surg. 1998;16:1155.
9. Lewis RJ, Caccavale N, Boncage JP, et al. Video-assisted thoracic surgical non-rib spreading simultaneously stapled lobectomy: a more patient-friendly oncologic resection. Chest. 1999;116:1119.
10. Lewis RJ. Simultaneously stapled lobectomy: a safe technique for video-assisted thoracic surgery. J Thorac Cardiovasc Surg. 1995;109:619–25.
11. Gharagozloo F, Tempesta B, Margolis M, et al. Video-assisted thoracic surgery lobectomy for stage I lung cancer. Ann Thorac Surg. 2003;76:1009–15.
12. Gharagozloo F, Margolis M, Tempesta B. One hundred consecutive cases of robotic video-assisted lobectomy for lung cancer. Ann Thorac Surg. 2008;85:1880–6.
13. Gharagozloo F, Margolis M, Najam F. Robotic completely endoscopic lobectomy, evolution from VATS to RAVS. In: Gharagozloo F, Najam F, editors. Robotic surgery: theory and operative technique. New York: McGraw Hill; 2008.
14. Emslie RG. Perspectives in the development of esophageal surgery. In: Jamieson GG, editor. Surgery of the esophagus. Melbourne: Churchill Livingstone; 1988. p. 3–8.
15. Earlam R, Cunha-Melo JR. Esophageal squamous cell carcinoma: I—a critical review of surgery. Br J Surg. 1980;67:381.
16. Muller JM, Erasmi H, Stelzner M, et al. Surgical therapy of esophageal carcinoma. Br J Surg. 1990;77:845.
17. Patti MG, Costantini M, Godwin DH, et al. A hospital's annual rate of esophagectomy influences the operative mortality rates. J Gastrointest Surg. 1998;2:186.
18. Gharagozloo F, Margolis M, Najam F. Robotic Ivor Lewis esophagogastrectomy. In: Gharagozloo F, Najam F, editors. Robotic surgery: theory and operative technique. New York: McGraw Hill; 2008.
19. Bodner J, Wykypiel H, Greiner A. Early experience with robot-assisted surgery for mediastinal masses. Ann Thorac Surg. 2004;78:259–65.
20. Margolis M, Gharagozloo F, Najam F. Robotic mediastinal surgery. In: Gharagozloo F, Najam F, editors. Robotic surgery: theory and operative technique. New York: McGraw Hill; 2008.
21. Shimi S, Nathanson LK, Cushieri A. Laparoscopic cardiomyotomy for achalasia. J R Coll Surg Edinb. 1991;36:152.
22. Pelligrini CA, Leichter R, Patti M. Thoracoscopic esophageal myotomy in the treatment of achalasia. Ann Thorac Surg. 1993;56:680–2.
23. Patti MG, Pelligrini CA, Arcerito M. Comparison of medical and minimally invasive surgical therapy for primary esophageal motility disorders. Arch Surg. 1995;130:609–16.
24. Patti MG, Pelligrini CA, Horgan S. Minimally invasive surgery for achalasia. Ann Surg. 1999;230:587.
25. Finley RJ, Clifton JC, Stewart KC, et al. Laparoscopic Heller myotomy for achalasia: a clinical and scintigraphic swallowing follow-up. Can J Surg. 1999; 42(suppl):25.
26. Kc S, Finley RJ, Clifton JC, et al. Thoracoscopic versus laparoscopic modified Heller myotomy for achalasia: efficacy and safety in 87 patients. J Am Coll Surg. 1999;189:164–70.
27. Gharagozloo F, Margolis M, Tempesta B. Robotic thoracoscopic Heller myotomy for achalasia. Chest. 2008;134:82006.
28. Gharagozloo F, Margolis M. Video-assisted thoracic surgical esophageal myotomy with intraoperative manometry for achalasia. Chest. 2007;132:660c.

25 Cardiac Surgery Advances: Do We Still Remember How to Do the Open Bypass?

Soroosh Kiani and Robert S. Poston

Strengths and Weakness of Traditional CABG

Traditional coronary artery bypass grafting (CABG), characterized by a full sternotomy and harvest of venous conduits, is one of the most thoroughly performed and investigated surgical procedures in medical history. CABG volume exceeds 200,000 cases/year only in the USA and has been the subject of multiple randomized controlled prospective clinical trials and retrospective analyses. Based on this extensive experience, this procedure has been continuously improved, optimized, and streamlined and now lends itself to rigorous statistical comparisons of outcomes against well-defined benchmarks from the Society of Thoracic Surgeons (STS) national database. CABG programs have followed methods analogous to those of efficient manufacturing [1] to exploit this strong evidence base in order to create detailed and reproducible management protocols that minimize error and reduce costs. At the same time, CABG has evolved into a fungible *commodity* capable of being provided with reproducible outcomes by most board-certified CT surgeons. Reproducibility enables quality to be tracked with credible metrics that are publically reported and linked to reimbursement through pay-for-performance initiatives. All these issues have been good for healthcare policy. Patients at rural settings that have limited ability to travel have been able to obtain CABG as safely at smaller facilities as the large-volume centers. Moreover, efficiency drives cost containment, which has major implications to our healthcare system given estimated annual expenditures for CABG that exceed $10 billion [2].

A strong value network has developed around CABG based on its stability and familiarity which, paradoxically, poses an important barrier to innovation. Significant changes in surgical technique obligate a learning curve that is associated with transient period of inefficiency. Surgeons have been reluctant to accept this learning period even in the face of competition with nonsurgical options to treat severe coronary diseases such as percutaneous interventions (PCI) [3, 4]. While it is estimated that at least 30 % of all heart surgeons have attempted less invasive approaches to CABG, most have not persisted long enough to get through the learning curve and these techniques are used in less than 0.5 % of all CABG cases in the USA [5]. Even modest innovations have failed to achieve wide-

S. Kiani, M.D., M.S., M.A.
Department of Internal Medicine, University of Virginia, Charlottesville, VA, USA
e-mail: soroosh@bu.edu

R.S. Poston, M.D. (✉)
Department of Cardiothoracic Surgery, St Francis Medical Center, Trenton, NJ, USA
e-mail: postonlab@gmail.com

R. Latifi et al. (eds.), *Technological Advances in Surgery, Trauma and Critical Care*,
DOI 10.1007/978-1-4939-2671-8_25

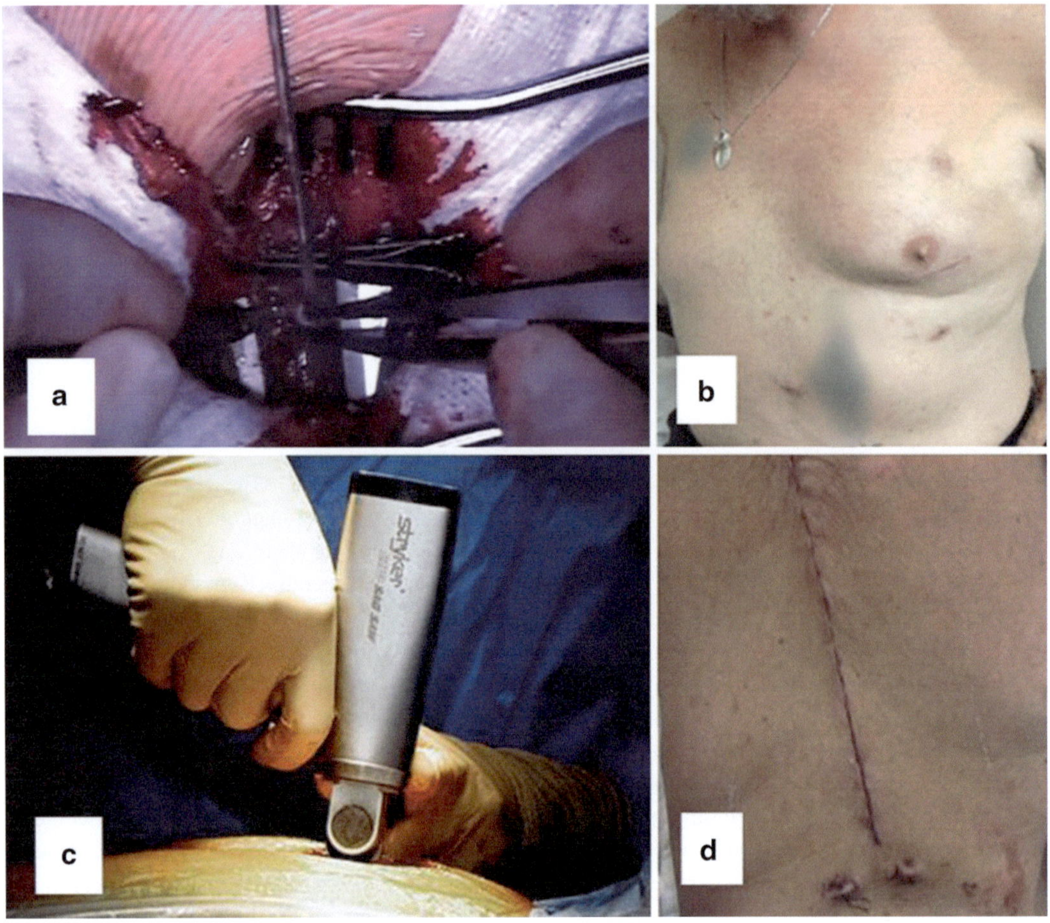

Fig. 25.1 In the less invasive approach, the surgeon can perform a direct, hand-sewn anastomosis of the LIMA to the LAD via a minithoracotomy using the same surgical instruments that would be used in the standard approach (**a**). A sternotomy is avoided by inserting robotic instruments through incisions in the left chest (**b**). In contrast, the standard incision for CABG utilizes a sternal saw (Stryker, Kalamazoo, MI) to widely open the chest cavity via a sternotomy (**c**, **d**)

spread adoption. For example, off-pump CABG via full sternotomy (OPCAB) to avoid side effects from cardiopulmonary bypass (CPB) is done by less than 20 % of surgeons [6]. As of 2014, the mainstay of surgical therapy for coronary heart disease remains fundamentally the same approach to CABG developed 20 years ago: complete CPB, an arrested heart, full median sternotomy, and grafts mainly consisting of saphenous veins.

Strengths and Weaknesses of Less Invasive Surgical Alternatives

Robotic assistance enables less invasive CABG without a median sternotomy (rCABG). Distal anastomoses during rCABG are performed by hand (i.e., minimally invasive direct coronary artery bypass grafting, MIDCAB) or totally endoscopically (TECAB) (Fig. 25.1a–d). Single-center reports about rCABG suggest attenuation of the bleeding and infection risk, reduced postoperative recovery times and convalescence, and shortening of the duration required for pain to resolve [7]. Many of these advantages were anticipated from the sternotomy OPCAB approach, but did not materialize. This suggests that the surgical incision is a more important (and previously underappreciated) driver of morbidity and recovery time than the use of CPB.

An important advantage of rCABG is the ability of this approach to interface with and take advantage of rapidly advancing technology in the field of computers and robotics to further improve surgical outcomes. For example, surgical loupes are used during standard CABG to enhance visualization of the microvascular anastomoses. Loupes provide limited magnification and ability to integrate visual data and represent relatively terminal technology with diminished prospects for future advances. On the other hand, a robotic workstation enables the surgeon to zoom in and out on the relevant anatomy, enhance magnification, and optimize lighting and resolution without sacrificing three-dimensional vision. Dexterity and tremor can be improved by translating larger, choppier movements of the human hand in smaller, better controlled movements of the instruments that interact at the patient end. While learning to perform the entire less invasive procedure is complex, the skills required to use robotic technology itself are acquired far quicker than those required for laparoscopy. This difference from laparoscopy has given robotics the reputation as a "democratizing tool" because it provides a wider range of surgeons with the ability to complete the technical tasks of less invasive procedures.

Further developments in imaging technologies may one day offer the surgeon the ability to detail surgical anatomy or identify other problems beyond what is visible to the human eye. While the existing surgical robot lacks tactile feedback—as subsequent advances in robotics are made, technology is under development that will actually *enhance* tactile feedback when using robotics compared to the human hand. Moreover, as new and competitive companies generating technologies for robotics emerge, the rate of further technological advancement is expected to grow as well. A potential caveat of all these advances is that surgeons may become too accustomed to having these new tools available, making it possible to forget how to do the open approach.

Strength: Patient Satisfaction

Regardless of the surgical approach that predominates, a successful CABG program drives patient traffic and acceptable levels of patient satisfaction because of the impact of this procedure on patient quality of life. Nevertheless, patients have shown a strong preference to know about less invasive surgery. Oftentimes, patients that require referral to a cardiac surgeon learn about their options from their medical providers and the surgeons to whom they are referred. Wide variability in the use of less invasive techniques suggests that centers only offering the traditional approach may not notify patients about all surgical alternatives [1, 2]. This lack of disclosure may result because physicians are unable to provide confident advice about a procedure for which they have no personal experience. Alternatively, the perceived advantages of r-CABG may be less meaningful to physicians than they are to patients. In either case, the assumption that a physician's rank order of priorities to be achieved from surgery is always the same as the patient's undermines patient decision making for preference-sensitive conditions. Instead, preferences of the surgeon and their referral sources have led r-CABG to be underutilized compared to what patients would otherwise demand [8, 9].

Because most patients referred for elective CABG have sufficient time to participate in the decision about where they receive their care [4], knowledge about r-CABG drives patients into programs offering this distinctive service that otherwise would not have come. As a result, these patients appreciate the clinical benefits derived from the procedure itself and that they were provided with information that might not have been discussed at other centers. Such a discussion is meaningful because it alleviates their vulnerability caused by asymmetry of information and empowers them with alternatives relevant to their personal needs, principles on which patient-centered care is based [5]. Patients and their families often become engaged in the idea that success for these novel programs helps foster transparency and beneficial competition in healthcare. For all these reasons, initiating a robotic cardiac surgical program drives up patient satisfaction scores and creates loyal advocates of the program. Supplemental strategies are also effective at improving satisfaction scores such as communicating with respect, sitting instead of standing at the bedside, the AIDET tool, face cards given to patients that describe the members of their care team, and follow-up phone calls. While these tools enhance the patient experience, none have the same fundamental impact of providing patients with a distinctive option that they highly value but cannot get elsewhere.

Patient satisfaction scores have become increasingly relevant because these data are publically reported [10] and influence pay-for-performance programs. Moreover, high scores have been shown to reduce legal exposure to malpractice suits [11]. Patient have demonstrated strong preferences for less invasive surgery [12], underscoring the role for surgical innovation as key part of a strategy for achieving patient-centered care [7, 13–17]. In addition to technical aspects of care (such as whether surgery is performed less invasively), overall patient satisfaction is also driven by ambiguous issues such as hospital experience, access to care, personality of the physician, and honest communication and other. Because ambiguous issues are difficult for the patient to judge, many patients will assimilate their opinions on these other issues to fit with their favorable first impressions about a distinctive service like rCABG, driving up satisfaction scores across the board.

Weakness: The Learning Curve

A prolonged period of inefficiency that must be endured before the team establishes proficiency at r-CABG is known as the "learning curve." A major weakness of rCABG is that difficulties with the learning curve can translate into more risk for the cardiac surgical patient than in other surgical specialties. Complications during the learning curve that occur often could have been prevented by more experience with technique and/or communication. This creates a stark contrast to the incumbent procedure where few are deemed to be preventable [18]. Despite the inherent bias from comparing a nascent r-CABG program in its early stages against a mature sternotomy CABG program, such comparisons often occur and lead critics to conclude that the challenges of r-CABG are not safely surmountable.

Because of the vulnerability that the learning curve causes for patients and the program, an important focus for the r-CABG team is to make rapid progress during this period. There are many examples of complex cardiovascular procedures that have endured lengthy learning curves to become accepted alternatives that compare quite favorably with the incumbent procedure. However, current training paradigms require at least 100 cases of experience that accumulate within time frames often exceeding a year in order to demonstrate proficiency [13]. The predominant training strategy has been experiential learning, or "learning by doing" on actual clinical cases. Under normal circumstances, educational theory suggests that experiential learning is more effective than other formal methods of training [19]. But team morale can be affected by preventable complications during the learning curve, which creates a poor learning environment [19]. Ineffective team learning aggravates the risks of the new rCABG program and limits the chances for sustainable success.

Evidence that programs have been able to shorten the learning curve has revealed some strategies that consistently work. The process starts with articulating how progress during this learning period will be measured, i.e., metrics of success. Standard quality assurance tools of conventional cardiac surgery include the review of incident reports, chart audits, autopsy findings, morbidity and mortality conferences, administrative data, and patient complaints. These are insensitive measures of progress with the learning curve of r-CABG. Successful programs use a much broader array of metrics that reflect performance of the surgeon (e.g., prolonged operative times, markers of myocardial injury), perioperative team (e.g., rates of postoperative morbidity or re-intubation, poor pain control, excess transfusions), and hospital (e.g., prolonged hospital stay, higher costs). Review of these data will likely reveal that the learning curve is impacted by stakeholders that extend well beyond the OR team. These team members are not passive observers of the robotic surgeon but actively influence the learning curve by accommodating their tasks to the new program. Evidence from the US Military has demonstrated that even the best teams typically have limited capacity to address the burdens of change during high tempo periods and require team debriefings to optimize learning [20]. Emulating this model with regular, multidisciplinary review of the data outside the OR is required to identify areas that need improvement and create specific action plans. These meetings signal to the team that there is the "psychological safety" needed for members to learn from mistakes and actively engage in troubleshooting [17].

Based on the irreplaceable role of the lead surgeon, it is tempting to conclude that the technical ability and experience of the surgeon are sufficient for the success of rCABG programs. However, Dhawan et al. showed that a lead surgeon with >300 cases of prior r-CABG experience at the outset when he initiated a new program was unable to avoid a substantial de novo learning curve [21]. Surrogates of the technical skill of a surgeon such as dexterity on simulators or how quickly their procedure times decline over time have not been found to correlate with the sustainability of robotic programs [21]. Instead, there are many nontechnical skills required to manage and lead change at the level of the organization that appear to be critical for success [22].

An often overlooked challenge posed by rCABG is a significant "forgetting curve." Early cases are often scheduled infrequently until the procedure becomes recognized and popularized among those that are appropriate candidates. If the frequency of scheduling early cases is too long, skills acquired from previous cases lapse and the learning curve becomes longer than it would with higher caseloads. This leaves surgical programs in a conundrum—the requirement of up-front volume in order to solidify training in a program that is new and requires time to ramp up its volume of referrals. The forgetting curve may be mitigated to some degree by training programs, including virtual reality simulator and cadaveric training. One benefit of the robotic console is the ability to use it to create "virtual environments." Utilizing available virtual simulators, as well as animal and human cadaveric training labs can be helpful to improve surgeon and team skill without exposing clinical patients to additional risk [23, 24]. Despite the promise of this approach and demonstrated utility in other surgical specialties, a validated curriculum for rCABG training has not been established and funding for these programs can be a challenge.

Weakness: Additional Safety Concerns

Likewise, the technical complexity of operating on the heart within the relatively tight and constrained chest cavity has given rise to safety concerns. The potential for sudden bleeding, either from the heart or vascular sources such as the IMA, cardiac fibrillation, ischemia, and hemodynamic collapse, is difficult to address when working in a closed chest and with the bulky arms of the robot hindering patient access (Fig. 25.2a, b). Indeed, to adequately address these concerns, best practices must be developed that facilitate early identification and appropriate responses to impending decompensation in the absence of direct inspection of the heart. This may include

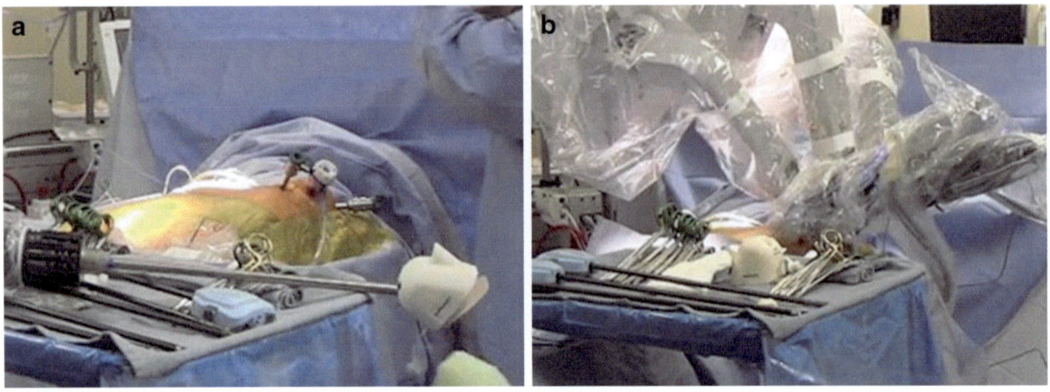

Fig. 25.2 Robotic cases are initiated by inserting ports (diameter 8–12 mm) in between the ribs in the left chest (a). The robot is then brought into the field, covered by sterile drapes, and docked to these ports. Docking enables the robotic instruments and camera to be inserted into the ports and controlled by the surgeon sitting at the console. An important risk of this setup is that access to the patient is limited after docking (**b**). If a patient were to develop the type of catastrophe that can happen during CABG (e.g., fibrillation or sudden hemodynamic collapse), the rapid access required to deal with these circumstances is hindered after docking

better utilizing TEE data, hemodynamics, better team communication, heightened "situational awareness," and standardized and reliable protocols to respond to those changes. While a learning curve for physicians performing the procedure has been clearly identified, staff must also undergo technically complex training. It is often argued that the inherent complexity of the robotic approach will never afford the surgical team the ability to achieve results equivalent to those seen with a sternotomy, leading to a fixed higher risk of error. The associated learning curve and concerns about overall safety may also be demoralizing to the team which can be a latent risk factor for preventable complications. Team morale, therefore, is a critical focus of improving the safety of the procedure. Developing and validating strategies for rapid progress through the learning curve and gaining "buy-in" about the benefits of less invasive surgery will be critical in enabling programmatic success.

Weakness: Cost Concerns

The added costs of less invasive CABG are widely perceived to be a disadvantage that limits its adoption. The additional time and expertise required for preparing the robotic apparatus prolong operating room times and alter the efficiency of the OR staff. Even after the learning curve is complete, multivessel revascularization by rCABG usually takes longer than sternotomy CABG. This may pose a significant hurdle to success at those hospitals where OR capacity is already a bottleneck for revenue generation and would be understandably reluctant to use this precious resource inefficiently.

The literature has demonstrated the cost-effectiveness of surgical robotics versus the standard approach for multiple cardiothoracic procedures. Most of these analyses have shown higher variable costs in the OR (e.g., longer operative times, more costs for disposable supplies) offset by less postoperative costs (e.g., shorter length of stay, less blood loss, less postoperative complications). However, any technically complex new procedure will have a learning curve period that reduces cost efficiency. Costs per case during the learning curve are dynamic—initial cost/case is high but declines as experience accrues for the surgeon and staff. In addition, case volumes increase as the robotic program becomes recognized, which reduces fixed costs/case by an effect known as economies of scale. Therefore, innovation in surgery must be met with innovation in accounting practices such as the designation of costs from capital expenses and the learning curve as sunk costs. This designation is rational because it eliminates the use of these costs to influence forecasts of future profitability of the r-CABG program after the learning curve is completed.

Much of the value created by rCABG is not directly measured by the hospital. For instance, a quick convalescence might a minimal impact on patients' hospital recovery but substantial impact on their need to take leave from work, request sick pay and return to work underemployed [19]. These are benefits to society but do not influence hospital costs or profitability. Other advantages become apparent when assessing the incremental cost-effectiveness of rCABG relative to conventional CABG. Unfortunately these advantages are often overlooked. This is because standard profit-loss statements that provide the basis for most hospital's strategic decision making do not often include an assessment of opportunity costs. The following are examples of these relative advantages of r-CABG:

1. *Reduce "never events"*: A sternal infection has been designated as a "never event" by Medicare [25]. This offers a strong incentive for developing non-sternal splitting procedures for cardiac surgery in order to reduce the risk of this complication. Many patients referred for cardiac surgery often have diabetes, obesity, lung disease, and other risk factors for sternal infection and mediastinitis. This "never event" in a patient with Medicare, regardless of pre-existing conditions, leads to unreimbursed costs that range from $50,000 to 100,000 per case of sternal infection.
2. *Improved performance on quality rating scores*: By avoiding aortic manipulation and the sternotomy, r-CABG consistently reduces the risk of stroke and mediastinitis. These major complications are publically reported as part of the composite quality rating score from the STS. In addition, less invasive surgery improves patient satisfaction, which is a metric of the quality measurement program called value-based purchasing. Many insurance plans (UnitedHealth, Blue Cross/Blue Shield) designate CT surgery programs as a "center of excellence" (COE) based on their ratings from these quality scores. COE designation can be leveraged by the hospital to negotiate higher reimbursement rates for other cardiac procedures.
3. *Improved operational efficiencies*: Shorter recovery time after less invasive surgery allows the hospital to leverage operational efficiencies in bed utilization and ICU resources, thereby capturing a larger share of DRG reimbursements as revenue. In a hospital that is near or at full capacity, an early discharge also frees up an available bed so that another patient can be admitted that might not otherwise been able to in the case of a bed shortage. Many hospitals find this enhanced efficiency particularly valuable for their cardiac and telemetry units.
4. *Improved payer mix*: Less invasive cardiac surgery is a distinctive program that is able to recruit patients via word of mouth and other social media that are outside the primary service area of the hospital. These patients are characterized by having more education, higher incomes, and commercial rather than public insurance coverage. The influx of these types of patients can improve the payer mix, allowing the hospital to capture a greater proportion of charges as revenue.

Weakness: Competitive Landscape

A common roadblock to widespread adoption of rCABG is a lack of acceptance by local stakeholders. On one hand, a new rCABG is controversial because it challenges a well-entrenched status quo. On the other hand, new rCABG programs are competitively positioned compared to the sternotomy option because of strong patient demand. In addition, introduction of an rCABG program creates a "first-mover" advantage that heightens barrier to entry from local competitors. First movers can capitalize on lower risk cases necessary for gaining the high volume of initial experience required for successful team learning. In contrast, later entrants are forced to accept a

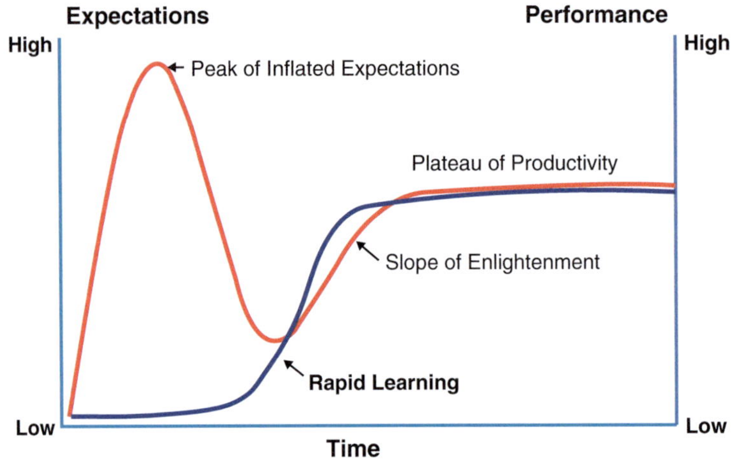

Fig. 25.3 A comparison of the change over time in local expectations about r-CABG (*red curve*) versus actual performance (*blue curve*) demonstrates an early phase where a large gap develops between expectations and performance. After this early phase, there is a period in which performance and expectations become aligned ("slope of enlightenment")

smaller subset of potential candidates. Incorporating rCABG with other less invasive revascularization procedures offered by interventional cardiologists (i.e., "hybrid procedure") avoids the typical "zero-sum" competition that exists between these specialties. In terms of the competitive landscape, this collaborative approach can alter the bargaining power of an influential supplier of patients.

The community response to a new rCABG program often occurs in a predictable manner similar to a pattern seen with other disruptive technologies [26]. There is often initial excitement surrounding any new technology after its introduction that peaks very early in its adoption. The timing of this heightened (or "hyped") expectation coincides with the learning curve period when performance tends to be lowest (Fig. 25.3). This combination of high expectations during a learning curve results in a very vulnerable period when the innovation is often criticized on the basis of this large gap between expectations and reality. Indeed, much of the criticism of rCABG that exists today was generated by the results of its early adoption in the late 1990s when both the field and practitioners were still in their learning phase and equipment in its initial versions. Subsequently, rCABG has been demonstrated to be safe and effective in expert hands, but the perceptions of these early experiences have been difficult to change and remain a persistent hindrance to widespread acceptance of this approach.

Weakness: Marketing of rCABG

Robotic heart surgery is a highly marketable topic. However, any form of advertising for innovative surgical procedures, particularly a complex one like robotic heart surgery, has been universally greeted with great skepticism and concern. It must be remembered that many patients that are appropriate candidates for r-CABG undergo traditional CABG because they either are not informed or learn about the robotic alternative at a stage that is too late in their workup. While the exact reasons why such information would not be shared are unclear, oftentimes it is merely because patients' healthcare providers are unable to provide confident advice about a novel procedure for which they have no personal experience. Extensive research has documented that variation in the use of "preference-sensitive" therapies is often based on preferences of the surgeon and their referral sources rather than those of the patient [8, 9]. In this context, marketing of rCABG can serve an important information

Table 25.1 Minithoracotomy over TECAB: based on the consensus from a discussion group of eight experienced rCABG surgeons who utilized either approach

Evaluation criteria	Rank	Weight	Minithoracotomy	TECAB
Acceptable "learning curve"; risk of forgetting	1	30	70 %=21	30 %=9
Ease of distal anastomoses	2	20	50 %=10	50 %=10
Safety (CO_2 insufflation, access)	3	15	70 %=10.5	30 %=4.5
Operative times	4	15	80 %=12	20 %=3
Increase revenue	5	5	35 %=1.75	65 %=3.25
Reduce costs	6	5	80 %=4	20 %=1
Patient satisfaction	7	5	10 %=0.5	90 %=4.5
Broad acceptance among stakeholders	8	5	60 %=3	40 %=2
Total	–	100	57 %=62.75	43 %=37.25

purpose to the community. Patient surveys have been consistently favorable about the usefulness of direct-to-consumer advertising towards mitigating the adverse effects of information asymmetry. Ads are particularly empowering when they include a "call to action" that engages patients to become more involved in obtaining a second opinion or visiting a website with credible information about rCABG.

It must be pointed out that, at least in the experience of the authors, members of the status quo usually initiate their own marketing efforts as a response to a new robotic, less invasive program. Their "campaign" is not directed to consumers but instead to internal stakeholders in cardiac surgery (e.g., cardiologists, administrators, nurses). Absent unambiguous evidence that the traditional CABG is superior, cardiac surgeons faced with competition from rCABG develop defensive strategies designed to discourage patients and their providers to investigate this alternative. A surgeon cannot prevent consumers from hearing claims about rCABG, but can stress the logic of "why change if it works" and emphasize the risks of experimentation. Incidentally, this is a classic marketing strategy used in the past by general surgeons objecting to laparoscopic cholecystectomy in the early 1990s and many market leaders responding to new entrants in industries outside of healthcare [27].

While effective, this defensive strategy deserves reconsideration and possibly revision in light of growing interest in patient empowerment and shared decision making. At a minimum, the notion of shared decision making requires practitioners to discuss all therapeutic options that a "reasonable patient" would want to know. It is clear based on the growth of PCI that patients have a strong interest in less invasive means of coronary revascularization.

Future Directions

While rCABG has already been demonstrated to be safe and effective, it remains novel with many "best practices" recommendations that have not yet been established. To date, there is no clear consensus on the best approach to performing the distal anastomoses, whether by minithoracotomy or totally endoscopic, TECAB. We have utilized a multicriteria decision analysis tool that allows practitioners to rank multiple criteria to achieve a weighted score to the overall influence that each criteria would have on the sustainable success of an rCABG program. The distribution of points between the minithoracotomy approach versus TECAB was based on the consensus from a discussion group of eight experienced rCABG surgeons who utilized either approach. This analysis favored minithoracotomy over TECAB (Table 25.1). However, further developments in technology to facilitate TECAB are likely to change many of these calculations.

Many systematic roadblocks need to be overcome in order for rCABG to succeed. A concerted effort is required to allow patients and institutions to take full advantage of rCABG.

The combination of shared decision making for patients, strategic accounting practices for administrators, and team development strategies for OR and ICU staff has been helpful. Ultimately, a leader with experience and skill with dynamics of change at the level of the organization is critical for sustainable success.

References

1. Womack JP, Jones DT. Lean thinking: banish waste and create wealth in your corporation. 1st ed. New York: Free Press; 2003.
2. Members WC, Hillis LD, Smith PK, et al. ACCF/AHA guideline for coronary artery bypass graft surgery: a report of the American College of Cardiology Foundation/American Heart Association Task Force on practice guidelines. Circulation. 2011;124(23):e652–735.
3. Molina JA, Heng BH. Global trends in cardiology and cardiothoracic surgery—an opportunity or a threat? Ann Acad Med Singapore. 2009;38(6):541–5.
4. Wilson CT, Fisher ES, Welch HG, Siewers AE, Lucas FL. U.S. trends in CABG hospital volume: the effect of adding cardiac surgery programs. Health Aff. 2007;26(1):162–8.
5. Harskamp RE, Brennan JM, Xian Y, et al. Practice patterns and clinical outcomes after hybrid coronary revascularization in the United States: an analysis from the society of thoracic surgeons adult cardiac database. Circulation. 2014;130(11):872–9.
6. Lazar HL. Should off-pump coronary artery bypass grafting be abandoned? Circulation. 2013;128(4):406–13.
7. Poston RS, Tran R, Collins M, et al. Comparison of economic and patient outcomes with minimally invasive versus traditional off-pump coronary artery bypass grafting techniques. Ann Surg. 2008;248(4):638–46.
8. Nattinger AB, Gottlieb MS, Veum J, Yahnke D, Goodwin JS. Geographic variation in the use of breast-conserving treatment for breast cancer. New Engl J Med. 1992;326(17):1102–7.
9. Wilson CT, Woloshin S, Schwartz LM. Choosing where to have major surgery: who makes the decision? Arch Surg. 2007;142(3):242–6.
10. Rowland C. Hospitals blitz airwaves with ad campaigns. Stiff competition as consumers gain more say in care. The Boston Globe. February 21, 2006.
11. Hickson GB, Federspiel CF, Pichert JW, Miller CS, Gauld-Jaeger J, Bost P. Patient complaints and malpractice risk. JAMA. 2002;287(22):2951–7.
12. Hornberger J, Bloch DA, Hlatky MA, Baumgartner W. Patient preferences in coronary revascularization. Am Heart J. 1999;137(6):1153–62.
13. Bonatti J, Schachner T, Bonaros N, et al. Effectiveness and safety of total endoscopic left internal mammary artery bypass graft to the left anterior descending artery. Am J Cardiol. 2009;104(12):1684–8.
14. Jones B, Desai P, Poston R. Establishing the case for minimally invasive, robotic-assisted CABG in the treatment of multivessel coronary artery disease. Heart Surg Forum. 2009;12(3):E147–9.
15. de Canniere D, Wimmer-Greinecker G, Cichon R, et al. Feasibility, safety, and efficacy of totally endoscopic coronary artery bypass grafting: multicenter European experience. J Thorac Cardiovasc Surg. 2007;134(3):710–6.
16. Damiano Jr RJ, Tabaie HA, Mack MJ, et al. Initial prospective multicenter clinical trial of robotically-assisted coronary artery bypass grafting. Ann Thorac Surg. 2001;72(4):1263–8. discussion 1268–1269.
17. Argenziano M, Katz M, Bonatti J, et al. Results of the prospective multicenter trial of robotically assisted totally endoscopic coronary artery bypass grafting. Ann Thorac Surg. 2006;81(5):1666–74. discussion 1674-1665.
18. Guru V, Tu JV, Etchells E, et al. Relationship between preventability of death after coronary artery bypass graft surgery and all-cause risk-adjusted mortality rates. Circulation. 2008;117(23):2969–76.
19. Cook RI, Woods DD. Adapting to new technology in the operating room. Hum Factors. 1996;38(4):593–613.
20. Rochlin GI, La Porte TR, Roberts KH. The self-designing high-reliability organization: aircraft carrier flight operations at sea. Nav War Coll Rev. 1987;40(4):76–90.
21. Dhawan R, Roberts JD, Wroblewski K, Katz JA, Raman J, Chaney MA. Multivessel beating heart robotic myocardial revascularization increases morbidity and mortality. J Thorac Cardiovasc Surg. 2012;143(5):1056–61.
22. Pisano GP, Bohmer RMJ, Edmondson AC. Organizational differences in rates of learning: evidence from the adoption of minimally invasive cardiac surgery. Manag Sci. 2001;47(6):752–68.
23. Aggarwal R, Ward J, Balasundaram I, Sains P, Athanasiou T, Darzi A. Proving the effectiveness of virtual reality simulation for training in laparoscopic surgery. Ann Surg. 2007;246(5):771–9.
24. Kanumuri P, Ganai S, Wohaibi EM, Bush RW, Grow DR, Seymour NE. Virtual reality and computer-enhanced training devices equally improve laparoscopic surgical skill in novices. JSLS. 2008;12(3):219–26.
25. Centers for M, Medicaid Services HHS. Medicaid program; payment adjustment for provider-preventable conditions including health care-acquired conditions Final rule. Fed Regist. 2011;76(108):32816–38.
26. Christensen CM. The innovator's dilemma: when new technologies cause great firms to fail. Boston: Harvard Business Review Press; 2013.
27. Alford BL. Affect, attribution, and disconfirmation: their impact on health care services evaluation. Health Mark Q. 1998;15(4):55–74.

26 Artificial Hearts and Cardiac Assist Devices: The Spectrum of the New Era

Jamshid H. Karimov, Nader Moazami, and Kiyotaka Fukamachi

Introduction

Heart failure (HF) is a serious healthcare issue and a primary contributor to cardiovascular mortality affecting about 23 million people worldwide [1, 2], and the prevalence of HF is rising rapidly even in developing nations [3]. More than 5.1 million Americans ≥20 years of age have HF, and its prevalence has recently been forecast to increase by 25 %, from 2.42 % in 2012 to 2.97 % in 2030 (with the total number of patients diagnosed with HF to increase by 46 %). By 2030, therefore, >8 million Americans will be living with HF, two million of whom will be >80 years of age (>26 % of the total HF population) [1, 4]. Direct medical costs associated with HF are projected to increase from $21 billion to $53 billion [4].

Heart transplantation can provide a remarkable improvement in quality of life and survival in selected patients with end-stage heart disease [5, 6], but a shortage of donor hearts will always limit this option [7]. In the USA, an estimated 50,000–100,000 patients need heart transplantation or mechanical circulatory support (MCS), but actual transplantation is performed in only 2,000–3,000 cases per year.

Such support is usually provided by left ventricular assist devices (LVADs), the most widely used means for improving the hemodynamic status of both transplant-eligible patients and those who do not meet criteria for heart transplantation [6]. LVADs have revolutionized the clinician's options for managing end-stage HF, and this technology continues to bring us closer to a true alternative to heart transplantation. In the past 5 years, the LVAD landscape has rapidly evolved in an opposite direction, that is, away from volume-displacement pulsatile-flow technology toward continuous-flow (CF) rotary pumps. The simple, elegant designs of CF pumps provide increased mechanical reliability, smaller size, improved durability, and better patient outcomes [7]. Since its approval by the US Food and Drug Administration (FDA) in April 2008, the HeartMate II® (Thoratec Corp., Pleasanton, CA) (the device of choice, implanted in >16,000 implants worldwide) has enjoyed a 25 % annual growth in the number of LVAD implants throughout the world (1,900 cases in 2007 versus 4,650 cases in 2011). It is expected that ~10,000 LVAD implants per year will be in

J.H. Karimov, M.D., Ph.D.
K. Fukamachi, M.D., Ph.D. (✉)
Department of Biomedical Engineering, Lerner Research Institute, Cleveland Clinic, Cleveland, OH, USA
e-mail: karimoj@ccf.org; fukamak@ccf.org

N. Moazami, M.D.
Department of Thoracic and Cardiovascular Surgery, Kaufman Center for Heart Failure, Cardiac Transplantation and Mechanical Circulatory Support, Miller Family Heart and Vascular Institute, Cleveland Clinic, Cleveland, OH, USA
e-mail: Moazamn@ccf.org

R. Latifi et al. (eds.), *Technological Advances in Surgery, Trauma and Critical Care*,
DOI 10.1007/978-1-4939-2671-8_26

place by 2015. Based on the fourth annual report of the Interagency Registry for Mechanically Assisted Circulatory Support, 99 % of LVADs implanted in the first half of 2011 were CF LVADs [8], which clearly indicates the future direction this therapy is taking.

Despite the many significant technological and therapeutic advances that have been achieved with prolonged duration of support (i.e., enhanced survival with less morbidity), there is room for significant improvements in the technology, and newer devices are being introduced. In this chapter, we center on the latest developments in the implantable MCS pumps currently used in clinical practice and investigational devices that are or will be undergoing evaluation in clinical trials.

Indications for Mechanical Circulatory Support and Treatment Limitations

MCS therapy is a treatment option for two major indications: "bridge to transplantation" (BTT), for heart transplant candidates who must have temporary support with an LVAD until a suitable donor organ can be found, and "destination therapy" (DT), for patients who are not candidates for transplant and in whom LVADs serve as a permanent support for the diseased myopathic heart [9]. LVAD implantation as a "bridge to decision" is another option for patients in whom heart transplantation or permanent LVAD implantation is considered to be the most viable option at the time of implant. In a "bridge to decision" setting, if relative contraindications are corrected, the patient may become transplant eligible. All BTT and DT patients must demonstrate the anatomic, psychosocial, and economic requirements necessary for these procedures. What distinguishes BTT from DT patients is whether the patient meets selection criteria for heart transplantation and the likelihood that a particular transplant-eligible patient will actually get a heart [7]. Additional criteria for DT candidates is a life expectancy without MCS placement of less than 2 years, with anticipated increase in life expectancy/quality of life with MCS placement (more than 2 years), and the absence of (a) comorbid pathology that would significantly limit the patient's rehabilitation potential on LVAD; (b) active drug or alcohol abuse, precluding compliance with medical therapy on MCS; and (c) active infection without appropriate treatment. The presence of relative contraindications to heart transplantation that are potentially reversible or otherwise amenable to cure or other intervention allows for eligibility for transplantation at a later date. These contraindications can include drug and/or alcohol abuse, smoking, pulmonary hypertension, recently remitted malignancy, lack of social support, or renal disease.

Implantable Mechanical Circulatory Support Technology

The development of CF rotary pump technology represents a milestone based on a novel pump design concept. These pumps have now almost completely replaced pulsatile, volume-displacement devices. CF rotary pumps have the advantages of a smaller design and potential for greater long-term mechanical reliability by eliminating the blood sac and valves needed by pulsatile pumps. CF rotary blood pumps are typically designed with an "axial" or "centrifugal" blood flow path featuring an internal rotor within that path [5].

HeartMate II®

The HeartMate II (Thoratec Corp., Pleasanton, CA) is an LVAD (Fig. 26.1) that had its origin in the early 1990s. This CF rotary pump provides continuous unloading of the left ventricle (LV) throughout the cardiac cycle. The HeartMate II received FDA approval as a DT device in January 2010, after obtaining the FDA approval as a BTT device in April 2008. The pump is axially configured; the path of blood flow through the rotor is parallel to the pump's axis. The HeartMate II is significantly smaller in size and weight compared with the older pulsatile LVADs, thanks to the elimination of the need for a blood sac or chamber. The HeartMate II weighs 290 g, with a length of 7.0 cm, a diameter of 4.0 cm, and an implant

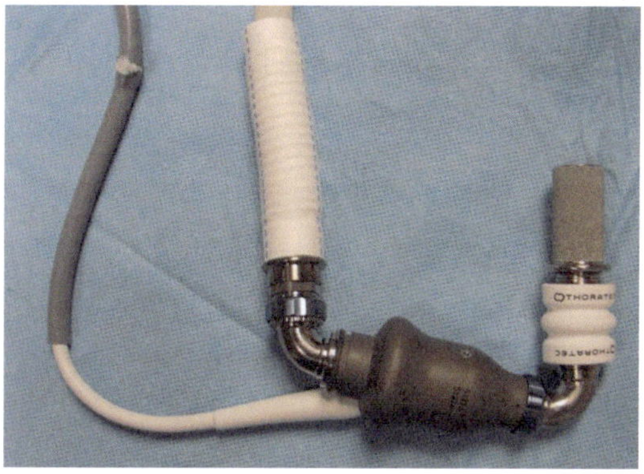

Fig. 26.1 The HeartMate II® (Thoratec Corp., Pleasanton, CA) is currently the device of choice for cardiac assist applications worldwide

volume of 63 mL. The rotor is the only moving part, which provides superior device durability. More than 16,000 implants of the HeartMate II have been performed worldwide, making the HeartMate II the most successful pump on the market today.

The HeartMate II contains a rotor capable of producing flow rates greater than 10 L/min at resolutions ranging from 8,000 to 15,000 rpm [5]. The blood pump itself is made of titanium with a ruby bearing; the straight pump tube is 12 mm in diameter and contains the inlet stator, pump rotor, and outlet stator. The stators are fixed components that form the pivots of the rotor. The rotor contains a magnet, and a magnetic field is generated between the rotor and the motor, which results in rotary motion and torque leading to blood flow. Blood from the LV's apex is carried to the inflow conduit via the inlet cannula. Blood enters the outflow graft (and then the ascending aorta) via the outflow elbow. The inner surfaces of the inflow elbow, inlet cannula, and outflow elbow contain a textured surface to stimulate a natural endothelial surface for blood flow. When blood enters the HeartMate II, it passes through the inlet stator, where the course that the blood follows is straightened out via three guide vanes. The LVAD rotor's three curving blades impart kinetic energy to the blood while also generating a radial velocity to the blood flow. Blood flow exits the pump rotor through the outlet stator, which contains three vanes with a twisted shape that convert the radial velocity of the blood flow to an axial velocity [9]. As in other axial-flow pumps, there is a risk of the pump's generating negative intraventricular pressure, causing the ventricle to collapse. As a result, inflow cannula positioning and ventricular preload are important. In the HeartMate II, the intraventricular portion of the inflow tract has been elongated and, as a result, tends to stent open the middle of the ventricle, thus improving reliability of CF throughout the cardiac cycle [5, 7].

Anticoagulation medication is, at present, recommended to prevent thrombosis by keeping the international normalized ratio of the blood between 2.0 and 2.5. The HeartMate II is placed either above the peritoneum or above the posterior rectus sheath in the left upper quadrant below the diaphragm. Power and control are delivered through a percutaneous cable that is attached to a controller.

A multicenter randomized trial (conducted at 38 US centers) reported results from the CF HeartMate II ($n=133$) and the pulsatile HeartMate XVE ($n=59$) implanted in almost 200 patients with similar baseline characteristics and DT risk scores [10]. The median duration of support was 1.7 years (range, 0.0–3.7) for the HeartMate II and 0.6 years (range, 0.0–2.1) for the pulsatile XVE, with a cumulative follow-up of 211 and 41 patient-years, correspondingly. All patients were followed up for at least 2 years, or until death, transplant, or device explant. The primary endpoint was a composite survival at 2 years, free of disabling stroke or reoperation to replace the device. The HeartMate II group was superior to the pulsatile device in terms of survival, with estimated 1- and 2-year survival rates of 68 and 58 %.

The functional class and quality of life in BTT ($n=281$) and DT ($n=374$) patients have been assessed at baseline and post-implant [11]. Post-implant, 82 % (BTT) and 80 % (DT) of patients at 6 months and 79 % (DT) at 24 months improved to NYHA functional class I or II. Mean 6-min walk distance of 204 m (DT) was improved to 350 and 360 m at 6 and 24 months.

Despite the improvements in survival since the approval of the HeartMate II for BTT and DT, there are still adverse effects associated with device use that must be considered [7]. The risk of pump thrombosis and thromboembolism is the biggest concern with the use of CF rotary pumps. An apparent increase in the rate of device thrombosis among patients who had received the HeartMate II, with substantial morbidity and mortality, has recently been observed [12]; this setback makes the search for the causes of thrombosis mandatory so that physicians can predict and prevent this daunting complication. Data from a multicenter clinical trial in 895 patients revealed 72 confirmed pump thromboses (in 66 patients), with 36 incidences of thrombosis. The estimated occurrence of thrombosis in the HeartMate II was reported to be 4.7 %, 7.5 %, and 12.3 %, correspondingly at 6, 12, and 24 months of support [13]. The causes of thrombosis seem multifactorial and yet remain uncertain (among the possibilities are hypercoagulability leading to thrombus deposition, hemodynamic compromise, flow reduction, heat dissipation from the bearing, inadequate anticoagulation, aortic regurgitation, hypovolemia, kinking of the outflow graft, or inflow cannula malposition). Therefore, careful recommendations for LVAD therapy should account for each patient's risk-benefit profile. Early perioperative pump power elevations can occur frequently, and this observation has been concerning; however, the relationship between early power elevations and subsequent development of stroke and pump thrombosis has yet to be defined [14].

HVAD®

The HVAD® (HeartWare International, Framingham, MA) CF pump weighs 160 g and has a displacement volume of 50 mL and an external diameter of 53 mm (Fig. 26.2). The HVAD operates within the range of 1,800–4,000 rpm and can pump up to 10 L/min of blood. Within its titanium pump housing, the HVAD has a unique wide-blade impeller (a single moving component), suspended by hybrid magnetic/hydrodynamic forces for frictionless rotation [15]. There are no points of mechanical contact within the pump, effectively ensuring a "wearless" system. The design integrates two motor stators for single-motor fault protection to increase reliability. An integrated inflow cannula is inserted into the LV and is held in position by a sewing ring; the pump is positioned in the pericardial space. The 10-mm outflow graft is anastomosed to the ascending aorta. Communication from the pump to the external power and control components is provided by a flexible, polyurethane-covered driveline that is externalized through the abdominal

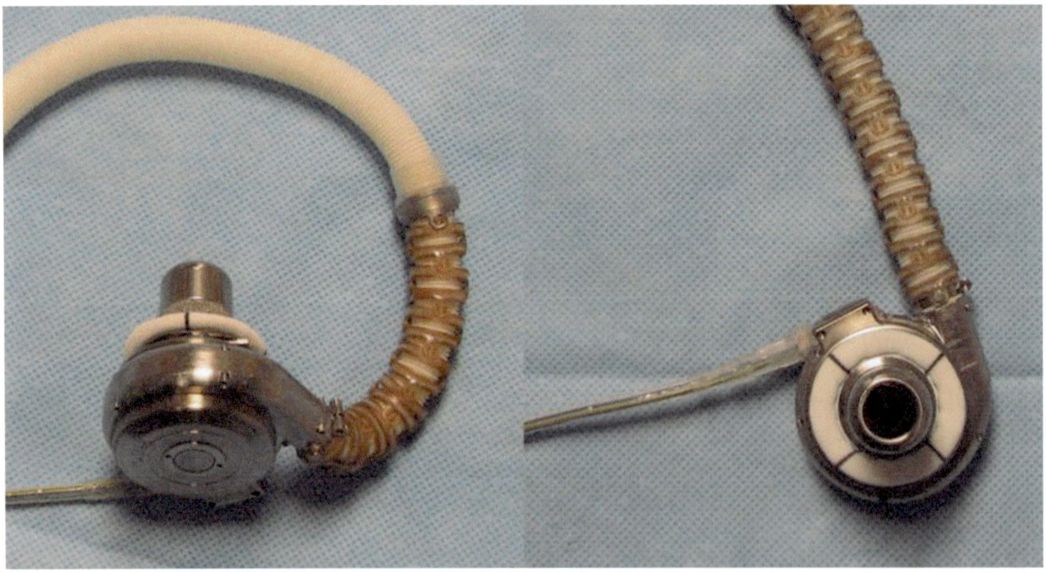

Fig. 26.2 The HVAD® (HeartWare International, Framingham, MA) pump

wall. A microprocessor-based controller monitors pump function and regulates power to dual motors within the pump. The controller displays pump speed, blood flow rate, power, alarm conditions, and instructions for resolving such conditions. A continuous power supply is provided by either alternating or direct current (AC or DC) sources, including lithium-ion batteries for portable operation. A system monitor provides a means for adjusting pump operating parameters, monitoring pump function, and storing data. External system components include the microprocessor-based controller, a monitor, lithium-ion battery packs, AC and DC power adapters, and a battery charger. Physiologic control algorithms are incorporated for safe operation.

The biventricular use of two HVADs has been described, but is as yet an "off-label" use. In such cases, the investigators have cautioned that even the lowest deliverable device flow (2,400 rpm) would still be too high in the pulmonary circulation without a systemic afterload and that, theoretically, use of the device would result in pulmonary edema [16]. Therefore, additional modifications, such as narrowing of the outflow graft, may be necessary to increase the afterload when the HVAD is used for right ventricular (RV) assist. The optimal anatomic sites for device insertion have yet to be established.

A large multicenter study (30 US centers) presented post-implant survival in 322 patients with the HVAD [17]. Patients were monitored for 180 days or more, or until heart transplantation or death. The study revealed survival rates at 60, 180, and 360 days as 97 %, 91 %, and 84 %, respectively. The study showed that 67.1 % of patients were alive 180 days after the HVAD was originally implanted, and 21.4 % had either received a donor heart or the device had been explanted during recovery within 6 months post-implant. Survival of patients in these latter groups (transplant or explant) was 90 % at 180 days and 89 % at 360 days. A smaller multicenter HVAD trial conducted in Europe and Australia reported an actuarial survival of 91 % at 6 months and 86 % at 12 months [18]. All pumps were implanted intrapericardially. From a total of 23 patients, at 1-year follow-up, a mean duration of support of 305 ± 105 days and total support of 19.2 patient-years have been reported.

Recently, the analysis of outcomes in 382 patients who underwent an HVAD implantation as part of a HeartWare BTT trial reported that pump thromboses were observed in 8.1 % (34 thrombotic events) of patients ($n=31$) [19]. These events occurred at an average of about 1 year (353 ± 329 days) after implant. The freedom from any pump thrombosis was 98 %, 96 %, and 92 %, respectively, at 3, 6, and 12 months. The investigators found no statistically significant difference ($p=0.21$) in survival at 1 year between the groups with thrombus (85.4 %) and without thrombus (69.4 %). Unexpected power increases and flow estimation beyond that predicted from power consumption were observed. Fibrin or clot on the surface of the impeller may have caused an increase in power consumption, resulting in a decrease in pump efficiency. Depending on the severity and formation characteristics of the thrombus, an increased trend and rapid rise in LVAD power consumption were noted.

Jarvik 2000

The Jarvik 2000 FlowMaker® LVAD (Jarvik Heart, Inc., New York, NY) is a compact axial-flow pump (Fig. 26.3) that provides continuous blood flow from the LV to the descending or ascending aorta [20]. The device for adults mea-

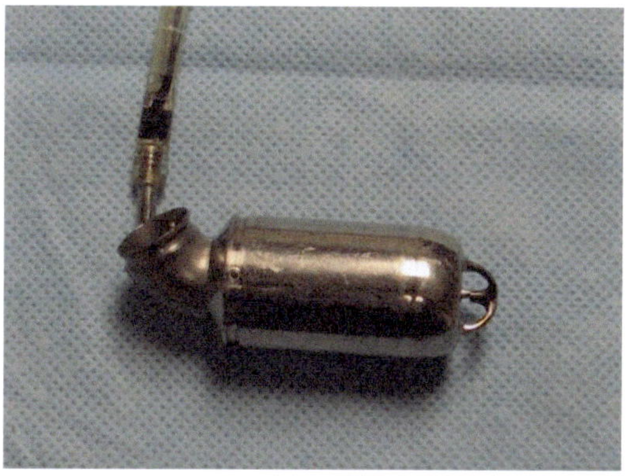

Fig. 26.3 The Jarvik 2000 FlowMaker® (Jarvik Heart, Inc., New York) axial continuous-flow pump. The device is inserted into the LV apex

sures 2.6 cm in diameter by 7.8 cm in length and weighs 85 g (90 g with a pre-attached 16-mm Hemashield outflow graft and small-bore percutaneous lead) and is about the size of a common C-cell battery. The pump has a volume of 30 mL and a priming volume of 7 mL [21]. The apical cuffed sewing ring secures the pump in place. The Jarvik 2000 is the only blood pump to be placed *within* the native heart's ventricle, and thus no inflow cannula is required. The blood-contacting surfaces within the pump are made of smooth titanium. The pump comprises a single rotating impeller, located in the center of the titanium housing. A brushless DC motor, also positioned within the housing, creates the electromagnetic force necessary to rotate the impeller. The impeller consists of a neodymium-iron-boron magnet and two titanium impeller blades that are suspended by ceramic cone bearings. Blood is directed through the outflow graft by stator blades located near the pump outlet. In addition to the blood pump, the Jarvik 2000 system comprises a 16-mm outflow graft, percutaneous power cable, speed controller, and DC power supply. The external speed controller powers the pump via a series of wires contained in a silicone tube, which is covered with Dacron. The pump can be operated at 8,000–12,000 rpm and can generate an average flow rate of 3–7 L/min at 4–8 W of power under optimal conditions [22].

Two smaller versions of the device are in development for pediatric patients. Specifications for the child and infant pumps are, respectively, as follows: diameter, 17.5 and 10.5 mm; length, 5.2 and 3.2 mm; displacement volume, 10 and 3 mL; and flow 1.0–1.5 L/min and 0.25–0.75 L/min [21].

The simplified configuration of the Jarvik 2000 makes an off-pump implantation feasible. The ability of the pump to be inserted through a thoracotomy has been reported as one of the key surgical advantages in patients who have not had previous cardiac surgery [23]. However, the difficulty of explanting the device implanted through a left thoracotomy may become very challenging after a median sternotomy at the time of transplantation.

Several trials have reported the safety and effectiveness of Jarvik 2000 for HF patients, both as a BTT and as DT. The device has been associated with a low incidence of thrombosis [24, 25], which is believed to be a result of the high-flow blood stream that washes the miniature bearings of the device [22].

New Devices and Concepts

MVAD®

HeartWare (HeartWare International, Framingham, MA) has in preclinical testing a next-generation device, the MVAD, a wide-blade axial CF pump (Fig. 26.4). The MVAD is approximately half the size of the HVAD, with 22 mL of displacement volume and 5 mL of priming volume. The MVAD is designed for versatility: it can be used as partial or full support for left, right, or biventricular applications, via either sternotomy or thoracotomy. The MVAD features a magnetic axial rotor and uses a combination of passive permanent magnets and hydrodynamic bearing surfaces to totally suspend the rotor in operation, with a displacement volume of only 15 mL. This is accomplished by a unique rotor with impeller blades that are wider than the blood flow channel between them, affording sufficient surface area for passive hydrodynamic radial rotor suspension. This design eliminates the mechanical pivot bearings typical of axial pumps and significantly reduces pump size by using pas-

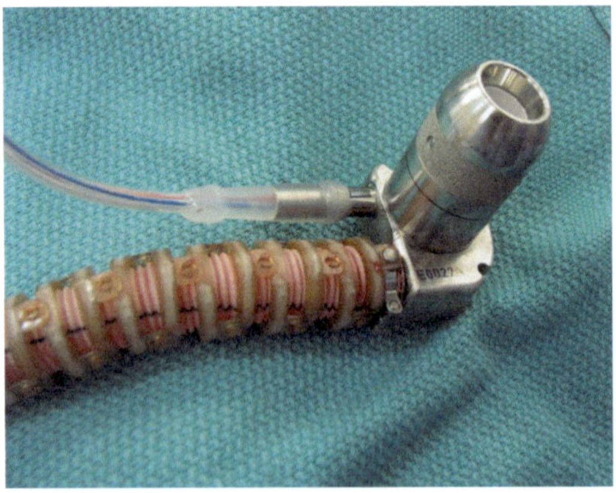

Fig. 26.4 Miniature ventricular assist device (MVAD®; HeartWare International, Framingham, MA). The inflow cannula, the largest portion of the device, is placed completely inside the ventricle

sive rotor suspension rather than the larger and more complex active electromagnetic bearing designs. Also not typical of axial pump design is an outflow port, angled 90° from the pump housing inlet port, similar to centrifugal pump designs [26]. Various versions of the MVAD are being tested, implanted within the LV or at the LV apex, in animal studies (Fig. 26.5). The MVAD is currently not available for clinical application, but a clinical trial is planned soon for this investigational device.

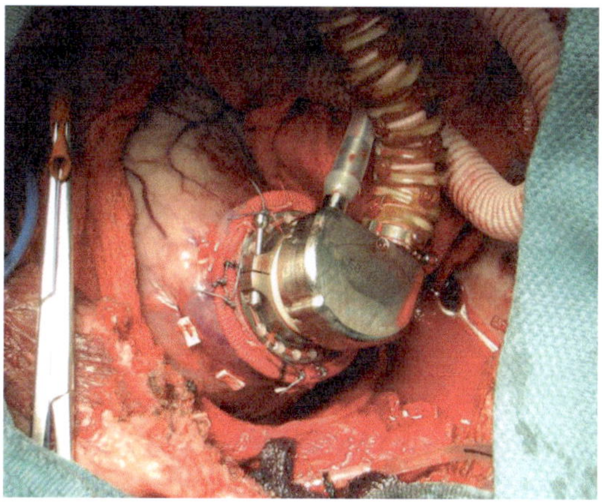

Fig. 26.5 The MVAD® (HeartWare International, Framingham, MA). The extremely small and low-profile pump design may enable its implantation using a minimally invasive approach

HeartMate III™

The HeartMate III (Thoratec Corp., Pleasanton, CA) centrifugal CF rotary pump (Fig. 26.6) is now in preparation for clinical testing and Conformité Européenne mark clinical trials (expected to start by the last quarter of 2014). The pump incorporates many critical family design elements of the HeartMate II (e.g., large gaps and textured blood-contacting surfaces) and has been designed to reduce the potential for adverse events (aortic insufficiency, bleeding, thrombus, and stroke). Its large gaps also enable rapid speed changes used by the artificial pulse feature without rotor and/or housing contact. The HeartMate III addresses many of the limitations of axial pump design: it features a bearingless magnetic levitation of the pump rotor (rather than mechanical pivot bearings) to increase reliability out to 10 years, has an accurate sensorless flow estimator, and incorporates a pulse mode to increase the

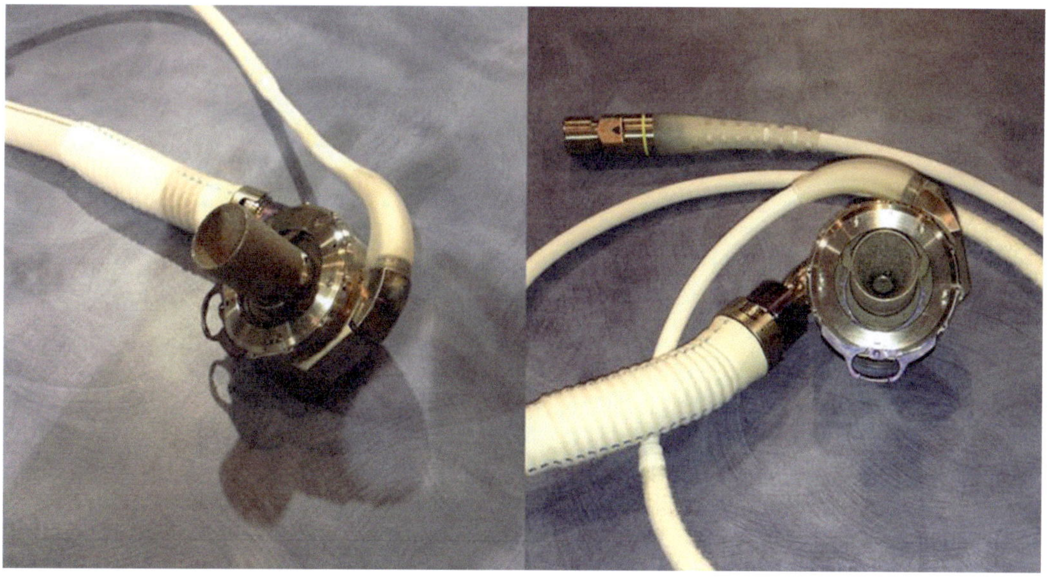

Fig. 26.6 The new centrifugal HeartMate III™ (Thoratec Corp, Pleasanton, CA) device. The inflow cannula design (*concave*) is similar to the one used in its predecessor

level of pulsatility and even produce physiological pulse pressures. This new pump may potentially reduce the need for anticoagulation agents. Wedging surfaces and other features required for hydrodynamic bearings are not required. The device's rotor and volute have been designed to minimize shear and avoid stasis over the entire range of operation (2–10 L/min). Rotor levitation is independent of rotor speed; levitation is maintained at any rotor speed, even zero. Rotor speed independence permits flexibility in operating speeds, which could in the future enable use of the HeartMate III under low-speed conditions, e.g., pulmonary circulation and weaning protocols. These features make it feasible to implement physiologic control algorithms based on accurate flow estimates. In addition, centrifugal pumps have characteristics that generate lower pressures over a wider flow range. This capability translates to more favorable outcomes owing to much lower inlet suction at low flows; lower outlet pressures at high levels of systemic vascular resistance, preventing the creation of exceedingly high systemic arterial pressures; higher flow pulsatility that is more sensitive to LV pressure swings, providing both a more sensitive pre-suction detection capability and increased diagnostic feedback about the functional status of the LV; and safer chronic management of pump speed and output optimization. These features suggest that centrifugal rotary pumps may overtake axial-flow rotary pumps in the CF rotary pump revolution that has made first-generation pulsatile pumps all but obsolete [7].

HeartMate X

The HeartMate X (Thoratec Corp., Pleasanton, CA), a highly energy-efficient axial-flow pump, leverages core HeartMate II bearing technology with a dramatic size reduction for rapid, less invasive implantation. The HeartMate X offers versatile cannulation options and, in this ultra-compact dimension, is considered suitable for partial to full ventricular support configurations for patients needing LVADs as well as the populations needing right or bi-ventricular assist devices (RVADs or BiVADs) [27]. The device can provide a stable 8 L/min of CF. The HeartMate X may thus further expand potential approaches for truly minimally invasive implantation techniques, especially in small size and younger patient populations.

SYNERGY®

In 2013, HeartWare International announced that it had acquired CircuLite®, Inc. (Saddle Brook, NJ), developer of the SYNERGY® Circulatory Support System, a "micro-pump" designed to treat less sick, ambulatory patients with chronic HF who are not yet inotrope dependent. The CircuLite Synergy LVAD (HeartWare) is a novel pump that combines axial, centrifugal, and orthogonal flow paths at a 7.5 mL volume and operating speeds of 20,000–28,000 rpm. The device is the size of a double-A battery, connects to the heart via an inflow cannula (8 mm diameter by 20 cm long), has a pumping capacity of up to 4.25 L/min, and is small enough to be placed in a subcutaneous pocket. The blood passes through narrow channels around the motor (which serves to cool the motor) and leaves the pump at a right angle to the inlet [28]. It uses a magnetically and hydrodynamically stabilized rotor design. The Synergy's pump body is implanted via a small right-sided thoracotomy into a subcutaneous pacemaker-like pocket in the right subclavian groove. It is implanted without the use of extracorporeal circulation, with the inflow cannula placed into the left atrium and the outflow graft connected to the right subclavian artery. The device has been implanted in 25 patients on the waiting list for a heart transplant as a partial support device. With flows recorded between 2.3 and 3.5 L/min, the applications of the pump may be extended for support in less sick patients (those considered in New York Heart Association functional class III) [29].

Although clinical experience is currently limited to pumping blood from the left atrium to the subclavian artery, recent cadaveric research has indicated that this micropump can also be easily positioned as an RVAD.

The SYNERGY® Circulatory Support System is currently undergoing a redesigning process related to such issues as device thrombosis and mechanical fractures of the inflow cannula portion. The additional device development and optimization will be critical to provide proper pump reliability and function. However, the US clinical trial that has been put on the company's agenda will most likely be further delayed.

Future Perspectives

Options for RVAD/BiVAD

The application of CF LVADs for refractory end-stage HF is increasing. When LV filling remains inadequate despite pharmacotherapy to enhance RV function and lower pulmonary vascular resistance, an RVAD may be required [20, 30]. The primary reason VADs have not been designed specifically for RVAD applications is that there is much less clinical need (and therefore a limited market) compared with that for LVADs [7, 30]. Although clinically approved implantable LVADs are not designed for right-sided support, LVAD implantation for right heart support is being considered simply because an effective, easily implantable RVAD is not yet available. The absence of a dedicated, clinically evaluated, long-term RVAD significantly diminishes the treatment options for patients with isolated and post-LVAD RV failure, as well as for those with biventricular HF requiring two pumps (BiVADs) [31–33]. The inherent CF pump mechanics and translation of clinical features, pump selection, and patient management issues have previously been detailed [26].

The first use of an implantable CF pump for RV support was reported in 2004; a 21-year-old patient with worsened RV failure and elevated peripheral vascular resistance after implantation of a Jarvik 2000 FlowMaker was treated by implanting a second one [20]. By directing the inlet toward the inferior vena caval-right atrial junction and keeping right atrial pressures at 5–10 cm H_2O, surgeons achieved stable RV unloading and satisfactory blood flow to the left-sided pump. Other groups consecutively reported on limited, off-label, clinical use of two LVADs. Saito et al. [34] converted a 6-month survival patient from a Toyobo paracorporeal device (Toyobo-Nipro, Osaka, Japan) to a Jarvik 2000 as RVAD and a DuraHeart (Terumo Heart, Inc., Ann Arbor, MI) for LVAD support.

Successful application of two HVADs for treatment of severe biventricular failure was reported by Strueber et al. [15] and Hetzer and collaborators [35]. Additional case reports of intrapericardial implantation of the HVAD followed, the surgeons using a similar technique of placing the pump on the RV diaphragmatic surface just below the acute margin. Two additional silicone rings were placed under the fixation ring. Artificial restriction applied to the outlet graft of the pump may compensate for the lower outlet pressures seen at the pulmonary artery [36]. HeartWare is currently working to obtain regulatory approval for modifications to the HVAD for use as RVAD support [7]. Potapov et al. [37] from the German Heart Institute in Berlin reported on ten patients with idiopathic dilated cardiomyopathy patients who received biventricular HVADs. In three of these patients, physicians have been able to turn the RVAD off following long-term biventricular support, having confirmed via echocardiography that the patients had stable hemodynamics and that no thromboembolic events and no regurgitation through the right pump had occurred. Krabatsch et al. [38] reported implantation of an HVAD, first on the RV free wall at the maximal distance from the interventricular septum. Because severe compression of the RV caused low flow of the right pump of maximally 2 L/min, the RVAD was reimplanted to the right atrium through the layer of pericardium (opening created from the right pleura) and by using two silicone rings (to prevent the inflow cannula being introduced too deeply into the chamber). That group subsequently reported 17 patients implanted with two HVADs [16]. Deuse at al. [39] recently reported the HVAD use for permanent RV support with no spacers (rings) used.

Recently, Schmitto et al. [28] investigated the use of two Synergy Micro-Pumps (CircuLite

Inc., Saddle Brook, NJ) for full biventricular support in ovine models. Such use may provide another option for partial (biventricular) support in patients and, as the authors stated, for full support in small adults and children.

Currently, temporary support via RVADs/BiVADs is available by CF extracorporeal or paracorporeal circulation support systems [30, 33] such as the CentriMag® (Thoratec Corp., Pleasanton, CA), the Bio-Pump (Medtronic, Minneapolis, MN), and the TandemHeart (CardiacAssist, Inc., Pittsburgh, PA). Progress in the development of clinically available rotary pumps now permits physicians to choose a hybrid approach for BiVAD placement, using both an implantable LVAD and temporary extracorporeal RVAD [33, 40, 41]. Since the first reported application of two Jarvik 2000 FlowMaker pumps [20], several groups have adopted this approach for biventricular assist. The adaptation of an LVAD to function as an RVAD is a technical challenge because of both ventricular distinctions and pump characteristics [30, 42].

RVAD design challenges involve pump dimensions and fit, as well as adaptability to operating flows. RVADs operate at much lower afterloads (pulmonary arterial pressures) than LVADs do and at significantly reduced hydraulic loads and power consumption rates. Because of its low-pressure working conditions and complex geometry, the RV stands in stark contrast to the LV. Under normal baseline conditions, the unique anatomy, myocardial ultrastructure, and coronary physiology of the RV reflect a high-volume, low-pressure pump. Once surgeons introduce an LVAD, they raise the expected output of the RV to that of the LVAD [43].

Based on our own previous experience evaluating the Cleveland Clinic DexAide CF RVAD (Arrow International, Reading, PA), we have validated that the operating range of an RVAD necessitates a range of 2–6 L/min of pump flow while raising the pump outlet pressure by 20–50 mmHg from that at the pump inlet port [30]. Even though the RVAD operating range may seem to exceed the requirements for even the most severe cardiovascular pulmonary pathophysiology, a pump flow of around 2 L/min must be provided, especially with compromised RV and during transient conditions of very high pulmonary vascular resistance. Use of an LVAD for RV support would certainly provide the hydraulic capability to exceed 2 L/min, but this application could lead to a further increase in the already high pulmonary arterial pressure [30].

It is important to note that CF pumps empty the ventricle during both systole and diastole, with higher flow rates during ventricular systole due to a lower delta pressure across the pump and lower flow rates during diastole due to higher delta pressure. Pumps generate variable degrees of pulsatility in the flow waveform based on the type of device and the degree to which the device unloads the ventricular chamber. Because RVADs empty a low-pressure ventricle, the degree of flow pulsatility is much lower than that seen in CF LVAD devices [26, 30]. Nonetheless, the management of RV failure continues to be non-evidence based. Biventricular support can be effective but is associated with lower survival and a worse quality of life than LV support alone [44]. The introduction of smaller rotary blood pumps should soon make biventricular support more attractive [43].

Total Artificial Hearts

Research into the total artificial heart (TAH) began in the USA in 1963 under the impetus of the American Congress. The studies soon encountered a myriad of difficulties related to biocompatibility, autoregulation, device dimensions, practicality of implant and post-implant lifestyle, energy delivery, and long-term durability. Significant advances have been made in our understanding of the progression and pathophysiology of HF since the initial conceptualization of TAH using the mechanical device from the laboratory of Dr. Willem Kolff. Advanced support systems can be implanted relatively earlier in patients with end-stage HF, with the perceived advantages of promoting ventricular remodeling and thus potentially reversing the severity of HF. In the twenty-first century, TAHs are used in patients with end-stage HF to replace cardiac function so that adequate viable perfusion can be restored. Experience with the available versions of volume-displacement TAHs has been encouraging when the TAH is used as a BTT in this subset of patients. However, clinical experience with the TAH as a DT has thus far been limited.

CardioWest and AbioCor

The CardioWest™ TAH (SynCardia Systems, Inc., Tucson, AZ) as a pneumatic system and the AbioCor® TAH (Abiomed, Inc., Danvers, MA) as a permanent pulsatile implantable system are the only two TAHs approved by the FDA for use in the USA. The story of the AbioCor heart is remarkable: over three decades, investors spent nearly $200 million to develop the world's first fully implantable TAH, but this device was found to be too impractical and too large and did not work long enough [45]. Clinical experience with the AbioCor is still limited, as this TAH has been implanted in just 14 patients. The CardioWest TAH, in contrast, has been implanted in more than 1,300 patients worldwide, with a successful BTT rate of 79 % [46]. The longest implant lasted for 1,374 days (nearly 4 years) in a 54-year-old male patient prior to his successful heart transplant [47]. However, both approved TAHs are large pulsatile devices and require the operation of four valves.

CARMAT

One of the latest artificial heart technologies is the recently introduced TAH from CARMAT (Vélizy-Villacoublay, France) (Fig. 26.7), an implantable, electrohydraulically driven, pulsatile-flow device with four bioprosthetic valves [48]. The CARMAT TAH operates by means of two pumping chambers. It consists of two ventricular cavities, right and left, containing two volume spaces, each separated by a flexible biomembrane, one for blood and one for the biocompatible actioning fluid (in this case, 300 mL of silicone oil). A flexible external bag contains the actioning fluid and beats at the same rate as a native heart would. The device has a displacement of 1,000 mL and weighs more than 1,300 g.

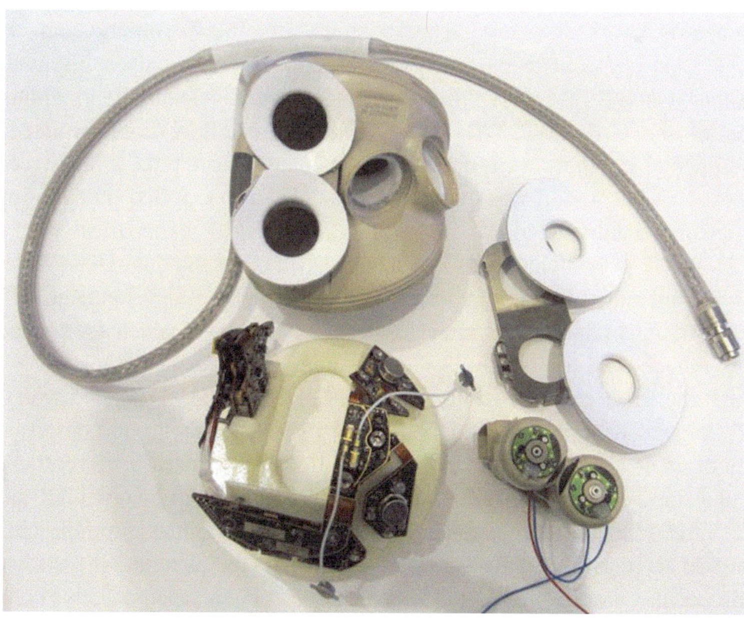

Fig. 26.7 The CARMAT TAH (Vélizy-Villacoublay, France)

Through hydraulic action via two miniature motorized DC pump sets, the actioning fluid displaces this biomembrane, reproducing the movement of the ventricular wall of the human heart during contraction. This movement causes filling and ejection of blood under optimal conditions: usual movement, and contact only with biologically compatible materials [49]. Each DC pump is designed to back the function of another, in case of failure.

An integrated electronic device regulates how the prosthesis operates according to patients' needs, using information from two independent pressure sensors and processed by a microprocessor. The internal layout of the CARMAT TAH has been the subject of continuous optimization to minimize the space occupied by the components and to maximize ventricular volume, thus ensuring the necessary blood flow in all circumstances without artificially increasing the operating frequency. The implantation method is also very similar to that of a heart transplant. A biocompatible interface device is sutured to the auricles, and the prosthesis is then simply connected to the device.

The blood-pumping surfaces consist of processed pericardial tissue and expanded polytetrafluorethylene, which lessens the need for anticoagulation agents.

The CARMAT TAH is meant to be an end-stage solution rather than a BTT device. Prior to the implantation of the CARMAT TAH in a patient, 19 experimental implants were done in calves; the longest survival period was 10 days (J.H. Karimov, personal communication).

In late 2013, the first patient received a CARMAT TAH implant and at first was reported to be doing well [50]. The patient died after 75 days, which was longer than the trial's 30-day endpoint; although the exact cause of death was not immediately known, it appeared that there was a possibility of an electronic malfunction in the pump that may have occurred. Three more such CARMAT TAH implants are planned in France, which would serve as a basis for seeking Conformité Européenne certification for the device, allowing it to be sold commercially in Europe. The US FDA application for device clearance may also be considered, but only after the initial 20 implants the company has planned. The projected lifetime of the current CARMAT TAH design is around 5 years (230 million beats).

Continuous-Flow Total Artificial Heart Using Dual-Continuous-Flow Pumps

The feasibility of native heart replacement with a CF TAH using two separate CF pumps has been reported; this was in the context of severe biventricular failure with the native ventricles left intact. The Texas Heart Institute's report of its initial experience with total cardiac replacement using dual-HeartMate II CF LVADs underscored the importance of controlling right pump speed to prevent pulmonary edema and the partial collapse of the right "neoatrium." A total of 63 chronic calf CF TAH experiments have been performed since 2004 [51, 52]. Investigators used two independent axial or centrifugal pumps, and 27 of the 63 calves survived for more than 7 days; the longest duration was 3 months. The two CF VADs did provide stable hemodynamic support, with mean right and left pump flows of 9.4 ± 2.0 L/ min and 9.6 ± 2.2 L/min, respectively, and with mean right and left atrial pressures of 15 ± 7 mmHg and 16 ± 7 mmHg, respectively. The calves implanted with a CF TAH were physically well maintained with continuous blood flow (nonmodulated [nonpulsatile] or via an induced pulse). More recently, Strueber et al. [15] also reported encouraging data for their initial clinical experience with total cardiac replacement using dual-HeartWare HVADs.

The ongoing development of CF TAHs to replace the native ventricles is expected to help a unique HF patient population who cannot be served by CF BiVAD support with the native heart left in place. This group comprises patients with multiple valve disease or ventricular wall aneurysms, intractable ventricular tachyarrhythmia, large intraventricular thrombi, and complications from myocardial infarction, such as post-infarction ventricular septal defects [7], which are common indications for TAH eligibility. Complex CF TAH control schemes and/or pressure/flow sensors will likely be needed to provide safe and effective cardiac replacement with dual-CF LVAD pumps for the chronic treatment of biventricular HF. The match of right- and left-side pump outputs while balancing atrial pressures has proven to be much more difficult for CF devices than for their pulsatile TAH predecessors when the native ventricle is not available to compensate for flow and pressure mismatches.

BiVACOR® TAH

An Australian team of collaborators [53] is evaluating a similar single-pump CF TAH concept for total heart replacement (BiVACOR BV Replace; BiVACOR, Wilston, QLD, Australia). It uses a magnetic field, a spinning disc, and centrifugal force to pump blood. Because it has only a single moving part and no friction is generated, this device is expected to be extremely durable. However, it requires significant input from sensors, as its rotating element requires electromagnetic suspension and must be actively positioned in the pump housing to balance flows. The team of inventors and research associates has joined with the Texas Heart Institute for device development and in vivo studies [45].

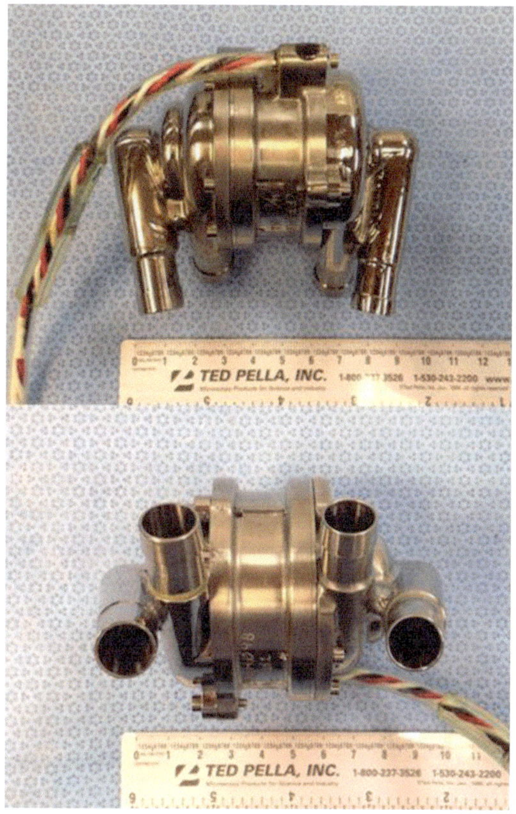

Fig. 26.8 The Cleveland Clinic continuous-flow total artificial heart (CF TAH)

Cleveland Clinic CF-TAH

Our team's progress with the Cleveland Clinic CF TAH (Fig. 26.8), which is designed to operate with the patient's native ventricles removed, was recently reported [54]. This device uses a single, centrally located, rotating assembly that has impellers for both left and right centrifugal pumps. It achieves passive, sensorless autoregulation of pump flows and filling pressures by varying relative left and right pump efficiencies, based on the position of its single moving part, to balance the left and right pump filling pressures and pump outputs [55].

The position of the centrally located rotating assembly is primarily determined by the differential force between the right and left pump filling pressures acting on this part. With the first successful chronic animal study conducted in early 2012, our in vivo experiments in calves ($n=12$, 77–93.9 kg) demonstrated good hemodynamic performance (pump flow, 7.5 ± 1 L/min; left atrial pressure, 15 ± 3 mmHg; right atrial pressure, 16 ± 3 mmHg; right-left atrial pressure difference, 1.2 ± 2.4 mmHg; mean arterial pressure, 104 ± 7 mmHg; arterial pulse pressure, 30 ± 13 mmHg; pulmonary arterial pressure, 32 ± 3 mmHg) and biocompatibility [56]. In all cases, the native ventricles had been fully removed. Teflon strips were sutured to right and left atrial stumps, and atrial cuffs were sutured to the corresponding stumps. Left and right outflow grafts were sutured to the pulmonary artery and aorta, respectively (Fig. 26.9). In all cases, we delivered the CF TAH pre-filled with saline and after a simple but meticulous de-airing procedure, the pump was connected to designated inflows

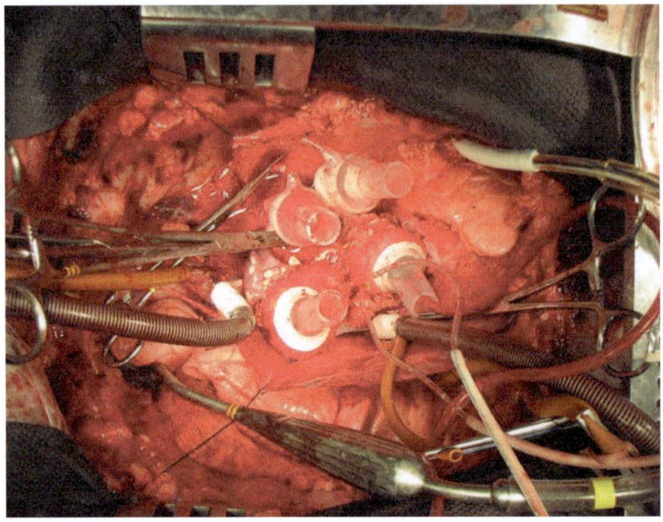

Fig. 26.9 The Cleveland Clinic CF TAH inflow and outflow conduits are in place before the pump connection

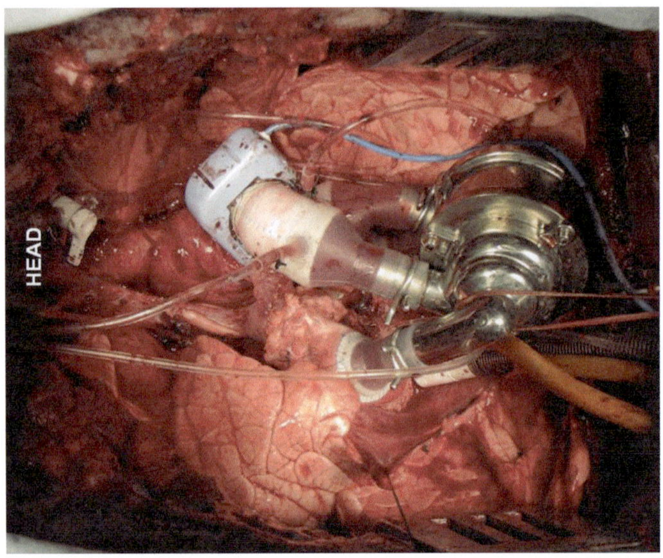

Fig. 26.10 The Cleveland Clinic CF TAH is placed inside the chest and connected

and outflows (Fig. 26.10). Recently (May, 2014), one calf was sacrificed after a planned duration of 30 days, still exhibiting excellent hemodynamic conditions and with no physical or pump-related complications. Most recently, two 90-day (November 2014) biocompatibility studies in calves were successfully completed at the planned durations and showed remarkable pump performance and biocompatibility. Device development and biocompatibility studies at Cleveland Clinic are ongoing.

Summary

Despite tremendous clinical advances in MCS over the last 25 years, the field is still considered to be in its infancy, and there is significant room for improvements in circulatory support technology. Given the potential number of patients who can benefit from this technology—an estimated 50,000–100,000 are in need of heart transplantation or MCS in the USA alone—

industry is vested in continuing to optimize the existing technology and bring new devices closer to clinical application. Over the next 3–5 years, we should expect to see transcutaneous energy delivery systems that, for at least some patients, will obviate the need for a driveline and allow 1–3 h of untethered time for showering, swimming, and other activities.

The theoretical advantages of centrifugal pumps over axial flow pumps could move the field more toward centrifugal pump design in the future. Centrifugal pumps have better flow characteristics that can minimize hemolysis and perhaps also lead to less need for anticoagulation therapy. In addition, such pumps have a greater degree of "pulsatility" inherent in their design, which may translate into reduced problems with aortic insufficiency, aortic valve fusion, and gastrointestinal bleeding. Finally, the particular pressure/flow characteristics of these pumps and their inherently more accurate flow estimation will likely lead to development of automatic speed control algorithms that may provide a much safer, more effective way of operating these pumps compared with the fixed-speed mode of operation that is currently practiced.

The issues surrounding management of RV failure are still at the crux of every decision that is made for LVAD implantation. Better techniques need to be developed to identify those who will not benefit from LVAD therapy alone. Development of a dedicated permanently implanted RVAD or of safe, effective conduit and pump speed modifications to current LVAD technology will greatly expand BiVAD application for chronic biventricular failure. Complete cardiac replacement with CF TAHs, while currently in early development and application, will play a key role in addressing a subset of chronic biventricular failure patients. Smaller, simpler CF TAHs that are proven reliable may even move the field completely in this direction. Biocompatible, subcutaneously implanted, percutaneously delivered intravascular pumps capable of providing permanent circulatory support at more than 3.0 L/min minimum may appear to be the new Holy Grail of the rapidly expanding market of cardiac circulatory support devices.

Issues surrounding the management of the ever-growing LVAD patient population are important for continued growth of the field and wider application of this technology. Although centers of excellence for LVADs will continue to develop, the only way that DT can truly become a preferred option is for more centers to obtain or expand their capability to implant LVADs. As the field moves toward treating the less sick HF patient population—those with fewer comorbidities and lesser degree of RV failure—and shifting its focus to improving quality of life, many more centers can become involved in LVAD implantation. This trend will provide patients with a wider access to centers of expertise and decongest some of the current high-volume implant centers, which will continue to concentrate their efforts on patients at higher risk. Furthermore, development of remote monitoring systems will allow improved assessment of patients with interventions implemented earlier to avert the high current readmission rates for those who have had VAD or TAH implantation.

Remarkable advances in the MCS field have revolutionized our thinking about the treatment of end-stage HF in patients who are not eligible for transplant. Despite much progress in performing randomized trials, which have consistently shown the benefits of this technology, commercial growth has been slow, and many surgeons and medical centers have yet to embrace this technology. It is expected that continued advances in this area will increase use of this therapy and perhaps replace heart transplantation either as the therapy of choice or as a strategy to delay transplantation in younger patients. Enthusiasm in the field of MCS will continue for years to come.

In the near future, we will be able to observe the HeartMate III, a centrifugal rotary pump replacement for the axial HeartMate II, and a series of miniaturized MVAD devices that can be placed for either intracardiac or intrapericardial implantation via a thoracotomy, off pump, in a beating heart. Miniaturized microaxial partial cardiac support pumps such as the Synergy LVAD and the Impella® cVAD (Abiomed), MVAD, and HeartMate X will be evaluated to determine their role in clinical HF treatment, and their limitations will be better defined. Permanent biventricular CF support and cardiac replacement with dual-CF TAH systems as well as single-piece CF TAHs are close to being introduced as a valid therapeutic option.

It is expected that advancement in the field of MCS will expand the use of these devices in patient numbers that will make heart transplantation a limited therapeutic option for a minority of terminally ill HF patients or will become a full long-term substitute in terms of quality of life. A consequence of the advances in pharmacotherapy, electrophysiology, and interventional procedures to treat HF is that these improvements increase the number of patients with end-stage HF who are unresponsive to conventional therapies, thus increasing the need for effective and safe MCS therapy.

It is worthwhile to realize that surgical indications continue to be updated and expanded as more innovative devices emerge. The most effective, durable, reliable, and fully autoregulated devices will save lives. However, until the ideal pump has been created and brought into accepted clinical practice, patient survival will continue to be primarily determined by an early decision to implant univentricular or biventricular devices and not by choice of device type.

Abbreviations

AC	Alternating current
BiVAD	Biventricular assist device
BTT	Bridge to transplant
CF	Continuous flow
DC	Direct current
DT	Destination therapy
HF	Heart failure
LVAD	Left ventricular assist device
MCS	Mechanical circulatory support
RV	Right ventricle
RVAD	Right ventricular assist device
TAH	Total artificial heart

References

1. Go AS, Mozaffarian D, Roger VL, Benjamin EJ, Berry JD, Borden WB, et al. Executive summary: heart disease and stroke statistics–2013 update: a report from the American Heart Association. Circulation. 2013;127(1):143–52.
2. McMurray JJ, Petrie MC, Murdoch DR, Davie AP. Clinical epidemiology of heart failure: public and private health burden. Eur Heart J. 1998;19 Suppl P:P9–16.
3. Braunwald E. Research advances in heart failure: a compendium. Circ Res. 2013;113(6):633–45.
4. Heidenreich PA, Albert NM, Allen LA, Bluemke DA, Butler J, Fonarow GC, et al. Forecasting the impact of heart failure in the United States: a policy statement from the American Heart Association. Circ Heart Fail. 2013;6(3):606–19.
5. Garbade J, Bittner HB, Barten MJ, Mohr FW. Current trends in implantable left ventricular assist devices. Cardiol Res Pract. 2011;2011:290561.
6. Wever-Pinzon O, Drakos SG, Kfoury AG, Nativi JN, Gilbert EM, Everitt M, et al. Morbidity and mortality in heart transplant candidates supported with mechanical circulatory support: is reappraisal of the current United network for organ sharing thoracic organ allocation policy justified? Circulation. 2013;127(4):452–62.
7. Moazami N, Hoercher KJ, Fukamachi K, Kobayashi M, Smedira NG, Massiello A, et al. Mechanical circulatory support for heart failure: past, present and a look at the future. Expert Rev Med Devices. 2013;10(1):55–71. Review.
8. Kirklin JK, Naftel DC, Pagani FD, Kormos RL, Stevenson L, Miller M, et al. Long-term mechanical circulatory support (destination therapy): on track to compete with heart transplantation? J Thorac Cardiovasc Surg. 2012;144(3):584–603. discussion 597–8.
9. Sheikh FH, Russell SD. HeartMate(R) II continuous-flow left ventricular assist system. Expert Rev Med Devices. 2011;8(1):11–21. Review.
10. Slaughter MS, Rogers JG, Milano CA, Russell SD, Conte JV, Feldman D, et al. Advanced heart failure treated with continuous-flow left ventricular assist device. N Engl J Med. 2009;361(23):2241–51.
11. Rogers JG, Aaronson KD, Boyle AJ, Russell SD, Milano CA, Pagani FD, et al. Continuous flow left ventricular assist device improves functional capacity and quality of life of advanced heart failure patients. J Am Coll Cardiol. 2010;55(17):1826–34.
12. Kounis NG, Soufras GD, Davlouros P, Tsigkas G, Hahalis G. Thrombus formation patterns in HeartMate II continuous-flow left ventricular assist devices: a multifactorial phenomenon involving Kounis syndrome? ASAIO J. 2014;60(4):369–71.
13. Starling RC, Moazami N, Silvestry SC, Ewald G, Rogers JG, Milano CA, et al. Unexpected abrupt increase in left ventricular assist device thrombosis. N Engl J Med. 2014;370(1):33–40.

14. Salerno CT, Sundareswaran KS, Schleeter TP, Moanie SL, Farrar DJ, Walsh MN. Early elevations in pump power with the HeartMate II left ventricular assist device do not predict late adverse events. J Heart Lung Transplant. 2014;33(8):809–15.
15. Strueber M, Meyer AL, Malehsa D, Haverich A. Successful use of the HeartWare HVAD rotary blood pump for biventricular support. J Thorac Cardiovasc Surg. 2010;140(4):936–7. Case Report.
16. Krabatsch T, Potapov E, Stepanenko A, Schweiger M, Kukucka M, Huebler M, et al. Biventricular circulatory support with two miniaturized implantable assist devices. Circulation. 2011;124(11 Suppl):S179–86.
17. Slaughter MS, Pagani FD, McGee EC, Birks EJ, Cotts WG, Gregoric I, et al. HeartWare ventricular assist system for bridge to transplant: combined results of the bridge to transplant and continued access protocol trial. J Heart Lung Transplant. 2013;32(7):675–83.
18. Wieselthaler GM, O-Driscoll G, Jansz P, Khaghani A, Strueber M, HVAD Clinical Investigators. Initial clinical experience with a novel left ventricular assist device with a magnetically levitated rotor in a multi-institutional trial. J Heart Lung Transplant. 2010; 29(11):1218–25.
19. Najjar SS, Slaughter MS, Pagani FD, Starling RC, McGee EC, Eckman P, et al. An analysis of pump thrombus events in patients in the HeartWare ADVANCE bridge to transplant and continued access protocol trial. J Heart Lung Transplant. 2014;33(1): 23–34.
20. Frazier OH, Myers TJ, Gregoric I. Biventricular assistance with the Jarvik FlowMaker: a case report. J Thorac Cardiovasc Surg. 2004;128(4):625–6.
21. Jarvik R. Jarvik 2000 pump technology and miniaturization. Heart Fail Clin. 2014;10(1 Suppl):S27–38.
22. John R. Current axial-flow devices—the HeartMate II and Jarvik 2000 left ventricular assist devices. Semin Thorac Cardiovasc Surg. 2008;20(3):264–72.
23. Sorensen EN, Pierson 3rd RN, Feller ED, Griffith BP. University of Maryland surgical experience with the Jarvik 2000 axial flow ventricular assist device. Ann Thorac Surg. 2012;93(1):133–40.
24. Myers TJ, Robertson K, Pool T, Shah N, Gregoric I, Frazier OH. Continuous flow pumps and total artificial hearts: management issues. Ann Thorac Surg. 2003;75(6 Suppl):S79–85.
25. Frazier OH, Myers TJ, Westaby S, Gregoric ID. Use of the Jarvik 2000 left ventricular assist system as a bridge to heart transplantation or as destination therapy for patients with chronic heart failure. Ann Surg. 2003;237(5):631–6. discussion 636–7.
26. Moazami N, Fukamachi K, Kobayashi M, Smedira NG, Hoercher KJ, Massiello A, et al. Axial and centrifugal continuous-flow rotary pumps: a translation from pump mechanics to clinical practice. J Heart Lung Transplant. 2013;32(1):1–11.
27. Fukamachi K. Current status of artificial heart (assist/replacement) development in the United States. Artif Organs. 2013;37(8):675–6.
28. Schmitto JD, Burkhoff D, Avsar M, Fey O, Ziehme P, Buechler G, et al. Two axial-flow Synergy Micro-Pumps as a biventricular assist device in an ovine animal model. J Heart Lung Transplant. 2012;31(11): 1223–9.
29. Klotz S, Meyns B, Simon A, Wittwer T, Rahmanian P, Schlensak C, et al. Partial mechanical long-term support with the CircuLite Synergy pump as bridge-to-transplant in congestive heart failure. Thorac Cardiovasc Surg. 2010;58 Suppl 2:S173–8.
30. Fukamachi K, Shiose A, Massiello AL, Horvath DJ, Golding LA, Lee S, et al. Implantable continuous-flow right ventricular assist device: lessons learned in the development of a Cleveland Clinic device. Ann Thorac Surg. 2012;93(5):1746–52.
31. Timms D, Gude E, Gaddum N, Lim E, Greatrex N, Wong K, et al. Assessment of right pump outflow banding and speed changes on pulmonary hemodynamics during biventricular support with two rotary left ventricular assist devices. Artif Organs. 2011; 35(8):807–13.
32. Loforte A, Stepanenko A, Potapov EV, Musumeci F, Dranishnikov N, Schweiger M, et al. Temporary right ventricular mechanical support in high-risk left ventricular assist device recipients versus permanent biventricular or total artificial heart support. Artif Organs. 2013;37(6):523–30.
33. Kaczorowski DJ, Woo YJ. Who needs an RVAD in addition to an LVAD? Cardiol Clin. 2011;29(4): 599–605.
34. Saito S, Sakaguchi T, Miyagawa S, Yoshikawa Y, Yamauchi T, Ueno T, et al. Biventricular support using implantable continuous-flow ventricular assist devices. J Heart Lung Transplant. 2011;30(4):475–8.
35. Hetzer R, Krabatsch T, Stepanenko A, Hennig E, Potapov EV. Long-term biventricular support with the heartware implantable continuous flow pump. J Heart Lung Transplant. 2010;29(7):822–4.
36. Loforte A, Monica PL, Montalto A, Musumeci F. HeartWare third-generation implantable continuous flow pump as biventricular support: mid-term follow-up. Interact Cardiovasc Thorac Surg. 2011; 12(3):458–60.
37. Potapov E, Schweiger M, Vierecke J, Dandel M, Stepanenko A, Kukucka M, et al. Discontinuation of HeartWare RVAD support without device removal in chronic BIVAD patients. ASAIO J. 2012;58(1):15–8.
38. Krabatsch T, Stepanenko A, Schweiger M, Kukucka M, Ewert P, Hetzer R, et al. Alternative technique for implantation of biventricular support with HeartWare implantable continuous flow pump. ASAIO J. 2011; 57(4):333–5.
39. Deuse T, Schirmer J, Kubik M, Reichenspurner H. Isolated permanent right ventricular assistance using the HVAD continuous-flow pump. Ann Thorac Surg. 2013;95(4):1434–6.
40. Chen JM, Levin HR, Rose EA, Addonizio LJ, Landry DW, Sistino JJ, et al. Experience with right ventricular assist devices for perioperative right-sided circulatory failure. Ann Thorac Surg. 1996;61(1):305–10. discussion 311–3.
41. Lazar JF, Swartz MF, Schiralli MP, Schneider M, Pisula B, Hallinan W, et al. Survival after left ventricular assist

device with and without temporary right ventricular support. Ann Thorac Surg. 2013;96(6):2155–9.
42. Meineri M, Van Rensburg AE, Vegas A. Right ventricular failure after LVAD implantation: prevention and treatment. Best Pract Res Clin Anaesthesiol. 2012;26(2):217–29.
43. Kormos RL. The right heart failure dilemma in the era of left ventricular assist devices. J Heart Lung Transplant. 2014;33(2):134–5.
44. Aissaoui N, Morshuis M, Schoenbrodt M, Hakim Meibodi K, Kizner L, Borgermann J, et al. Temporary right ventricular mechanical circulatory support for the management of right ventricular failure in critically ill patients. J Thorac Cardiovasc Surg. 2013; 146(1):186–91.
45. Berger E. Donor brings inventor of artificial heart closer to Houston. [*Houston Chronicle* (Houston, TX) Web site] January 14, 2013. http://www.chron.com/news/health/article/Donor-brings-of-artificial-heart-closer-to-Houston-4189733.php#photo-4023246. Accessed 29 June 2014.
46. Copeland JG, Smith RG, Arabia FA, Nolan PE, Sethi GK, Tsau PH, et al. Cardiac replacement with a total artificial heart as a bridge to transplantation. N Engl J Med. 2004;351(9):859–67.
47. Italian man surpasses 1,000 days of support with SynCardia's total artificial heart. [Press release, Syncardia Systems, Inc., Web site] October 12, 2010. http://www.syncardia.com/2010-press-release/italian-man-surpasses-1000-days-of-support-with-syncardias-total-artificial-heart.html. Accessed 29 June 2014.
48. Jansen P, van Oeveren W, Capel A, Carpentier A. In vitro haemocompatibility of a novel bioprosthetic total artificial heart. Eur J Cardiothorac Surg. 2012; 41(6):e166–72.
49. carmatsa.com [Internet, Web site of CARMAT, Velizy Villacoublay, France]. Available (in English): http://www.carmatsa.com/index.php?&lang=en. Accessed 29 June 2014.
50. Irish J. Heart maker Carmat to wait before next transplant: founder. [*Reuters* Web site] March 16, 2014. http://www.reuters.com/article/2014/03/16/us-carmat-heart-trials-idUSBREA2F0K920140316. Accessed 29 June 2014.
51. Cohn WE, Winkler JA, Parnis S, Costas GG, Beathard S, Conger J, et al. Ninety-day survival of a calf implanted with a continuous-flow total artificial heart. ASAIO J. 2014;60(1):15–8.
52. Cohn WE, Handy KM, Parnis SM, Conger JL, Winkler JA, Frazier OH. Eight-year experience with a continuous-flow total artificial heart in calves. ASAIO J. 2014;60(1):25–30.
53. Timms D, Fraser J, Hayne M, Dunning J, McNeil K, Pearcy M. The BiVACOR rotary biventricular assist device: concept and in vitro investigation. Artif Organs. 2008;32(10):816–9.
54. Kobayashi M, Horvath DJ, Mielke N, Shiose A, Kuban B, Goodin M, et al. Progress on the design and development of the continuous-flow total artificial heart. Artif Organs. 2012;36(8):705–13.
55. Fukamachi K, Horvath DJ, Massiello AL, Fumoto H, Horai T, Rao S, et al. An innovative, sensorless, pulsatile, continuous-flow total artificial heart: device design and initial in vitro study. J Heart Lung Transplant. 2010;29(1):13–20.
56. Karimov JH, Fukamachi K, Moazami N, Kobayashi M, Sale S, Mielke N, et al. In vivo evaluation of the Cleveland clinic continuous-flow total artificial heart in calves. J Heart Lung Transplant. 2014;33(4 Suppl): S165–6.

New Valves: Where Do We Stand?

27

Jochen Reinöhl, Manfred Zehender, and Christoph Bode

Introduction

Percutaneous, catheter-based systems were tested in animal models as early as the mid-1960s [1–3]. However, 30 years of further development of frame and valve technology was necessary before the first transcatheter implantation of a balloon-expandable prosthesis was successfully performed in a pig model [4]. In 2000, Bonhoeffer and his team achieved the first percutaneous cardiac valve implantation in humans with implantation of a stent-mounted, bovine jugular vein valve in the position of the pulmonary valve [5]. For the first time worldwide, Alain Cribier successfully treated a high-grade, calcified aortic valve stenosis using a balloon-expandable aortic valve in 2002 [6]. Numerous smaller mono- and multicenter studies later confirmed the technical feasibility of this procedure. Its true value as an important alternative to open heart surgery in inoperable and high-risk patients was not confirmed until 2010 by broad multicenter registers and the prospective, randomized PARTNER Study (Placement of Aortic Transcatheter Valves) [7–9].

J. Reinöhl, M.D. (✉) • M. Zehender, M.D.
C. Bode, M.D.
Department of Cardiology and Angiology I, Heart Center of Freiburg University, Freiburg, Germany
e-mail: Jochen.reinoehl@universitaets-herzzentrum.de; Manfred.zehender@universitaets-herzzentrum.de; Christoph.bode@universitaets-herzzentrum.de

Indication and Patient Selection

Stringent patient selection and thorough assessment of the technical feasibility are decisive for the procedural success and safety of TAVR (Transcatheter Aortic Valve Replacement). The clinical indication for TAVR is set forth in the appropriate guidelines of the specialist societies [10]. In addition to native aortic valve stenosis, TAVR can be nowadays used in selected patients for both pure aortic valve regurgitation and the treatment of degenerative bioprostheses (i.e., valve-in-valve procedure). In accordance to the guidelines, TAVR should only be undertaken in patients with contraindication for conventional aortic valve replacement (such as porcelain aorta) and/or high operative risk. Surgical risk scores, such as the EuroSCORE or the STS Score, are used to assess the risk of SAVR (Surgical Aortic Valve Replacement). Once the clinical indication has been made and the patient has been identified as a possible TAVR candidate, the technical feasibility and absence of contraindications must be clarified. The diagnostic procedures and their significance within the scope of the TAVR screening are summarized in Table 27.1.

Aortic Valve Anatomy and Morphology

Precise measurement of the aortic annulus is decisive for transcatheter heart valve (THV) size selection. Due to the complex, frequently oval

R. Latifi et al. (eds.), *Technological Advances in Surgery, Trauma and Critical Care*,
DOI 10.1007/978-1-4939-2671-8_27

Table 27.1 Diagnostic procedures and their significance for the TAVI screening

Screening parameters	Diagnostic procedure TTE	TEE (3D-TEE)	CT	R/L catheter
Severity of the aortic valve stenosis	++	++	+	++
Fixated vs. functional stenosis	++ (Dobutamine)		–	–
Aortic valve anatomy and morphology	+	++	++	±
Aortic annulus	–	+	++	±
Vascular access	–	–	++	+
Catheter passage	–	±	++	+
Coronary heart disease	–	–	±	++

– not helpful, ± somewhat helpful, + helpful, ++ very helpful (selection method)

With permission from Delgado V, Ng AC, Shanks M, van der Kley F, Schuijf JD, van de Veire NR, Kroft L, de Roos A, Schalij MJ, Bax JJ. Transcatheter aortic valve implantation: Role of multimodality cardiac imaging. Expert Rev Cardiovasc Ther. 2010;8:113–123

anatomy of the aortic annulus, three-dimensional transesophageal echocardiography (3D-TEE) and/or computed tomography (CT) do provide decisive additional information and should be used in supplement to transthoracic echocardiography (TTE) and/or angiography [11, 12]. Minimal, maximal, and the annulus area derived diameter help to understand the annulus anatomy and enable an optimal prosthesis selection [13]. Moreover, the assessment of aortic valve anatomy and the severity as well as localization of the aortic valve calcification are important components of TAVR screening. Due to the danger of an implantation-associated aortic rupture, a bicuspid aortic valve is a typical contraindication, which must be reliably ruled out during screening [14].

Aortic Root and Coronary Ostia Distance

Assessment of the aortic root is particularly important for implantation of the self-expandable Medtronic (Minneapolis, MN) CoreValve® System. Because of the directional and fixation mechanism of the prosthesis, extremely narrow or broad aortic roots are contraindications. These limitations do not apply to the balloon-expandable Edwards THVs. Measurements of the aortic annulus, the sinus of Valsalva, and the ascending aorta are necessary. CT and MRI are considered the gold standard as a result of the potential for multiplane reconstruction with orthogonal measurement in all segments [15]. Both procedures also enable a thorough assessment of the degree of calcification of the aortic root and may therefore be helpful in selecting the path of access. Moreover, in assessing the risk of the rare but often fatal coronary ostia obstruction, determination of the spacing of coronary orifices at the level of the aortic valve is essential [16].

Vascular Access and Catheter Passage

In planning the vascular access, evaluation of the size, the degree of calcification, and the vascular tortuosity of the peripheral arteries and of the abdominal and thoracic aorta is essential [17]. The coincidence of symptomatic aortic valve stenosis and peripheral vascular disease is known and increases the risk of complications [18]. Therefore, a transapical procedure should be preferred in the case of small-caliber femoral arteries (<5.5–6 mm), extremely calcified and tortuous iliacal or femoral vessels, or in the presence of a porcelain aorta [16]. In addition to the invasive angiography, CT and MRI are available for the assessment. The latter not only enable measurement of the endoluminal diameter but also provide information for determination of the extent and site of calcifications and stenosis.

Supplemental Diagnostics

In addition to the examination procedures already listed, TAVR screening is completed by right/left coronary catheter (including AOA determination, coronary angiography, bulbus and iliacal/femoral artery angiography), lung function testing, and laboratory tests. Important information on accompanying diseases of the heart, lungs, kidneys, or liver can thus be collected and used for therapy decisions for the individual patient. Serious secondary findings are not infrequently disclosed which may in part explain the patient's symptoms (e.g., coronary heart disease as a cause of dyspnoea), and sometimes require re-evaluation of the life expectancy and indication for TAVR (e.g., neoplasia of the pancreas).

Implantation Technique

The basic principle of the procedure is the percutaneous, transcatheter implantation of a bioprosthesis anchored in a metal frame (THV). After balloon aortic valvuloplastie or immediately, the THV affixed to the tip of the catheter is positioned retrograde or anterograde in the aortic annulus of the native aortic valve and is then expanded. To date, there are primarily two types of transcatheter aortic valve prostheses in broad clinical use: the balloon-expandable Edwards-Bioprosthesis (Edwards Lifesciences Corporation, Irvine, CA) and the self-expanding CoreValve System (Medtronic Inc., Irvine, CA). The technical details and anatomic prerequisites of both are summarized in Table 27.2.

Balloon-Expandable Bioprostheses

The current generation of the Edwards-THV, the SAPIEN XT® (Edwards Lifesciences Corporation, Irvine, CA) (Fig. 27.1a), consists of a cobalt-chrome frame with integrated tricuspid bovine pericardial valve. Analogous to coronary stent implantation, implantation of the prosthesis is performed by balloon inflation. A high-frequency, right ventricular stimulation (180–220 bpm) for minimizing the transaortic flow stabilizes the prosthesis during the expansion phase and prevents prosthesis dislocation. The SAPIEN XT® is available in three sizes (23, 26, and 29 mm) and can be used in aortic annuli from 20 to 27 mm. Currently, the third generation THV (SAPIEN 3®, Fig. 27.1b) is just being introduced in Europe. It is mainly characterized by a new frame design, intended for a lower delivery profile, and an outer skirt designed to reduce paravalvular leakage. The first two generations of the Edwards-Bioprosthesis (Cribier-Edwards and

Table 27.2 Technical details and anatomic prerequisites of the Edwards SAPIEN XT® (Edwards Lifesciences, Irvine, CA) and Medtronic CoreValve® prosthesis (Medtronic, Minneapolis, MN)

	Edwards SAPIEN XT THV			Medtronic CoreValve		
Technical details	Cobalt chromium stent			Nitinol frame		
	Tricuspid bovine pericardial valve			Tricuspid porcine pericardial valve		
Prosthesis						
Size (mm)	23	26	29	26	29	31
Catheter system						
Transfemoral (Fr)	16[a]	18	20	18	18	18
Transapical (Fr)	24	24	26	–	–	–
Anatomic prerequisites						
Aortic annulus (mm)	18–22	21–25	24–27	20–23	23–27	26–29
Coronary ostia distance (mm)	≥10	≥10	≥10	–	–	–
Height of the sinus of Valsalva (mm)	–	–	–	≥15	≥15	≥15
Vascular diameter of catheter passage (mm)	≥6	≥6.5	≥7	≥6	≥6	≥6

[a]Edward Nova Flex Plus System with eSheath (expandable sheath)

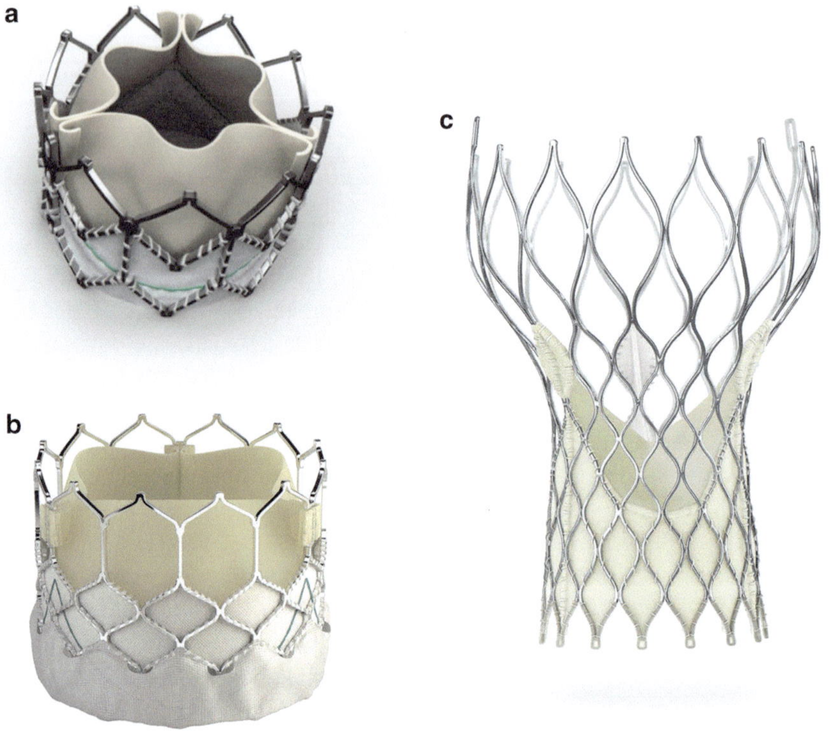

Fig. 27.1 (**a**, **b**) Balloon-expandable Edwards SAPIEN XT® and SAPIEN 3® THV (Courtesy of Edwards Lifesciences, Irvine, CA). (**c**) Self-expanding Medtronic CoreValve® bioprosthesis (Courtesy of Medtronic, Minneapolis, MN)

Edwards SAPIEN®) were tested in randomized studies for transfemoral and transapical procedures.

Self-Expandable Bioprostheses

The present third generation of the CoreValve bioprosthesis (Fig. 27.1c) is constructed of an optimized (maximal radial force, anatomic adaptation), self-expandable nitinol frame with integrated tricuspid porcine pericardial valve. It is released by withdrawing the outer catheter sheath. Contrary to balloon-expandable systems, no tachycardic pacing is required during prosthesis expansion. The valve is available in sizes of 23, 26, 29, and 31 mm for a retrograde procedure, via the femoral/subclavian/axillary artery, or via a direct transaortic access. Whereas the first prosthesis generation required a 25F sheath, the procedure is performed now using an 18F sheath.

Approaches

Supported by the catheter, the valve prosthesis can be brought to the native aortic valve via two different routes: (1) anterograde, i.e., following blood flow, from the left ventricle via a transapical access; or (2) retrograde, i.e., via the ascending aorta applying a transarterial procedure. Transarterial, i.e., the transfemoral procedure or access via A. subclavia or A. axillaris or as an alternative the direct, transaortic procedure have proven valuable.

The transapical approach (TA-AVR; Fig. 27.2) requires a small left lateral minithoracotomy with direct puncture of the left ventricular apex and was first described in 2006 by Litchenstein et al. [19]. Advantages of the TA-AVR are (1) the very good control of the prosthesis during positioning and implantation due to the very short distance between the vascular access and the native aortic valve, and (2) that there is no need for peripheral arterial catheter passage, especially with pre-existing peripheral artery disease. TA-AVR is mainly performed under general anesthesia in the operating room or in a hybrid-OR. Case reports have been published on high epidural anesthesia in TA-AVR, but these are not widely used [20, 21].

With the continuous reduction of sheath size and improvement in closure devices used, transfemoral TAVR (TF-AVR; Fig. 27.2) has developed nowadays in most centers to the preferred procedure. As a purely percutaneous procedure, TF-AVR is performed under local or general anesthesia primarily in the cardiac catheter laboratory or in the hybrid-OR. The access via the subclavian or axillary artery (TS-AVR; Fig. 27.2) is considered as an alternative to the transfemoral approach [21] and is reported in a proportion of 20 % in an Italian registry. Due to the anatomical site, TS-AVR usually requires surgical exposure of the artery. An advantage of the axillary over the subclavian approach is that vascular injuries can be treated more easily.

Direct, transaortic access through a small right or medial sternotomy (TAO-AVR; Fig. 27.2) was first presented in 2009 as a retrograde alternative [22]. Analogous to the TA- and TS-AVR, the short distance to the aortic valve enables optimal catheter control. Moreover, there is an advantage that no peripheral arterial catheter passage or apical puncture is necessary. However, due to the risk of severe intrathoracic bleeding, TAO-AVR is indicated only for a few selected patients (e.g., if alternative access routes are not feasible).

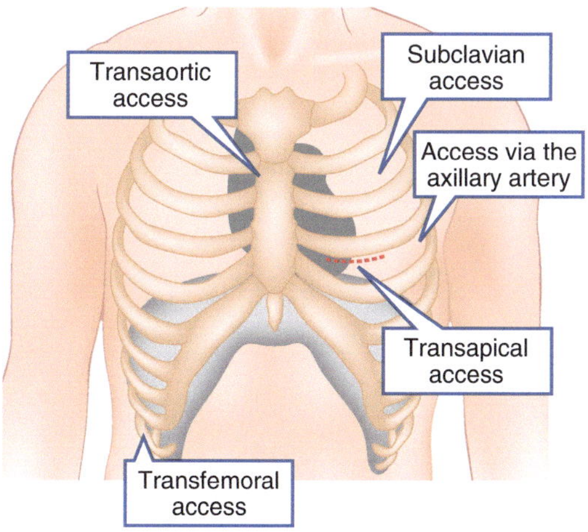

Fig. 27.2 Illustration of the different TAVR approaches

Clinical Studies and Results

The PARTNER trial and the CoreValve High Risk Study are currently the only prospective, randomized TAVR studies. The most important results are shown in Table 27.3. In the CoreValve High Risk Study, only patients with severe aortic valve stenosis who were at increased risk were included. In PARTNER patients were enrolled who were either at increased operative risk (Cohort A) or inoperable (Cohort B). Cohort A compared TF- and TA-AVR with surgical aortic valve replacement (SAVR) [23, 24]. In Cohort B, TF-AVR was tested in comparison with a standard therapy [13]. Moreover, several multicenter registries have been published in recent years. An overview of the registries with the largest number of patients is found in Table 27.3. It should be noted that the registries consist primarily of inoperable and high-risk patients (EuroSCORE >20 %, STS Score >8 %) [8, 9, 25–29]. Furthermore, most patients present with a mean age above 80 years and with numerous comorbidities, like coronary (>50 %) and peripheral artery disease, as well as chronic kidney and pulmonary disease (>20 %).

Procedural Success and Hemodynamics

The feasibility of the procedure is clearly demonstrated in clinical practice with a procedural success rate of >90 % and an extremely low conversion rate to SAVR (0.5–2.3 %). The short- and long-term hemodynamic results after TAVR are also convincing, with a mean gradient of <15 mmHg and an orifice area >1.5 cm [2] (Fig. 27.3) [6–9, 16, 23–26, 28–40]. Moreover, hemodynamics after TAVR, analogous to SAVR, result in an improvement of left ventricular function in most patients, especially in patients with LVEF

Table 27.3 Randomized controlled trials and multicenter registries

Study	*n*	Approach (*n*)	Valve type	Euro Score I (%)	Success rate (%)	30-day mortality (%)	1-year mortality (%)	Stroke (%)	Major vascular complications (%)	Permanent pacemaker (%)
Randomized controlled trials										
PARTNER A [17, 18] (inoperable cohort)	358	TF: 179	SAPIEN®	26.4 ± 17.2	98.8	5	30.7	6.7	16.2	3.4
PARTNER B [1] (high-risk cohort)	699	TF: 244	SAPIEN®	29.3 ± 16.5	N/A	3.4 (TF: 3.3; TA: 3.8)	24.2 (TF: 22.2; TA: 29)	4.6	11	3.8
		TA: 104								
CoreValve High Risk Study	795	TF	CoreValve®	17.6 ± 13.0	N/A	N/A	14.2 % vs. 19.1 %	N/A	5.9 % vs. 1.7 %	19.8 % vs. 7.1 %
Registries										
Canadian [24]	339	TF: 162	Cribier-Edwards: 57	27.7 ± 16.3	93.3	10.4	24	2.3	13	4.9
					TF: 90.5	TF: 9.5	TF: 25	TF: 3.0	TF: 13.1	TF: 3.6
			SAPIEN®: 275	TF: 25.8 ± 14.9	TA: 96.1	TA: 11.3	TA: 22	TA: 1.7	TA: 13.0	TA: 6.2
		TA: 177	SAPIEN XT®: 7	TA: 29.4 ± 17.2						
European [19]	646	All TF	CoreValve®	TF: 23.1 ± 13.8	TF: 97.2	TF: 8.0	N/A	TF: 1.9	TF: 1.9	TF: 9.3
German [22]	697	TF: 644	SAPIEN®: 109	20.5 ± 13.2	98.4	12.4	N/A	2.8	19.5	39.3
										SAPIEN®: 22.0
		TS: 22	CoreValve®: 588							CoreValve®:42.5
		TA: 26								
		TAO: 5								
Italian [20]	663	TF: 599	CoreValve®	23.0 ± 13.7	98	5.4	15	1.2	2	16.6
		TS: 64								
SOURCE [3]	1038	TF: 463	SAPIEN®	TF: 25.7 ± 14.5	93.8	8.5	23.9	2.5	7	7
		TA: 575			TF: 95.2	TF: 6.3	TF: 18.9	TF: 2.4	TF: 10.6	TF: 6.7
				TA: 29.1 ± 16.3	TA: 92.7	TA: 10.3	TA: 27.9	TA: 2.6	TA: 2.4	TA: 7.3
UK [23]	870	TF: 599	SAPIEN®: 410	N/A	97.2	7.1	21.4	4.1	6.3	16.3
		Others: 271	CoreValve®: 452							

SAPIEN®, SAPIEN XT®, Cribier-Edwards: Edwards Lifesciences Corporation, Irvine, CA; CoreValve®: Medtronic, Minneapolis, MN
Abbreviations: *TAVI* transcatheter aortic valve implantation, *TF* transfemoral, *TS* subclavian, *TA* transapical, *TAO* transaortic, *N/A* data not available

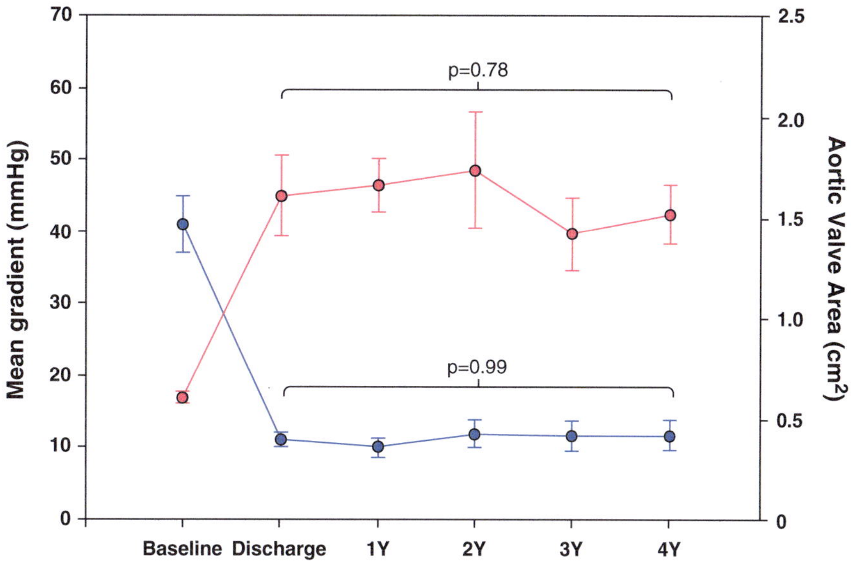

Fig. 27.3 Short- and long-term hemodynamic results after TAVR, with a mean residual gradient of < 15 mmHg and an orifice area >1.5 cm². Data from Rodes-Cabau J, Webb J, Cheung A, Ye J, Dumont E, Chris F, Osten M, Natarajan M, Velianou JL, Martucci G, DeVarennes B, Thompson CR, Chisholm R, Peterson M, Lichtenstein S, Toggweiler S, Doyle D, DeLarochelli R, Dumesnil J, Teoh K, Chu V, Cheema A, Wood D, Pibarot P, Horlick E. Long-term outcomes following transcatheter aortic valve implantation: Insights on prognostic factors and valve durability from the Canadian multicenter experience. Journal of the American College of Cardiology. 2012;59:E10–E10

<50 % [41–43]. It is, however, decisive that the current results do not indicate any basic long-term problems for TAVR.

NYHA Class and Quality of Life

TAVR improves the patient's symptoms and NYHA Class, respectively [6–9, 16, 23–26, 28–40]. While most patients have NYHA Class III prior to the procedure, NYHA Class I or II could be attained even in the mid-term course [7, 9, 44]. Improvement in exercise capacity was objectified using the standardized 6-min walking test [44]. Several studies have also shown a positive effect on the quality of life [45–48]. Due to the numerous, sometimes serious secondary comorbidities (cardiomyopathy, mitral valve regurgitation, COPD, stroke, dialysis) and also because of the advanced age, not all patients benefit from TAVR [47, 49]. Future studies will help to identify patients with a positive benefit-risk ratio.

Mortality

PARTNER B (inoperable patients) showed a clear survival advantage for transcatheter aortic valve replacement [7]. The 1-year mortality was 30.7 % vs. 50.7 % in the conservative treatment group ($p<0.01$). Patients treated with the SAPIEN THV (exclusively TF-AVR) had an absolute reduction in mortality at 1 year of 20 %, with a number needed to treat (NNT) of 5. PARTNER A, designed to prove the non-inferiority of TAVR compared to SAVR, confirmed this with respect to the 30-day (TAVR: 3.4 % vs. SAVR: 6.5 %; $p=0.07$) and 1-year mortality (TAVR: 24.2 % vs. SAVR: 26.8 %; $p=0.44$) [23, 24]. Analogous, the CoreValve High Risk study showed that TAVR with a self-expanding THV is associated with a significantly higher rate of survival at 1 year than surgical aortic valve replacement (14.2 % vs. 19.2 %).

The published studies and registry data systematically show a 30-day mortality of <10 % for the transfemoral and <17 % for the transapical approach [8, 9, 25–29, 40, 50, 51]. It can be assumed that the difference between the two approaches is most likely due to the higher risk profile of the patients undergoing the transapical procedure. The mortality after 1 year was 20 % (TF-AVR: 15–25 %), respectively 30 % (TA-AVR: 22–37 %).

To date, there are only few long-term data on TAVR. In the PARTNER A Cohort, Kodali et al. showed a mortality after 2 years of 33.9 % for TAVR and 35 % for SAVR ($p=0.78$) [24]. In the 2-year follow-up, the PARTNER B Cohort confirmed the significant survival advantage found after 1 year for TAVR compared to conservative treatment (TF-AVR: 56.7 % vs. Standard therapy: 32.4 %; $p<0.01$) [52]. Buellesfeld et al. reported a 2-year survival rate of 72 % for the CoreValve System [53]. A small Edwards collective (88 patients, treated with the Cribier-Edwards or Edwards SAPIEN valves) showed a survival rate of 51 % after 3 years [54]. Comparable results with survival rates of 52 % after 3 years and 50 % after 4 years are found in the Canadian Registry [55]. When one considers the learning curve effect and the technical advances, further improvement can be expected in the future [56, 57].

Complications

In assessing TAVR complications, it must be remembered that a standardized consensus definition of the relevant clinical endpoints and complications was not made by the Valve Academic Research Consortium (VARC) until 2011 [58]. Differences in the published complication rates may thus sometimes be attributed to this situation. In addition, the continuous technical advances (such as smaller catheter systems, prosthesis design) and the learning curve effect may explain discrepancies encountered over time. The most important complications associated with TAVR are listed in Table 27.3.

Cerebrovascular Events

A decisive factor for the acceptance and future expansion of the indication spectrum for TAVR is certainly the frequency of cerebrovascular events. A meta-analysis of 10,037 published cases showed an event rate (TIA and stroke) of 3.3 % in the first 30 days after TAVR [59]. In the majority of cases, serious stroke occurred. These were accompanied by a 3.5-fold higher mortality. MRI studies also show postinterventional "silent" cerebral insults in 66–84 % of TAVR patients, occurring independently of valve type and route of access [60–62]. Decisive, predisposing factors for the occurrence of stroke are a newly occurring atrial fibrillation and a higher-grade mitral valve insufficiency [63]. Moreover, the antithrombotic and anticoagulatory regime appear to play a major role. There are presently no clear recommendations from the specialist societies in this respect.

Solutions and Prevention Strategies

Several protection systems have been developed in recent years to prevent cerebrovascular events during TAVR [64]. Additional studies are needed, however, to confirm the benefit and safety of these systems. With respect to postinterventional drug treatment, Ussia et al. demonstrated in a smaller series that dual antiplatelet therapy (combination of ASS and clopidogrel), which is used at most centers, is not superior to administration of aspirin alone [65]. There are as yet no larger studies on antithrombotic or anticoagulatory therapy.

Vascular Complications

Vascular complications occur frequently in TAVR, particularly in the transfemoral procedure, and are an independent predictor of the 30-day mortality [26, 66, 67]. The incidence varies in the published studies and registries between 2 and 26 % in TF-AVR, and 5 and 7 % in TA-AVR [26, 27, 68, 69]. The causes are (1) the use of large catheter and tube systems (18–24 French) and (2) marked atherosclerosis in the usually >80-year-old patients [70]. The extent and localization of vascular calcification and kinking, the relationship between sheath and vascular diameter, but also the degree of experience at the center and of the individual operator have also been proven to affect the frequency of occurrence [67, 70]. Whereas in the past exposure of the access vessel was often made in TF-AVR, most centers perform this procedure these days purely percutaneously, using closure systems such as Prostar® or Perclose® (both Abbott Vascular Inc., Red City, CA) [71–73].

Solution and Prevention Strategies

Essential in avoiding vascular complications is the accurate, preprocedural assessment of the available access routes, and the interdisciplinary decision concerning the type of access [67, 74]. Future technical improvements, with considerably smaller catheter and tube systems will also have a positive effect on the complication rates (complication rate of the CoreValve System: <5 % with 18F-sheath vs. >20 % with 24F-sheath) [73].

Cardiac Arrhythmias

Due to the anatomical proximity of the conduction system to the aortic valve and the septal segment of the left ventricular outflow tract, there are frequently intraventricular conduction disruptions after TAVR. Potential causes are the direct mechanical impairment of the stimulus conduction systems and inflammatory processes. The onset of a new left bundle branch block occurs in 7–18 % with the balloon-expandable Edwards prosthesis and in 30–80 % with the self-expandable CoreValve prosthesis; the permanent pacemaker rate for CoreValve is ~20 % (in some studies up to ~40 %), respectively ~3 % for the Edwards prosthesis [75–83].

Solutions and Prevention Strategies

Some centers use a smaller balloon for valvuloplasty prior to implantation of the prosthesis, others dispense entirely with the BAV in CoreValve-Procedures [84]. The extent to which these measures result in a lower rate of cardiac arrhythmias and overall to better results after TAVR has not yet been completely elucidated.

Paravalvular Regurgitation

Suboptimal positioning of the prosthesis, with implantation too low or too high, and high-grade calcification of the native aortic valve with resultant incomplete prosthesis expansion are the most common reasons for paravalvular regurgitation [85–87]. Moderate to high-grade regurgitation occurs with TAVR in ca. 10 % (5–17 %) of cases and is demonstrably associated with higher hospital mortality and a poorer long-term survival rate [24, 88]. Differences between the two types of prostheses are found in the subanalysis of the British TAVR-Registry: after CoreValve implantation there was more frequently moderate to higher-grade paravalvular regurgitation (CoreValve: 17.3 % Edwards: 9.6 %) [28].

Solutions and Prevention Strategies

In addition to the accurate measurement of the aortic annulus (see above) on which selection of the optimal prosthesis depends, the prosthesis design and the exact and stable positioning of the prosthesis during the expansion phase are essential in avoiding paravalvular regurgitation. Prostheses of the latest generation address these points and already lead to a clearly lower complication rates these days.

Myocardial Infarction

The combination of a low coronary ostia branching with (1) too high implantation of the prosthesis; (2) a pronounced, usually eccentric calcification of the native aortic valve; or (3) calcification of the ascending aorta near to the ostia may lead to coronary obstruction during TAVR. Though this is rare (incidence <1 %), this complication is life-threatening [8, 9, 18, 24, 26, 27, 50–52, 89].

Solution and Prevention Strategies

The accurate preprocedural estimation of the risk of coronary occlusion, quantified via the severity and distribution of aortic valve calcification, along with the distance between coronary ostia and native aortic valve, is mandatory as part of the screening process. Moreover, TAVR centers should have experience with complex coronary interventions in general and at least in coronary angiography in TAVR patients. Some successful rescue coronary interventions after TAVR have already been described [90, 91].

Acute Kidney Failure

With a prevalence up to 50 %, chronic kidney failure is a common comorbidity in TAVR patients [8, 9, 25–29, 50]. As is to be expected, the extent of preprocedural kidney dysfunction correlates closely with the incidence of acute kidney failure after TAVR [92, 93]. This, or the necessity for postinterventional hemodialysis, ranges between 11.7 % and 28 %, respectively between 1.4 and 15.75 % [92–96].

The Future Outlook

The immediate future will be characterized by further technical improvements in the prosthesis design and implantation technique with the aim of preventing TAVR-associated complications. Coupled with growing experience in pre-, peri- and postinterventional management, expansion of the indication spectrum will be indispensable.

Moreover, TAVR could be the routine treatment of surgical bioprosthesis dysfunction in the future. The limited durability of surgical bioprostheses requires valve replacement in a large number of SAVR patients over time. The advantage of this purely percutaneous procedure could thus be that re-operation is not necessary. Some reports have already presented the technical feasibility [97–99]. Larger studies are needed, however, to prove the value of this valve-in-valve technique. The extent to which TAVR will alter the general treatment strategy of symptomatic aortic valve stenosis remains unclear at present.

Summary

The rapid development of transcatheter therapy procedures has characterized interventional cardiology, as well as cardiac surgery in recent years, and decisively altered the treatment of symptomatic aortic valve stenosis. TAVR is now considered the therapy of choice for inoperable patients and as a valuable therapeutic alternative to surgical aortic valve replacement in high-risk patients. Even without considering the positive PARTNER data and the good short-, middle- and long-term registry results, cardiologists and cardiovascular surgeons should work in close interdisciplinary cooperation to promote the further development of the technique. The short-term goal must be to reduce TAVR-associated complications by exchanging experience and increasing competence, as well as by means of standardized patient selection and optimal periprocedural management and the long-term goal to maintain the quality of life. The current limitations in the indication spectrum could then be dropped and new therapy strategies developed.

References

1. Moulopoulos SD, Anthopoulos L, Stamatelopoulos S, Stefadouros M. Catheter-mounted aortic valves. Ann Thorac Surg. 1971;11:423–30.
2. Paniagua D, Condado JA, Besso J, Velez M, Burger B, Bibbo S, Cedeno D, Acquatella H, Mejia C, Induni E, Fish RD. First human case of retrograde transcatheter implantation of an aortic valve prosthesis. Tex Heart Inst J. 2005;32:393–8.
3. Davies H. Catheter mounted valve for temporary relief of aortic insufficiency. Lancet. 1965;1.
4. Andersen HR, Knudsen LL, Hasenkam JM. Transluminal implantation of artificial heart valves. Description of a new expandable aortic valve and initial results with implantation by catheter technique in closed chest pigs. Eur Heart J. 1992;13: 704–8.
5. Bonhoeffer P, Boudjemline Y, Saliba Z, Merckx J, Aggoun Y, Bonnet D, Acar P, Le Bidois J, Sidi D, Kachaner J. Percutaneous replacement of pulmonary valve in a right-ventricle to pulmonary-artery prosthetic conduit with valve dysfunction. Lancet. 2000;356:1403–5.
6. Cribier A, Eltchaninoff H, Bash A, Borenstein N, Tron C, Bauer F, Derumeaux G, Anselme F, Laborde F, Leon MB. Percutaneous transcatheter implantation of an aortic valve prosthesis for calcific aortic stenosis: first human case description. Circulation. 2002;106:3006–8.
7. Leon MB, Smith CR, Mack M, Miller DC, Moses JW, Svensson LG, Tuzcu EM, Webb JG, Fontana GP, Makkar RR, Brown DL, Block PC, Guyton RA, Pichard AD, Bavaria JE, Herrmann HC, Douglas PS, Petersen JL, Akin JJ, Anderson WN, Wang D, Pocock S. Transcatheter aortic-valve implantation for aortic stenosis in patients who cannot undergo surgery. N Engl J Med. 2010;363:1597–607.
8. Eltchaninoff H, Prat A, Gilard M, Leguerrier A, Blanchard D, Fournial G, Iung B, Donzeau-Gouge P, Tribouilloy C, Debrux JL, Pavie A, Gueret P. Transcatheter aortic valve implantation: early results of the FRANCE (French Aortic National CoreValve and Edwards) registry. Eur Heart J. 2011;32(2):191–7.
9. Thomas M, Schymik G, Walther T, Himbert D, Lefevre T, Treede H, Eggebrecht H, Rubino P, Michev I, Lange

R, Anderson WN, Wendler O. Thirty-day results of the SAPIEN aortic Bioprosthesis European Outcome (source) Registry: a European registry of transcatheter aortic valve implantation using the Edwards SAPIEN valve. Circulation. 2010;122:62–9.
10. Vahanian A, Baumgartner H, Bax J, Butchart E, Dion R, Filippatos G, Flachskampf F, Hall R, Iung B, Kasprzak J, Nataf P, Tornos P, Torracca L, Wenink A. Guidelines on the management of valvular heart disease: the task force on the management of valvular heart disease of the European Society of Cardiology. Eur Heart J. 2007;28:230–68.
11. Smid M, Ferda J, Baxa J, Cech J, Hajek T, Kreuzberg B, Rokyta R. Aortic annulus and ascending aorta: comparison of preoperative and perioperative measurement in patients with aortic stenosis. Eur J Radiol. 2010;74:152–5.
12. Ng AC, Delgado V, van der Kley F, Shanks M, van de Veire NR, Bertini M, Nucifora G, van Bommel RJ, Tops LF, de Weger A, Tavrlla G, de Roos A, Kroft LJ, Leung DY, Schuijf J, Schalij MJ, Bax JJ. Comparison of aortic root dimensions and geometries before and after transcatheter aortic valve implantation by 2- and 3-dimensional transesophageal echocardiography and multislice computed tomography. Circ Cardiovasc Imaging. 2010;3:94–102.
13. Blanke P, Siepe M, Reinohl J, Zehender M, Beyersdorf F, Schlensak C, Langer M, Pache G. Assessment of aortic annulus dimensions for Edwards SAPIEN Transapical Heart Valve implantation by computed tomography: calculating average diameter using a virtual ring method. Eur J Cardiothorac Surg. 2010;38(6):750–8.
14. Vahanian A, Alfieri OR, Al-Attar N, Antunes MJ, Bax J, Cormier B, Cribier A, De Jaegere P, Fournial G, Kappetein AP, Kovac J, Ludgate S, Maisano F, Moat N, Mohr FW, Nataf P, Pierard L, Pomar JL, Schofer J, Tornos P, Tuzcu M, van Hout B, von Segesser LK, Walther T. Transcatheter valve implantation for patients with aortic stenosis: a position statement from the European association of cardio-thoracic surgery (eacts) and the European society of cardiology (esc), in collaboration with the European association of percutaneous cardiovascular interventions (eapci). Eur J Cardiothorac Surg. 2008;34:1–8.
15. Delgado V, Ng AC, Shanks M, van der Kley F, Schuijf JD, van de Veire NR, Kroft L, de Roos A, Schalij MJ, Bax JJ. Transcatheter aortic valve implantation: role of multimodality cardiac imaging. Expert Rev Cardiovasc Ther. 2010;8:113–23.
16. Webb JG, Chandavimol M, Thompson CR, Ricci DR, Carere RG, Munt BI, Buller CE, Pasupati S, Lichtenstein S. Percutaneous aortic valve implantation retrograde from the femoral artery. Circulation. 2006;113:842–50.
17. Kaleschke G, Seifarth H, Kerckhoff G, Reinecke H, Baumgartner H. Imaging decision-making for transfemoral or transapical approach of transcatheter aortic valve implantation. EuroIntervention. 2010;6(Suppl G):G20–7.
18. Masson JB, Kovac J, Schuler G, Ye J, Cheung A, Kapadia S, Tuzcu ME, Kodali S, Leon MB, Webb JG. Transcatheter aortic valve implantation: review of the nature, management, and avoidance of procedural complications. JACC Cardiovasc Interv. 2009;2:811–20.
19. Lichtenstein SV, Cheung A, Ye J, Thompson CR, Carere RG, Pasupati S, Webb JG. Transapical transcatheter aortic valve implantation in humans: initial clinical experience. Circulation. 2006;114:591–6.
20. Mukherjee C, Walther T, Borger MA, Kempfert J, Schuler G, Mohr FW, Ender J. Awake transapical aortic valve implantation using thoracic epidural anesthesia. Ann Thorac Surg. 2009;88:992–4.
21. Petronio AS, De Carlo M, Bedogni F, Marzocchi A, Klugmann S, Maisano F, Ramondo A, Ussia GP, Ettori F, Poli A, Brambilla N, Saia F, De Marco F, Colombo A. Safety and efficacy of the subclavian approach for transcatheter aortic valve implantation with the CoreValve revalving system. Circ Cardiovasc Interv. 2010;3:359–66.
22. Bauernschmitt R, Schreiber C, Bleiziffer S, Ruge H, Mazzitelli D, Hutter A, Tassani P, Lange R. Transcatheter aortic valve implantation through the ascending aorta: an alternative option for no-access patients. Heart Surg Forum. 2009;12:E63–4.
23. Smith CR, Leon MB, Mack MJ, Miller DC, Moses JW, Svensson LG, Tuzcu EM, Webb JG, Fontana GP, Makkar RR, Williams M, Dewey T, Kapadia S, Babaliaros V, Thourani VH, Corso P, Pichard AD, Bavaria JE, Herrmann HC, Akin JJ, Anderson WN, Wang D, Pocock SJ. Transcatheter versus surgical aortic-valve replacement in high-risk patients. N Engl J Med. 2011;364:2187–98.
24. Kodali SK, Williams MR, Smith CR, Svensson LG, Webb JG, Makkar RR, Fontana GP, Dewey TM, Thourani VH, Pichard AD, Fischbein M, Szeto WY, Lim S, Greason KL, Teirstein PS, Malaisrie SC, Douglas PS, Hahn RT, Whisenant B, Zajarias A, Wang D, Akin JJ, Anderson WN, Leon MB. Two-year outcomes after transcatheter or surgical aortic-valve replacement. N Engl J Med. 2012;366:1686–95.
25. Piazza N, Grube E, Gerckens U, den Heijer P, Linke A, Luha O, Ramondo A, Ussia G, Wenaweser P, Windecker S, Laborde JC, de Jaegere P, Serruys PW. Procedural and 30-day outcomes following transcatheter aortic valve implantation using the third generation (18 fr) corevalve revalving system: results from the multicentre, expanded evaluation registry 1-year following ce mark approval. EuroIntervention. 2008;4:242–9.
26. Tamburino C, Capodanno D, Ramondo A, Petronio AS, Ettori F, Santoro G, Klugmann S, Bedogni F, Maisano F, Marzocchi A, Poli A, Antoniucci D, Napodano M, De Carlo M, Fiorina C, Ussia GP. Incidence and predictors of early and late mortality after transcatheter aortic valve implantation in 663 patients with severe aortic stenosis. Circulation. 2011;123:299–308.

27. Zahn R, Gerckens U, Grube E, Linke A, Sievert H, Eggebrecht H, Hambrecht R, Sack S, Hauptmann KE, Richardt G, Figulla HR, Senges J. Transcatheter aortic valve implantation: first results from a multi-centre real-world registry. Eur Heart J. 2011;32(2):198–204.
28. Moat NE, Ludman P, de Belder MA, Bridgewater B, Cunningham AD, Young CP, Thomas M, Kovac J, Spyt T, MacCarthy PA, Wendler O, Hildick-Smith D, Davies SW, Trivedi U, Blackman DJ, Levy RD, Brecker SJ, Baumbach A, Daniel T, Gray H, Mullen MJ. Long-term outcomes after transcatheter aortic valve implantation in high-risk patients with severe aortic stenosis: the U.K. TAVR (United Kingdom transcatheter aortic valve implantation) registry. J Am Coll Cardiol. 2011;58:2130–8.
29. Rodes-Cabau J, Webb JG, Cheung A, Ye J, Dumont E, Feindel CM, Osten M, Natarajan MK, Velianou JL, Martucci G, DeVarennes B, Chisholm R, Peterson MD, Lichtenstein SV, Nietlispach F, Doyle D, DeLarochelliere R, Teoh K, Chu V, Dancea A, Lachapelle K, Cheema A, Latter D, Horlick E. Transcatheter aortic valve implantation for the treatment of severe symptomatic aortic stenosis in patients at very high or prohibitive surgical risk: acute and late outcomes of the multicenter Canadian experience. J Am Coll Cardiol. 2010;55:1080–90.
30. Cribier A, Eltchaninoff H, Tron C, Bauer F, Agatiello C, Sebagh L, Bash A, Nusimovici D, Litzler PY, Bessou JP, Leon MB. Early experience with percutaneous transcatheter implantation of heart valve prosthesis for the treatment of end-stage inoperable patients with calcific aortic stenosis. J Am Coll Cardiol. 2004;43:698–703.
31. Webb JG, Pasupati S, Humphries K, Thompson C, Altwegg L, Moss R, Sinhal A, Carere RG, Munt B, Ricci D, Ye J, Cheung A, Lichtenstein SV. Percutaneous transarterial aortic valve replacement in selected high-risk patients with aortic stenosis. Circulation. 2007;116:755–63.
32. Walther T, Simon P, Dewey T, Wimmer-Greinecker G, Falk V, Kasimir MT, Doss M, Borger MA, Schuler G, Glogar D, Fehske W, Wolner E, Mohr FW, Mack M. Transapical minimally invasive aortic valve implantation: multicenter experience. Circulation. 2007;116:I240–5.
33. Svensson LG, Dewey T, Kapadia S, Roselli EE, Stewart A, Williams M, Anderson WN, Brown D, Leon M, Lytle B, Moses J, Mack M, Tuzcu M, Smith C. United states feasibility study of transcatheter insertion of a stented aortic valve by the left ventricular apex. Ann Thorac Surg. 2008;86:46–54. Discussion 54–45.
34. Walther T, Kasimir MT, Doss M, Schuler G, Simon P, Schachinger V, Mohr FW, Wimmer-Greinecker G. One-year interim follow-up results of the TRAVERCE trial: the initial feasibility study for trans-apical aortic-valve implantation. Eur J Cardiothoracic Surg. 2011;39:532–7.
35. Rodes-Cabau J, Dumont E, De LaRochelliere R, Doyle D, Lemieux J, Bergeron S, Clavel MA, Villeneuve J, Raby K, Bertrand OF, Pibarot P. Feasibility and initial results of percutaneous aortic valve implantation including selection of the transfemoral or transapical approach in patients with severe aortic stenosis. Am J Cardiol. 2008;102:1240–6.
36. Lefevre T, Kappetein AP, Wolner E, Nataf P, Thomas M, Schachinger V, De Bruyne B, Eltchaninoff H, Thielmann M, Himbert D, Romano M, Serruys P, Wimmer-Greinecker G. One year follow-up of the multi-centre european partner transcatheter heart valve study. Eur Heart J. 2011;32:148–57.
37. Grube E, Laborde JC, Zickmann B, Gerckens U, Felderhoff T, Sauren B, Bootsveld A, Buellesfeld L, Iversen S. First report on a human percutaneous transluminal implantation of a self-expanding valve prosthesis for interventional treatment of aortic valve stenosis. Catheter Cardiovasc Interv. 2005;66:465–9.
38. Grube E, Laborde JC, Gerckens U, Felderhoff T, Sauren B, Buellesfeld L, Mueller R, Menichelli M, Schmidt T, Zickmann B, Iversen S, Stone GW. Percutaneous implantation of the CoreValve self-expanding valve prosthesis in high-risk patients with aortic valve disease: the Siegburg first-in-man study. Circulation. 2006;114:1616–24.
39. Grube E, Schuler G, Buellesfeld L, Gerckens U, Linke A, Wenaweser P, Sauren B, Mohr FW, Walther T, Zickmann B, Iversen S, Felderhoff T, Cartier R, Bonan R. Percutaneous aortic valve replacement for severe aortic stenosis in high-risk patients using the second- and current third-generation self-expanding CoreValve prosthesis: device success and 30-day clinical outcome. J Am Coll Cardiol. 2007;50:69–76.
40. Bosmans JM, Kefer J, De Bruyne B, Herijgers P, Dubois C, Legrand V, Verheye S, Rodrigus I. Procedural, 30-day and one year outcome following CoreValve or Edwards transcatheter aortic valve implantation: results of the Belgian national registry. Interact Cardiovasc Thorac Surg. 2011;12:762–7.
41. Clavel MA, Webb JG, Rodes-Cabau J, Masson JB, Dumont E, De Larochelliere R, Doyle D, Bergeron S, Baumgartner H, Burwash IG, Dumesnil JG, Mundigler G, Moss R, Kempny A, Bagur R, Bergler-Klein J, Gurvitch R, Mathieu P, Pibarot P. Comparison between transcatheter and surgical prosthetic valve implantation in patients with severe aortic stenosis and reduced left ventricular ejection fraction. Circulation. 2010;122:1928–36.
42. Clavel MA, Webb JG, Pibarot P, Altwegg L, Dumont E, Thompson C, De Larochelliere R, Doyle D, Masson JB, Bergeron S, Bertrand OF, Rodes-Cabau J. Comparison of the hemodynamic performance of percutaneous and surgical bioprostheses for the treatment of severe aortic stenosis. J Am Coll Cardiol. 2009;53:1883–91.
43. Bauer F, Eltchaninoff H, Tron C, Lesault PF, Agatiello C, Nercolini D, Derumeaux G, Cribier A. Acute improvement in global and regional left ventricular systolic function after percutaneous heart valve implantation in patients with symptomatic aortic stenosis. Circulation. 2004;110:1473–6.
44. Bagur R, Rodes-Cabau J, Dumont E, Larochelliere RD, Doyle D, Bertrand OF, Cote M, Poirier P, Pibarot

P. Exercise capacity in patients with severe symptomatic aortic stenosis before and six months after transcatheter aortic valve implantation. Am J Cardiol. 2011;108:258–64.
45. Reynolds MR, Magnuson EA, Lei Y, Leon MB, Smith CR, Svensson LG, Webb JG, Babaliaros VC, Bowers BS, Fearon WF, Herrmann HC, Kapadia S, Kodali SK, Makkar RR, Pichard AD, Cohen DJ. Health-related quality of life after transcatheter aortic valve replacement in inoperable patients with severe aortic stenosis. Circulation. 2011;124:1964–72.
46. Goncalves A, Marcos-Alberca P, Almeria C, Feltes G, Hernandez-Antolin RA, Rodriguez E, Rodrigo JL, Cobiella J, Maroto L, Cardoso JC, Macaya C, Zamorano JL. Quality of life improvement at midterm follow-up after transcatheter aortic valve implantation. Int J Cardiol. 2013;162(2):117–22.
47. Bagur R, Rodes-Cabau J, Dumont E, De Larochelliere R, Doyle D, Pibarot P, Cote M, Clavel MA, Villeneuve J, Gutierrez M, Poirier P, Bertrand OF. Performance-based functional assessment of patients undergoing transcatheter aortic valve implantation. Am Heart J. 2011;161:726–34.
48. Ussia GP, Mule M, Barbanti M, Cammalleri V, Scarabelli M, Imme S, Capodanno D, Ciriminna S, Tamburino C. Quality of life assessment after percutaneous aortic valve implantation. Eur Heart J. 2009;30:1790–6.
49. Gotzmann M, Pljakic A, Bojara W, Lindstaedt M, Ewers A, Germing A, Mugge A. Transcatheter aortic valve implantation in patients with severe symptomatic aortic valve stenosis-predictors of mortality and poor treatment response. Am Heart J. 2011;162:238–45.
50. Thomas M, Schymik G, Walther T, Himbert D, Lefevre T, Treede H, Eggebrecht H, Rubino P, Colombo A, Lange R, Schwarz RR, Wendler O. One-year outcomes of cohort 1 in the Edwards SAPIEN Aortic Bioprosthesis European Outcome (source) registry: the European registry of transcatheter aortic valve implantation using the Edwards SAPIEN valve. Circulation. 2011;124:425–33.
51. Gilard M, Eltchaninoff H, Iung B, Donzeau-Gouge P, Chevreul K, Fajadet J, Leprince P, Leguerrier A, Lievre M, Prat A, Teiger E, Lefevre T, Himbert D, Tchetche D, Carrie D, Albat B, Cribier A, Rioufol G, Sudre A, Blanchard D, Collet F, Dos Santos P, Meneveau N, Tirouvanziam A, Caussin C, Guyon P, Boschat J, Le Breton H, Collart F, Houel R, Delpine S, Souteyrand G, Favereau X, Ohlmann P, Doisy V, Grollier G, Gommeaux A, Claudel JP, Bourlon F, Bertrand B, Van Belle E, Laskar M. Registry of transcatheter aortic-valve implantation in high-risk patients. N Engl J Med. 2012;366:1705–15.
52. Makkar RR, Fontana GP, Jilaihawi H, Kapadia S, Pichard AD, Douglas PS, Thourani VH, Babaliaros VC, Webb JG, Herrmann HC, Bavaria JE, Kodali S, Brown DL, Bowers B, Dewey TM, Svensson LG, Tuzcu M, Moses JW, Williams MR, Siegel RJ, Akin JJ, Anderson WN, Pocock S, Smith CR, Leon MB. Transcatheter aortic-valve replacement for inoperable severe aortic stenosis. N Engl J Med. 2012;366:1696–704.
53. Buellesfeld L, Gerckens U, Schuler G, Bonan R, Kovac J, Serruys PW, Labinaz M, den Heijer P, Mullen M, Tymchak W, Windecker S, Mueller R, Grube E. 2-year follow-up of patients undergoing transcatheter aortic valve implantation using a self-expanding valve prosthesis. J Am Coll Cardiol. 2011;57:1650–7.
54. Gurvitch R, Wood DA, Tay EL, Leipsic J, Ye J, Lichtenstein SV, Thompson CR, Carere RG, Wijesinghe N, Nietlispach F, Boone RH, Lauck S, Cheung A, Webb JG. Transcatheter aortic valve implantation: durability of clinical and hemodynamic outcomes beyond 3 years in a large patient cohort. Circulation. 2010;122:1319–27.
55. Rodes-Cabau J, Webb J, Cheung A, Ye J, Dumont E, Chris F, Osten M, Natarajan M, Velianou JL, Martucci G, DeVarennes B, Thompson CR, Chisholm R, Peterson M, Lichtenstein S, Toggweiler S, Doyle D, DeLarochelli R, Dumesnil J, Teoh K, Chu V, Cheema A, Wood D, Pibarot P, Horlick E. Long-term outcomes following transcatheter aortic valve implantation: Insights on prognostic factors and valve durability from the Canadian multicenter experience. J the Am Coll Cardiol. 2012;59:E10–E10.
56. Alli OO, Booker JD, Lennon RJ, Greason KL, Rihal CS, Holmes Jr DR. Transcatheter aortic valve implantation: assessing the learning curve. J Am Coll Cardiol Intv. 2012;5:72–9.
57. Nuis RJ, van Mieghem NM, van der Boon RM, van Geuns RJ, Schultz CJ, Oei FB, Galema TW, Raap GB, Koudstaal PJ, Geleijnse ML, Kappetein AP, Serruys PW, de Jaegere PP. Effect of experience on results of transcatheter aortic valve implantation using a Medtronic CoreValve system. Am J Cardiol. 2011; 107:1824–9.
58. Leon MB, Piazza N, Nikolsky E, Blackstone EH, Cutlip DE, Kappetein AP, Krucoff MW, Mack M, Mehran R, Miller C, Morel MA, Petersen J, Popma JJ, Takkenberg JJ, Vahanian A, van Es GA, Vranckx P, Webb JG, Windecker S, Serruys PW. Standardized endpoint definitions for transcatheter aortic valve implantation clinical trials: a consensus report from the valve academic research consortium. Eur Heart J. 2011;32:205–17.
59. Eggebrecht H, Schmermund A, Voigtlander T, Kahlert P, Erbel R, Mehta RH. Risk of stroke after transcatheter aortic valve implantation (TAVR): a meta-analysis of 10,037 published patients. EuroIntervention. 2012;8:129–38.
60. Kahlert P, Knipp SC, Schlamann M, Thielmann M, Al-Rashid F, Weber M, Johansson U, Wendt D, Jakob HG, Forsting M, Sack S, Erbel R, Eggebrecht H. Silent and apparent cerebral ischemia after percutaneous transfemoral aortic valve implantation: a diffusion-weighted magnetic resonance imaging study. Circulation. 2010;121:870–8.
61. Ghanem A, Muller A, Nahle CP, Kocurek J, Werner N, Hammerstingl C, Schild HH, Schwab JO, Mellert F, Fimmers R, Nickenig G, Thomas D. Risk and fate

of cerebral embolism after transfemoral aortic valve implantation: a prospective pilot study with diffusion-weighted magnetic resonance imaging. J Am Coll Cardiol. 2010;55:1427–32.
62. Rodes-Cabau J, Dumont E, Boone RH, Larose E, Bagur R, Gurvitch R, Bedard F, Doyle D, De Larochelliere R, Jayasuria C, Villeneuve J, Marrero A, Cote M, Pibarot P, Webb JG. Cerebral embolism following transcatheter aortic valve implantation: comparison of transfemoral and transapical approaches. J Am Coll Cardiol. 2011;57:18–28.
63. Nuis RJ, Piazza N, Van Mieghem NM, Otten AM, Tzikas A, Schultz CJ, van der Boon R, van Geuns RJ, van Domburg RT, Koudstaal PJ, Kappetein AP, Serruys PW, de Jaegere PP. In-hospital complications after transcatheter aortic valve implantation revisited according to the valve academic research consortium definitions. Catheter Cardiovasc Interv. 2011;78:457–67.
64. Nietlispach F, Wijesinghe N, Gurvitch R, Tay E, Carpenter JP, Burns C, Wood DA, Webb JG. An embolic deflection device for aortic valve interventions. J Am Coll Cardiol Intv. 2010;3:1133–8.
65. Ussia GP, Scarabelli M, Mule M, Barbanti M, Sarkar K, Cammalleri V, Imme S, Aruta P, Pistritto AM, Gulino S, Deste W, Capodanno D, Tamburino C. Dual antiplatelet therapy versus aspirin alone in patients undergoing transcatheter aortic valve implantation. Am J Cardiol. 2011;108:1772–6.
66. Wenaweser P, Pilgrim T, Roth N, Kadner A, Stortecky S, Kalesan B, Meuli F, Bullesfeld L, Khattab AA, Huber C, Eberle B, Erdos G, Meier B, Juni P, Carrel T, Windecker S. Clinical outcome and predictors for adverse events after transcatheter aortic valve implantation with the use of different devices and access routes. Am Heart J. 2011;161:1114–24.
67. Hayashida K, Lefevre T, Chevalier B, Hovasse T, Romano M, Garot P, Mylotte D, Uribe J, Farge A, Donzeau-Gouge P, Bouvier E, Cormier B, Morice MC. Transfemoral aortic valve implantation new criteria to predict vascular complications. J Am Coll Cardiol Intv. 2011;4:851–8.
68. Godino C, Maisano F, Montorfano M, Latib A, Chieffo A, Michev I, Al-Lamee R, Bande M, Mussardo M, Arioli F, Ielasi A, Cioni M, Taramasso M, Arendar I, Grimaldi A, Spagnolo P, Zangrillo A, La Canna G, Alfieri O, Colombo A. Outcomes after transcatheter aortic valve implantation with both Edwards-SAPIEN and CoreValve devices in a single center: the Milan experience. J Am Coll Cardiol Intv. 2010;3:1110–21.
69. Moynagh AM, Scott DJ, Baumbach A, Khavandi A, Brecker SJ, Laborde JC, Brown S, Chowdhary S, Saravanan D, Crean PA, Teehan S, Hildick-Smith D, Trivedi U, Khogali SS, Bhabra MS, Roberts DH, Morgan KP, Blackman DJ. CoreValve transcatheter aortic valve implantation via the subclavian artery: comparison with the transfemoral approach. J Am Coll Cardiol. 2011;57:634–5.
70. Kahlert P, Al-Rashid F, Weber M, Wendt D, Heine T, Kottenberg E, Thielmann M, Kuhl H, Peters J, Jakob HG, Sack S, Erbel R, Eggebrecht H. Vascular access site complications after percutaneous transfemoral aortic valve implantation. Herz. 2009;34:398–408.
71. Cockburn J, de Belder A, Brooks M, Hutchinson N, Hill A, Trivedi U, Hildick-Smith D. Large calibre arterial access device closure for percutaneous aortic valve interventions: use of the Prostar system in 118 cases. Catheter Cardiovasc Interv. 2012;79:143–9.
72. Van Mieghem NM, Nuis RJ, Piazza N, Apostolos T, Ligthart J, Schultz C, de Jaegere PP, Serruys PW. Vascular complications with transcatheter aortic valve implantation using the 18 fr Medtronic CoreValve System: the Rotterdam experience. EuroIntervention. 2010;5:673–9.
73. Sharp AS, Michev I, Maisano F, Taramasso M, Godino C, Latib A, Denti P, Dorigo E, Giacomini A, Iaci G, Manca M, Ielasi A, Montorfano M, Alfieri O, Colombo A. A new technique for vascular access management in transcatheter aortic valve implantation. Catheter Cardiovasc Interv. 2010;75:784–93.
74. Saia F, Bordoni B, Marrozzini C, Ciuca C, Moretti C, Branzi A, Marzocchi A. Incidence, prognostic value and management of vascular complications with transfemoral transcatheter aortic valve implantation. Future Cardiol. 2011;7:321–31.
75. Sinhal A, Altwegg L, Pasupati S, Humphries KH, Allard M, Martin P, Cheung A, Ye J, Kerr C, Lichtenstein SV, Webb JG. Atrioventricular block after transcatheter balloon expandable aortic valve implantation. J Am Coll Cardiol Intv. 2008;1:305–9.
76. Gutierrez M, Rodes-Cabau J, Bagur R, Doyle D, DeLarochelliere R, Bergeron S, Lemieux J, Villeneuve J, Cote M, Bertrand OF, Poirier P, Clavel MA, Pibarot P, Dumont E. Electrocardiographic changes and clinical outcomes after transapical aortic valve implantation. Am Heart J. 2009;158:302–8.
77. Godin M, Eltchaninoff H, Furuta A, Tron C, Anselme F, Bejar K, Sanchez-Giron C, Bauer F, Litzler PY, Bessou JP, Cribier A. Frequency of conduction disturbances after transcatheter implantation of an Edwards SAPIEN aortic valve prosthesis. Am J Cardiol. 2010;106:707–12.
78. Piazza N, Onuma Y, Jesserun E, Kint PP, Maugenest AM, Anderson RH, de Jaegere PP, Serruys PW. Early and persistent intraventricular conduction abnormalities and requirements for pacemaking after percutaneous replacement of the aortic valve. JACC Cardiovasc Interv. 2008;1:310–6.
79. Jilaihawi H, Chin D, Vasa-Nicotera M, Jeilan M, Spyt T, Ng GA, Bence J, Logtens E, Kovac J. Predictors for permanent pacemaker requirement after transcatheter aortic valve implantation with the CoreValve bioprosthesis. Am Heart J. 2009;157:860–6.
80. Erkapic D, Kim WK, Weber M, Mollmann H, Berkowitsch A, Zaltsberg S, Pajitnev DJ, Rixe J, Neumann T, Kuniss M, Sperzel J, Hamm CW, Pitschner HF. Electrocardiographic and further predictors for permanent pacemaker requirement after transcatheter aortic valve implantation. Europace. 2010;12:1188–90.
81. Nuis RJ, Van Mieghem NM, Schultz CJ, Tzikas A, Van der Boon RM, Maugenest AM, Cheng J, Piazza

N, van Domburg RT, Serruys PW, de Jaegere PP. Timing and potential mechanisms of new conduction abnormalities during the implantation of the Medtronic CoreValve System in patients with aortic stenosis. Eur Heart J. 2011;32:2067–74.
82. Baan Jr J, Yong ZY, Koch KT, Henriques JP, Bouma BJ, Vis MM, Cocchieri R, Piek JJ, de Mol BA. Factors associated with cardiac conduction disorders and permanent pacemaker implantation after percutaneous aortic valve implantation with the CoreValve prosthesis. Am Heart J. 2010;159:497–503.
83. Fraccaro C, Buja G, Tarantini G, Gasparetto V, Leoni L, Razzolini R, Corrado D, Bonato R, Basso C, Thiene G, Gerosa G, Isabella G, Iliceto S, Napodano M. Incidence, predictors, and outcome of conduction disorders after transcatheter self-expandable aortic valve implantation. Am J Cardiol. 2011;107:747–54.
84. Grube E, Naber C, Abizaid A, Sousa E, Mendiz O, Lemos P, Kalil Filho R, Mangione J, Buellesfeld L. Feasibility of transcatheter aortic valve implantation without balloon pre-dilation: a pilot study. J Am Coll Cardiol Intv. 2011;4:751–7.
85. John D, Buellesfeld L, Yuecel S, Mueller R, Latsios G, Beucher H, Gerckens U, Grube E. Correlation of device landing zone calcification and acute procedural success in patients undergoing transcatheter aortic valve implantations with the self-expanding CoreValve prosthesis. JACC Cardiovasc Interv. 2010;3:233–43.
86. Sherif MA, Abdel-Wahab M, Stocker B, Geist V, Richardt D, Tolg R, Richardt G. Anatomic and procedural predictors of paravalvular aortic regurgitation after implantation of the Medtronic CoreValve bioprosthesis. J Am Coll Cardiol. 2010;56:1623–9.
87. Detaint D, Lepage L, Himbert D, Brochet E, Messika-Zeitoun D, Iung B, Vahanian A. Determinants of significant paravalvular regurgitation after transcatheter aortic valve: implantation impact of device and annulus discongruence. J Am Coll Cardiol Intv. 2009; 2:821–7.
88. Abdel-Wahab M, Zahn R, Horack M, Gerckens U, Schuler G, Sievert H, Eggebrecht H, Senges J, Richardt G. Aortic regurgitation after transcatheter aortic valve implantation: incidence and early outcome. Results from the German transcatheter aortic valve interventions registry. Heart. 2011;97:899–906.
89. Stabile E, Sorropago G, Cioppa A, Cota L, Agrusta M, Lucchetti V, Rubino P. Acute left main obstructions following TAVR. EuroIntervention. 2010;6:100–5.
90. Kapadia SR, Svensson L, Tuzcu EM. Successful percutaneous management of left main trunk occlusion during percutaneous aortic valve replacement. Catheter Cardiovasc Interv. 2009;73:966–72.
91. Bagur R, Dumont E, Doyle D, Larose E, Lemieux J, Bergeron S, Bilodeau S, Bertrand OF, De Larochelliere R, Rodes-Cabau J. Coronary ostia stenosis after transcatheter aortic valve implantation. JACC Cardiol Interv. 2010;3:253–5.
92. Elhmidi Y, Bleiziffer S, Piazza N, Hutter A, Opitz A, Hettich I, Kornek M, Ruge H, Brockmann G, Mazzitelli D, Lange R. Incidence and predictors of acute kidney injury in patients undergoing transcatheter aortic valve implantation. Am Heart J. 2011; 161:735–9.
93. Van Linden A, Kempfert J, Rastan AJ, Holzhey D, Blumenstein J, Schuler G, Mohr FW, Walther T. Risk of acute kidney injury after minimally invasive transapical aortic valve implantation in 270 patients. Eur J Cardiothoracic Surg. 2011;39:835–42. Discussion 842–3.
94. Nuis RJ, Van Mieghem NM, Tzikas A, Piazza N, Otten AM, Cheng J, van Domburg RT, Betjes M, Serruys PW, de Jaegere PP. Frequency, determinants, and prognostic effects of acute kidney injury and red blood cell transfusion in patients undergoing transcatheter aortic valve implantation. Catheter Cardiovasc Interv. 2011;77:881–9.
95. Sinning JM, Ghanem A, Steinhauser H, Adenauer V, Hammerstingl C, Nickenig G, Werner N. Renal function as predictor of mortality in patients after percutaneous transcatheter aortic valve implantation. J Am Coll Cardiol Intv. 2010;3:1141–9.
96. Bagur R, Webb JG, Nietlispach F, Dumont E, De Larochelliere R, Doyle D, Masson JB, Gutierrez MJ, Clavel MA, Bertrand OF, Pibarot P, Rodes-Cabau J. Acute kidney injury following transcatheter aortic valve implantation: predictive factors, prognostic value, and comparison with surgical aortic valve replacement. Eur Heart J. 2010;31:865–74.
97. Webb JG, Wood DA, Ye J, Gurvitch R, Masson JB, Rodes-Cabau J, Osten M, Horlick E, Wendler O, Dumont E, Carere RG, Wijesinghe N, Nietlispach F, Johnson M, Thompson CR, Moss R, Leipsic J, Munt B, Lichtenstein SV, Cheung A. Transcatheter valve-in-valve implantation for failed bioprosthetic heart valves. Circulation. 2010;121:1848–57.
98. Pasic M, Unbehaun A, Dreysse S, Buz S, Drews T, Kukucka M, Hetzer R. Transapical aortic valve implantation after previous aortic valve replacement: clinical proof of the "valve-in-valve" concept. J Thorac Cardiovasc Surg. 2011;142:270–7.
99. Kempfert J, Van Linden A, Linke A, Borger MA, Rastan A, Mukherjee C, Ender J, Schuler G, Mohr FW, Walther T. Transapical off-pump valve-in-valve implantation in patients with degenerated aortic xenografts. Ann Thorac Surg. 2010;89:1934–41.

Bibliography

Baumgartner H. Hemodynamic assessment of aortic stenosis: are there still lessons to learn? J Am Coll Cardiol. 2006;47:138–40.
Bonow RO, Carabello BA, Kanu C, de Leon AC Jr, Faxon DP, Freed MD, Gaasch WH, Lytle BW, Nishimura RA, O'Gara PT, O'Rourke RA, Otto CM, Shah PM, Shanewise JS, Smith SC Jr, Jacobs AK, Adams CD, Anderson JL, Antman EM, Fuster V, Halperin JL, Hiratzka LF, Hunt SA, Nishimura R, Page RL, Riegel

B. Acc/aha 2006 guidelines for the management of patients with valvular heart disease: a report of the american college of cardiology/american heart association task force on practice guidelines (writing committee to revise the 1998 guidelines for the management of patients with valvular heart disease): developed in collaboration with the society of cardiovascular anesthesiologists: endorsed by the society for cardiovascular angiography and interventions and the society of thoracic surgeons. Circulation 2006;114:e84–231.

Buellesfeld L, Gerckens U, Grube E. Percutaneous implantation of the first repositionable aortic valve prosthesis in a patient with severe aortic stenosis. Catheter Cardiovasc Interv. 2008;71:579–84.

Charlson E, Legedza AT, Hamel MB. Decision-making and outcomes in severe symptomatic aortic stenosis. J Heart Valve Dis. 2006;15:312–21.

Dewey TM, Brown DL, Herbert MA, Culica D, Smith CR, Leon MB, Svensson LG, Tuzcu M, Webb JG, Cribier A, Mack MJ. Effect of concomitant coronary artery disease on procedural and late outcomes of transcatheter aortic valve implantation. Ann Thorac Surg. 2010;89:758–67. discussion 767.

Falk V, Schwammenthal EE, Kempfert J, Linke A, Schuler G, Mohr FW, Walther T. New anatomically oriented transapical aortic valve implantation. Ann Thorac Surg. 2009;87:925–6.

Falk V, Walther T, Schwammenthal E, Strauch J, Aicher D, Wahlers T, Schafers J, Linke A, Mohr FW. Transapical aortic valve implantation with a self-expanding anatomically oriented valve. Eur Heart J. 2011;32:878–87.

Gaia DF, Palma JH, Ferreira CB, Souza JA, Agreli G, Guilhen JC, Telis A, Buffolo E. Transapical aortic valve implantation: results of a Brazilian prosthesis. Rev Bras Cir Cardiovasc. 2010;25:293–302.

Gaia DF, Palma JH, Souza JA, Guilhen JC, Telis A, Fischer CH, Ferreira CB, Buffolo E. Off-pump transapical balloon-expandable aortic valve endoprosthesis implantation. Rev Bras Cir Cardiovasc. 2009;24:233–8.

Iung B, Cachier A, Baron G, Messika-Zeitoun D, Delahaye F, Tornos P, Gohlke-Barwolf C, Boersma E, Ravaud P, Vahanian A. Decision-making in elderly patients with severe aortic stenosis: why are so many denied surgery? Eur Heart J. 2005;26:2714–20.

Kempfert J, Rastan AJ, Mohr FW, Walther T. A new self-expanding transcatheter aortic valve for transapical implantation—first in man implantation of the JenaValve. Eur J cardiothoracic Surg. 2011;40:761–3.

Kolh P, Kerzmann A, Lahaye L, Gerard P, Limet R. Cardiac surgery in octogenarians; peri-operative outcome and long-term results. Eur Heart J. 2001;22:1235–43.

Latib A, Michev I, Laborde JC, Montorfano M, Colombo A. Post-implantation repositioning of the CoreValve percutaneous aortic valve. JACC Cardiovasc Interv. 2010;3:119–21.

Piazza N, Nuis RJ, Tzikas A, Otten A, Onuma Y, Garcia-Garcia H, Schultz C, van Domburg R, van Es GA, van Geuns R, de Jaegere P, Serruys PW. Persistent conduction abnormalities and requirements for pacemaking six months after transcatheter aortic valve implantation. EuroIntervention. 2010;6:475–84.

Rodes-Cabau J. Transcatheter aortic valve implantation: current and future approaches. Nat Rev Cardiol. 2012;9:15–29.

Rodes-Cabau J, Dumont E, Doyle D. "Valve-in-valve" for the treatment of paravalvular leaks following transcatheter aortic valve implantation. Catheter Cardiovasc Interv. 2009;74:1116–9.

Rodes-Cabau J, Gutierrez M, Bagur R, De Larochelliere R, Doyle D, Cote M, Villeneuve J, Bertrand OF, Larose E, Manazzoni J, Pibarot P, Dumont E. Incidence, predictive factors, and prognostic value of myocardial injury following uncomplicated transcatheter aortic valve implantation. J Am Coll Cardiol. 2011;57:1988–99.

Szeto WY, Augoustides JG, Desai ND, Moeller P, McGarvey ML, Walsh E, Bannan A, Herrmann HC, Bavaria JE. Cerebral embolic exposure during transfemoral and transapical transcatheter aortic valve replacement. J Card Surg. 2011;26:348–54.

Tamburino C, Barbanti M, Capodanno D, Sarkar K, Cammalleri V, Scarabelli M, Mule M, Imme S, Aruta P, Ussia GP. Early- and mid-term outcomes of transcatheter aortic valve implantation in patients with logistic EuroSCORE less than 20%: a comparative analysis between different risk strata. Catheter Cardiovasc Interv. 2012;79:132–40.

Taylor J. The time has come for a syntax-like trial for transcatheter aortic valve implantation. Eur Heart J. 2011;32:128–9.

Ussia GP, Barbanti M, Ramondo A, Petronio AS, Ettori F, Santoro G, Klugmann S, Bedogni F, Maisano F, Marzocchi A, Poli A, Napodano M, Tamburino C. The valve-in-valve technique for treatment of aortic bioprosthesis malposition an analysis of incidence and 1-year clinical outcomes from the Italian CoreValve registry. J Am Coll Cardiol. 2011;57:1062–8.

Webb JG, Altwegg L, Boone RH, Cheung A, Ye J, Lichtenstein S, Lee M, Masson JB, Thompson C, Moss R, Carere R, Munt B, Nietlispach F, Humphries K. Transcatheter aortic valve implantation: impact on clinical and valve-related outcomes. Circulation. 2009;119:3009–16.

Part V

System-Oriented Technological Advances: Section C—Vascular Surgery

28 Technological Advances in Endovascular Surgery

Miguel Montero-Baker, Jonathan D. Braun, Craig Weinkauf, and Luis R. Leon Jr.

Brief History of the Development of Endovascular Tools

In 1964, Dr. Charles Theodore Dotter, a radiologist from the Oregon Health Sciences Center, published the first report on peripheral arterial disease (PAD) interventions [1]. To our knowledge, this is the first publication of a lower extremity endovascular intervention; although only very primitive tools (a combination of stiff wires and Teflon dilators) were used, the article was nonetheless amazingly visionary [1]. Dotter's work started years earlier. He was unable to develop significant collaboration with the surgical community at the time, perhaps because he was viewed as eccentric and abrasive. Based on documented interviews by Dr. Thomas Fogarty, he did modestly participate in Dotter's work against the expressed wishes of his superiors. Most of his collaboration was in the form of surgical cutdowns to treat some patients collaboratively, but also provided Dotter with his novel balloon catheters, which although originally created as embolectomy devices, were also apt for percutaneous balloon angioplasty.

While Dotter and Judkins were among the few in the USA who advocated such catheter-based procedures, they were more rapidly adopted into practice in Europe. By March 1977, a total of 1,800 cases were discussed at an international meeting devoted to transluminal angioplasty [2]. At that same meeting, Dotter contributed 322 cases of his own.

A publication in 1979, authored by Andreas Grüntzig and David Kumpe, [2] provided an in depth description of the construction of the "Grüntzig Balloon Catheter," which served as the model for the devices we utilize to the present day. Interestingly, they detailed clinical scenarios that still prove problematic in the current era: "… only occlusions less than 10 cm are treated because of low patency rates for longer recanalizations…" Katzen, Freiman and Colapinto soon

M. Montero-Baker, M.D.
Pima Vascular Group, Department of Vascular and Endovascular Surgery, University of Arizona Health Sciences, Tucson, AZ, USA
e-mail: mmontero@pimavascular.com

J.D. Braun, M.D.
Division of Vascular Surgery, Department of Vascular and Endovascular Surgery, Arizona Health Sciences Center, University of Arizona Medical Center, Tucson, AZ, USA
e-mail: Jonathan.d.braun@gmail.com

C. Weinkauf, M.D., Ph.D.
Division of Vascular Surgery, Department of Surgery, University of Arizona Medical Center, Tucson, AZ, USA
e-mail: ccweinkauf@gmail.com

L.R. Leon Jr., M.D., R.V.T., F.A.C.S. (✉)
Pima Heart PC, Department of Vascular and Endovascular Surgery, Tucson Medical Center, Tucson, AZ, USA
e-mail: Luisrleon1@gmail.com

R. Latifi et al. (eds.), *Technological Advances in Surgery, Trauma and Critical Care*,
DOI 10.1007/978-1-4939-2671-8_28

published their initial experiences with the technique in peripheral vessels, mainly the iliac arteries, at about the same time. Early results were promising; with better patency rates noted for treatment of lesions in larger caliber iliac arteries than for more distal and complex disease in the femoropopliteal segments [3–5].

The next three decades in the history of lower extremity endovascular therapy can be summarized as a combination of greatly accelerated technical and technological advancement. Physicians have more aggressively sought to validate the concept, improve techniques and identify the most appropriate clinical scenarios to apply endovascular therapy as a favorable risk-benefit solution for the patient. Industry has pushed the envelope regarding miniaturization of the technology, which now allows one to reach and treat even the most distal vessels of the foot.

Regarding endovascular therapy of aneurysmal disease, Dr. Juan Parodi began working on a less invasive procedure around 1976 at the Cleveland Clinic. During the same time, Nicholas Volodos began similar work in Kharkov, Soviet Union and introduced in an article written in 1988 [6]. The article describes the first endovascular repair of a thoracic aneurysm: a false aneurysm that likely developed from a motor vehicle accident three decades before. The procedure was successful and the patient died of unrelated causes 18 years later.

Dr. Parodi performed the first successful endovascular repair (EVAR) of an abdominal aortic aneurysm (AAA) in 1990 in Buenos Aires, Argentina. Volodos attempted an EVAR 1 year before but the twisting and occlusion of the endograft, required immediate conversion to traditional open surgical AAA repair. In 1992, Parodi and Claudio Schonholz visited Montefiore Medical Center in New York (lead at the time by Dr. Frank Veith) to perform the first endovascular AAA repair to be done in the USA [7].

The modern endovascular device used to repair AAAs, which is bifurcated and modular, was pioneered and first employed by Dr. Timothy Chuter while a fellow at the University of Rochester [8]. The first clinical series of this device, as well as its use in an emergency setting for ruptured AAAs was published by Yusuf et al. from Nottingham in 1994 [9, 10].

From the Battlefield to the Outpatient Operating Suite

The practice of vascular surgery has drastically changed during the last century not only in what relates to technology and methods of therapy, but also in the location where vascular procedures are performed. Long gone are the times when vascular surgery interventions were mostly performed to aid wounded soldiers in the battlefield. Vascular procedures are nowadays being increasingly performed in the outpatient office (Fig. 28.1). This change has been motivated by different factors. Among the most important of them is the financial factor. The US Health Care System is the most expensive in the world and yet, it is thought to deliver an extremely poor product. Health care practitioners are pressured to provide better care, in a more efficient, cost-constrained manner, in the midst of rising medical litigation cases. Furthermore, government and private payers continuously implement new rules to limit expenses. Among them, reducing reimbursement for providers and facilities is an important measurement. Practitioners found better reimbursement rates when the same exact procedures were performed at office-based laboratories (OBLs). This dramatically changed the dynamics of surgical care, and, by 1970 and onward, ambulatory surgery centers began to proliferate. Vascular Surgery followed suit and several OBLs have been created within this subspecialty.

This change was not exempt from controversy. Critics cite that, since the actual practitioners who staff them own most of these OBLs (and among them, practitioners belong to multiple subspecialties, i.e., interventional radiology, interventional cardiology, vascular surgeons), the financial incentives inherent to owning an OBL have been alleged to affect practitioner behavior. In our personal opinion, we strongly believe that a key requisite to embark into such a financial and professional endeavor, the high moral and ethical behavior that the practitioners abided

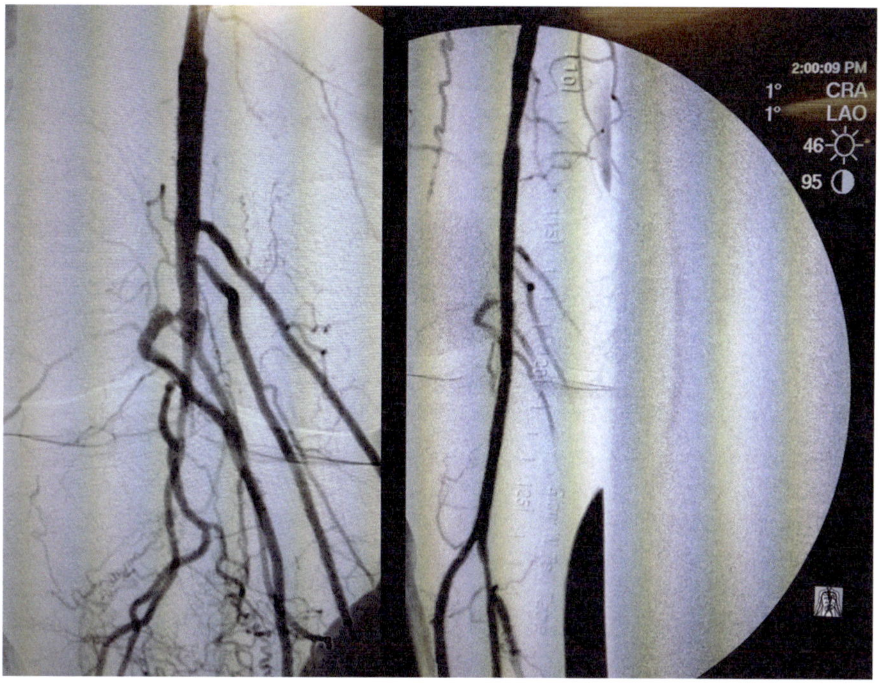

Fig. 28.1 Case of a 68-year-old diabetic gentleman with severe tissue loss and Duplex ultrasound evidence of a popliteal artery occlusion at the below-the-knee segment. Successful revascularization was performed, with restoration of palpable pedal pulses and excellent angiographic results, fully percutaneous and in an office-based laboratory in Tucson, Arizona. Such highly selected cases can be safely performed in the outpatient setting, with comparable morbidity as in the hospital venue, and significantly less financial charges to the health care system

while they use to perform procedures in the hospital setting need to remain absolutely unchanged when changing operating room scenarios, in line with the Hippocratic Oath. As important of a requisite, is a full knowledge of the natural history of PAD, so that the indication to intervene is based on solid scientific foundations, which could never be questioned. This requires appropriate education of vascular interventionists, regardless of the subspecialty that these practitioners are certified on. Lastly, external peer-review systems and internal measurements of safety and compliance need to be in effect to guarantee adhesion to standards of care.

As strong as our beliefs above, we feel that a vascular surgery practice can strongly benefit from office-based procedures. Ideal Duplex scanning performed by properly trained technicians along with technical advances in endovascular tools allow vascular interventionists to safely and effectively perform arterial and venous peripheral interventions in the ambulatory setting [11]. They allow providers to better manage their schedules, thus permitting scheduling more cases per day while improving the quality of life of the practitioners; as well as significant savings to the health care system, since fees are paid directly to the provider, bypassing overhead costs charged for the exact same procedure in a hospital setting. Several publications and the authors' own experience have attested that carefully selected peripheral vascular interventions can be performed in the outpatient setting with low complication rates [11].

Advances in Aortic Diseases

Aneurysmal Disease

Aneurysms are arterial dilations to more than 50 % of the diameter of adjacent non-diseased proximal or distal artery. Although aneurysms are found throughout the arterial vasculature, infrarenal AAAs are the most common. They represent the 13th leading cause of mortality in the USA in men older than 65 years [12]. Their etiology is an area of ongoing research. It is thought that there is an initial vessel wall insult (possibly atherosclerosis or smoking-related damage) followed by a pathophysiologic response that results in vessel wall weakening and dilation [13]. Matrix metalloproteinases (MMPs), which are enzymes that degrade arterial wall matrix molecules responsible for arterial wall integrity, are also thought to play a key role in AAA formation and progression [14]. More rarely, AAAs are secondary to autoimmune and collagen-vascular diseases.

Because of the high mortality associated with aneurysm rupture, newly developed guidelines recommend a one-time screening for AAA in males who ever smoked between the ages of 65–75 years old [15]. Current Society for Vascular Surgery (SVS) guidelines suggest surgical repair (open or endovascular) for abdominal aneurysms with a diameter of 5.5 cm and thoracic aneurysms with a diameter 6.5 cm or if the aneurysm has a rapid growth of >1.0 cm/year [16].

Repair of AAAs include both endovascular and open surgical options. However, since Parodi and colleagues placed the first endograft for repair of an AAA in 1991 [17], adoption of this technique has been rapid—over 80 % of AAAs are now repaired endovascularly in the USA.

Whereas no major technological advances have been reported during the last century in the open aneurysm repair technique, major improvements in the endovascular arena have been reported. Successful placement of an aortic endograft depends on: having adequate arterial access; having adequate proximal and distal landing zones for the graft to interface with arterial wall and; and having ideal aneurysm characteristics, specifically the angle of the neck and the amount of wall calcium and thrombus. Improvements in these key factors that govern successful aneurysm repair are listed and explained herewith:

- *Access Vessels*: An exclusion device must fit through an access vessel (primarily the common femoral and iliac arteries), which limits treatment because of access vessel diameter, tortuosity and calcification. The average external iliac artery of men is 9-mm and women is 7-mm. To accommodate, device manufacturers have evolved towards increasingly streamlined products with a smaller profile (smaller diameter). For instance, in November 2011, The US Food and Drug Administration (FDA) approved a stent graft system that provides patients with small arteries the option of endovascular AAA repair. The Ovation Abdominal Stent Graft System (20 millimeter diameter), manufactured by TriVascular Inc. (Santa Rosa, CA) (Fig. 28.2), uses a narrow delivery system, of about 4.7 mm in diameter. This new device differs from other stent grafts in that a portion of the metal stent is replaced with ring-shaped channels, which are injected with a polymer after the device is in place in the aorta, expanding the endograft against the aorta to create a seal.

This is a very useful addition to the already existing techniques to deal with poor access vessels, including conduits sutured into the common iliac artery or endoconduits lining the native vessel. In the former technique, extra-anatomic prosthetic conduits can be anastomosed to more proximal vessels, such as the common iliac artery, to provide for device delivery. The distal end of the conduit is then often anastomosed to the common femoral artery, which adds the benefit of bypassing often diseased or occluded iliac vessels. With the latter technique, "endoconduits" provide an entirely endovascular option when covered stent grafts with a sufficient diameter are deployed in the common or external iliac arteries to provide conduit for graft access. This technique developed by the vascular group in Malmo, Sweden, is referred to as "crack and pave" because vessels are lined with "endoconduit" and balloon angioplasty then "cracks" the native vessel to allow sufficient diameter for device passage [18].

- *Proximal Landing Zones*: Certain proximal landing zones are compromised by acute neck angulation or neck lengths that are short but not so short as to require fenestration or snorkel,

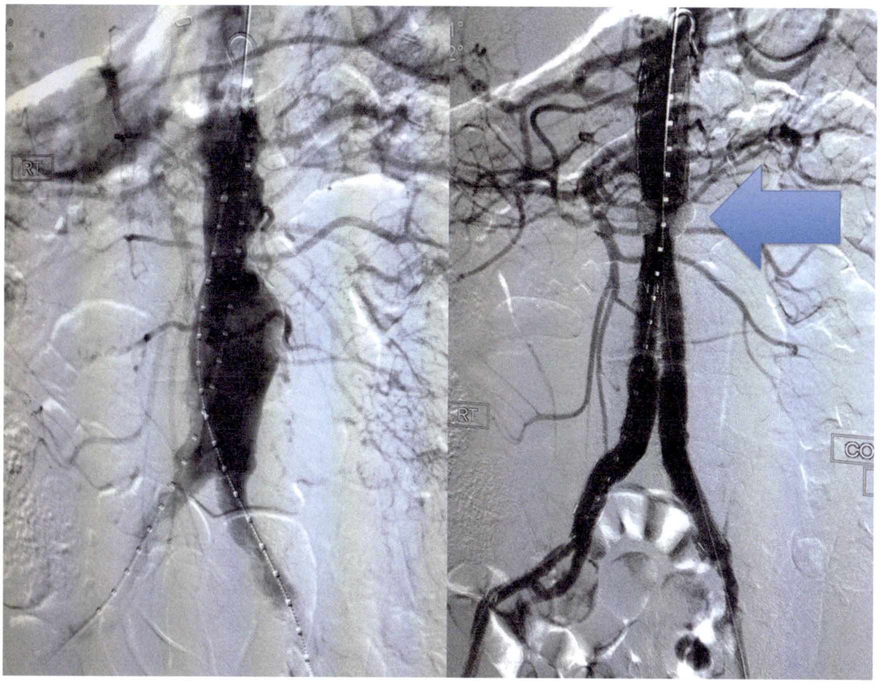

Fig. 28.2 This is a 78-year-old male patient who had a history of a 5.8-cm infrarenal abdominal aortic aneurysm, who had successful placement of an endovascular percutaneous placement of an Ovation Abdominal Stent Graft System (TriVascular Inc., Santa Rosa, CA) by the authors. The ring-shaped channel can be seen inflated with polymer (*blue arrow*), providing adequate seal for the endograft

as we will describe later. In such instances, some endorse fixation of the endovascular exclusion device via tacking to the arterial wall. Endofixation using endoanchors is thought to increase the force of fixation and decrease stent graft shifting. The Heli-FX™ EndoAnchor System (Aptus Endosystems, Sunnyvale, CA) is thought to improve fixation and endograft sealing within the infrarenal aortic neck, mimicking a surgical anastomosis. As a results, the force required to displace an endograft is higher, potentially: (1) diminishing the risk of proximal aortic neck complications with difficult aortic necks; (2) treating endoleaks and migration when these complications occurred with a previously placed endograft; (3) increasing eligibility for EVAR to those with more complex aortic neck anatomy, and; (4) improving the durability of endovascular repair through a more robust attachment between the endograft and the aorta. In a recent trial that implanted EndoAnchors in 319 patients with type IA endoleaks, 91 % of endoleaks resolved and at the end of published follow-up, 95 % of patients did not require additional intervention [19]. Results of the ANCHOR prospective, multicenter registry of EndoAnchors for type Ia endoleaks and endograft migration in patients with challenging anatomy [19]. Inadequate neck lengths are seen with juxtarenal and pararenal aneurysms. In such cases, sufficient sealing zones could be created with coverage one or two renal arteries or in some cases large accessory renal arteries. To accomplish this and preserve renal blood flow, fenestrated grafts can be deployed, or alternatively the "snorkel" technique is used when appropriate. For this technique, a covered stent graft is deployed into the artery to be preserved and the proximal end is advanced to above where the top of the AAA exclusion graft will need to be deployed. As such, blood flow is maintained to the preserved artery via a "snorkel." The snorkel technique is a 95 % patency at 2 years in experienced hands. Direct comparison of snorkel vs fenestrated EVAR (fEVAR) has not been made, but preliminary results from both techniques suggest both have adequate short-term outcomes [20, 21].

- *Neck Configuration*: Aneurysm neck angulation can prevent endograft devices from maintaining arterial wall approximation, which leads to endoleaks and aneurysm sac pressurization. In addition, as aneurysms undergo natural remodeling after EVAR; neck angulation can increase and lengthen which often results in endoleak creation. Required neck angulation has typically been considered <60°, but, increasingly, devices are able to conform to more acute neck angles. Last February 2013, the FDA completed its review of the Aorfix™ AAA Flexible Stent Graft System (Lombard Medical, Didcot, UK). This new device is a highly conformable modular nitinol and polyester stent which combines circular and helical structures that provide the flexibility needed to treat tortuous aortic anatomies. It is indicated for the treatment of patients with abdominal aortic and aorto-iliac aneurysms having vascular morphology suitable for endovascular repair, including infrarenal aortic neck angulations including those up to and including 90°.
- *Distal Landing Zones*: During EVAR, the common iliac artery represents the distal site for stent-graft implantation. The benefit of EVAR could be compromised if an adequate distal seal is not obtained. Concomitant common iliac artery aneurysms are present in 15–40 % of patients with AAA [22]. One solution is to deploy stent-graft extensions into the external iliac artery, but this is thought to compromise the long-term patency of the repair [23]. Furthermore, IIA coverage can result in buttock claudication and/or erectile dysfunction. The actual frequency of such complications is not well defined. In younger populations (with fewer collaterals and who have greater oxygen demand because they are more active), these complications can occur in 30 % of single vessel coverage and 35 % if both hypogastric arteries are covered [24]. But the frequency of buttock claudication in the majority of patients is much lower, but still occurs.

The distal seal zone is quite important for successful AAA exclusion [25, 26]. In fact, difficulties with the distal landing zone represent a more important reason for reintervention than those with the proximal zone. Progressive iliac artery aneurysm formation and iliac limb thrombosis are among the most important reasons for reintervention in a series of 832 EVAR patients [25]. Hypogastric arterial preservation can be achieved to good success using branched endografts that provide flow both into the hypogastric and the external iliac artery [27]. Another useful technique is the "bell-bottom," where the distal graft flares to create wall apposition with an aneurysmal distal common iliac artery [28].

Next, we present a succinct review of more advanced techniques involved in EVAR. AAA anatomy dictates the feasibility and difficulty of their repair, and multiple adjunctive procedures have evolved during the last century to expand the number of aneurysms amenable to EVAR.

Percutaneous EVAR (pEVAR)

Open exposure of femoral vessels has historically been the preferred method to gain arterial access for AAA endograft deployment because percutaneous access resulted in high complications rates including bleeding and iliofemoral dissection compared to open exposure [29]. Open exposure requires approximately 5–8 cm groin incisions (often bilaterally) and is a safe way to access vessels with direct arterial control. However, this technique results in a small (~1–2 %) but present risk of wound infection. Two factors have allowed for increased utilization of pEVAR (Fig. 28.3): exclusion devices with smaller profiles and improved percutaneous arterial closure devices [30]. A recent multicenter RCT determined pEVAR has decreased surgical site infections and no increase in access vessel complications. However, the study excluded "hostile" groins [31]. Femoral artery calcification is a major predictor of pEVAR success because calcifications can prevent closure devices from proper functioning [32].

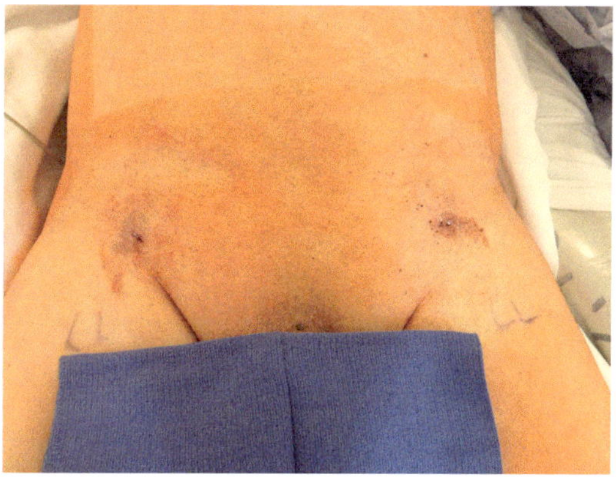

Fig. 28.3 Postoperative photography of a patient after successful percutaneous endovascular aneurysm repair. His body habitus, lack of calcification of femoral vessels, and a small profile endograft made him a perfect candidate for a completely percutaneous approach

In summary, pEVAR vs. open arterial exposure is the surgeon's preference, but preparedness for open cut-down is necessary.

Fenestrated EVAR (fEVAR)

The proximal aortic neck remains an important limitation of endovascular treatment of AAAs. Roughly 20 % of aneurysms are not candidates for standard endovascular repair due to poor proximal neck anatomy [33]. As discussed above, appropriate infra-renal landing zones of 10–15 mm is required for proximal graft seal. A recent meta-analysis including 1,559 patients retrospectively reviewed found that patients with hostile AAA neck anatomy had a fourfold increased rate of Type I endoleak and a ninefold increase in 1-year aneurysm-related death [34]. Endografts can be fenestrated for renal, superior mesenteric and celiac artery accommodation. This technique started with graft modification (cauterizing a hole in a prefabricated graft), but pre-fenestrated grafts are now available at specific study centers in the USA. Useful comparison between fEVAR and open repair of juxtarenal and visceral aneurysms are not useful because the patient populations in the two arms are so disparate [35]. Assuming that patients selected for fEVAR have greater comorbidities than those who are candidates for open repair, the results that indicate equivalent 30-day mortality (4.1 %) between the two groups is encouraging [36]. Although data is limited, the technical feasibility of fEVAR has been shown and the method is increasing.

EndoVascular Aneurysm Sealing (EVAS) system

It is thought that up to 40 % of infrarenal AAA are not suitable for EVAR due to hostile proximal neck anatomy (e.g., highly angulated, dilated, short, or encroaching on or involving the renal arteries [12, 37, 38]). In most EVAR studies, the infrarenal non-aneurysmal neck length and angulation to the aneurysm sac requirements are ≥15 mm and ≤60°, respectively; shorter or more angled necks have been reported to increase the risk of migration, endoleaks and associated need for intervention [38, 39]. When selecting the specific stent graft to be used for EVAR, the characteristics of the graft must be considered in light of the patient's anatomic and physiologic characteristics. Most of the currently available devices seal aneurysm by proximal and distal fixation of the stent graft by either active fixation (anchoring pins) or stent oversizing for increased radial force thereby achieving seal and excluding the aneurysm sac. Greater than 25 % of subjects develop an endoleak (mostly type II, due to back-bleeding of branch arteries within the aneurysm sac) within the first 2 years following EVAR [40].

Endovascular aneurysm sealing (EVAS), the Nellix® system (Endologix, Irvine, CA) was designed to exclude the aneurysm with two ePTFE balloon-expandable covered stents creating pathways to each common iliac artery. In addition, the system deploys an "Endobag" filled with polymer that surround the two stents and fills the aneurysm sac (Fig. 28.4). This is a unique, "out of the box thinking" kind of device. In theory, this Endobag promotes graft stability, prevents aneurysm degeneration and diminishes possibility of all types of endoleaks. A clinical trial has been performed to assess the safety and effectiveness of the first generation Nellix system for EVAR and results serve as the basis for CE Mark approval in October 2012. Initial results showed that the Nellix System is quite versatile in treating a variety of AAA anatomies, including

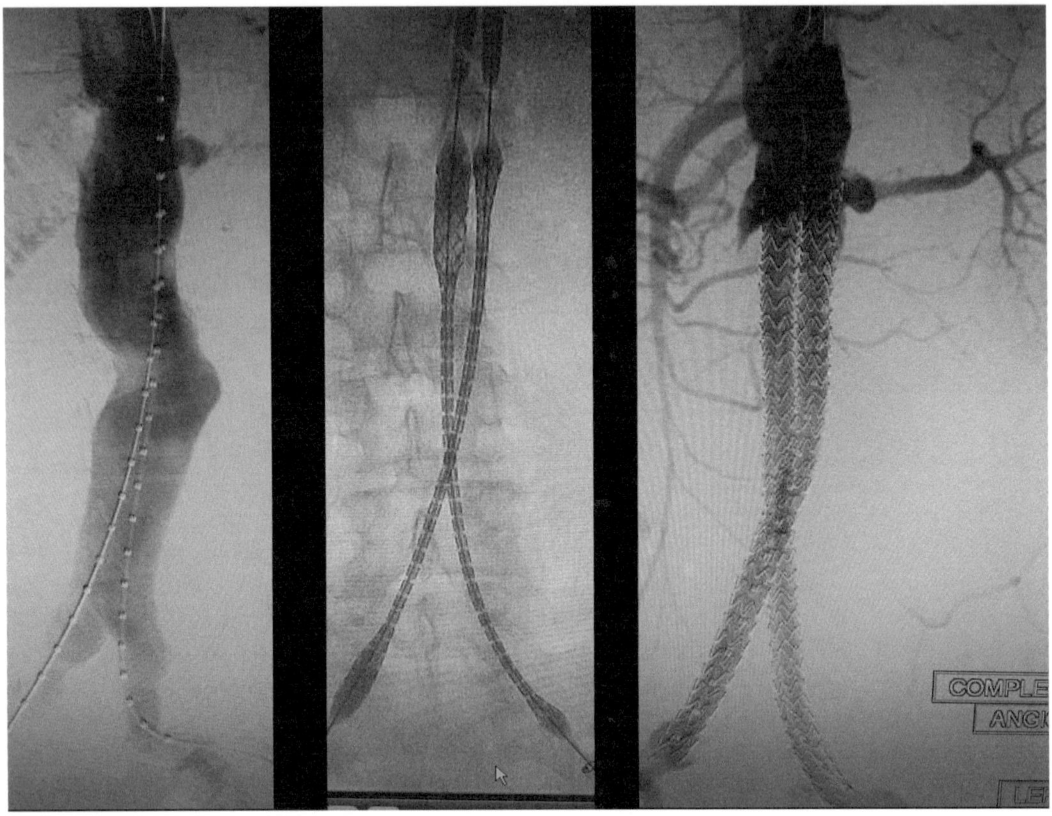

Fig. 28.4 These are intra-operative angiographic images of a patient enrolled in the EVAS Nellix® (Endologix, Irvine, CA) trial by the authors. Patient is an 83-year-old Caucasian male with a 6.8-cm infrarenal abdominal aortic aneurysm, with ideal features for an endovascular repair (*left panel*). The two e-PTFE balloon-expandable covered stents of the Nellix system are being deployed (*middle panel*), with the final result showed in the *right panel*, with successful exclusion of the aneurysm sac

those with common iliac artery involvement bilaterally. An ongoing trial with the Nellix System in a broader group of institutions and physicians was then begun to assess its safety and effectiveness. This is a multicenter, prospective, single arm clinical study. Subjects with infrarenal AAA who are suitable candidates for EVAR were considered for enrollment. Up to 30 sites in the EU, Canada, and the US enrolled patients for endpoint analysis. The enrollment phase has closed and now the trial is in the follow-up stage.

In summary, AAAs are an important disease and a common cause of death in our aging population, especially in those who have ever smoked. Disease treatment is aimed at prevention of AAA rupture, and the techniques to achieve this are ever increasing and complex. The available technology generally outpaces our ability to thoroughly evaluate it and determine their long-term (5–10 year) success. As such, this requires experts who stay abreast of technology and consider such technology with a discerning and critical eye using years of experience with aneurysm anatomy and physiology to make judgments of how best to deal with each patient's anatomy.

Acute Aortic Syndromes

Endovascular Management of Ruptured AAA

One of the most immediately life-threatening challenges in vascular surgery is repair of a ruptured aneurysm involving the aorta and/or iliac vessels. Classically this has been addressed with an open abdominal approach and a perioperative mortality rate of nearly 50 % [41]. While this has been slowly decreasing at about 3.5 % per decade, an exciting development in the twenty-first century is the increasing body of data on the use of endovascular grafts and devices for not just elective aneurysm repair, but also in cases of rupture.

Multiple centers have demonstrated and published the feasibility of endovascular repair of ruptured aneurysms in the emergent setting with reduced rates of perioperative mortality [42–46]. By analyzing data from the National Surgery Quality Improvement Project (NSQIP) database, a real-world comparison of open repair vs. EVAR could be made [47]. While the 30-day mortality risk was increased with open repair vs. EVAR, this was not statistically significant in this study. However, those treated with open repair had significantly higher rates of blood transfusion, overall morbidity and rates of pulmonary adverse events.

Utilizing femoral access for endovascular techniques as opposed to open laparotomy results in smaller incisions and lower rates of morbidity, but one of the limitations of endovascular repair instead of open repair are endoleaks that result in continued pressurization of the aneurysm sac. This may be particularly challenging in the emergent setting as device options may be more limited and the usual planning is more rushed. Along with a good stock of endografts for treating ruptures, the development of techniques to deal with endoleaks is helpful an assuring depressurization of the aneurysm. If needed for seal, embolization of the internal iliac arteries is more easily achieved before deploying a device across them as is sometimes performed in elective repairs, and type II endoleaks are not always easy to cannulate and occlude. However, published techniques such as direct sac puncture via translumbar approach appear to provide viable solutions to these problems [48, 49] Still, quick planning and an armamentarium of wires, catheters, embolization coils and vascular plugs can make control of these branch vessels feasible even in the setting of rupture.

Type B Aortic Dissections

The gold standard in the therapy of acute type B Aortic dissections (AAD) remains medical therapy. Despite progress in surgical techniques for open repair, the morbidity and mortality associated to this procedure remains high. Thoracic endovascular dissection repair (TEDR) has emerged as a less morbid procedure with potential clinical benefit [50].

Recently the task force for the diagnosis and treatment of Aortic disease of the European Society of Cardiology agreed on TEDR as the treatment of choice for complicated ADD. The term complicated refers to persistent or recurrent pain, uncontrolled hypertension despite full medication, early aortic expansion, malperfusion and signs of rupture (hemothorax, increasing periaortic and mediastinal hematoma) [51].

In uncomplicated patients, there seems to be a trend toward more aggressive TEDR. The intention of expanding interventional therapy in this subgroup is to stabilize the dissected aorta and prevent late complications by inducing aortic remodeling. From the technical standpoint, the operator should attempt to close the proximal intimal tear by implanting a stent-graft and redirecting blood flow from the false lumen to the true lumen [52].

The INSTEAD trial randomized a total of 140 patients with subacute (>14 days) uncomplicated ADD to receive either best medical management or endografting. Two-year follow-up results indicated that TEDR was an effective tool regarding successful Aortic remodeling. The TEDR group had 91.3 % vs. 19.4 % remodeling in the medical cohort. That said, TEDR demonstrated no clinical benefit over medical therapy from the survival standpoint (88.9 ± 3.7 % with TEDR vs. 95.6 ± 2.5 % with optimal medical therapy; $p = 0.15$) [53].

Upon extended follow-up and statistical analysis at 5-years (INSTEAD-XL trial) the aorta-related mortality (6.9 % vs. 19.3 %; $p = 0.04$) and disease progression (defined as aneurysmal dilation or further dissection) were significantly lower on the TEDR subgroup. There was no difference in overall mortality [54]. The IRAD registry, a multicenter international ADD registry, has also published similar results and has further identified factors that may help risk-stratify these patients and tailor the aggressiveness of the therapy [55, 56].

The role of preventive TEDR in uncomplicated but high risk ADD is yet to be definitively proven, but the following are clinical scenarios that selected authors advocate merit a more aggressive primary-TEDR approach: primary entry tear with a diameter greater than 10 mm; primary entry location at the lesser curvature of the arch ("concave" side); total Aortic diameter greater or equal to 4 cm; false lumen diameter greater or equal to 22 mm; partial false lumen thrombosis and Marui Fusiform Index greater than 0.64; Marui et al. developed this indicator: Maximum total diameter (including the false lumen) of the descending Aorta divided by the sum of the diameters of the Aortic arch and descending Aorta at the level of the pulmonary artery [57, 58].

Advances in Peripheral Arterial Disease

An estimated 12–20 million people in the USA alone have PAD [59]. PAD symptoms and signs include walking impairment (fatigue, aching, numbness, and pain), ischemic pain at rest, and chronic non-healing wound. The most common presenting symptom of lower extremity PAD is ambulation-induced muscle pain, or claudication. PAD is characterized by occlusive lesions in the lower extremity and portends an increased cardiovascular risk. [60]. Atherosclerotic lesions occur throughout the arterial tree in vessels from the aorta to pedal arteries. The location of arterial disease has important clinical implications for both prognosis and management [61].

Patients with critical limb ischemia (CLI) typically have multilevel arterial occlusive disease and significant comorbidities that increase their perioperative risk. Successful revascularization and limb salvage traditionally required lengthy, often staged interventions with significant associated morbidity and mortality. Endovascular techniques present an attractive alternative to open interventions especially in high-risk patients. Balloon angioplasty and/or stenting for TASC A and B (and perhaps for TASC C) iliac lesions have proven very good patency rates and have become the preferred initial treatment [61]. CLI, however, has long been considered an indication for bypass surgery [62]. The growing experience with endovascular techniques has helped to better identify patients and lesions that are best-treated by percutaneous interventions. Kudo et al. [63] described this change in practice over a 12-year period showing that balloon angioplasty could be the procedure of choice for CLI therapy.

Advances in the Diagnosis and Assessment of Peripheral Arterial Disease

The etiology of PAD in the vascular practice appears to be undergoing a change along with the changing population of the USA. The usual vascular risk factors are still present (i.e., age, smoking, hypertension, hyperlipidemia); however, the prevalence of diabetes in the USA and around the world has been increasing in the twenty-first century. The sensory and autonomic neuropathy, increased rates of chronic kidney disease, immunosuppressive and wound-healing inhibitory effects of diabetes make it much more challenging than the pure-ischemia model described in the term critical limb ischemia originally defined in 1982 [64]. Recognizing these complexities, the authors of that paper explicitly excluded diabetics from assessment by this method. Diabetes also appears to change the pattern of disease from the classic proximal distribution (aortoiliac and femoropopliteal) to a more distal distribution of tibial vessels and intrinsic foot vessels. This often results in medial calcinosis of these vessels making it difficult to assess severity of disease and response to treatment with conventional methods of ankle-brachial index and toe pressure as medial calcinosis causes false elevation of these pressures and intrinsic foot disease combined with tibial occlusions may cause regionalized ischemia of the foot even with normal pressure in one of the other tibial vessels. For this reason, alternative methods of assessing tissue perfusion are being investigated. One of these methods is using Indocyanine Green (ICG) dye injected intravascularly and visualizing the fluorescence using a charge-coupled device camera. The dye stays intravascularly and the intensity of the fluorescence in the tissue corresponds to the degree of perfusion of the tissue. It therefore does not assess blood flow based pressure but is an assessment of end-perfusion. This technology has been used for decades in ophthalmology, cardiothoracic surgery, plastic surgery, liver transplantation, bowel resections and surgical oncology. Its use in assessing foot perfusion in patients with PAD and foot wounds is still in the early stages but multiple series have been published in the USA and around the world on this topic. It requires an IV to test, which is more invasive than traditional noninvasive tests of ABI/Toe pressure and duplex ultrasound; however, it is available for use even when traditional noninvasive tests are unreliable or unobtainable due to medial calcinosis, active wounds, prior amputations or other conditions. Multiple criteria have been proposed as surrogates for adequate perfusion for healing [65–67] but as of now, no accepted standard has been adopted.

Another technology for monitoring tissue perfusion is implantable micro-oxygen sensors. A first-in-man study has been published recently based on technology from PROFUSA, Inc. (South San Francisco, CA) [68]. The eventual hope is that an implantable, biodegradable tissue oxygen sensor could be implanted in the foot & serial monitoring be done either at the physician's office or via an app on a hand-held device, allowing earlier detections of change that may signal worsening arterial stenosis or impending occlusion at a time when it is easier to repair than when the vessels have occluded. While this technology is still well away from mass use, it may fill a gap left by current vascular assessments.

Advances in the Therapy of Peripheral Arterial Disease

Aortoiliac Arterial Disease

Endovascular therapy of the aorto-iliac system has far developed since the initial results by Kichikawa et al. in 1990 [69]. The Dutch trial further analyzed the impact of metal scaffolding, concluding that simple (TASC A/B) lesions respond well to plain old balloon angioplasty reserving stenting as a bail-out plan [70].

The widespread use of endovascular therapies has lead operators to tackle more complex lesions (TASC C/D). Within this specific complexity, some of the preliminary data suggests an advantage of PTFE-covered stents over BM-stents [71]. Sabri et al. concluded that the use of covered balloon-expandable kissing stents for atherosclerotic aortic bifurcation occlusive disease provides superior patency at 2 years when compared with bare meal balloon-expandable stent in a small number of patients [72].

In 2011, the COBEST (Covered versus balloon expandable stent trial) trial revealed its early data. Aortoiliac lesions treated with a PTFE-covered stent were significantly more likely to remain free from binary restenosis than those that were treated with a bare-metal stent (hazard ratio [HR], 0.35; 95 % confidence interval (CI), 0.15–0.82; $p=0.02$). Freedom from occlusion was also higher in lesions treated with covered stents than in those treated with a bare-metal stent (HR, 0.28; 95 % CI, 0.07–1.09); however, this did not reach statistical significance ($p=0.07$) [73].

Femoropopliteal Arterial Disease

Contemporary treatment of femoropopliteal occlusive arterial disease is most frequently via an endovascular approach. When comparing inpatient vascular procedures in the USA from 1997 to 2008, open peripheral reconstruction declined by 24.5 %, whereas percutaneous interventions dramatically increased by 296.8 % [74]. Unfortunately, the combination of a wide array of available endovascular tools, inconsistent outcomes data, and differing training paradigms, have produced uninformed and highly variable endovascular practice patterns.

The lack of consensus regarding reporting standards leaves the practitioner with inadequate data to formulate evidence-based clinical decisions. Some authors have attempted to create uniformity [75, 76] but there are as yet no broadly accepted and applied practice standards. Moreover, most of the randomized controlled data available to date are industry driven.

Restenosis of femoropopliteal therapy has been certainly the main concern during the past 10 years of practice. There is not one device that has proven to be far superior to others, yet there are evolving technologies that have added value and a potential role in this segment. Amongst the most notorious advances in the field are: new fracture-free, vasculo-mimetic stents; drug-coated stents; drug-coated balloons; advanced drug-delivery systems; and newer generation atherectomy (plaque debulking) devices.

Fracture-Free, Vasculo-mimetic Stents

The Supera® (Abbott Vascular, Santa Clara, CA) self-expanding, interwoven, nitinol-stent received FDA approval for use in the femoropopliteal early in year 2014. The study that led to the FDA approval is known as the SUPERB registry. The primary patency rate achieved in this pivotal trial was 86.3 % (Kaplan–Meier) with 1-year freedom from reintervention at 89 % and 3-year freedom from reintervention (TLR) at 83 %, despite having 45 % of patients with severe calcium and 25 % with total occlusions.

A subset analysis of the SUPERB trial was conducted to determine the impact of lesion length on restenosis. In both short lesions (3.5 cm) and long lesions (12 cm), the percentage of patients without restenosis was the same at 88 %, which was dramatically different than other investigational device exemption trials such as STROLL (S.M.A.R.T.® Control®, Cordis Corporation, East Bridgewater, NJ) or DURABILITY II (EverFlex™, Covidien, Minneapolis, MN), which showed a decline in patency as lesion lengths increased.

The main issue with inter-woven technology is the potential to mis-deploy resulting in an elongated or compressed conformation. In proper deployments of Supera® (Abbott, Abbott Park, IL) (nominal length deployments), primary patency was 90.5 % at 12 months. In addition, 97 % and 94 % freedom from reintervention rates were achieved at 1 and 3 years, respectively, in nominal deployments. Lower primary patency and freedom from reintervention rates were associated with severely elongated deployments.

Drug-Coated Stents

One of the major factors causing recurrent stenosis in peripheral artery interventions is the development of neo-intimal hyperplasia. This is an overgrowth as a result of the vessel's response to injury. Original investigations into this problem were conducted in the coronaries, and the first drug-eluting stent (DES) was approved in Europe in 2002 with FDA approval in 2003 initially for treatment of in-stent restenosis [77]. Drug-eluting stents cause a time-released local application of a drug (generally a chemotherapeutic drug such as sirolimus, paclitaxel or everolimus) to the tissue abutting the stent in order to inhibit the inflammatory response and neointimal hyperplasia, thereby reducing rates of restenosis and thrombosis. Since initial approval, the use of drug-eluting stents has expanded profoundly in coronary artery disease.

Given that the same neointimal hyperplasia process occurs in the periphery as well as in the coronary bed, eventual research looked into using drug-eluting stents for peripheral artery disease. The first DES approved for use in the superficial femoral and popliteal arteries was the Zilver® PTX stent by Cook (Cook Inc, Bloomington, IL) [78, 79], which received FDA approval in 2012. The Zilver PTX stent elutes paclitaxel from a polymer-free laser-cut nitinol stent. Dake et al. led the Zilver PTX stent trial which initial results were published in 2011 [78]. This was a prospective, multinational randomized controlled trial and a complementary single-arm study evaluated the 2-year safety and effectiveness of the implant in patients with superficial femoral artery lesions. The trial compared the DES with percutaneous transluminal angioplasty and provisional bare-metal stent placement.

The trial showed an unsurprising superiority of drug-eluting stent over balloon angioplasty in terms of primary patency (74.8 % vs. 26.5 %, $p<0.01$). However, it also showed superiority in the use of drug-eluting stent over bare-metal stent in patients who had initial failure of primary angioplasty (83.4 % vs. 64.1 %, $p<0.01$). This corresponds to a number needed to treat (NNT) of 5 to prevent 1 re-thrombosis at 2 years. There is an up-front higher cost to the drug-eluting stents, which is one of the reasons why it has not replaced bare-metal or covered-stent technology in the primary treatment of PAD. In addition, the provisional DES group achieved higher sustained clinical benefit (83.9 % vs. 68.4 %, $p<0.05$). Two-year freedom from target lesion revascularization with primary DES placement was 80.5 % in the single-arm study and 86.6 % in the Randomized Control Trial [79].

Even though these new-generation devices have proven to be superior to older scaffolds, the presence of a non-absorbable implant still perpetuates a constant inflammatory process that may lead to intimal hyperplasia. Tepe et al. attempted to introduce a new paradigm of care with the publication of the THUNDER trial. The preliminary results of these trial concluded that the use of paclitaxel-coated angioplasty balloons during percutaneous treatment of femoropopliteal disease is associated with significant reductions in late lumen loss and target-lesion revascularization without leaving any implant behind [80].

Drug-Coated Balloons

Another area of ongoing interest is the use of drug-coated balloons (DCBs) for treatment of lower extremity arterial stenosis (Fig. 28.5). The rationale is that if a drug-eluting balloon can provide improved patency results without the need for leaving a stent in place, it might help avoid some of the other problems of stents such as fracture or ongoing stress leading to neointimal hyperplasia. Late in 2014, the FDA approved the Lutonix® paclitaxel DCB (Bard PV Inc, Phoenix, AZ) for use in the USA. The primary composite safety endpoint for Lutonix was noninferiority to PTA. For the primary effectiveness endpoint, utilizing duplex scan evaluation with a lax peak-systolic velocity (PSVR) of 2.5, Lutonix demonstrated superior 12-month patency rates to

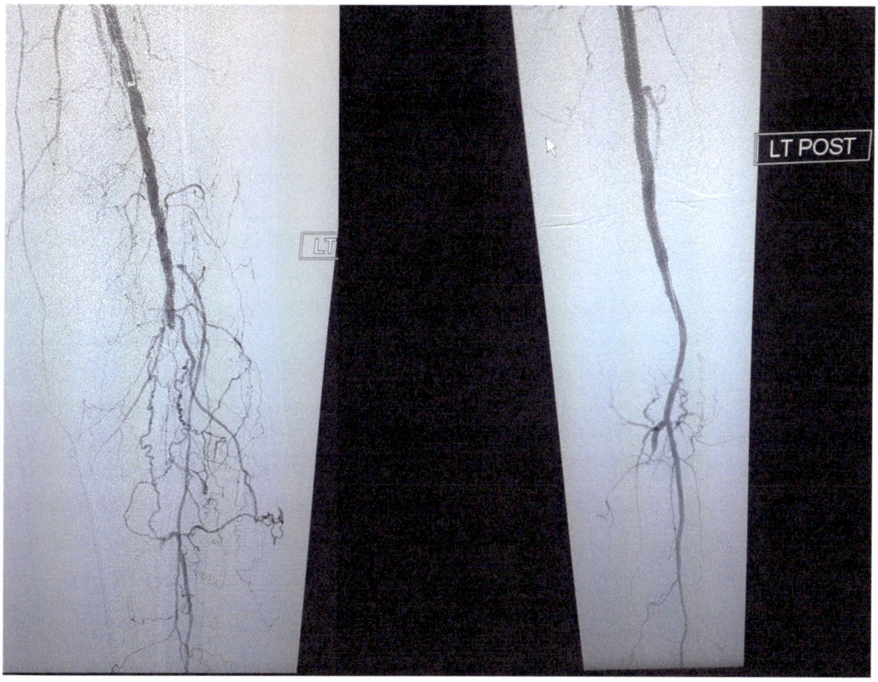

Fig. 28.5 Patient is a 79-year-old diabetic female with advanced gangrene of the foot and severe ischemic cardiomyopathy. Successful endovascular revascularization was performed by using a drug-eluting balloon, with outstanding angiographic results and restoration of palpable pedal pulses

PTA using Kaplan–Meier estimates (73.5 % vs. 56.8 %). However, when using a standard PSVR of 2.0, as used in the SUPERB and ZILVER PTX pivotal trials for primary patency assessment, there was no significant difference between Lutonix and plain old balloon angioplasty ($P=0.13$). Moreover, the Lutonix freedom from TLR dataset demonstrated no significant difference with balloon angioplasty alone at 12 months. Despite the lower-than-expected patency rates, Lutonix's results did show a favorable trend over PTA on several endpoints, suggesting that there is a benefit conferred from the paclitaxel coating [81].

Most recently, in early 2015, the FDA has approved the use of the IN.PACT balloon by Medtronic (Minneapolis, MN), which is a paclitaxel-coated balloon, for the treatment of SFA and popliteal disease [82]. It has been in use in Europe since 2009. The paclitaxel-coated balloon resulted in higher 1 year-patency rate compared to non-coated balloon angioplasty (82.2 % vs. 52.4 %, $p<0.001$) and a lower rate of clinically driven target lesion revascularization (2.4 % vs. 20.6 %, $p<0.001$). Of note, the patients in this study had predominately claudication as their indication with only 5 % of the DCB arm had rest pain along with 5.4 % of those in the PTA arm along with 0.9 % in the PTA arm with minor tissue loss. Therefore, the lack of amputations eventual amputations in the 1-year follow-up was not surprising. Robust data on other clinical endpoints such as wound-healing and amputation-free survival in patients with tissue loss is lacking for this technology, but further research is ongoing. Combining local pharmacologic effects and biomechanical effects of balloons/stents is on the cutting-edge of PAD treatment.

Advanced Drug-Delivery Systems

Concern has grown as to the potential downstream loss of cytotoxic drugs in patients with ischemic foot ulcers. Development of novel tools to directly allocate drugs in a safe and efficacious manner is being set in motion. The patented, proprietary and FDA-cleared Bullfrog® Micro-Infusion Device (Mercator MedSystems Inc, San Leandro, CA) delivers drugs directly to the adventitia. Inflation of the balloon safely slides a micro needle through the vessel wall, where agents are delivered and diffuse to bathe the vessel cylindrically (circumferentially, longitudinally and transmurally). Delivering drugs through the blood vessel wall into the perivascular space and adventitia allows for direct, highly controllable and concentrated treatment, minimizing the toxicity of systemic administration, while avoiding the dilution of drug in the bloodstream. The DANCE study—a US-based, multicenter, prospective registry is in the process of recruiting patients to evaluate the use of this device as means to dose steroids to the deep arterial layers.

The TAPAS ("Targeted Adjusted Pharmaceutical Administration System") catheter (ThermopeutiX® Inc., San Diego, CA) is another newly introduced device, with FDA clearance and CE mark (Fig. 28.6). This device features two occlusion balloons that allow targeted local delivery of any pharmaceutical agent, i.e., chemotherapy drugs, thormbolysis medications, sclerotherapy, anti-inflammatory agents, etc. The distance between the balloons determines the treatment zone, and this can be adjusted from 15 to 300-mm due to its coaxial design. The medication can be aspirated out of the catheter after therapy if desired. Research is planned to prove the safety and efficacy of this technology in the peripheral circulation.

New Generation Atherectomy Devices

These have emerged as additional alternatives for plaque debulking. For instance, the Volcano's Phoenix® Atherectomy System (Menlo Park, CA) is a novel device which has a front-cutting design, with its housing capturing atherectomy debris by a helical blade that cuts inward, mechanism known as "Continuous Mechanical Conveyance." In this manner, the debulked plaque is removed without vessel suck down or excessive aspiration of blood. It is a single insertion, single-operator device. There is no need to remove catheter to purge the collected material during the procedure. There is no capital equipment component or tableside infusion pump required. The distal cutting element rotates at 12,000 RPM. The cutting element is made of stainless steel alloy with proprietary coating. In theory, the front cutting design

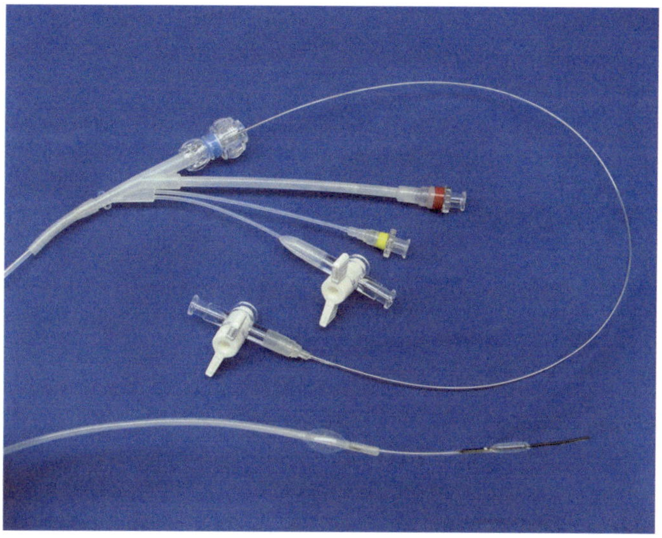

Fig. 28.6 The TAPAS® ("Targeted Adjusted Pharmaceutical Administration System") catheter. (Courtesy of ThermopeutiX® Inc., San Diego, CA)

eliminates the need to pass the device nosecone through a disease segment prior to treatment. This, along with its mechanism of cutting, capturing and clearing, could potentially reduce the risk of distal embolization. The device has been designed to treat a wide range of disease types, from soft plaques to calcified arteries. In addition, it has the ability to actively deflect its direction, thus being able to cut a lumen larger than the catheter diameter. A small 5 F profile optimizes treatment of disease located below the knee. Lastly, being an over-the-wire device, its pushable design maximizes deliverability. There are several devices, both for femoropopliteal and for tibial applications (5–7 French profile, 1.8–2.4 mm of luminal gain depending on the device used). The femoropopliteal device has a deflecting tip, which allows the interventionist to guide the helical blade as needed. The EASE Study (Endovascular Atherectomy Safety and Effectiveness Study) was designed for the clinical evaluation of the safety and effectiveness of Volcano's Phoenix® Atherectomy System in atherectomy of the peripheral vasculature in an IDE Study. It was a prospective, single arm, multicenter, FDA-approved IDE study in the USA and Germany. This included lower limb atherectomy with or without adjunctive therapies. This cohort included one-third of patients afflicted with critical limb ischemia and 70 % of the lesions were located at or below the knee level. More than half of these patients were diabetic. With a follow-up at 30 days and 6 months, the Phoenix Atherectomy System proved to be a safe and effective atherectomy solution for peripheral arteries. The study met predefined performance goals in safety and effectiveness; it had a high technical success, (95.1 %) low clinical complications and major adverse events (5.7 % at 30 days). These results were consistent with pivotal trials for predicate devices. FDA clearance was received on January 23, 2014.

Tibial Arterial Disease

The first published successful experience using a retrograde approach to recanalize a tibial vessel was by Iyer et al. in 1990, via cutdown of the posterior tibial artery [83]. The suspected hypothetical benefit of using alternative retrograde wire passage was first well described by Ozawa et al. in 2006 [84]. Although this article exemplifies retrograde chronic total occlusion (rCTO) crossing in the coronary arteries, the fundamental, physiopathologic principles can likely be extrapolated, with some caveats, to tibial-pedal artery procedures. Briefly, the technical hurdle with antegrade guidewire passage is failure to penetrate the proximal cap or failure to accomplish true-lumen distal reentry, primarily due to differential fibrotic cap composition. A complex and hard proximal fibrotic cap will prevent the wire from crossing or quickly divert it into the subadventitial space. In contrast, the distal fibrotic cap is said to be "either very thin or nonexistent" [83]. Moreover, there are potentially invisible residual true lumen channels that taper proximally to their narrowest area, which, as a result, are invisible on angiography. In general terms, the objective of retrograde access is to aid in lesion traversability. Once the lesion is crossed and the wire is secured in the proximal true lumen, most operators recommend recapturing the wire from a proximal, conventional access site and then using it as a rail (a through-and-through configuration that is achieved by establishing the wire from the pedal to the groin access site). Finally, once the lesion is crossed in an antegrade fashion with a support catheter or a balloon catheter, the wire is pulled out of the pedal access site and repositioned in the usual antegrade configuration. Hemostasis of the pedal puncture site is achieved with a combination of simple direct pressure and endohemostasis (inflation at the level of the puncture site of an angioplasty balloon sized one-to-one to the vessel at a low atmospheric pressure for 2–4 min). The development of newer devices with lower profiles has allowed operators to utilize retrograde access not only to cross the lesion, but also to effectively treat it [85].

Retrograde access should be secured close to the area of access artery reconstitution. Long areas of non-diseased vessel will hinder force vectors and minimize wire and balloon pushability. Moreover, vessel spasm is not infrequent, and the interventionalist must always abide by the general principle to minimize unnecessary contact between a healthy vessel and the wire or catheter. With these principles in mind there will be two groups: proximal (or high) and distal (or low pedal) retrograde access.

Initial experience in the 1990s described cutdown as a means of accessing pedal vessels, and although bailout surgical cutdown might be useful on rare occasions, the experienced operator will rarely need to resort to it. More recent published experiences have demonstrated the safety of percutaneous vessel access across a multitude of publications [86]. Recently, an industry-sponsored multicenter registry of nearly 200 patients who underwent rCTO therapy also concluded that the technique was safe and associated with high, initial technical success rates (tibiopedal study sponsored by Cook Medical; unpublished data).

Once the access is secure, there are two basic options: a sheathless or micropedal sheath technique. Historically, complications associated with pedal access were related to large-bore sheaths and these should be avoided [87].

The sheathless technique was used initially and has the theoretical advantage of creating a smaller arteriotomy. Operators secure a long wire in the vessels via the usual Seldinger technique, but then support the wire with either a low-profile balloon or catheter directly through the skin. The drawbacks associated with this are the potential risk of losing access during device exchange and the lack of a port that can be used to administer medications (i.e., antivasospastic drugs) or to inject contrast to obtain angiographic control images.

Current best practice is to secure the access with use of a 2.9-F micropuncture pedal access set. This approach secures low-profile access during the entire procedure. Operators can freely change devices and wires without compromising access, and there is a port to inject medications or contrast. Although most balloons on the market are not compatible with an extremely small inner lumen diameter, the Micro™ 14 (Cook Inc, Bloomington, IL) is a newly approved device that overcomes this hurdle.

Devices for Nonsurgical Management of Peripheral Arterial Disease

Claudication is normally a nonsurgical, medically treated problem. PAD can be improved in many patients with medical treatments [88]. In the absence of heart failure, cilostazol should be considered in patients with claudication pain [88]. Ischemic ulcers are among the most difficult to treat successfully and almost as a rule they typically require surgical interventions for their therapy.

High-pressure, rapid sequence, intermittent pneumatic calf and foot compression (HPIPC) devices apply compression to the foot, ankle and calf using cuffs attached to the leg. This compression regimen simulates the beneficial effects of brisk walking, without pain or tissue trauma. In 1917 Sinkowich and Gottlieb [89] were the first to report the benefits of intermittent compression for the treatment of thromboangiitis obliterans (Burger's Disease). In 1934, Herman and Reid [90] demonstrated that pneumatic compression improved tissue perfusion in patients with PAOD. Since 1993, several trials on the effects of HPIPC for the treatment of arterial claudication and CLI have been reported [91–94]. In all of these studies the investigators reported significant beneficial effects on walking distance, symptoms and systolic blood pressure measurements on both upper and lower limbs with therapy.

The foot, ankle and calf veins are almost completely emptied in the sitting position by using pressures that are much higher than those typically used in intermittent pneumatic compression (IPC) devices designed for instance, for deep venous thrombus (DVT) prevention. By compressing tissues below the knee, venous blood is almost completely emptied with venous pressures reaching almost zero. The increased arterial–venous pressure gradient results in greater arterial flow. Greater arterial flow alters the shear rate and may stimulate endothelial cell function causing the release of nitric oxide along with tissue factor pathway inhibitors that cause dilation and anticoagulation [95]. Several studies using HPIPC have shown improvement in perfusion, claudication (resting) pain, and wound healing in patients with PAOD and CLI [96–98]. HPIPC therapy appears to significantly improved peak walking time, resting pain, healing rates and physical function in most studies, along with a low device-related complication rate. HPIPC appears to be safe and effective and is an important adjunct to the medical treatment of PAD and CLI.

Advances in Venous Disease

Advances in Superficial Venous Disease

Superficial chronic vein disease is one of the most common entities encountered in a typical vascular surgery practice. Its symptoms can be as trivial as minor cosmetic complaints or as devastating as chronic venous non-healing ulcers. This is seen more as the population age increases and this problem is more prevalent in female patients than males. Anatomically, great saphenous vein (GSV) insufficiency accounts for most cases, whereas in about 15 % of patients, small saphenous vein (SSV) insufficiency is the main cause [99–101]. Surgical therapy of superficial venous insufficiency was the standard of care during the last century. However, surgery has been associated with recurrence rates as high as 60 %, as well as nerve injuries and other significant postoperative complications [102–104]. During the last few years, minimally invasive catheter-based, endovenous techniques took over the role of surgical therapy in the treatment of saphenous vein insufficiency. Success rates after such techniques as endovenous laser ablation (EVLA) and radiofrequency ablation (RFA) are high (88 % of anatomical success rate at 1 year follow-up) [102], and RFA is associated with less pain and bruising than surgery, superior cosmetic results and earlier resumption of daily activities compared to traditional surgery [105, 106].

Endovenous techniques are not exempt of caveats and complications. First, tumescent anesthesia is a must. Second, heat-induced skin and/or nerve injury are possibilities that can become chronic and can be severe. Nerve damage is one of the most common causes of litigation after varicose vein surgery [107].

These problems with traditional endovenous procedures led to the development of ablative methods that do not require heat or tumescent anesthesia for their performance. Mechanochemical endovenous ablation (MOCA™), using the ClariVein™ system (Vascular Insights LLC, Madison, CT) produces mechanical endovenous injury by a rotating wire at the tip of a catheter. Simultaneously, liquid sclerosant agents are injected to the treated vein to aid in the ablation process. This technique was introduced in Europe in 2010. The first results of MOCA™ showed excellent occlusion rates, significant improvements in Venous Clinical Severity Score (VCSS), an objective measure for varicose vein-specific symptoms, and no major complications, including nerve injury. These clinical results were retained at 1 year after treatment [108–110].

Cyanoacrylate is a strong, fast acting adhesive that have industrial and household uses. It has been successfully used in medicine for several years to treat bleeding duodenal varices, orbital varices, arteriovenous malformations and intracranial aneurysms. The first human use of endovenous cyanoacrylate for closure of insufficient GSVs in 38 patients, using injections under ultrasound guidance without tumescent anesthesia or graduated compression stockings proved to be feasible, safe and effective [111]. With a 2-year follow-up, complete GSV occlusion was sonographically documented in all patients except for one complete and two partial recanalizations observed at, 1, 3, and 6 months of follow-up, respectively. Kaplan–Meier analysis yielded an occlusion rate of 92.0 % (95 % CI 0.836–1.0) at 24 months follow-up. Venous Clinical Severity Score improved in all patients ($p<0.0001$). This commercially available VenaSeal™ Sapheon (Sapheon, Santa Rose, CA) closure system is used in Europe following CE Mark approval in September 2012.

Varithena ™ (polidocanol injectable foam) (BTG International, London, UK) is indicated for the therapy of saphenous vein incompetence, incompetence of its accessory veins and visible varicose veins of the GSV above and below the knee. It is supplied as polidocanol solution (10 mg/mL) in 18 mL. The medication must be activated before its use, using the Varithena™ oxygen canister and polidocanol canister. Once activated, Varithena™ is a white, injectable foam delivering a 1 % polidocanol solution. Each mL of Varithena™ injectable foam contains 1.3 mg of polidocanol. (For intravenous use under ultrasound guidance only, up to 5 mL per injection and 15 mL per treatment session are used.) The injectable foam must be given within 75 s of extraction from its canister to maintain injectable foam properties. In clinical trials, the most common related adverse events (occurring in ≥3 % of patients treated with Varithena™) were discomfort in the treated extremity, infusion site thrombosis, hematoma or pain, superficial thrombophlebitis and extravasation.

Advances in Deep Venous Disease

Acute Deep Venous Thrombosis

Deep vein thrombosis (DVT) is a very common problem affecting between 250,000 and 2 million patients every year in the USA [112]. Its most common complication is post-thrombotic syndrome (PTS), which can affect up to two-thirds of patients initially affected by DVT, despite systemic anticoagulation and compression stocking therapy (ECS) [113]. PTS may lead to significant limitations in their quality of life [114–116]. The chronic vein lumen obstruction caused by DVT produces venous hypertension, which is considered to be the main pathophysiological feature of PTS. Recanalization of chronically occlusive DVT, restoring flow in the occluded venous segment and decreasing venous pressure, can be safely and successfully performed to provide significant venous flow improvement, symptoms relief, and quality of life improvement [117].

The last few years have witnessed a more aggressive approach toward the therapy of patients with DVT, in order to prevent its devastating complications including PTS, limb loss and death. A recent retrospective study showed that iliofemoral DVT is associated with significant post-thrombotic morbidity if treated with early anticoagulation alone [118]. Previous authors have reported that 90 % of patients treated with anticoagulation alone will develop chronic venous insufficiency, 15 % will develop venous ulcers and 15 % will show symptoms of venous claudication [119]. The financial cost and morbidity associated with these adverse effects illustrates the importance in developing better methods in treating this disease process.

Present therapies for the treatment of acute DVT have ranged from conservative treatment with heparin or heparinoids to surgical thrombectomy. While somewhat effective, the morbidity associated with open venous thrombectomy fueled an interest in percutaneous venous thrombectomy procedures. Presently, catheter-based endovenous therapies have emerged as an important alternative option in the treatment of these patients. CDT either alone or in combination with venous stenting has proved to be reasonably safe and effective in treating patients with acute DVT based on case series or isolated case reports [120]. Successful thrombolysis maintains venous valve function and clears luminal obstruction. These two factors have been found to be associated with the most severe cases of PTS morbidity [121]. Pharmacomechanical options have included CDT in combination with mechanical thrombus debulking therapies. This combination therapy has the distinct advantage of rapid clot dissolution while minimizing thrombolytic drug requirement.

Percutaneous pharmacomechanical thrombectomy (PMT) techniques, catheter directed thrombolysis (CDT) and adjunctive endovascular modalities are now widely used in the management of these patients. Currently in the USA, the PMT devices most frequently used include the Trellis-8™ system (Covidien, Mansfield, MA), the Angiojet® Ultra Thrombectomy System (MEDRAD Interventional/Possis, Minneapolis, MN) and the EKOS ultrasound accelerated thrombolysis device (EKOS Corporation, Bothell, WA). The use of the Trellis-8™ peripheral infusion system during single-session PMT combined with tissue plasminogen activator (Alteplase, tPA) administration is our preferred approach for the treatment of patients with acute iliofemoral DVT.

The Trellis-8™ Peripheral Infusion System is an isolated thrombolysis catheter with two occluding balloons, drug infusion holes between the balloons, and mechanical drug dispersion capabilities. The initial use of the Trellis-8™ device has been criticized by some because in most hands, the typical duration of therapy is often over 24 h, thus requiring access to a monitored bed, multiple trips to the suite to assess progress, prolonged bed rest, patient discomfort, large doses of tPA and multiple laboratory blood work evaluations. During the last 3 years, our group modified the utilization of this device, in order to minimize those shortcomings. In fact, this modification has allowed us to perform some of these procedures in the ambulatory setting. Starting on July 2008, we have followed our modified protocol in over 140 patients affected by DVT in both upper and lower extremities. More often than not, large amounts of subacute thrombi are seen after the initial Trellis application. These are in need of removal in order to obtain optimal results. With this in mind, an 8-French multipurpose catheter (MPC, Cook, Bloomington, IN) is used to perform suction of the more organized thrombi. A 60-cc syringe is attached at the end of the MPC and several passes are made through the entire thrombosed segment under constant suction, with frequent contrast injection checks in between suctions to monitor our progress. These passes need to be very careful, keeping in mind the orientation of the venous valve cusps. After each pass, the collected blood and clots are strained by using 4×4 gauzes, capturing the clot in them. The unclotted blood is returned to the patient's veins to avoid exsanguination. The use of the MPC to extract thrombi may cause them to fragment, thereby resulting in PE. An IVCF previously placed could protect from this catastrophic event and this is done in selected cases. To further reduce the risk of PE during catheter passage, the patient is asked to perform Valsalva's maneuver, if awake, to increase central venous pressure. At this point, any residual venous defects (i.e., stenosis, extrinsic venous compression) are treated with angioplasty or stenting as indicated.

The ATTRACT (Acute Venous Thrombosis: Thrombus Removal with Adjunctive Catheter Directed Thrombolysis) randomized trial is currently underway to examine the outcomes of patients with acute symptomatic DVT undergoing conventional therapeutic anticoagulation versus pharmacomechanical catheter directed lysis in addition to therapeutic anticoagulation [122]. The results of this trial may help establish guidelines for treating DVT of the lower extremity.

The ATTRACT Steering Committee just recently announced the successful accrual of 100 % of the study's original target sample, precisely in January 2015. The trial accrued its originally planned cohort of 692 patients, who were enrolled at 56 hospitals, since its start in September 2008.

Combined ultrasound and thrombolytic therapy was developed to accelerate thrombolysis and rapidly achieve complete clot lysis while reducing the risk of serious complications such as bleeding. High frequency, low power ultrasound accelerates thrombolysis both in vitro and in vivo. This idea was pioneered by Kudo and confirmed by other investigators [123–126]. Ultrasound temporarily alters the local architecture of the fibrin clot, thereby enhancing its permeability by reducing the diameter of the fibrin strands and increasing the pore size of the fibrin mesh [127]. Ultrasound energy also provides an acoustic pressure gradient to enable transportation of a greater quantity of thrombolytic drug into the clot itself. The resulting faster, more complete clot lysis is due to increased diffusion of the thrombolytic agent into the clot and not mechanical disruption. The EkoSonic System (EKOS Corp, Bothell, WA) is an FDA cleared drug delivery catheter that uses ultrasound delivered through the catheter core to speed the delivery of thrombolytic drug into the interstices of the clot and increase the speed of lysis. By making the clot more permeable and pushing the drug into the fibrin mesh, the EKOS System has the potential to reduce time to lysis, increase the efficacy of lysis, reduce drug dose and thereby reduce the risk of bleeding complications (Fig. 28.7a, b).

The adoption of these novel modalities allowed our group to treat challenging venous occlusive situations. For instance, acute thrombosis of the inferior vena cava can be a devastating problem. It is uncommon and its current treatment options are not well defined. These include anticoagulation, systemic thrombolytic therapy, and open surgical thrombectomy. These modalities have been shown to be minimally effective and carry significant risks [128, 129]. If left untreated, IVC thrombosis can lead to chronic venous stasis, limb loss or pulmonary embolism (PE) [128, 130]. The long-term morbidity in patients with inferior vena cava thrombosis is largely unknown [131].

More recently, with the increasing use of caval interruption devices (IVC filters), the number of cases of caval occlusion appears to be on the rise. Recent studies have demonstrated that up to 30 % of these patients present with significant symptoms including bilateral lower extremity swelling and pain [132, 133]. The presence or absence of an IVC filter is important as it will frequently impact on both the methods as well as the outcomes of treatment.

Two groups have published a case report each on managing IVC thrombosis using the Trellis-8 system. In 2011, Kamel Abdel Aal and colleagues [134] used two simultaneously operated Trellis-8 devices in a "kissing" fashion in a 62-year-old man with a thrombosed IVC secondary to a non-functioning hemodialysis catheter placed in the right femoral vein. The authors were able to successfully debulk the thrombus in the IVC and the patient was free of thromboembolic complications at a 3-month follow-up. The second case published by Saettele et al. [135] reported a 62-year-old woman with extensive venous clot involving the infrarenal segment of a duplicated IVC; she underwent pharmacomechanical thrombolysis using the Trellis-8 device with complete deep venous thrombosis resolution. We have recently published our experience in the subject [136]. Between January 1, 2009, and November 30, 2013, we treated 11 consecutive cases of IVC filter thrombotic acute total occlusion. IVC thrombotic occlusion was diagnosed by CT imaging and/or duplex ultrasonography and confirmed by standard contrast venography. Of those patients, three were minimally symptomatic and underwent medical management with anticoagulation. The remaining eight symptomatic patients (6 men; mean age 57.4 years, range 34–78 years) were managed using the Trellis-8 system. The access site was selected based on anatomical extension of the clot. Ultrasound-guided venous access was employed in all cases. Access was obtained through bilateral popliteal or common femoral veins. Then, 11-cm long, 8-F sheaths were placed. Two 0.035-in. glidewires (Terumo Medical Corporation, Somerset, NJ) were then

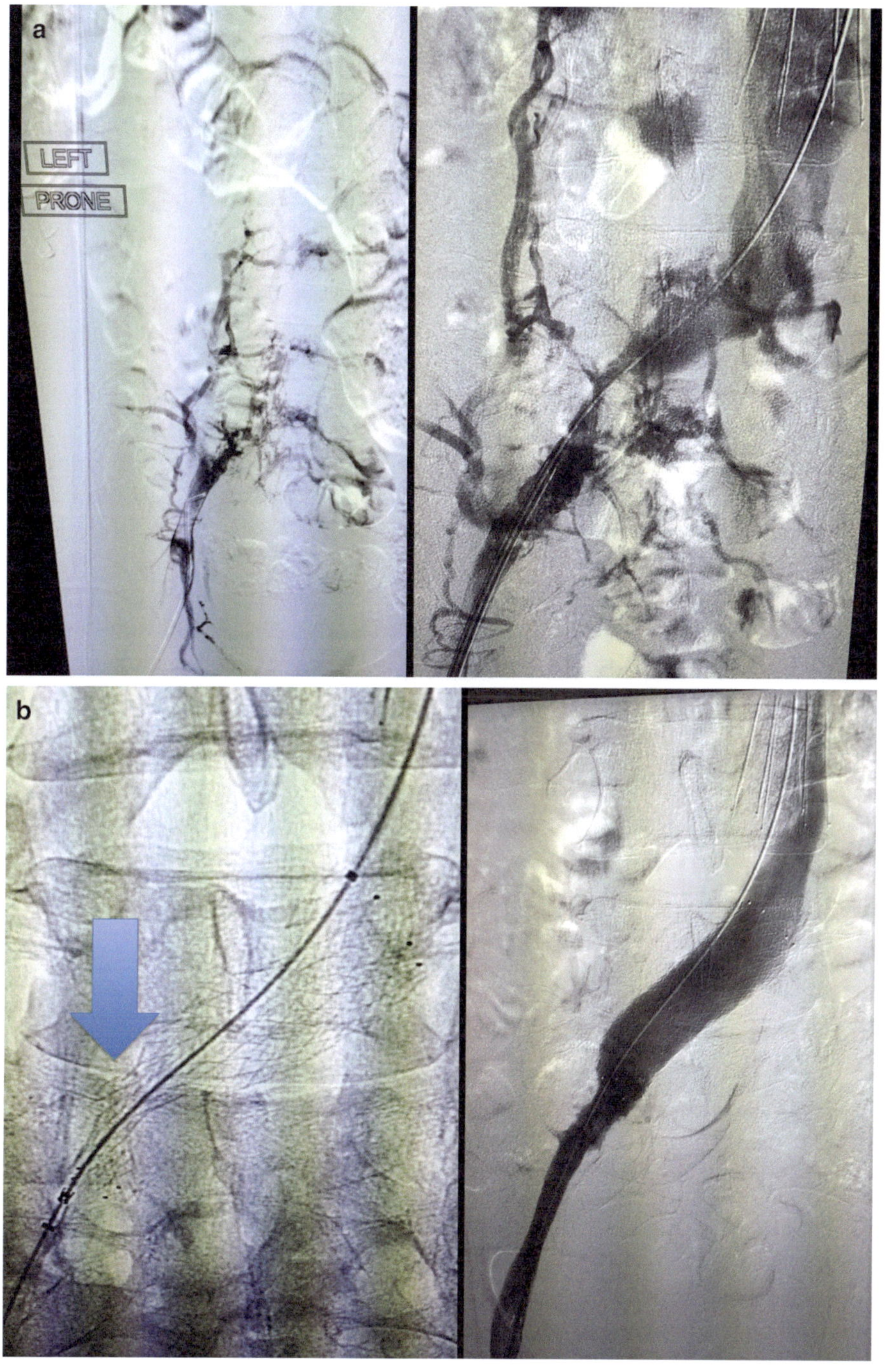

Fig. 28.7 (**a**, **b**) These are venographic images of a 53-year-old Hispanic male with a diagnosis of colon carcinoma and who presented with a 48 h history of massive left lower extremity swelling. (**a**) *Left panel* shows a complete thrombotic occlusion of the left iliofemoral venous segment. Decision was made to use the EkoSonic® System (EKOS Corp, Bothell, WA) after inferior vena cava filter placement (Option™ Elite, Argon, Medical Devices, Plano, TX). After 24 h of thrombolysis (**a**, *right panel*), significant clearance of thrombotic material was seen but a clear area of extrinsic compression over the left common iliac vein, consistent with May–Thurner syndrome. This was also evident by the use of intravascular ultrasound. (**b**) Shows stent deformity immediately after placement (*left panel*), corrected by balloon angioplasty. Completion venography is shown in the *right panel*

used to traverse the thrombosed venous segments, advancing the wires past the point of occlusion in the IVC. Two Trellis-8 systems were then advanced into the occluded IVC, positioning the distal occlusive balloons past the IVC filter in a kissing balloon manner. The two Trellis-8 systems were then operated simultaneously. In this limited performance and safety evaluation, the Trellis-8 thrombectomy system combined with adjunctive therapies, such as mechanical thrombectomy and balloon angioplasty, was effective in 75 % of patients with IVC filter-related acute caval occlusion. There were two (25 %) unsuccessful attempts to use the Trellis-8 system, both due to inability to cross the occlusion with guidewires. These patients were managed with anticoagulation. No thromboembolic complications developed during the follow-up period.

Chronic Deep Venous Thrombosis and Post-thrombotic Syndrome

Chronic venous insufficiency has devastating sequelae in terms of patients' lifestyles and negative economic impact on society. Traditional surgical procedures have yielded variable patency results, and follow-up has not always been reported.

Venous stenting has introduced a minimally invasive and safe technique. The procedure can be performed with low morbidity, low mortality, long-term high patency rate, and low rate of in-stent restenosis. It has replaced bypass surgery as the primary treatment. It is applicable in a wide spectrum of patients with chronic venous disease with disabling symptoms. Long-term patency and clinical outcome are excellent even when associated reflux is present and left untreated. The need for open surgery to correct reflux or obstruction has been drastically reduced. In 2007, the American Venous Forum stated that, "iliocaval venoplasty and stenting has emerged as the "method of choice" in relieving proximal iliofemoral obstruction." Although the data available indicate that stenting for chronic obstructive iliofemoral lesions comes with a very low risk, there are still no randomized or multicenter trials on venous stenting. The literature to date consists mainly of retrospective single center trials. However, such procedures can still be carried out later in the event of stent occlusion or failure to relieve symptoms.

The Zilver vena stent is the only stent currently indicated and designed specifically for treating symptomatic iliofemoral venous outflow obstruction [137]. O'Sullivan et al. studied 20 patients in which Zilver stents were used to treat chronic venous occlusive disorders. There were 12 women, and the mean age of all patients was 59 years ± 17 years. There were 10 patients with active malignancy. This center is a large referral center for oncology patients; this number of cancer patients is atypical of many previous reports on iliofemoral stenting, where these types of patients are often excluded from treatment. They also included patients who had previously failed conservative therapy and patients with iliofemoral vein obstruction from any other cause (May–Thurner, acute thrombosis, malignant mass, etc.). They excluded patients with IVC occlusion, active infection or life expectancy of less than 6 months. Almost all patients suffered from leg discomfort and edema whereas only one of them reported venous claudication. All patients had symptoms on one side; most patients (85 %) had symptoms on their left side. The lesions were isolated to the iliac veins in 35 % of patients. These lesions included the iliac and femoral veins in 65 % of patients, and were occlusive in half of these patients. The thrombus was managed via pharmacomechanical thrombectomy, pharmacological thrombolysis, or mechanical thrombectomy. Four of the 20 patients required IVC filter placement. All vessels were reopened at procedure end. In one patient, wire access was inadvertently lost in an attempt to post-dilate a Zilver Vena stent which had been successfully placed in a very tight lesion (associated with a malignant tumor whose size was not fully appreciated on pre-procedure imaging). Ultimately, a Wallstent was placed inside the Zilver Vena. The stents extended into IVC in 45 % of patients and extended under the inguinal ligament in 65 % of them. Post-stent placement observations: stents were nonuniformly expanded in 10 % of patients, both associated with an iliopsoas mass. There was immediate in-stent thrombus in 5 % of patients, successfully treated with thrombolysis. On follow-up imaging, early (less than 30 days) thrombosis was seen in 15 % of patients. The clinical patency rate was 85 %. (Note: stent patency was assumed unless clinical symptoms and/or imagine results suggested otherwise.) In this study, the Zilver Vena was associated with very few procedural complications and favorable outcomes. This was however a very small retrospective evaluation, without standard imaging follow-up and a short-term follow-up. Additional studies are needed to establish device performance.

The Veniti VIRTUS study is a randomized multicenter trial designed to assess the safety and efficacy of the VENITI™ VICI™ Venous Stent System (VENITI, Inc., St. Louis, MO) when used to treat clinically significant chronic nonmalignant obstruction of the Iliofemoral venous segment. This study is unique in that it is prospective, has three core labs, and will have the safety data adjudicated by a DSMB and CEC. The study will recruit up to 200 patients at up to 30 global centers. Primary patency at the 12-month follow-up is the efficacy endpoint. The primary safety endpoint for this study will be a composite endpoint of any major adverse event within 30 days. The trial will look at several QoL scales such as CIVQ2 and VCSS as secondary endpoints and will include a specific algorithm for antiplatelet/anti-coagulation post stenting. Patients will be followed for up to 5 years.

In contrast with the relatively solid data on stenting iliofemoral venous segments for chronic DVT patients, to date there has only been a limited report of stenting the femoralpopliteal veins. In the Deep Venous Registry, the authors reported that five patients had a bare metal stent placed in the femoral-popliteal segment. Four of these five stents thrombosed within a mean of 42 days (range 17–70 days). Some have suggested that the thrombosis rate would likely decrease significantly with the use of a stent with an anticoagulant bioactive surface, and suggested the use of Gore® Viabahn® Endoprosthesis (Gore Medical, Newark, DE) with a heparin bioactive surface to treat venous occlusions. A physician-sponsored IDE study was designed to determine the safety and feasibility of using the Viabahn endoprosthesis with a heparin bioactive surface to treat venous occlusions and stenosis in locations that have demonstrated poor patency rates with bare metal stents. These locations include the popliteal vein, femoral vein, brachial vein, axillary vein, subclavian vein, and jugular vein. The primary endpoints included decrease in pain (visual analog scale) and swelling of affected extremity. The study however, was closed due to limited enrollment. There were a few factors that contributed to limited enrollment. The first is that many patients present also with iliofemoral disease. Once this was treated, the patients were relatively asymptomatic and thus ethically, patients were not enrolled then to treat the more peripheral disease. Second, there were some patients that would have required stenting over either the deep femoral vein orifice and thus, it was not felt appropriate to block the origin of that vessel. The use of covered stents in the venous system is not supported by the available scientific literature at this time.

More recently, the use of ultrasound accelerated thrombolysis in patients with chronic proximal venous obstruction after DVT and PTS has been suggested. In the case of chronic venous obstruction, it is hypothesized that the effects of ultrasound allow the infused thrombolytic agent to act on any fibrin remaining in retracted, chronic thrombus. The ACCESS DVT is an ongoing prospective, single arm, multicenter study, intended to describe relevant clinical and imaging outcomes of patients with chronic proximal venous obstruction after DVT and the PTS who are treated with thrombolytic infusion using the EkoSonic System. Up to 200 symptomatic DVT patients that are objectively diagnosed by duplex imaging at least 6 months previously will be enrolled at up to 30 sites. After successful and complete passage of the guide wire through the occlusion, an appropriate sized angioplasty balloon shall be placed and then dilated across the entire occlusive segment to promote enlargement of the channel to allow passage of the EkoSonic device. Ultrasound accelerated EKOS thrombolysis will be initiated. Follow-up venographic evaluation shall be performed of the entire affected limb once the EKOS thrombolysis procedure is completed. At the discretion of the investigator, adjunctive treatments such as angioplasty or stenting can be performed as necessary to enhance venous flow after EKOS treatment. Venography images are sent to a core lab for analysis. Post-procedure (baseline) Duplex imaging of the treated venous segments shall be performed within 24 h of completing the interventional procedure (thrombolysis and any adjunctive therapy). Follow-up evaluation shall occur at 1, 3, 6 and 12 months using Duplex imaging as well as clinical evaluation including the Villalta scale, the SF-36 generic quality of life measure and the Clinical Etiologic Anatomic and Pathophysiologic (CEAP) and Venous Clinical Severity Score (VCSS) scales. It is anticipated that the clinical study duration will be 44 months.

Inferior Vena Cava Filters

Inferior vena cava filters (IVCFs) were originally developed for caval interruption in patients afflicted by venous thromboembolism (VTE) who had a contraindication to anticoagulation or in whom failure of anticoagulation was demonstrated. Since the inception of retrievable IVCFs, there appears to be an increase in their use, with the presumption that the filter will be removed, thus theoretically resulting in fewer long-term complications in comparison to permanent IVCFs [138]. Disappointingly, the literature demonstrates that the majority of retrievable IVCFs are not removed [139, 140] For instance, a study of trauma patients showed that over 75 % of retrievable IVCFs are not removed, mainly because several patients are lost to follow-up [140].

Consequently, both early and delayed complications associated with IVCFs still persist with retrievable devices and range from local complications related to insertion site to IVC thrombosis and perforation [141–146].

The insertion of IVC filters have increased over the last several years, with the rate of prophylactic IVC filter placement increasing at a significantly higher rate than filter placement for associated DVT or PE [147]. Corriere et al. have described four cases of vena cava thrombosis following IVC filter placement in 189 patients. The incidence of filter thrombosis differed according to the specific filter device they deployed. In their series, all observed vena cava thromboses were associated with patients who received opposed biconical filter designs [148]. The Trapease device was the most commonly thrombosed filter (60 %) seen in our review. The rate of IVC thrombosis from these biconical designed devices range from 6 to 28 % [133, 149–151]. With a wide variety of filter types currently available, no one specific type seemed to impose a greater risk although large case reports implicate certain types [149–151]. Early filter retrieval when feasible should be practiced to avoid the increased incidence of AT-IVC in patients with filters.

Several new designs of retrievable filters have been produced. For instance, two of the most recent developed designs are the Option Elite® (Argon, Medical Devices, Plano, TX) and the Crux® (Volcano Corp, San Diego, CA) filters. The Option Elite filter is made of a single piece of nitinol construction and has an open lumen, enabling its delivery over a guidewire. Its apex is designed for easy snare capture at retrieval and the filter is electro-polished for increased fracture resistance. It has curved anchors for cephalad migration prevention, anchor grips for caudal migration prevention and anchor extensions for perforation prevention. The delivery sheath is 70-cm long and has a 6.5 Fr outer diameter, one of the smallest profiles currently available. The filter comes in a dual delivery system for a femoral or jugular delivery from a single kit. The sheath dilator has a 32 mm spaced radiopaque markers for accurate cava diameter measurement. It has dilator side holes arranged in a helix formation compatible with power injectors up to 800 psi. The delivery system has a curved pusher to aid centering and resist tilt during delivery. In addition, its filter base is designed to conform to the caval anatomy aiding in centering filter and reducing caval penetration [152] in vena cavas up to 30 mm.

The Crux® Vena Cava Filter is another novel clot trapping design, with a helical nitinol wire form, tissue anchors and an e PTFE filter web. The nitinol wire form is designed to distribute the radial force equally along the vessel lumen and along with multiplanar tissue anchors, which were designed to prevent tilting. The Crux filter provides trans-luminal filtering via a thin, e PTFE web. A tilted vena cava filter is not ideal because it disrupts the flow through and around the filter [153]. In the RETRIEVE 2, 3, and 4 trials [154], the Crux filter caval occlusion was 0 % post-implant, measured up to 6 months post-implant. In the same RETRIEVE 2, 3, and 4 trials, the Crux filter had a low incidence of PE post-implant (2.4 %), also measured up to 6 months post-implant. With zero incidence of filter tilt post-implant during the RETRIEVE 2, 3, and 4 trials. These results were however, based on a nonrandomized single-arm design, with a short follow-up period of only 6 months, and the potential for biases associated with the manufacturer funding of the regulatory device trial.

Several investigational IVC filter prototypes are being evaluated for safety, feasibility and long-term retrievability. For instance, resorbable inferior vena cava (IVC) filters are currently being studied. Thors and Muck [155] reported results with ten of these designs in a porcine model (Yorkshire-type pigs). These were dual-filtration cones made of was polyglycolic acid polymer strands oriented in a staggered cone formation with the apex of the cone in a cephalad orientation in relation to the IVC. IVC fixation was accomplished using a nitinol Z-stent, which was not resorbable. The IVC filters were operatively removed en bloc 6 weeks after implantation, and the pigs were euthanized. The IVC specimens were subsequently analyzed grossly and using light microscopy. In nine of the ten retrieved devices, the filtration cones were completely dissolved. One device had a retained strand of filtration cone material completely incorporated into the caval wall, excluded from luminal flow. Significant inflammatory response was appreciated from the specimen histology, and significant collagen deposition was observed, especially on trichrome staining. The intima and media of nine of ten specimens were two to three times normal thickness. Significant reactive change was also appreciated in the pericaval lymph nodes that were taken in the specimen.

Pulmonary Embolism

Acute massive pulmonary embolism (PE) is a life-threatening episode. Before the time of cardiopulmonary bypass (CPB), pulmonary embolectomy was indicated in patients with severe hemodynamic compromise, as a last treatment option in already dying patients. Currently, the role of pulmonary embolectomy is not clearly defined. Even though this is true, with current technology this procedure can be still life saving in selected situations. Recently published guidelines suggest thrombolysis as the treatment of choice for PE in high-risk patients (acute massive PE who present or developed hemodynamic shock). If contraindications do exist, pulmonary embolectomy is indicated [156]. Previously reported series described survival rates of 50–70.4 % [157, 158]. More recently published data revealed survival rates at 1- and 3-year follow-up of 86 % and 83 %, respectively, probably improved by inclusion of intermediate risk patients (more stable patients but with echocardiographic evidence of right ventricular strain preoperatively) [159]. The surgical approach is rendered easier in the last few years, due to the availability and routine use of CPB, but still carries significant perioperative morbidity and mortality.

The role of surgery should be discussed and probably redefined, as it is actually limited as a secondary treatment alternative to thrombolysis in PE related high-risk mortality group (acute massive PE). Comparative studies of an operative approach versus thrombolysis and their impact of post procedural cardiac function have not been undertaken. Ideally, these treatments should be compared in randomized studies in high volume centers with availability of both approaches, in a short lapse of time in order to create final treatment algorithms. However, such comparison has not been performed and logistically, it would be quite difficult. Following the line of minimally invasive technologies, pulmonary thrombolysis has gained a wide terrain in this arena.

Minimally invasive techniques for the therapy of PE date back to the development of the Greenfield suction catheter in the 1960s [160]. A more recent improvement of the same idea

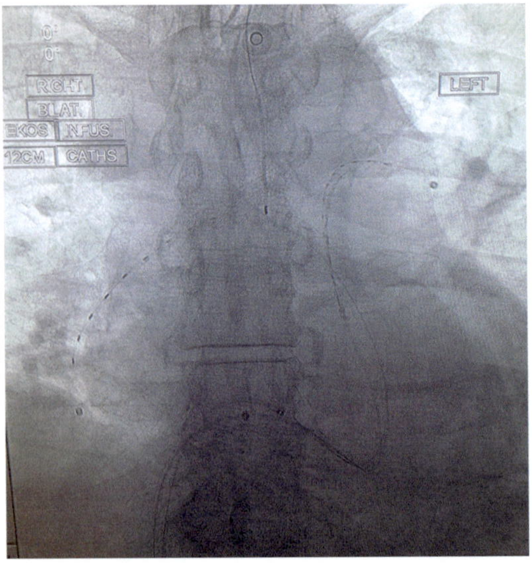

Fig. 28.8 Typical catheter configuration after placement of EKOS devices (EkoSonic® Endovascular, EKOS Corp, Bothell, WA) in the right and left main pulmonary arteries

is the Angiovac catheter (Vortex Medical, Angiodynamics, Latham, NY), which has been approved by the FDA for removal of vascular debris, and consists of a large-caliber catheter with an expandable funnel at its tip that is connected to a circuit resembling a cardiopulmonary bypass system, where a pump generates suction of 3 L/min, filters the blood, and returns it via another catheter. The large caliber size requires either surgical cut-down or a large-bore sheath insertion.

Technical advances in endovascular devices now allow for combining ultrasonic thrombus disruption and thrombolysis. This is called pharmacomechanical ultrasound-accelerated thrombolysis therapy. This technique allows rapid right ventricular after load reduction in patients with massive and sub-massive PE. This is our choice of therapy for patients with massive and sub-massive PE, by the use of the EKOS device (EkoSonic Endovascular). Ultrasound energy has been shown to disrupt the thrombus structure, rendering it more susceptible to thrombolysis with ensuing shorter and lower-dose administration. We use this catheter as standalone strategy of ultrasound-assisted, catheter-directed thrombolysis (Fig. 28.8). This technique can achieve complete thrombus resolution in 76 % of patients and near-complete resolution in an additional 18 % [161].

References

1. Dotter CT, Judkins MP. Transluminal treatment of arteriosclerotic obstruction description of a new technic and a preliminary report of its application. Circulation. 1964;30:654–70.
2. Gruntzig A, Kumpe DA. Technique of percutaneous transluminal angioplasty with the Gruntzig ballon catheter. AJR Am J Roentgenol. 1979;132:547–52.
3. Katzen BT, Chang J. Percutaneous transluminal angioplasty with the Grüntzig balloon catheter. Radiology. 1979;130:623–6.
4. Freiman DB, Ring EJ, Oleaga JA, Berkowitz H. Transluminal angioplasty of the iliac, femoral, and popliteal arteries. Radiology. 1979;132:285–8.
5. Colapinto RF, Harries-Jones EP, Johnston KW. Percutaneous transluminal dilatation and recanalization in the treatment of peripheral vascular disease. Radiology. 1980;135:583–7.
6. Volodos NL, Karpovich IP, Shekhanin VE. A case of distant transfemoral endoprosthesis of the thoracic artery using a self-fixing synthetic prosthesis in traumatic aneurysm. Grudn Khir. 1988;6:84–6.
7. Veith FJ, Marin ML, Cynamon J, Schonholz C, Parodi J. 1992: Parodi, Montefiore, and the first abdominal aortic aneurysm stent graft in the United States. Ann Vasc Surg. 2005;19:749–51.
8. Chuter T, Green RM, Ouriel K, Fiore WM. Transfemoral endovascular aortic graft placement. J Vasc Surg. 1993;18:185–97.
9. Yusuf SW, Baker DM, Chuter TA, Whitaker SC, Wenham PW, Hopkinson BR. Transfemoral endoluminal repair of abdominal aortic aneurysm with bifurcated graft. Lancet. 1994;344:650–1.
10. Yusuf SW, Whitaker SC, Chuter TA, Wenham PW, Hopkinson BR. Emergency endovascular repair of leaking aortic aneurysm. Lancet. 1994;344:1645.
11. Jain KM, Munn J, Rummel M, Vaddineni S, Longton C. Future of vascular surgery is in the office. J Vasc Surg. 2010;51:509–13.
12. Semenciew R, Morrison H, Wigle D, Cole W, Hill G. Recent trends in morbidity and mortality rates for abdominal aortic aneurysms. Rev Can Santé Publique. 1992;83:274–6.
13. Pearce WH, Shively VP. Abdominal aortic aneurysm as a complex multifactorial disease: interactions of polymorphisms of inflammatory genes, features of autoimmunity, and current status of MMPs. Ann N Y Acad Sci. 2006;1085:117–32.
14. Morris DR, Biros E, Cronin O, Kuivaniemi H, Golledge J. The association of genetic variants of matrix metalloproteinases with abdominal aortic

aneurysm: a systematic review and meta-analysis. Heart. 2014;100:295–302.
15. LeFevre ML. U.S. Preventive Services Task Force. Screening for abdominal aortic aneurysm: U.S. Preventive Services Task Force recommendation statement. Ann Intern Med. 2014;161:281–90.
16. The UK Small Aneurysm Trial Participants. Mortality results for randomised controlled trial of early elective surgery or ultrasonographic surveillance for small abdominal aortic aneurysms. Lancet. 1998;352:1649–55.
17. Parodi JC, Palmaz JC, Barone HD. Transfemoral intraluminal graft implantation for abdominal aortic aneurysms. Ann Vasc Surg. 1991;5:491–9.
18. Hinchliffe RJ, Ivancev K, Sonesson B, Malina M. "Paving and Cracking": an endovascular technique to facilitate the introduction of aortic stent-grafts through stenosed iliac arteries. J Endovasc Ther. 2007;14:630–3.
19. Jordan Jr WD, Mehta M, Varnagy D, Moore Jr WM, Arko FR, Joye J, et al. Aneurysm treatment using the Heli-FX aortic securement system global registry (ANCHOR) workgroup members. J Vasc Surg. 2014;60:885–92.
20. Lee JT, Lee GK, Chandra V, Dalman RL. Comparison of fenestrated endografts and the snorkel/chimney technique. J Vasc Surg. 2014;60:849–56.
21. Lee JT, Varu VN, Tran K, Dalman RL. Renal function changes after snorkel/chimney repair of juxtarenal aneurysms. J Vasc Surg. 2014;60:563–70.
22. Kirkwood ML, Saunders A, Jackson BM, Wang GJ, Fairman RM, Woo EY. Aneurysmal iliac arteries do not portend future iliac aneurysmal enlargement after endovascular aneurysm repair for abdominal aortic aneurysm. J Vasc Surg. 2011;53:269–73.
23. Hobo R, Laheij RJ, Buth J. The influence of aortic cuffs and iliac limb extensions on the outcome of endovascular abdominal aortic aneurysm repair. J Vasc Surg. 2007;45:79–85.
24. Rayt HS, Bown MJ, Lambert KV, Fishwick NG, McCarthy MJ, London NJ, et al. Buttock claudication and erectile dysfunction after internal iliac artery embolization in patients prior to endovascular aortic aneurysm repair. Cardiovasc Intervent Radiol. 2008;31:728e34.
25. Conrad MF, Adams AB, Guest JM, Paruchuri V, Brewster DC, LaMuraglia GM, et al. Secondary intervention after endovascular abdominal aortic aneurysm repair. Ann Surg. 2009;250:383–9.
26. Mehta M, Sternbach Y, Taggert JB, Kreienberg PB, Roddy SP, Paty PS, et al. Long-term outcomes of secondary procedures after endovascular aneurysm repair. J Vasc Surg. 2010;52:1442–9.
27. Karthikesalingam A, Hinchliffe RJ, Holt PJ, Boyle JR, Loftus IM, Thompson MM. Endovascular aneurysm repair with preservation of the internal iliac artery using the iliac branch graft device. Eur J Vasc Endovasc Surg. 2010;39:285–94.
28. Naughton PA, Park MS, Kheirelseid EA, O'Neill SM, Rodriguez HE, Morasch MD, et al. A comparative study of bell-bottom technique versus hypogastric exclusion for the treatment of aneurysmal extension to the iliac bifurcation. J Vasc Surg. 2012; 55:956–62.
29. Traul DK, Clair DG, Gray B, O'Hara PJ, Ouriel K. Percutaneous endovascular repair of infrarenal abdominal aortic aneurysms: a feasibility study. J Vasc Surg. 2000;32:770–6.
30. Malkawi AH, Hinchliffe RJ, Holt PJ, Loftus IM, Thompson MM. Percutaneous access for endovascular aneurysm repair: a systematic review. Eur J Vasc Endovasc Surg. 2010;39:676–82.
31. Nelson PR, Kracjer Z, Kansal N, Rao V, Bianchi C, Hashemi H, et al. A multicenter, randomized, controlled trial of totally percutaneous access versus open femoral exposure for endovascular aortic aneurysm repair (the PEVAR trial). J Vasc Surg. 2014; 59:1181–94.
32. Manunga JM, Gloviczki P, Oderich GS, Kalra M, Duncan AA, Fleming MD, et al. Femoral artery calcification as a determinant of success for percutaneous access for endovascular abdominal aortic aneurysm repair. J Vasc Surg. 2013;58:1208–12.
33. Malina M, Resch T, Sonesson B. EVAR and complex anatomy: an update on fenestrated and branched stent grafts. Scand J Surg. 2008;97:195–204.
34. Antoniou GA, Georgiadis GS, Antoniou SA, Kuhan G, Murray D. A meta-analysis of outcomes of endovascular abdominal aortic aneurysm repair in patients with hostile and friendly neck anatomy. J Vasc Surg. 2013;57:527–38.
35. Armstrong N, Burgers L, Deshpande S, Al M, Riemsma R, Vallabhaneni SR, et al. The use of fenestrated and branched endovascular aneurysm repair for juxtarenal and thoracoabdominal aneurysms: a systematic review and cost-effectiveness analysis. Health Technol Assess. 2014;18(70): 1–66.
36. Rao R, Lane TR, Franklin IJ, Davies AH. Open repair versus fenestrated endovascular aneurysm repair of juxtarenal aneurysms. J Vasc Surg. 2015; 61:242–55.
37. Lelienfeld DE, Gurdenson PD, Sprafka JM, et al. Epidemiology of aortic aneurysms: mortality trends in the United States 1951–1981. Atherosclerosis. 1987;7:637–43.
38. Fowkes FRG, Macintyre CCA, Rucjerley CV. Increasing incidence of aortic aneurysms in England and Wales. Brit Med J. 1989;298:33–5.
39. Quil DS, Colgan MP, Summer DS. Ultrasonic screening for the detection of abdominal aortic aneurysms. Surg Clin North Am. 1989;69:713–20.
40. Bengtsson H, Bergqvist D. Ruptured abdominal aortic aneurysm: a population-based study. J Vasc Surg. 1993;18:74–80.
41. Brown MJ, Sutton AJ, Bell PR, Sayers RD. A meta-analysis of 50 years of ruptured abdominal aortic aneurysm repair. Br J Surg. 2002;89:714–30.
42. Veith FJ, Ohki T, Lipsitz EC, Suggs WD, Cynamon J. Endovascular grafts and other catheter directed

techniques in the management of ruptured abdominal aortic aneurysms. Semin Vasc Surg. 2003;16: 326–31.
43. Veith FJ, Lachat M, Mayer D, Malina M, Holst J, Mehta M, et al. Collected world and single center experience with endovascular treatment of ruptured abdominal aortic aneurysms. Ann Surg. 2009;250: 818–24.
44. Larzon T, Lindgren R, Norgren L. Endovascular treatment of ruptured abdominal aortic aneurysms: a shift of the paradigm? J Endovasc Ther. 2005;12: 548–55.
45. Hinchliffe RJ, Braithwaite BD, Hopkinson BR. The endovascular management of ruptured abdominal aortic aneurysms. Eur J Vasc Endovasc Surg. 2003;25:191–201.
46. Hechelhammer L, Lachat ML, Wildermuth S, Bettex D, Mayer D, Pfammatter T. Midterm outcome of endovascular repair of ruptured abdominal aortic aneurysms. J Vasc Surg. 2005;41:752–7.
47. Davenport DL, O'Keeffe SD, Minion DJ, Sorial EE, Endean ED, Xenos ES. Thirty-day NSQIP database outcomes of open versus endoluminal repair of ruptured abdominal aortic aneurysms. J Vasc Surg. 2010;51(2):305–9.
48. Rial R, Serrano Fj F, Vega M, Rodriguez R, Martin A, Mendez J, et al. Treatment of type II endoleaks after endovascular repair of abdominal aortic aneurysms: translumbar puncture and injection of thrombin into the aneurysm sac. Eur J Vasc Endovasc Surg. 2004;27:333–5.
49. Gambaro E, Abou-Zamzam Jr AM, Teruya TH, Bianchi C, Hopewell J, Ballard JL. Ischemic colitis following translumbar thrombin injection for treatment of endoleak. Ann Vasc Surg. 2004;18:74–8.
50. Evangelista A, Nienaber CA, editors. Pharmacotherapy in aortic disease, current cardiovascular therapy, vol. 7. Springer, Switzerland; 2015. P. 213–38.
51. Authors/Task Force members, Erbel R, Aboyans V, Boileau C, Bossone E, Bartolomeo RD, et al. ESC Guidelines on the diagnosis and treatment of aortic diseases: document covering acute and chronic aortic diseases of the thoracic and abdominal aorta of the adult * The Task Force for the Diagnosis and Treatment of Aortic Diseases of the European Society of Cardiology (ESC). Eur Heart J. 2014; 35:2873–926.
52. Xu SD, Huang FJ, Yang JF, Li ZZ, Wang XY. Endovascular repair of acute type B aortic dissection: early and mid-term results. J Vasc Surg. 2006;43:1090–5.
53. Nienaber CA, Kische S, Akin I, Rousseau H, Eggebrecht H, Fattori R, Rehders TC, Kundt G, Scheinert D, Czerny M, Kleinfeldt T, Zipfel B, Labrousse L, Ince H. Strategies for subacute/chronic type B aortic dissection: the Investigation Of Stent Grafts in Patients with type B Aortic Dissection (INSTEAD) trial 1-year outcome. J Thorac Cardiovasc Surg. 2010;140(6 Suppl):S101–8.
54. Nienaber CA, Kische S, Rousseau H, Eggebrecht H, Rehders TC, Kundt G, Glass A, Scheinert D, Czerny M, Kleinfeldt T, Zipfel B, Labrousse L, Fattori R. Ince H; INSTEAD-XL trial. Endovascular repair of type B aortic dissection: long-term results of the randomized investigation of stent grafts in aortic dissection trial. Circ Cardiovasc Interv. 2013;6:407–16.
55. Hagan PG, Nienaber CA, Isselbacher EM, Bruckman D, Karavite DJ, Russman PL, Evangelista A, Fattori R, Suzuki T, Oh JK, Moore AG, Malouf JF, Pape LA, Gaca C, Sechtem U, Lenferink S, Deutsch HJ, Diedrichs H, Marcos y Robles J, Llovet A, Gilon D, Das SK, Armstrong WF, Deeb GM, Eagle KA. The International Registry of Acute Aortic Dissection (IRAD): new insights into an old disease. JAMA. 2000;283:897–903.
56. Baliga RR, Nienaber C, Isselbacher EM, Eagle KA. Aortic dissection and related syndromes. New York: Springer Science & Business Media; 2007. p. 1.
57. Dake MD. An algorithmic strategy for the evaluation and management of type B dissections. Endovasc Today 2014;13:1–8
58. Kudo T, Mikamo A, Kurazumi H, Suzuki R, Morikage N, Hamano K. Predictors of late aortic events after Stanford type B acute aortic dissection. J Thorac Cardiovasc Surg. 2014;148:98–104.
59. Hackman DG. Medical management of peripheral arterial disease. JAMA. 2006;296:41–2.
60. Hirsch AT, Haskal ZJ, Hertzer NR, Bakal CW, Creager MA, Halperin JL, et al. ACC/AHA 2005 Practice Guidelines for the management of patients with peripheral arterial disease (lower extremity, renal, mesenteric, and abdominal aortic). Circulation. 2006;113:e463–654.
61. Norgren L, Hiatt WR, Dormandy JA, Nehler MR, Harris KA, Fowkes FG. Inter-Society consensus for the management of peripheral arterial disease (TASC II). J Vasc Surg. 2007;45(Suppl S):S5–67.
62. Blair JM, Gewertz BL, Moosa H, Lu CT, Zarins CK. Percutaneous transluminal angioplasty vs. surgery for limb-threatening ischemia. J Vasc Surg. 1989;9:698–703.
63. Kudo T, Chandra F, Kwun WH, Haas B, Ahn S. Changing pattern of surgical revascularization for critical limb ischemia over 12 years: endovascular vs. open bypass surgery. J Vasc Surg. 2006;44:304–13.
64. Jamieson C. The definition of critical ischaemia of a limb. Br J Surg. 1982;69:S2.
65. Igari K, Kudo T, Uchiyama H, Toyofuku T, Inoue Y. Indocyanine green angiography for the diagnosis of peripheral arterial disease with isolated infrapopliteal lesions. Ann Vasc Surg. 2014;28:1479–84.
66. Braun JD, Trinidad-Hernandez M, Perry D, Armstrong DG, Mills JL. Early quantitative evaluation of indocyanine green angiography in patients with critical limb ischemia. J Vasc Surg. 2013;57: 1213–8.
67. Braun JD, Rajguru P, Armstrong DG, Mills JL. Indocyanine green angiographic criteria using

ingress and ingress rate to detect SVS lower extremity threatened limb classification (WIfI) grade 3 ischemia. J Vasc Surg. 2013;60(2):538.
68. Montero-Baker M, Morelli-Alvarez L, Helton K, Au-Yeu KY. The use of micro-oxygen sensors (MOXYs) to determine dynamic relative oxygen indices in the foot of patients with critical limb ischemia (CLI) during an endovascular therapy: the first-in-man "Si Se Puede" study. J Vasc Surg. 2014;60(2):548–9.
69. Kichikawa K, Uchida H, Yoshioka T, Maeda M, Nishimine K, Kubota Y, et al. Iliac artery stenosis and occlusion: preliminary results of treatment with Gianturco expandable metallic stents. Radiology. 1990;177:799–802.
70. Klein WM, Graaf YVD, Seegers J, Spithoven JH, Buskens E, Baal JGV, et al. Dutch iliac stent trial: long-term results in patients randomized for primary or selective stent placement 1. Radiol Radiol Soc N Am. 2006;238:734–44.
71. Rzucidlo EM, Powell RJ, Zwolak RM, Fillinger MF, Walsh DB, Schermerhorn ML, et al. Early results of stent-grafting to treat diffuse aortoiliac occlusive disease. YMVA. 2003;37:1175–80.
72. Sabri SS, Choudhri A, Orgera G, Arslan B, Turba UC, Harthun NL, et al. Outcomes of covered kissing stent placement compared with bare metal stent placement in the treatment of atherosclerotic occlusive disease at the aortic bifurcation. J Vasc Interv Radiol. 2010;21:995–1003.
73. Mwipatayi BP, Thomas S, Wong J, Temple SEL, Vijayan V, Jackson M, et al. A comparison of covered vs bare expandable stents for the treatment of aortoiliac occlusive disease. J Vasc Surg. 2011;54: 1561–70.
74. Jim J, Owens PL, Sanchez LA, Rubin BG. Population-based analysis of inpatient vascular procedures and predicting future workload and implications for training. YMVA. J Vasc Surg. 2012;55:1394–9. Discussion: 1399–400.
75. Rocha-Singh KJ, Jaff MR, Crabtree TR, Bloch DA, Ansel G, On Behalf of VIVA Physicians. Inc Performance goals and endpoint assessments for clinical trials of femoropopliteal bare nitinol stents in patients with symptomatic peripheral arterial disease. Cathet Cardiovasc Intervent. 2007;69:910–9.
76. Conte MS, Geraghty PJ, Bradbury AW, Hevelone ND, Lipsitz SR, Moneta GL, et al. Suggested objective performance goals and clinical trial design for evaluating catheter-based treatment of critical limb ischemia. J Vasc Surg. 2009;50:1462–3.
77. Moses JW, et al. Sirolimus-eluting stents versus standard stents in patients with stenosis in a native coronary artery. N Engl J Med. 2003;349:1315–23.
78. Dake MD, Ansel GM, Jaff MR, Ohki T, Saxon RR, Smouse HB, et al. Paclitaxel-eluting stents show superiority to balloon angioplasty and bare metal stents in femoropopliteal disease: twelve-month Zilver PTX randomized study results. Circ Cardiovasc Interv. 2011;4:495–504.
79. Dake MD, Ansel GM, Jaff MR, Ohki T, Saxon RR, Smouse HB, et al. Sustained safety and effectiveness of paclitaxel-eluting stents for femoropopliteal lesions: 2-year follow-up from the Zilver PTX randomized and single-arm clinical studies. JAC J Am Coll Cardiol. 2013;61:2417–27.
80. Tepe G, Zeller T, Albrecht T, Heller S, Schwarzwälder U, Beregi J-P, et al. Local delivery of paclitaxel to inhibit restenosis during angioplasty of the leg. N Engl J Med. 2008;358:689–99.
81. Ansel G. Drug elution, data, and decisions. In Phillips JA, editor. Entovascular Today; 2014. p. 1–6.
82. Tepe G, Laird J, Schneider P, Brodmann M, Krishnan P, Micari A, et al. Drug-coated balloon versus standard percutaneous transluminal angioplasty for the treatment of superficial femoral and/or popliteal peripheral artery disease: 12-month results from the IN.PACT SFA randomized trial. Circulation. 2015;131:495–502.
83. Iyer SS, Dorros G, Zaitoun R, Lewin RF. Retrograde Recanalization of an occluded posterior tibial artery by using a posterior tibial cutdown: two case reports. Cathet Cardiovasc Diagn. 1990;20:251–3.
84. Ozawa N. A new understanding of chronic total occlusion from a novel PCI technique that involves a retrograde approach to the right coronary artery via a septal branch and passing of the guidewire to a guiding catheter on the other side of the lesion. Catheter Cardiovasc Interv. 2006;68:907–13.
85. Mustapha JA, Saab F, McGoff T, Heaney C, Diaz-Sandoval L, Sevensma M, Karenko B. Tibio-pedal arterial minimally invasive retrograde revascularization in patients with advanced peripheral vascular disease: The TAMI technique, original case series. Catheter Cardiovasc Interv. 2014;83:987–94.
86. El-Sayed HF. Retrograde pedal/tibial artery access for treatment of infragenicular arterial occlusive disease. Methodist Debakey Cardiovasc J. 2013;9:73–8.
87. Montero-Baker M, Schmidt A, Bräunlich S, Ulrich M, Thieme M, Biamino G, et al. Retrograde approach for complex popliteal and tibioperoneal occlusions. J Endovasc Ther. 2008;15:594–604.
88. Hirsch AT, Haskal CJ, Hertzer NR, Bakal CW, et al. ACC/AHA Guidelines for the Management of Patients with Peripheral Arterial Disease (lower extremity, renal, mesenteric, and abdominal aortic): a collaborative report from the American Associations for Vascular Surgery/Society for Vascular Surgery, Society for Cardiovascular Angiography and Interventions, Society for Vascular Medicine and Biology, Society of Interventional Radiology, and the ACC/AHA Task Force on Practice Guidelines (writing committee to develop guidelines for the management of patients with peripheral arterial disease)—summary of recommendation. J Vasc Interv Radiol. 2006;17:1383–97.
89. Sinkowich SJ, Gottlieb I. Thromboangiitis obliterans—the conservative treatment by Bier's hyperemia suction apparatus. JAMA. 1917;68:961–3.

90. Herrmann LG, Reid MR. The conservative treatment of arteriosclerotic peripheral vascular diseases. Ann Surg. 1934;100:750–60.
91. Mehlsen J, Himmelstrup H, Himmelstrup B, Winther K, Trap-Jensen J. Beneficial effects of intermittent suction and pressure treatment in intermittent claudication. Angiology. 1993;44:16–20.
92. Delis KT, Nicolaides AN, Wolfe JHN, Stansby G. Improved walking ability and ankle brachial pressure indices in symptomatic peripheral vascular disease with intermittent pneumatic compression: a prospective controlled study with one-year follow-up. J Vasc Surg. 2000;31:650–61.
93. Kakkos S, Geroulakos G, Nicolaides A. Improvement in the walking ability in intermittent claudication with supervised exercise and pneumatic foot and calf compression : results at 6 months of a randomized controlled trial. Presented at the 18th Annual meeting of the European Society of Vascular Surgery, Innisbruck, Austria; 2004.
94. Delis KT, Nicolaides AN. Effect of intermittent pneumatic compression in patients with arterial claudication: a prospective randomized controlled study with 1-year follow up. Ann Surg. 2005;241:431–41.
95. Provost P, Lam JY, Lacoste L, Merhi Y, Waters D. Endothelium-derived nitric oxide attenuates neutrophil adhesion to endothelium under arterial flow conditions. Arterioscler Thromb. 1994;14:331–5.
96. Konstantinos D, Nicolaides AN. Effect of intermittent pneumatic compression of foot and calf on walking distance, hemodynamics, and quality od life in patients with arterial claudication. Ann Surg. 2005;241:39.
97. Ramaswami G, D'Ayala M, Hollier LH, Deutsch R, McElhinney AJ. Rapid foot and calf compression increases walking distance in patients with intermittent claudication: Results of a randomized study. J Vasc Surg. 2005;41(5):794–800.
98. Labropoulos N, Leon RL, Bhatti A, Melton S, Kang SS, Mansour AM, Borge M. Hemodynamics effects of intermittent pneumatic compression in patients with critical limb ischemia. J Vasc Surg. 2005; 42:710–6.
99. Andreozzi GM, Cordova RM, Scomparin A, Martini R, D'Eri A, Andreozzi F. Quality of life working group on vascular medicine of SIAPAV. Quality of life in chronic venous insufficiency. an Italian pilot study of the Triveneto Region. Int Angiol. 2005;24:272–7.
100. Callam MJ. Epidemiology of varicose veins. Br J Surg. 1994;81:167–73.
101. Almgren B, Eriksson E. Valvular incompetence in superficial, deep and perforator veins of limbs with varicose veins. Acta Chir Scand. 1990;156:69–74.
102. Van den Bos R, Arends L, Kockaert M, Neumann M, Nijsten T. Endovenous therapy of lower extremity varicosities: a meta-analysis. J Vasc Surg. 2009;49: 230–9.
103. O'Hare JL, Vandenbroeck CP, Whitman B, Campbell B, Heather BP, Earnshaw JJ. Joint Vascular Research Group: a prospective evaluation of the outcome after small saphenous varicose vein surgery with one-year follow-up. J Vasc Surg. 2008;48:669–73.
104. Allegra C, Antignani PL, Carlizza A. Recurrent varicose veins following surgical treatment: our experience with five years follow-up. Eur J Vasc Endovasc Surg. 2007;33:751–6.
105. Shepherd AC, Gohel MS, Brown LC, Metcalfe MJ, Hamish M, Davies AH. Randomized clinic trial of VNUS ClosureFAST radiofrequency ablation versus laser for varicose veins. Br J Surg. 2010;97:810–8.
106. Proebstle TM, Gul D, Kargl A, Knop J. Endovenous laser treatment of the lesser saphenous vein with a 940-nm diode laser: early results. Dermatol Surg. 2003;29:357–61.
107. Creton D, Pichot O, Sessa C, Proebstle TM. Radiofrequency-powered segmental thermal obliteration carried out with the ClosureFast procedure: results at 1 year. Ann Vasc Surg. 2010;24:360–6.
108. Boersma D, Van Eekeren RRJP, Werson DAB, De Vries JPPM, Reijnen MMJP. Mechanochemical endovenous ablation of small saphenous vein insufficiency using the ClariVein® device: one-year results of a prospective series. Eur J Vasc Endovasc Surg. 2013;45:299–303.
109. Van Eekeren RRJP, Boersma D, Elias S, Holewijn S, Werson DAB, De Vries JPPM, Reijnen MMJP. Mechanochemical endovenous ablation of great saphenous vein incompetence using the ClariVein® device: a safety study. J Endovasc Ther. 2011;18:328–34.
110. Bishawi M, Bernstein R, Boter M, Draugh D, Gould C, Hamilton C, Koziarski J. Mechanochemical ablation in patients with chronic venous disease: a prospective multicenter report. Phlebology. 2013;29: 397–400.
111. Almeida JI, Javier JJ, Mackay EG, Bautista C, Cher DJ, Proebstle TM. Two-year follow-up of first human use of cyanoacrylate adhesive for treatment of saphenous vein incompetence. Phlebology. 2014 Apr 30 [Epub ahead of print].
112. Goldhaber S, Morrison R. Pulmonary embolism and deep vein thrombosis. Circulation. 2002;106:1436.
113. Ashrani AA, Heit JA. Incidence and cost burden of post-thrombotic syndrome. J Thromb Thrombolysis. 2009;28:465–76.
114. Brandjes DP, Büller HR, Heijboer H, Huisman MV, de Rijk M, Jagt H. Randomized trial of effect of compression stocking in patients with symptomatic proximal vein thrombosis. Lancet. 1996;349: 759–62.
115. Prandoni P, Lensing AWA, Cogo A, Cuppini S, Villalta S, Carta M, et al. The long-term clinical course of acute deep venous thrombosis. Ann Intern Med. 1996;125:1–7.
116. Kahn SR, Solymoss S, Lamping DL, Abenhaim L. Long-term outcomes after deep vein thrombosis: postphlebetic syndrome and quality of life. J Gen Intern Med. 2000;15:425–9.
117. Grilli CJ, McGarry M, Ali M, et al. Aggressive management of chronic DVT: technical and clinical

outcomes. Presented at: SIR 37th Annual Scientific Meeting; March 24–29, 2012; San Francisco, CA.
118. Delis KT, Bountouroglou D, Mansfield AO. Venous claudication in iliofemoral thrombosis: long-term effects on venous hemodynamics, clinical status, and quality of life. Ann Surg. 2004;239:118–26.
119. Akesson H, Brudin L, Dahlstrom JA, Eklof B, Ohlin P, Plate G. Venous function assessed during a 5 year period after acute ilio-femoral venous thrombosis treated with anticoagulation. Eur J Vasc Surg. 1990;4:43–8.
120. Comerota AJ, Gravett MH. Iliofemoral venous thrombosis. J Vasc Surg. 2007;46:1065–76.
121. Meissner MH, Manzo RA, Bergelin RO, Markel A, Strandness Jr DE. Deep venous insufficiency: the relationship between lysis and subsequent reflux. J Vasc Surg. 1993;18:596–605.
122. Comerota AJ. The ATTRACT trial: rationale for early intervention for iliofemoral DVT. Perspect Vasc Surg Endovasc Ther. 2009;21:221–4.
123. Kudo S. Thrombolysis with ultrasound effect. Tokyo Jikeikai Med J. 1989;104:1005.
124. Blinc A, Francis CW, Trudnowski JL, Carstensen EL. Characterization of ultrasound-potentiated fibrinolysis in vitro. Blood. 1993;81:2636–43.
125. Braaten JV, Goss RA, Francis CW. Ultrasound reversibly disaggregates fibrin fibers. Thromb Haemost. 1997;78:1063–8.
126. Tachibana K, Tachibana S. Ultrasound energy for enhancement of fibrinolysis and drug delivery: special emphasis on the use of a transducer-tipped ultrasound system. In: Siegel RJ, editor. Ultrasound angioplasty. Boston: Kluwer; 1996. p. 121–33.
127. Atar S, Luo H, Nagai T, Sahm R, Fishbein M, Siegel R. Arterial thrombus dissolution in vivo using a transducer-tipped, high frequency ultrasound catheter and local low dose urokinase delivery. J Endovasc Ther. 2001;8:282–90.
128. Tarry WC, Makhoul RG, Tisnado J, Posner MP, Sobel M, Lee HM. Catheter-directed thrombolysis following vena cava filtration for severe deep venous thrombosis. Ann Vasc Surg. 1994;8:583–90.
129. Comerota AJ, Katz ML, White JV. Thrombolytic therapy for acute deep venous thrombosis: how much is enough? Cardiovasc Surg. 1996;4:101–4.
130. Radomski JS, Jarrell BE, Carabasi RA, Yang SL, Koolpe H. Risk of pulmonary embolus with inferior vena cava thrombosis. Am Surg. 1987;53:97–101.
131. Fink AM, Herzog N, Borst-Krafek B, Jurecka W, Steiner A. Long-term mortality in patients with thrombosis of the inferior vena cava, iliac and femoral veins. Eur J Vasc Endovasc Surg. 2006;31:200–3.
132. Usoh F, Hingorani A, Ascher E, Shiferson A, Patel N, Gopal K, et al. Prospective randomized study comparing the clinical outcomes between inferior vena cava Greenfield and TrapEase filters. J Vasc Surg. 2010;52:394–9.
133. Ray Jr CE, Kaufman JA. Complications of inferior vena cava filters. Abdom Imaging. 1996;21:368–74.
134. Kamel Abdel Aal AM, Hamed MF, Saddekni S, Osman S, Zarzour J. Treatment of acute inferior vena cava and iliac vein thrombosis with pharmacomechanical thrombectomy using simultaneously operating "kissing" Trellis-8 thrombolysis catheters. J Endovasc Ther. 2011;18:739–43.
135. Saettele MR, Morelli JN, Chesis P, Wible BC. Use of a Trellis device for endovascular treatment of venous thrombosis involving a duplicated inferior vena cava. Cardiovasc Intervent Radiol. 2013;36:1699–703.
136. Branco BC, Montero-Baker M, Espinoza E, Gamero M, Zea R, Labropoulos N, León LR. Pharmacomechanical thrombolysis in the management of acute inferior vena cava filter occlusion using the Trellis-8 device. J Endovas Ther. 2015;22(1):99–104.
137. O'Sullivan GJ, Sheehan J, Lohan D, McCann-Brown JA. Iliofemoral venous stenting extending into the femoral region: initial clinical experience with the purpose-designed Zilver Vena stent. J Cardiovasc Surg. 2013;54:255–61.
138. Rutherford RB. Prophylactic indications for vena cava filters: critical appraisal. Semin Vasc Surg. 2005;18:158–65.
139. Tschoe M, Kim HS, Brotman DJ, Streiff MB. Retrievable vena cava filters: a clinical review. J Hosp Med. 2009;4:441–8.
140. Grande WJ, Trerotola SO, Reilly PM, Grande WJ, Trerotola SO, Reilly PM, Clark TW, Soulen MC, Patel A, et al. Experience with the recovery filter as a retrievable inferior vena cava filter. J Vasc Interv Radiol. 2005;16:1189–93.
141. Looby S, Given MF, Geoghegan T, McErlean A, Lee MJ. Gunther Tulip retrievable inferior vena caval filters: indications, efficacy, retrieval, and complications. Cardiovasc Intervent Radiol. 2007;30:59–65.
142. Dentali F, Ageno W, Imberti D. Retrievable vena cava filters: clinical experience. Curr Opin Pulm Med. 2006;12:304–9.
143. Joels CS, Sing RF, Heniford BT. Complications of inferior vena cava filters. Am Surg. 2003;69:654.
144. Becker DM, Philbrick JT, Selby JB. Inferior vena cava filters. Indications, safety, effectiveness. Arch Intern Med. 1992;152:1985.
145. Doody O, Given MF, Kavnoudias H, Street M, Thomson KR, Lyon SM. Initial experience in 115 patients with the retrievable Cook Celect vena cava filter. J Med Imaging Radiat Oncol. 2009;53:64–8.
146. Durack JC, Westphalen AC, Kekulawela S, Bhanu SB, Avrin DE, Gordon RL, et al. Perforation of the IVC: Rule rather than exception after longer indwelling times for the Gunther Tulip and Celect retrievable filters. Cardiovasc Intervent Radiol. 2012;35(2):299–308.
147. Moore PS, Andrews JS, Craven TE, Davis RP, Corriere MA, Godshall CJ, et al. Trends in vena caval interruption. J Vasc Surg. 2010;52:118–25.
148. Corriere MA, Sauve KJ, Ayerdi J, Craven BL, Stafford JM, Geary RL, et al. Vena cava filters and inferior vena cava thrombosis. J Vasc Surg. 2007;45:789–94.

149. Kalva SP, Wicky S, Waltman AC, Athanasoulis CA. TrapEase vena cava filter: experience in 751 patients. J Endovasc Ther. 2006;13:365–72.
150. Nazzal M, Chan E, Nazzal M, Abbas J, Erikson G, Sediqe S, et al. Complications related to inferior vena cava filters: a single-center experience. Ann Vasc Surg. 2010;24:480–6.
151. Kim HS, Young MJ, Narayan AK, Hong K, Liddell RP, Streiff MB. A comparison of clinical outcomes with retrievable and permanent inferior vena cava filters. J Vasc Interv Radiol. 2008;19:393–9.
152. Johnson MS, Benenati JF, Kaufman JA, et al. The safety and effectiveness of the retrievable OptionTM vena cava filter: a United States, Prospective Multicenter Clinical Study. J Vasc Intervent Radiol. 2010;21:1173–84.
153. Singer M, Wang S. Modeling flow past a tilted vena cava filter. J Med Dev 2009. https://e-reports-ext.llnl.gov/pdf/375100.pdf.
154. Smouse HB, Mendes R, Bosiers M, Van Ha TG, Crabtree T. The RETRIEVE Trial: safety and effectiveness of the retrievable Crux Vena Cava Filter. J Vasc Interv Radiol. 2013;24:609–62.
155. Thors A, Muck P. Resorbable inferior vena cava filters: trial in an in-vivo porcine model. J Vasc Interv Radiol. 2011;22:330–5.
156. Torbicki A, Perrier A, Konstantinides S, Agnelli G, Galiè N, Pruszczyk P, et al. The Task Force for the Diagnosis and Management of Acute Pulmonary Embolism of the European Society of Cardiology (ESC). Guidelines on the diagnosis and management of acute pulmonary embolism. Eur Heart J. 2008; 29:2276–315.
157. Gray HH, Morgan JM, Paneth M, Miller GA. Pulmonary embolectomy for acute massive pulmonary embolism: an analysis of 71 cases. Br Heart J. 1988;60:196–200.
158. Mattox KL, Feldtman RW, Beall AC, DeBakey ME. Pulmonary embolectomy for acute massive pulmonary embolism. Ann Surg. 1982;195:726–31.
159. Leacche M, Unic D, Goldhaber SZ, et al. Modern surgical treatment of massive pulmonary embolism: results in 47 consecutive patients after rapid diagnosis and aggressive surgical approach. J Thorac Cardiovasc Surg. 2006;131:503–4.
160. Greenfield LJ, Kimmell GO, McCurdy 3rd WC. Transvenous removal of pulmonary emboli by vacuum-cup catheter technique. J Surg Res. 1969; 9:347–52.
161. Chamsuddin A, Nazzal L, Kang B, Best I, Peters G, Panah S, Martin L, Lewis C, Zeinati C, Ho JW, Venbrux AC. Catheter-directed thrombolysis with the Endowave system in the treatment of acute massive pulmonary embolism: a retrospective multicenter case series. J Vasc Interv Radiol. 2008;19: 372–6.

Carotid Disease: The Stents and the Evidence-Based Medicine: What Happened to the Old Surgery?

29

David W. Birchley, Catherine E. Western, and Alison Guy

Introduction

Carotid arterial stenotic disease is a manifestation of peripheral arterial occlusive disease and is of relevance when it affects the internal carotid artery. The fundamental pathophysiology is deposition of lipid-rich material within the arterial wall, complicated by a local inflammatory response. In addition to flow-related phenomena, the disease carries the risk of plaque rupture with activation of platelets and the formation of adherent platelet thrombi which may embolize. The disease may be asymptomatic and detected incidentally (e.g. on general screening for vascular disease or specifically prior to cardiac surgery) or symptomatic. Untreated the disease carries risks related to thrombosis and embolism.

The symptomatic patient will manifest symptoms and signs of end-organ ischaemia—retinal ischaemia with the classical "shutter coming down" of amaurosis fugax or true cortical infarction with symptoms and signs relating to the laterality and precise anatomical territory affected. Cortical symptoms may be in the form of a Transient Ischaemic Attack (TIA—cortical symptoms resolving completely within 24 h) or an established stroke (persistent deficit beyond 24 h).

It is established that the risk of thromboembolic complications relates to the degree of stenosis with two standards being used: the European and North American standards. Due to differences in the measurements made, the cut-off for "Significance" in terms of stenosis is 70 % for the former and 50 % for the latter.

Furthermore, carotid disease exists as a dynamic spectrum. Asymptomatic disease becomes symptomatic when a thromboembolic complication occurs. There is then a period of greatest risk of further thromboembolic events, which lasts for approximately 4–6 weeks. After this period, it may be argued that the "Symptomatic" stenosis had become "Asymptomatic" if no further ischaemic events have occurred.

Carotid arterial stenotic disease may be treated (in addition to Best Medical Therapy - see below) with either open carotid endarterectomy or endovascular stenting. The former involves exposure and control of the common, internal and external carotid arteries with clamping and formal surgical endarterectomy using either a longitudinal arteriotomy or an eversion technique. Closure is either primary suture or patching if eversion is not used.

Endovascular stenting invariably involves the use of a cerebral protection device to prevent intraprocedural embolization of the cerebral

D.W. Birchley, M.B.B.S., F.R.C.S., M.Sc. (✉)
C.E. Western, M.B.B.S., B.Sc.
A. Guy, M.B.Ch.B., M.R.C.S.
Department of Vascular Surgery, Royal Devon and Exeter Hospital, Barrack Road, Exeter, Devon EX2 5DW, UK
e-mail: David.birchley@nhs.net; Catherine.western@nhs.net; alisonguy@doctors.net.uk

R. Latifi et al. (eds.), *Technological Advances in Surgery, Trauma and Critical Care*, DOI 10.1007/978-1-4939-2671-8_29

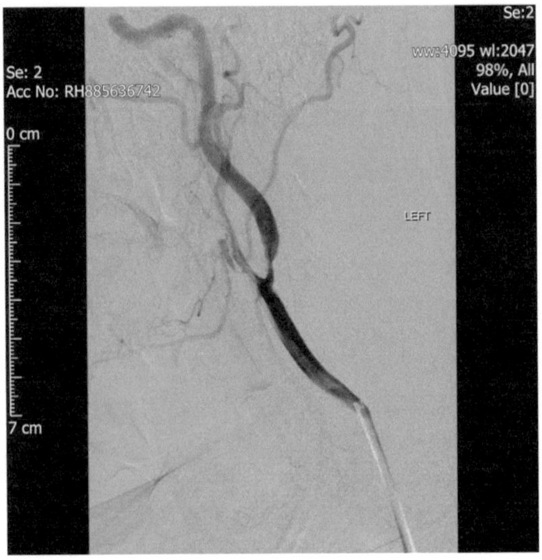

Fig. 29.1 Pre-stent angiogram

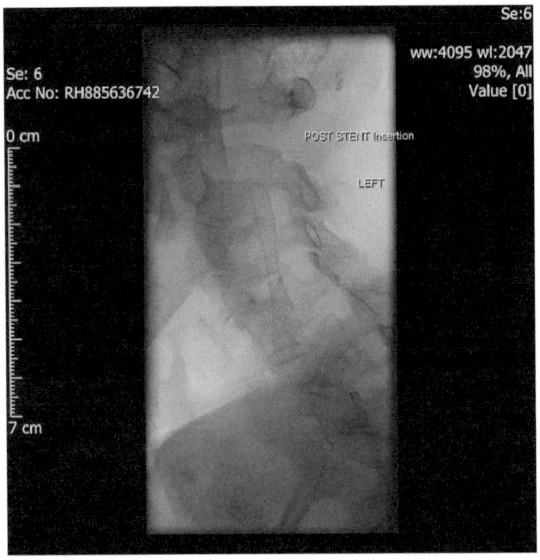

Fig. 29.2 Stent in situ

circulation. Following passage of a guide-wire, the stent is deployed (Figs. 29.1, 29.2 and 29.3).

Irrespective of treatment modality (open or endovascular), there is a per procedural stroke and death risk which needs to be balanced against the risk of further thromboembolic events in the patient who receives Best Medical Therapy alone. Given that the risk of events is so low for asymptomatic disease, the threshold for intervention must be much higher; conversely, the risk of

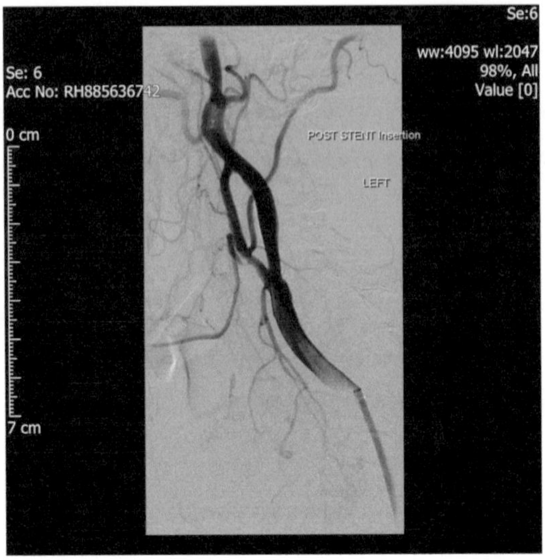

Fig. 29.3 Post stenting

further events after symptoms can greatly outweigh the risk of per procedural complications.

It is also a central tenet of treatment in symptomatic disease that endarterectomy does not reverse established ischaemic damage (or the related symptoms); it is an exercise in future risk reduction. Similarly, there is no indication for treating occlusive internal carotid disease as there can by definition be no thromboembolic risk through the occluded vessel.

Best Medical Therapy

The aspects of Best Medical Therapy (BMT) are well established: the cessation of cigarette smoking, statin therapy to lower LDL cholesterol, control of hypertension, glycaemic control in diabetes and the provision of antiplatelet therapy.

Questions to Be Answered

In consideration of a patient with internal carotid stenotic disease above the threshold for significance (50 % or 70 % dependent on the system used) and who is established on BMT, we have fundamental questions that need to be addressed in terms of guiding our management decisions:

Is a patient with carotid disease better treated with Best Medical Therapy (BMT) or intervention plus BMT? Which is superior—carotid endarterectomy (CEA) or carotid artery stenting (CAS)? Does the presentation (symptomatic or asymptomatic carotid disease) influence the best therapy? What do we consider "Significant" in terms of treatment failure? Is it any stroke? Death? Stroke sub-types? Myocardial infarction? Cranial nerve injury? A combination of the above?

It would therefore seem reasonable to propose a prospective randomized-controlled trial of treatment in carotid disease, which is powered to evaluate significant outcomes between three modalities (BMT, CEA plus BMT and CAS plus BMT) for—ideally—symptomatic and asymptomatic disease with pre-agreed outcomes (any stroke and death). So why do we still not have definitive answers despite the multiplicity of trials addressing precisely these issues?

The aim of this chapter is not to exhaustively review the details of every trial, systematic review and pooled meta-analysis; rather it is to identify the difficulties in answering the above questions based on the major trials subsequent to the Cochrane Collaborative Review of 2005. The major outcome of interest throughout all the presented studies is death and stroke of all types.

The Cochrane Review 2005 [1]

This was an attempt to definitively answer—through systematic review and meta-analysis—the questions of who and how to treat in terms of open and endovascular therapy. Five trials including 1,269 patients were reviewed (being a mix of symptomatic and asymptomatic in presentation). Outcomes were reviewed at 30 days and 1 year with the major end-points being any stroke or death and myocardial infarction (30 days) and any stroke or death/cranial nerve injury (1 year). At both 30 days and 1 year there were no significant differences in the Odds Ratios for either any stroke or death (Odds Ratio for stenting 1.33 range 0.86–2.04). There was (as might be expected from the procedural details) a significantly lower Odds Ratio for cranial nerve injury during carotid stenting compared with open surgery (OR 0.13 range 0.06–0.25). We therefore start from the position of neither treatment being superior in terms of the primary end-points, with an advantage in terms of reduced cranial nerve injury. Due to the small numbers and resultant wide confidence intervals, superiority could not be established for either therapy and the recommendation was made to continue with stenting only in the context of controlled trials.

Endarterectomy Versus Angioplasty in Patients with Symptomatic Severe Stenosis (EVA-3S) 2008 [2]

Published in 2008, EVA-3S randomized 527 patients with symptomatic disease of 50 % or greater (using the North American Carotid Surgery Trial criteria and defined as an event within 120 days) to either CEA or CAS. Results have been published up to 4 years of follow-up based on an early end to the trial due to safety concerns.

At 30 days the risk of any stroke or death was 3.9 % in the CEA group and 9.6 % in the CAS group, giving a relative risk of the primary end-point in the CAS group of 2.5; an absolute risk increase of 5.7 %. At 6 months the risk of the same end-point was 6.1 % in the CEA group and 11.7 % in the CAS group. Overall the risk of cranial nerve injury was 1.1 % with CAS and 7.7 % with CEA. At 4 years the risk of the primary end-point was 6.2 % for CEA and 11.1 % for CAS. It may therefore be concluded at this stage that the greatest risk of the primary end-point (any stroke or death) occurs in the early perioperative period, and that there is a clear benefit to CEA over CAS in this population. It is also clear, however, that there are multiple outcomes, which may be presented either alone or in combination:

- Nonfatal stroke
- Death (including fatal stroke)
- Any stroke or death
- Any disabling stroke or death
- TIA
- Myocardial infarction (MI)

Stent Protected Angioplasty Versus Carotid Endarterectomy (SPACE) 2008 [3]

SPACE was designed to evaluate outcomes in patients with a symptomatic stenosis of >70 % (using European Carotid Surgery Trial criteria) and an event within the preceding 6 months. Of the 1,214 patients randomized, there were 60 exclusions from the 30-days results. The risk of death or any stroke was 5.5 % for CEA and 6.8 % for CAS. At 2 years the risk had increased to 8.8 % for CEA and 9.5 % for CAS. It was also highlighted that the risk of a 70 % or greater restenosis at 2 years was 4.6 % for CEA and 10.7 % for CAS. In addition to the previous points, it may now be noted that: A significant proportion of patients in both groups will return to their high-risk disease state within 2 years. It is possible in comparing the two sets of results to overlook the fact that neither is particularly satisfactory when compared to current thinking in terms of acceptable perioperative stroke risk.

The definition of symptomatic in terms of time since event may be argued to have changed significantly since publication.

Carotid Revascularization Endarterectomy Versus Stenting Trial (CREST) 2010 [4]

CREST differs from EVA-3S and SPACE in that it studied outcomes in both symptomatic and asymptomatic patients with 2,522 being randomized (predominantly symptomatic). Follow-up was presented at 30 days and up to 4 years. At 30 days the risk of any stroke or death in the CEA group was 2.3 %, compared with 4.4 % for CAS. At 4 years, the risk had increased to 4.7 % for CEA and 6.4 % for CAS. Furthermore, the results were sub-divided into symptomatic and asymptomatic disease. Symptomatic patients had a 6.4 % risk with CEA as opposed to 8 % with CAS. Asymptomatic patients had (as would be expected) lower risk of 2.7 % (CEA) and 4.5 % (CAS). We therefore now have a measure of the reduced risk of the primary outcome in asymptomatic disease although again this does not stand well against current estimate of acceptable perioperative stroke risk for asymptomatic disease.

International Carotid Stenting Study (ICSS) [5]

Although the trial is yet to publish final outcome data, a 120-day interim analysis has been produced for this study of CEA versus CAS in symptomatic disease of >50 % (NASCET) with 1,713 patients randomized. The 30-day Hazard Ratio for any stroke for CAS relative to CEA was 1.92 (range 1.27–2.89); for all cause death 2.76 (range 1.16–6.56).

Trial Synthesis: Symptomatic Carotid Disease [6]

As stated, the relatively small numbers per trial make clear judgments difficult and therefore meta-analysis has been used to pool and re-analyse the data from EVA-3S, SPACE and ICSS in terms of short-term outcomes at 30 days (per protocol) up to 120 days (intention to treat). A maximum of 3,433 patients were included in the analysis at two points in time: 1,679 CAS and 1,645 CEA analysed per protocol at 30 days; 1,725 CAS and 1,708 CEA analysed by intention to treat at 120 days. The primary outcome was all-type stroke and death. At 30 days, the risk of the primary outcome was 2.6 % for CEA and 3.9 % for CAS. By 120 days the risks had increased to 5.8 % for CEA and 8.9 % for CAS. It was also noted that the risk of the primary outcome was far worse in patients over 70 undergoing CAS (12 % vs. 5.9 %). On this basis, it was concluded that: The risk of stenting exceeded the risk of open endarterectomy. Age was significant in terms of treatment outcome.

Systematic Review and Meta-analysis: Symptomatic and Asymptomatic

Carotid Disease [7]

In their review and re-analysis of the literature, Murad et al. re-evaluated 13 randomized controlled trials of stenting versus endarterectomy including a total of 7,484 patients of which 80 % were symptomatic for carotid disease. Due to the low numbers of asymptomatic patients and the inherent low number of primary outcomes, no clear conclusions can be drawn for this group. In terms of the symptomatic patients, the Relative Risk of any stroke for CAS was 1.45 (range 1.06–1.99). The Relative Risk of per procedural MI was 0.43 (range 0.26–0.71). This was summarized as "...stenting would lead to 19 more strokes and 10 fewer MIs per 1,000 treated patients" for CAS relative to CEA.

Summary of Study Findings

Based on the selected studies presented (and without attempts to critique each in detail) certain observations may be made: The landscape of carotid disease has changed rapidly over the period that the studies have taken place in terms of degrees of stenosis considered significant, the definition of symptomatic disease relative to the index symptoms, the role of best medical therapy and the experience of CAS within trial centres.

Carotid endarterectomy carries a lower periprocedural risk of stroke at the risk of a higher incidence of per procedural myocardial infarction. The risk/benefit profile may not favour CAS in asymptomatic or indeed symptomatic primary disease, but the increased complexity of open surgery for recurrent disease or disease in the presence of previous surgery would logically seem to favour CAS. Carotid stenting carries lower per procedural risks of cranial nerve injury.

Why the Need for Further Studies?

To return to the original questions: Is a patient with carotid disease better treated with Best Medical Therapy (BMT) or intervention plus BMT? Which is superior—carotid endarterectomy (CEA) or carotid artery stenting (CAS)? Does the presentation (symptomatic or asymptomatic carotid disease) influence the best therapy?

The first question simply has not been addressed to date. The second depends on your perception of "Superior" and the presence (and definition of) symptoms in the context of the patient with carotid disease. There is insufficient data to answer the third question for asymptomatic disease.

Future Studies

At least four studies have been proposed to further investigate the roles of CEA and CAS in patients with carotid disease: ACT-1, ACST-2, SPACE-2 and CREST-2. ACT-1 was designed to demonstrate the non-inferiority of CAS relative to CEA using a specific device in asymptomatic patients. Since inception, it has been terminated without recruitment. ACST-2 is designed to answer the question: "Which is better in the management of a patient with asymptomatic, significant carotid disease on Best Medical Therapy: CAE or CAS?" Patients deemed suitable at risk for treatment of their asymptomatic disease are randomized to CEA or CAS in addition to BMT. It is, however, unclear as to what criteria will be used to decide between high and low risk asymptomatic patients.

SPACE-2 on the other hand proposes to answer the question "Which is better in the management of a patient with asymptomatic, significant carotid disease: Best Medical Therapy alone, in combination with CEA or CAS?" Patients in this study will be allocated to groups based on the re-design of the study. SPACE 2a will randomize patients to BMT alone or BMT plus CEA; SPACE-2b will randomize to BMT alone or BMT and CAS. CREST-2 is proposed to have the same format as SPACE-2.

Conclusion

There is still no clear answer to the question "Which is better" because of the multiple variables and nuances. The risk is that, as our knowledge of the disease process develops, so do the proposed trials become outdated before they have completed recruitment and follow-up. Ultimately, it is clear that BMT is the mainstay of disease management in the patient with peripheral arterial stenotic disease. It may become apparent that the benefits of aggressive risk management are such that there can be no demonstrable benefit to either CEA or CAS in the context of asymptomatic disease. The evidence would seem to favour CEA for symptomatic primary disease with the very different risk/benefit profile supporting CAS in more complex recurrent disease/hostile anatomy. It may therefore be suggested that the Old Surgery is alive and well, whilst the New Stenting is striving to define its role in contemporary management of carotid stenotic disease.

References

1. Chambers BR, Donnan G. Carotid endarterectomy for asymptomatic carotid stenosis. Cochrane Database Syst Rev. 2005;(4). Art. No.: CD001923.
2. EVA-3S Investigators. Endarterectomy versus angioplasty in patients with symptomatic severe carotid stenosis (EVA-3S) trial: results up to 4 years from a randomised, multicentre trial. Lancet Neurol. 2008; 7(10):885–92.
3. Eckstein HH, Ringleb P, Allenberg JR, et al. Results of the stent-protected angioplasty versus carotid endarterectomy (SPACE) study to treat symptomatic stenoses at 2 years: a multinational, prospective, randomised trial. Lancet Neurol. 2008;7(10):893–902.
4. Mas JL, Brown MM, Ringleb PA, Carotid Stenting Trialists Collaboration. N Engl J Med. 2010; 363(18):1766–7.
5. Bonati LH, Fraedrich G, Carotid Stenting Trialists' Collaboration. Carotid artery stenting compared with endarterectomy in patients with symptomatic carotid stenosis (International Carotid Stenting Study): an interim analysis of a randomised controlled trial. Lancet. 2010;375(9719):985–97.
6. Carotid Stenting Trialists' Collaboration. Short-term outcome after stenting versus endarterectomy for symptomatic carotid stenosis: a preplanned meta-analysis of individual patient data. Lancet. 2010;376(9746):1062–73.
7. Murad MH, Shahrour A, Shah ND, Montori VM, Ricotta JJ. A systematic review and meta-analysis of randomized trials of carotid endarterectomy vs stenting. J Vasc Surg. 2011;53(3):792–7.

Part VI

System-Oriented Technological Advances: Section D—Abdomen and Pelvis

Laparoscopic Approaches in General Surgery: Is There Anything New?

30

Timothy G. Johnson and William W. Hope

Introduction

Laparoscopic surgery has become the standard for many general surgical procedures and is commonplace in most operating rooms. As is true with the pioneers who began laparoscopic and endoscopic procedures, surgeons continue to innovate and improve on technical aspects of these surgeries. With advancement in technology, many surgeries can employ minimally invasive techniques, and surgeons continue to minimize trauma related to surgical incisions and operations.

Traditional Laparoscopy

Traditional laparoscopic surgery was initially based on attempting to recreate all the technical aspects of an open procedure. Successful laparoscopic procedures that recreated these open procedures were not too difficult for the surgeon to perform. With improvement in instrumentation and training, surgeons have applied minimally invasive techniques to most general surgical procedures. With these improvements, surgeons have begun to question some of the principles of laparoscopic surgery such as the need for triangulation of instruments and, in some instances, have altered the surgical techniques from the open procedure based on successes using the laparoscopic technique. Despite the potential advantage of the many new techniques and technologies discussed in this chapter, traditional multiport laparoscopy remains the standard for many surgical procedures and is the basis of comparing new techniques.

Laparoscopic Access

One of the most important steps in any laparoscopic surgery is the ability to obtain laparoscopic access. The goals of laparoscopic access should be a safe, reproducible, and an efficient procedure that is comfortable for the surgeon and inexpensive. Trocar or abdominal access injuries are some of the most feared and catastrophic injuries associated with laparoscopic surgery. Multiple different options are available for gaining access to the abdominal cavity and range from open techniques such as the Hasson technique to closed techniques such as the use of a Veress needle or an optical trocar entry. Surgeons should use the technique that they feel most comfortable with and must have expertise in many different techniques, as there are advantages and disadvantages

T.G. Johnson, M.D. • W.W. Hope, M.D. (✉)
Department of Surgery, New Hanover Regional Medical Center, 2131 South 17th Street, Wilmington, NC 28401, USA
e-mail: Timothy.johnson@seahec.net; William.hope@seahec.net

R. Latifi et al. (eds.), *Technological Advances in Surgery, Trauma and Critical Care*,
DOI 10.1007/978-1-4939-2671-8_30

to all techniques. A recent Cochrane review reported on 28 randomized trials relating to laparoscopic access techniques. The review showed no advantages in terms of major vascular or visceral injury with any particular technique; however, there was a lower rate of failed entry, omental injury, and extraperitoneal insufflation with the open technique compared to the Veress needle [1].

Hand-Assisted Surgery

Although not a new technique, hand-assisted surgery is a valuable tool and has allowed surgeons who are learning laparoscopy or performing challenging laparoscopic procedures some of the advantages of open surgery. The concept of hand-assisted surgery was to marry the technology of laparoscopic surgery with the ability to have tactile feedback by using the surgeon's hand and, therefore, allowing complex surgeries to be performed in a minimally invasive fashion. In the early era of laparoscopic surgery, hand-assisted surgery was often a bridge or a way to facilitate the transition from open to laparoscopic surgery for many surgeons. While there remains controversy on the indications and benefits of hand-assisted laparoscopic surgery compared with pure laparoscopic surgery, it is a valuable adjunct in the armamentarium of the minimally invasive surgeon and can be an efficient technique when surgeries require large organ extractions or in complex operations.

Hand-assisted surgery entails placing a small incision, often recommended to be approximately 1 cm less than the surgeon's glove size, at the initiation of the surgery. Commercially available hand-assisted sealing devices can then be placed into the incision allowing for the surgeon to place his hand intra-abdominally without losing pneumoperitoneum (Fig. 30.1). Following this, additional laparoscopic trocars can be added as needed, and the hand allows for increased tactile feedback and can aid in retraction (Fig. 30.2). Despite the assumption that because the hand is used the surgery mimics an open procedure, the ability to use the hand efficiently and without interfering with the laparoscopic instruments or visualization is a skill that needs to be mastered to maximize the benefits of hand-assisted surgery.

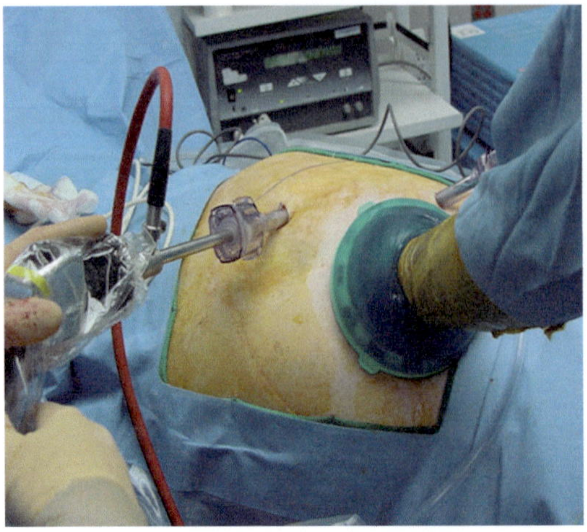

Fig. 30.1 Hand-assisted surgery setup with surgeon using nondominant hand in port and additional laparoscopic trocars using instruments and camera

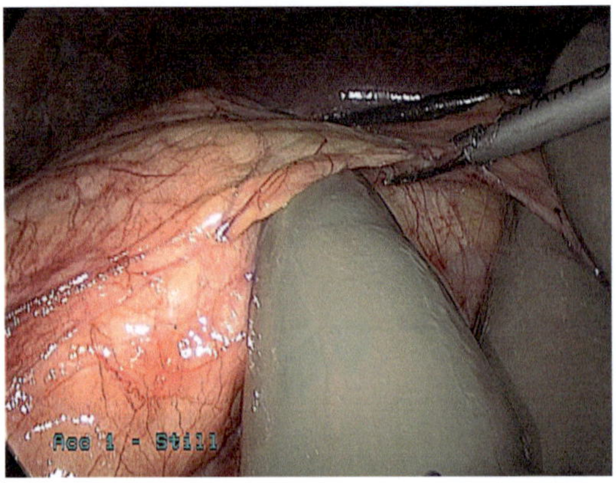

Fig. 30.2 Intraoperative picture showing the use of the hand intra-abdominally to retract and allow for dissection

Hand-assisted surgery has been used in many different general surgical cases but is best suited for complex cases where removal of organs mandates a larger incision than the traditional laparoscopic port site. One particular general surgical arena where hand-assisted surgery is often used is in colorectal surgery. Laparoscopic colorectal surgery is a difficult laparoscopic case that often requires the removal of the colon with associated mesentery and lymph nodes. The extraction incision used by many surgeons is often several centimeters and, in some cases, the procedure can be performed more efficiently using the hand-assisted approach. Recent systematic reviews comparing the use of hand-assist and conventional laparoscopy for colorectal surgery showed decreased conversion rates with the use of hand-assisted surgery [2, 3] and no difference in outcomes [2]. These systemic reviews had mixed reports on operating times with one reporting decreased time with hand-assisted surgery [3] and the other showing no difference [2].

Microlaparoscopy/Needlescopic Surgery

After surgeons applied minimally invasive techniques to most commonly performed general surgical procedures, innovators in laparoscopic surgery began work to make the surgeries more minimally invasive. The initial enthusiasm involved single incision surgeries using special access cannulas and instruments that allowed abdominal entry through one incision. This enthusiasm in single incision surgery has rekindled the interest in microlaparoscopic and needlescopic techniques. Needlescopy employs the use of very small trocars and instruments no larger than 3 mm in diameter (Fig. 30.3).

The reasons surgeons began to experiment with needlescopy are the same reasons surgeons initially started using laparoscopes instead of open incisions; less tissue damage and less patient pain with better cosmesis and less fascial disruption, which potentially produces fewer hernias. Needlescopic instruments are smaller than traditional laparoscopic trocars and result in less tissue damage and thus potentially produce these beneficial patient endpoints.

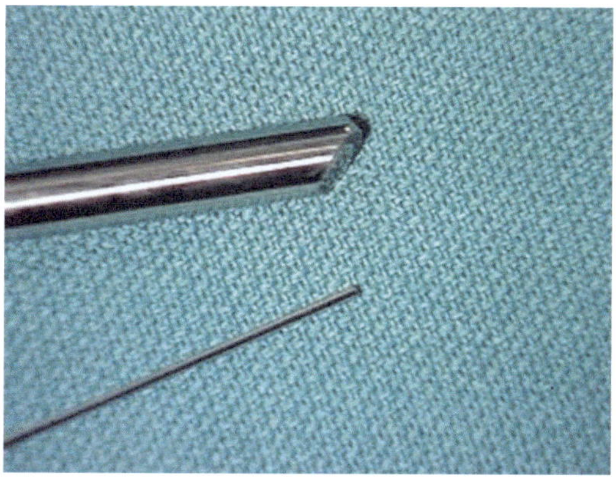

Fig. 30.3 Size comparison of traditional 10 mm laparoscopic versus the 3 mm laparoscope used in needlescopic surgery

Early studies in the surgical literature in the mid- to late 1990s initially assessed the feasibility of some basic laparoscopic procedures such as appendectomy, cholecystectomy, and diagnostic laparoscopy (Figs. 30.4 and 30.5). Other more complicated procedures were reviewed, such as Heller myotomy, splenectomy, cyst marsupialization, adrenalectomy, colon resection, sympathectomy, Nissen fundoplication, and inguinal herniorrhaphy.

Larger studies emerged comparing needlescopy and laparoscopy with appendectomies and cholecystectomies. These are two of the most common laparoscopic procedures performed in America and are easily mastered by the general surgeon, making them good procedures to embark with a potentially technically challenging advancement. Naturally studies started out as retrospective comparisons and moved to small prospective studies and eventually larger controlled, randomized trials. Primary endpoints for early studies included operative time, technical feasibility, cosmesis, postoperative pain, complications, hospital stay, and conversion rates. As expected, the results of these studies were sometimes contradictory.

Two large systematic reviews comparing needlescopic and laparoscopic cholecystectomies showed that needlescopy is feasible and as safe as laparoscopy with similar hospital stays. Postoperative pain and cosmesis were improved with needlescopy in one study, while there was only a trend toward improvement in the other. Both studies found that conversion to open was higher in the needlescopy group. The results of a review comparing needlescopic and laparoscopic appendectomies mirrored those of the cholecystectomy reviews. Some of the results were in line with their expectations, such as the safety of the procedure, the longer operative times as the new technology is mastered, and improved cosmesis since the length of one or more incisions is reduced by nearly half [4, 5].

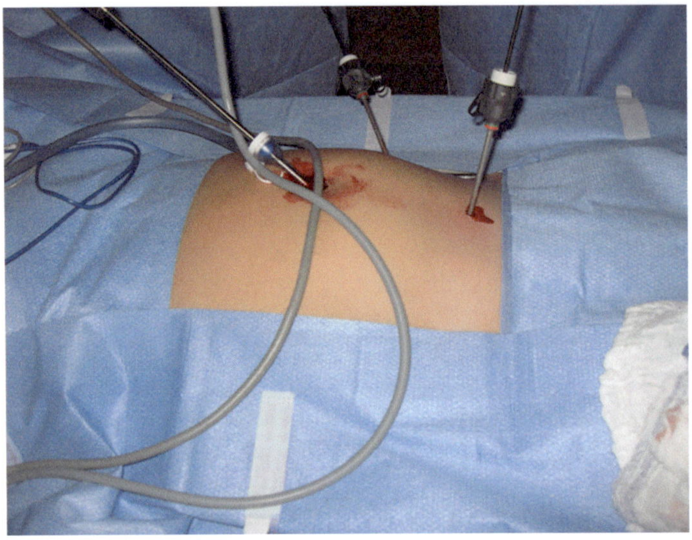

Fig. 30.4 Laparoscopic appendectomy utilizing two 3 mm needlescopic ports and an additional 5 mm port

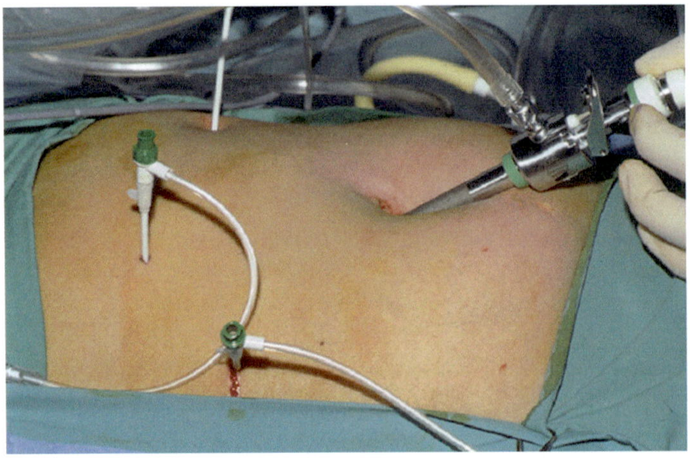

Fig. 30.5 Laparoscopic cholecystectomy utilizing three 3 mm needlescopic ports and one 11 mm camera port

With smaller instruments and tissue damage, one would expect less postoperative pain, but only one of the reviews found less postoperative pain while the other did not, and the individual studies correspond to these findings [6–9]. One potential reason for the pain outcome is the use of some traditional sized trocars during needlescopic surgery, since the laparoscopic ports for the studied procedures were not entirely replaced with needlescopic instruments. Five millimeter ports are needed for modern laparoscopes as adequate optics for laparoscopes smaller than 5 mm are still being developed. Ten millimeter or even in some cases 12 mm ports are still required for specimen retrieval. These ports are also required for some advanced laparoscopic tools that are only available in 10 mm size, and surgical staplers require 12 mm ports as well. As a result of these unchanged port sizes, the patient's pain is unlikely to change, as these larger port sites are the source of considerable postoperative pain. Similarly, the hospital stay is unchanged with patient pain remaining unchanged. Furthermore, the hospital stay for appendectomies and cholecystectomies is so short that any statistical diminution in that time would be difficult to show in studies.

Needlescopy is a safe alternative to traditional laparoscopy but still has limitations in many general surgery cases. Lack of sufficient technology to this point has limited significant conversion from normal laparoscopic trocars to needlescopic instruments. Advances in needlescopic technology continue and are focused on firmer instruments and adequate 3 mm camera optics. As we advance our knowledge and skill in laparoscopy, needlescopic advancements are sure to follow and may allow many general surgical procedures to employ 3 mm or smaller instruments and cameras that are as useful as the 5 and 10 mm instruments we use today.

Single Incision Surgery

Multiport laparoscopy has been the gold standard for minimally invasive surgery and has allowed surgeons to perform many complex laparoscopic surgeries using the cornerstone concepts of triangulation of ports. The ability to triangulate ports and access allowed surgeons to work ergonomically with good visualization of the target organ.

As was the case with the advent of laparoscopic surgery, the beginnings of the use of single incision surgery started with cholecystectomy. With the introduction of the possibility of removing gallbladders through the colon or vagina [10, 11], surgeons became more interested in more minimally invasive ways to remove gallbladders and noticed some of the shortcomings of the NOTES approach. Navarra had initially hypothesized the use of a single incision for cholecystectomy in 1997 [12], but this did not gain wide acceptance until approximately 10 years later. Since 2008, single incision surgery, which has been referred to as laparoendoscopic single site surgery (LESS), single port access (SPA), transumbilical endoscopic surgery (TUES), and single incision surgery (SILS), has gained modest popularity and use and been applied to most abdominal general surgical procedures.

Cholecystectomy has been the most common procedure performed using the single incision technique and has the most data supporting its use. Initial reports of single incision cholecystectomy showed feasibility and safety, and many different techniques have been described. Initially, techniques involved multiple trocars being placed at slightly extended umbilical incisions and use of conventional instrumentation. As technology improved, commercially available platforms for placement of three to four trocars became available as well as specially designed instruments and cameras that assisted with these procedures including flexible tip laparoscopes and curved instruments (Fig. 30.6). During early experience and with the learning curve of single incision surgery, additional trocars were sometimes required and recommended to aid in completion and achieve a safe laparoscopic surgery (Fig. 30.7). Some of the initial criticism and concern regarding using single incision techniques included the potential for more hernia formations with larger umbilical incisions, the potential for more bile duct injuries, and, for those performing the technique by placing sutures through the gallbladder for assistance in retraction, the possibility of spillage of tumor in unsuspected gallbladder cancer cases. Other concerns related to the thoroughness of the dissection and ability to obtain the critical view as well as the feasibility of performing cholangiograms, which were addressed by several authors [13–15].

Since many different techniques were initially described for single incision laparoscopic cholecystectomy and since many surgeons found the technique to be challenging with a steep learning curve, a consensus statement was published in an attempt to standardize the technique based on high volume experienced surgeons who had mastered the learning curve. They recommended a 12 mm vertical incision through the existing anatomic scar of the umbilicus followed by insertion of a single 4-trocar port and the use of a 5 mm deflectable tip laparoscope [16]. Their proposed technique included placing the laparoscope at the 8 O'clock position, a bariatric length rigid grasper at the 4 O'clock position to grab the fundus, and a rigid bent grasper placed at the 2 O'clock position to grab the infundibulum, and at the 10 O'clock position a dissector of the surgeon's

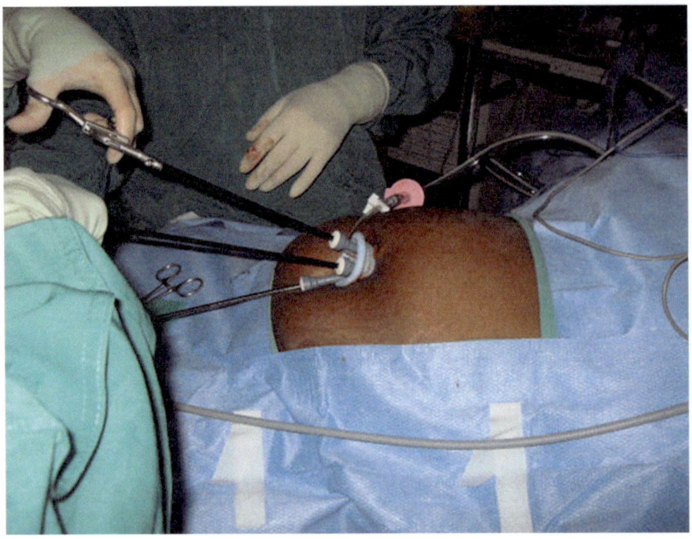

Fig. 30.6 Single incision laparoscopic cholecystectomy utilizing a commercially available single incision port allowing four instruments to be placed. Flexible tip laparoscopes greatly aid in single incision surgery allowing better visualization and ergonomics

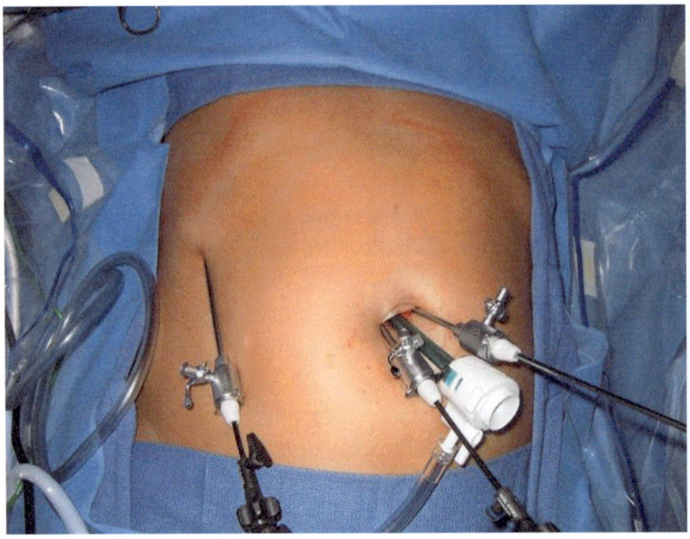

Fig. 30.7 Single incision laparoscopic cholecystectomy with ports placed within umbilical incision and additional 3 mm needlescopic port used for retraction

choice placed as the working port [16]. This configuration, per their report, allows retraction of the gallbladder in the cephalad and lateral direction, provides triangulation, and facilitates dissection of the cystic artery and duct to allow for the critical view, which is the standard technique for a four-port cholecystectomy [16].

As the data for single incision laparoscopic cholecystectomy has matured from safety and feasibility to comparative studies with four-port cholecystectomy, some of the enthusiasm for this technique has tempered. In a randomized clinical trial and two meta-analyses, single incision cholecystectomy was reported to be safe but had only modest benefits of possible decreased postoperative vomiting and some improvement in cosmesis with no significant benefit of decreased pain, shorter length of stay, or decreased complication rate [17–19]. A recent Cochrane review evaluated nine trials with 855 total patients comparing 4-port and fewer than 4-port cholecystectomy. The review showed insufficient data and low quality evidence to show clinical benefit of reduced port cholecystectomy and recommended less than 4-port cholecystectomy surgeries be reserved for well-designed randomized clinical trials [20].

Robotic Surgery

As robotic surgery is covered in detail in another chapter, only a brief overview is presented here. Few areas of laparoscopic surgery generate more controversy and interest than surgical robotics. Although laparoscopic surgery has penetrated nearly every procedure in general surgery, there are still some limits associated with the techniques and technology that fail to make it universal. Limitations associated with current laparoscopic surgery include rigid/inflexible instruments that provide only finite movements, two-dimensional visualization, fatigue and poor ergonomics associated with some procedures, and amplification of tremors. Advances in surgical robotics have attempted to lessen some of these limitations allowing surgeons flexibility in instrument motions, 3-D vision, and the ability to perform surgeries in a comfortable position. Currently the da Vinci® Surgical System (Intuitive Surgical Inc; Sunnyvale CA) is the only available robotic system approved by the Food and Drug Administration (FDA). This system consists of a control console, a tower for the insufflator and video electronics, and the patient side cart (Fig. 30.8a–c).

Robotic surgery was initially adopted by urologists predominantly for the use in prostatectomy, but gynecologists were also early adopters of this technology. Only recently have general surgeons seen the potential value of robotic surgery. The slow adoption into general surgery is mostly related to the cases being performed by general surgeons and to some of the limitations of the current robot. The advantages of robotic surgery including improved visualization, the ability to work in confined spaces, and the need for complex motor tasks and suturing were sometimes outweighed by the limitations of the current surgical robot, which limits working in multiple abdominal quadrants, which is often needed for general surgical cases.

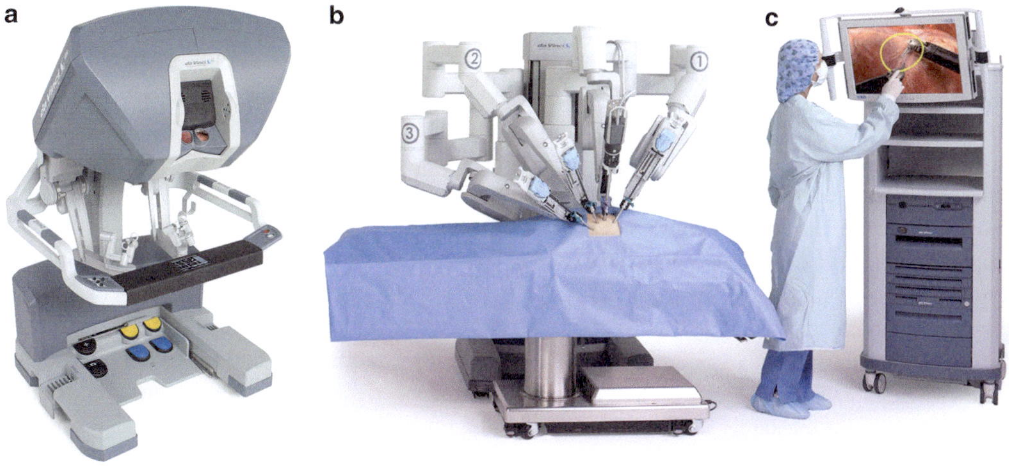

Fig. 30.8 (**a**–**c**) da Vinci® Si system (Intuitive Surgical Inc; Sunnyvale CA) with control console (**a**), the patient cart (**b**), and a tower for the insufflator and video electronics (**c**). (All: Used by permission. Copyright © 2015 Intuitive Surgical, Inc.)

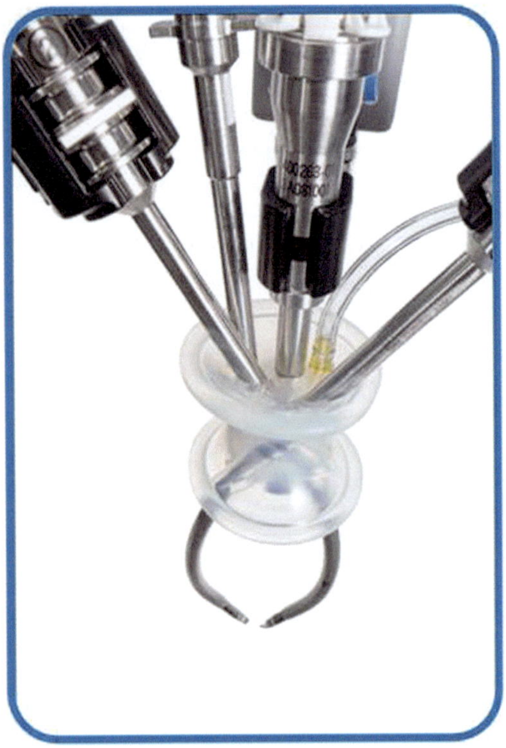

Fig. 30.9 da Vinci® Single site platform (Intuitive Surgical Inc; Sunnyvale CA) allowing four robotic flexible instruments to be placed through small 2.5 cm umbilical incision. (Used by permission. Copyright © 2015 Intuitive Surgical, Inc.)

One new robotic technology that has gained clinical interest is the single incision platform (Fig. 30.9). As previously mentioned, adoption of the single incision surgery has been slow due to the learning curve, clashing of instruments, loss of triangulation and poor visualization, and surgeon fatigue associated with this technique. The robotic single incision platform was designed to help overcome some of the challenges and learning curve associated with single incision surgery by allowing triangulation of instruments and improving ergonomics.

In 2011, the first human experience with the robotic single incision cholecystectomy was reported and showed the safety and feasibility in 13 patients [21]. Two larger series of 82 and 100 patients have subsequently been published reporting low conversion rates, low complications rates, and short learning curves deemed easier than traditional single incision cholecystectomy [22, 23]. Another study compared the traditional single incision cholecystectomy and robotic single incision cholecystectomy and reported the robotic procedure to be safe with outcomes similar to the traditional technique but with shorter operative times [24].

Apart from the traditional robotic platform currently used for surgical procedures, some have experimented with the use of miniature robots for intra-abdominal placement. This concept differs from some of the current focus and technology of using robotic arms or flexible endoscopic platforms and relies on placement of multiple, independent miniature robots that can be inserted into the abdominal cavity through the abdominal wall or a natural orifice application [25]. This approach, while still in its infancy, may build on and be a potentially complimentary adjunct to single incision and NOTES surgery by helping to overcome some of the constraints such as dexterity, visualization, orientation, retraction, and triangulation.

Natural Orifice Transluminal Endoscopic Surgery

Perhaps no minimally invasive technique since the introduction of laparoscopic surgery has led to more of a paradigm shift in thinking than the Natural Orifice Transluminal Endoscopic Surgery (NOTES). Although it should come as no surprise that the marriage of gastroenterologists and surgeons and the endoscope and laparoscope would eventually occur, many were surprised when videos of appendixes being taken out using upper endoscopy and endoscopes emerged. This concept of using natural orifices, most commonly stomach, colon, or vagina, instead of the abdominal wall to access the abdomen elicited much excitement and concern. Due to the many concerns and potential for harm associated with these techniques, leadership associated with the creation of these techniques met in 2005 under the sponsorship of the American Society of Gastrointestinal Endoscopy (ASGE) and the Society of American Gastrointestinal and

Endoscopic Surgeons (SAGES) to further evaluate these techniques. Since this time, much research has evaluated the safety of NOTES in preclinical studies and this technology. The details of the development and application of NOTES are discussed elsewhere in this book but a brief introduction is essential for this chapter's completeness.

The concept of NOTES stems from the thought that using natural human orifices, which would avoid incisions through the skin, subcutaneous tissue, and fascia, would result in some obvious benefits to the patient. Less pain, essentially no risk of hernia, shorter hospital stays, quicker return to work, and improved cosmesis are some of the benefits that were thought to result from NOTES.

Initially gastroenterologists believed that using pre-existing endoscopes with slight variations would be all that was needed to perform many common procedures, as these scopes already had cautery, balloon dilators, clips, graspers, endo-loops, retrieval nets, and snares. In fact, some gastroenterologists and surgeons have been performing some fairly complex procedures, such as endoscopic mucosal resection, repair of perforated ulcers, drainage of pancreatic pseudocysts, and transanal endoscopic microsurgery with current endoscopes. The adaptation of basic endoscopy to perform these more complex procedures was the precursor to the development of NOTES.

Inevitably, the development of NOTES led to advancements in flexible endoscope technology, as many of the NOTES proponents, particularly surgeons, believed that the existing flexible endoscopes lacked sufficient adaptability to the needs of complex intraperitoneal surgery. Some of the advancements that have been adapted to newer flexible endoscopes for NOTES include multiple large-instrument channels, horizon-correcting optics, an insufflation port that connects to modern laparoscopic insufflators, and the ability to firmly fix the scope in a single position.

The development of new endoscopes specifically for NOTES has led to multiple laboratory reports and even human cases in the surgical literature. There have been multiple animal studies including complex cases such as distal pancreatectomy, ventral hernia repair, gastric sleeve resection, and right and left colectomies. Some human cases have included transgastric appendectomy and cholecystectomy, transvaginal and transrectal cholecystectomy, and cancer staging. Many of these procedures to date have required the use of at least one retracting instrument that is placed transabdominally, but with the advent of the needlescopic instruments previously mentioned, these can be inserted through a tiny skin incision without much blunt dissection created by the port itself.

One challenge to NOTES continues to be visual guidance during the operation, as traditional endoscopes were not designed to stabilize the horizon like modern laparoscopes are. As a result, an adaptation of the NOTES procedure has been developed and has been dubbed hybrid NOTES. During a hybrid NOTES procedure, a single incision is created near the umbilicus, and a port, usually 5 mm, is placed in the abdomen and a standard laparoscope is placed into the insufflated abdomen. The procedure is then performed with the endoscope through the natural orifice, using the laparoscopic camera as visual guidance and providing superior spatial orientation. Some recent studies have shown successful use of this hybrid technique to remove the gallbladder, appendix, and repair incisional hernias. Since its inception in the mid-2000s, NOTES has generated more than 2,000 clinical studies across many surgical subspecialties and continues to be a field of intense clinical and experimental research.

Another concept related to NOTES has been the ability to remove organs through a natural orifice or the natural orifice specimen extraction (NOSE). This technique was created because of the disadvantages of laparoscopic surgeries requiring large specimen extraction whereby the surgery could be performed completely laparoscopically until, at the end of the case, a moderate sized incision had to be made for specimen extraction, which potentially nullified the benefits of the minimally invasive approach. The NOSE concept has largely been centered on colorectal surgery as a way to remove colon specimens but could be used in any laparoscopic surgery where larger organs need to be removed intact.

Laparoscopy in Trauma, Critical Care, and Acute Care Surgery

As surgeons became more comfortable with laparoscopy for elective cases, they began to adapt their new skill to the acute and emergent setting. Nowhere is this more evident than with appendectomies. However, laparoscopy is being employed in the emergency setting for more and more complex procedures in acute surgery settings, and as technology has been improving and laparoscopy has become more portable, its use for both diagnostic and therapeutic in the intensive care setting has become common.

Though our reliance on imaging for diagnosis of the acute abdomen has increased recently, there is still a role for laparoscopy when assessing the acute abdomen. Laparoscopy can be both diagnostic and therapeutic in many cases of an acute abdomen, which can be caused by basic problems such as appendicitis and cholecystitis but can also be caused by more complicated pathology such as gastroduodenal perforation. Small bowel obstructions are now even being treated laparoscopically in some patients. Conversion to open surgery is low, under 3 %, during the diagnosis and treatment of these surgical problems. Urgent and emergent treatment of colorectal pathology is also treatable laparoscopically. Conversion to open for these cases is also low at about 6 %, and laparoscopic cases have a shorter length of stay than open cases and better short-term outcomes.

Perhaps no greater diagnostic conundrum exists than the critically ill patient with possible abdominal pathology. Diagnosing these patients can be difficult as their severe illness can make their lab values and radiological findings equivocal; sometimes they are even too sick for transport to the radiology department for their diagnostic evaluation. In cases such as these, laparoscopy has been shown to be a safe bedside diagnostic tool. These procedures have even been performed with mini, 3 mm laparoscopes. Some common pathologic causes of these critically ill patients are acute acalculous cholecystitis, bowel perforation, and bowel ischemia. Bedside laparoscopy can be used to identify these common problems to allow more directed treatment. It can also spare patients a nontherapeutic laparotomy when no pathology is found or if cholecystitis is found and is treated with a percutaneous cholecystostomy tube.

To date, laparoscopy for trauma has been limited to evaluation of peritoneal violation from abdominal stab wounds, tangential gunshot wounds, or evaluations for diaphragmatic injuries. Yet even with these limited indications, many patients have been spared nontherapeutic and negative laparotomies. The traditional role of the use of laparoscopy in the trauma setting has been for diagnosis, and this is being expanded to the possibility of using this technology outside of the operating room and in places such as the trauma bay or intensive care units. In the past, evaluation of the peritoneal cavity was done with diagnostic peritoneal lavage. This has largely been replaced with ultrasonography and the focused abdominal sonography for trauma (FAST) exam. In some institutions, laparoscopy is being added to the end of the diagnostic algorithm for patients who will either be observed or undergo surgical intervention. Indications for laparoscopy in trauma have been expanded to include those previously mentioned and for suspicion of injury on imaging studies, herniation of omentum through abdominal wounds, and equivocal exam findings in penetrating trauma. In all cases, these patients must be hemodynamically stable to safely undergo laparoscopy.

The use of therapeutic laparoscopy in trauma is somewhat limited due to the inherent nature of trauma patients and associated critical illness. However, as surgeons become more comfortable with complex laparoscopic techniques, there may be increasing indications for their use and increasing indications for therapeutic laparoscopy in isolated intestinal injuries (Figs. 30.10 and 30.11), diaphragmatic injuries (Figs. 30.12 and 30.13), or for hemostasis in selected hemodynamically stable patients [26, 27].

Although the use of laparoscopy is sometimes limited in trauma and acute care surgery, as technology, surgical technique, and anesthetic efforts continue to improve, some of the previous contraindications for use of laparoscopy in critical ill patients may slowly wane, and these skills should remain in the surgeon's armamentarium.

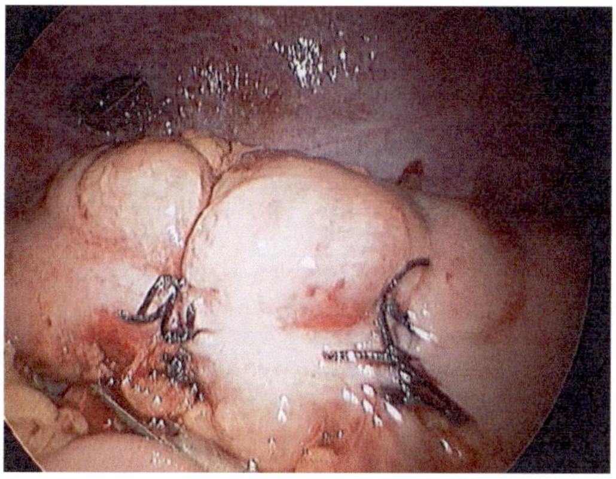

Fig. 30.10 Laparoscopic repair of isolated colonic injury secondary to penetrating trauma. Colostomies were sutured laparoscopically and abdominal wall defect from entrance wound in upper left portion of picture was also sutured closed

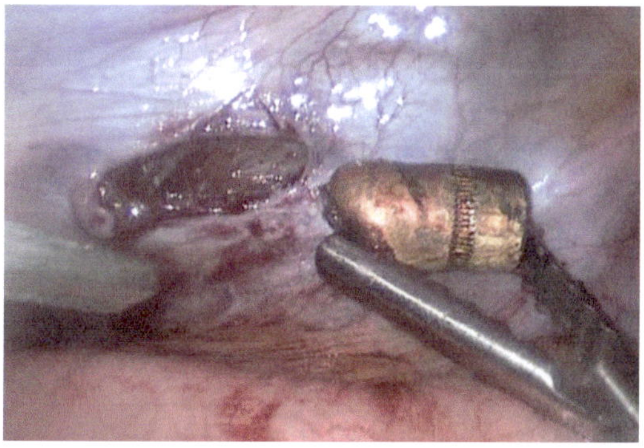

Fig. 30.11 Laparoscopic evaluation for gunshot wound to abdomen with bullet retrieved

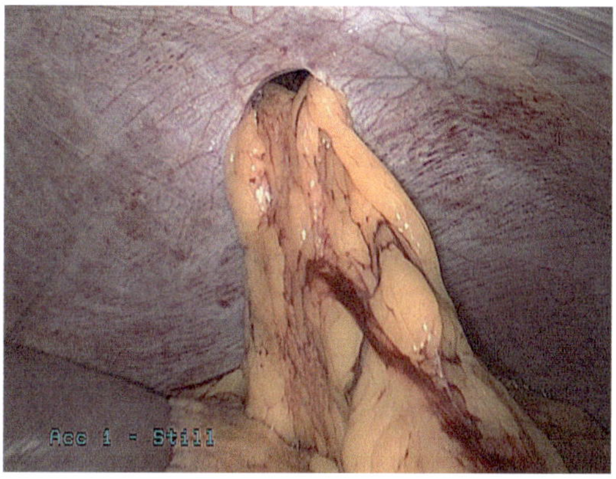

Fig. 30.12 Laparoscopic evaluation of stab wound to chest with isolated diaphragm injury

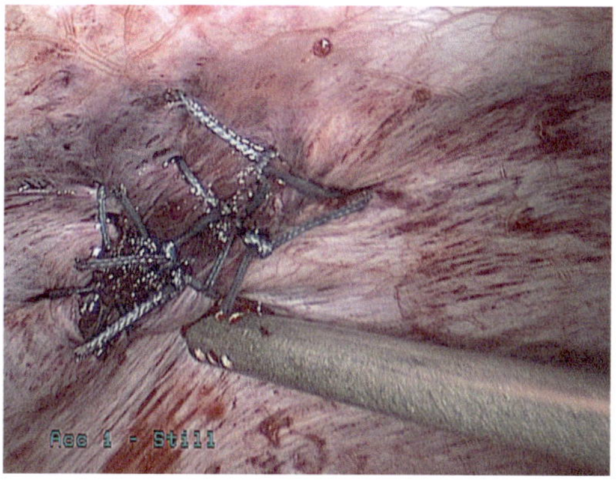

Fig. 30.13 Laparoscopic suture repair of traumatic diaphragm injury with interrupted sutures

Future Directions

As evidenced in this chapter, the future of laparoscopy and minimally invasive surgery is quite bright, and the possibilities appear almost limitless. Ongoing collaboration between surgeons, gastroenterologists, and interventional radiologists and the marrying of techniques will no doubt allow surgeons to perform increasingly complex operations with minimal trauma in ways akin to those read about in science fiction novels and seen in visual media. Disease-based multispecialty teams will likely evolve combining hybrid procedures that use image guidance, minimally invasive surgery, and endoscopy to perform targeted and precise operations.

Many of the techniques discussed in this chapter will be improved using instruments and technology becoming smaller, easier to work with, less expensive, and applicable to all general surgeons and general surgical procedures. Robotic systems will be improved to facilitate haptic feedback, smaller and more flexible instruments, and the ability to perform procedures intraluminally, through NOTES applications, or through small incisions in the abdominal wall. The surgeon will likely be based at a console where he/she can perform operations and have access to imaging and telemedicine technology. Virtual reality may allow surgeons to plan operations before performing them and help in training surgeons for new technologies and complex cases. Improvements in imaging may allow surgeons to better evaluate operative anatomy or see structures not visible in the operative field. Although many of these techniques have not been proven and remain experimental, they have a promising future. As it has been throughout history, surgeons will continue to be innovators while improving patient care and minimizing trauma from their surgical procedures so that the cure will not be more harmful than the disease.

Disclosure Dr. Hope has the following disclosures: research support, Ethicon, Inc.; honorarium, eMedicine; consultant, C.R. Bard.

References

1. Ahmad G, O'Flynn H, Duffy JM, Phillips K, Watson A. Laparoscopic entry techniques. Cochrane Database Syst Rev. 2012;2, CD006583.
2. Moloo H, Haggar F, Coyle D, Hutton B, Duhaime S, Mamazza J, et al. Hand assisted laparoscopic surgery versus conventional laparoscopy for colorectal surgery. Cochrane Database Syst Rev. 2010;10, CD006585.
3. Aalbers AG, Doeksen A, Van Berge Henegouwen MI, Bemelman WA. Hand-assisted laparoscopic versus open approach in colorectal surgery: a systematic review. Colorectal Dis. 2010;12(4):287–95.
4. Sajid MS, Khan MA, Cheek E, Baig MK. Needlescopic versus laparoscopic appendectomy: a systematic review. Can J Surg. 2009;52(2):129–34.
5. Sajid MS, Khan MA, Ray K, Cheek E, Baig MK. Needlescopic versus laparoscopic cholecystectomy: a meta-analysis. ANZ J Surg. 2009;79(6):437–42.
6. Lee PC, Lai IR, Yu SC. Minilaparoscopic (needlescopic) cholecystectomy: a study of 1,011 cases. Surg Endosc. 2004;18(10):1480–4.
7. Lai EC, Fok M, Chan AS. Needlescopic cholecystectomy: prospective study of 150 patients. Hong Kong Med J. 2003;9(4):238–42.
8. Novitsky YW, Kercher KW, Czerniach DR, Kaban GK, Khera S, Gallagher-Dorval KA, et al. Advantages of mini-laparoscopic vs conventional laparoscopic cholecystectomy: results of a prospective randomized trial. Arch Surg. 2005;140(12):1178–83.
9. Mostafa G, Matthews BD, Sing RF, Kercher KW, Heniford BT. Mini-laparoscopic versus laparoscopic approach to appendectomy. BMC Surg. 2001;1:4.
10. Scott DJ, Tang SJ, Fernandez R, Bergs R, Goova MT, Zeltser I, et al. Completely transvaginal NOTES cholecystectomy using magnetically anchored instruments. Surg Endosc. 2007;21(12):2308–16.
11. Auyang ED, Hungness ES, Vaziri K, Martin JA, Soper NJ. Natural orifice translumenal endoscopic surgery (NOTES): dissection for the critical view of safety during transcolonic cholecystectomy. Surg Endosc. 2009;23(5):1117–8.
12. Navarra G, Pozza E, Occhionorelli S, Carcoforo P, Donini I. One-wound laparoscopic cholecystectomy. Br J Surg. 1997;84(5):695.
13. Horisberger K, Grossen E, Schob O. How to meet the challenge of flexible exposure of the Calot triangle in SILS cholecystectomy. Surg Laparosc Endosc Percutan Tech. 2012;22(2):e63–5.
14. Rawlings A, Hodgett SE, Matthews BD, Strasberg SM, Quasebarth M, Brunt LM. Single-incision laparoscopic cholecystectomy: initial experience with critical view of safety dissection and routine intraoperative cholangiography. J Am Coll Surg. 2010; 211(1):1–7.
15. Yeo D, Mackay S, Martin D. Single-incision laparoscopic cholecystectomy with routine intraoperative cholangiography and common bile duct exploration via the umbilical port. Surg Endosc. 2012;26(4): 1122–7.
16. Ross S, Rosemurgy A, Albrink M, Choung E, Dapri G, Gallagher S, et al. Consensus statement of the consortium for LESS cholecystectomy. Surg Endosc. 2012;26(10):2711–6.
17. Garg P, Thakur JD, Garg M, Menon GR. Single-incision laparoscopic cholecystectomy vs. conventional laparoscopic cholecystectomy: a meta-analysis of randomized controlled trials. J Gastrointest Surg. 2012;16(8):1618–28.
18. Markar SR, Karthikesalingam A, Thrumurthy S, Muirhead L, Kinross J, Paraskeva P. Single-incision laparoscopic surgery (SILS) vs. conventional multiport cholecystectomy: systematic review and meta-analysis. Surg Endosc. 2012;26(5):1205–13.
19. Jorgensen LN, Rosenberg J, Al-Tayar H, Assaadzadeh S, Helgstrand F, Bisgaard T. Randomized clinical trial of single- versus multi-incision laparoscopic cholecystectomy. Br J Surg. 2014;101(4):347–55.
20. Gurusamy KS, Vaughan J, Rossi M, Davidson BR. Fewer-than-four ports versus four ports for laparoscopic cholecystectomy. Cochrane Database Syst Rev. 2014;2, CD007109.
21. Kroh M, El-Hayek K, Rosenblatt S, Chand B, Escobar P, Kaouk J, et al. First human surgery with a novel single-port robotic system: cholecystectomy using the da Vinci Single-Site platform. Surg Endosc. 2011;25(11):3566–73.
22. Pietrabissa A, Sbrana F, Morelli L, Badessi F, Pugliese L, Vinci A, et al. Overcoming the challenges of single-incision cholecystectomy with robotic single-site technology. Arch Surg. 2012;147(8):709–14.
23. Morel P, Buchs NC, Iranmanesh P, Pugin F, Buehler L, Azagury DE, et al. Robotic single-site cholecystectomy. J Hepatobiliary Pancreat Sci. 2014;21(1): 18–25.
24. Spinoglio G, Lenti LM, Maglione V, Lucido FS, Priora F, Bianchi PP, et al. Single-site robotic cholecystectomy (SSRC) versus single-incision laparoscopic cholecystectomy (SILC): comparison of

learning curves. First European experience. Surg Endosc. 2012;26(6):1648–55.
25. Tiwari MM, Reynoso JF, Lehman AC, Tsang AW, Farritor SM, Oleynikov D. In vivo miniature robots for natural orifice surgery: state of the art and future perspectives. World J Gastrointest Surg. 2010;2(6):217–23.
26. Barzana DC, Kotwall CA, Clancy TV, Hope WW. Use of laparoscopy in trauma at a level II trauma center. JSLS. 2011;15(2):179–81.
27. Lin HF, Wu JM, Tu CC, Chen HA, Shih HC. Value of diagnostic and therapeutic laparoscopy for abdominal stab wounds. World J Surg. 2010;34(7):1653–62.

31 Robotic Applications in Advancing General Surgery

Monika E. Hagen, William M. Tauxe, and Philippe Morel

History of Robotics for General Surgery

Considering the general expectations triggered by the history of robotics, their present applications in everyday life, as well as the robotic scenes from many science fiction movies of our days, the term "Robotic Surgery" prompts the false impression (at least until this point in time) that an autonomic system might perform surgical procedures without the direct interaction of a physician. As of today, surgical procedures—particularly involving continuous soft tissue deformation—are too dynamic and complex for a machine to perform all of them without human control. As such, the only autonomous surgical robots in use today are those applied for a specific surgical subtask such as taking a biopsy or aligning and positioning joint implants. However, nonautonomous robots, directed by human hands in real time, are gaining popularity for applications in the field of General Surgery. These are the "master-slave" machines where a surgeon controls the movements of the "robotic" device in real time and might therefore rather be categorized as remote manipulators, similar to the much larger machines used to deal with hazardous material.

The dawning of robotics for Digestive Surgery traces back to transdisciplinary co-operations in the Silicon Valley, located just outside San Francisco, California: During the 1980s the National Aeronautics and Space Administration (NASA) Ames Research Group developed one of the first versions of a head-mounted display, designed to transmit great amounts of data from NASA space missions to on-the-ground controllers [1]. In the same geographical area and around the same time, VPL Inc. invented "virtual reality" through the development of the DataGlove—a wired glove that allowed physical interaction with virtual scenes. These two innovative groups envisioned the potential of robotic surgery using the combination of their technologies. While necessary tools were already at hand for vision and control, a robotic end-effector needed to be developed. Since both groups lacked robotic expertise, the Stanford Research Institute (SRI) which possessed extensive robotic knowledge was invited to join the collaboration and a highly dexterous telemanipulator was produced. Under medical advice from local Stanford University, this

M.E. Hagen, M.D., M.B.A. (✉) • P. Morel, M.D.
Department of Surgery, Geneva University Hospital, 4 Rue Gabrielle-Perret-Gentil, Geneva 1211, Switzerland
e-mail: monikahagen@aol.com; philippe.morel@hcuge.ch

W.M. Tauxe, M.S.T.
Emory University School of Medicine, Atlanta, GA, USA
e-mail: wtauxe@emory.edu

R. Latifi et al. (eds.), *Technological Advances in Surgery, Trauma and Critical Care*,
DOI 10.1007/978-1-4939-2671-8_31

original system was intended to perform complex microsurgery such as hand transplantation.

However, other developments made the group turn to the application of robotics for General Surgery: The world's first laparoscopic appendectomy was performed by Kurt Semm in 1981 and it quickly became applied to many of the most common general surgical procedures within the next decade. Around the same time, the US Department of Defense developed an interest in funding research into tele-macro-surgery to provide surgical intervention to critically wounded service personnel during CASEVAC or MEDEVAC operations. This resulted in heavy funding by DARPA for several research groups including the above mentioned hand. Thus Ames, VPL, and SRI refocused their program to develop a robot suitable for laparoscopic surgery controlled by their telepresence system. This collaboration became very successful over the following years and produced a robotic system for minimally invasive surgery which was further refined and later commercialized by Intuitive Surgical Incorporation (Sunnyvale, CA, USA) as the da Vinci® Surgical System [2].

While the da Vinci Surgical System is currently the most commonly used robotic device for General Surgery, the earliest device in this category was the Automated Endoscopic System for Optimal Positioning (AESOP) which was developed by Computer Motion (Santa Barbara, CA, USA). AESOP was a system that allowed the surgeon to control the movement and position of a laparoscopic camera held by a robotic arm via voice recognition software eliminating the need for a surgical assistant to hold the camera. This allowed a steadier view with more consistent and precise camera movements. AESOP received clearance by the Food and Drug Administration (FDA) in 1993 shortly after its first human use [3]. In the years to follow, Computer Motion developed an entire robotic surgical system that was based on the design of the AESOP arm. The final product named ZEUS consisted of three arms arranged so that two held surgical instruments and one held the endoscopic camera. Much like the da Vinci Surgical System, the Zeus was a master-slave tool with remote manipulators telecontrolled from a surgical console. Early clinical work with the ZEUS commenced in 1998 and final FDA approval for this product was received in 2001. During the same year, ZEUS was used for the famous "Operation Lindberg" during which a patient in Strasbourg, France, underwent a robotic cholecystectomy by a surgeon working from a ZEUS console in New York City [4].

Although Intuitive Surgical and Computer Motion initially shared a competitive marketplace, the similarities between their designs led them to become embroiled in a legal dispute over intellectual property. This lawsuit, which diverted a great deal of corporate effort and funds from product research, finally ended when Intuitive Surgical claimed victory as well as the assets of Computer Motion, Inc. The distribution of ZEUS and AESOP was eventually discontinued and Intuitive took over the control of the market. Since then, Intuitive Surgical continued to market the da Vinci Surgical System which thus far has no serious competition in the field of laparoscopic robotics (June 2014).

The original da Vinci Standard System—which was introduced in 1999—was matured into the da Vinci S System which was released in 2006. Further enhancements resulted in the commercialization of the da Vinci Si in 2009 [5] (Fig. 31.1). This system was upgraded with a several features including dual-console capability, enhanced high-definition 3D vision, improved ergonomics, an updated user interface, and extensibility for digital OR integration. Several advanced instruments such as surgical staplers with wristed articulation and Single Site Instrumentation were exclusively developed for this model.

The latest version, the da Vinci Xi Surgical System, was released for the US market in early 2014. This system is designed to facilitate the process of surgical access with a newly designed, more flexible robotic arm configuration (Fig. 31.2). The Xi surgical cart can thus access all four surgical quadrants from a single position, which greatly simplifies setup. The arms of the Xi system are also thinner and provide a greater range of motion when compared to the previous models. This novel arm design in combination

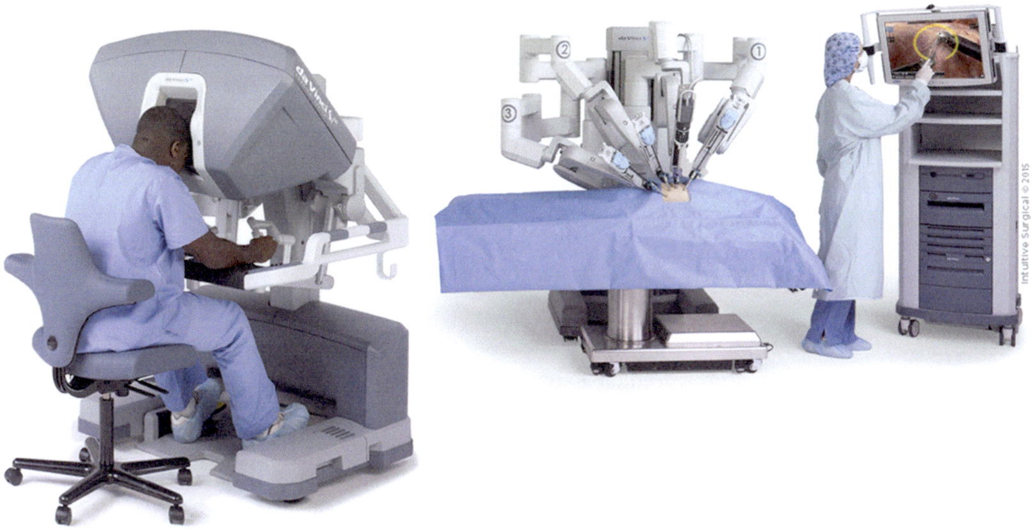

Fig. 31.1 The da Vinci® Si Surgical System. (Used with permission. Copyright © 2015 Intuitive Surgical Inc.)

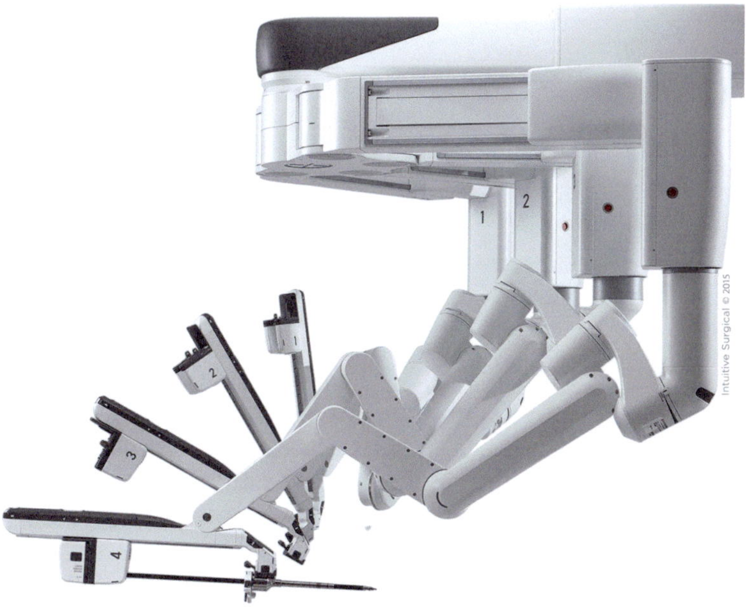

Fig. 31.2 Robotics arms of the da Vinci® Xi System with improved flexibility. (Used with permission. Copyright © 2015 Intuitive Surgical Inc.)

with instruments of longer reach offers a more flexible port placement. The surgical cart hosts a number of new features including a guided setup process with voice assistance to facilitate a quick and precise setup. A laser targeting system is used to help arrange the surgical cart and the robotic arms in an optimal configuration around the targeted anatomy [6].

While the technology of the da Vinci Surgical Systems has been progressively updated, all systems remain are very similar in their basic components and contain a surgeon's console, a surgical cart, and a vision cart. They share the following core features as major differences to conventional laparoscopy:

- All systems are designed in a master-slave configuration with physical separation of the surgeon and the patient.
- Vision system with a true 3-dimensional image with up to ten times magnification streamed into the stereo viewer of the surgical console resulting in a panoramic view of the surgical field (Fig. 31.3).
- Wristed instruments (Fig. 31.4) with seven degrees of freedom and intuitive control (Fig. 31.5) due to the humanoid design of the robotic anatomy (robotic arm and instruments mimic the human upper extremity—movements of surgeon's hands are followed by surgical instruments).
- All systems are equipped with distinct software feature including motion scaling and tremor filtration.

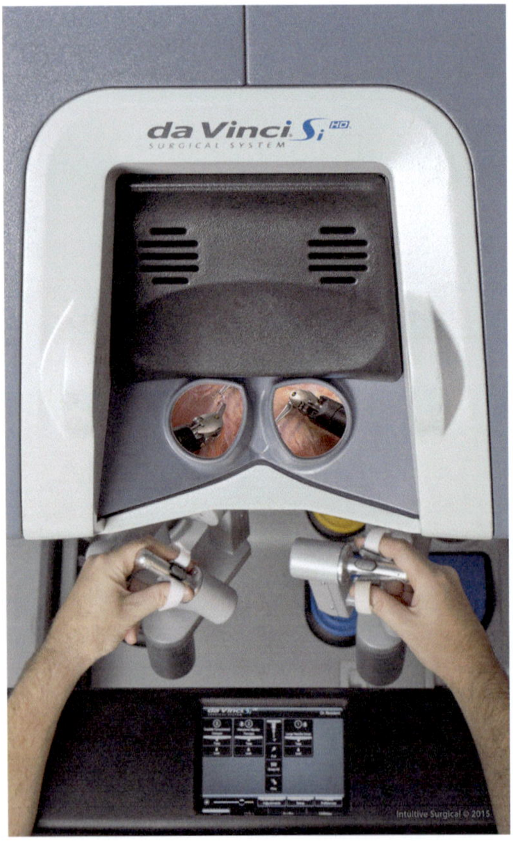

Fig. 31.3 The da Vinci® stereo viewer. (Used with permission. Copyright © 2015 Intuitive Surgical Inc.)

Considering the above descriptions of the da Vinci Surgical System, it seems apparent that this robotic system offers distinct technical advantages when compared to conventional laparoscopy. Since its first clinical application for a cholecystectomy in 1997 and its market launch in 1999, the system has been used for an increasing amount of surgical procedures including operations from many fields of surgery [7–9]. With growing clinical experience, it soon became evident that the da Vinci could enable advanced surgical procedures to be performed in a minimally invasive fashion [10]. Perioperative parameters are usually improved for almost all surgical procedures when performed via minimally invasive surgery versus an open approach. Although an initial goal of the da Vinci was to perform complex cardiac surgeries, a group of German surgeons found particular value in the system when working in the tight confines of the male pelvis and developed a robotic approach to radical prostatectomy [11]. This insight led to a growing adoption of the da Vinci for this challenging procedure. At the time of this publication, the value of robotic technology for radical prostatectomy has been clearly established by numerous high-level-of-evidence manuscripts, including prospectively randomized trials and meta-analyses. It is the recommended surgical method for this procedure by several clinical guidelines as well as Health Technology Assessments [12].

In continuous pursuit of improving techniques and reduced invasiveness, abdominal surgeons also developed interest in this technology. Reports can be found in the literature of many robotic digestive surgical procedures that have been performed successfully including benign and malignant foregut surgery, colorectal surgery, bariatric surgery, endocrine surgery, hepato-biliary-pancreatic surgery as well as many others.

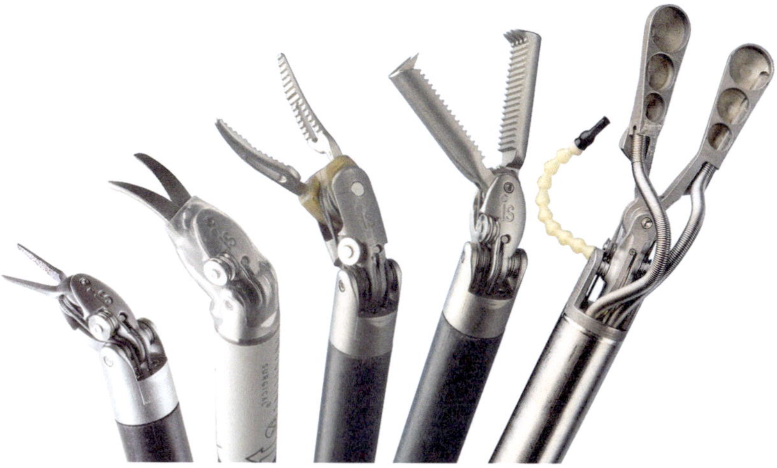

Fig. 31.4 da Vinci® wristed instruments. (Used with permission. Copyright © 2015 Intuitive Surgical Inc.)

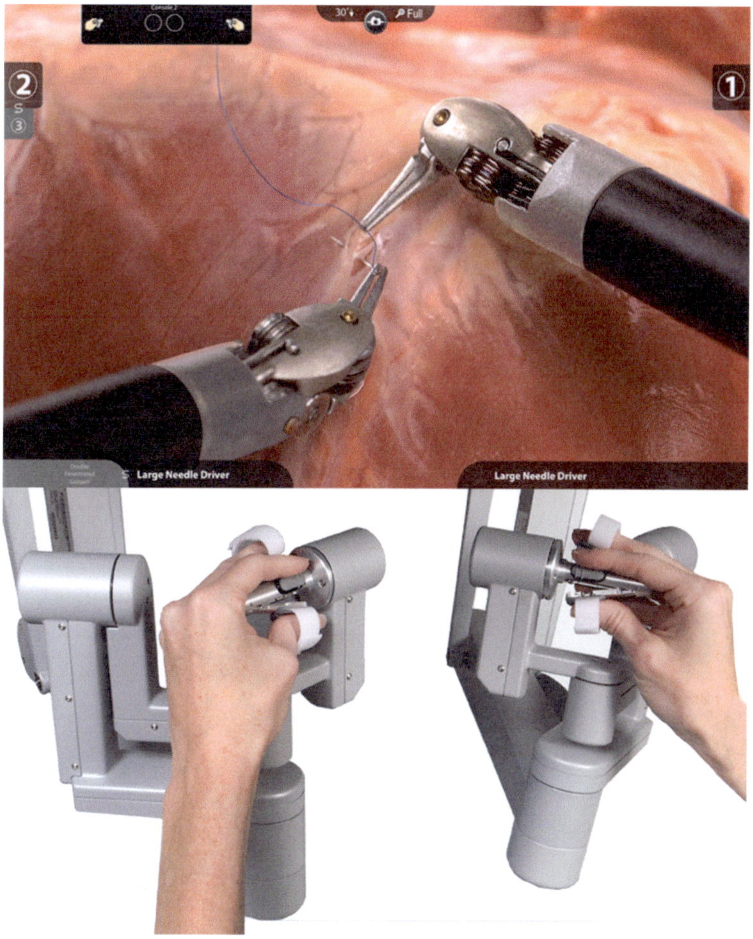

Fig. 31.5 Intuitive control of robotic instruments achieved by humanoid design of the da Vinci® Surgical System and hand-eye alignment. (Used with permission. Copyright © 2015 Intuitive Surgical Inc.)

Clinical Applications of Robotics in General Surgery

Upper Gastrointestinal Tract

Early reports of robotic anti-reflux surgery can be found in the literature of the performance of *fundoplication*. While many reports demonstrate the general feasibility of the robotic approach for this procedure, no clear clinical advantages over a laparoscopic approach can be derived from the current literature. However, several studies suggest it entails increased operative time and costs of surgery [13, 14].

A similar conclusion can be arrived at for the procedure of robotic *Heller myotomy*. While some publications suggest a lower rate of perforations with the robotic application, the overall data indicate general feasibility of a robotic approach to Heller myotomy with no clear clinical advantage over laparoscopic technique [15–17].

While many procedures of the field of *bariatric surgery* are most commonly performed with conventional laparoscopy, several distinct anatomical challenges often exist, including a thick abdominal wall, hepatomegaly, and increased amounts of intra-abdominal fat. These constraints produce a limited workspace, which results in reduced surgical dexterity and impaired ergonomics during conventional laparoscopy. Several publications from other fields of surgery indicate that robotics may facilitate surgery in the obese population [18, 19] and the number of clinical reports of robotic applications for a variety of bariatric procedures is growing.

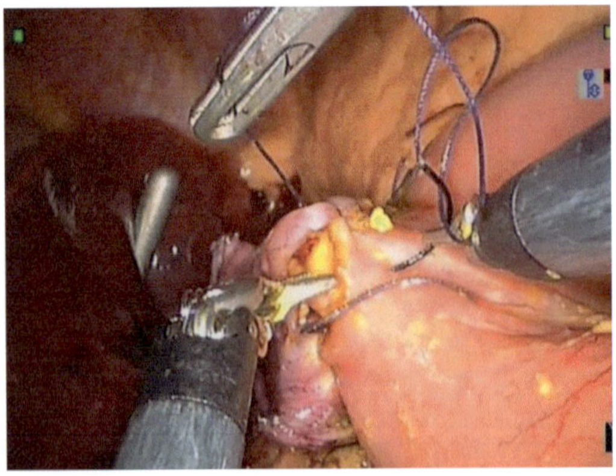

Fig. 31.6 da Vinci® (Intuitive Surgical Inc; Sunnyvale, CA) sutured gastrojejunal anastomosis

At this point, the largest body of clinical evidence on robotic use for bariatric indications can be found for *Roux-en-Y gastric bypass* (RYGB) with early reports beginning in 2003. Since that time, multiple groups have published their clinical outcomes with a variety of surgical methods including hybrid and total robotic approaches to RYGB. While some of the early articles reported challenges of the robotic technology, mainly around the absence of force feedback leading to bowel injuries [20], more recent comparative studies [21–23] as well as systematic reviews [24, 25] do offer some evidence supporting the clinical advantages of robotic RYGB surgery including low rates of anastomotic strictures and leaks. These potential clinical advantages of robotic technique can be explained by the different techniques usually used for the creation of a laparoscopic gastrojejunal anastomosis. While the technical challenges of creating a sutured anastomosis laparoscopically caused a shift towards stapled technique during conventional laparoscopy, the robotic technology enables a return to the hand-sutured style of gastrojejunal anastomosis (Fig. 31.6) which is believed to be superior when compared to stapling. In support of this theory, several comparative studies have shown a lower leak and stricture rate of the gastrojejunal anastomosis when using a robotically sutured technique compared to laparoscopic stapling [21, 23]. A meta-analysis further recognized an advantage regarding postoperative strictures after robotic RYGB when compared to the laparoscopic technique [25].

While the clinical data of RYGB show some clear indications in regard to the clinical value of the robotic technology, the value of a robotic approach to *sleeve gastrectomy* (SG) seems less clear. Although the robotic approach may facilitate the mobilization of the stomach and enable suturing of the previously stapled tissue, the most critical element of this procedure is currently still most commonly performed using laparoscopic staplers. Robotic staplers have just recently been released in the United States only, and exclusively for the da Vinci Si System. Further experience with the robotic staplers will show whether this procedure might gain significance as a robotic approach. To date, literature on robotic SG indicates general feasibility and safety with longer operative times [26, 27]. One research group analyzed their series of robotic assisted SGs and compared data to a systematic review of laparoscopic sleeve gastrectomies (LSG): Lower leak and stricture rates were found with the robotic approach to SG [28].

The first robotic bariatric procedure performed was a robotic placement of an *adjustable gastric band* (AGB) by Cadiere and Himpens in 1998 [29]. Subsequently, other authors have reported on the feasibility and safety of performing robotic AGB placement [30, 31]. Although it seems apparent that robotic technology can provide advantages during some parts of the dissection and suturing the anterior gastric plication, the lack of tactile feedback may be a disadvantage during the "blind" preparation of the posterior gastric tunnel. In addition, AGB is a surgical procedure of low complexity and few perioperative complications occur when it is performed laparoscopically. Therefore, the incremental clinical value of robotics to this procedure might be limited considering the added cost.

Besides these common bariatric procedures, robotics has also been applied to some more advanced procedures including *biliopancreatic diversion with duodenal switch* (BPD/DS) and *revisional surgery* (RS) [32]. While both procedures are of advanced complexity and therefore have the potential to benefit significantly from the technical advantages of a robotic approach, a very limited number of reports of its application can be found in the literature. Due to its limited application and the extensive need for multiquadrant access (from stomach to ileocecal valve), BPD/DS will most likely not develop into a dominating robotic indication. The new da Vinci Xi system is designed for four-quadrant access and may demonstrate increased suitability for this procedure in the future. Revisional surgery is currently significantly increasing in terms of case numbers and the complex nature of these procedures makes it ideal for the robotic approach. It is expected that the body of evidence in regard to robotic RS will increase over the next few years and shed more light on the value of robotics for this bariatric procedure.

Several reports can be found in the robotic application for early *gastric cancer* with similar indications as for a laparoscopic approach. Overall data suggest that robotic surgery for gastric cancer is safe, feasible, and results in similar perioperative outcomes when compared to conventional laparoscopy [33–35]. In addition, it has been suggested that the technical specifications of the robotic technology enable a minimally invasive approach to D-2 lymphadenectomy [35]. This procedure has been established as the gold standard of treatment, with improved long-term oncological outcomes for the patients when compared to a limited D-1 lymphadenectomy [36]. More systematic data is needed to verify this potentially very meaningful advantage of robotics over conventional laparoscopy.

Colorectal Surgery

Besides evidence of general feasibility, the role of robotics in *colon surgery* remains undetermined at this point: While the technical advantages of robotics could play a role during more complex maneuvers including extended lymphadenectomy (D3 for right colectomy) and the formation of intra-corporeal anastomoses, more substantial clinical evidence is needed to verify clinical advantages of robotic technology for colon surgery.

A greater body of evidence can be found for the application of robotics in *rectal surgery*, particularly regarding the treatment of rectal cancer (Fig. 31.7). While conventional laparoscopy can be safe and effective for the resection of rectal cancer by experienced hands, relatively high rates of conversions and circumferential margin positivity have been demonstrated by systematic research [37–39]. Therefore, the laparoscopic approach has not yet been established as the gold standard approach for patients with rectal cancer [40, 41]. The technical superiority of robotics holds the promise to overcome the limitations of

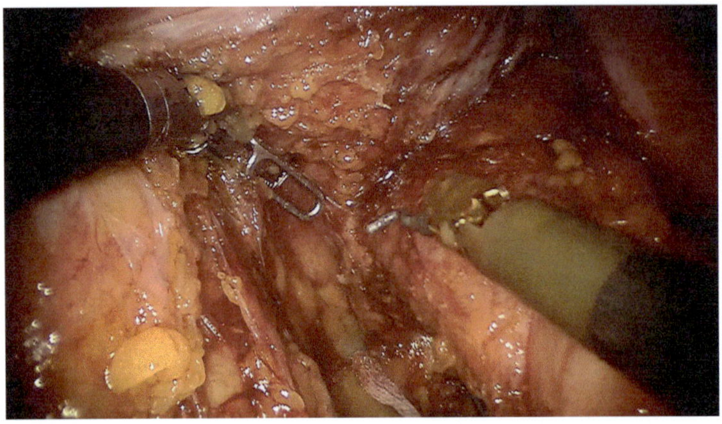

Fig. 31.7 da Vinci® (Intuitive Surgical Inc; Sunnyvale, CA) low anterior resection

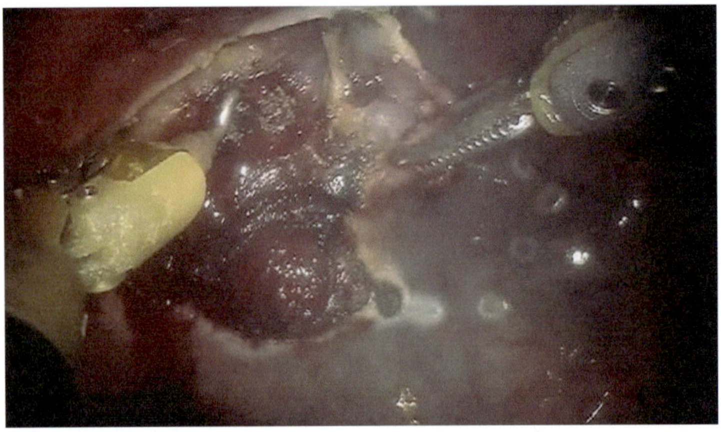

Fig. 31.8 da Vinci® (Intuitive Surgical Inc; Sunnyvale, CA) transanal surgery

conventional laparoscopy in this setting and may result in fewer conversions and reduced rates of positive margins when compared to conventional laparoscopy [10]. While most of the studies of this sort which have been performed to date are of limited quality and therefore prone to bias, more systematic research of the field of robotics for rectal cancer is currently under way and first results are expected soon.

An emerging and highly interesting novel procedure is a robotic application in *transanal resection* of low-risk rectal cancers and benign conditions (Fig. 31.8). Several research groups have published their laboratory experience as well as initial clinical experience of transanal robotic surgery for local excisions and retrograde total mesorectal excision [42, 43].

A number of reports from the field of robotic *hepatobiliary surgery* can be found. Robotic pancreatic resections have been performed for a variety of procedures including distal, central, and total pancreatectomy as well as for pancreaticoduodenectomy [44, 45]. Current literature suggests the feasibility of robotic pancreatic resection with potential advantages over open and laparoscopic surgery in terms of short-term outcomes. However, quality of these studies is limited and more systematic research is needed to verify these positive early findings. Similarly, robotic liver resections have been reported to be safe and feasible in experienced hands [46, 47]. While robotic technology seems to have advantages that facilitate a variety of surgical maneuvers that are needed during liver resection, more advanced robotic instrumentation will be needed to enable widespread application.

Single-Site Surgery

While some groups reported their early experience with robotic surgery through a single incision using the conventional da Vinci instruments in unconventional arrangements [48], a dedicated set of semi-rigid instruments and curved cannulae for robotic *single-site surgery* was released in 2011 [49]. This platform was predominantly used for cholecystectomy (Fig. 31.9). Literature shows the general safety and feasibility of the technique with potentially shorter OR times and facilitated learning curves when compared to conventional single-incision laparoscopy [50, 51]. Several reports can be found on the application of robotic single-site surgery for other procedures [52].

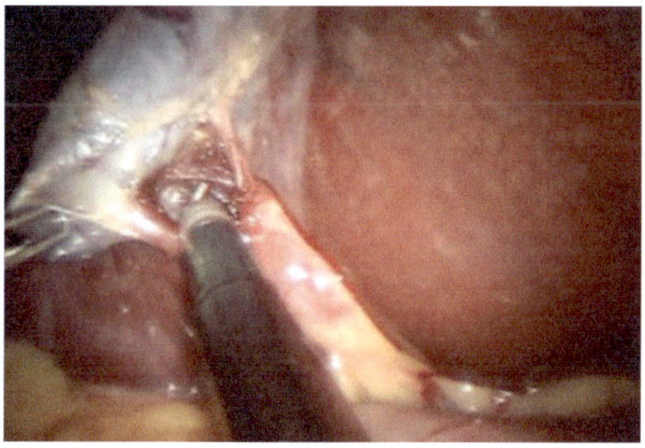

Fig. 31.9 da Vinci® (Intuitive Surgical Inc; Sunnyvale, CA) Single-Site cholecystectomy

Fluorescence Imaging

Recently, an intraoperative *near infrared fluorescence imaging system* has been developed for the use with the da Vinci Si system. The technology has been used during a variety of surgical procedures to visualize blood flow (Fig. 31.10), lymph node mapping, intraoperative cholangiography and to identify anatomy of the surgical field [53–55]. Systematic research will be needed to determine the impact of this technology on clinical outcomes.

Limitations of Current Robotic Systems for General Surgery

Despite the clear technological advance represented by surgical robotics and potential it holds to overcome several limitations of conventional laparoscopy, the use of robotic systems in the present day does not come without controversy: There is abundant data to suggest that robotics are safe and feasible for many procedures in General Surgery, but overall clinical outcomes are often not superior when compared to conventional laparoscopy and/or open surgery.

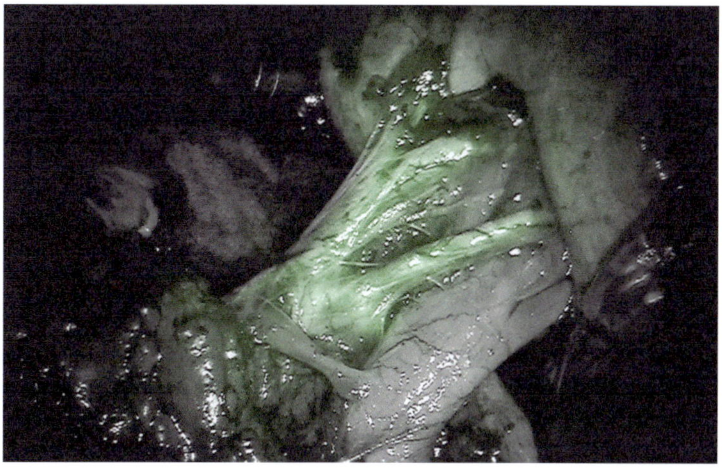

Fig. 31.10 da Vinci® (Intuitive Surgical Inc; Sunnyvale, CA) fluorescence imaging of renal hilum

While some studies suggest clinical advantages in certain applications, the clear value of robotics and its role in General Surgery remains undefined. Robotics entails increased costs due to capital investment, system maintenance, and reposable instruments, so it must prove it can deliver short- and long-term patient benefits by providing unique solutions to otherwise unobtainable clinical demands in order to be cost effective. Unfortunately, current published studies on this topic are low-level-of-evidence and are therefore prone to bias. Various prospectively randomized trials from different fields of General Surgery are currently underway to answer some of these important questions that stand in the way of robotics becoming the gold standard for numerous procedures of the field of General Surgery.

Future and Alternative Robotic Systems for General Surgery

In addition to the da Vinci family, a variety of other robotic surgical systems are being developed and implemented at the present time. Some are master-slave robots with operator consoles and instrument carts which will provide competition for the da Vinci. Another group of robots finding surgical applications is direct image-guided robots. These rely on imaging of the patient to calculate their motions and usually specialized to a particular task, such as reaming cavities in bone for precision-fit implants. Additionally, research and development of miniaturized self-propelled devices capable of operating within the body via remote control offers the potential for a true quantum leap in surgical technique in the future.

Console-and-Cart Systems

These systems share many of the essential features of the da Vinci and may be thought of as two-piece sets of matching surgical furniture. The surgeon is seated at the control console and observes the camera feed on a computer screen and controls the manipulator arms using hand and/or foot controls. The patient lies on a bed locked to the surgical cart on which are mounted the manipulator arms which conduct the operation. A persistent bottleneck in the efficient operation of console-and-cart systems is the lengthy setup process required to arrange the patient and the cart respective to each other and insert the endoscopic arms into the body cavity. Additionally, the cost of sterile single-use disposable robotic components can be significant. However, console-and-cart systems are intrinsically suited to teleoperation and telementoring as has been described in the da Vinci Si system.

Because of Intuitive's established dominance in the field of surgical robotic intellectual property, development of other general-purpose robotics platforms has been driven by innovation. Although no comparable system has yet been released for widespread commercial distribution, several products are anticipated to be available soon. Each offers a different strategy to refine and improve the existing technology in hopes of creating superior patient outcomes. A common complaint about the da Vinci system is the lack of tactile feedback in the motor controllers which can lead to unnecessary strain on tissues. This has provided an avenue for new development. The Verro Touch is a product under development at the University of Pennsylvania, Philadelphia, PA, to add haptic capabilities to the da Vinci system. It provides tactile and auditory feedback to a da Vinci operator based on instrument vibration. An analogous accessory potentially familiar to the reader is the Nintendo® Rumble Pak (Kyoto, Japan).

The ALF-X Telelap system, developed by SOFAR s.p.a. in Milano, Italy, is a four-arm system which seeks to streamline the robotic surgical experience using enhanced tactile and visual feedback for the surgeon as well as a cheaper and faster setup. Their console system uses eye-tracking technology to allow surgeons to better control their camera view without taking their hands from the manipulator controls.

Titan Medical, Inc. in Toronto, Canada, is developing a single-incision system slated for release pending FDA approval in 2015. The cart unit uses small flexible endoscopic instruments sharing a common 25 mm cannula with the camera. The single-incision approach is anticipated to contribute to increased setup speed and improved patient outcomes.

The DLR MIRO is a modular system being developed by the Institute of Robotics and Mechatronics in Oberpfaffenhofen, Germany. The MIRO is a multi-jointed surgical arm which can be used alone or in groups to perform a wide variety of surgical tasks. Thus, a single MIRO might be used in conjunction with a human surgeon to perform specific visualization or manipulation tasks.

Direct Image-Guided Robots

Another developing field of surgical robotics involves the use of robots whose movements are not controlled by the surgeon in real time. Instead, their motions are controlled by a computer to precisely fit anatomical constraints determined from imaging. Because they are guided directly by the patient's anatomy, they are called "Direct Image-Guided Robots"; however, they might also be thought of as "smart power tools." These robots are intended for extremely specific tasks where close tolerances are desirable.

The first such system was the Cyberknife® (Accuray, Sunnyvale, CA), approved by the FDA for human use in 2001 and used to deliver precision dosages of radiation to tissue. The system uses an articulated emitter arm as well as a sensing system to adjust the emitter arm's actions to allow for patient motion due to breathing, etc. Using imaging data, the Cyberknife bathes the desired site in radiation from multiple angles, reducing the effect on surrounding tissue. It has a demonstrated track record of successful use on a wide variety of tumors in locations throughout the body. Other DIGRs have been approved for use as well. The SpineAssist® by Mazor Robotics of Caesarea, Israel, is designed for assisting in orthopedic spinal procedures to ensure precise drilling of implant holes. The Robotic Arm Interactive Orthopedic System (RIO®) by MAKO Surgical Corp in Fort Lauderdale, FL, uses pre-obtained imaging to delineate the motion of its cutting arm for resurfacing bone during arthroplastic procedures. Much current DIGR development is focused on magnetic resonance imaging to guide access to specific regions such as the prostate, but no such robotic systems have been approved to date.

Miniaturized Surgical Robotics

Advances in miniaturization offer the opportunity to design small autonomous robots capable of operating within the patient's body under remote control. Such an approach would minimize tissue manipulation and afford improved access to sensitive or difficult-to-reach targets such as the heart or retroperitoneum. Although the promise of such technology is great, clinical applications are still thin on the ground.

The PillCam® series from Given Imaging of Yoqneam, Israel, offers real-time imaging and pH monitoring of the gastrointestinal tract. The PillCam is a self-contained passive sensor system which is moved through the gut by peristalsis. Unlike endoscopy, the PillCam does not require the use of lavage or laxative preparation which can result in dysbiosis. It also permits easy visualization of the complete small intestine, including regions not accessible via endoscopy.

The PillCam already offers some clear advantages over endoscopic techniques, and future advances are predicted. One approach is to make a PillCam with a ferromagnetic core. Using an external 3D electromagnetic field, it will then be possible to control the orientation and movement of the PillCam within the patient. With this capability, a more active interventional role is possible if other miniaturized systems like electrocautery tips, biopsy forceps, or pharmaceutical dispensers are included in the design.

Other miniaturized robotic systems are still under development using a variety of movement techniques. The Heartlander, under development at the Robotics Institute of Carnegie Mellon University, Pittsburgh, PA, uses an inchworm-like locomotion system to gently move around on the epicardium. Researchers at Hanyang University in Seoul, South Korea, have developed a microbot intended to crawl inside blood vessels to address occlusive disease. This system uses an external electromagnetic system to power the actuators that allow it to move; this avoids the need for carrying a bulky onboard power source. Although these systems are not ready for clinical application in humans, they have shown promise in animal trials and give a glimpse of the capabilities this technology may eventually offer.

Future Perspective for Robotic Applications in General Surgery

Besides the concrete technical advantages that robotic systems bring today, the true future value of surgical robotic systems lies in the fact that they are information-based systems. This allows them to uniquely integrate many other technologies that are currently or could be used in or around surgery. This could include, for example, the superimposition of preoperative imaging over the surgeon's real-time view of the anatomy. The fusion of such data with the surgical video and its integration with surgical instrumentation control will result in increased precision of surgical dissection and many other tasks. With further expected advances in soft tissue deformation calculations, it will be possible to load preoperative data sets including patient imaging into surgical robots for preoperative planning and rehearsals of the procedure using simulation technologies. As a final step in the logical progression of this thought it is conceivable that 1 day, robotic procedures will first be performed virtually by surgeons on a simulation of the patient's anatomy, allowing them to stop, rewind, or restart the procedure as they desire. When the surgeon is satisfied with the surgical run, the robot is programmed to perform the same procedure on the patient, using the same unerring motions but in a fraction of the time required by a well-trained but unpracticed human surgeon. In addition, the computerized element of robotic surgery has an immense potential for long distance surgery and the remote surgical training and telementoring. In considering such possibilities, it becomes apparent that the future of robotic surgery is limited only by our imagination and the ultimate possibilities of this technology are endless. Robotics will profoundly transform the practice of surgery and we are only just beginning to see the revolutionary changes it will bring to how we care for our patients in the years to come.

References

1. Fisher SS, McGreevy M, Humphries J, et al. Virtual environment display system. In: Crow F, Pizer S, editors. Proceedings of the workshop on interactive 3-dimensional graphics. New York: AMC; 1986. p. 1–12.
2. Satava RM. Robotic surgery: from past to future – a personal journey. Surg Clin North Am. 2003;83(6): 1491–500. 6.
3. Ewing DR, Pigazzi A, Wang Y, Ballantyne GH. Robots in the operating room – the history. Semin Laparosc Surg. 2004;11(2):63–71.
4. Marescaux J. Code name: "Lindbergh operation". Ann Chir. 2002;127(1):2–4.
5. http://www.intuitivesurgical.com/products/.
6. Abboudi H, Khan MS, Aboumarzouk O, Guru KA, Challacombe B, Dasgupta P, et al. Current status of validation for robotic surgery simulators – a systematic review. BJU Int. 2013;111(2):194–205.
7. Baek SJ, Kim SH. Robotics in general surgery: an evidence-based review. Asian J Endosc Surg. 2014;7(2):117–23.
8. Augustin F, Bodner J, Wykypiel H, Schwinghammer C, Schmid T. Perioperative results of robotic lung lobectomy: summary of literature. Surg Endosc. 2012;26(4):1190–1.
9. Genden EM, O'Malley Jr BW, Weinstein GS, Stucken CL, Selber JC, Rinaldo A, et al. Transoral robotic surgery: role in the management of upper aerodigestive tract tumors. Head Neck. 2012;34(6):886–93.
10. Collinson FJ, Jayne DG, Pigazzi A, Tsang C, Barrie JM, Edlin R, et al. An international, multicentre, prospective, randomised, controlled, unblinded, parallel-group trial of robotic-assisted versus standard laparoscopic surgery for the curative treatment of rectal cancer. Int J Colorectal Dis. 2012;27(2):233–41.
11. Binder J, Kramer W. Robotically-assisted laparoscopic radical prostatectomy. BJU Int. 2001;87(4): 408–10.
12. (DGU) DGfU. Interdisziplinäre Leitlinie der Qualität S3 zur Früherkennung, Diagnose und Therapie der verschiedenen Stadien des Prostatakarzinoms Version 1.03 – März 2011.
13. Nakadi IE, Melot C, Closset J, DeMoor V, Betroune K, Feron P, et al. Evaluation of da Vinci Nissen fundoplication clinical results and cost minimization. World J Surg. 2006;30(6):1050–4.
14. Markar SR, Karthikesalingam AP, Hagen ME, Talamini M, Horgan S, Wagner OJ. Robotic vs. laparoscopic Nissen fundoplication for gastro-oesophageal reflux disease: systematic review and meta-analysis. Int J Med Robot. 2010;6(2):125–31.

15. Galvani C, Gorodner MV, Moser F, Baptista M, Donahue P, Horgan S. Laparoscopic Heller myotomy for achalasia facilitated by robotic assistance. Surg Endosc. 2006;20(7):1105–12.
16. Horgan S, Galvani C, Gorodner MV, Omelanczuck P, Elli F, Moser F, et al. Robotic-assisted Heller myotomy versus laparoscopic Heller myotomy for the treatment of esophageal achalasia: multicenter study. J Gastrointest Surg. 2005;9(8):1020–9. discussion 9–30.
17. Shaligram A, Unnirevi J, Simorov A, Kothari VM, Oleynikov D. How does the robot affect outcomes? A retrospective review of open, laparoscopic, and robotic Heller myotomy for achalasia. Surg Endosc. 2012;26(4):1047–50.
18. Gallo T, Kashani S, Patel DA, Elsahwi K, Silasi DA, Azodi M. Robotic-assisted laparoscopic hysterectomy: outcomes in obese and morbidly obese patients. JSLS. 2012;16(3):421–7.
19. Hemli JM, Darla LS, Panetta CR, Jennings J, Subramanian VA, Patel NC. Does body mass index affect outcomes in robotic-assisted coronary artery bypass procedures? Innovations (Phila). 2012;7(5): 350–3.
20. Hubens G, Balliu L, Ruppert M, Gypen B, Van Tu T, Vaneerdeweg W. Roux-en-Y gastric bypass procedure performed with the da Vinci robot system: is it worth it? Surg Endosc. 2008;22(7):1690–6.
21. Hagen ME, Pugin F, Chassot G, Huber O, Buchs N, Iranmanesh P, et al. Reducing cost of surgery by avoiding complications: the model of robotic Roux-en-Y gastric bypass. Obes Surg. 2012;22(1):52–61.
22. Ayloo SM, Addeo P, Buchs NC, Shah G, Giulianotti PC. Robot-assisted versus laparoscopic Roux-en-Y gastric bypass: is there a difference in outcomes? World J Surg. 2011;35(3):637–42.
23. Park CW, Lam EC, Walsh TM, Karimoto M, Ma AT, Koo M, et al. Robotic-assisted Roux-en-Y gastric bypass performed in a community hospital setting: the future of bariatric surgery? Surg Endosc. 2011;25(10): 3312–21.
24. Fourman MM, Saber AA. Robotic bariatric surgery: a systematic review. Surg Obes Relat Dis. 2012;8(4): 483–8.
25. Markar SR, Karthikesalingam AP, Venkat-Ramen V, Kinross J, Ziprin P. Robotic vs. laparoscopic Roux-en-Y gastric bypass in morbidly obese patients: systematic review and pooled analysis. Int J Med Robot. 2011;7(4):393–400.
26. Ayloo S, Buchs NC, Addeo P, Bianco FM, Giulianotti PC. Robot-assisted sleeve gastrectomy for super-morbidly obese patients. J Laparoendosc Adv Surg Tech A. 2011;21(4):295–9.
27. Diamantis T, Alexandrou A, Nikiteas N, Giannopoulos A, Papalambros E. Initial experience with robotic sleeve gastrectomy for morbid obesity. Obes Surg. 2011;21(8):1172–9.
28. Romero RJ, Kosanovic R, Rabaza JR, Seetharamaiah R, Donkor C, Gallas M, et al. Robotic sleeve gastrectomy: experience of 134 cases and comparison with a systematic review of the laparoscopic approach. Obes Surg. 2013;23(11):1743–52.
29. Cadiere GB, Himpens J, Vertruyen M, Favretti F. The world's first obesity surgery performed by a surgeon at a distance. Obes Surg. 1999;9(2):206–9.
30. Muhlmann G, Klaus A, Kirchmayr W, Wykypiel H, Unger A, Holler E, et al. DaVinci robotic-assisted laparoscopic bariatric surgery: is it justified in a routine setting? Obes Surg. 2003;13(6):848–54.
31. Edelson PK, Dumon KR, Sonnad SS, Shafi BM, Williams NN. Robotic vs. conventional laparoscopic gastric banding: a comparison of 407 cases. Surg Endosc. 2011;25(5):1402–8.
32. Sudan R, Puri V, Sudan D. Robotically assisted biliary pancreatic diversion with a duodenal switch: a new technique. Surg Endosc. 2007;21(5):729–33.
33. Anderson C, Ellenhorn J, Hellan M, Pigazzi A. Pilot series of robot-assisted laparoscopic subtotal gastrectomy with extended lymphadenectomy for gastric cancer. Surg Endosc. 2007;21(9):1662–6.
34. Baek SJ, Lee DW, Park SS, Kim SH. Current status of robot-assisted gastric surgery. World J Gastrointest Oncol. 2011;3(10):137–43.
35. D'Annibale A, Pende V, Pernazza G, Monsellato I, Mazzocchi P, Lucandri G, et al. Full robotic gastrectomy with extended (D2) lymphadenectomy for gastric cancer: surgical technique and preliminary results. J Surg Res. 2011;166(2):e113–20.
36. Songun I, Putter H, Kranenbarg EM, Sasako M, van de Velde CJ. Surgical treatment of gastric cancer: 15-year follow-up results of the randomised nationwide Dutch D1D2 trial. Lancet Oncol. 2010;11(5): 439–49.
37. Agha A, Benseler V, Hornung M, Gerken M, Iesalnieks I, Furst A, et al. Long-term oncologic outcome after laparoscopic surgery for rectal cancer. Surg Endosc. 2014;28(4):1119–25.
38. Dulucq JL, Wintringer P, Stabilini C, Mahajna A. Laparoscopic rectal resection with anal sphincter preservation for rectal cancer: long-term outcome. Surg Endosc. 2005;19(11):1468–74.
39. Guillou PJ, Quirke P, Thorpe H, Walker J, Jayne DG, Smith AM, et al. Short-term endpoints of conventional versus laparoscopic-assisted surgery in patients with colorectal cancer (MRC CLASICC trial): multicentre, randomised controlled trial. Lancet. 2005; 365(9472):1718–26.
40. Row D, Weiser MR. An update on laparoscopic resection for rectal cancer. Cancer Control. 2010;17(1): 16–24.
41. Pox C, Aretz S, Bischoff SC, Graeven U, Hass M, Heussner P, et al. S3-guideline colorectal cancer version 1.0. Z Gastroenterol. 2013;51(8):753–854.
42. Buchs NC, Pugin F, Volonte F, Hagen ME, Morel P, Ris F. Robotic transanal endoscopic microsurgery: technical details for the lateral approach. Dis Colon Rectum. 2013;56(10):1194–8.

43. Hompes R, Rauh SM, Hagen ME, Mortensen NJ. Preclinical cadaveric study of transanal endoscopic da Vinci(R) surgery. Br J Surg. 2012;99(8):1144–8.
44. Giulianotti PC, Addeo P, Buchs NC, Ayloo SM, Bianco FM. Robotic extended pancreatectomy with vascular resection for locally advanced pancreatic tumors. Pancreas. 2011;40(8):1264–70.
45. Giulianotti PC, Addeo P, Buchs NC, Bianco FM, Ayloo SM. Early experience with robotic total pancreatectomy. Pancreas. 2011;40(2):311–3.
46. Giulianotti PC, Coratti A, Sbrana F, Addeo P, Bianco FM, Buchs NC, et al. Robotic liver surgery: results for 70 resections. Surgery. 2011;149(1):29–39.
47. Buchs NC, Oldani G, Orci LA, Majno PE, Mentha G, Morel P, et al. Current status of robotic liver resection: a systematic review. Expert Rev Anticancer Ther. 2014;14(2):237–46.
48. Hagen ME, Wagner OJ, Inan I, Morel P, Fasel J, Jacobsen G, et al. Robotic single-incision transabdominal and transvaginal surgery: initial experience with intersecting robotic arms. Int J Med Robot. 2010;6(3):251–5.
49. Kroh M, El-Hayek K, Rosenblatt S, Chand B, Escobar P, Kaouk J, et al. First human surgery with a novel single-port robotic system: cholecystectomy using the da Vinci Single-Site platform. Surg Endosc. 2011; 25(11):3566–73.
50. Morel P, Hagen ME, Bucher P, Buchs NC, Pugin F. Robotic single-port cholecystectomy using a new platform: initial clinical experience. J Gastrointest Surg. 2011;15(12):2182–6.
51. Spinoglio G, Lenti LM, Maglione V, Lucido FS, Priora F, Bianchi PP, et al. Single-site robotic cholecystectomy (SSRC) versus single-incision laparoscopic cholecystectomy (SILC): comparison of learning curves. First European experience. Surg Endosc. 2012;26(6):1648–55.
52. Morelli L, Guadagni S, Caprili G, Candio GD, Boggi U, Mosca F. Robotic right colectomy using the Da Vinci Single-Site(R) platform: case report. Int J Med Robot. 2013;9(3):258–61.
53. Hellan M, Spinoglio G, Pigazzi A, Lagares-Garcia JA. The influence of fluorescence imaging on the location of bowel transection during robotic left-sided colorectal surgery. Surg Endosc. 2014;28(5): 1695–702.
54. Buchs NC, Hagen ME, Pugin F, Volonte F, Bucher P, Schiffer E, et al. Intra-operative fluorescent cholangiography using indocyanin green during robotic single site cholecystectomy. Int J Med Robot. 2012;8(4): 436–40.
55. Holloway RW, Bravo RA, Rakowski JA, James JA, Jeppson CN, Ingersoll SB, et al. Detection of sentinel lymph nodes in patients with endometrial cancer undergoing robotic-assisted staging: a comparison of colorimetric and fluorescence imaging. Gynecol Oncol. 2012;126(1):25–9.

Natural Orifice Transluminal Endoscopic Surgery (NOTES)

32

Mehmet Mahir Ozmen

Introduction

Natural Orifice Transluminal Endoscopic Surgery (NOTES) is defined as surgery without a skin incision utilizing flexible endoscopes passing through natural orifices (*vagina, mouth, anus, and urethra*). Therefore, procedures may be performed through *transvaginal, transesophageal, transgastric, transrectal*, or *transvesical* approaches. As a scar-free surgery, this technique avoids complications related to incisions including wound infections, incisional hernias, and postoperative pain, which might result in shorter recovery time and better quality of life.

NOTES is considered a logical evolution in minimally invasive surgery. The purpose of this chapter is to summarize the progress of NOTES in humans to date and try to answer the question whether it is a necessary evolution or not.

Terminology

There are a number of terms that have been reported to describe NOTES. When NOTES is performed using transluminal approach without any percutaneous assistance or visualization, it is called totally NOTES (*T-NOTES*); when NOTES uses mixed technologies including transabdominal instrumentation and flexible tools through natural orifices, it is called "*Hybrid*" NOTES; if only visualization is performed through a natural orifice during an endoscopic procedure, the procedure is called as NOTES-*assisted*; and, finally, if only the specimen is extracted through a natural orifice after a standard laparoscopic procedure, then it is named *Natural Orifice Specimen Extraction* (NOSE) [1].

History

Although Kalloo et al. performed the first successful peroral transgastric approach for peritoneoscopy for a liver biopsy and presented in a meeting in 2000, the concept of NOTES gained greater attention only after their published paper in 2004 [2, 3]. One year after their report, Reddy and Rao reported the first human transgastric appendectomy in India [4].

For the most part, animal models have been used and studies have focused on intra-abdominal applications, including tubal ligation, cholecystectomy, splenectomy, gastrojejunostomy, distal pancreatectomy, and oophorectomy with tubectomy; however, intrathoracic procedures such as mediastinoscopy, thoracoscopy, and lymph node dissections have also been performed [5–7].

M.M. Ozmen, M.D., M.S., F.A.C.S., F.R.C.S. (✉)
Professor of Surgery, Department of Surgery,
Hacettepe University Medical School,
Ankara, Turkey
e-mail: Mahir.ozmen@hacettepe.edu.tr

R. Latifi et al. (eds.), *Technological Advances in Surgery, Trauma and Critical Care*,
DOI 10.1007/978-1-4939-2671-8_32

Table 32.1 Challenges to be addressed about NOTES outlined by NOSCAR's first White Paper

• Peritoneal access
• Gastric closure
• Prevention of infection
• Suturing and anastomotic devices
• Maintaining spatial orientation
• Development of a multitasking platform
• Management of intraperitoneal complications and hemorrhage
• Physiologic untoward events caused by NOTES
• Training

With permission from Rattner D, Kalloo A. ASGE/SAGES Working Group on Natural Orifice translumenal Endoscopic Surgery. October 2005. Surg Endosc 2006;20: 329–333

The *Natural Orifice Surgery Consortium for Assessment and Research* [NOSCAR] was founded by surgeons and gastroenterologist in 2005. Two white papers by NOSCAR addressed challenges including the physiologic implications of the procedure (Table 32.1) [8] and established clinical guidelines [9].

Since the first description of the procedure, *more than* 2,000 clinical NOTES have been reported. Transvaginal route has been the most common followed by transgastric approach, while cholecystectomy and appendectomy have been the most popular procedures reported. Meta-analyses and single-center studies of NOTES in humans have revealed that cholecystectomy, appendectomy, mediastinoscopy, and peritoneoscopy procedures for intestinal and renal cancers are all feasible [10–12].

Instrumentation

Access

Technical complications encountered during NOTES have revealed that there is a need for new endoscopic instruments, in order to safely perform these procedures.

Initially published papers led to believe that NOTES would be done primarily as transgastric procedures. However, peritoneal cavity could safely be accessed through a variety of other transluminal routes. Gynecologists had been accessing pelvic organs transvaginally since the early twentieth century. In fact, the first transvaginal cholecystectomy had been performed by Tsin et al. long before the White Paper by NOSCAR [12]. Currently most human NOTES procedures use transvaginal access since this route is well established and vaginal closure is safe, secure, and easy to perform. On the other hand, transgastric access still seems to be a better approach as it is more universally available than transvaginal and often more appealing to the patients. However, despite the availability of variety of closure devices and techniques, endoluminal method of determining closure security at the end of a transgastric or transrectal procedure remains an unresolved issue.

Transvaginal NOTES access devices have been initially reported on by Gettman et al. [13]. In their technique following a posterior colpotomy, modified 24–30F dilators were inserted over a 24F dilating balloon as access ports. Further reports, including the first reported transvaginal cholecystectomy in the USA, either used standard laparoscopic ports (12 or 15 mm) or rigid ports with outer diameter between 21 and 26 mm as transvaginal access sites into the abdomen. Clayman et al. performed hybrid nephrectomy in a porcine model using the most novel system [14]. Furthermore, 12 mm laparoscopic ports were used for both transcolonic and transvesical access.

However, NOTES without any laparoscopic assistance have not been achieved yet. Limitations of technology for the access still need further development in instrumentations. Therefore, the ideal matchup between access, pathology, and patient preference has yet to be determined.

Operating Instruments

In addition to the access, there are still some other limitations in current NOTES instrumentation, including minimal traction-countertraction that is required. In order to overcome these limitations, multitasking endoscopic platforms and new instruments have been developed and used to achieve better triangulation with promising results. Magnetic anchoring and guidance system (MAGS) has been used widely to facilitate especially single-port NOTES-assisted nephrectomies [15]. Multitasking platforms such as TransPort® (USGI Medical San Clemente, CA), Cobra™ (USGI Medical, San Clemente, CA), R-scope (XGIF-2TQ160R; Olympus Corp, Tokyo, Japan), the Endo-SAMURAI™ (Olympus Corp, Tokyo, Japan), and the Direct Drive Endoscopic System (DDES) (Boston Scientific, Natick, MA) each have a common flexible endoscopic design with some differences on channel system, motion, angulations, and suturing being used [16–20].

Clinical Applications

Autorino et al. analyzed the published literature between 2006 and 2012 and found 644 publications [21]. More than half were original articles, around 30 % were review articles, and 12 % were case reports. Half of the articles were animal studies. Eighty percent of the papers originated from Europe and the USA only. When they divided the time period in two eras as early (2006–2008) and late (2009–2011), they found a significant increase in the number of clinical cases reported per article (2 vs. 6, $p=0.008$) and a significant increase in the number of randomized controlled trials (RCTs, 5.6 % vs. 7.2 %) or non-randomized but comparative studies (5.6 % vs. 22.9 %, $p<0.001$) from the early to the late period.

Table 32.2 shows the distribution of published articles, procedures, access route, and the technique used between early and late period.

A review paper by Keller and Delaney covering the period between 2004 and 2013 [11] found that with the abundance of safety and feasibility studies, only 43 reports covering 432 cases were reported in humans. Cholecystectomy (84 %) and appendectomy (7 %) were the most popular procedures reported. Therefore, they concluded that the question why NOTES has not progressed

Table 32.2 The distribution of published articles, procedures, access route, and the technique used between early and late period

	Early (2006–2008)	Late (2009–2011)
Publications n (%)	138 (54.1)	220 (56.6)
Original article	36 (14.1)	44 (11.3)
Case report	81 (31.8)	125 (32.1)
Review, consensus		
Procedures n (%)	28 (18.1)	49 (18.4)
Cholecystectomy	9 (5.8)	32 (12.0)
Colorectal resection	18 (11.6)	34 (12.7)
Gastric surgery	32 (20.6)	21 (7.9)
Peritoneoscopy	7 (4.5)	19 (7.1)
Nephrectomy	29 (18.7)	38 (14.2)
Access (*closure, creation*)	32 (20.6)	74 (27.7)
Others		
Access route n (%)	77 (53.8)	133 (51.8)
Transgastric/transesophageal	16 (11.2)	33 (12.8)
Transcolonic/transanal	24 (16.8)	18 (7.0)
Transvaginal	10 (7.0)	40 (15.6)
Transvesical	16 (11.2)	33 (12.8)
>1 Access, or other access		
Technique n (%)	221 (90.6)	304 (81.3)
NOTES	17 (7.0)	29 (7.8)
Hybrid NOTES	6 (2.5)	32 (8.6)
NOTES-assisted laparoscopy	0	9 (2.4)
>1 Technique		

With permission from Autorino R, Yakoubi R, White WM, Gettman M et al. Natural orifice transluminal endoscopic surgery (NOTES): where are we going? A bibliometric assessment. BJU International.2012; 111:11–16 further into the clinical practice remains unanswered. However, one should take into consideration that the progress of NOTES is directly related to the developments in instrumentation, its worldwide availability, and of course acceptability by practitioners.

Hybrid NOTES is the combination of laparoscopic and endoscopic techniques which may allow operations beyond cholecystectomy. Therefore, currently, it is more common than novel NOTES in humans, comprising over 50 % of the reported cases. Hybrid approach is also thought to be safer enabling better visibility of the abdomen and standard suturing [22].

In their current review, Bingener et al. have evaluated all published reports on NOTES in emergency situations and concluded that although appendectomy is one of the most common NOTES procedure, the value of NOTES in patients with diverticulitis, ulcer perforation, and infected pancreatic necrosis is not clear yet [23]. They have found NOTES quite useful for gastrostomy tube insertion in the ICU and repair of iatrogenic perforations during colonoscopy as it might save the patients from unnecessary laparotomy.

Challenges

Technical

NOTES still has some unresolved issues identified and published by working group of NOSCAR, including access, closure, devices, spatial orientation, etc. as shown in Table 32.1.

Many different access routes to peritoneal cavity including transgastric, transvesical, transcolonic, transvaginal, and combined have been described. Main access routes in humans are transvaginal and followed by transgastric, transesophageal, and transrectal, respectively [24–26]. The transgastric approach requires creation and dilatation of a hole on the anterior stomach wall for the introduction of the operating platform. Therefore, there is a certain level of risk of bleeding, leak, or injuring the adjacent organs or tissues. In order to decrease the risk, some devices, such as endoscopic ultrasound, have been reported to be used but its efficacy needs to be evaluated in humans [27].

The incision for transvaginal approach can be achieved under direct visualization without an intra-abdominal scope; on the other hand, it requires working deep in the pelvis, is only applicable in 50 % of the population, and carries the risk of injuries to adjacent organs [26]. Transvesical approach might also be used but its major limitation is working against the long male urethra.

Both transvaginal and transvesical approaches have potential reduction in morbidity compared to transgastric access [25].

Transrectal approach allows direct access to upper quadrants without retroflexion and permits the removal of large specimens and secure closure.

The ideal tool for optimal visceral closure after NOTES must be easy to use, applicable to multiple organs, reproducible, reliable, and safe. However, there is no such tool at the moment. Current options include clips, endoscopic tubes, T fasteners, endoscopic suturing devices including tissue apposition system (TAS), and novel closure devices, such as the SPIDER® (TransEnterix Surgical, Durham, NC) [28, 29].

Current instruments exist for hybrid NOTES with a transabdominal port, but flexible endoscopic instrumentation is much more limited. Moreover, the choice of endoscope and dissection tools differs greatly between pure and hybrid NOTES even within the same procedure.

Ergonomics

Surgeons must have good visualization, ability of tissue manipulation, and ability to independently perform tasks. NOTES introduces ergonomic challenges to surgeons [30]. These ergonomic issues are due to the fact that surgical tools and instrumentation used for NOTES are actually borrowed from the laparoscopic tool box, which have not been developed to meet the increased task demands. Therefore, it remains to be determined whether complications associated with NOTES are a result of an early learning curve or inherent procedure and likely to occur at unacceptable rates even after the learning curve.

Practicality

As reported by Dunkin, success in NOTES includes proper hands-on training, close monitoring of performance to confirm procedural competence of surgeon, and mentoring through their initial procedures [22].

The adaption of NOTES has been directly influenced both by surgeon and public attitude. Studies revealed that NOTES would only be considered by patients if there was no additional risk and if it was better than laparoscopy in pain, operative time, and cost [31]. Studies evaluating surgeon's choice between NOTES and laparoscopy both for their patients and their own care are still lacking.

Complications of NOTES

Although multiple potential benefits have been suggested for NOTES, Clark et al. evaluated studies in humans between 2007 and 2011 and found that the most common reported complications were sepsis, hematoma, laceration, perforation, and biliary leakage [1]. Transvaginal cholecystectomy was the most common procedure with the complication rate of 1.5–25 %. However, the main limitation is the lack of comparative data from trials comparing one approach with another in a prospective manner.

Justification

As pointed out by Swain P, the three main justifications for natural orifice transluminal endoscopic surgery (NOTES) are improved cosmetic appearance, ease of access, and the concept that human ingenuity and technological advance can continue to reduce the trauma and discomfort associated with effective surgery [32].

In order to be preferable for patients, NOTES procedures do not have to be "better" than laparoscopic or open surgical procedures. If the procedures are judged by comparing the cosmetic effect, NOTES procedures will always be superior to laparoscopic or open surgery, as they do not produce scarring while other procedures always do [33].

NOTES might also be preferable in obese patients, in patients with sepsis in the ICU, and in patients unfit for laparotomy.

There are real advantages of ease of access. Flexible endoscopy can easily reach, from the inside, structures that are difficult to reach with conventional laparoscopes passing through the abdominal wall [34]. It may stimulate a great deal of innovation and development in flexible endosurgical device. This is likely to result in the delivery of more effective flexible endo-surgical tools, which are frankly poor at present. Suturing is in its infancy and the devices are difficult to use and are too expensive. Flexible stapling barely exists. This competition may also improve laparoscopic surgery, encourage the development of operations with smaller skin incisions, and combine transgastric surgical procedures with laparoscopic techniques. Another important advance will be the development of thinner, more effective flexible endoscopic instruments that can be used readily in small children.

Conclusions

NOTES is a promising evolution in surgery, in which endoscopic intervention is performed through existing orifices with the purpose of eliminating abdominal incisions. Although the potential for NOTES technology seems endless, technical challenges have limited its use and many of the procedures are hybrid. I believe that, currently, we are far from drawing certain conclusions on its overall safety, efficacy, or superiority over current minimally invasive techniques due to lack of evidence and the immaturity of the technique in humans.

References

1. Clark PM, Qayed ES, Kooby DA, Maithel SK, Willingham FF. Natural orifice transluminal endoscopic surgery in humans: a review. Minim Invasive Surg. 2012; Article ID 189296, 8 p; http://dx.doi.org/10.1155/2012/189296.
2. Kalloo A, Kantsevoy SV, Singh VK, et al. Flexible transgastric peritoneoscopy: a novel approach to diagnostic and therapeutic interventions in the peritoneal cavity. Gastroenterology. 2000;118:A1039.
3. Kalloo AN, Singh VK, Jagannath SB, et al. Flexible transgastric peritoneoscopy: a novel approach to diagnostic and therapeutic interventions in the peritoneal cavity. Gastrointest Endosc. 2004;60:114–7.
4. Reddy N, Rao P. Per oral transgastric endoscopic appendectomy in human. In: Proceedings of the 45th Annual Conference of the Society of Gastrointestinal Endoscopy of India, p. 28–29, Jaipur, India; 2004.
5. Park PO, Bergstrom M, Ikeda K, Fritscher-Ravens A, Swain P. Experimental studies of transgastric gallbladder surgery: cholecystectomy and cholecystogastric anastomosis (videos). Gastrointest Endosc. 2005;61:601–6.
6. Wagh MS, Merrifield BF, Thompson CC. Endoscopic transgastric abdominal exploration and organ resection: initial experience in a porcine model. Clin Gastroenterol Hepatol. 2005;3:892–6.
7. USGI Medical, Inc. USGI medical announces first NOTES transgastric cholecystectomy procedures performed by Dr. Lee Swanstrom at Legacy Hospital. 2007.
8. Rattner D, Kalloo A. ASGE/SAGES Working Group on natural orifice translumenal endoscopic surgery. Surg Endosc. 2006;20:329–33.
9. Rattner DW, Hawes R, Schwaitzberg S, Kochman M, Swanstrom L. The Second SAGES/ASGE White Paper on natural orifice transluminal endoscopic surgery: 5 years of progress. Surg Endosc. 2011;25:2441–8.
10. Mohan HM, O'Riordan JM, Winter DC. Natural-orifice translumenal endoscopic surgery (NOTES): minimally invasive evolution or revolution? Surg Laparosc Endosc Percutan Tech. 2013;23:244–50.
11. Keller DS, Delaney CP. Current evidence in gastrointestinal surgery: natural orifice transluminal endoscopic surgery (NOTES). J Gastrointest Surg. 2013;17:1857–62.
12. Tsin DA, Sequeria RJ, Giannikas G. Culdolaparoscopic oophorectomy with vaginal hysterectomy: an optional minimal access surgical technique. J Laparoendosc Adv Surg Tech A. 2003;12(4):269–71.
13. Gettman MT, Lotan Y, Napper CA, Cadeddu JA. Transvaginal laparoscopic nephrectomy: development and feasibility in the porcine model. Urology. 2002;59:446–50.
14. Clayman RV, Box GN, Abraham J. Rapid communication: transvaginal single-port NOTES nephrectomy: initial laboratory experience. J Endourol. 2007;21:640–4.
15. Scott DJ, Tang S, Fernandez R, et al. Completely transvaginal NOTES cholecystectomy using magnetically anchored instruments. Surg Endosc. 2007;21:2308–16.
16. Best SL, Cadeddu JA. Use of magnetic anchoring and guidance systems to facilitate single trocar laparoscopy. Curr Urol Rep. 2010;11:29–32.
17. Raman JD, Scott DJ, Cadeddu JA. Role of magnetic anchors during laparoendoscopic single site surgery and NOTES. J Endourol. 2009;23:781–6.
18. Bardaro SJ, Swanström L. Development of advanced endoscopes for natural orifice transluminal endoscopic surgery (NOTES). Minim Invasive Ther Allied Technol. 2006;15:378–83.
19. Astudillo JA, Sporn E, Bachman S, et al. Transgastric cholecystectomy using a prototype endoscope with 2 deflecting working channels (with video). Gastrointest Endosc. 2009;69:297–302.
20. Shaikh SN, Thompson CC. Natural orifice translumenal surgery: flexible platform review. J Gastrointest Surg. 2010;2:177–8.
21. Autorino R, Yakoubi R, White WM, Gettman M, et al. Natural orifice transluminal endoscopic surgery (NOTES): where are we going? A bibliometric assessment. BJU Int. 2012;111:11–6.
22. Dunkin BJ. Natural orifice transluminal endoscopic surgery: educational challenge. World J Gastrointest Surg. 2010;2(6):224–30.
23. Bingener J, Ibrahim-zada I. Natural orifice transluminal endoscopic surgery for intra-abdominal emergency conditions. BJS. 2014;101:e80–9.
24. Khashab MA, Kalloo AN. Notes: current status and new horizons. Gastroenterology. 2012;142:704–10.
25. Liu L, Chiu PWY, Reddy N, et al. Natural orifice transluminal endoscopic surgery (NOTES) for clinical management of intra-abdominal diseases. Dig Endosc. 2013;25:565–77.
26. Moris DN, Bramis KJ, Mantonakis EI, et al. Surgery via natural orifices in human beings: yesterday, today, tomorrow. Am J Surg. 2012;204:93–102.
27. Fritscher-Ravens A, Ghanbari A, Cuming T, et al. Comparative study of NOTES alone vs EUS-guided NOTES procedures. Endoscopy. 2008;40:925–30.
28. Sylla P. Current experience and future directions of completely NOTES colorectal resection. World J Gastrointest Surg. 2010;2:193–8.
29. Flora ED, Wilson TG, Martin IJ, O'Rourke NA, Maddern GJ. A review of natural orifice translumenal endoscopic surgery (NOTES) for intra-abdominal surgery: experimental models, techniques, and applicability to the clinical setting. Ann Surg. 2008;247:583–602.
30. Tessier C, Zhang L, Cao CG. Ergonomic considerations in natural orifice translumenal endoscopic surgery (NOTES): a case study. Work. 2012;41 Suppl 1:4683–8.
31. Hucl T, Saglova A, Benes M, et al. Patient and physician perception of natural orifice transluminal endoscopic appendectomy. World J Gastroenterol. 2012;18:1800–5.
32. Swain P. A justification for NOTES – natural orifice transluminal endosurgery. Gastrointest Endosc. 2007;65(3):514–6.
33. Meining A, Spaun G, Fernández-Esparrach G, Arezzo A, Wilhelm D. NOTES in Europe: summary of the working group reports of the 2012 EURO-NOTES meeting. Endoscopy. 2013;45:214–7.
34. Morgan M, Olweny EO, Cadeddu JA. LESS and NOTES instrumentation: future. Curr Opin Urol. 2014;24:58–65.

Bariatric Surgery: The Less, The Better

33

Julia Samamé and Carlos A. Galvani

Introduction

Obesity has become a serious health problem in the USA and around the world. Seventy-eight million adults are overweight (defined as a Body Mass Index (BMI) greater than or equal to 25) or obese (defined as a BMI greater than or equal to 30) in the USA. The prevalence of obesity is steadily growing every year; from 1960 to 2010, the number of overweight and obese people has increased by 54.9 % in both the adult and pediatric population [1]. During 2011–2012, 34.9 % of adults and 17 % of adolescents were obese in the USA [2], and although those numbers have not changed significantly from previous years, there was a shift to the right in the BMI distribution which is greatest at the upper percentiles, meaning that the increased prevalence was larger for those patients who were extremely obese [3].

Worldwide, the situation is not very different. According to the numbers reviewed by the World Health Organization in 2014, obesity has nearly doubled since 1980 with more than 1.4 billon adults being overweight and in 2012 more than 40 million children under the age of five were overweight or obese [4].

The negative implications of being overweight or obese are well known. Around 3.4 million adults die each year as a result of obesity-related conditions with more deaths occurring than those caused in individuals that are underweight. The increased risk of comorbidities such as diabetes, hypertension, coronary artery disease, sleep apnea, hyperlipidemia, and stroke and certain types of cancer are a direct consequence of overweight and obesity [4–6].

Weight loss surgery, known as bariatric surgery, has proven to be the only effective and durable treatment currently available for morbid obesity. Bariatric surgery consistently induced sustained weight loss and improvement or remission of the comorbid conditions [7–9].

The Evolution of Bariatric Surgery

The Open Era

Although the first bariatric surgical intervention could be traced back to the early 1950s, when Henrikson performed a small bowel resection to treat a woman suffering from obesity [10], it was not until two decades ago that bariatric surgery

J. Samamé, M.D.
Department of Surgery, University of Arizona, 1501 N. Campbell Avenue, Tucson, AZ 85724, USA
e-mail: jsamame@surgery.arizona.edu

C.A. Galvani, M.D. (✉)
Department of Surgery, University of Arizona Medical Center, 1501 N. Campbell Avenue, Tucson, AZ 85724, USA
e-mail: cgalvani@surgery.arizona.edu

R. Latifi et al. (eds.), *Technological Advances in Surgery, Trauma and Critical Care*,
DOI 10.1007/978-1-4939-2671-8_33

steadily increased its popularity and become a field in rapid and constant evolution. The trend adheres to several factors that can be reduced to two. Obesity has become the epidemic with the greatest prevalence and incidence in the USA, and second bariatric surgeries are now very safe, they are better tolerated, and 90 % of the cases are performed by a minimally invasive approach.

Bariatric surgery evolved from the jejunoileal bypass, a purely malabsorptive procedure described by Varco in 1953, which then underwent several modifications over the next two decades. Due to its significant morbidity and mortality associated with the development of both blind loop and short bowel syndrome, the jejunoileal bypass was left behind for other less morbid bariatric procedures [11].

In the 1960s, the gastric bypass was developed by Mason and Ito, a combined malabsorptive with gastric restriction procedure that also evolved from their original description. As a consequence of its reduced long-term complication profile and equivalent weight loss as a jejunoileal bypass, the malabsorptive/restrictive procedures had become the most popular bariatric surgery in the 1970s and early 1980s [11].

By the mid-1970s, the modern malabsorptive procedure era began when Scopinaro and colleagues described the biliopancreatic diversion. More than a decade later Hess and Marceau described a modification of the biliopancreatic diversion, the duodenal switch (BPD/DS), which involved the preservation of the pylorus and proximal duodenum; doing so they avoided postgastrectomy complications such as dumping diarrhea and marginal ulcers [11].

During the 1970s and 1980s, several purely restrictive procedures were introduced, such as gastroplasties, gastric partitioning, banded or ringed vertical gastroplasties, and gastric banding. Of those, only gastric banding remains popular nowadays [12, 13].

The newest bariatric surgery developed was another restrictive procedure, the sleeve gastrectomy. Originally described as the restrictive component of the BPD/DS [14], its true origin as a stand-alone surgery was described in the late 1980s as the Magenstrasse and Mill procedure [15].

The Minimally Invasive Era

The first description of a successful laparoscopic bariatric procedure in humans took place in Australia in 1993, when Broadbent and colleagues reported the placement of a nonadjustable gastric band [10]. This initial report entailed without any doubt the beginning of the biggest contribution to growing the field of bariatric surgery. Also in 1993 the first adjustable gastric band was performed and later that same year [13], Wittgrove and Clark completed the first laparoscopic Roux-en-Y gastric bypass (RYGB) [10]. Several variations and refinements to the original technique were described for the gastrojejunostomy and those changes are a result of the development of the new laparoscopic instruments and supplies.

Despite a learning curve, the introduction of laparoscopy resulted in an improvement of outcomes over time, equaling and then surpassing the results obtained during the open era. The occurrence of less morbidity, shorter hospital stay, improved postoperative quality of life, and reduction in mortality promptly generated an increased demand of laparoscopic procedures, which considerably surpassed the number of open procedures that had been performed annually [11, 14–17].

The State-of-the-Art Bariatric Procedures

Bariatric surgical procedures are intended to reduce caloric intake by a reversible or permanent modification of the gastrointestinal tract. Based on the mechanisms through which they achieve this reduction, they are classified by malabsorptive, restrictive, or a combination of malabsorptive/restrictive (Fig. 33.1). There is no superior bariatric surgical procedure; therefore, the selection of a particular surgery should be specific to each individual patient and their needs.

Based on estimated bariatric surgery numbers for 2013 published by the American Society for Metabolic and Bariatric Surgery (ASMBS),

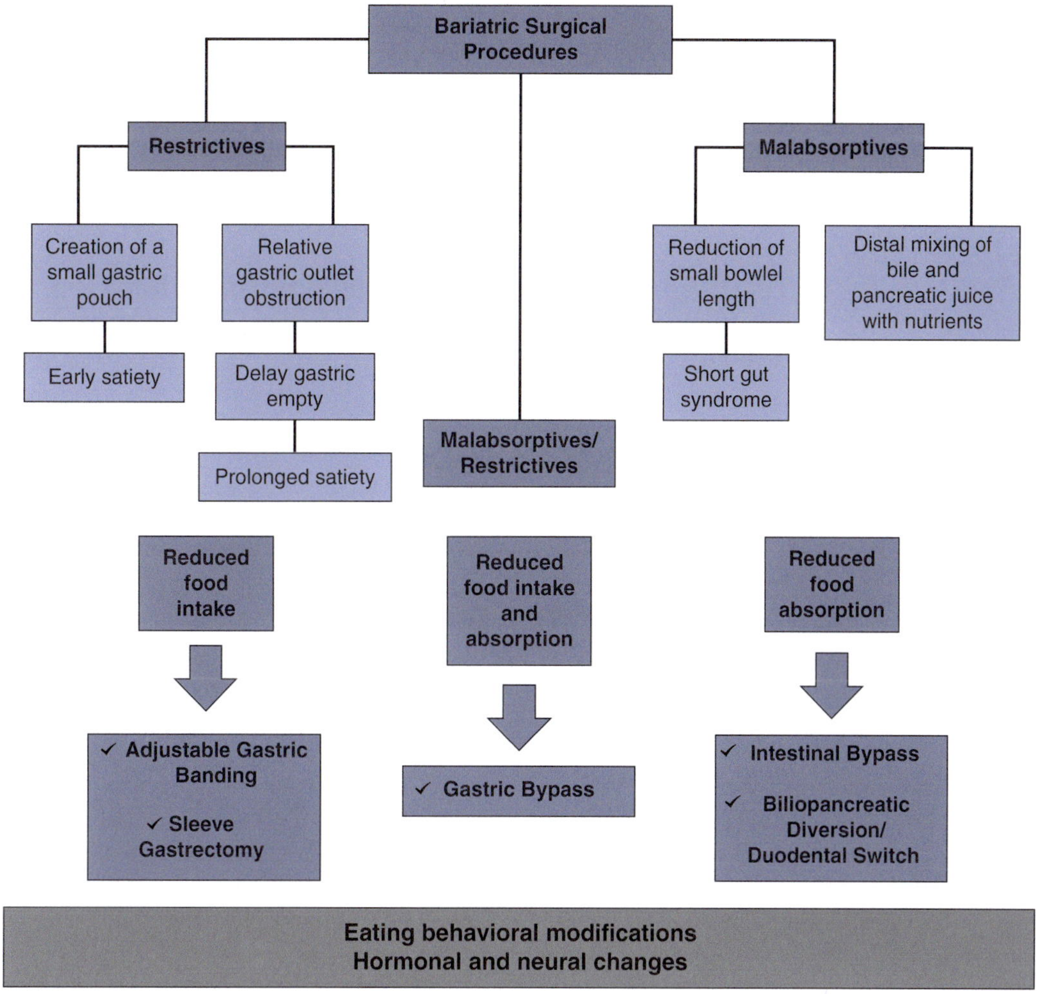

Fig. 33.1 Mechanism of action of surgical bariatric procedures

Roux-en-Y gastric bypass (RYGB), adjustable gastric band (AGB), and sleeve gastrectomy (SG) account for 90.3 % of all of the bariatric procedures performed in 2013 [17]. Of those, 88.9 % are performed laparoscopically, an approach that now represents the standard of care for bariatric surgery [16]. Although very good outcomes in terms of morbidity and mortality are achieved with this approach, many of these procedures are complex and can only be carried out by highly skilled surgeons after a steep learning curve.

Adjustable Gastric Band

Its use was primarily widespread in Australia and European countries due to its relative simplicity, reversibility, and safety profile [12]. Since the approval of the LAP-BAND® (Apollo Endosurgery, Austin, TX) system in the USA in 2001, its use has grown significantly and is now considered a well-established bariatric procedure with good medium and long-term results in terms of sustained weight loss [18, 19]. LAGB is a purely restrictive procedure that can be routinely performed in an outpatient setting; however, gastric banding is an implantable device that can be associated with late complications such as band slippage or erosion, gastric prolapse, pouch enlargement, and tubing/access port complication, which in the long term will require either band revision or explantation in a high percentage of patients [20–23].

Roux-en-Y Gastric Bypass

Laparoscopic roux-en-Y gastric bypass (RYGB) is considered the gold standard for the surgical treatment of morbid obesity due to its greater weight loss and lower rates of weight regain when compared with other bariatric procedures, becoming one of the most commonly performed bariatric surgeries in the USA [17]. This combined, malabsorptive/restrictive procedure induces weight loss by several mechanisms: by gastric restriction and early satiety, the volume of food to be consumed is decreased and ultimately the amount of caloric intake and by malabsorption which is created by bypassing the foregut delivering enteral nutrition directly into the mid small intestine avoiding the nutrient absorptive circuit. Bypassing the foregut also induces anorexia by alteration of hormone secretion [24].

Sleeve Gastrectomy

Sleeve Gastrectomy (SG), which is the fastest growing procedure in bariatric surgery [17], was first performed laparoscopically in 1999 [11]. Subsequently it was used as a first step in a staged concept for high-risk patients undergoing bariatric surgery. The rationale for this approach was to lower the morbidity of a complex surgical procedure by offering a less challenging operation, decreasing operative time, and allowing patients to lose weight before proceeding with the second stage. However, as a consequence of the proven outcomes in terms of excellent weight loss and resolution of comorbidities, it is now being increasingly favored as a stand-alone procedure [25–27]. Initially conceived of as a purely restrictive surgery, it has been shown that laparoscopic sleeve gastrectomy (LSG) has strong metabolic effects probably due to accelerated gastric emptying, early satiety, reduction of the ghrelin-producing cell mass after resection of the gastric fundus, and complex neurohormonal regulation of intestinal hormones [14, 28].

Novel Technologies in Bariatric Surgery

The Role of Robotics

The most significant impact in robotically assisted surgery was the possibility to extend the already well-known benefits achieved with minimally invasive surgery to difficult procedures often performed in an open manner. Its application in bariatric surgery amplified the benefits of minimally invasive access without increasing complication risks and with a lower learning curve.

The first bariatric procedure with robotic assistance was described by Cadière who performed a robotic-assisted adjustable gastric band placement in 1999 [29], and after that in 2001, Horgan and Vanuno published the first series of robotic-assisted RYGB [30]. Robotic technology is now applied to complex primary and revisional bariatric procedures without increasing complication risks as a result of the learning curve and overcoming the drawbacks inherent to a laparoscopic approach especially in the morbidly obese population.

Major advantages of the use of robotic technology for bariatric surgery are the greater exposure and visualization particularly useful in morbidly obese patients with excessive intra-abdominal fat deposition and oversized and fatty livers, which makes maneuverability difficult. Larger, more rigid and articulated instruments that avoid bending are an additional benefit while operating on patients with thicker abdominal walls (Fig. 33.2a, b). The possibility to perform precise maneuvers despite increased torque pressure facilitates the completion of hand-sewn gastrointestinal anastomosis, which can reduce the risk of leaks and future anastomotic strictures (Fig. 33.3a–c).

The major disadvantage is the higher operational costs compared with laparoscopic surgery [27].

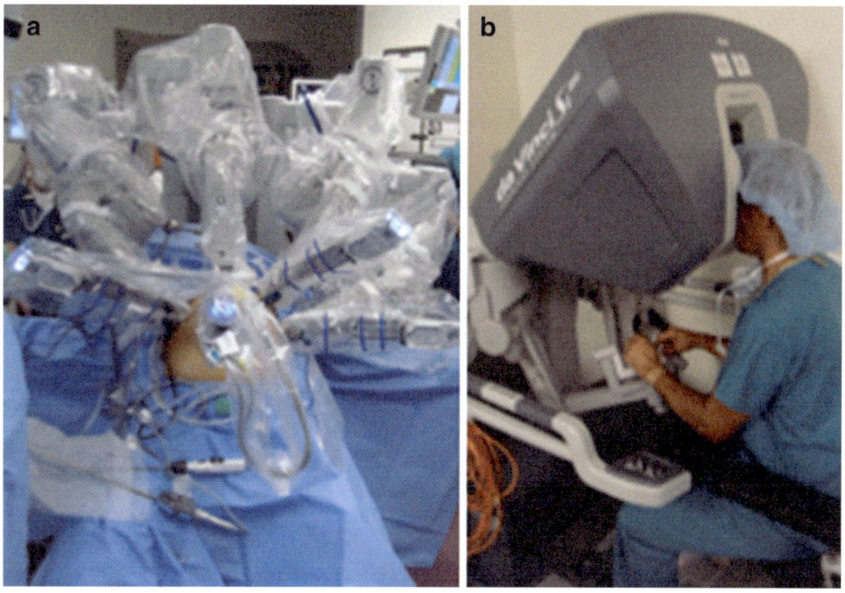

Fig. 33.2 (**a**, **b**) Robotic-assisted bariatric surgery. (**a**) Surgical cart over the head of the patient. (**b**) Surgeon at the robotic console

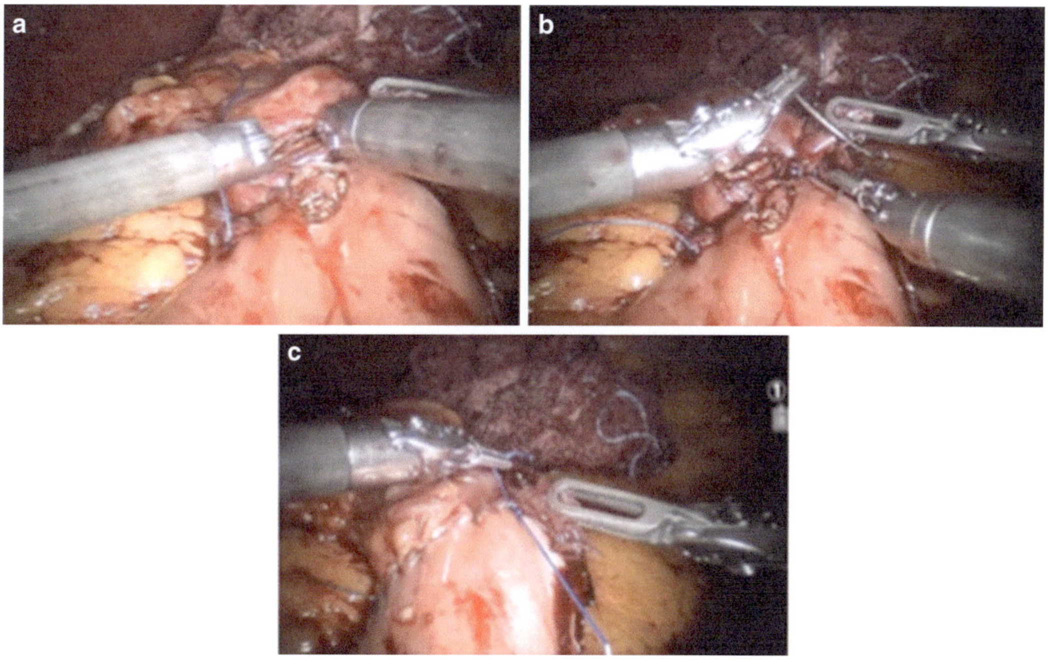

Fig. 33.3 (**a**–**c**) Robotic-assisted Roux-en-Y gastric bypass. (**a**) Creation of the gastrostomy and jejunostomy in preparation for the gastrojejunal anastomosis. (**b**) Running suture of the posterior outer layer of the gastrojejunal anastomosis. (**c**) Completed gastrojejunostomy

Robotic Lap Band

Few studies followed the first publication of robotic-assisted lap band [31–33]. Due to the safety and effectiveness of the laparoscopic approach, the adoption of robotic-assisted LAGB continues to be scarce; however, its use for patients with preoperative BMI >50 kg/m^2 was suggested to be advantageous owing to the characteristics of the robotic instruments that are longer and stiffer and with greater mechanical power. Also operative time in these patients proved to be shorter than laparoscopic counterparts [33]. Another application of the robotic platform is in the case of revisions for band slippage.

Robotic Roux-en-Y Gastric Bypass

Robotic-assisted RYGB was first introduced in 2001 [30], but its acceptance rapidly increased as its feasibility and safety have been clearly proven especially for difficult cases such as high-risk and super obese patients [33, 34]. Several systematic reviews and comparative studies reported similar or better outcomes thanks to robotic technology. Main advantages of its use for RYGB were the shorter learning curve and a lower overall complication rate but specifically for the gastrojejunostomy leak rate [31, 34].

A recent comparative study which included 389 laparoscopic and 388 robotic RYGB also showed a significantly reduced conversion rate in the robotic arm compared with the laparoscopic arm (<1 % vs. almost 5 %) although operative time was longer [34]. The same study group reported their cost analysis, which showed a clear advantage of the robotic approach by reducing complication rate and the need for postoperative radiologic studies.

Along the same line, Hagen et al. evaluated the costs of robotic versus laparoscopic RYGB. An increase in costs was observed for the laparoscopic approach, with contributing factors such as length of hospital stay, time in the ICU, complication rates, such as anastomotic leak and the use of laparoscopic staplers [35]. The robotic platform is also showing promising results in revisional surgery, where cases are considerably more complex and challenging due to the frequent occurrence of previous open approach, multiple adhesions, altered anatomy, erosions, and fistulas.

Robotic Sleeve Gastrectomy

Robotic technology for SG has not been widely adopted among bariatric surgeons due to its relatively straightforward acceptance to perform it laparoscopically; however, few series with encouraging results have been published [36–38]. The main indication for robotic assistance is represented by super and super-super obese patients, where the accomplishment of the procedure by laparoscopic approach implies a greater challenge because of the previously mentioned characteristics of the laparoscopic instruments and the patients' abdomen [39, 40]. Although there are no reports about middle and long-term follow-up, results of robotic SG seem to be comparable to laparoscopic approach in terms of excess weight loss but with technical advantages and a reduced learning curve [36–38]. Also, this procedure represents a helpful training model for bariatric fellows and residents [38].

The Role of Single-Incision Surgery

In an effort to progress toward a less invasive and more innovative approach, the so-called scarless surgery emerged in an attempt to allow surgeons to perform laparoscopic procedures with virtually no visible scars. Those procedures were single-incision laparoscopic surgery (SILS) and natural orifice translumenal endoscopic surgery (NOTES).

Potential advantages include additional reduction of wound morbidity such as infection, hematoma, and incisional hernia, less postoperative pain, faster recovery, and further enhancing of cosmetic results (Fig. 33.4a–f).

Although SILS proved to be feasible, surgeons faced several challenges: the lack of instrument triangulation, the lack of optimal visualization of the operative field, internal and external friction between the instrument, and inadequate internal retraction. Hence, the widespread application of this technique came with different developments from the industry to overcome these issues such as articulating instruments, multiple access lumen, and multichannel operative platform among others.

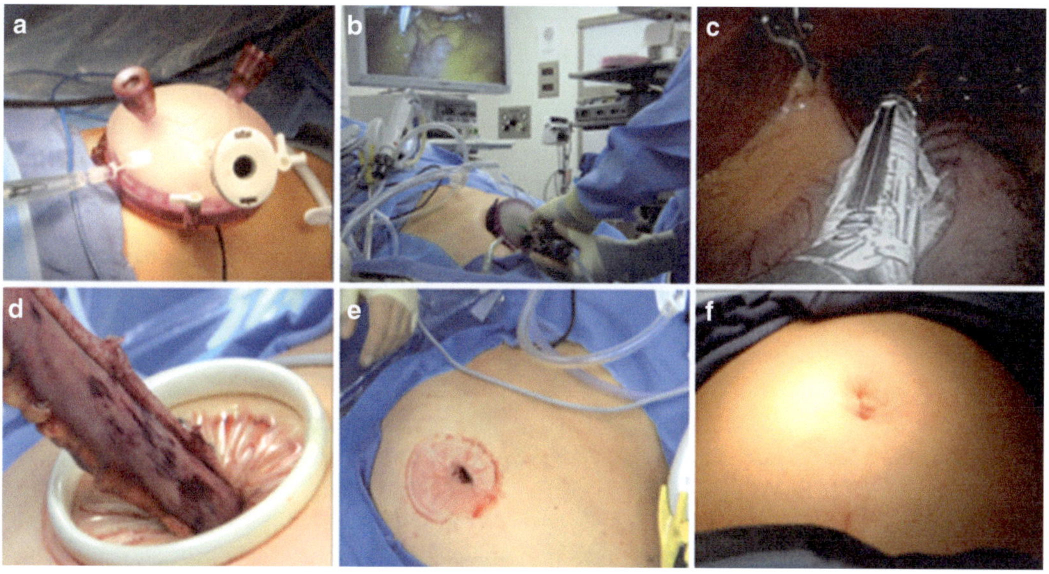

Fig. 33.4 (**a–f**) Single-incision laparoscopic sleeve gastrectomy. (**a**) Ports placement. (**b**) Laparoscopic instruments introduced through the single-port platform. (**c**) Gastric transection. The left lobe of the liver is lifted by a laparoscopic internal retractor. (**d**) Extraction of resected stomach after sleeve completion through the umbilical incision. (**e**) Umbilical incision after the single-port platform was extracted. (**f**) Immediate postoperative cosmetic result

Beginning in 2008, many groups started to report the application of a single-incision technique for bariatric procedures [41–43]. Several series demonstrated that single-incision LAGB and single-incision SG can be performed safely even with the challenges that entail operating on a morbidly obese patient. The technique was proven to be as effective and safe as conventional multiport laparoscopic approach with equivalent outcomes for weight loss [44–46]. However, patient selection is of paramount importance when performing SILS, particularly in bariatric patients. As was shown by a systematic review published in 2014 [44], the presence of super obesity, concomitant incisional hernias, previous abdominal surgeries, and a xiphoid-umbilicus distance longer than 20 cm may represent exclusion criteria for the application of this approach. Also, the common presence of an enlarged and fatty liver and its retraction are still a true challenge [46–48].

The single-incision approach was also described for more complex procedures such as RYGB, reported by Huang and colleagues in 2009 [49]. Later, in 2012 the same author published the first series with promising outcomes [50]. However, no other authors have published anything else other than case reports or technique descriptions.

Novel Technologies Outcomes

The latest systematic review and meta-analyses of robotic-assisted bariatric surgery was published in 2013 [51]. Two previous systematic reviews were published in 2011 [51] and 2012 [52], but the first one did not include SG in their analysis.

Even though the last systematic review and meta-analysis has major limitations such as the low quality of the studies, sample size, and lack of important information such as bariatric and metabolic outcomes, the study suggests that robotic bariatric surgery is feasible independently of the type of procedure performed and safe based on complications, reoperations, and 30-day postoperative mortality rates.

A lower complication profile, specifically anastomotic leak, strictures, and bleeding, a shorter learning curve, and the ease to carry out complex maneuvers such as gastrointestinal anastomosis in RYGB and vertical gastric resection in SG are named as the main advantages of robotic surgery over open and laparoscopic approaches. The main disadvantage was the cost of the robotic platform.

Thirty-day postoperative mortality was zero regardless of the procedure and the rate of postoperative complications was 4.26 % for major and 1 % for minor in RYGB and 1.2 and 0 % for SG. An updated systematic review and meta-analysis of laparoscopic and open bariatric surgery published in 2014 [53] showed a 30-day postoperative mortality rate between 0.11 and 0.07 % for RYGB and 0.50 and 0.29 % for SG. Complication rate for laparoscopic and open RYGB was 21 and 13 % for SG. Specific surgical complications were not mentioned in this meta-analysis.

The systematic review published in 2012 by Fourman and Saber compared the outcomes of robotic bariatric surgery versus laparoscopic bariatric surgery [52]. They found a mean complication rate for all robotic procedures of 10.2 % versus 12.6 % for the conventional laparoscopic approach. The learning curve was measured for RYGB and proved to be shorter for robotic than laparoscopic approach (10–15 vs. ≥100). No major differences were observed for mean hospital stay or excess body weight loss when these variables were reported. The strongest advantages of robotic surgery found in this study were the shorter learning curve, lower leak rate for gastrojejunal anastomosis, improved ergonomics, and less operator fatigue. The major drawback was also the cost of the robotic system and its maintenance.

The most recent systematic review of single-incision bariatric surgery was published by Moreno-Sanz and colleagues in 2014, and included 13 observational studies and 1 randomized control study with a total of 2,357 patients analyzed [52]. The study concluded that single-incision bariatric surgery is a feasible option when the patients are correctly selected and the procedure is carried out by an expert bariatric surgeon knowledgeable in single-incision techniques. Conversion rate to laparoscopic approach was 2.4 % for LAGB and 1.83 % for SG. No conversions were observed among the RYGB cases. The use of an additional trocar to complete the case was reported in 3 of 8 studies of LAGB, in 1 of 4 of SG, and in 1 of 2 studies for RYGB. Overall morbidity rate was 4.8 % for single-incision versus 5 % for conventional laparoscopic approach, and the predominance was for minor complications. Interestingly, no differences were observed in terms of wound complications. Mortality was 0.005 % of all single-incision cases and was represented by one case in the AGB group.

No differences were observed on percentage of weight loss and improvement of comorbidities.

The main advantages observed with single-incision approach were reduced analgesic consumption and improved cosmesis. Disadvantages were longer operative times in almost all single-incision groups. In terms of costs, no significant differences were found between groups; however, if lower morbidity rates, necessity of reoperations, and reduced length of stay associated with single-incision access are achieved, this technique could be more cost-effective.

The Future of Bariatrics

Bariatric surgery has been continually evolving to shift from open procedures to minimally invasive approaches, considering laparoscopy as the gold standard nowadays. The state-of-the-art surgeries are still changing to improve their safety profile and technique, as the case of the laparoscopic gastric plication, a similar procedure to laparoscopic sleeve gastrectomy, which involves the creation of gastric folds by a suture line to reduce the size of the stomach.

Research interests are now focused on approaches and procedures that have similar mechanisms to surgery but less invasiveness aiming at developing durable, reversible, easier, and safer treatment options. Current and ongoing studies have delivered promising results with endoscopy, endoluminal surgery, and natural orifice translumenal endoscopic surgery; however, many of those techniques are still in there study phase or are considered as experimental due to the lack of controlled data, even when they have been used for several years already (Table 33.1).

Named advantages besides less invasiveness are a reduce risk of complications, particularly anastomotic leak, reversibility, and the possibility of an ambulatory weight loss procedure.

Table 33.1 Summary of bariatric emerging procedures

Procedure	Device	Indication	Status
Restrictive			
Gastric volume reduction			
Endolumenal vertical gastroplasty	EndoCinch™ (C.R. Bard, Murray Hill, NJ)	Primary/revision	On market
Intragastric restrictive implant	TERIS (BaroSense, Redwood City, CA)	Primary	Investigational not FDA approved
Transoral gastroplasty	Sleeve stapler (TOGA®) (Satiety, Inc., Palo Alto, CA)	Primary	Investigational not FDA approved
Endolumenal suturing	OverStitch™ (Apollo Endosurgery, Austin, TX)	Primary/revision	Clinical trials
Endolumenal suturing	Incisionless operating platform (IPO; USGI Medical Inc., San Clemente, CA)	Primary/revision	Clinical trials
Intragastric space occupying			
Intragastric balloon	BioEnterics® BIB (Carpinteria, CA), Orbera® (Apollo Endosurgery, Austin, TX)	Primary	Investigational not FDA approved
Intragastric balloon	Heliosphere bag system	Primary	Premarket approval (PAM) application
Intragastric balloon	Silimed gastric balloon (Rio de Janeiro, Brazil)	Primary	Investigational not FDA approved
Intragastric balloon	Spatz™ 3 adjustable balloon system (Great Neck, NY)	Primary	Clinical trials
Malabsorptive			
Duodenojejunal bypass sleeve	EndoBarrier® (GI Dynamics Inc, Lexington, MA)	Primary/T2 diabetes	Clinical trials
Malabsorptive/restrictive			
Gastroduodenojejunal bypass sleeve	ValenTx (Maple Grove, NJ)	Primary	Clinical trials
Regulating gastric emptying			
Gastric electrical stimulation	Transcend® IGS (Medtronics, Minneapolis, MN)	Primary	Investigational not FDA approved
Vagal nerve blockade	V-Bloc®/Maestro® (EnteroMedics, St. Paul, MN)	Primary/revision	Investigational not FDA approved
Reducing gastric emptying	Botox injection	Primary	Investigational not FDA approved
Gastric outlet obstruction	TransPyloric shuttle® (BAROnova Inc., Goleta, CA)	Primary/revision	Investigational not FDA approved

FDA food and drug administration

Endoscopic Procedures

Mimicking the mechanism of action of bariatric surgery, endoscopic weight loss modalities can also be divided into restrictive, malabsorptive, and a combination of both. Restrictive procedures are intended to decrease gastric volume by placing space-occupying devices or by suturing or stapling devices that alter gastric anatomy. Malabsorptive procedures tend to create malabsorption by preventing food contact with the duodenum and proximal jejunum.

Gastric Volume Reduction Devices

Several endoscopic suturing devices were developed in order to decrease gastric volume by creating tissue plication.

- The *EndoCinch™ Suturing System* (C.R. Bard, Murray Hill, NJ) for endoluminal vertical gastroplasty is a suturing device mounted on the tip of the endoscope, which uses a suction chamber to enclose the gastric wall and creates pleats by tagged sutures to reduce gastric volume [54].

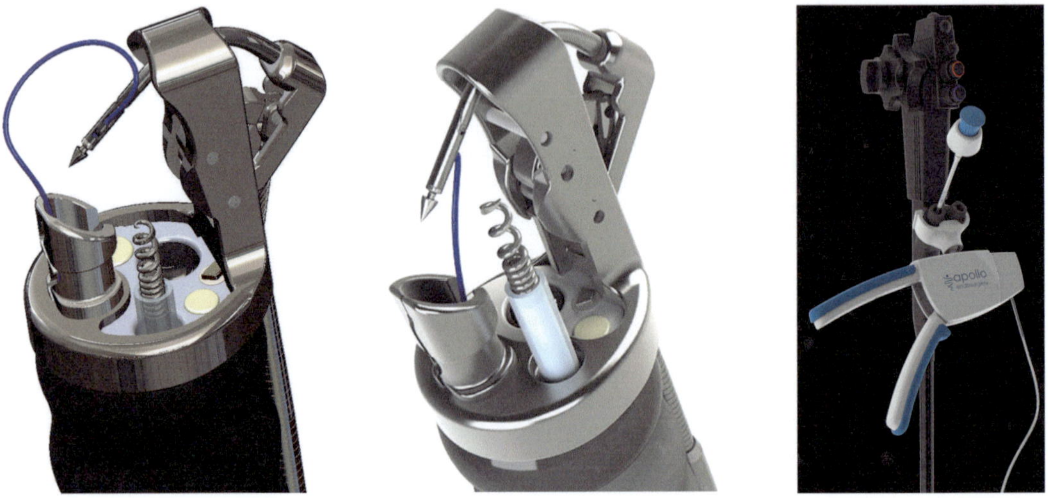

Fig. 33.5 OverStitch™. (Reproduced with permission of Apollo Endosurgery, Austin, TX)

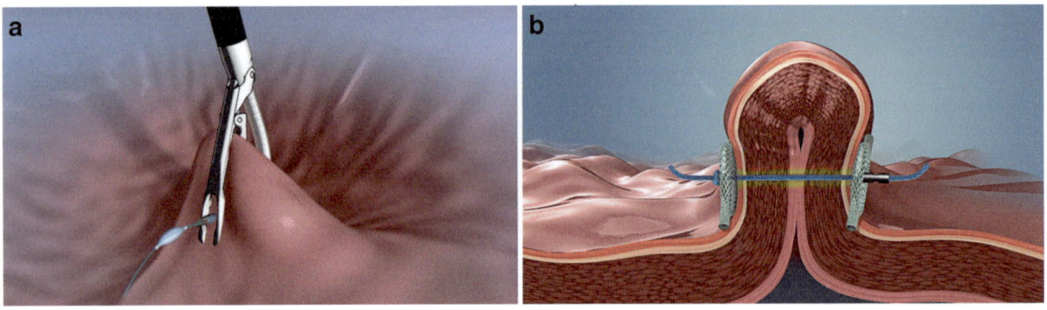

Fig. 33.6 (**a**, **b**) Incisionless operating platform. (**a**) Specialized grasper creating a tissue fold. (**b**) Deployed suture anchor fastening the tissue folds together. (Reproduced with permission of USGI Medical, San Clemente, CA)

- *Transoral Endoscopic Restrictive Implant System* (TERIS; BaroSense, Redwood City, CA) is a restrictive implant that creates a narrow lumen by multiple gastric plications around the cardia of the stomach in a circular fashion and subsequent attachment via anchors to stapled plications of a prosthetic restrictor diaphragm [55].
- The *Tans-oral Gastroplasty System* (TOGA®; Satiety, Inc., Palo Alto, CA) is an endoscopic full-thickness stapling device, which uses vacuum suction to oppose the anterior and posterior wall of the stomach prior to fire the staples in order to create a narrow pouch from the esophagus along the lesser curvature [54].
- The *Overstitch™* (Apollo Endosurgery, Austin, TX) is a suturing device that contains a curved needle and opposable jaws and is premounted alongside a standard endoscope. The device deploys running stitch as well as interrupted sutures and can be reloaded without scope removal. The suturing system can be used as a primary procedure or to restore a dilated gastric sleeve as a revisional procedure [54, 56] (Fig. 33.5).
- The Incisionless Operating Platform (IPO; USGI Medical Inc., San Clemente, CA) is a multifunctional endoscopic platform that utilized four large channels, which allows the use of multiple instruments (the endoscope and three endoscopic instruments) for two-handed operation for primary (Primary Obesity Surgery Endolumenal, POSE) and revisional bariatric procedures (Restorative Obesity Surgery Endolumenal, ROSE). One of the instruments is a grasper that allows the creation of full-thickness tissue plications [57] (Fig. 33.6a, b).

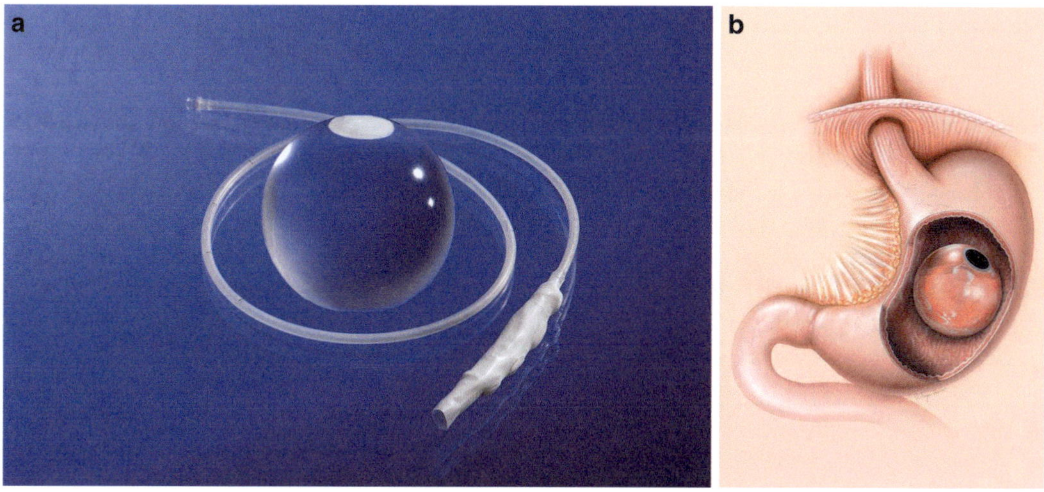

Fig. 33.7 (**a**, **b**) Intragastric balloon, Orbera®. (**a**) Intragastric filled balloon and an uninflated system in the foreground. (**b**) Inflated balloon after deployment into the stomach. (**a**, **b**: Reproduced with permission of Apollo Endosurgery, Austin, TX)

Intragastric Space-Occupying Devices

Intragastric balloons have been in use since the 1980s when the Garran-Edwards gastric bubble was approved by the FDA; however, their use has been discontinued due to associated significant complications such as intolerance, gastric erosion, and intestinal obstruction [54]. Many modifications were introduced to the newer balloons, which have larger capacity, a smoother surface to prevent mucosal erosion, they contain a marker to detect balloon rupture, and they can be filled with either saline solution or air. However, none of them has FDA approval so far, due to limited efficacy and the risk of severe complications. Multiple trials have been carried out in the USA primarily on the BioEnterics® Intragastric Balloon (Carpinteria, CA) and worldwide with uncertain outcomes in terms of weight loss and resolution of comorbidities. However they proved to be safe and effective when they are used as a prebariatric procedure or as a primary procedure in obese population, for less than 6 months, with appropriate volumes and under supervision [54, 55] (Fig. 33.7a, b).

Malabsorptive Devices

The *Endobarrier® Gastrointestinal Liner* (GI Dynamics Inc, Lexington, MA) is a device that is endoscopically deployed and consists of an impermeable, self-expanding, 60-cm long sleeve that is anchored in the duodenal bulb and extents into the proximal jejunum with drawstrings in the proximal end for removal. By doing so, it creates a barrier to absorption and delays the mixing of food with pancreatic and bile juices. The indications for its use have been weight loss prior to bariatric surgery and improvement of type 2 diabetes. The main concern about its use is the poor tolerability with nausea and abdominal pain as the most common adverse events reported, particularly with longer use. Small studies suggested that the duodenojejunal bypass sleeve might be effective but poorly tolerated in its current design [54, 55].

Malabsorptive/Restrictive Devices

The *ValenTx Endoluminal Bypass* (ValenTx Inc., Maple Grove, MN) is an implantable sleeve (120-cm long) that is inserted endoscopically beginning at the gastroesophageal junction and extended into the jejunum. The device was designed to mimic the mechanism of action of the traditional RYGB by restricting the amount of food intake, excluding food from the stomach and small bowel, and leaving undigested food exposed to the jejunum. A prospective human trial demonstrated that the device and the procedure are safe and effective for both weight loss and improvement of comorbidities. No major complications were observed, patient adaptation was favorable, and the device was retrieved without difficulties proving the reversibility of the procedure. However, first generation products required laparoscopic assistance in attaching the product to the gastroesophageal junction [54, 57]. The company has since developed a fully transoral delivery method (Fig. 33.8).

Regulating Gastric Emptying Devices

- Gastric electrical stimulation has been suggested and is actually investigated as a potential therapeutic option for obesity. The implantable gastric stimulation devices that can be delivered endoscopically act by inducing food intake reduction, gastric emptying delay, and decreasing the appetite-stimulating gut hormones and increasing the appetite-inhibiting gut hormones in gastric and duodenal tissues [54].
- The application of Botulinum toxin A (BTXA) injection is also novel in the filed of bariatrics. Its intraparietal administration in the antrum and fundus of the stomach may reduce gastric emptying and increase satiety as a result of cholinergic denervation, with no significant side effects [55].
- The TransPyloric Shuttle® (BAROnova Inc., Goleta, CA) is a removable endoscopically delivered device that is deployed into the stomach. Once in there, the device is intended to work in concert with the natural cycles of peristalsis to self-position across the pylorus. By doing so, it creates an intermittent pyloric obstruction that delays gastric emptying and generates early satiety and prolonged satiety (Fig. 33.9a, b).

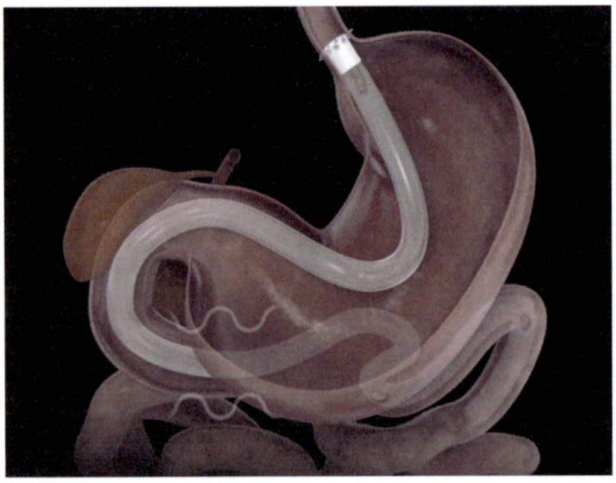

Fig. 33.8 ValenTx endoluminal bypass. (Reproduced with permission of ValenTx, Maple Grove, MN)

Natural Orifice Translumenal Endoscopic Surgery (NOTES)

The attractiveness of endoscopic access through natural orifices for performance of traditional surgical procedures is based mainly on the possibility

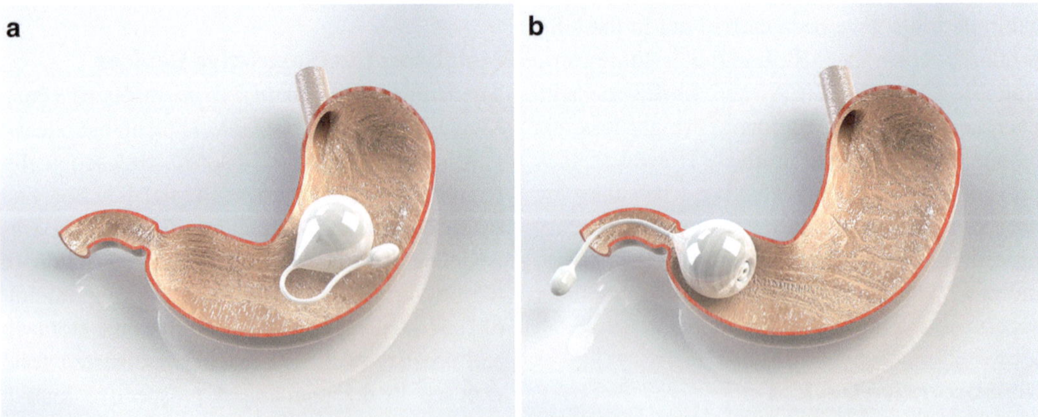

Fig. 33.9 (**a**, **b**) TransPyloric Shuttle®. (**a**) Gastric position. (**b**) Transpyloric position. (**a**, **b**: Reproduced with permission of BAROnova Inc., Goleta, CA)

to perform surgery without any externally visible incisions. Original descriptions of the approach dated back to 1979 and although the application of NOTES to bariatric procedures has been very recent and scarce, it represents an attractive option due to the potential to reduce the incidence of wound-related complications in the obese population.

Sleeve gastrectomy was carried out in porcine models as well as more complex surgeries such as RYGB, described in human cadaver models as pure and hybrid procedures [58].

Although with a promising future, NOTES is still in its infancy and several major hurdles should be overcome to increase its application related to instrumentation, improved techniques, and costs. The combination of NOTES with robotic technology is also an attractive option that opens a new horizon for the management of bariatric patients.

Summary

Due to the worsening epidemic of obesity, bariatric surgery is a field continuously evolving with an exponential increase in popularity. The state-of-the-art surgical procedures with laparoscopy as the gold standard approach are still the only proven long-term effective treatment for morbid obesity, yet a great portion of the qualifying candidates is excluded from therapy. Although the application of robotic technology in bariatric surgery is still evolving, it is likely that they will be widely adopted due to their ability to compensate for the limitations encountered with laparoscopic approach especially in the morbidly obese population. The continuing goal set to reduce invasiveness is greatly expanding the research on emerging technologies and new procedures in the fields of therapeutic endoscopy and minimally invasive surgery. Recently developed minimally invasive techniques and devices with promising results may potentially pave the unmet needs of many obese populations; however, they should be considered as experimental until strong published data becomes available.

References

1. Ogden CL, Carroll MD, Kit BK, Flegal KM. Prevalence of obesity among adults: United States 2001-2012. NCHS Data Brief. 2013;131:1–8.
2. Ogden CL, Carroll MD, Kit BK, Flegal KM. Prevalence of obesity in the United States, 2009-2010. NCHS Data Brief. 2012;82:1–8.
3. Ogden CL, Carroll MD, McDowell MA, Flegal KM. Obesity among adults in the United States- no statistically significant change since 2003-2004. NCHS Data Brief. 2007;1:1–8.
4. www.who.int/mediacentre/factsheets/fs311/en/.
5. Haslam DW, James WP. Obesity. Lancet. 2005; 366(9492):1197–209.
6. Li Z, Bowerman S, Heber D. Health ramifications of the obesity epidemic. Surg Clin North Am. 2005;85(4):681–701. v. Review.
7. Gastrointestinal surgery for severe obesity: National Institutes of Health consensus development conference statement. Am J Clin Nutr. 1992;55(2 Suppl): 615s–619s.
8. O'Brien PE. Bariatric surgery: mechanisms, indications and outcomes. J Gastroenterol Hepatol. 2010; 25(8):1358–65.
9. Karlsson J, Taft C, Rydén A, et al. Ten-year trends in health related quality of life after surgical and conventional treatment for severe obesity: the SOS intervention study. Int J Obes. 2007;31(8):1248–61.
10. Baker MT. The history and evolution of bariatric surgical procedures. Surg Clin North Am. 2011;91(6):1181–201.
11. Buchwald H, Buchwald JN. Evolution of operative procedures for the management of morbid obesity 1950-2000. Obes Surg. 2002;12(5):705–17.
12. McBride CL, Kothari V. Evolution of laparoscopic adjustable gastric banding. Surg Clin North Am. 2011;91(6):1239–47.
13. Marceau P, Biron S, St Georges R, et al. Biliopancreatic diversion with gastrectomy as surgical treatment of morbid obesity. Obes Surg. 1991;1(4):381–7.
14. Brethauer SA. Sleeve gastrectomy. Surg Clin North Am. 2011;91(6):1265–79.
15. Zhao Y, Encinosa W. Bariatric surgery utilization and outcomes in 1998 and 2004: statistical brief #23. Healthcare Cost and Utilization Project (HCUP) Statistical Briefs. Rockville (MD): Agency for Health Care Policy and Research (US); 2006–2007. http://www.hcup-us.ahrq.gov/reports/statbriefs/sb23.pdf.
16. DeMaria EJ, Pate V, Warthen M, Winegar DA. Baseline data from American Society for Metabolic and Bariatric Surgery-designated Bariatric Surgery Centers of Excellence using the Bariatric Outcomes Longitudinal Database. Surg Obes Relat Dis. 2010;6(4):347–55.
17. ASMBS total bariatric procedures numbers from 2011, 2012 and 2013 based on the best estimation from available data (BOLD, ASC/MBSAQIP, National Inpatient Sample data and outpatient estimations).

http://asmbs.org/2014/03/estimate-of-bariatric-surgery-numbers/.
18. Cobourn C, Chapman MA, Ali A, Amrhein J. Five-year weight loss experience of outpatients receiving laparoscopic adjustable gastric band surgery. Obes Surg. 2013;23(7):903–10.
19. O'Brien PE, MacDonlad L, Anderson M, et al. Long-term outcomes after bariatric surgery: fifteen-year follow-up of adjustable gastric banding and a systematic review of the bariatric surgical literature. Ann Surg. 2013;257(1):87–94.
20. Owers C, Ackroyd R. A study examining the complications associated with gastric banding. Obes Surg. 2013;23(1):56–9.
21. Boza C, Gamboa C, Perez G, et al. Laparoscopic adjustable gastric banding (LAGB): surgical results and 5-year follow-up. Surg Endosc. 2011;25(1):292–7.
22. Nguyen NT, Hohmann S, Nguyen XM, et al. Outcome of laparoscopic adjustable gastric banding and prevalence of band revision and explantation at academic centers: 2007-2009. Surg Obes Relat Dis. 2012;8(6): 724–7.
23. Himpens J, Cadière GB, Bazi M, et al. Long-term outcomes of laparoscopic adjustable gastric banding. Arch Surg. 2011;146(7):802–7.
24. Needelman BJ, Happel LC. Bariatric surgery: choosing the optimal procedure. Surg Clin North Am. 2008;88(5):991–1007.
25. Rosenthal RJ, International Sleeve Gastrectomy Expert Panel. International sleeve gastrectomy expert panel consensus statement: best practice guidelines based on experience of >12,000 cases. Surg Obes Relat Dis. 2012;8(1):8–19.
26. ASMBS Clinical Issues Committee. Updated position statement on sleeve gastrectomy as a bariatric procedure. Surg Obes Relat Dis. 2012;8(3):e21–6.
27. Diamantis T, Apostolou KG, Alexandrou A, et al. Review of long-term results after laparoscopic sleeve gastrectomy. Surg Obes Relat Dis. 2014;10(1):177–83.
28. Sieber P, Gass M, Kern B, et al. Five-year results of laparoscopic sleeve gastrectomy. Surg Obes Relat Dis. 2014;10(2):243–9.
29. Cadière GB, Himpens J, Vertruyen M, Favretti F. The world's first obesity surgery performed by a surgeon at a distance. Obes Surg. 1999;9(2):206–9.
30. Horgan S, Vanuno D. Robots in laparoscopic surgery. J Laparoendosc Adv Surg Tech A. 2011;11(6):415–9.
31. Moser F, Horgan S. Robotically assisted bariatric surgery. Am J Surg. 2004;188(4A Suppl):38S–44.
32. Nguyen NT, Hinojosa MW, Finley D, et al. Application of robotics in general surgery: initial experience. Am Surg. 2004;70(10):914–7.
33. Edelson PK, Dumon KR, Sonnad SS, et al. Robotic vs. conventional laparoscopic gastric banding, a comparison of a 407 cases. Surg Endosc. 2011;25(5): 1402–8.
34. Buchs NC, Morel P, Azagury DE, et al. Laparoscopic versus robotic Roux-en-Y gastric bypass: lessons and long-term follow-up learned from a large prospective monocentric study. Obes Surg. 2014;24(12):2031–9.
35. Hagen ME, Inan I, Pugin F, Morel P. The da Vinci surgical system in digestive surgery. Rev Med Suisse. 2007;3(117):1622–6.
36. Ayloo S, Buchs NC, Addeo P, et al. Robot-assisted sleeve gastrectomy for super-morbidly obese patients. J Laparoendosc Adv Surg Tech A. 2011;21(4):295–9.
37. Diamantis T, Alexandrou A, Nikiteas N, et al. Initial experience with robotic sleeve gastrectomy for morbid obesity. Obes Surg. 2011;21(8):1172–9.
38. Vilallonga R, Fort JM, Gonzalez O, et al. The initial learning curve for robot-assisted sleeve gastrectomy: a surgeon's experience while introducing the robotic technology in a bariatric surgery department. Minim Invasive Surg. 2012;2012:347131.
39. Stephens DJ, Saunders JK, Belsley S, et al. Short-term outcomes for super-super obese (BMI $\geq$60 kg/m^2) patients undergoing weight loss surgery at a high-volume bariatric surgery center: laparoscopic adjustable gastric banding, laparoscopic gastric bypass, and open tubular gastric bypass. Surg Obes Relat Dis. 2008;4(3):408–15.
40. Parikh MS, Shen R, Weiner M, et al. Laparoscopic bariatric surgery in super-obese patients (BMI>50) is safe and effective: a review of 332 patients. Obes Surg. 2005;15(6):858–63.
41. Nguyen NT, Hinojosa MW, Smith BR, Reavis KM. Single laparoscopic incision transabdominal (SLIT) surgery-adjustable gastric banding: a novel minimally invasive surgical approach. Obes Surg. 2008;18(12):1628–31.
42. Saber AA, El-Ghazaly TH. Early experience with single-access transumbilical adjustable laparoscopic gastric banding. Obes Surg. 2009;19(10):1442–6.
43. Teixeira J, McGill K, Binenbaum S, Forrester G. Laparoscopic single-site surgery for placement of an adjustable gastric band: initial experience. Surg Endosc. 2009;23(6):1409–14.
44. Moreno-Sanz C, Morandeira-Rivas A, Sedano-Vizcaino C et al. Single-incision laparoscopic bariatric surgery: a systematic review. Surg Obes Relat Dis. 2013; pii: S1550-7289(13)00390-0.
45. Gomberawalla A, Salamat A, Lutfi R. Outcome analysis of single incision vs traditional multiport sleeve gastrectomy: a matched cohort study. Obes Surg. 2014;24(11):1870–4.
46. Sucher R, Resch T, Mohr E, et al. Single-incision laparoscopic sleeve gastrectomy, analysis of 80 cases in a single center. J Laparoendosc Adv Surg Tech A. 2014;24(2):83–8.
47. Lakdawala MA, Muda NH, Goeal S, Bhasker A. Single-incision gastrectomy versus conventional laparoscopic sleeve gastrectomy – a randomised pilot study. Obes Surg. 2011;21(11):1664–70.
48. Galvani CA, Choh M, Gorodner MV. Single-incision sleeve gastrectomy using a novel technique for liver retraction. JSLS. 2010;14(2):228–33.
49. Huang CK, Houng JY, Chiang CJ, et al. Single incision transumbilical laparoscopic Roux-en-Y gastric bypass: a first case report. Obes Surg. 2009;19(12):1711–5.
50. Huang CK, Lo CH, Houng JY, et al. Surgical results of single-incision transumbilical laparoscopic Roux-en-Y gastric bypass. Surg Obes Relat Dis. 2012;8(2):201–7.

51. Cirocchi R, Boselli C, Santoro A, et al. Current status of robotic bariatric surgery: a systematic review. BMC Surg. 2013;13:53.
52. Gill R, Al-Adra DP, Birch D, et al. Robotic-assisted bariatric surgery: a systematic review. Int J Med Robotics Comput Assist Surg. 2011;7:249–55.
53. Chang SH, Stoll CR, Song J, et al. The effectiveness and risks of bariatric surgery: an updated systematic review and meta-analysis, 2003-2012. JAMA Surg. 2014;149(3):275–87.
54. Singhal S, Le DL, Duddempudi S, Anand S. The role of endoscopy in bariatrics: past, present, and future. J Laparoendosc Adv Surg Tech A. 2012;22:802–11.
55. ASGE Technology Committee, Kethu SR, BAnjeree S, Barth BA, et al. Endoluminal bariatric techniques. Gastrointest Endosc. 2012;76:1–7.
56. Hu B, Chung SCS, Sun LCL, et al. Transoral obesity surgery: endoluminal gastroplasty with an endoscopic suture device. Endoscopy. 2005;37:411–4.
57. Majumder S, Birk J. A review of the current status of endoluminal therapy as a primary approach to obesity management. Surg Endosc. 2013;27:2305–11.
58. Tsemelli N, Coumaros D. The future of bariatrics: endoscopy, endoluminal surgery, and natural orifice translumenal endoscopic surgery. Endoscopy. 2010; 42:155–62.

New Minimally Invasive Treatments for Acid Reflux

34

Prashant Sukharamwala, Sharona Ross, and Alexander Rosemurgy

Introduction

In the USA, approximately 10–20 % of the population suffers from gastroesophageal reflux. Many factors contribute to the development of gastroesophageal reflux include pregnancy, obesity, increasing age, smoking, and alcohol consumption. Gastroesophageal reflux disease (GERD) is a chronic form of gastroesophageal reflux, whether it is gastric acid or bile, and the term implies morbidity, maybe just symptomatic, due to the reflux. The conventional treatment of GERD includes lifestyle modification (e.g., weight loss, cessation of smoking, elevating the head of the bed at night) and medical therapy with H-2 blockers or proton pump inhibitors (PPI) to decrease gastric acid secretion. While the first line of treatment for GERD involves medical therapy, many question the long-term use of H-2 blockers and PPIs as there is a plausible cause-effect relationship with these medications and osteoporosis, bone fractures, hypomagnesaemia, development of gastric polyps, enteric infections, interstitial nephritis, pneumonia, and more [1, 2]. The medications are "anti-acid" medications and, thereby, do not impact, inhibit, or cease gastroesophageal reflux. Inherent in this concern is that, under the best of circumstances, effective "anti-acid" therapy leads to ongoing nonacidic reflux (i.e., unconjugated bile salts refluxing into the esophagus) which is carcinogenic. As a result of 30 plus years of uncontrolled "anti-acid" therapy in our population, esophageal cancer in the USA is approaching epidemic proportions [3]. Unlike medical therapy, anti-reflux surgery provides a solution for GERD and in its current laparoscopic format has been widely applied for more than 20 years with results supporting further ongoing application. However, conventional laparoscopic fundoplication may not be an optimal option for some patients. In the last decade, several endoscopic solutions have been introduced and are increasingly widely applied. Herein, we detail the evolving endoscopic and new laparoscopic approaches, including "scarless surgery," for treating GERD.

Minimally Invasive Surgical Approach

In 1991, Dallemagne et al. presented their data on laparoscopic Nissen fundoplication in the treatment of GERD. Since then, laparoscopic fundoplication has been embraced by surgeons as the "gold standard" in treating GERD [4].

P. Sukharamwala, M.D. • S. Ross, M.D., F.A.C.S. (✉)
A. Rosemurgy, M.D., F.A.C.S.
Florida Hospital Tampa, 3000 Medical Park Drive, Suite 310, Tampa, FL 33613, USA
e-mail: prashantsukharamwala@yahoo.com; Sharona.ross@yahoo.com; arosemurgy@hotmail.com

R. Latifi et al. (eds.), *Technological Advances in Surgery, Trauma and Critical Care*,
DOI 10.1007/978-1-4939-2671-8_34

For appropriate and good reasons (stated above), some patients with GERD do not want to commit themselves to a lifelong consumption of "anti-acid" medications or undergo what they perceive to be a "major" operation, and therefore, they seek and are willing to undergo a less invasive endoscopic procedure. The endoscopic approach for the treatment of GERD is also attractive for patients who experience recurrence of excessive gastroesophageal reflux following an operative fundoplication. The principles applied to endoscopic solutions over the past 15 years have been purveyed through plication at the gastroesophageal (GE) junction, injection of bulking agents at the gastroesophageal junction, application of radiofrequency energy at the GE junction, electrical stimulation of the lower esophageal sphincter (LES) mechanism, and the placement of a ring of magnets (i.e., magnetic band application) around the GE junction.

Endoscopic suturing and plicating approaches for treating GERD began to be introduced in the early 2000s. One of the first developed endoscopic "solutions" was a plication device named EndoCinch™ (C.R. Bard Inc., Murray Hill, NJ), which facilitated endoscopic suturing at and near the GE junction to augment the LES mechanism. This involved very superficial suturing and the application of the plication was not durable. It has fallen out of favor and into disuse because of insufficient long-term efficacy [5]. It is no longer commercially available. In the last decade, several novel endoscopic anti-reflux devices to treat GERD have been introduced; however, the application of these devices has been hindered by the lack of long-term data documenting their amelioration of GERD and GERD symptoms and the generally nihilistic view of gastroenterologists in treating GERD beyond "open-ended" PPI therapy.

Endoscopic treatment of symptomatic chronic GERD seems best indicated for patients with excessive gastroesophageal reflux who do not have a hiatal hernia greater than 2 cm. Patients who are at high risk for an abdominal operation, or have had an operative fundoplication specifically, should also be considered for endoscopic therapy, as it avoids violation of the coelomic cavity and a reoperative field. This includes patients with severe cardiorespiratory comorbidities and patients with a history of previous intra-abdominal surgery, especially previous anti-reflux surgery or gastric bypass or sleeve gastrectomy.

Only a handful of patients will qualify to undergo endoscopic treatment for GERD as the incidence of hiatal hernia increases with age and approximately 60 % of patients above 50 years of age have hiatal hernia greater than 2 cm [6]. With increasing awareness among patients of long-term consequences of "anti-acid" medications, patients are seeking endoscopic treatments as a means to avoid lifelong medications and transabdominal operative therapy, with potential complications perceived (and propagated) by nonsurgeons to be unique complications and ramifications following surgery, including dysphagia, bloating, diarrhea, and inability to vomit. However, the possible, but very infrequent, complications of endoscopic therapy must be made clear to patients, including hematoma, mediastinal abscess, and esophageal perforation. Patients with a BMI more than 35 kg/m^2, a hiatal hernia more than 2 cm, esophageal ulcers, portal hypertension, and varices should not be considered for endoscopic treatment of GERD.

Transoral Incisionless Fundoplication: EsophyX® (EndoGastric Solutions, Inc., Redmond, WA)

Transoral Incisionless Fundoplication (TIF), as the name implies, is undertaken transorally rather than through an abdominal incision like laparoscopy. It results in a 270° valve constructed over an endoscope which is 2–3 cm in length. The FDA approved the use of the EsophyX® device to undertake TIF (Fig. 34.1) in the USA after Cadiere et al. reported its safety and efficacy through a prospective multicenter trial [7]. The 12-month results proved EsophyX®, and the resultant TIF, was safe and effective in improving quality of life, ameliorating symptoms of acid reflux, reducing PPIs use, preventing esophagitis, and increasing the LES resting pressure in

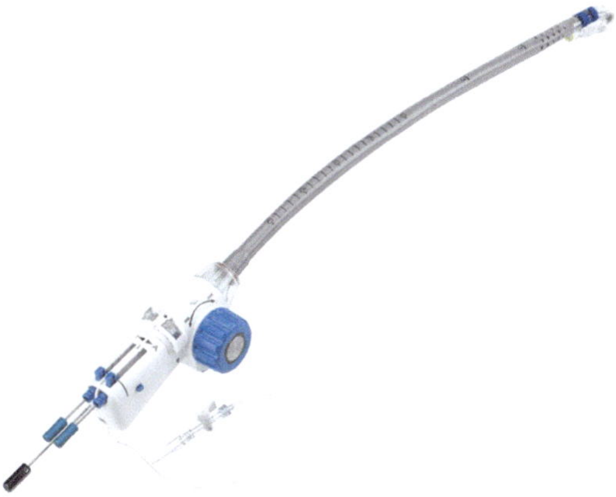

Fig. 34.1 EsophyX® device. (Reprinted with permission of EndoGastric Solutions, Inc., Redmond, WA. Copyright © 2014 EndoGastric Solutions, Inc.)

patients. To date, EsophyX® has been undertaken in over 10,000 patients worldwide.

TIF involves an endoscopically guided transoral insertion of the EsophyX® device to create a 270°, 2–3 cm esophagogastric valve by placing 12–20 full-thickness polypropylene H-fasteners. This approach augments the gastroesophageal flap valve, the valve visualized in the stomach which correlates to the angle of His on external view of the stomach. To undertake TIF, a flexible video endoscope is passed through the EsophyX® device, and both are passed transorally into the stomach. The entire procedure is undertaken with endoscopic guidance. Through the EsophyX® device a helical screw device is deployed and anchored into the deficient gastroesophageal flap valve and the screw is used to draw the deficient gastroesophageal valve into the device. The device is then closed and the gastric fundus and the deficient gastroesophageal valve is compressed allowing polypropylene H-fasteners to be passed across the esophagus and the gastric fundus, anchoring these structures together and augmenting the valve. A total of 12 H-fasteners are used to construct the fundoplication. The procedure may also result in reduction of all small hiatal hernias up to 2 cm in size [7]. Factors that affect positive outcomes after TIF include a large number of fasteners and hiatal hernia less than or equal to 2 cm. Presence of esophageal dysmotility and hiatal hernia may increase the risk of recurrence of GERD symptoms [8].

Longer-term data suggest 70–80 % of patients are completely off PPIs following TIF and only a small group of patients have to take PPIs daily, which would suggest the TIF has failed [9, 10]. Following TIF, DeMeester scores were reduced and normalized in 60–70 % of patients. The average number of acid reflux episodes per 24-h testing period was also significantly reduced following TIF and normalized in 80–90 % of patients [10]. Most patients who underwent TIF report amelioration of symptoms of heartburn and regurgitation. For patients with failed TIF, revisional laparoscopic fundoplication was found to be safe and efficacious resulting in objective reflux control [11]. Complications noted by various published series indicate hemorrhage as the most common complication; however, the risk is less than 1 % and amenable to endoscopic control of bleeding. There is a 0.7 % risk for esophageal perforation associated with TIF. TIF appears to consistently provide symptomatic relief with promising levels of patient satisfaction [11, 12].

In patients with erosive esophagitis or Barrett's esophagus, TIF may not be considered adequate anti-reflux therapy, as normalization of esophageal pH is of utmost importance [10].

The Stretta System (Curon Medical, Fremont, CA)

The Stretta system (Fig. 34.2a, b) is another endoscopic endoluminal system utilized for treating GERD. It has been available for more than a decade. This unique system applies radiofrequency ablation energy (RFA) to the muscularis propria in the LES without causing a significant thermal burn to the mucosa. This device utilizes an inflatable balloon through which four electrodes emanate; these electrodes deliver RFA energy under a controlled temperature to cause inflammation and healing by fibrosis. Stretta works by reducing the relaxation pressure of the LES, reducing tissue compliance without fibrosis, and increasing the smooth muscle fiber size with more muscle fibers per muscle bundle resulting in

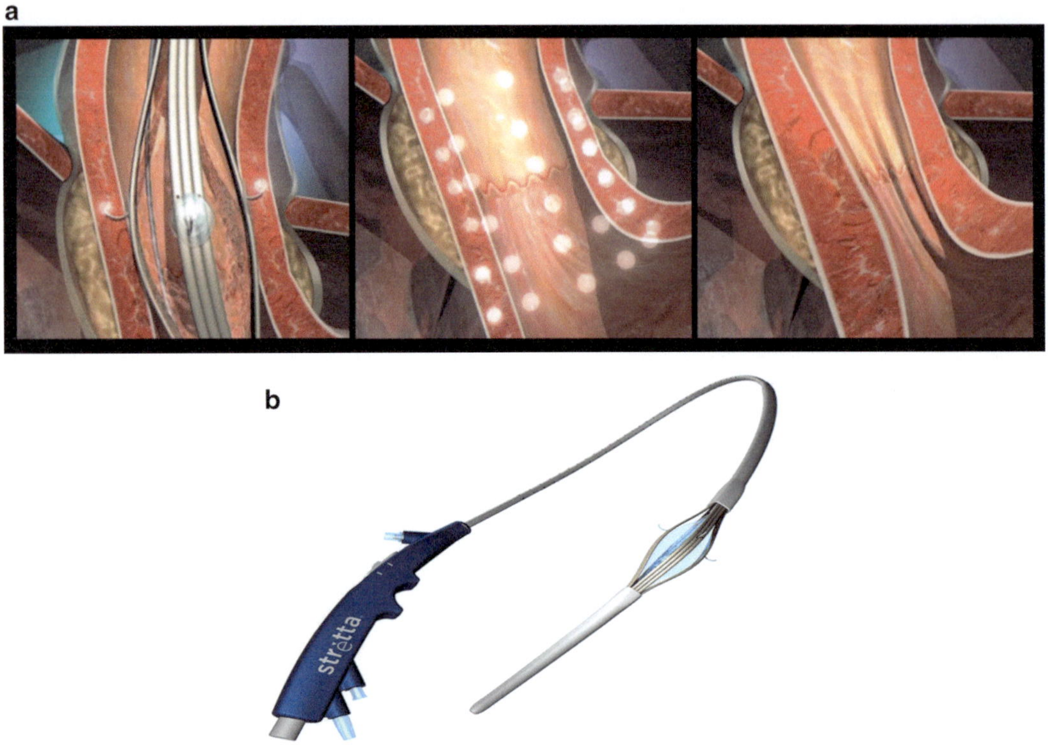

Fig. 34.2 (**a**, **b**) Stretta device. (Reprinted with permission of Mederi Therapeutics, Norwalk, CT. Copyright © 2014 Mederi Therapeutics, Inc.)

lengthening and thickening of the sphincter, thereby improving the barrier function of the LES mechanism [13]. To minimize collateral injury, the device utilizes continuous saline irrigation while continuously monitoring the temperature of the mucosa and muscularis propria.

Although the Stretta procedure has shown promise in the ability to improve heartburn and decrease PPI usage over a 12 months period and up to 5 years after application, only a small number of studies have long-term outcomes [7, 14, 15]. Abdel Aziz et al. reported through a prospective randomized trial that the total esophageal acid exposure was reduced after the Stretta procedure and this effect was sustained through the 12 months of follow-up [16]. The Stretta system alleviated GERD symptoms, including heartburn, and reduced PPI requirements in nearly two-thirds of patients. Reymunde and Santiago reported a 4-year follow-up with sustained improvements in symptoms, quality of life, and PPI use after Stretta [17]. The efficacy was again demonstrated by Dughera et al. as they documented that 72.3 % of patients with GERD remained PPI-free at 48 months [18]. A meta-analysis of 18 studies reporting data on 1,441 patients was reported by Perry et al. [19]. This meta-analysis showed significant improvement in symptoms of reflux, improved quality of life measured by GERD QOL scale, and significantly reduced DeMeester scores. While pre-procedure DeMeester scores were reduced from 44.4 to 28.5, they did not normalize (normal being <14.7).

In four randomized controlled trials comparing sham Stretta or PPI versus Stretta alone, patients who underwent Stretta had significantly reduced GERD health related quality of life complications, reduced use of PPIs, reduced esophageal acid exposure, normalization of LES pressures, and improved grades of esophagitis [15, 16, 20, 21]. Noar et al. prospectively followed 217 patients with 10-year follow-up after

Stretta. Interestingly, the most common short-term side effect reported was chest pain. Seventy-two percent of patients reported normalization of GERD-HRQL and more than 50 % reported reduction in PPI use with 41 % of patients completely off of PPIs. In this series, no esophageal perforations were noted; other series have reported esophageal perforation as a dreaded, albeit very infrequent, complication [22]. No data is available for the use of Stretta in patients with severe esophagitis, hiatal hernias more than 2 cm (this is a contraindication to the procedure), Barrett's esophagus, or with a history of autoimmune disease, collagen vascular disease, and/or coagulation disorders. Based on the available literature, Stretta can be recommended for patients with acid reflux, but without hiatal hernia more than 2 cm. Stretta seems best applied to patients with excess gastroesophageal reflux who have had operations which have reduced gastric volume, such as sleeve gastrectomy or gastric bypass for weight loss.

The LINX® Reflux Management System (Torax Medical, Inc., Shoreview, MN)

In 2012, the FDA approved the LINX® system (Fig. 34.3) for the treatment of GERD. The LINX® system consists of a small band with interlinked titanium beads with magnetic cores. Utilizing laparoscopy, the band is placed around the GE junction in such a way that the magnetic attraction between the beads works to keep the GE junction closed at rest. With swallowing, as the food bolus reaches the LES, esophageal generated swallowing forces push the food and liquid through the GE junction as the magnetic beads separate. After the food bolus passes the GE junction, the magnetic force causes the LES to close immediately preventing acid reflux.

In a feasibility trial, 44 patients with GERD were enrolled between 2008 and 2009 and 2-year follow-up results were reported [23]. At 1 and 2 years, 77 and 90 % of patients had normal esophageal acid exposure. The trial documented that the mean percentage of time with a pH less than 4 decreased from a baseline of 11.9–3.1 % ($p<0.0001$) at 1 year and to 2.4 % ($p<0.0001$) at 2 years. Patient satisfaction was 87 % at 1 year and 86 % at 2 years. Based in part on this data, the FDA approved the use of the LINX® system for the treatment of GERD. Patients excluded from this trial had a hiatal hernia more than 3 cm, dysphagia, greater than grade A esophagitis, and Barrett's esophagus. In 2013, Bonavina et al. reported a prospective case series of 100 consecutive patients, who underwent laparoscopic LINX® placement. With median implant duration of 3 years, this series reported improved total acid exposure time and improved GERD HRQL scores with no long-term complications such as device migration or erosion. However, three patient had the device removed for persistent dysphagia or GERD [24].

The LINX® system is a new approach for treating acid reflux. Long-term data about efficacy

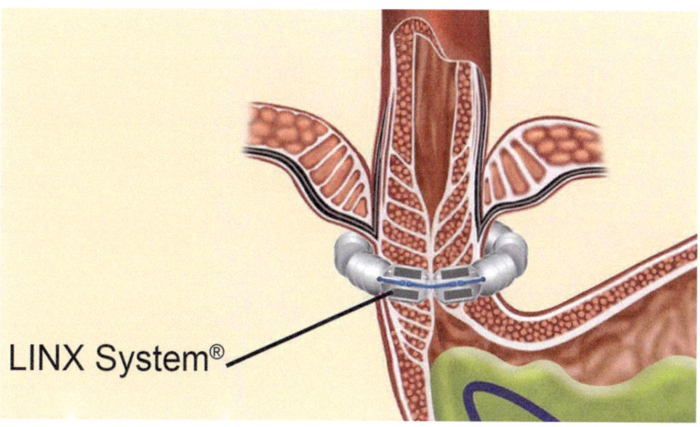

Fig. 34.3 The LINX® system. (Reprinted with permission of Torax Medical, Inc., Shoreview, MN)

and complications are lacking. Therefore, the LINX® reflux management system can only be recommended with caution as a first-line therapy in treating GERD.

EndoStim (EndoStim®, St. Louis, Missouri, and The Hague, The Netherlands)

The EndoStim system is a new device focusing on increasing lower esophageal sphincter tone by delivering electric stimulation to the lower esophagus. This system is proposed as a long-term treatment option for patients with severe GERD.

EndoStim's Stimulation System involves laparoscopic placement of electrodes on the lower esophagus which are connected to an electrical simulator placed in the subcutaneous pocket made in the abdominal wall. It delivers low-energy electrical pulses to the gastroesophageal junction. Rodriguez et al. [25] reported 2 years outcome of electrical stimulation therapy in 25 patients. They reported significant and sustained improvement in symptoms and reduction in PPI use. This group reported improved GERD Health Related Quality of Life improvement off PPI. Possible complications of the EndoStim system include esophageal perforation during the placement of the electrodes which may lead to removal of the device.

The EndoStim is a new system, and the data are evolving. Due to the paucity of convincing data in long-term treatment of acid reflux, the EndoStim system is not approved for use in the USA by the FDA.

Laparo-Endoscopic Single Site (LESS) Fundoplication

The long-term outcomes associated with laparoscopic fundoplication for treating GERD are well documented in the literature. Its mention in any discussion about efficacious therapy for GERD is warranted given its proven safety and efficacy. Laparoscopic fundoplication is the "first-line" surgical therapy for treating GERD.

With laparoscopy, operative techniques and technology are continuously evolving. The evolution of conventional laparoscopy to LESS surgery began with the observation that a laparoscopic cholecystectomy could be safely undertaken with fewer port sites and trocars [26]. The most recent innovative laparoscopic approach for treating GERD has been the Laparo-Endoscopic Single Site (LESS) fundoplication. This operation is undertaken through a single 8–12 mm incision at the umbilicus, preserving the umbilical ring [27] (Fig. 34.4). The fundoplication constructed and the conduct of the operation in general are not different than when laparoscopic fundoplication is

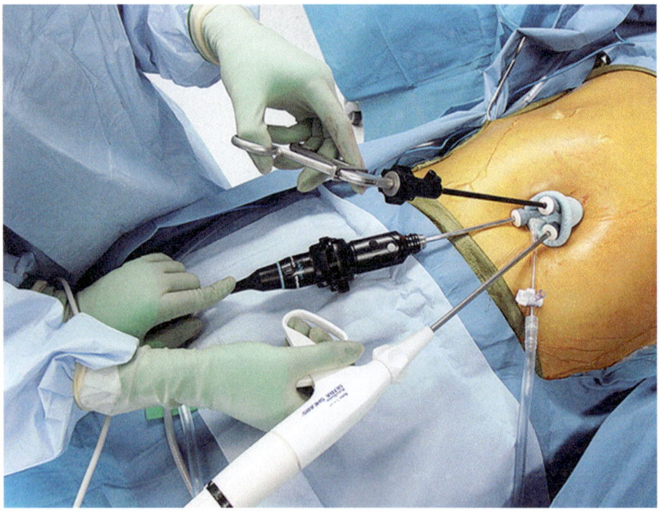

Fig. 34.4 Port placement for laparoendoscopic single site fundoplication

undertaken. Because the approach is "scarless," LESS surgery is a cosmetically superior approach to treating gastroesophageal reflux compared to multi-incision laparoscopic surgery, which usually involves five or more ports each through its own incision to complete. The "scar" with LESS surgery is hidden at the umbilicus, itself a scar; therein the operative approach is "scarless" (Fig. 34.5). As well, this single incision laparoscopic may lead to reduced postoperative pain, a reduced incidence of wound infections and complications, and a shorter length of stay.

The learning curve for LESS fundoplication is documented in the literature. The learning curve for LESS fundoplication is definable, short, and safe [28]. In the early part of the learning curve, LESS fundoplication may take longer and additional ports may be required, but as more operations are undertaken operative time with LESS fundoplication will converge with operative time required for the conventional laparoscopic approach. However, the caveat is that to undertake LESS fundoplication surgeons must have basic and advanced laparoscopic skills and must have developed proficiency in undertaking fundoplication with conventional laparoscopy. Not surprisingly, surgeon experience with anti-reflux surgery has been linked to better outcomes after fundoplication [29].

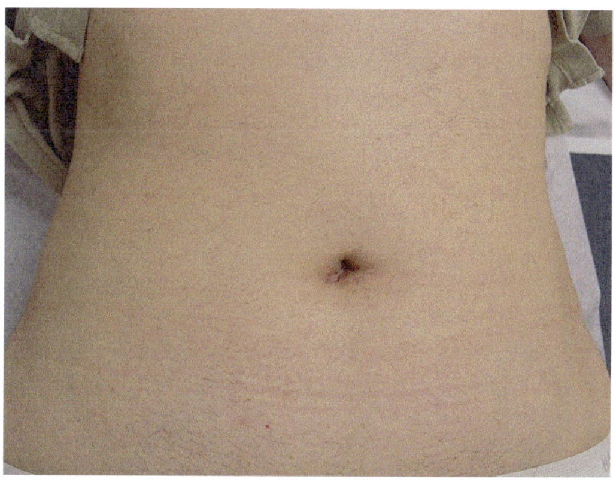

Fig. 34.5 Postoperative LESS scar

It is well known that laparoscopic fundoplication durably provides high patient satisfaction with long-term amelioration of the frequency and severity of symptoms of gastroesophageal reflux disease [30]. Relative to conventional laparoscopic fundoplication, LESS fundoplication provides excellent resolution of symptoms without apparent scaring. In comparison to conventional laparoscopic fundoplication, LESS fundoplication is as safe with similar symptom improvement and superior cosmesis [31] (Table 34.1). Given that the steps for laparoscopic fundoplication are the same as for LESS fundoplication, the long-term resolution of acid reflux symptoms should be similarly preserved [31]. If given a choice, patients inherently will choose the most minimally invasive option (i.e., single incision laparoscopy); LESS surgery is perceived

Table 34.1 Demographic data, hospital course, and complications for patients undergoing LESS fundoplication versus laparoscopic fundoplication

	LESS fundoplication	Laparoscopic fundoplication	*p* value
No. of patients	130	130	NS
Male/female ratio	44/86	46/84	NS
Age (year)	61 (57 ± 14.6)	57 (57 ± 13.2)	NS
BMI (kg/m^2)	27 (27 ± 4.1)	27 (27 ± 3.9)	NS
Length of stay (days)	1 (2 ± 1.2)	1 (2 ± 1.8)	NS
Length of operation (min)	146 (154 ± 54.5)	101 (126 ± 74)	0.0009
Blood loss (mL)	128 < 100 cc, 2 = 150 cc	117 < 100 cc, 13 ≥ 150 cc	NS
Preoperative DeMeester score	31 (37 ± 30.8)	30 (38 ± 35)	NS
Nissen/Toupet	107/23	106/24	NS
Total complications—intraoperative	2 (2 %)	5 (4 %)	NS
Total complications—postoperative	9 (7 %)	20 (15 %)	0.04
Conversions to open	0	7	0.01

by patients to provide a better cosmetic outcome. Furthermore, satisfaction is greater after LESS fundoplication because patients can return to normal activity sooner due to a shorter recovery time [31]. Several authors have noted better pain profiles and lower analgesia requirements in patients who undergo LESS surgery compared to those who undergo conventional laparoscopy. In addition patients have a shorter median return to work time when they underwent the LESS approach [25, 31–33]. Given the benefits of LESS fundoplication compared to conventional laparoscopy, it seems to be a very desirable approach for treatment of acid reflux.

Summary

With exponential growth of newer technology available for the treatment of acid reflux, there are an increasing number of patients presenting with reflux symptoms who seek minimally invasive approaches to acid reflux. A thorough evaluation and diagnostic workup are necessary to diagnose GERD and tailor an effective definitive solution. All patients should be counseled about the available endoscopic and surgical treatment options for acid reflux. Endoscopic treatment of symptomatic chronic GERD should be considered in patients who do not have a hiatal hernia greater than 2 cm and who have failed or require open-ended pharmacologic therapy. Transoral Incisionless Fundoplication and the Stretta system provide a robust long-term benefit from acid reflux in appropriate high-risk patients, who wish to discontinue daily medications and want to avoid laparoscopic fundoplication. At our institution, Laparo-Endoscopic Single Site fundoplication remains the procedure of choice for the treatment of gastroesophageal acid reflux.

References

1. Howlader N, Noone AM, Krapcho M, Neyman N, Aminou R, Altekruse SF, Kosary CL, Ruhl J, Tatalovich Z, Cho H, Mariotto A, Eisner MP, Lewis DR, Chen HS, Feuer EJ, Cronin KA (eds) SEER cancer statistics review, 1975–2009 (Vintage 2009 Populations) http://seer.cancer.gov/csr/1975_2009_pops09/2012. http://seer.cancer.gov/csr/1975_2009_pops09/.
2. Ito T, Jensen R. Association of long-term proton pump inhibitor therapy with bone fractures and effects on absorption of calcium, vitamin B12, iron, and magnesium. Curr Gastroenterol Rep. 2010;12(6):448–57.
3. Siegel R, Naishadham D, Jemal A. Cancer statistics. CA Cancer J Clin. 2012;62(1):10–29.
4. Dallemagne B, Weerts J, Jehaes C, Markiewicz S, Lombard R. Laparoscopic Nissen fundoplication: preliminary report. Surg Laparosc Endosc. 1991;1(3):138–43.
5. Schiefke I, Zabel-Langhennig A, Neumann S, Feisthammel J, Moessner J, Caca K. Long term failure of endoscopic gastroplication (EndoCinch). Gut. 2005;54(6):752–8.
6. Goyal R. Dysphagia. In: Harrison's principles of internal medicine. New York: McGraw-Hill; 2008. p. 17e
7. Cadière G, Buset M, Muls V, Rajan A, Rösch T, Eckardt A, et al. Antireflux transoral incisionless fundoplication using EsophyX: 12-month results of a prospective multicenter study. World J Surg. 2008; 32(8):1676–88.
8. Testoni P, Vailati C, Testoni S, Corsetti M. Transoral incisionless fundoplication (TIF 2.0) with EsophyX for gastroesophageal reflux disease: long-term results and findings affecting outcome. Surg Endosc. 2012; 26(5):1425–35.
9. Trad K, Turgeon D, Deljkich E. Long-term outcomes after transoral incisionless fundoplication in patients with GERD and LPR symptoms. Surg Endosc. 2012;26(3):650–60.
10. Bell R, Freeman K. Clinical and pH-metric outcomes of transoral esophagogastric fundoplication for the treatment of gastroesophageal reflux disease. Surg Endosc. 2011;25(6):1975–84.
11. Witteman B, Kessing B, Snijders G, Koek G, Conchillo J, Bouvy N. Revisional laparoscopic antireflux surgery after unsuccessful endoscopic fundoplication. Surg Endosc. 2013;27(6):2231–6.
12. Wilson E, Barnes W, Mavrelis P, Carter B, Bell R, Sewell R, et al. The effects of transoral incisionless fundoplication on chronic GERD patients: 12-month prospective multicenter experience. Surg Laparosc Endosc Percutan Tech. 2014;24(1):36–46.
13. Tam W, Schoeman M, Zhang Q, Dent J, Rigda R, Utley D, et al. Delivery of radiofrequency energy to the lower oesophageal sphincter and gastric cardia inhibits transient lower oesophageal sphincter relaxations and gastro-oesophageal reflux in patients with reflux disease. Gut. 2003;52(4):479–85.
14. Herman R, Berho M, Murawski M, Nowakowski M, Rys J, Schwarz T, et al. Non ablative radiofrequency (RF) application to smooth muscle of internal anal sphincter (IAS): a tissue study. Surg Endosc. 2013;27.
15. Arts J, Bisschops R, Blondeau K, Farré R, Vos R, Holvoet L, et al. A double-blind sham-controlled study of the effect of radiofrequency energy on symptoms and distensibility of the gastro-esophageal junction in GERD. Am J Gastroenterol. 2012;107(2):222–30.

16. Aziz A, El-Khayat H, Sadek A, Mattar S, McNulty G, Kongkam P, et al. A prospective randomized trial of sham, single-dose Stretta, and double-dose Stretta for the treatment of gastroesophageal reflux disease. Surg Endosc. 2010;24(4):818–25.
17. Reymunde A, Santiago N. Long-term results of radiofrequency energy delivery for the treatment of GERD: sustained improvements in symptoms, quality of life, and drug use at 4-year follow-up. Gastrointest Endosc. 2007;35(3):361–6.
18. Dughera L, Navino M, Cassolino P, De Cento M, Cacciotella L, Cisarò F, et al. Long-term results of radiofrequency energy delivery for the treatment of GERD: results of a prospective 48-month study. Diagn Ther Endosc. 2011;2011:507157.
19. Perry K, Banerjee A, Melvin W. Radiofrequency energy delivery to the lower esophageal sphincter reduces esophageal acid exposure and improves GERD symptoms: a systematic review and meta-analysis. Surg Laparosc Endosc Percutan Tech. 2012; 22(4):283–8.
20. Coron E, Sebille V, Cadiot G, Zerbib F, Ducrotte P, Ducrot F, et al. Clinical trial: radiofrequency energy delivery in proton pump inhibitor-dependent gastro-oesophageal reflux disease patients. Aliment Pharmacol Ther. 2008;28(9):1147–58.
21. Corley D, Katz P, Wo J, Stefan A, Patti M, Rothstein R, et al. Improvement of gastroesophageal reflux symptoms after radiofrequency energy: a randomized, sham-controlled trial. Gastroenterology. 2003;125(3): 668–76.
22. Noar M, Squires P, Noar E, Lee M. Long-term maintenance effect of radiofrequency energy delivery for refractory GERD: a decade later. Surg Endosc. 2014;28(8):2323–33.
23. Bonavina L, DeMeester T, Fockens P, Dunn D, Saino G, Bona D, et al. Laparoscopic sphincter augmentation device eliminates reflux symptoms and normalizes esophageal acid exposure: one- and 2-year results of a feasibility trial. Ann Surg. 2010;252(5):857–62.
24. Bonavina L, Saino G, Bona D, Sironi A, Lazzari V. One hundred consecutive patients treated with magnetic sphincter augmentation for gastroesophageal reflux disease: 6 years of clinical experience from a single center. J Am Coll Surg. 2013;217(4):577–85.
25. Rodriguez L, Rodriguez P, Gomez B, Galvao M, Soffer E, Crowell M. Electrical simulation therapy (EST) of the lower esophageal sphincter (LES) is successful in treating GERD – long-term two year results. Am J Gastroenterol. 2013;108:S27.
26. Bucher P, Pugin F, Buchs N, Ostermann S, Morel P. Randomized clinical trial of laparoendoscopic single-site versus conventional laparoscopic cholecystectomy. Br J Surg. 2011;98(12):1695–702.
27. Hernandez J, Morton C, Ross S, Albrink M, Rosemurgy A. Laparoendoscopic single site cholecystectomy: the first 100 patients. Am Surg. 2009; 75(8):681–5.
28. Ross S, Choung E, Teta A, Colibao L, Luberice K, Paul H, et al. The learning curve of laparo-endoscopic single site (LESS) fundoplication: definable, short, and safe. JSLS. 2013;17(3):376–84.
29. Watson D, Baigrie R, Jamieson G. A learning curve for laparoscopic fundoplication. Definable, avoidable, or a waste of time? Ann Surg. 1996;224(2):198–203.
30. Cowgill S, Gillman R, Kraemer E, Al-Saadi S, Vailladolid D, Rosemurgy A. Ten-year follow-up after laparoscopic Nissen fundoplication for gastroesophageal reflux disease. Am Surg. 2007;73(8):748–52.
31. Ross S, Roddenbery A, Luberice K, Paul H, Farrior T, Vice M, et al. Laparoendoscopic single site (LESS) vs. conventional laparoscopic fundoplication for GERD: is there a difference. Surg Endosc. 2013;27(2):538–47.
32. Tsimoyiannis E, Tsimogiannis K, Pappas-Gogos G, Farantos C, Benetatos N, Mavridou P, et al. Different pain scores in single transumbilical incision laparoscopic cholecystectomy versus classic laparoscopic cholecystectomy: a randomized controlled trial. Surg Endosc. 2010;24:1842–8.
33. Marks J, Tacchino R, Robers K, Onders R, Denoto G, Paraskeva P, et al. Prospective randomized controlled trial of traditional laparoscopic cholecystectomy versus single-incision laparoscopic cholecystectomy: report of preliminary data. Am J Surg. 2011;201:369–72.

35 Minimally Invasive Hepato-Pancreato-Biliary Surgery and Associated GI Interventions

Ramanathan M. Seshadri, Russell C. Kirks Jr., and David A. Iannitti

Introduction

The historical advances in hepatobiliary surgery have taken an interesting course over the last century. Elliot in 1897 described the liver being "so friable, so full of gaping vessels and so evidently incapable of being sutured that it seems impossible to manage large wounds of its substance." The major issue at that time was the extensive bleeding encountered during parenchymal transection. Kousnetzoff and Pensky in 1896 had described techniques to reduce bleeding by passing ligatures in the liver substance and pulling up on them during the transection period [1]. The method of packing the liver to temporize major bleeding was described by Garre in 1907 [2]. He was also instrumental in advocating the use of the crush clamp technique prior to dividing liver parenchyma. Another significant contribution towards liver surgery was made by Pringle in 1908, who described the method of inflow control to reduce the bleeding during surgery [3]. In time, the sentinel work by Couinand in 1954 describing the segmental anatomy of the liver led to further advancements in hepatobiliary surgery with the ability to control the major vascular pedicles of the liver [4]. The first person to perform a major liver resection was Wendell in 1911 but it was not until 1952 that the procedure gained substantial momentum when Lortat-Jacob and Robert performed the first true anatomic liver resection [5, 6]. Soon enough, the ability of the liver to regenerate was widely published based on the research by Pack et al. in 1962 and Lin and Chen in 1965 [7, 8]. This made larger resections possible without the fear of sending patients into liver failure.

The first laparoscopic cholecystectomy was performed by Professor Dr. Med Erich Muhe in Germany in 1985 [9]. This marked the beginning of using minimally invasive techniques in Hepatobiliary Surgery. The initial laparoscopic liver resections and techniques (left lateral sectionectomies) were described by Gagner et al., Ferzli et al., and Azagra et al. [10–12]. Since first being described in the late twentieth century, there has been an exponential rise in the number of resections being performed laparoscopically. The availability of several instruments used in open liver surgery such as surgical staplers and bipolar electrosurgical devices now designed for laparoscopic use has made major liver resections possible in a minimally invasive fashion.

R.M. Seshadri, M.D. • D.A. Iannitti, M.D., F.A.C.S. (✉)
Department of Hepatopancreatobiliary Surgery, Carolinas Medical Center, 1025 Morehead Medical Drive, Suite 600, Charlotte, NC 28204, USA
e-mail: Ramanathan.seshadri@carolinashealthcare.org; David.iannitti@carolinashealthcare.org

R.C. Kirks Jr., M.D.
Department of General Surgery, Carolinas Medical Center, 1000 Blythe Blvd, Charlotte, NC 28203, USA
e-mail: Russell.kirks@carolinashealthcare.org

R. Latifi et al. (eds.), *Technological Advances in Surgery, Trauma and Critical Care*,
DOI 10.1007/978-1-4939-2671-8_35

Minimally Invasive Liver Resections

The most commonly performed laparoscopic liver procedure is wedge resection followed by left lateral sectionectomy. These procedures are usually associated with minimal morbidity and can be safely performed by a surgeon with a sound knowledge of liver anatomy and laparoscopy. In large tertiary care referral centers, major liver resections are increasingly being performed in a minimally invasive manner. In these cases, the use of a hand port to aid in tactile feedback has been extremely useful. Some centers perform the procedure in a hybrid fashion where the initial dissection is carried out laparoscopically and the remainder of the procedure is completed in an open fashion. When performed laparoscopically, these procedures have been shown to have acceptable degree of morbidity and mortality and comply with the standards of oncologic resections in cases dealing with malignancy.

Several papers have been published addressing the safety and efficacy of performing liver surgery in a minimally invasive fashion. A meta-analysis by Nguyen et al. analyzed all the published literature on laparoscopic liver resections. A total of 127 articles were reviewed and accounted for 2,804 patients. The major indication for surgery was malignancy (50 %) followed by benign lesions (45 %) and live donor hepatectomies (1.7 %). Seventy-five percent of the cases were performed totally laparoscopically, 17 % were hand assisted, and 2 % were done using the hybrid technique. The most common procedure performed was a wedge resection or segmentectomy (45 %) followed by left lateral sectionectomy (20 %) and lobectomy (9 % right; 7 % left). The overall mortality and morbidity were 0.3 and 10.5 %, respectively [13]. A major consensus statement published from Louisville in 2008 as a collaborative effort by 45 experts in hepatobiliary surgery concluded that laparoscopic liver surgery was a safe and effective approach to manage surgical liver disease in the hands of trained surgeons with experience in hepatobiliary and laparoscopic surgery [14].

Vigano and colleagues in their single institution retrospective study from 1996 thru 2008 were able to demonstrate the increasing use of laparoscopy in liver surgery. They had divided the patient cohort ($n=174$) into three groups based on the time period. The variables for analysis included number of cases, indications for procedure, conversion rate, operating time, blood loss, and pedicle clamping time (Pringle maneuver). The group was able to show the increase in the number of cases done laparoscopically with lower conversion rates, operating time, and blood loss over the period of time chosen for the study [15].

With the advent of robotic surgery in the latter half of the twentieth century, this minimally invasive technique has recently been used to perform minor and major liver resections at experienced centers. The sheer advantage of the six axis control and real-time 3D visualization of the surgical field via the surgeon console has made the use of robotics in liver surgery effective and feasible with similar outcomes as laparoscopy.

Surgical Technique

At Carolinas Medical Center, the division of HPB surgery has performed over 250 laparoscopic and robotic liver resections over the last 5 years. All minor resections (wedge and left lateral sectionectomies) are performed in a pure laparoscopic fashion. The major liver resections are performed either purely laparoscopically or with the use of a hand port. The surgical technique employed is standard and usually involves placing the patient in a supine fashion. For posterior sectionectomies (segment 6 and 7) and right hepatic lobectomies, the patient is placed in a 45° left lateral decubitus position. Pneumoinsufflation is achieved with carbon dioxide with a maximum intraabdominal pressure of 15 mmHg. There are usually three to five laparoscopic ports placed to perform the surgery (see Fig. 35.1a, b). A 30° laparoscope is used for visualization and a routine laparoscopic ultrasound is performed in all cases. The decision to place a hand port is made during the procedure. Bipolar shears are used for the parenchymal transection and laparoscopic linear staplers are used for division of major vascular pedicles.

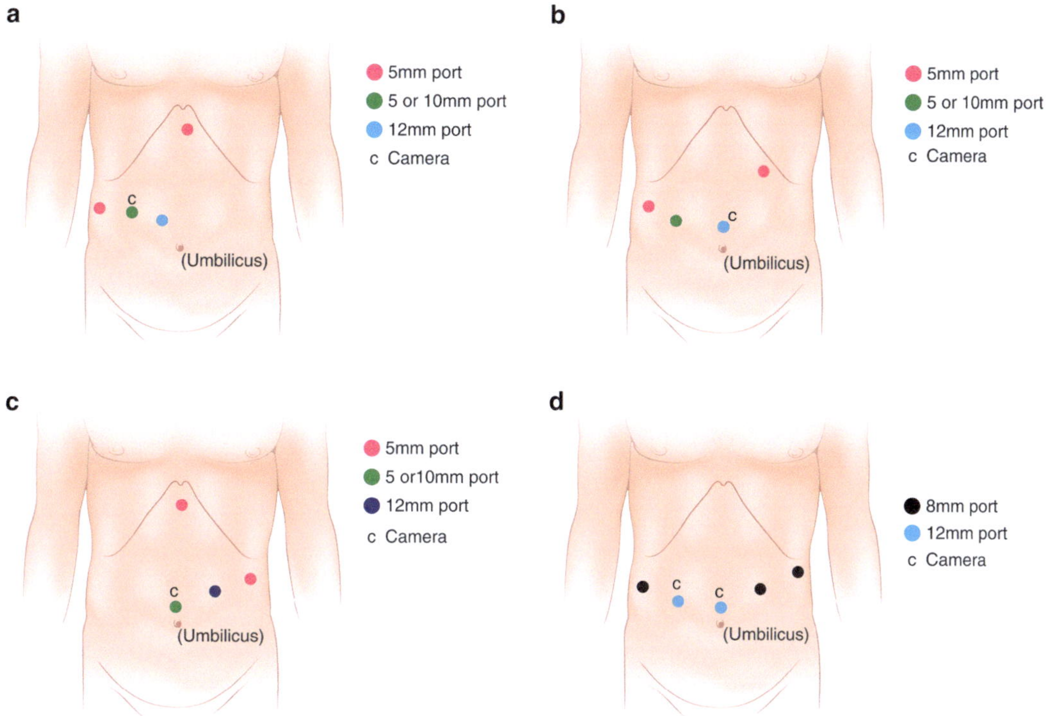

Fig. 35.1 (**a–d**) (**a**) Port placement for laparoscopic right hepatectomy. (**b**) Port placement for laparoscopic left hepatectomy. (**c**) Port placement for laparoscopic distal pancreatectomy and splenectomy. (**d**) Port placement for robotic pancreaticoduodenectomy

Hemostasis is obtained with electrocautery and saline-coupled radiofrequency electrosurgery devices as needed. The cut surface is checked carefully for any bile leaks and then covered with a fibrin sealant. Closed suction drains are selectively placed along the cut surface of the liver. The specimen may be removed via the hand port incision if one is employed, one of the port sites may be enlarged to retrieve the specimen, or the specimen is morcellated and removed via an existing laparoscopic port site.

Laparoscopic and Robotic Distal Pancreatectomy and Splenectomy

The term "distal pancreatectomy" applies to resection of the body and tail of the pancreas (left of the portal vein). Distal pancreatectomy is performed for various indications ranging from inflammatory processes such as chronic pancreatitis, trauma, as well as for benign and malignant neoplasms. Left-sided pancreatectomy was first performed in the late nineteenth century in Europe, notably in 1882 and 1884 by Trendelenburg and Billroth, respectively [16]. Von Mickulicz-Radecki attributed the slow development of pancreatic surgery to factors that remain relevant today: difficulty with exposure and access to the gland as well as difficulty with early diagnosis of pancreatic lesions. With advances in axial imaging and endoscopic and surgical techniques, pancreatic lesions can be diagnosed at an earlier stage and this has provided the ability to perform pancreatic resections in a minimally invasive fashion. Laparoscopic-assisted distal pancreatectomy was first described in the early 1990s by Sussman et al. for treatment of an insulinoma located in the tail of the pancreas [16]. Gagner and Pomp also reported their experience in minimally invasive pancreatic surgery in 1992; their described series included distal pancreatectomies as well as enucleation procedures performed laparoscopically for islet cell tumors of the left pancreas [16, 17].

Pancreatic lesions arising in the head and uncinate process have a greater chance for producing symptoms via mass effect at smaller sizes than do lesions of the body and tail of the pancreas [18]. Right-sided lesions and periampullary lesions commonly obstruct the common bile duct and lead to jaundice. The duodenum and distal pancreatic duct can also become obstructed. For this reason, new-onset pancreatitis in an older patient without gallstones or ethanol abuse necessitates pancreatic imaging to rule out a mass. Lacking these classic obstructive symptoms seen in comparatively smaller right-sided tumors, left-sided pancreatic masses have been historically diagnosed only at a larger size than those on the right [18, 19]. Retrospective reviews of pancreatic resections performed at high-volume pancreatic surgical centers continue to show statistically larger left-sided lesions compared to those on the right [18]. Vague symptoms including a dull abdominal pain may be present; less common manifestations such as new-onset diabetes mellitus, pancreatitis in the absence of gallstones or ethanol use, and fat malabsorption are also described. Given the typically larger size of left-sided lesions at the time of diagnosis, there is a higher chance of locally advanced tumors with invasion or compression of surrounding vascular, neural, and visceral structures.

Distal pancreatectomy has classically been performed with concomitant splenectomy for multiple reasons. The splenic vasculature travels along the length of the pancreatic body and tail with the splenic vein closely adherent to the posterior parenchyma of the gland; veins from the body and tail of the pancreas drain directly into the splenic vein. The splenic artery lies posterior to the pancreas but follows a more variable and ectatic course than the vein. The tail of the pancreas terminates in the hilum of the spleen in many patients and tail lesions may involve the vessels within the hilum or the spleen itself from direct extension. Resection of the tail for these reasons may risk splenic devascularization or incomplete pancreatic parenchymal resection from the hilum. The lymphatic drainage of the pancreas is perhaps the most crucial factor considered in splenectomy for malignant lesions of the body and tail of the pancreas [20, 21].

Distal pancreatectomy with splenectomy is currently being performed more commonly via a laparoscopic technique since this procedure was introduced in the early 1990s. A spleen-preserving technique can be considered for benign lesions and for traumatic injuries to the pancreas if the splenic vascular structures can be preserved. With increasing experience in performing this procedure laparoscopically, morbidity rates and other postoperative factors seem to mirror the benefits seen in other laparoscopic surgeries [22].

Another procedure developed for traumatic parenchymal injury with ductal disruption or low-grade neoplastic processes such as islet cell tumors is the central pancreatectomy. Central pancreatectomy removes a central segment of the body and results in two exposed portions of the pancreatic duct. This is a parenchyma-sparing procedure compared with a distal pancreatectomy performed for a discrete lesion in the pancreatic body. The right-sided duct can be oversewn as described in the description of a distal pancreatectomy with a Roux limb of bowel anastomosed to the distal duct to facilitate drainage; the wall of the Roux limb can be used as a seromuscular patch to the proximal stump.

For malignant lesions of the distal pancreas, Strasberg et al. in 2003 described the radical antegrade modular pancreatosplenectomy (RAMPS), a procedure designed to resect tumors arising from the left pancreas using existing fascial planes to achieve a negative margin and to include all draining lymph nodes [20]. Dissecting within retroperitoneal fascial planes and including all draining lymph nodes was proposed to emulate the surgical techniques that had been developed for pancreaticoduodenectomy for treatment of right-sided pancreatic malignancy. Unlike the traditional distal pancreatectomy, the dissection for a RAMPS procedure begins by dissecting around the neck of the pancreas and proceeds in a right-to-left direction. Two versions of the procedure are described, anterior and posterior, and differ based on tumor penetration of the posterior capsule of the pancreas; when penetration is not seen on preoperative imaging, the dissection is performed anterior to the left adrenal and proceeds along the anterior aspect of Gerota's fascia. In cases of tumor extension beyond the posterior capsule of the pancreas, the dissection is taken through Gerota's fascia, sacrifices the left adrenal gland, and is carried down to the capsule of the left kidney itself. The dissection includes the peri-pancreatic nodes as well as the para-aortic and celiac nodes that serve as primary and secondary drainage for the body and tail of the pancreas. This procedure was originally described as an open procedure and is now being performed laparoscopically.

For malignant tumors of the body of the pancreas that have invaded the celiac axis, distal pancreatectomy with resection of the celiac axis (DP-CAR), commonly referred to as the modified Appleby procedure, is described. The original Appleby procedure was performed in 1953 for locally advanced gastric adenocarcinoma with extension into the celiac axis. This procedure purposefully occludes and ligates the celiac artery, an action that acutely halts the usual pattern of arterial blood flow to the stomach and liver. The celiac and common hepatic arteries are ligated in this step, and blood flow to the liver is maintained via collateral circulation from the SMA and the pancreatoduodenal arcade that restores blood flow to the proper hepatic artery through the gastroduodenal artery. Some centers perform preoperative embolization of the common hepatic artery to induce maturation of the pancreatoduodenal collaterals. Bypass grafts from the aorta and iliac artery to the common hepatic have also been performed primarily or when poor pulsation or lack of back-bleeding has been observed intraoperatively. Though many series have evaluated the immediate postoperative period of patients undergoing the modified Appleby procedure, little data is present on long-term survival and evidence of disease recurrence [18, 20].

Surgical Technique

The laparoscopic technique follows the same principles as the open procedure and we prefer to do our dissection from the medial to lateral aspect. After gaining access into the patient's abdomen and obtaining adequate pneumoinsufflation (Fig. 35.1c), the abdominal cavity is carefully inspected for evidence of metastatic spread. Once the disease is confirmed to be involving only the pancreas, the lesser sac is entered by dividing the attachments between the greater curvature of the stomach and the transverse colon to expose the anterior surface of the pancreas. A laparoscopic vessel-sealing device is used for this purpose. The peritoneal attachments to the inferior and superior borders of the pancreas are divided with care taken to identify the inferior mesenteric vein in the inferior peritoneal attachments. An intraoperative ultrasound is routinely performed to confirm the location of the tumor. Alternatively, a hand port can be placed and the gland is palpated for the tumor. The splenic artery is identified by intraoperative ultrasound to the left of the celiac; the hepatic arteries and other branches from the celiac axis are also identified and traced via ultrasound prior to arterial ligation. Meticulous dissection is performed to adequately mobilize the pancreas from its retroperitoneal attachments. The inferior mesenteric vein on the inferior border of the pancreas is exposed and ligated. The splenic vein is also visualized at this point in time and it is carefully dissected off the inferior aspect of the pancreas prior to dividing it with a vascular stapler at its junction with the portal vein. As the dissection continues from a medial to lateral aspect, the left adrenal gland is commonly encountered. Dissection anterior to the adrenal or posterior to the adrenal with inclusion of the gland in the resected specimen depends on the gross involvement of the gland by tumor seen at the time of surgery or based on preoperative imaging showing preservation or loss of the plane between the pancreas and adrenal. In cases of a posterior tumor, the adrenal may be resected en bloc with the pancreas. The spleen is mobilized by dividing the gastrosplenic ligament which includes the short gastric vessels as well as the splenocolic attachments. For a known malignancy, ligation of the ligament is performed close to the wall of the stomach to include all nodes within the ligament. The pancreas is generally transected with a stapling device at the level of the portal vein. Sometimes, the gland is divided using laparoscopic bipolar electrosurgery device and the pancreatic duct is oversewn with nonabsorbable suture. The specimen is retrieved via the hand port site or one of the laparoscopic ports is enlarged to do the same. Hemostasis is obtained and a closed suction drain is left adjacent to the cut end of the pancreas.

Minimally Invasive Pancreaticoduodenectomy

The first laparoscopic pancreaticoduodenectomy was performed in 1994 by Ganger and Pomp for a patient with chronic pancreatitis [23]. The operation took about 10 h to complete. The next case series to come out with outcomes in ten patients was in 1997 by Ganger and Pomp again [24]. There was a 40 % conversion rate which made the surgeons question the benefit of laparoscopy for pancreaticoduodenectomy. With the advancement in technology (laparoscopy and robotics) and refinement of surgical instruments including enhanced optics, there was a renewed interest amongst surgeons. The first case series on robotic pancreatic resections by Giulianotti et al. was published in 2003 in Europe [25]. Melvin and Needleman reported their experience with robotic resection of a pancreatic neuroendocrine tumor in the United States at the same time [26]. Kendrick et al. published their series from the Mayo Clinic in Rochester on the safety and efficacy of total laparoscopic pancreaticoduodenectomy. Their case series involved a total of 65 patients with a mean age of 66 years. The average operative time was 368 min and median blood loss was 240 ml. The perioperative morbidity mainly consisted of delayed gastric emptying ($n=9$), pancreatic fistula ($n=11$), and bleeding ($n=5$). The median length of stay was 7 days. Based on the results, they concluded that laparoscopic pancreaticoduodenectomy was feasible, safe, and effective [27]. The recent systemic review and meta-analysis of studies comparing minimally invasive pancreaticoduodenectomy to open pancreaticoduodenectomy by Camilo Correa-Gallego et al. concluded that the minimally invasive approach was feasible in select patients at select centers. The outcomes were comparable to that of the open procedure based on the 6 studies that included 542 patients (169 minimally invasive and 373 open) [28].

Based on the current literature published, it is safe to say that minimally invasive pancreaticoduodenectomy is technically feasible and has similar outcomes as the open procedure. Further studies are warranted to determine patient recovery and quality of life especially in the group of patients that require adjuvant therapy after surgery.

Surgical Technique

At our institution the robot is used to perform minimally invasive pancreaticoduodenectomies. Our technique usually involves the patient being positioned in a supine fashion. After intubation and prepping and draping the field, pneumoinsufflation is obtained with a Veress needle at the umbilicus and subsequently upsized to a 12 mm port three additional 8 mm cannulas as well as an additional 12 mm camera port (in the right midclavicular line) are placed under direct vision (Fig. 35.1d). The umbilical trocar site serves as the assistant port during most of the resection portion of the procedure. Upon initial entry the abdominal cavity is always inspected for evidence of metastatic disease. The robotic shears are then used to mobilize the round and falciform ligaments off of the anterior abdominal wall. These are used at the end of the case as a vascularized pedicle flap with which we wrap the pancreaticojejunostomy for reinforcement [29]. The inferior border of the distal gastric antrum and proximal duodenum is mobilized with care to avoid injury to the distal gastric antrum or the pylorus.

We then identify the origin of the right gastroepiploic blood vessels. These are dissected out and then sealed and divided using the robotic vessel-sealing device. Similarly, the superior border of the distal gastric antrum is identified and the right gastric artery pedicle is sealed with a vessel-sealing device and divided at its origin from the proper hepatic artery. We then mobilize the remainder of the proximal duodenum which is subsequently stapled and divided using a laparoscopic 60 mm linear stapler. The stomach is placed in the left upper quadrant for reconstruction at the end of the case. The hepatic flexure and transverse colon and omentum are mobilized away from the anterior face of the pancreas and the duodenum. An extended Kocher maneuver is performed by mobilizing the duodenum away from its retroperitoneal attachments until the duodenum and pancreas are freed from the inferior vena cava and the aorta. The ligament of Treitz is mobilized using the robotic vessel-sealing device to facilitate the small bowel to flip up underneath the mesenteric vessels to the right upper quadrant. The common hepatic artery is dissected out and the portal and celiac lymph nodes are mobilized off the blood vessels. An extensive lymphadenectomy is performed along the posterior and medial aspect of the porta hepatis and sent separately for permanent pathological examination. Similarly, the common hepatic artery lymph node and the proximal celiac lymph nodes are dissected off the blood vessels and sent separately for pathological examination. An intraoperative ultrasound is performed to confirm the vascular anatomy of the porta hepatis. The gastroduodenal artery is identified and then clipped and divided using locking plastic clips. This allows one to mobilize hepatic artery proper away from the common hepatic duct. The inferior border of the pancreas and the neck are dissected out and mobilized. A tunnel is created underneath the neck of the pancreas, anterior to the superior mesenteric and portal vein to the superior aspect of the pancreas. An umbilical tape is passed beneath the pancreas. At this point, the neck of the pancreas is transected using the robotic monopolar scissors coupled with saline irrigation to minimize charring of the tissue.

The small bowel is transected approximately 20 cm distal to the ligament of Treitz, and the small bowel mesentery is taken with a robotic vessel-sealing device towards the base of the uncinate process. Finally, the uncinate process is mobilized away from the superior mesenteric vein and the superior mesenteric artery. The common hepatic duct is then transected just above the cystic duct takeoff. The cystic artery is identified as a discrete branch coming off the right hepatic artery. This is sealed and divided using the vessel-sealing device. The gallbladder is then taken off the undersurface of the liver using the monopolar robotic shears. The entire specimen is then placed into an Endo Catch™ bag (Covidien, Minneapolis, MN) and retrieved from the abdominal cavity from the slightly enlarged umbilical trocar site. The trocar site is closed using interrupted figure-of-eight 0 PDS sutures.

For the reconstruction phase of the procedure, the stapled end of the jejunum is brought alongside the transected surface of the pancreas. The posterior pancreaticojejunostomy layer is performed using 4-0 absorbable suture in a running fashion. A small enterotomy matching the diameter of the pancreatic duct is created in the jejunum with the and a duct to mucosal anastomosis is performed using interrupted 6-0 absorbable sutures over an 8 French pediatric feeding tube cut to approximately 6 cm. The anterior pancreaticojejunostomy is completed using an additional 4-0 absorbable suture in a running fashion. The entire anastomosis is then wrapped with the round ligament pedicle flap and reinforced with a fibrin sealant.

The hepaticojejunostomy is performed approximately 10–15 cm distal to the pancreaticojejunostomy using a 4-0 absorbable suture in a running or interrupted fashion, depending on the size of the duct. The antecolic duodenojejunostomy is performed approximately 50 cm from the biliary anastomosis using absorbable suture. A 19 French closed suction drain is placed in the right upper quadrant close to the biliary and pancreatic anastomoses. All the port sites are closed with absorbable suture.

Thermal Ablation and Chemical Injection

Ablation technology, which involves the destruction of tumor in situ, has become a mainstay form of treatment of tumors in the liver, kidney, lungs, and other solid organs. Ablative modalities for hepatic malignancy include chemical injection (via alcohol and acetic acid) and thermal methods (cryoablation using liquid nitrogen and argon, coagulative destruction using radiofrequency, microwave, laser, and HIFU). The newer technology includes irreversible electroporation which causes destruction of tumor by cellular reprogramming.

Ablation is primarily indicated for unresectable hepatic tumors though this concept is changing with the advancements in ablation technology and published literature showing excellent survival rates and low rates of recurrence in patients with potentially resectable tumors [30]. It has become one of the primary modalities of choice in patients with hepatocellular carcinoma and underlying cirrhosis who are awaiting a transplant. As the experience in ablating HCC has grown, the technology has also been used for other liver tumors such as adenomas, cholangiocarcinoma, and metastatic lesions with results equivalent to resection. There is no actual size limit on the lesion chosen for ablation but expert advise applying the technology to lesions 4 cm or less and those not in close proximity to major bile ducts for the best oncological response.

Cryoablation

From a historical perspective, ablation was first started in combination with cryogenics. In 1963 Cooper used cryosurgery to treat Parkinson's disease [31, 32]. Soon, the idea of treating primary and metastatic liver tumors using a vacuum insulated probe cooled by liquid nitrogen was conceived. The theory behind the application was that the probe would make rapid extraction of heat possible while freezing the tumor in situ. Despite the promising results achieved initially, cryoablation was limited to use on superficial tumors since there was no way to visualize deep seated tumors or surrounding structures in real time. The advent of intraoperative ultrasound in the 1990s made precise identification and ablation of intrahepatic tumors possible. As the technology improved over the next decade, laparoscopy was introduced into the world of surgery and soon enough with newly designed probes, ablation was made possible in conjunction with laparoscopy [33].

Cryoablation has its set of limitations. The time taken to complete a single ablation is close to 30–40 min. Some of the complications associated with cryoablation include bile leaks and excess bleeding. One of the major complications is termed "cryoshock" where a patient develops acute renal failure, acute respiratory distress syndrome, disseminated intravascular coagulation, and liver failure. With the advancement in ablation technology using radiofrequency and microwaves, cryotherapy has fallen out of favor amongst liver surgeons. Nonetheless, the technology is currently being used in conjunction with immunotherapy in the treatment of unresectable breast and hepatocellular cancer in a few centers [34, 35].

Radiofrequency Ablation

Radiofrequency ablation was first approved for use in the liver by the FDA in 1997 though its clinical applications had started two decades earlier. The main mechanism of tissue destruction is causing hyperthermia via radiofrequency waves. The technology relies on the interaction of an alternating current with tissue during which ions become agitated secondary to the high frequency waves (460–480 kHz), and the heat generated in the process causes coagulative necrosis [36, 37]. The entire process is controlled via an external generator based on continuous real-time measurement of tissue impedance. The radiofrequency probes have various designs the most common ones being needle electrodes with multiple extendable metal tines and single or clusters of internally cooled straight needles that pass electricity through the tissues between grounding pads applied to the patient (monopolar) or to a second probe inserted a short distance away (bipolar).

The incidence of bile leaks and bleeding is minimal when performed carefully under ultrasound guidance and there is no phenomenon similar to cryoshock that exists with radiofrequency. On the other hand, one of the major limitations is the "heat sink" effect where the hyperthermia caused by the antenna is reduced at the periphery by the blood flowing through the tissue. This raises the concern of leaving viable tumor cells behind at the periphery and between tines. The result of the effect can be negated by performing overlapping ablations and ensuring the complete destruction of the tumor. Radiofrequency ablation remains the most common thermal ablation technique used currently to treat primary and metastatic tumors.

Microwave Ablation

Microwave ablation was the next technology to follow radiofrequency for treating solid tumors. The first use of microwave technology in the treatment of liver tumors was in Japan in the early 1980s but did not gain adequate momentum due to the relative small ablation volumes obtained at that point in time. Subsequently as the technology developed and the use of clustered antennae became possible, it was adopted by surgeons and radiologists for ablating tumors in solid organs [38].

The tumor destruction is primarily achieved by placing an antenna within the tumor and passing high frequency electromagnetic radiation through the tissue. The water molecules within the cells absorb the electromagnetic waves which in turn cause the molecules' poles to rapidly align and realign in a phenomenon termed di-electric hysteresis which causes heat production [39]. The term "Near field" is of significant importance in microwave ablation. It represents the first 2–3 cm of tissue in a radial fashion from the antenna tip. This is the zone that has 100 % coagulative necrosis secondary to hyperthermia via microwaves. Microwaves generated at a higher frequency have lower tissue penetrance. The two common frequencies used commercially for thermal ablation are 915 MHz and 2.45 GHz. Some of the key advantages of using microwave technology in comparison to the more widely used radiofrequency technology is the reduced "heat sink" effect which makes it a more effective modality in treating tumors next to large vessels. The normal follow-up for patients is 4 weeks from the time of the initial ablation with a triphasic liver CT scan (Fig. 35.2a, b). This is our institution's preferred method of ablation and we describe our technique below.

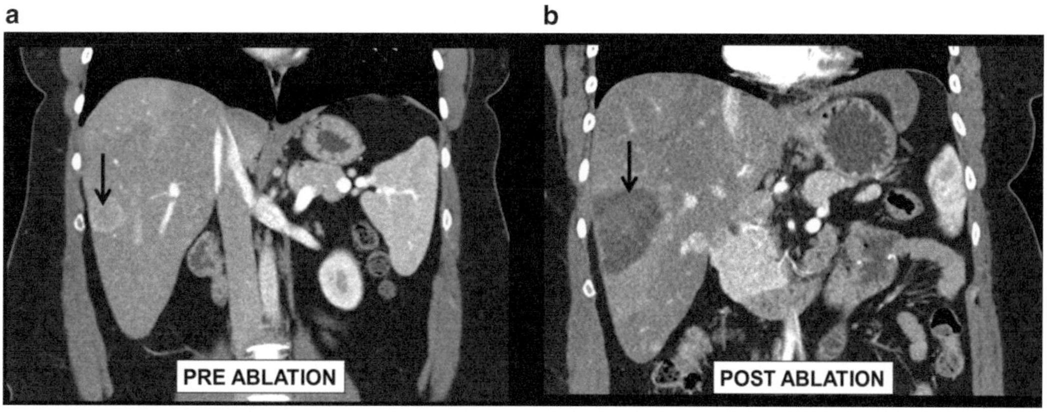

Fig. 35.2 (**a**, **b**) Coronal plan images of a hepatocellular carcinoma prior to and 4 weeks following laparoscopic microwave ablation. The site of the tumor is now fluid filled with some edema around it

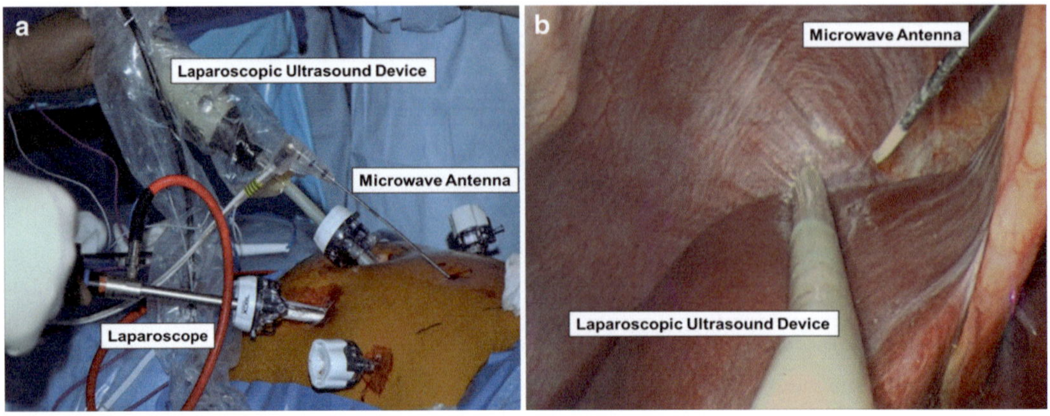

Fig. 35.3 (**a**, **b**) External and laparoscopic views illustrating typical port placement for laparoscopic liver ultrasound and microwave ablation. Concomitant laparoscopic and ultrasonographic guidance is used to target the lesion with the microwave antenna

Surgical Technique

The patient is placed in a supine position unless the lesion of interest is located in the right posterior section in which case they are positioned in an oblique fashion with the right side elevated. Following administration of general anesthesia and intubation, access into the abdomen is gained via a hasson trocar and the abdomen is insufflated. A 30° laparoscope is generally used for visualization and a thorough inspection of the entire abdominal cavity is made to rule out extrahepatic disease which might make the ablation procedure unnecessary. A second port of sufficient size (usually 10 mm to accommodate the laparoscopic ultrasound probe) is inserted into the abdominal cavity (Fig. 35.3a). The liver is sometimes mobilized to facilitate easier targeting of the lesion and to protect surrounding structures from thermal damage.

Once the lesion has been identified with the ultrasound probe, a small skin incision is made to facilitate the insertion of the microwave antenna. No port is needed given the fact that the antenna has a cooled shaft (no concern for skin burns) and is only a few millimeters in diameter. The antenna is then inserted into the tumor under ultrasound guidance using the in plane technique and, when needed, in the out of plane fashion to enable complete destruction of the tumor (Figs. 35.3b and 35.4a). The duration of ablation is based on the size of the lesion targeted. For a 2–3 cm lesion, a 4–5 min ablation at 140 W using a 2.45 GHz generator is sufficient to achieve complete destruction of the tumor. One of the methods employed to ensure the near field is located precisely on the targeted lesion is the use of Doppler on the ultrasound. The ablation can be visualized as a sphere filled with blue and red colored dots due to the Doppler shifts caused by the microwaves (Fig. 35.4b). The antenna is withdrawn while active to cauterize the tract and obtain hemostasis.

Irreversible Electroporation

Irreversible electroporation (IRE) is one of the newer modalities used to ablate solid tumors. Unlike thermal ablation, IRE employs low energy, unipolar electric pulses that pass through electrodes inserted directly into the tumor. These pulses induce nanoscale defects (pores) in the plasma membrane that remain after the stimulus is removed. In this compromised state the cell is rendered unable to function and apoptotic cell death is initiated. Because cell death following IRE is not necrotic, post-ablation immune responses are less severe and the underlying architecture (biliary structure) is preserved.

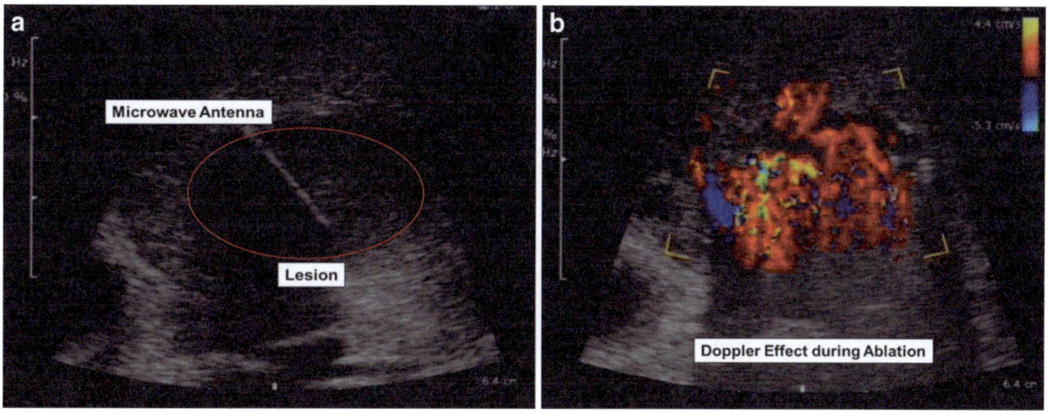

Fig. 35.4 (**a**, **b**) (**a**) Intraoperative ultrasound imaging demonstrating the microwave antenna being guided into the center of a liver lesion. (**b**) Intraoperative ultrasound view of the liver tumor being ablated. The ablation can be visualized as a sphere filled with *blue* and *red* colored dots due to the Doppler shifts caused by the microwaves

A sentinel publication on the outcomes of IRE in treating biopsy proven early stage HCC was a prospective multicenter trial by Lencioni et al. The results of the study were very favorable with the complete response rates being close to 79 % with no major complications or mortality [40]. The use of IRE in treating patients with locally advanced pancreatic cancer has been recently studied by Martin et al. [41]. The study was a prospective multi-institutional trial evaluating the overall survival of patients with stage III unresectable pancreatic cancer. Fifty-four patients underwent the procedure and the results were compared to 85 matched patients who were treated with chemotherapy and radiation. The local progression-free survival was 14 months in IRE-treated patients compared to standard therapy patients, and the overall survival was 20 months in the IRE group versus 9 months in the standard group. It should be noted that 90 % of the IRE patients had undergone chemotherapy or chemoradiation prior to IRE and 73 % underwent post IRE chemotherapy or chemoradiation. The conclusion of the study was that IRE in combination with standard therapy for stage III unresectable pancreas cancer patients improved overall survival compared to standard therapy alone. The validation of the results is currently underway as part of the Phase 2 IDE study [41].

As with other ablation approaches, the potential drawbacks associated with IRE cannot be overlooked. These include the need to pulse IRE in synchronization with cardiac rhythm to avoid cardiac arrest. While this is accomplished by timing the generator with an EKG output, it also means the time to perform the ablation is increased as IRE can only be applied during a portion of the cardiac rhythm. Additionally, IRE patients must receive intraoperative paralytics and, unlike thermal ablation, cell death following IRE cannot be easily visualized during follow-up leading to concerns regarding the completeness of ablation and risk of local recurrence (lesions <5 cm).

Interventional GI Procedures

Since the first description of flexible fiberoptics and its visualization of the intraluminal stomach and duodenum in 1957 by Hirschowitz, esophagogastroduodenoscopy (EGD) has become a widespread modality used in the diagnosis and management of upper gastrointestinal disease [42]. The technique advanced rapidly when in 1968 McCune presented the first endoscopic retrograde pancreatogram [43]. This initial demonstration of cannulation of the pancreatobiliary ductal system has evolved into the modern endoscopic retrograde cholangiopancreatography

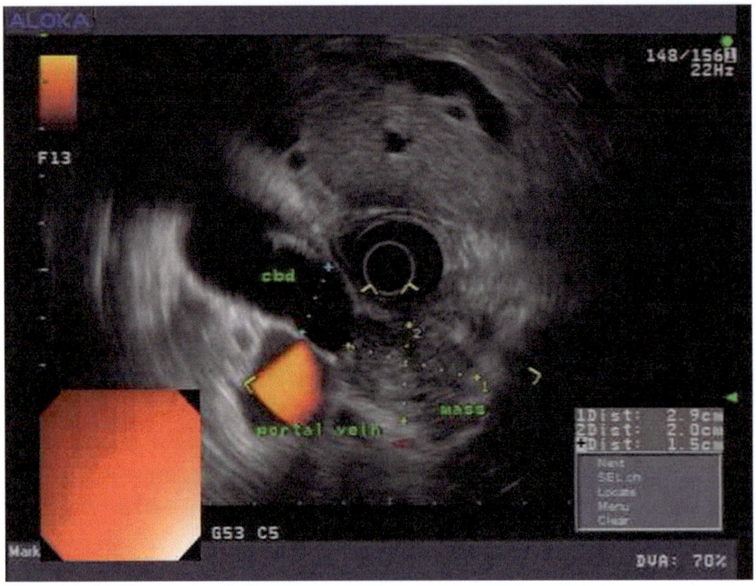

Fig. 35.5 Endoscopic ultrasound evaluating a pancreatic head mass. The common bile duct is markedly dilated and the pancreatic head mass appears to abut the portal vein

(ERCP) that is now being used for diagnostic and therapeutic management of hepatopancreatobiliary disorders. Combined with endoscopic ultrasound (EUS) that allows for identification and description of structures outside of the bowel wall, advances in device technology and increasing experience with the technique of ERCP have vastly expanded the range of endoscopic therapies that can be performed for both benign and malignant diseases of the foregut and pancreatobiliary system.

The diagnostic capabilities of ERCP are multifactorial and rely on visual inspection, radiographic interpretation of ductography following contrast injection, and the ability to perform sampling [44]. EUS expands on this by allowing real-time evaluation of extraluminal lesions that do not directly invade or compress the bowel and do not cause extrinsic ductal stenosis that would be detected on ductography. The definition of locoregional tumor spread and involvement of lymphoid and vascular structures is a key diagnostic application of EUS (see Fig. 35.5).

Early studies of EUS compared it to transabdominal ultrasound and axial imaging in the form of computed tomography (CT) and later magnetic resonance (MRI). Amouyal et al. compared transabdominal ultrasound, EUS, and CT and found EUS significantly more sensitive in identifying the presence and etiology of extrahepatic cholestasis as well as locoregional lymphatic invasion [45]. EUS allows biliary drainage without direct visualization. Since it was first described in 2001 by Giovannini et al. [46], multiple approaches to EUS-guided transluminal biliary drainage have been described and vary based on the available anatomy and the level of biliary obstruction (Fig. 35.6). Ultrasound and CT remain more appropriate methods for surveying the entire hepatic parenchyma.

Though more recent advances in CT technology and specialized biliary and pancreatic protocols have improved the sensitivity and specificity of CT in detecting mesenteric vascular invasion by pancreatic adenocarcinoma [47], EUS remains a more sensitive technique for detecting nodal involvement and determining the nodal stage of pancreatic adenocarcinoma. Smaller nodes can be detected with EUS compared to CT and malignant disruption of the internal structure and density of the node can be detected in a node that may be of a normal size when visualized by CT. An added advantage of EUS compared to axial imaging is the ability to perform transluminal fine needle aspiration (FNA) to obtain tissue samples, often with bedside cytopathological diagnosis.

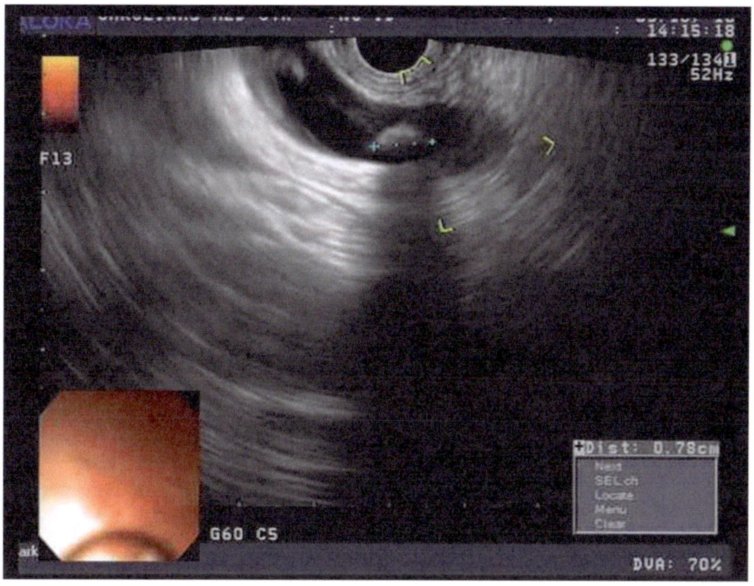

Fig. 35.6 Endoscopic ultrasound demonstrating a hyperechoic gallstone in the distal common bile duct in a patient with choledocholithiasis and obstructive jaundice

Limitations of EUS in evaluation of pancreatic masses and biliary or pancreatic obstruction are encountered in patients with chronic pancreatitis or with diffusely infiltrative tumors. In cases where parenchymal echogenicity has been homogenized by chronic inflammation or in a gland replaced by tumor infiltration, adjuncts to EUS such as a contrast-enhanced approach and computer-interpreted differences in tissue compressibility can aid in detection and characterization of a mass. The contrast-enhanced EUS is based on neovascularization of a mass and ultrasonographic visualization of intravascular contrast with increased flow to a mass compared with the surrounding tissue. EUS elastography compares the differential displacement of tissue when pressure is applied by the ultrasound probe. The differences in tissue displacement by pressure are displayed with color overlay in early versions and later with quantitative values to show differences in parenchymal texture. Elastography has shown promising sensitivity in differentiating benign from malignant masses when firmer tissues are examined with both color and quantitative comparisons are used but sensitivity decreases when softer tissues are examined [48].

ERCP is now a common method employed in biliary drainage. This practice has been used in benign processes such as cholangitis and choledocholithiasis but is also used to decompress the biliary system in cases of malignant obstruction (Fig. 35.7). ERCP by definition utilizes a retrograde approach and requires visualization and access to the duodenum and the Ampulla of Vater to cannulate the biliary ductal system; this can be complicated by gastric outlet obstruction, duodenal diverticulum, periampullary tumor involvement, inability to visualize the ampulla, and surgically altered anatomy such as that

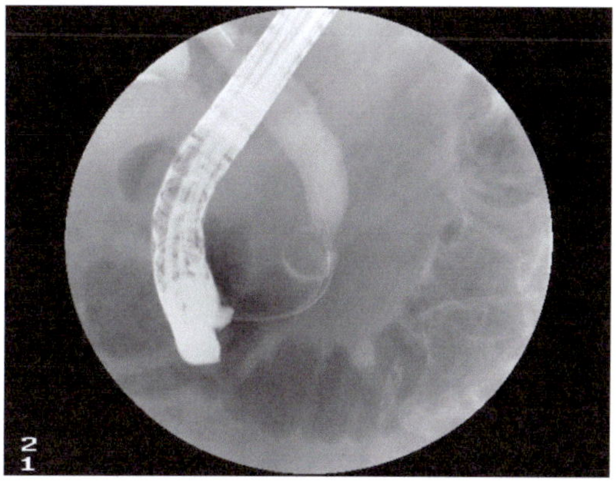

Fig. 35.7 ERCP cholangiogram demonstrating severe dilatation of the distal common bile duct with a structure in the pancreatic head

encountered in patients who have undergone gastric bypass surgery or pancreaticoduodenectomy [44]. In cases where the duodenum is accessible but the ampulla is not visualized or could not be cannulated, the Rendezvous procedure (RV) can be performed. The intrahepatic bile ducts (IHBD) can be located endosonographically via the stomach and the extrahepatic bile duct (EHBD) via the duodenum. Under US guidance, a needle and then a wire are introduced into the biliary system and passed antegrade through the ampulla into the duodenum [42, 44]. Standard ERCP is then attempted with assistance of the wire passing through the ampulla as a guide. In patients with a proximal biliary obstruction whose duodenum cannot be accessed (e.g., gastric outlet obstruction, previous pancreaticoduodenectomy, or gastric bypass), the biliary system can be accessed in an antegrade fashion via the IHBD. The bile ducts within the left lateral lobe are accessed under US guidance and a temporary fistula created through which wires, balloons, and stents can be passed and later manipulated with radiographic visualization. Hepaticogastrostomy and hepaticoesophagostomy have been described, though a transgastric approach is preferred as it avoids the possibility of mediastinitis and esophageal perforation [44].

A retrograde approach can also be performed for very distal obstructions with access to the EHBD performed from D1 via the posterior wall or at D2 at the level of the ampulla itself for an ampullary obstruction. Many centers performing these ultrasound-guided transluminal drainage procedures prefer the RV procedure as an initial alternative to failed ERCP based on previous experience with ERCP and the avoidance of a temporary bilioenteric fistula which can lead to biliary leak into the peritoneal cavity. When transluminal drainage is required (usually due to duodenal obstruction); transgastric access to the IHBD theoretically allows for tamponade of bile by the hepatic parenchyma but requires a higher grade obstruction to facilitate intrahepatic biliary ductal dilatation. Failure of the transluminal methods to gain biliary ductal access would necessitate a percutaneous transhepatic approach, laparoscopic-assisted ERCP for patients who have had a gastric bypass, or surgical biliary drainage. Similar US-guided transluminal techniques are described for endoscopic drainage of biloma, the gallbladder, and hepatic abscesses [46].

In addition to the diagnosis of pancreatic cancer and biliary drainage, palliative endoscopic techniques and novel therapies have been developed. Biliary stent decompression of obstructive jaundice has multiple benefits including relief from pruritis, nutritional improvement, immune function, and overall quality of life for patients with locally advanced or metastatic disease who are not candidates for resection [6]. Preoperative stenting in those planning to undergo resection has the above benefits and is also intended to improve the tolerance of a full course of neoadjuvant chemotherapy. The stent diameter and composition, plastic or metal, determine the time to stent occlusion; in those who will likely not receive surgical intervention, self-expandable metal stents (SEMS) increase the time to stent occlusion and maximize the duration of benefit from stent placement. Patients expecting to undergo resection often receive plastic stents that typically provide 3 months of drainage prior to occlusion [49].

Other palliative procedures used in the management of pancreatic cancer include duodenal wall stenting for treatment of gastric outlet or duodenal obstruction. Previous techniques used to treat enteric obstruction included endoscopic balloon dilatation and surgical bypass. Though surgical bypass in the form of gastrojejunostomy provides a longer period of relief from obstruction, it is associated with greater short-term morbidity than with endoscopic duodenal stenting [49]. In cases of duodenal obstruction, concomitant biliary drainage is often required since the ampulla of Vater is often included in the portion of duodenum that will be stented. The biliopancreatic ductal system is usually stented prior to duodenal stent deployment or the ampulla can occasionally be placed into one of the interstices of the SEMS to allow continued drainage [49, 50]. Silicone-covered metal stents do not allow for this and require careful placement of the stent or alternative biliary drainage (see Fig. 35.8a, b).

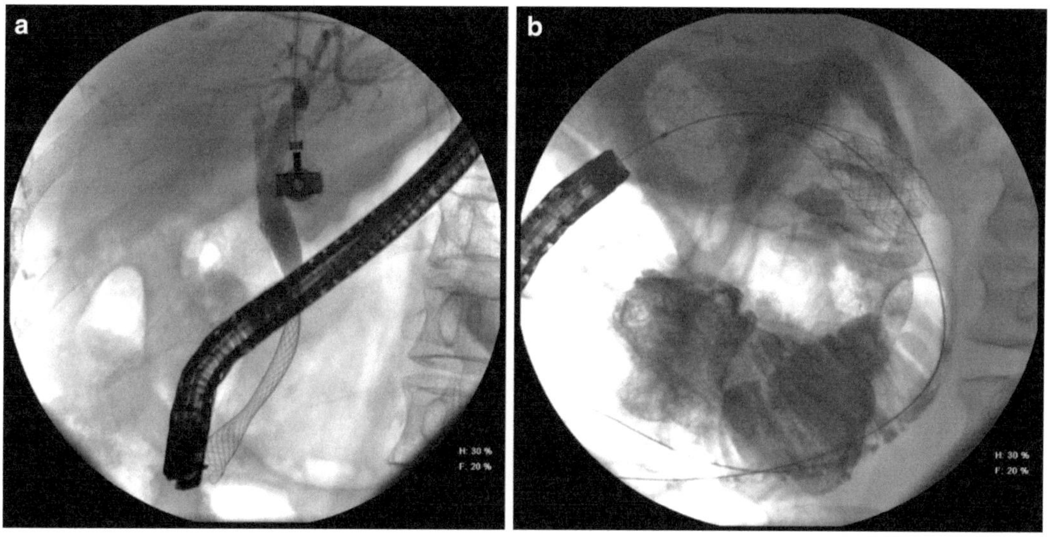

Fig. 35.8 (**a**, **b**) (**a**) ERCP with deployment of a self-expanding metal wall stent in the common bile duct. Note the intrahepatic biliary dilatation and distal stenosis of the stent. (**b**) Endoscopic deployment of a self-expanding duodenal metal wall stent (SEMS) for a duodenal obstruction related to pancreatic adenocarcinoma invading the duodenum

Unremitting abdominal pain is characteristic of advanced pancreatic cancer, and many require increasing doses of narcotic analgesics over the course of the disease. EUS-guided celiac ganglion neurolysis is performed transgastrically due to the ganglion's proximity to the posterior wall of the stomach. Ultrasound allows the visualization of the ganglion but in cases where it is not visualized, the regions lateral to the takeoff of the celiac artery are injected with local anesthetics, neurolytic agents such as ethanol, or a combination of both. Direct visualization and guidance of the injection needle results in much higher rates of analgesia with up to 85 % of those undergoing blockade having decreased pain and opiate requirement in some series [49].

Multiple new and emerging endoscopic therapeutic strategies have been developed for the treatment of pancreatic adenocarcinoma and other hepatobiliary malignancies. EUS can be used to place radio-opaque markers to guide external beam radiation therapy and narrow the field of delivery, allowing maximal doses into the field of the malignancy while excluding surrounding structures [48, 49]. EUS guidance has also been used for tumor chemotherapeutic injection with paclitaxel and gemcitabine. Placement of radiofrequency ablation probes has also been performed endoscopically. Novel therapies including antitumor lymphocyte infusions as well as genetically modified adenovirus cultures that sensitize pancreatic adenocarcinoma cells to radiation have also been developed. Many of these new antitumor infusions and local delivery of antineoplastic drugs or ablation probes are currently under study and in the early phases of clinical trials [48, 49]. Their development underscores the evolution of endoscopy and its progression from a diagnostic method to one with the potential to treat pancreatic malignancy.

What the Future Holds

The advancement in technology to push minimally invasive surgery to the next frontier is very promising. Some of the common devices used in laparoscopic HPB surgery are the surgical stapling device and the vessel-sealing device. One of the recent advances in the stapling technology was the introduction of varied-height staple loads which are designed to deliver graduated compression of tissue and preserve vascular flow. The availability of articulating tissue allows surgeons to access tissue in deep spaces with minimal difficulty when compared to the traditional tissue sealers available in the market.

With respect to ablation, the devices of the next generation would have permittivity matched algorithm output control and multifrequency options. This will make the use of ablation more feasible amongst surgeons in the community who are new to this technology. The other aspect of using ablation technology is the associated level of comfort with intraoperative ultrasound targeting. 3D visualization of lesions in real time is a work in progress which again would facilitate extending ablation technologies to novice users in order to perform ablations in a safe and effective manner.

References

1. Kousnetzoff M, Pensky J. Sur la resection partielle du foie. Rev Chir. 1896;16:954.
2. Garre C. On resection of the liver. Surg Gynecol Obstet. 1907;5:331.
3. Pringle JH. Notes on the arrest of hepatic hemorrhage due to trauma. Ann Surg. 1908;48:514–9.
4. Couinaud C. Bases anatomiques des hepatectomies gauche et droite réglées. J Chir. 1954;70:933–66.
5. Wendell W. Beiträge zur Chirurgie der Leber. Arch Klin Chir. 1911;95:887–92.
6. Lortat-Jacob J, Robert H. Hepatectomie droite réglée. Presse Med. 1952;60:549–51.
7. Pack GT. Regeneration of human liver after major hepatectomy. Surgery. 1962;52:617–23.
8. Lin TY, Chen CC. Metabolic function and regeneration of cirrhotic and non-cirrhotic livers after hepatic lobectomy in man. Ann Surg. 1965;162:959–72.
9. Muhe E. Die erste Cholecystectomie durch das Laparoskop. Langenbecks Arch Chir. 1986;369:804.
10. Gagner M. Laparoscopic partial hepatectomy for liver tumor. Surg Endosc. 1992;6:99.
11. Ferzli G. Laparoscopic resection of a large hepatic tumor. Surg Endosc. 1995;9:733–5.
12. Azagra JS. Laparoscopic anatomical left lateral segmentectomy: technical aspects. Surg Endosc. 1996; 10:758–61.
13. Buell JF, Cherqui D, Geller DA, O'Rourke N, Iannitti D, Dagher I, et al. The international position on laparoscopic liver surgery: the Louisville Statement, 2008. Ann Surg. 2009;250(5):825–30.
14. Nguyen KT, Gamblin TC, Geller DA. World review of laparoscopic liver resection-2,804 patients. Ann Surg. 2009;250(5):831–41.
15. Vigano L, Laurent A, Tayar C, Tomatis M, Ponti A, Cherqui D. The learning curve in laparoscopic liver resection: improved feasibility and reproducibility. Ann Surg. 2009;250(5):772–82.
16. Beger HG, et al., editors. Diseases of the pancreas: current surgical therapy. Heidelberg, Berlin: Springer; 2008.
17. Gagner M, Pomp A, Herrera MF. Early experience with laparoscopic resections of islet cell tumors. Surgery. 1996;120(6):1051–4.
18. Blumgart LH, et al., editors. Surgery of the liver, biliary tract, and pancreas. 4th ed. Philadelphia: Saunders-Elsevier; 2007.
19. Sohn TA, et al. Resected adenocarcinoma of the pancreas – 616 patients: results, outcomes, and prognostic indicators. J Gastrointest Surg. 2000;4(6):567–79.
20. Strasberg SM, Field R. Left-sided pancreatic cancer. distal pancreatectomy and its variants: radical antegrade modular pancreatosplenectomy and distal pancreatectomy with celiac axis resection. Cancer J. 2011;18(6):562–9.
21. O'Morchoe CC. Lymphatic system of the pancreas. Microsc Res Tech. 1997;37:456–77.
22. Lillemoe KD, et al. Distal pancreatectomy: indications and outcomes in 235 patients. Ann Surg. 1999; 229(5):693–700.
23. Gagner M, Pomp A. Laparoscopic pylorus-preserving pancreaticoduodenectomy. Surg Endosc. 1994;8: 408–10.
24. Gagner M, Pomp A. Laparoscopic pancreatic resection: is it worthwhile? J Gastrointest Surg. 1997;1(1): 20–5.
25. Giulianotti PC, Coratti A, Angelini M, Sbrana F, Cecconi S, Balestracci T, Caravaglios G. Robotics in general surgery: personal experience in a large community hospital. Arch Surg. 2003;138(7):777–84.
26. Melvin WS, Needleman BJ, Krause KR, Ellison EC. Robotic resection of pancreatic neuroendocrine tumor. J Laparoendosc Adv Surg Tech A. 2003;13(1):33–6.
27. Kendrick M, Cusati D. Total laparoscopic pancreaticoduodenectomy: feasibility and outcome in an early experience. Arch Surg. 2010;145:19–23.
28. Correa-Gallego C, et al. Minimally invasive vs open pancreaticoduodenectomy: systematic review and meta-analysis. JACS. 2014;218:129–39.
29. Iannitti DA, Coburn NG, Somberg J, Ryder BA, Monchik J, Cioffi WG. Use of the round ligament of the liver to decrease pancreatic fistulas: a novel technique. J Am Coll Surg. 2006;203(6):857–64.
30. Groeschl RT, Pilgrim CH, Hanna EM, Simo KA, Swan RZ, Sindram D, et al. Microwave ablation for hepatic malignancies: a multiinstitutional analysis. Ann Surg. 2014;259(6):1195–200.
31. Rubinsky B, Lee CY, Bastacky J, Onik G. The process of freezing and the mechanism of damage during hepatic cryosurgery. Cryobiology. 1990;27(1):85–97.
32. Gage A. History of cryosurgery. Semin Surg Oncol. 1998;14:99–109.
33. Iannitti DA, Heniford T, Hale J, Grundfest-Broniatowski S, Gagner M. Laparoscopic cryoablation

of hepatic metastases. Arch Surg. 1998;133(9): 1011–5.
34. Niu L-Z, Li J-L, Zeng J-Y, Feng M, Liao M-T, Yoa F, et al. Combination treatment with comprehensive cryoablation and immunotherapy in metastatic hepatocellular cancer. World J Gastrornterol. 2013;19(22): 3473–80.
35. Niu L, Mu F, Zhang C, Li Y, Liu W, Jiang F, et al. Cryotherapy protocols for metastatic breast cancer after failure of radical surgery. Cryobiology. 2013; 67(1):17–22.
36. Simo KA, Sereika SE, Newton KN, Gerber DA. Laparoscopic-assisted microwave ablation for hepatocellular carcinoma: safety and efficacy in comparison with radiofrequency ablation. J Surg Oncol. 2011;104(7):822–9.
37. Poon RT, Fan ST, Tsang FH, Wong J. Locoregional therapies for hepatocellular carcinoma: a critical review from the surgeon's perspective. Ann Surg. 2002;235(4):466–86.
38. Iannitti DA, Martin RC, Simon CJ, et al. Hepatic tumor ablation with clustered microwave antennae: the US Phase II trial. HPB (Oxford). 2007;9(2):120–4.
39. Swan R, Tsirline V, Sindram D, Martinie JB, Iannitti DA. Fundamentals of microwave physics: application to hepatic ablation. J Microwave Surg. 2012;30:25–40.
40. Lencioni R, Izzo F, Crocetti L, Vilgrain V, Abdel-Rehim M, Bianchi L, Ricke J, Pech M, Bruix J. A prospective, multicenter phase II clinical trial using irreversible electroporation for the treatment of early stage HCC. J Vasc Interv Radiol. 2012;23(3):1114.
41. Martin II RC, Mcfarland K, Ellis S, Velanovich V. Irreversible electroporation therapy in the management of locally advanced pancreatic adenocarcinoma. J Am Coll Surg. 2012;215(3):361–9.
42. Baron T. Endoscopic management of biliary disorders. Surg Clin North Am. 2014;94:395–411.
43. McCune W, Shorb P, Moscovitz H. Endoscopic cannulation of the ampulla of vater: a preliminary report. Ann Surg. 1968;167(5):752–6.
44. Iwashita T, et al. Endoscopic ultrasound-guided biliary drainage: a review. Clin J Gastroenterol. 2014;7: 94–102.
45. Amouyal P, et al. Endosonography: promising method for diagnosis of extrahepatic cholestasis. Lancet. 1989;2:1195–8.
46. Giovannini M, et al. Endoscopic ultrasound-guided bilioduodenal anastomosis: a new technique for biliary drainage. Endoscopy. 2001;33(10):898–900.
47. Cotton P, et al. Cannulation of papilla of vater via fiber-duodenoscope. Assessment of retrograde cholangiopancreatography in 60 patients. Lancet. 1972;1:53–8.
48. Othman M, Wallace M. The role of endoscopic ultrasonography in the diagnosis and management of pancreatic cancer. Gastroenterol Clin North Am. 2012;41:179–88.
49. Coté G, Sherman S. Endoscopic palliation of pancreatic cancer. Cancer J. 2012;18(6):584–90.
50. Khashab M, Varadarajulu S. Endoscopic ultrasonography as a therapeutic modality. Curr Opin Gastroenterol. 2012;28:467–76.

36 Pancreatic Advances

John A. Stauffer and Horacio J. Asbun

Introduction

Pancreatic surgery has undergone a progressive evolution over the past 125 years, which has transformed the operation from a rarely performed and highly morbid procedure to a highly studied and safe procedure that is commonly performed in major institutions. Pancreatic surgeons have often earned reputations as technically adept, skilled, and progressive surgeons who are constantly challenged to make difficult and occasionally perilous operations safe for even the sickest of patients. The goal of the progression has continuously been to improve the outcomes for patients who require treatment of a wide range of pancreatic diseases, from the acute and dramatic processes (e.g., acute necrotizing pancreatitis) to the prolonged but highly lethal ones (e.g., pancreatic adenocarcinoma). The gastrointestinal and vascular complications that may arise even after surgical intervention of the primary disease are the most feared in all of abdominal surgery. These complications occur from attempting meticulous dissection of a retroperitoneally located organ or advanced reconstruction of intricate structures, often in an inflammatory setting. The ramifications of these complications or the inflammation of the pancreas itself can easily trigger systemic effects that can quickly deteriorate into a multiorgan downward spiral from which recovery is difficult and resource intensive. Therefore, it has been of vital importance to develop methods and techniques to deal with pancreatic disease that are of less harm to the patient than the patient's actual underlying disease. Most often, patients who undergo surgical treatment of their pancreas will never be the same again, and nearly all of these patients will have some loss in quality of life that may or may not be clinically relevant. Consequently, the goal of all pancreatic surgeons should be to cause minimal surgical impairment by avoiding nontherapeutic, overly aggressive, or ineffective methods and techniques.

In this chapter, we highlight major advances seen in the past two decades that have contributed to improved care for patients with pancreatic disease. While the actual pancreatic operations such as pancreaticoduodenectomy (PD), distal pancreatectomy (DP), total pancreatectomy (TP), enucleation, or drainage procedures performed in modern days are relatively similar in technique to the operations performed over 50 years ago, each operation has undergone numerous modifications with the goal of improved short- and long-term patient outcomes. We as surgeons are often limited in what

J.A. Stauffer (✉) • H.J. Asbun
Department of General Surgery, Mayo Clinic,
4500 San Pablo Road, Jacksonville, FL 32224, USA
e-mail: stauffer.john@mayo.edu;
asbun.horacio@mayo.edu

R. Latifi et al. (eds.), *Technological Advances in Surgery, Trauma and Critical Care*,
DOI 10.1007/978-1-4939-2671-8_36

can be done inside the operating room, so many of these modifications have also occurred outside of the operating room. We will discuss many of these innovations that have occurred in the preoperative, intraoperative, and postoperative setting in order to highlight their importance to the overall care of patients with pancreatic disease.

Evolution of Selected Concepts in Pancreatic Surgery

Preoperative Advances

Major pancreatic surgery in the United States began with Whipple's description of a two-stage pancreaticoduodenectomy procedure in 1935. Reports of additional pancreatic operations such as Priestley's total pancreatectomy in 1944 and DuVal's pancreaticojejunostomy for chronic pancreatitis in 1954 soon followed. However, this early era of pancreatic surgery was associated with very high morbidity and mortality, often of over 25 % for the latter. A significant drop in the risks to the patient was generally not seen until the 1980s and was first reported at high-volume institutions. Since then, many studies have demonstrated that results of pancreatic surgery are clearly improving over time and that the improvements are most pronounced in high-volume centers. In a report of the Nationwide Inpatient Sample from 1998 to 2003, the highest volume centers (>18 pancreatic resections/year) had a much lower mortality of 2.5 % in comparison to the medium volume (5–18 pancreatic resections/year) and low volume (<5 pancreatic resections/year) who experienced mortality rates of 5.9 % and 9.2 %, respectively [1]. In addition, this study also demonstrated a drop in overall nationwide mortality rates over the study time period from 7.8 % in 1998 to 4.6 % in 2003. Due to a multitude of reports showing similar volume-outcome relationships in morbidity and mortality, a slow shift towards regionalization of pancreatic surgery has been steadily occurring with an emphasis on major pancreatic operations being performed by the most experienced centers and surgeons.

While it may be difficult to pinpoint exactly which individual characteristics of a high-volume institution are the major contributors to this improved outcome, there are several elements that have recently gained prominence in improving the care of a patient with pancreatic disease. Tseng et al. provided strong evidence that a surgeon's operative experience had significant impact upon the safety of the operation, oncologic quality, and time to recovery for patients undergoing PD [2]. The results of this study lend support to the theory that surgeons who perform these operations more frequently are more likely to improve their operative techniques over time as well as to identify and treat complications at an earlier stage, which decreases the surgical impact on the patient. Additionally, the resource expenditure needed for care of these patients as a whole is decreased, providing value to the healthcare system. One can assume that the results of this study and others that have followed can be extrapolated to other pancreatic procedures that also greatly benefit from surgeon experience. Another defining characteristic of a high-volume institution is the use of multidisciplinary care for patients with pancreatic disease. This is most pronounced for patients with malignancy because coordinated care delivered by surgeons, medical/radiation oncologists, pathologists, radiologists, interventional radiologist, and gastroenterologists has been shown to improve treatment recommendations over individual or isolated single-physician treatment recommendations [3]. This pancreas-specific "tumor board" is frequently helpful when deciding treatment options for patients with benign or preneoplastic disease because input from dedicated radiologists and gastroenterologist skilled in advanced endoscopy is often essential for optimal outcome.

The most frequently utilized radiographic imaging of the pancreas has traditionally included computerized tomography (CT) for cross-sectional anatomy and endoscopic retrograde cholangiopancreatography (ERCP) for pancreaticobiliary ductal anatomy and for obtaining diagnostic cells. Pancreas-specific protocol CTs that involve fine cuts in the area of the pancreas with three-phase imaging acquisition result in excellent image quality with fine resolution and allow for very accurate and specific diagnostic information for a skilled radiologist. CT has the advantage of being widely available, having simple standardized protocols, and being relatively inexpensive and noninvasive in relation to other modalities. ERCP, in the hands of a skilled endoscopist, can be diagnostic as well as therapeutic with the option of placing biliary or pancreatic stents for a variety of pathology including biliary obstruction, duct disruption from acute pancreatitis, or for assistance in managing a pancreatic fistula after enucleation or distal pancreatectomy among others. While these studies continue to evolve and improve in quality, other modalities have distinct advantages when assessing specific types of pancreatic pathology. Magnetic resonance imaging (MRI) has become an incredibly valuable tool in the evaluation of hepatopancreaticobiliary disease. MRI has the advantage of being able to provide high-quality anatomic cross-sectional imaging of the pancreas with vascular detail and the option of combining cholangiopancreatography (Fig. 36.1a–d). Magnetic resonance cholangiopancreatography (MRCP) is a much less invasive diagnostic modality that can often replace the need for invasive ERCP, except for patients requiring therapeutic treatments. MCRP imaging quality is greatly facilitated by the co-administration of secretin analogues that stimulate pancreatic juice secretion, thereby filling the pancreatic duct with a high volume of fluid that can unmask subtle ductal abnormalities, which are normally very difficult to see in the miniscule pancreatic duct. Additionally, secretin analogue enhanced imaging can also give an experienced pancreatic radiologist physiologic information regarding

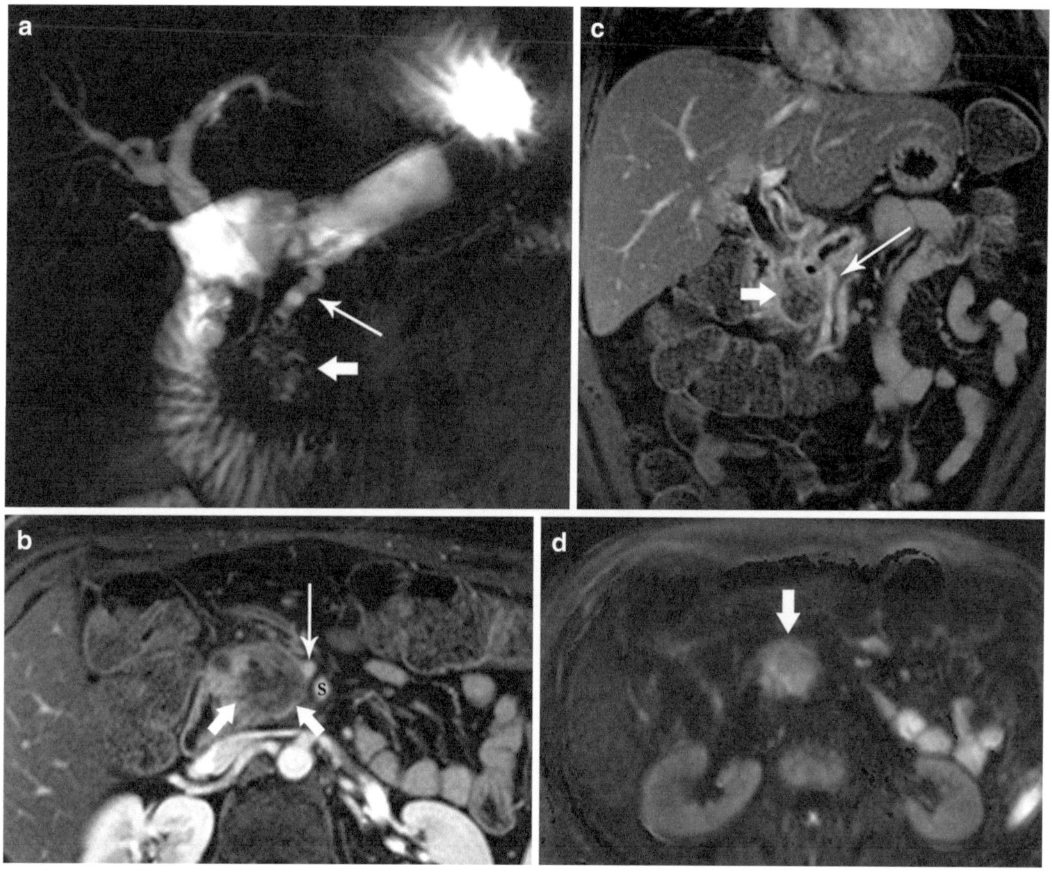

Fig. 36.1 (**a**) MRCP image reveals a dilated duct (*long arrow*) abruptly terminating as it descends into the pancreatic head. Presence of tumor hinted at by the cluster of minute cystic spaces (*short arrow*). (**b**, **c**) Axial and coronal enhanced images show the hypoenhancing tumor (*short arrows*) broadly abutting the superior mesenteric vein (*long arrow*) (*S* SMA). (**d**) Axial diffusion-weighted image highlights the mass (*arrow*)

pancreatic exocrine function that may have valuable clinical significance to the treating gastroenterologist or surgeon with regard to determining underlying disease pathology. In the case of pancreatic malignancy, MRI also has the advantage of providing excellent liver imaging. Due to its subtle presentation, pancreatic adenocarcinoma is more frequently found in a locally advanced or metastatic stage. Additionally, hepatic recurrence within as little as one year is not uncommon, indicating occult metastatic disease presence at the time of the operation. Therefore, to prevent an ultimately futile operation, it is of great importance to rule out the possibility of metastatic disease in the preoperative setting because palliative debulking has not at this time been shown to improve survival for patients with pancreatic adenocarcinoma. Contrast-enhanced MRI with diffusion sequence imaging, while clearly not foolproof, offers the greatest chance of finding metastatic involvement of the liver, which is generally the initial site of extrapancreatic disease (Fig. 36.2). The main disadvantage for MRI is its high cost and the expertise required to obtain high-quality imaging, from the radiologist protocoling and interpreting the study to the technicians who perform and assist patients throughout the procedure.

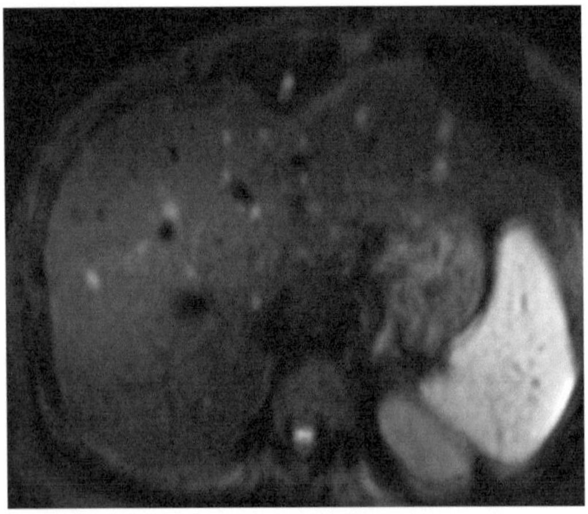

Fig. 36.2 A diffusion-weighted image (DWI) from a staging MRI revealing a number of hepatic metastases from pancreatic adenocarcinoma. DWI phase is extremely sensitive for liver metastases as these lesions were not discernible on triple phase pancreas protocol CT or PET/CT

Another diagnostic modality that has become invaluable in the workup and management of pancreatic disease is endoscopic ultrasonography (EUS). EUS is highly operator dependent and requires a skilled and experienced gastroenterologist to interpret the study in real time but has the ability to characterize pancreatic masses, cysts, and parenchymal architecture along with fine needle aspiration for cytopathologic evaluation (Fig. 36.3a–d). Utility is greatly increased by on-site determination of sample adequacy and preliminary diagnosis by an expert pathologist that is immediately available. In fact, this modality has replaced percutaneous needle biopsy as the preferred method for obtaining tissue diagnosis of pancreatic malignancy. EUS is a very safe and minimally invasive procedure that can also provide palliation for patients with surgically unresectable disease by performing celiac plexus neurolysis. EUS is highly accurate regarding T and N staging for pancreatic adenocarcinoma, pancreatic neuroendocrine tumors, and distal common bile duct cholangiocarcinoma [4]. Many surgeons argue that for resectable disease, EUS is unnecessary because tissue diagnosis is not mandatory for a patient with a pancreatic mass who is otherwise a good surgical candidate. The greatest value of EUS is that it permits high resolution imaging with simultaneous sampling. Therefore it is very useful in the evaluation of pancreatic cystic lesions, which are becoming more frequently incidentally found by the increasing use of highly sensitive cross-sectional imaging for other abdominal pathology. Information obtained by EUS can include surrounding inflammatory or fibrotic changes consistent with chronic pancreatitis, communication or involvement of the main pancreatic duct consistent with intraductal papillary mucinous neoplasm (IPMN), debris or mural nodules within the cyst wall, or fluid aspiration with tumor marker and enzyme evaluation, presence or absence of mucin, as well as biochemical fluid analysis [5].

Improved pancreatic imaging has led to lower rates of nontherapeutic laparotomies for pancreatic malignancies and pancreatic resections for benign indications. Additionally, accurate preoperative diagnostic imaging will assist the surgeon

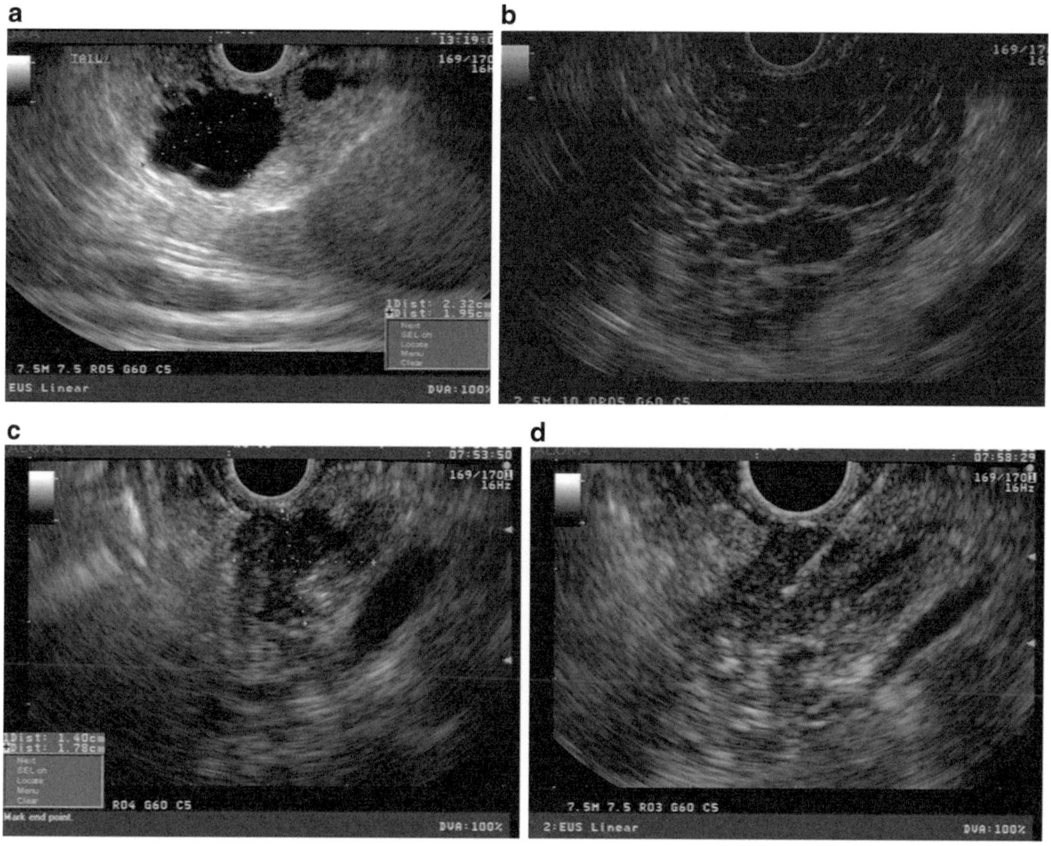

Fig. 36.3 (**a**) Endosonographic ultrasound image of a small side branch intraductal papillary mucinous neoplasm. (**b**) Endosonographic ultrasound image of a serous microcystic neoplasm of the pancreas. (**c**) Endosonographic ultrasound image of a T1 mass in the head of the pancreas. (**d**) Endosonographic ultrasound image of a fine needle aspiration biopsy verifying invasive adenocarcinoma

in identifying borderline or locally advanced disease prior to surgical exploration. Unresectable vascular involvement should be determined prior to entering the operating room because intraoperative surgical assessment of the extent of disease is difficult to determine even for experienced pancreatic surgeons due to the desmoplastic and inflammatory changes that often accompany benign and malignant pancreatic disease conditions. For the most part, nontherapeutic operations due to unresectable disease at experienced centers are mostly limited to patients with small volume peritoneal or surface liver disease, which is difficult for any imaging modality to find. Diagnostic laparoscopy prior to surgical resection still has a role for patients with malignant pancreatic disease, often most useful for patient presenting with back pain, weight loss, significantly elevated tumor markers, and lesions in the body/tail of the pancreas. Typically, however, the yield of this modality often inversely correlates with the quality of preoperative imaging.

Borderline resectable pancreatic tumors have received increased attention in the past several years. While at most centers patients with resectable disease will proceed directly to surgery and those with locally advanced or metastatic disease will undergo palliative treatments, patients with borderline tumors will be considered candidates for neoadjuvant treatment with chemotherapy, external beam radiation, or proton beam therapy. The clinical advantages of neoadjuvant treatment for these patients will include allowing for a time period of observing tumor biology and response to the treatment given. If very aggressive or metastatic disease is noted during restaging protocols, the patient is likely spared an operation that would have been associated with very little chance of success or benefit. Additionally, preoperative treatment for patients with borderline disease may downsize the tumor, allowing for a less aggressive vascular resection and fewer postoperative complications as well as helping to decrease the risk of an R1 margin positive resection, which has been shown to have a negative impact on long-term survival. Pancreatic surgeons, however, have only recently come to define borderline resectable pancreatic tumors, and this definition varies based on the use of a single institutional classification or a consensus definition proposed through international societies and associations [6]. Regardless of what definition is used, for the most part, patients with borderline resectable pancreatic tumors are preferentially given neoadjuvant preoperative treatments and have a reasonable rate of eventually proceeding to surgery. On the other hand, patients with locally advanced disease, often characterized by circumferential involvement of the superior mesenteric artery or long segment occlusive disease of the portomesenteric venous system with non-reconstructible anatomy, are very rarely if ever downstaged to resectable disease (Fig. 36.4a, b).

Preoperative administration of neoadjuvant treatment for resectable pancreatic adenocarcinoma is becoming more frequently performed but has yet to significantly improve long-term survival of patients. Selection criteria, treatment protocols, chemotherapy agents, and the use of radiation vary widely between institutions and trials making meaningful analysis difficult [7]. However, it is important to note that patients undergoing treatment prior to pancreatic surgery have not experienced an increased rate of complications or mortality after surgery. Neoadjuvant treatment protocols clearly have the advantage of selection bias by avoiding surgical intervention for those with aggressive disease or those patients with poor performance during treatment administration. Perhaps the greatest value of this treatment, until more effective agents are discovered, is in resource allocation of the surgical procedure to those patients who will benefit the most.

Elderly patients, who often have more medical comorbidities than their younger counterparts, are being more frequently evaluated for surgical treatment of pancreatic pathology. Due to advances in perioperative anesthesia, postoperative care, and the increasing safety of the procedure, these patients are undergoing pancreatic surgery often without a significantly increased complication or mortality rate over younger patients. Studies have demonstrated that elderly patients can safely undergo pancreatic surgery and that age alone is not a contraindication [8]. Pancreatic surgeons continue to push the limits for

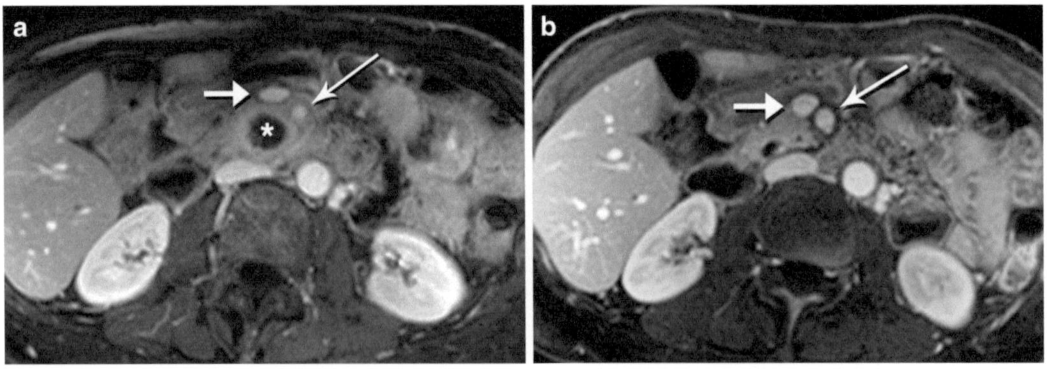

Fig. 36.4 (**a**) Markedly hypoenhancing tumor (*asterisk*) in association with complete encasement of the superior mesenteric artery (*long arrow*) (*Short arrow*=superior mesenteric vein). (**b**) After 7 months of neoadjuvant therapy, tumor tissue has receded from the SMA, with apparently clean margins. The patient underwent a complete resection with a margin negative pancreaticoduodenectomy. Tumor pathology showed significant treatment response

safe surgery for patients with cardiac, pulmonary, or other medical disease that were once thought to be associated with too much risk for postoperative complications.

Preoperative biliary stenting performed for obstruction within the head of the pancreas had previously been introduced as a method to decrease the risk of complications after PD as a way to improve liver dysfunction. However, multiple studies including a large multicenter randomized trial comparing preoperative biliary drainage versus proceeding directly to surgery indicate that this practice is not necessary and may actually increase the risk of infectious complications for these patients [9]. Generally, preoperative biliary drainage is used only for patients who are not proceeding directly to surgical resection within a reasonable time period and an endoscopic route is greatly preferred over a percutaneous route.

Pancreatic cystic lesions are becoming more frequently identified by the widespread use of cross-sectional imaging and are more frequently being referred for evaluation (Fig. 36.5a–d). Many of these lesions are mucinous cysts with the possibility of harboring preneoplastic or invasive disease. Therefore, multidisciplinary recommendations based on available literature have given treatment algorithms (Modified Sendai Criteria) for the evaluation, surgical treatment, and follow-up for these lesions [10]. In short, surgical resection is recommended for all fit patients

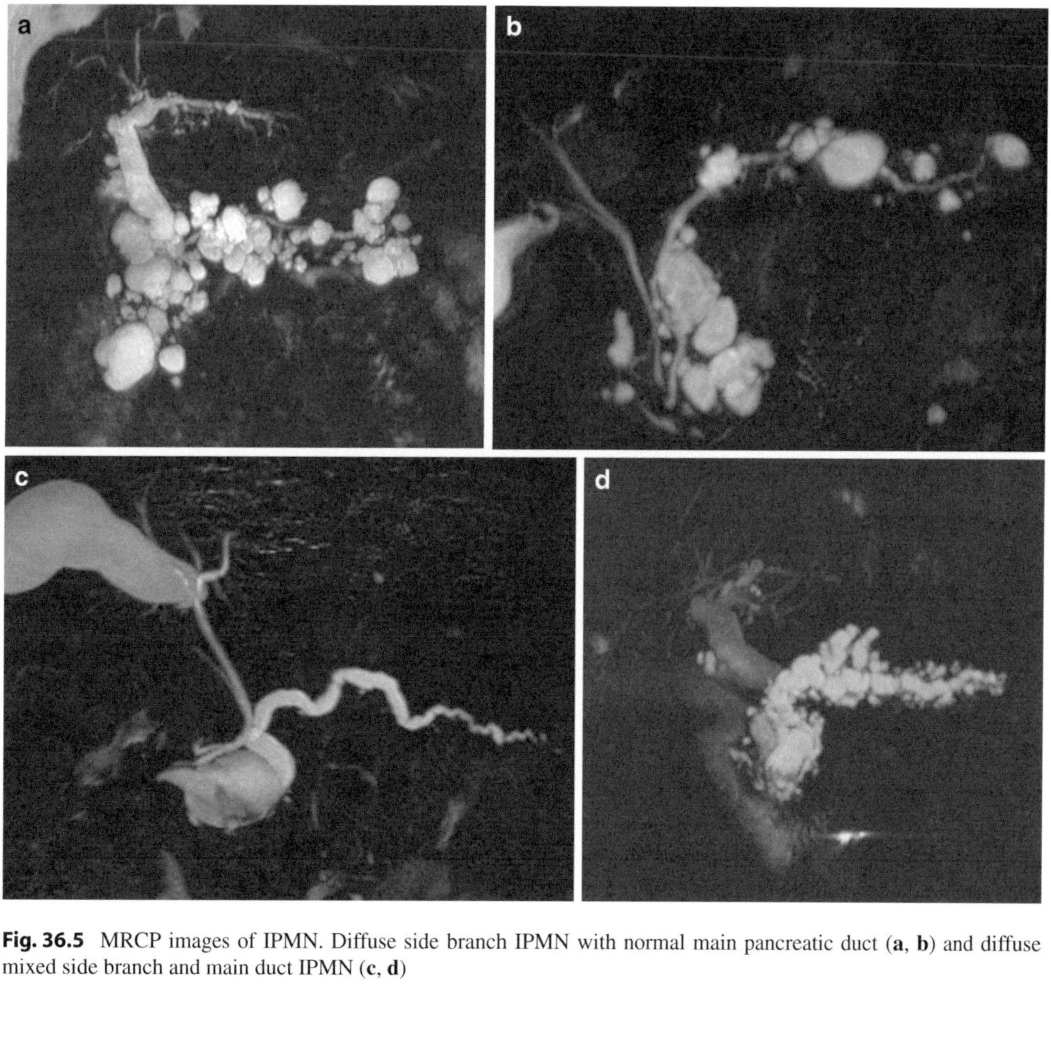

Fig. 36.5 MRCP images of IPMN. Diffuse side branch IPMN with normal main pancreatic duct (**a**, **b**) and diffuse mixed side branch and main duct IPMN (**c**, **d**)

with main duct intraductal papillary mucinous neoplasm (MD-IPMN) and mucinous cystic neoplasms (MCN). Branch duct intraductal papillary mucinous neoplasm (BD-IPMN) with high-risk characteristics including obstructive jaundice, enhancing mural nodules, dysplastic cytology, or main duct involvement should undergo surgical resection. Other worrisome features include size greater than 3 cm, thickened cyst wall, nonenhanced nodule, borderline main duct dilation, focal stricture, cyst growth, and other abdominal symptoms. Surgical treatment is often recommended for these patients, and if not, very aggressive close follow-up is recommended as the risk of malignancy is considerably higher for these patients over those who have none of these worrisome features.

Intraoperative Advances

Pancreatic adenocarcinoma is a highly lethal neoplasm, and disease control often fails even after apparent complete surgical resection. For this reason, investigation into more complete surgical clearance of disease has been performed in the past. Radical regional pancreatic resections including total pancreatectomy, extended lymphadenectomy, and extensive vascular resections have fallen out of favor and are not associated with an increase in patient survival. In fact, these extended regional resections are generally associated with greater frequency of postoperative complications with little additional benefit over other techniques. However, concepts proposed by these surgical strategies certainly have merit.

The surgical resection margin for patients with pancreatic adenocarcinoma has repeatedly been demonstrated as a major predictor of survival. The prognosis for patients with positive margin is often much poorer, and the average survival has historically not been much higher than for patients undergoing palliative treatment. Therefore, wide en bloc clearance of pancreatic adenocarcinoma encompassing regional vascular or contiguous organs to obtain these margins is favorable for patient survival. It is unknown whether additional re-resection of an initially positive margin has actual benefit towards long-term survival similar to that of an initially margin negative resection (R0). Therefore, as stated above, preoperative imaging is of vital importance to carefully assess the feasibility and plan for an R0 resection. A surgeon should not undertake an operation that is felt to have a low chance for an R0 margin, especially in the era of options that include neoadjuvant therapy.

Accurate margin analysis is considered to be of extreme importance when determining patient prognosis after resection. Microscopic margin positive rates (R1) have been reported at widely variable rates even at high-volume institutions due to variable pathologic processing methods and definitions of what constitutes an R0 versus R1 resection. The resection margins of the retroperitoneally located pancreatic gland are notoriously difficult for pathologists to assess, and the circumferential surfaces may have variable terminology between surgeons and pathologists. Verbeke has done considerable work to describe in detail the accurate and uniform assessment of a pancreaticoduodenal specimen [11]. An optimal situation is present when the surgeon and pathologist remain in clear communication regarding an accurate assessment of each pancreatic margin by frozen section analysis at the time of the operation. Many surgeons will be directly involved in marking different anatomic surfaces and providing the pathologist orientation of the specimen in this process.

For tumors in the head of the pancreas, mesenteric and portal venous resection may be required for complete en bloc tumor clearance. This too has been studied quite extensively and has been clearly shown to be a suitable method to assist in avoiding positive margins of the vascular groove, and retroperitoneum and has not been associated with worsened survival compared to patients who do not need vein resection. Multiple technical options for resection and reconstruction have been reported and include adjunctive intraoperative measures such as superior mesenteric artery occlusion and systemic heparinization [12]. In general, vascular involvement is ideally determined by high-quality preoperative imaging, neoadjuvant treatment is considered, and the surgeon is prepared to perform an en bloc vein resection with the necessary resources to perform suitable reconstruction in the operating room.

Pancreatic resection in combination with arterial resection, as opposed to vein resection, has not been associated with any significant survival benefit and is associated with increased complications. Resection of a long segment common hepatic artery, superior mesenteric artery, or celiac artery has been reported as technically feasible but is rarely if ever associated with any long-term survivors. Resection of the celiac artery with en bloc distal pancreatectomy and splenectomy (Appleby procedure) has been described as a surgical option for stage III pancreatic adenocarcinoma of the neck and body of the pancreas that has circumferential celiac artery involvement. Recently, this procedure has been described after neoadjuvant treatment and relies on the pancreaticoduodenal arterial collateral circulation to maintain hepatic and gastric circulation. Carefully selected patients can achieve an estimated median average survival up to 26 months but had a very short disease-free survival of only 21 weeks [13].

Lymph node analysis, like surgical margins, has received additional attention as a predictor of overall survival for patients with pancreatic adenocarcinoma. Nearly all studies show a significantly worsened survival for those with node positive (N1) disease versus those without node involvement (N0). In addition, data supports the notion that for N1 patients with pancreatic adenocarcinoma, the number of lymph nodes involved also seems to affect overall patient survival. The Hopkins group found that an increasing lymph node ratio (LNR) was highly predictive of poorer overall survival [14]. It remains to be seen whether surgical modifications in the operating room to increase the number of lymph nodes examined (thereby lowering the LNR) or increasing the robustness of the pathologic assessment evaluation will result in an increased survival or at least improved prognostic information. Regardless, lymph node harvest is a closely followed surrogate marker for oncologic appropriateness of a pancreatic resection for malignancy.

The magnitude of impact that operative blood loss and packed red blood cell transfusions have has recently come to light with reports indicating that increasing estimated blood loss [15] and the use of transfusions [16] significantly negatively impacts overall survival in patients with pancreatic adenocarcinoma after surgical resection. This factor may be the single most surgeon-controlled factor that can impact the patient's long-term outcome and has received attention as a quality control measure for optimal performance of pancreatic resection. Even for those patients without neoplastic disease, the short- and long-term detrimental effects of packed red blood cell transfusions are significant, and efforts should be made to avoid major hemorrhage during any pancreatic operation. Transfusion of packed red blood cells, while not always avoidable during major pancreatic surgery, is thought to have an immunosuppressive effect through a process that is not fully understood at this time.

Emphasis on obtaining a circumferentially negative margin resection for pancreas adenocarcinoma of the body and tail of the pancreas has led some surgeons to develop the procedure termed radical antegrade modular pancreatosplenectomy (RAMPS). This procedure emphasizes a deeper posterior margin to include an en bloc resection of the anterior renal fascia and, occasionally, the left adrenal gland and Gerota's fascia along with concomitant DP and splenectomy. Utilization of this particular modification has allowed patients with malignancy of the left-sided pancreas, historically associated with even poorer survival, to obtain impressive estimated median of 26 months and 5-year survival of 35 % [17]. Minimally invasive RAMPS is also feasible and allows for a meticulous dissection performed under magnified vision within noninvolved tissue planes to permit wide dissection around a neoplasm known for its locally invasive nature.

Total pancreatectomy (TP), while not the answer to improved survival for pancreatic adenocarcinoma localized within either the proximal or distal pancreas, has its place for treatment of certain disease states of the pancreas. This operation has recently become more commonly performed for several reasons. It is currently recognized that the malignant degeneration of MD-IPMN leads to adenocarcinoma and requires an aggressive resection of a dilated main duct which frequently involves the entire pancreas gland. Patients requiring complete removal of the pancreas will have instantaneous complete endocrine and exocrine insufficiency resulting from the loss of the entire organ, but the brittle diabetes and malnourishment seen in the past has been greatly improved by modern replacement therapy. Many centers have reported improved outcomes [18] and quality of life after TP for neoplastic disease, and it is no longer a dreaded operation for the patient.

Total pancreatectomy with islet autotransplantation (TP-IAT) has been proposed as an effective treatment for end-stage small duct chronic pancreatitis. This operation, for carefully selected patients at a limited number of centers in the United States, has been shown to improve quality of life while decreasing narcotic analgesia requirements [19]. The islet cells are harvested from the surgical specimen and infused into the patient's portal circulation. The yield and viability of the cells is greatly affected by the degree of pancreatic fibrosis as well as any previous pancreatic surgery. Known or suspected neoplastic or preneoplastic disease of the pancreas is considered a contraindication for this procedure. Generally, most patients have insulin requirements after surgery, but reasonable glycemic control is expected, and some patients achieve improved control from preoperative diabetic medication requirements. However, TP-IAT is not currently the first-line treatment for chronic pancreatitis due to operative morbidity and unpredictable outcomes. Resectional procedures are indicated for patients with disease isolated to the proximal or distal pancreas with anatomic abnormalities or worrisome lesions. Drainage procedures that relieve intraductal hypertension such as a longitudinal pancreaticojejunostomy are best for diffuse large duct chronic calcific pancreatitis. In general, surgical intervention for the treatment of pain in patients with chronic pancreatitis is reserved as last-line therapy. Medical and endoscopic therapies have become increasingly effective at palliation of this difficult to manage situation, and treatment algorithms incorporating these recent advances have increased the quality of care for these patients in recent times [20].

Management of acute pancreatitis has improved significantly with emphasis on nonsurgical treatment. Surgical intervention is generally only required for consequences of pancreatic necrosis. Sterile necrosis is best managed by watchful waiting during the evolution of the process. Avoidance of surgical or percutaneous intervention for at least 2–4 weeks from the inciting event is ideal to prevent infectious complications or pancreatic fistula. Pseudocyst formation is a late complication that may require surgical management including endoscopic cystogastrostomy (non-debris containing cysts) or surgical cystogastrostomy or cystojejunostomy (debris containing cysts). Patients with extensive pancreatic necrosis are a high risk to progress to infected pancreatic necrosis. Infected necrotizing pancreatitis can be associated with abdominal sepsis, hemorrhagic complications, intestinal perforation, or abdominal compartment syndrome and will require intervention with the goal of debridement of necrosis and infected devitalized tissue. Again, early aggressive conservative management with later necrosectomy is associated with improved results even in this setting [21]. The neck and body of the pancreas are particularly susceptible to ischemic changes resulting in pancreatic necrosis. Due to operative debridement or parenchymal atrophy, patients recovering from severe necrotizing pancreatitis can frequently be left with what is known as disconnected left pancreatic remnant (DLPR). Management of DLPR includes resection of the distal pancreas and spleen versus internal drainage of the remnant tail depending on the size and viability of the remnant and patency of the splenic vein [22].

Pancreatic fistula (PF) is the Achilles heel of pancreatic surgery, and investigations continue for methods to decrease its incidence. For PD, a wide range of PF rates have been reported based on heterogenous definitions. Somatostatin, an inhibitor of exocrine function, has not been proven to be an effective pharmacologic prophylaxis. Operative measures used to prevent PF during PD including internalized pancreatic stents, externalized stents, surgical drains, duct to mucosa or invaginating pancreaticojejunostomy, and pancreaticogastrostomy have been extensively studied

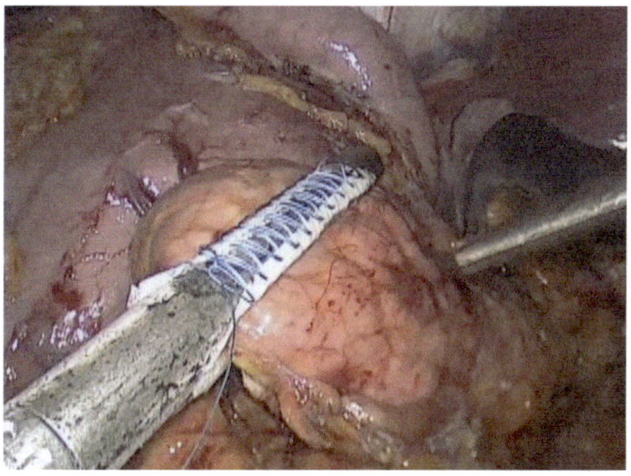

Fig. 36.6 Intraoperative photograph showing a stapled transection of the pancreas using a slow compression technique and staple line reinforcement during laparoscopic distal pancreatectomy

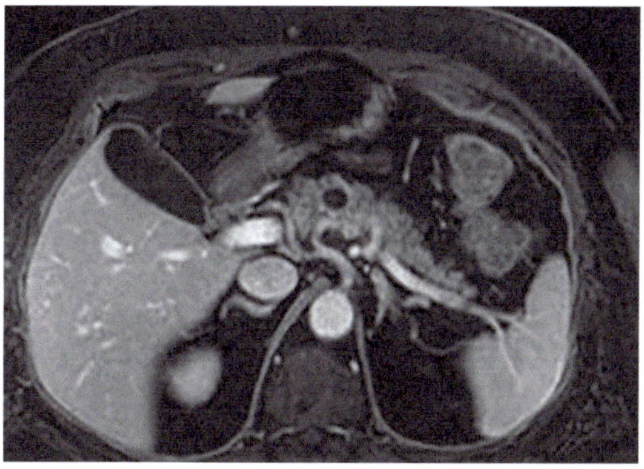

Fig. 36.7 MRI of a mucinous cystic neoplasm in the proximal body of the pancreas treated by central pancreatectomy

without definitive conclusions regarding the optimal method of reconstruction of the pancreas remnant [23]. Similar to proximal pancreatectomy, PF after DP is problematic. Measures used to control the cut surface of the pancreas include staplers, various energy sources, fibrin glue application, or suture techniques, but yet again, the optimal method to reliably prevent pancreatic fistula has been elusive to pancreatic surgeons and investigators. Nevertheless, using a stepwise compression technique with staple line reinforcement on left-sided pancreatectomies has been associated with a low rate of pancreatic fistulae [24] (Fig. 36.6).

Splenic preservation during DP for benign or low-grade neoplastic disease has been described and requires precise dissection of the body and tail of the pancreas away from the splenic artery and vein. Open, laparoscopic, or robotic spleen sparing DP has been reported with variable success rates. Many of these reports emphasize the dissection performed under the magnified view afforded by the laparoscope to aid in control of short vessels from the splenic vasculature with various energy sources or ligation techniques. Splenic preservation has been reported to be beneficial in decreasing the complications after surgery [25], but the long-term benefits are unclear. While technically possible, splenic preservation is contraindicated in cases of malignant disease.

Partial and nonstandard pancreatectomy techniques include pancreatic enucleation, central pancreatectomy, and duodenum-preserving pancreatic head resections. Enucleation of pancreatic lesions is mostly used for functioning and nonfunctioning pancreatic neuroendocrine tumors but has been described for other low-grade neoplastic or rare benign conditions. Disadvantages of this technique include lack of surrounding lymphatic clearance and a higher rate of PF than standard resection. Advantages of this procedure include salvage of pancreatic parenchyma and avoidance of altered gastrointestinal anatomy after PD. Patients who gain the most benefit include those with superficial lesions of the head, uncinate process, or proximal body of the pancreas without involvement of the main pancreatic duct, as this is a contraindication to enucleation. Central pancreatectomy is performed for similar indications for lesions of the neck and proximal body of the pancreas (Fig. 36.7). Again, PF is higher than standard resection, and reconstruction of the left-sided pancreas remnant to a jejunal limb or the stomach is required. Duodenum-preserving pancreatic head resection is more commonly performed in Europe for the treatment of intractable pain in chronic pancreatitis. This procedure involves transection of the pancreas at the neck with preservation of the duodenum and removal of the head and uncinate process of the pancreas. The common bile duct is preserved along with a small rim of pancreatic tissue at the proximal aspect of the head, and reconstruction is accomplished with a pancreaticojejunostomy or pancreaticogastrostomy to the pancreatic remnant. Variations of this procedure include common bile duct resection with hepaticojejunostomy for common bile duct obstruction or longitudinal pancreaticojejunostomy for large duct, "chain of lakes" chronic pancreatitis disease of the pancreatic remnant, both of which require a roux limb of jejunum.

Recently, minimally invasive approaches to all forms of pancreatic surgery have been applied with success to decrease the morbidity and recovery time required after surgery. The location of the pancreas, deep within the central retroperitoneum, makes access difficult even with standard open surgical techniques. However, advances in instrumentation and optics along with increasing experience and skill sets of surgeons have allowed for a more widespread adoption of laparoscopic or robotic pancreatic surgery. Minimally invasive DP has clear benefits over open surgery. Meta-analysis of literature and population based studies show significantly decreased morbidity, blood loss, and length of stay for a minimally invasive approach [26, 27]. While the use of this modality has been increasing, it appears to continue to be underutilized despite its significant advantages. All studies examining oncologic parameters for minimally invasive DP show at least similar long-term outcomes and many show decreased blood loss and increased lymph node harvest [28]. Laparoscopic [29] and robotic PD have also been shown to have similar advantages with less blood loss and decreased hospital stay. However, this is a very complex undertaking requiring considerable skills and experience that has not shown decreased complication rates at this time. However, at select centers this procedure is performed safely with the goal of eventually improving recovery, oncologic outcomes, and quality of life for patients requiring PD for pancreatic disease.

Minimally invasive surgical techniques have been applied to nonstandard resections such as enucleation and central pancreatectomy, as well as treatment for complications stemming from pancreatitis. Patients with necrotizing pancreatitis requiring operative debridement can undergo a "step up" approach that combines the use of interventionally placed drainage catheters followed by videoscopically aided debridement of necrotic pancreas debris. Use of these techniques significantly decreases the morbidity and mortality for these patients over open necrosectomy [30]. Surgical drainage procedures for chronic pancreatitis including cystogastrostomy and cystojejunostomy are feasible and generally require techniques to lavage debris from pancreatic pseudocysts.

Postoperative Advances

Pancreatic surgery has undergone thorough investigation throughout the years, especially in relation to the frequency in which it is performed. However, comparisons between studies were difficult to perform due to heterogeneity of definitions. Recent publications from the International Study Group of Pancreatic Surgery have allowed for standardized definitions regarding post-pancreatectomy hemorrhage [31], delayed gastric emptying [32], and pancreatic fistula [33]. The use of these pancreas-specific definitions, along with other standardized postoperative complication grading systems, has allowed for an improved understanding on how variations in technique can affect outcomes across a wide range of patients from multiple centers.

Complications after pancreatic surgery are nearly inevitable due to the complex nature of the operation and general poor health condition of the patient. As stated before, complications can be minimized by regionalization of these procedures to high-volume centers. Not only are complications decreased, but the effect of the complication on the patients seems to be minimized in centers experienced in treating patients undergoing complex gastrointestinal operations such as pancreatectomy [34]. This underscores the multidisciplinary management of a patient undergoing pancreatic surgery that goes well beyond that of the skill level and experience of the surgeon. Perioperative anesthetic management, availability of dedicated intensive care physicians, and experienced nursing care have under-recognized effects on the overall success of pancreatic surgery patients. Additionally, accessibility to proficient interventional radiologists is vital in the perioperative setting, especially for complications stemming from pancreatic fistula and post-pancreatectomy hemorrhage. In the past, reoperation with completion total pancreatectomy was a frequently used treatment method for severe fistula or hemorrhagic complications. Today, completion total pancreatectomy is rarely even considered [35] because interventional methods of percutaneous drainage or intravascular control are more effective and allow for a more expedient "rescue" from these complications.

Implementations of "fast track" or "enhanced recovery" pathways have been introduced throughout all facets of complex alimentary surgery and pancreas surgery. Critical pathways created to streamline recovery from surgical procedures have demonstrated a significant effect on patients undergoing pancreas surgery [36]. These recovery strategies generally include less invasive monitoring techniques and decreased use of nasogastric tube drainage. Minimization of crystalloid fluid administration, early mobilization, advanced pain control techniques, and patient education are some of the usual components of a successfully designed recovery pathway after pancreatic surgery.

Readmission after pancreas surgery remains a problem and continues to occur in nearly a quarter of patients, even at high-volume centers. Most readmissions are related to procedure-specific complications such as pancreatic fistula, delayed gastric emptying, intra-abdominal abscess, or hemorrhage, but medical deconditioning and failure to thrive are other common causes of readmission after pancreatic surgery. Strategies proposed to decrease this incidence include earlier recognition of those patients at high risk, including those who deviate from care pathways [37].

Conclusion

Surgical expertise, a multispecialty approach, and a strong commitment to excellence are keys for the success when treating these patients with complex pancreatic processes. Technical improvements regarding the surgical management of pancreatic disease such as minimally invasive surgery, parenchymal sparing resections, decreased blood loss during surgery, and recognizing and treating complications have made pancreatic surgery a much safer endeavor than it has ever been. Concepts regarding extended pancreatic resection, neoadjuvant treatment, management of pancreatic necrosis, and multidisciplinary decision making have made pancreatic surgery more effective for patients with pancreatic disease. Overall, it is likely that the need for safe and effective pancreatic surgery will remain, and investigators will continue thorough study to gain new understanding behind pancreas pathology. Evolving and advancing technical developments will continue to aid in the treatment of this pathology.

Abbreviations

BD-IPMN	Branch duct intraductal papillary mucinous neoplasm
CT	Computed tomography
DLPR	Disconnected left pancreatic remnant
DP	Distal pancreatectomy
ERCP	Endoscopic retrograde cholangio-pancreatography
EUS	Endoscopic ultrasonography
IPMN	Intraductal papillary mucinous neoplasm
LNR	Lymph node ratio
MCN	Mucinous cystic neoplasms
MD-IPMN	Main duct intraductal papillary mucinous neoplasm
MRCP	Magnetic resonance cholangio-pancreatography
MRI	Magnetic resonance imaging
N0	Node negative
N1	Node positive
PD	Pancreaticoduodenectomy
PF	Pancreatic fistula
R0	Negative margin
R1	Positive margin
RAMPS	Radical antegrade modular pancreatosplenectomy
TP	Total pancreatectomy
TP-IAT	Total pancreatectomy with islet autotransplantation

References

1. McPhee JT, Hill JS, Whalen GF, Zayaruzny M, Litwin DE, Sullivan ME, et al. Perioperative mortality for pancreatectomy: a national perspective. Ann Surg. 2007;246(2):246–53.
2. Tseng JF, Pisters PW, Lee JE, Wang H, Gomez HF, Sun CC, et al. The learning curve in pancreatic surgery. Surgery. 2007;141(4):456–63.
3. Pawlik TM, Laheru D, Hruban RH, Coleman J, Wolfgang CL, Campbell K, et al. Evaluating the impact of a single-day multidisciplinary clinic on the management of pancreatic cancer. Ann Surg Oncol. 2008;15(8):2081–8.
4. Varadarajulu S, Eloubeidi MA. The role of endoscopic ultrasonography in the evaluation of pancreatico-biliary cancer. Surg Clin North Am. 2010;90(2):251–63.
5. Thosani N, Thosani S, Qiao W, Fleming JB, Bhutani MS, Guha S. Role of EUS-FNA-based cytology in the diagnosis of mucinous pancreatic cystic lesions: a systematic review and meta-analysis. Dig Dis Sci. 2010;55(10):2756–66.
6. Papavasiliou P, Chun YS, Hoffman JP. How to define and manage borderline resectable pancreatic cancer. Surg Clin North Am. 2013;93(3):663–74.
7. Assifi MM, Lu X, Eibl G, Reber HA, Li G, Hines OJ. Neoadjuvant therapy in pancreatic adenocarcinoma: a meta-analysis of phase II trials. Surgery. 2011;150(3):466–73.
8. Oliveira-Cunha M, Malde DJ, Aldouri A, Morris-Stiff G, Menon KV, Smith AM. Results of pancreatic surgery in the elderly: is age a barrier? HPB (Oxford). 2013;15(1):24–30.
9. van der Gaag NA, Rauws EA, van Eijck CH, Bruno MJ, van der Harst E, Kubben FJ, et al. Preoperative biliary drainage for cancer of the head of the pancreas. N Engl J Med. 2010;362(2):129–37.
10. Tanaka M, Fernandez-del Castillo C, Adsay V, Chari S, Falconi M, Jang JY, et al. International consensus guidelines 2012 for the management of IPMN and MCN of the pancreas. Pancreatology. 2012;12(3):183–97.
11. Verbeke CS. Resection margins in pancreatic cancer. Surg Clin North Am. 2013;93(3):647–62.
12. Christians KK, Lal A, Pappas S, Quebbeman E, Evans DB. Portal vein resection. Surg Clin North Am. 2010;90(2):309–22.
13. Baumgartner JM, Krasinskas A, Daouadi M, Zureikat A, Marsh W, Lee K, et al. Distal pancreatectomy with en bloc celiac axis resection for locally advanced pancreatic adenocarcinoma following neoadjuvant therapy. J Gastrointest Surg. 2012;16(6):1152–9.
14. Pawlik TM, Gleisner AL, Cameron JL, Winter JM, Assumpcao L, Lillemoe KD, et al. Prognostic relevance of lymph node ratio following pancreaticoduodenectomy for pancreatic cancer. Surgery. 2007;141(5):610–8.
15. Kazanjian KK, Hines OJ, Duffy JP, Yoon DY, Cortina G, Reber HA. Improved survival following pancreaticoduodenectomy to treat adenocarcinoma of the pancreas: the influence of operative blood loss. Arch Surg. 2008;143(12):1166–71.
16. Yeh JJ, Gonen M, Tomlinson JS, Idrees K, Brennan MF, Fong Y. Effect of blood transfusion on outcome after pancreaticoduodenectomy for exocrine tumour of the pancreas. Br J Surg. 2007;94(4):466–72.
17. Mitchem JB, Hamilton N, Gao F, Hawkins WG, Linehan DC, Strasberg SM. Long-term results of resection of adenocarcinoma of the body and tail of the pancreas using radical antegrade modular pancreatosplenectomy procedure. J Am Coll Surg. 2012; 214(1):46–52.
18. Stauffer JA, Nguyen JH, Heckman MG, Grewal MS, Dougherty M, Gill KR, et al. Patient outcomes after total pancreatectomy: a single centre contemporary experience. HPB (Oxford). 2009;11(6):483–92.
19. Morgan K, Owczarski SM, Borckardt J, Madan A, Nishimura M, Adams DB. Pain control and quality of life after pancreatectomy with islet autotransplantation for chronic pancreatitis. J Gastrointest Surg. 2012;16(1):129–33. discussion 33–4.
20. Chauhan S, Forsmark CE. Pain management in chronic pancreatitis: a treatment algorithm. Best Pract Res Clin Gastroenterol. 2010;24(3):323–35.
21. Beger HG, Rau BM. New advances in pancreatic surgery. Curr Opin Gastroenterol. 2007;23(5):522–34.
22. Murage KP, Ball CG, Zyromski NJ, Nakeeb A, Ocampo C, Sandrasegaran K, et al. Clinical framework to guide operative decision making in disconnected left pancreatic remnant (DLPR) following acute or chronic pancreatitis. Surgery. 2010;148(4): 847–56. discussion 56–7.
23. Lai EC, Lau SH, Lau WY. Measures to prevent pancreatic fistula after pancreatoduodenectomy: a comprehensive review. Arch Surg. 2009;144(11): 1074–80.
24. Asbun HJ, Stauffer JA. Laparoscopic approach to distal and subtotal pancreatectomy: a clockwise technique. Surg Endosc. 2011;25(8):2643–9.
25. Shoup M, Brennan MF, McWhite K, Leung DH, Klimstra D, Conlon KC. The value of splenic preservation with distal pancreatectomy. Arch Surg. 2002;137(2):164–8.
26. Venkat R, Edil BH, Schulick RD, Lidor AO, Makary MA, Wolfgang CL. Laparoscopic distal pancreatectomy is associated with significantly less overall morbidity compared to the open technique: a systematic review and meta-analysis. Ann Surg. 2012;255(6): 1048–59.
27. Tran Cao HS, Lopez N, Chang DC, Lowy AM, Bouvet M, Baumgartner JM, et al. Improved perioperative outcomes with minimally invasive distal pancreatectomy: results from a population-based analysis. JAMA Surg. 2014;149(3):237–43.
28. Stauffer JA, Rosales-Velderrain A, Goldberg RF, Bowers SP, Asbun HJ. Comparison of open with laparoscopic distal pancreatectomy: a single institution's transition over a 7-year period. HPB (Oxford). 2013;15(2):149–55.

29. Asbun HJ, Stauffer JA. Laparoscopic vs open pancreaticoduodenectomy: overall outcomes and severity of complications using the Accordion Severity Grading System. J Am Coll Surg. 2012;215(6):810–9.
30. van Santvoort HC, Besselink MG, Bakker OJ, Hofker HS, Boermeester MA, Dejong CH, et al. A step-up approach or open necrosectomy for necrotizing pancreatitis. N Engl J Med. 2010;362(16):1491–502.
31. Wente MN, Veit JA, Bassi C, Dervenis C, Fingerhut A, Gouma DJ, et al. Postpancreatectomy hemorrhage (PPH): an International Study Group of Pancreatic Surgery (ISGPS) definition. Surgery. 2007;142(1):20–5.
32. Wente MN, Bassi C, Dervenis C, Fingerhut A, Gouma DJ, Izbicki JR, et al. Delayed gastric emptying (DGE) after pancreatic surgery: a suggested definition by the International Study Group of Pancreatic Surgery (ISGPS). Surgery. 2007;142(5):761–8.
33. Bassi C, Dervenis C, Butturini G, Fingerhut A, Yeo C, Izbicki J, et al. Postoperative pancreatic fistula: an international study group (ISGPF) definition. Surgery. 2005;138(1):8–13.
34. Ghaferi AA, Birkmeyer JD, Dimick JB. Hospital volume and failure to rescue with high-risk surgery. Med Care. 2011;49(12):1076–81.
35. Buchler MW, Wagner M, Schmied BM, Uhl W, Friess H, Z'Graggen K. Changes in morbidity after pancreatic resection: toward the end of completion pancreatectomy. Arch Surg. 2003;138(12):1310–4. discussion 5.
36. Kennedy EP, Rosato EL, Sauter PK, Rosenberg LM, Doria C, Marino IR, et al. Initiation of a critical pathway for pancreaticoduodenectomy at an academic institution—the first step in multidisciplinary team building. J Am Coll Surg. 2007;204(5):917–23. discussion 23–4.
37. Kent TS, Sachs TE, Callery MP, Vollmer Jr CM. Readmission after major pancreatic resection: a necessary evil? J Am Coll Surg. 2011;213(4):515–23.

Laparoscopic Liver Resection for Hepatocellular Carcinoma

37

Takeshi Takahara and Go Wakabayashi

Indications and Current Role of Laparoscopic Liver Resection

The advancements of laparoscopic procedures in liver surgery have proceeded slowly given the inherent morbidity associated with liver resection. Despite initial obstacles, Gagner et al. reported the first case of laparoscopic liver resection (LLR) in 1992 [1]. Subsequently, minimally invasive surgery has been embraced largely due to the reduction in abdominal wall morbidity and enhanced postoperative recovery. Earlier experiences with laparoscopic liver surgery were usually associated with staging procedures and non-anatomical or wedge liver resection such as cysts, adenomas, hemangiomas, and solitary liver metastases [2, 3]. The first laparoscopic anatomical resection (a left lateral sectionectomy (LLS)) was performed in February 1993 [4]. While minimally invasive surgery has been embraced in other fields, there have been several obstacles to its widespread use in LLR. Nevertheless, despite its lateness to embrace laparoscopy, liver surgery is now gaining momentum in this paradigm shift. Following improvements in technology and equipment, LLR should now be considered a safe option if performed by experienced surgeons. Additionally, dramatic improvements in the safety of hepatic resection, based on an increased understanding of liver anatomy and better preoperative radiologic imaging, have facilitated this transition. Thus, adoption of the laparoscopic approach for the surgical treatment of hepatic lesions is now progressively expanding. The advancements in high-definition optical technology in recent years have greatly enhanced visual preciseness in laparoscopic surgery, thus allowing the identification of vital structures in liver surgery.

A panel of experts at a conference in Louisville, Kentucky, in 2008, agreed that the best indications for laparoscopic hepatectomy were solitary lesions, under 5 cm, located in the anterior segments, and at a distance from the hepatic hilum and the vena cava [5]. This approach has since evolved to encompass more difficult anatomical resections, including right hepatectomy and central hepatectomy, as well as extended hepatectomies and living donor hepatectomies [6, 7]. Although the fear of uncontrollable bleeding or gas embolism explains the initial slow development of LLR, there were no intraoperative deaths reported in the largest study for major LLR [8, 9], and, though frequent embolisms of CO_2 [10] have occurred, these have been without any clinical repercussions in both animal and human studies [11].

T. Takahara, M.D., Ph.D. (✉)
Department of Surgery, Iwate Medical University School of Medicine, Morioka, Iwate, Japan
e-mail: takahara@iwate-med.ac.jp; takahara731026@yahoo.co.jp

G. Wakabayashi, M.D., Ph.D., F.A.C.S.
Department of Surgery, Ageo Central General Hospital, Ageo, Saitama, Japan
e-mail: gowaka@ach.or.jp

R. Latifi et al. (eds.), *Technological Advances in Surgery, Trauma and Critical Care*,
DOI 10.1007/978-1-4939-2671-8_37

Treatments for Hepatocellular Carcinoma

Hepatocellular carcinoma (HCC) is the most frequent primary liver tumor, especially in the Association of Southeast Asian Nations region, where the prevalence of hepatitis virus infection is high [12]. The potential treatment options for HCC include surgical resection, liver transplantation, chemotherapy, and local ablative therapy. Liver resection plays an important part in the treatment of this disease. The traditional surgical management for HCC is open hepatectomy. Nevertheless, liver resection for HCC is somewhat limited by the liver function reserve and the general condition of the patient, although it is excellent in terms of the efficacy of local control. Liver resection and liver transplantation can both achieve cure of HCC; however, less invasive therapeutic modalities, including percutaneous ablation therapy or transarterial chemoembolization (TACE) or systemic chemotherapy, are also effective.

The hepatectomy approach for HCC becomes an issue if repeated hepatectomies are necessary due to multicentric carcinogenesis. It is widely accepted that laparoscopy is suitable for performing subsequent surgical procedures since it leads to less intra-abdominal adhesions compared with open surgery. A recent report indicated that prior LLR for HCC compared to open liver resection (OLR) facilitated subsequent salvage liver transplantation with a lower morbidity [13]. Intra-abdominal adhesions after repeated hepatectomy for recurrent HCC after LLR were slight and were located only at the small surgical wound used to remove the resected specimen and port site [14]. A randomized clinical trial comparing laparoscopic to open hepatectomy for HCC has not been performed, but such a trial may not be feasible as patients expect to consider less invasive procedures if the oncological outcomes are equal to those offered by open procedures. A recent meta-analysis demonstrated that, in patients with solitary left lateral section or right peripheral subcapsular tumors treated with minor resection, LLR may have short-term advantages in terms of blood loss and postoperative morbidity for HCC compared to OLR, with similar long-term outcomes [15]. A review of the literature shows that LLR for HCC seems to be superior to OLR in terms of perioperative results without compromising the oncological outcomes, especially in cirrhotic patients in whom postoperative ascites are decreased due to reduced obstruction of the abdominal wall [16].

Technical Advancement of LLR

Herein, we describe the technical aspects of the various procedures of LLR for HCC available in our institute, including the new techniques available and the pitfalls experienced over the past 2 years.

Partial Hepatectomy

Pure laparoscopic partial liver resection is now readily available and considered the treatment of choice. However, the technical difficulties associated with laparoscopic partial resection are mainly attributed to the tumor size and location (upper lesions such as segment II, XII, or XIII). The operator stands to the right of the patient with the assistant and the scopist on the patient's left (Fig. 37.1).

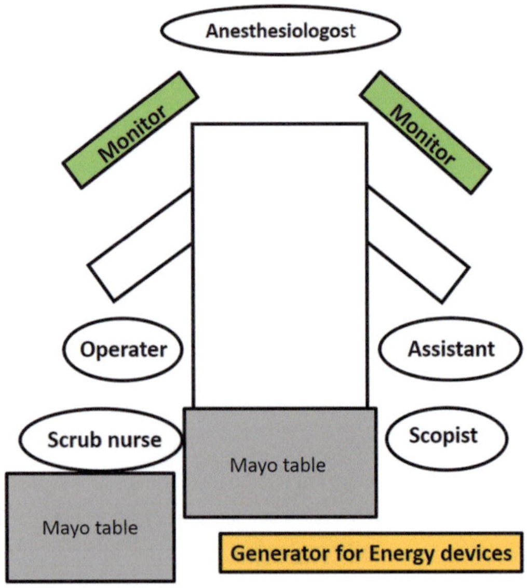

Fig. 37.1 Setting and placement of the various equipment in the operating room. This setting is the same for all procedures of laparoscopic liver resection

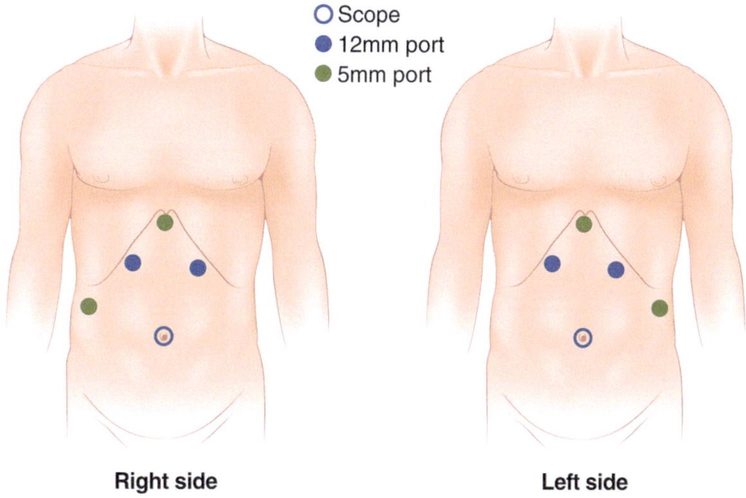

Fig. 37.2 Trocar placement for laparoscopic partial hepatectomy

Five trocars are placed as shown in Fig. 37.2. A CO_2 pneumoperitoneum was created and maintained at 10–12 mmHg. LLR for small HCC remains a challenge due to the limited tactile sensation and complex liver anatomy; therefore, intraoperative screening using Sonazoid ultrasound is important to delineate a safe surgical margin. The parenchymal dissection is performed using a vessel-sealing device, while monopolar coagulation is used for minor bleeding and larger structures are clipped and divided with endoclips.

In our initial experience of laparoscopic partial hepatectomy, precoagulation by radiofrequency ablation was used before hepatic parenchymal dissection in laparoscopic wedge resection, primarily to minimize hemorrhage, to coagulate tissue surrounding the tumor, and to secure the surgical margin. The understanding obtained from the recent laparoscopic partial hepatectomies performed at our institution led to the following conclusions (Fig. 37.3a–c):

- An intermittent Pringle maneuver is necessary to minimize hemorrhage during hepatic parenchymal dissection.
- In partial resection for HCC localized on the right lobe, mobilization of the right lobe by hanging it is necessary to control unexpected bleeding from the right hepatic vein.
- To secure the surgical margin, the parenchymal dissection should be performed along the tributaries of the main hepatic vein or the tumor-feeding Glissonean pedicle, which form the landmark for the deep transection line.

Left Lateral Sectionectomy

The procedure is conducted by placing the supine patient in the reverse Trendelenburg position. Four ports are placed as shown in Fig. 37.4. CO_2 pressure for pneumoperitoneum is kept at 8–10 mmHg during hepatic parenchymal transection. The round ligament and the falciform ligament are divided by a harmonic scalpel through the right port. The round ligament is grasped with Endoloop ligatures and pulled to the right using an Endo Close™ (Covidien, Dublin, Ireland) suturing device. The coronary ligament, the left triangular ligament, and the upper membrane of the hepatogastric ligament are divided with a harmonic scalpel to mobilize the left lateral section. The liver is then transected along the line near the left of the falciform ligament, using a harmonic scalpel. The liver parenchyma is transected to a depth of 2–3 cm by using a harmonic scalpel without the inflow occlusion to enable the insertion of an endoscopic linear stapler. Both portal pedicles, with the surrounding liver tissue, are divided using an Echelon Flex™ (Ethicon Endosurgery, Blue Ash, OH) stapler with a 60-mm gold cartridge. Thereafter,

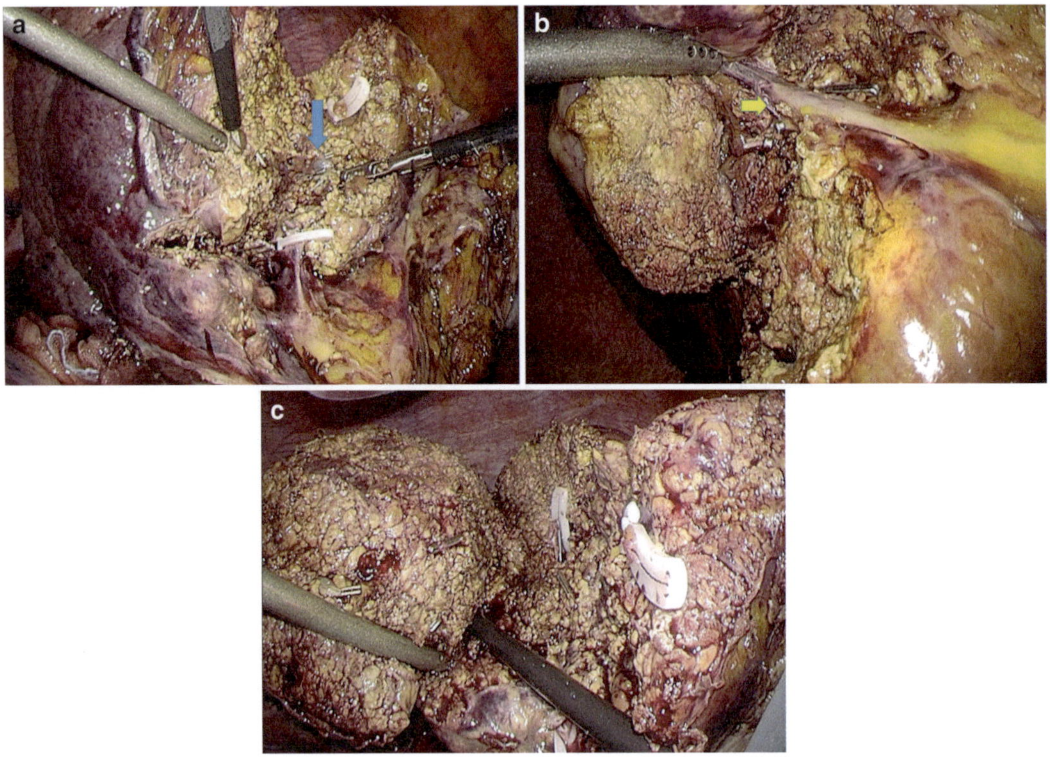

Fig. 37.3 (**a**–**c**) Laparoscopic partial hepatectomy. (**a**) To secure the surgical margin, perform the parenchymal dissection exposing the tributary of the middle hepatic vein (*blue arrow*). (**b**) Perform the partial hepatectomy of the segment XI along the posterior Glisson (*yellow arrow*). (**c**) Hanging up of the liver to prevent bleeding of the cut surface

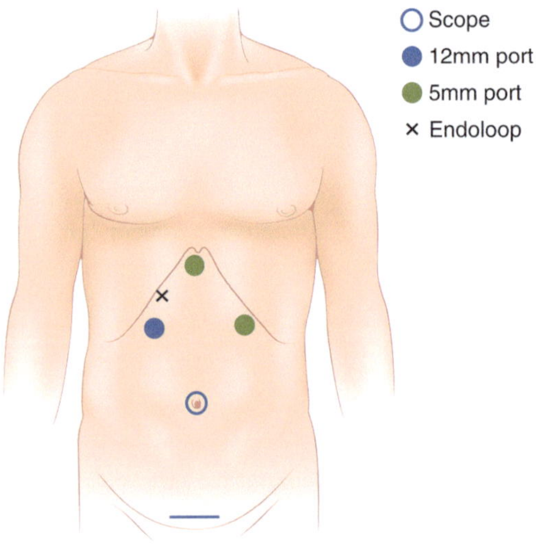

Fig. 37.4 Trocar placement for laparoscopic left lateral sectionectomy

the left hepatic vein, including the liver parenchyma, is divided using the Echelon Flex™ stapler with a 60-mm white cartridge. Finally, the specimen is extracted using a protective bag through a suprapubic incision or a previous surgical incision. The technical requirements to safely and routinely perform laparoscopic LLS are as follows (Fig. 37.5a–c):

- The surface of the hepatogastric ligament is divided with a harmonic scalpel to free the left lateral section.
- In performing the liver parenchyma, neither the left hepatic nor the portal pedicles of segments II and III are exposed.
- The branch form of the umbilical fissure vein [17] should be checked preoperatively.

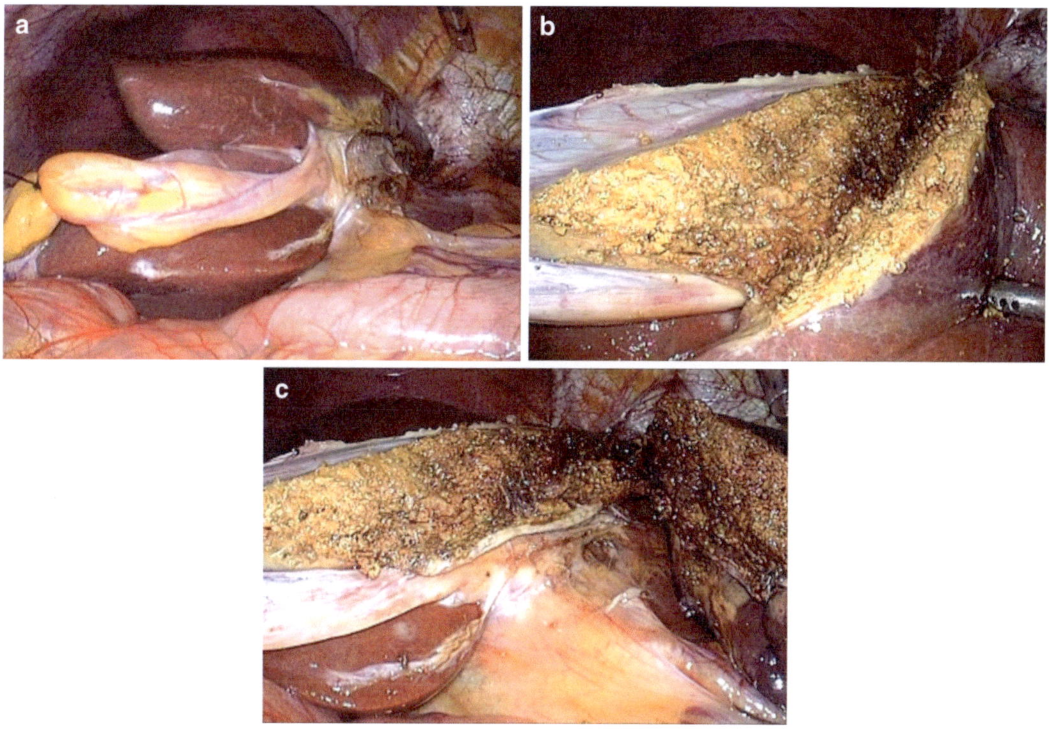

Fig. 37.5 (**a**–**c**) Laparoscopic left lateral sectionectomy. (**a**) After dividing the surface of the hepatogastric ligament, mobilize the left lateral section enough to detect the Arantius duct. (**b**) Perform the parenchymal dissection, not exposing the portal pedicles of segments II and III. (**c**) Completion of dividing both portal pedicles with the surrounding liver tissue, using an Echelon Flex™ (Ethicon Endosurgery, Blue Ash, OH) stapler with a 60-mm gold cartridge

Our procedure for pure LLS has been standardized and is reproducible. Hasegawa et al. reported that training new surgeons by allowing them to gain supervised experience with laparoscopic hepatectomy is both safe and feasible [18]. Further, they specified that LLS is a useful operation to train surgeons prior to more complex laparoscopic hepatectomy procedures [18]. Presently, there is a trend in favor of a pure laparoscopic approach for LLS for pediatric living donor liver transplantation, which can be considered as a safe procedure with potential advantages provided by the laparoscopic technique [19].

Major Hepatectomy

We have found a significant increase in the number of laparoscopic major hepatectomies performed over the past 2 years, with a concurrent reduction in the use of the hybrid method [20]. Initially, a laparoscopic trocar is inserted into the umbilicus using an open procedure and a 12-mm trocar is inserted under the xiphoid. Three further trocars are inserted in the subcostal region (Fig. 37.6), after which the supporting ligaments surrounding the resected side of the liver are resected and the liver is mobilized. Following cholecystectomy, the resected side of the hepatoduodenal ligament is skeletonized, and the right or left hepatic artery and the right or left portal vein are encircled with a piece of vessel tape, paying careful attention not to damage the branch for segment I and, if necessary, dividing it. Following division of the inflow vessels, the liver demarcation defines the transection line, marked on the liver surface with monopolar cautery, and intraoperative ultrasound is used to identify the middle hepatic vein, which is a deep resection line landmark. Once the parenchymal transection has begun over the hilar plate

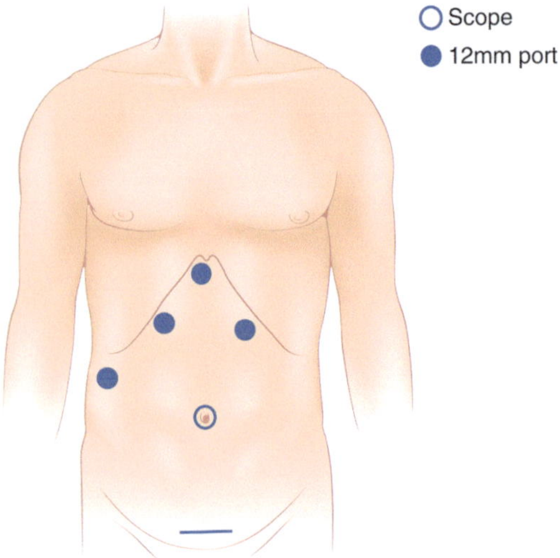

Fig. 37.6 Trocar placement and skin incision for laparoscopic major hepatectomy

to detect the middle hepatic vein, it continues by keeping the cut plane between the middle hepatic vein and the demarcation line on the liver surface. The hepatic parenchymal transection is performed using the vessel-sealing device and clips, while a CO_2 pneumoperitoneum is created and maintained at 12 mmHg. The specimen is externalized through a suprapubic incision in a section without muscle and placed in a large plastic bag. The incision is closed, the pneumoperitoneum reestablished, and hemostasis and biliostasis of the cut surface are checked. Finally, the drain is inserted near the cut surface from the trocar's hole.

Pure laparoscopic major hepatectomy is preferred over hybrid methods for the following reasons (Fig. 37.7a–c):

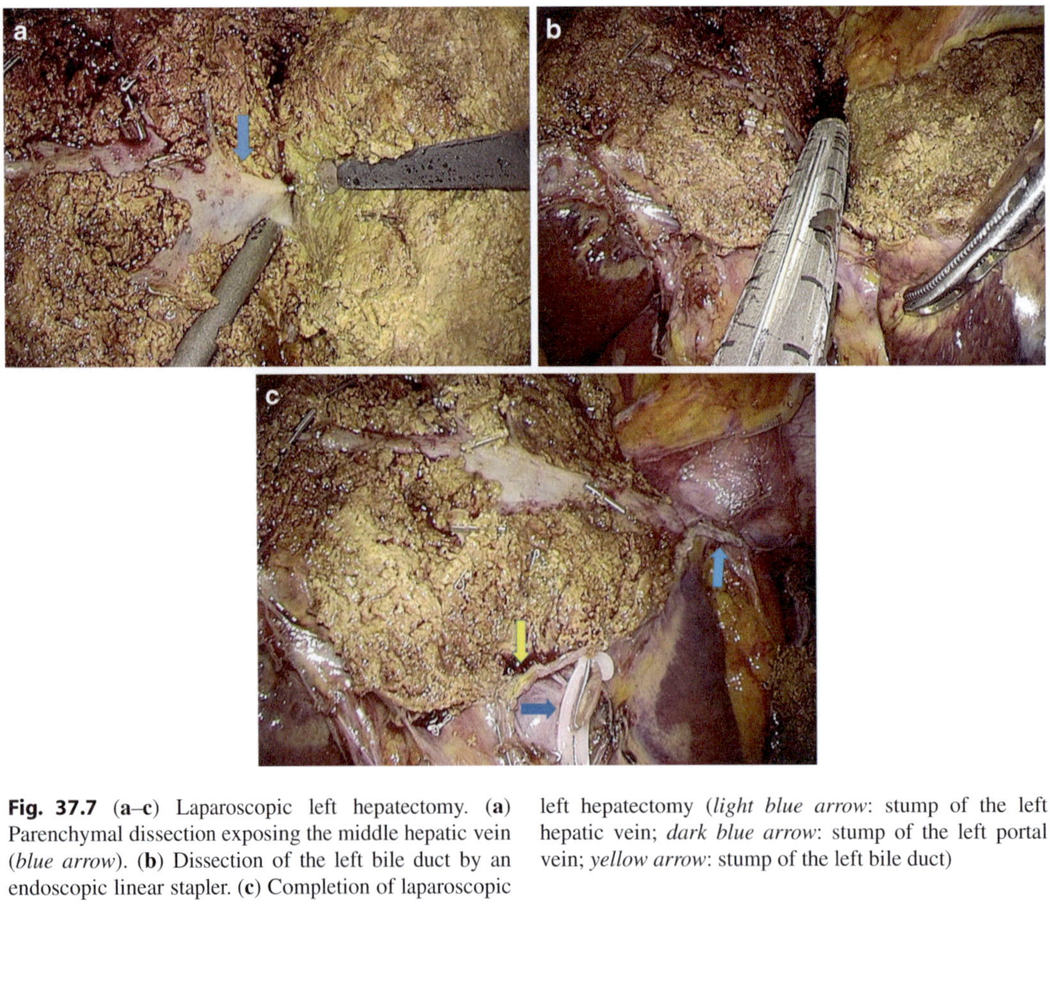

Fig. 37.7 (**a**–**c**) Laparoscopic left hepatectomy. (**a**) Parenchymal dissection exposing the middle hepatic vein (*blue arrow*). (**b**) Dissection of the left bile duct by an endoscopic linear stapler. (**c**) Completion of laparoscopic left hepatectomy (*light blue arrow*: stump of the left hepatic vein; *dark blue arrow*: stump of the left portal vein; *yellow arrow*: stump of the left bile duct)

- Based on animal experiments, a pneumoperitoneal pressure of around 12 mmHg reduces bleeding from the hepatic veins and vena cava [21]. Thus, a parenchymal dissection exposing the middle hepatic vein can be comfortably performed.
- A flexible laparoscope provides a better exposure with magnification deep inside the abdominal cavity and even behind the liver, thus allowing the liver to be safely mobilized near the vena cava.

Acknowledgements The authors declare no conflict of interest, funding, grant equipment, and drugs. The authors declare not having received funding for this work from any of the following organizations: National Institutes of Health (NIH); Wellcome Trust; Howard Hughes Medical Institute (HHMI); or other(s). All authors have seen and approved and are fully conversant with the contents of the manuscript. All authors are responsible for the accuracy of the manuscript.

References

1. Abecassis MM, Fisher RA, Olthoff KM, et al. Complications of living donor hepatic lobectomy–a comprehensive report. Am J Transplant. 2012;12(5):1208–17.
2. Nguyen KT, Laurent A, Dagher I, et al. Minimally invasive liver resection for metastatic colorectal cancer: a multi-institutional, international report of safety, feasibility, and early outcomes. Ann Surg. 2009;250(5):842–8.
3. Descottes B, Glineur D, Lachachi F, et al. Laparoscopic liver resection of benign liver tumors. Surg Endosc. 2003;17(1):23–30.
4. Azagra JS, Goergen M, Gilbart E, et al. Laparoscopic anatomical (hepatic) left lateral segmentectomy-technical aspects. Surg Endosc. 1996;10(7):758–61.
5. Buell JF, Cherqui D, Geller DA, et al. The international position on laparoscopic liver surgery: the Louisville Statement, 2008. Ann Surg. 2009;250(5):825–30.
6. Ishizawa T, Gumbs AA, Kokudo N, et al. Laparoscopic segmentectomy of the liver: from segment I to VIII. Ann Surg. 2012;256(6):959–64.
7. Ho CM, Wakabayashi G, Nitta H, et al. Total laparoscopic limited anatomical resection for centrally located hepatocellular carcinoma in cirrhotic liver. Surg Endosc. 2013;27(5):1820–5.
8. Dagher I, Di Giuro G, Dubrez J, et al. Laparoscopic versus open right hepatectomy: a comparative study. Am J Surg. 2009;198(2):173–7.
9. Abu Hilal M, Di Fabio F, Teng MJ, et al. Single-centre comparative study of laparoscopic versus open right hepatectomy. J Gastrointest Surg. 2011;15(5):818–23.
10. Schmandra TC, Mierdl S, Hollander D, et al. Risk of gas embolism in hand-assisted versus total laparoscopic hepatic resection. Surg Technol Int. 2004;12:137–43.
11. Poon JT, Law WL, Chow LC, et al. Outcome of laparoscopic resection for colorectal cancer in patients with high operative risk. Ann Surg Oncol. 2011;18(7):1884–90.
12. El-Serag HB, Rudolph KL. Hepatocellular carcinoma: epidemiology and molecular carcinogenesis. Gastroenterology. 2007;132(7):2557–76.
13. Laurent A, Tayar C, Andreoletti M, et al. Laparoscopic liver resection facilitates salvage liver transplantation for hepatocellular carcinoma. J Hepatobiliary Pancreat Surg. 2009;16(3):310–4.
14. Kanazawa A, Tsukamoto T, Shimizu S, et al. Laparoscopic liver resection for treating recurrent hepatocellular carcinoma. J Hepatobiliary Pancreat Sci. 2013;20(5):512–7.
15. Yin Z, Fan X, Ye H, et al. Short- and long-term outcomes after laparoscopic and open hepatectomy for hepatocellular carcinoma: a global systematic review and meta-analysis. Ann Surg Oncol. 2013;20(4):1203–15.
16. Gaillard M, Tranchart H, Dagher I. Laparoscopic liver resections for hepatocellular carcinoma: current role and limitations. World J Gastroenterol. 2014;20(17):4892–9.
17. Reichert PR, Renz JF, D'Albuquerque LA, et al. Surgical anatomy of the left lateral segment as applied to living-donor and split-liver transplantation: a clinicopathologic study. Ann Surg. 2000;232(5):658–64.
18. Hasegawa Y, Nitta H, Sasaki A, et al. Laparoscopic left lateral sectionectomy as a training procedure for surgeons learning laparoscopic hepatectomy. J Hepatobiliary Pancreat Sci. 2013;20(5):525–30.
19. Scatton O, Katsanos G, Boillot O, et al. Pure laparoscopic left lateral sectionectomy in living donors: from innovation to development in France. Ann Surg. 2015;261(3):506–12.
20. Nitta H, Sasaki A, Fujita T, et al. Laparoscopy-assisted major liver resections employing a hanging technique: the original procedure. Ann Surg. 2010;251(3):450–3.
21. Makabe K, Nitta H, Takahara T, et al. Efficacy of occlusion of hepatic artery and risk of carbon dioxide gas embolism during laparoscopic hepatectomy in a pig model. J Hepatobiliary Pancreat Sci. 2014;21(8):592–8.

38 Advances in Colorectal Surgery

Manuela Elía-Guedea, Jose Manuel Ramírez-Rodríguez, and Jose Antonio Gracia-Solanas

Introduction

This chapter aims to analyse the recent advances that have appeared on the scene in the last few years in the field of colorectal surgery. Obviously, we have selected those changes that have demonstrated an actual improvement in the treatment of the patient or at least have opened a door for new studies.

Haemorrhoidal disease, highly prevalent, benign, and affecting up to 50 % of the population, has always been surrounded by new therapies. Various treatments have presented themselves, none of them with a clear advantage over the rest. It is mandatory to apply common sense, looking for efficiency and quality of life.

The treatment of complex perianal fistulas remains a challenge even for the most experienced surgeon. The risk of incontinence and the high rate of recurrence must always be kept in mind, and less aggressive techniques are gaining in popularity. New therapies, such as fistuloscopy and platelet-rich plasma, as well as the use of laser, biological materials, adhesives, clips, lift technique, or stem cells have recently appeared in the armamentarium for the management of perianal fistula.

Faecal incontinence is considered an embarrassing problem that affects the quality of life of the patient very significantly. Bulking agents and nerve stimulation are both promising treatments.

In terms of malignant disease, the most important issue is to decrease clinical variability by means of enhanced recovery protocols. In any case, the results should be analysed in terms of morbidity, mortality, local recurrence rate, and disease-free survival. Local rectal surgery and the down-to-up technique have their indications in selected patients. In this chapter, we also review the latest data regarding the defunctioning stoma, the diagnosis and treatment of anastomotic leaks, the persistent fistula, and the anterior resection syndrome.

Benign Conditions

Haemorrhoidal Disease

Haemorrhoidal disease is highly prevalent and can affect up to 50 % of the population. Various treatments [1] have been described, and there are no clear boundaries between any of them. Patient treatments should be individualized according to symptoms. Generally, and no matter what the treatment

M. Elía-Guedea, M.D. (✉)
J.M. Ramírez-Rodríguez, M.D.
J.A. Gracia-Solanas, M.D.
Department of Surgery, Clinic University Hospital of Zaragoza, Zaragoza, Spain
e-mail: maguedea@hotmail.com; jramirez@unizar.es; joseantoniograciasolanas@hotmail.com

R. Latifi et al. (eds.), *Technological Advances in Surgery, Trauma and Critical Care*,
DOI 10.1007/978-1-4939-2671-8_38

applied, patients should be encouraged to follow a fibre-rich diet together with a high intake of fluids. If this is not sufficient, vasoactive drugs (usually a micronized combination of diosmin (90 %) and hesperidin (10 %)), which act by inhibiting some of the mechanisms of inflammatory response, may be added. These measures could result in success in up to 80–90 % of symptomatic patients. Hence, surgical treatment would be indicated in only 5–10 % of cases. The main indications for surgery are symptomatic haemorrhoids of the third or fourth degree. Surgery is also indicated when conservative management has failed.

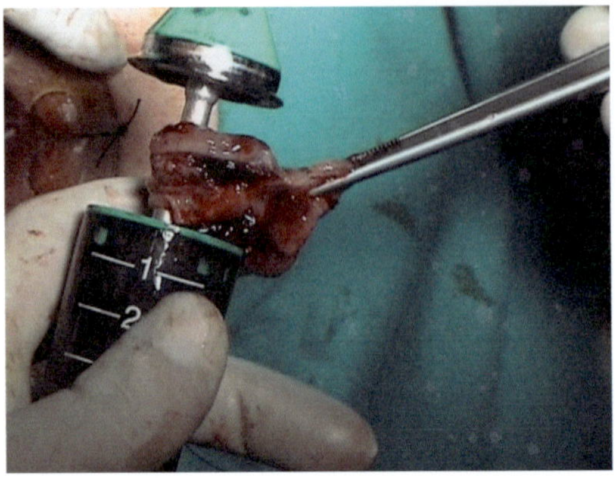

Fig. 38.1 Stapled haemorrhoidopexy

Haemorrhoidectomy

After analysing long-term surgical results, the haemorrhoidectomy according to Milligan and Morgan [2] remains the gold standard.

Since 2001, and in an attempt to decrease postoperative pain, the use of radiofrequency rather than diathermy for haemorrhoid removal has been popularized. Several randomized trials [3] comparing the use of the LigaSure™ (Covidien, Minneapolis, MN) instrument versus conventional diathermy haemorrhoidectomy have been published. In the majority of these studies, the number of patients enrolled was small; due to this and in the face of pain as the principal outcome, the results of these studies must be considered carefully.

Doppler-Guided Haemorrhoidal Artery Ligation

The proponents of the Doppler-guided artery ligation claim it is a "nearly" pain-free technique for the management of symptomatic grade III and grade IV haemorrhoids. According to the few other studies (none of them of high quality) that have been published on the subject, the best results have been achieved with this technique when treating grade III haemorrhoids [4]. Some authors recommend adding a mucopexy to the procedure in order to improve long-term results [5].

Stapled Haemorrhoidopexy (Fig. 38.1)

On the basis of the Thomson theory that proposes the deterioration of the anal supporting tissue and the consequent sliding downward of the anal lining as responsible for the development of haemorrhoids, the circular stapled anopexy was developed to cut the redundant tissue and to restore the anal canal anato-physiology. All surgery is done at a safe distance from the sensitive dentate line.

A prospective, randomized, multicentre study [6] comparing haemorrhoidal artery ligation versus circular stapled anopexy for grade III haemorrhoids shows significantly less pain after ligation, with shorter hospital stays but with higher recurrence rates.

Other Procedures

Embolization using coils in the terminal branches of the superior rectal artery has also been recently covered in published data [7]. The most commonly used other treatments are summarized in Table 38.1.

Evidence

There is no consensus regarding the optimal treatment to be applied to haemorrhoidal disease, given the low quality of the published studies. In general, conservative management must be the first choice. Surgery is elected if the first choice fails.

What's New in the Treatment of Perianal Fistulas?

Treatment of complex anal fistulas remains a challenge even for the most experienced surgeon. The risk of incontinence and the high rate of

Table 38.1 Commonly used treatments for haemorrhoidal disease

Technique	Grade	Complications/side effects	Results
Sclerosis	I and II	Fibrosis of other surrounding tissues	18 % recurrences (after 2 years of F-U)
Banding	I, II, III	Anal pain that can range from minor discomfort to severely incapacitating pain Bleeding Anal sepsis	77–80 % success
Infrared photocoagulation	I and II	Discomfort	81 % success 28 % recurrence
Laser photocoagulation	I and II	Mild pain	76–79 % success

recurrence show that the definitive solution has not yet been found. Keeping in mind the patient's quality of life, these are some of the therapies being suggested [8].

Fistuloscopy

New techniques such as the fistuloscopy have emerged in the therapeutic armamentarium. A small endoscope is inserted through the external opening of the fistula to identify the main and secondary tracts. Once the tracts have being identified, they are cauterized under direct vision. The internal opening is then treated by either a single suture or an advancement flap. This technique is reinforced by the use of cyanoacrylate. The authors describe up to a 70 % rate of success (6 months of follow-up).

Mucosal Advancement Flap Combined with Platelet-Rich Plasma

The long-term outcome results [9] of patients with primary and recurrent high cryptoglandular perianal fistulas treated with a loose seton followed by mucosal advancement flap and platelet-rich plasma show an 83 % rate of success after 2 years of follow-up, with a low incontinence rate.

Fistula Laser Closure (FiLaC™, Biolitic Biomedical Technology, Jena, Germany)

Another new technique for the treatment of complex fistulas is the so-called fistula laser closure (FiLaC™). Primary closure of the tract is achieved using laser energy emitted by a radial fibre connected to a diode laser. The energy causes shrinkage of the tissue around the radial fibre with the aim being to close the tract.

The internal opening must be eliminated by a flap. The authors report a 75 % success rate in terms of healing, and no patient reported incontinence postoperatively.

Plug

This technique involves the introduction of a plug of biological material in the fistula tract. The conical-shaped plug is anchored in the anal fistula and acts as a scaffold into which new tissue can grow. A prospective study [10] from four referral centres with a mean follow-up of 68 months reports a 56 % rate of recurrence. There are some ongoing clinical trials, but currently the evidence of efficacy of anal fistula plug treatment is quite limited.

Biological Sealants/Cyanoacrylate Glue

The use of fibrin glues shown in a multicentre study [11] demonstrates a success rate of 74 %, with a 26 % rate of recurrence (mean follow-up of 6 years). New biological glues such as Vivostat® (Vivostat, Alleroed, Denmark) have shown better results than the previously marketed glues.

OTSC® Proctology (Ovesco Endoscopy, Tűbingen, Germany)

EL OTSC® Proctology is a new treatment for fistula-in-ano based on the placement of a clip that closes the tract of the fistula. In a study with ten patients recruited [12], this device was shown to have a 90 % rate of success.

LIFT (Ligation of Inter-sphincter Fistula Tract)

Described by Rojanasakul in 2007 [13], LIFT is based on secure closure of the internal opening and removal of infected cryptoglandular tissue through the inter-sphincter approach. Essential steps of the procedure include incision at the groove, identification of the inter-sphincter tract, ligation of inter-sphincter tract, and closure of the internal. A prospective study of 26 patients [14] with high trans-sphincter fistula showed successful results in 77 % without postoperative incontinence.

Some others [15] have used this technique not only in high, trans-sphincter fistulas but also in supra-sphincter fistulas with a more than 70 % success rate.

Stem Cells

Using autologous adipose-derived stem cells is a novel approach for the management of complex fistula-in-ano. Human Adipose-Derived Stem Cells emerge as key regulators of immune/inflammatory responses in vivo and as attractive candidates for cell-based therapies to treat sepsis and hence to improve healing. In a phase II clinical trial [16] that included patients with Crohn's perianal fistulas, the success rate was of 71 %.

Faecal Incontinence

Faecal incontinence (FI) is defined as the inability to hold a bowel movement until one has reached a toilet as well as passing stool into one's underwear without being aware of this happening. Faecal incontinence ranges from an occasional leakage of stool while passing gas to a complete loss of bowel control. It affects men and women of all ages, and it is estimated to affect as much as 15 % of elderly people.

The most common cause of bowel incontinence is damage to the muscles around the anus due to obstetric injuries. Anal surgery can also damage the anal sphincters or nerves, leading to bowel incontinence. Throughout history, many treatments and techniques have been developed in an attempt to improve the quality of life of these patients.

The first step of any treatment for faecal incontinence is to modify dietary habits, to eat the right amount of fibre, and to start pelvic floor muscle training by means of biofeedback. Rectal sensitivity also improves with biofeedback.

Another new treatment for FI is the perianal injection of bulking agent. There are different substances that can be used; however, the ideal agent should be biologically compatible and easy to apply. The agent could be injected into the submucosal or inter-sphincter space, and some studies [17] have shown better results when the injection is ultrasound guided.

The major problem of these substances is the rejection of the agent with complications such as anal pain, ulceration, itching, sepsis, or even migration.

A Cochrane review [18] concluded that using Dextranomer in stabilized hyaluronic acid as a perianal injectable bulking agent improves continence for a little over half of patients in the short term.

Sacral neuro-modulation (also termed sacral nerve stimulation) was described in 1995 by Matzel et al. [19]. It has shown good results in terms of improvement of incontinence and quality of life. In addition, sacral neuro-modulation has been described for the management of low anterior resection syndrome after total mesorectal excision.

An alternative to sacral nerve stimulation that follows the same principles is transcutaneous electrical nerve stimulation. It was proposed in 1975 by Melzack [20] and Wall as a new pain treatment method. In 1983, Nakamura et al. [21] demonstrated the efficacy of transcutaneous stimulation of the posterior tibia nerve (PTN) in controlling urinary incontinence and the overactive bladder.

In the management of faecal incontinence, Shafiq [22] reported an improvement in 78.2 % of patients and Queralto [23] in 60 % of those patients that were treated by PTN. The main advantage of this approach is its simplicity. It is a non-invasive technique that can be performed by the patient at home.

Colon and Rectal Cancer

Surgery for Rectal Cancer and Evidence-Based Medicine (EBM)

Total Mesorectal Excision

In 1982, Heald et al. [24] published the results of the technique of total mesorectal excision (TME) for the management of rectal cancer. They reported a 4 % rate of local recurrence. Afterward, different multicentre studies showed that the implementation of the TME decreased the rate of local recurrence and improved survival. In short, TME became the gold standard surgical technique for tumours located in the middle and lower rectum. Currently, rectal cancer should be managed by a multidisciplinary team where each case is treated individually.

Surgical Reconstruction After Low Anterior Resection

One of the problems that arises after total mesorectal excision is determining what type of reconstruction should be carried out [25]. Over the years, anastomotic techniques have been refined. Keeping in mind that most of us are using primarily mechanical stapled colorectal anastomosis, the so-called Colon Ring, a staple-free technique based on a ring of titanium and nickel that produces compression with a consistent force at the end-to-end anastomosis, was marketed a few months ago.

First studies [26] on the subject show that the compression technique is surgically feasible, easy to use, and without significant complication rates; however, a large randomized controlled trial is needed in order to determine the actual benefits of the Colon Ring over traditional stapling techniques.

Colonic Pouch

Other important technical advances in rectal surgery thanks to the improvement of the anastomotic technique are the sphincter-saving procedures that have become the standard treatment in the surgical approach to most cancers of the middle and lower third of the rectum. When the total rectum is removed, straight colo-anal anastomosis is related to the well-known anterior resection syndrome characterized by increased stool frequency, urgency, and incontinence mostly due to loss of the reservoir function. In order to improve functional outcome, the construction of a colonic J-pouch from the distal colon was proposed. The distal section of the colon is formed into a J-shaped pouch in order to replace the function of the rectum and store stool until it can be eliminated. A significant number of studies [27] that compared the J-pouch with straight end-to-end colo-anal anastomosis have shown functional superiority of the pouch, especially in the first 2 years after surgery, with similar morbidity. However, up to one out of four patients complains of evacuator dysfunction which is related to an oversized reservoir. Currently, it is recommended that the reservoir be fashioned no larger than 5–6 cm. From a technical point of view, it is not difficult to make a colonic J-Pouch; what is sometimes a challenge is to down it through a narrow pelvis, which is the norm in obese male patients.

Transverse Coloplasty and Side-to-End Anastomosis

As seen before, while colonic J-pouch anastomosis is able to eliminate some of the functional problems of straight colo-anal anastomosis, it comes with the problem of pouch evacuation. Hence, in an attempt to improve functional results, alternative techniques, such as transverse coloplasty pouch and side-to-end colo-anal anastomosis, have been suggested.

In a randomized controlled study [28], transverse coloplasty reconstruction after rectal cancer resection and colo-anal anastomosis is functionally similar to colonic J-pouch both in short- and long-term outcomes. The coloplasty technique does not seem to improve significantly the incomplete defecation symptom with respect to the J-pouch. The same outcomes are reported when compared to side-to-end anastomosis. This last technique has as a major advantage in that it is the easiest and fastest to perform.

With reference to quality of life issues, it is very difficult to extract any conclusion. There are few studies, most of them based on a smaller number of patients. Studies such as that of Hallbook and Furst [29], using the NHP and EORTC questionnaires, respectively, found no differences when straight anastomosis was compared to colo-anal reservoir. On the contrary, more recent papers, such as the one by Sailer [30], that use the GIQL, C30, and CR38 questionnaires, found that patients with a reservoir presented with a better quality of life.

In any case, and keeping in mind the lack of proper evidence, it seems that those reconstructive techniques that offer a "neo-rectum" are associated with a better quality of life.

Is It Mandatory to Have a Protective Defunctioning Stoma After Rectal Resection?

If there is a major postoperative issue that all colorectal surgeons are afraid of, it is anastomotic dehiscence. It is very well known that the anastomotic leakage rate rises as it comes close to the pelvic floor. In order to minimize the morbidity, a protective ostomy is recommended for many. This preventive manoeuvre, however, is not free of morbidity by itself: in some studies nearly 50 % [31] of cases present a complication related to the protective ostomy. Hence, an ostomy should be performed when the risk of dehiscence is high enough to justify it. In this context, it seems reasonable to add a protective ostomy to the low anterior rectal resection if the patient has received neo-adjuvant treatment.

Whether to use a colostomy or an ileostomy to protect the anastomosis could be left to the surgeon's preferences. However, there are some RCT that point out that the ileostomy is linked to a lower morbidity rate in terms of prolapse and sepsis.

Lastly, some authors perform [32] the so-called ghost-ileostomy. It is done by placing a removable Silastic band (vascular loop) around the ileum which is exteriorized, through the abdominal wall, without tension, and secured to the skin on a rod. In case of an anastomotic complication, the ileostomy is performed under local anaesthesia. Ghost-ileostomy allows selective ileostomy formation; however, current evidence tells us that this kind of ileostomy should be reserved for instances in which the risk of leak is relatively low, such as anastomoses performed in the absence of neo-adjuvant therapy.

Another important concern the surgeon has to cope with when performing a DE functioning ostomy is the best timing for its withdrawal. Alves and Mengaux [33] recommend removing the ileostomy by the tenth postoperative day, as a way to improve the patient's quality of life. But most authors believe that the best timing is around the eighth week after surgery. In a significant number of cases, the time for ileostomy withdrawal is in the hands of the oncologist, since, if the patient is in chemotherapy, the recommendation is to wait until that treatment is completed.

Whatever the selected time, before the withdrawal, it is recommended to evaluate the anastomosis by means of a digital examination and sigmoidoscopy. If there is a suspicion of complication, a contrast CT would confirm it.

Low Anastomosis Leakage

After rectal cancer surgery, the reported anastomotic leakage varies between 2 and 23 % of cases, the higher rates in the low and colo-anal ones.

Currently, many centres do a routine PCR blood test (some also include Pro-calcitonin) at second and fourth postoperative days, due to its known value in detecting septic complications.

Once the leak appears, the management would depend on many factors, among them the anastomosis location, age of the patient, obesity, or whether there is a protective ileostomy or not.

In any case, as a mean, 30 % of patients with anastomotic dehiscence after rectal surgery will eventually have a permanent colostomy.

In some cases, abdominal surgery can be avoided and the anastomotic leak treated transanally, by a simple drainage or even with the TEM equipment to clean the space and re-make the anastomosis.

Another procedure for anastomotic leaks or low pelvic sepsis management is the vacuum sponge system. The sponge is endoscopically introduced in the septic cavity or fistula and connected to a vacuum machine. The reported success rate is approximately 60–70 % of cases, with a recurrence rate of nearly 25 %.

Abdominoperineal Resection

Unfortunately, even with the advent of the sphincter preserving techniques, approximately 25 % of patients complaining of rectal cancer will need an abdominal-perineal resection (APR) and a permanent colostomy [34]. In this context, recent studies [35] show that the overall prognosis for these patients is inferior to that of patients undergoing AR, and that the local recurrence rates are higher. One of the proposed ways to address this problem is to go with a more extensive surgical operation to get a cylindrical (without a waist) specimen, hence minimizing the risk of circumferential margin involvement. At the present time, there are few studies comparing both APR techniques and, even with promising results that favour the extralevator, the evidence is still of low quality as to recommend one of them. We should wait for well-designed controlled studies.

Another question that arises when discussing APR is patient position in the operating room. Traditionally, the lithotomy has been the preferred position, but the prone position, which claims to offer better access to the perianal and mesorectum area, is being adopted in a significant number of centres not only due to the access but also because of the better morbidity and recurrence outcomes. It is important to know that some studies have linked the prone and Trendelenburg positions to ocular hypertension, leading to perioperative reduction of visual acuity [36].

Local Surgery

In the 1980s, Buess described [37] Transanal Endoscopic Microsurgery (TEM), a technique that makes possible the excision of large adenomas located up to 20 cm from the anal verge. Before TEM (Figs. 38.2 and 38.3), local rectal surgery was limited to low tumours that could be reached using the Parks retractor.

With reference to rectal carcinoma, the local surgery must be restricted to carefully selected patients. Lymph node involvement could be seen in up to 10 % of stage I rectal cancer. This fact, together with the high rate of reported recurrence, makes local surgery for rectal cancer a current controversy.

Evidence is sparse, and until the results of the ongoing studies are available, most authors agree to offer local surgery for T1 tumours. For T2 lesions, some surgeons would choose this technique in addition of adyuvant therapy. Tumour size, grading,

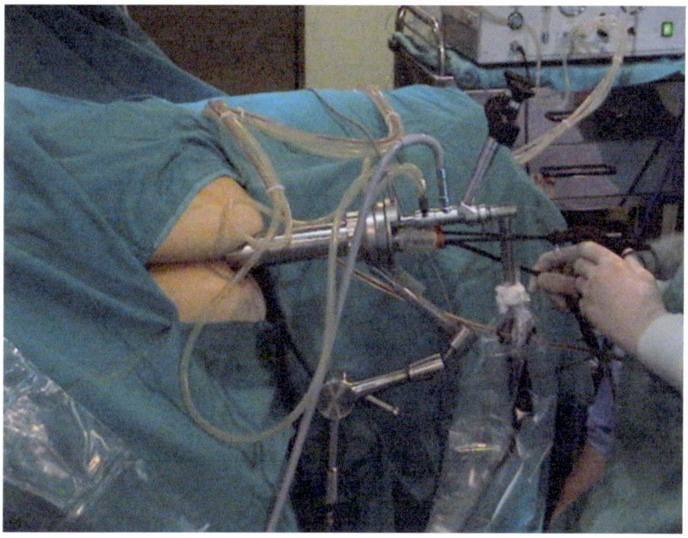

Fig. 38.2 Special equipment for transanal local surgery

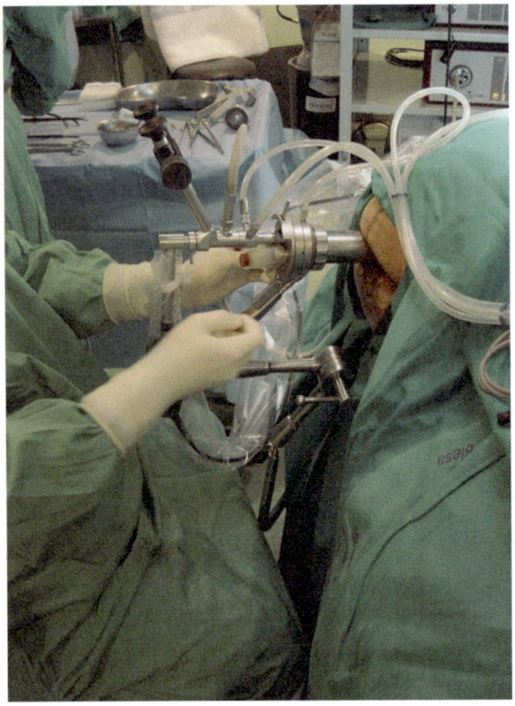

Fig. 38.3 Special equipment for transanal local surgery

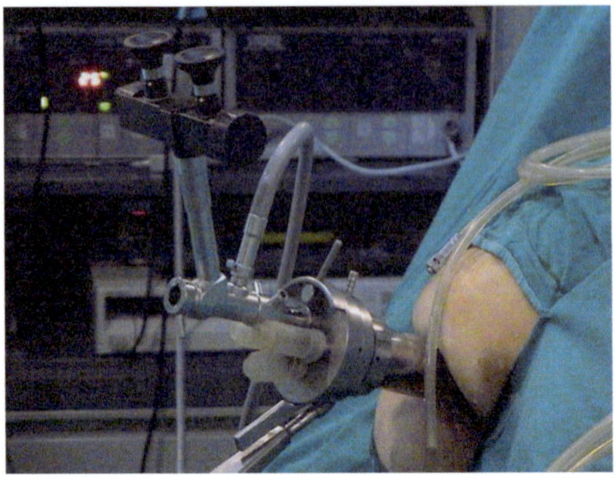

Fig. 38.4 Special equipment for transanal local surgery

and location within the rectum should be clearly defined before local surgery is indicated.

In 2009, the so-called TAMIS (Transanal minimally invasive surgery) appeared as a variation of abdominal single-port surgery [38]. Different companies are involved in marketing their transanal devices. In any case, the tool must be able to open widely the anal canal and allow the introduction of basic surgical instruments including the optic. TAMIS is gaining in popularity due to the fact that it is less expensive than TEM and has not been associated with anal incontinence. On the other hand, TEM gets better exposure of the rectal cavity and makes suturing easier.

Whatever the technique or instrument used (Fig. 38.4), in early rectal cancer, the recommendation is to get a full-thickness specimen with at least 1 cm of free margins. TEM has a longer learning curve than TAMIS, but both of these approaches must be in the repertoire of the experienced surgeons.

New Techniques for Abdominal Approach

Robotic Surgery

In the USA, it is estimated that 50 % of laparoscopic rectal resections are performed with robotic assistance. With few indications in colon surgery, in the treatment of rectal cancer (total mesorectal excision), the use of robotic surgery could provide benefits in terms of urinary and sexual function, and reduction of the learning curve. The ROLARR is a large ongoing randomized study that attempts to shed some light to this contested subject. The high cost of robotic surgery makes it mandatory to determine which procedures are cost efficient.

Notes/Nose

Natural orifice transluminal endoscopic surgery (NOTES) is an emerging field within gastrointestinal surgery. It is a natural evolution from flexible transluminal endoscopy. Though the initial approach was transgastric, nowadays NOTES is being performed through several other orifices, and in the last few years the number of procedures is growing rapidly. NOTES is creating a new scenario that changes our perceptions of how to approach abdominal surgery.

In laparoscopic colorectal surgery, specimen retrieval requires a mini-laparotomy wound, which can cause postoperative pain, wound infection, and incisional hernia. Thus, the benefits of minimally invasive surgery may be compromised. NOTES can completely abolish pain and wound complication. However, technological limitations of the current flexible platforms have been major challenges, and NOTES procedures remain, to date, available only in a few centres.

Another new approach is NOSE (natural orifice specimen extraction), for many an important step in the evolution towards "scar-less" surgery. While laparoscopic colorectal surgery is done in the conventional manner, the specimen is transanally or transvaginally retrieved.

Single-Port Colorectal Laparoscopic Surgery

Single-port laparoscopic surgery (SPLS) for colorectal pathology is an advanced technique wherein laparoscopic surgery is carried out through a single small incision hidden in the umbilicus. It has been suggested that this approach provides a better cosmetic outcome for patients than conventional laparoscopic surgery. However, with reference to morbidity and hospital stay, a study reviewing [39] 5 papers and 120 patients found no differences. SPLS is a feasible and safe procedure, but it is technically challenging, which prevents it from wider dissemination.

Transanal Down-to-Up Mesorectal Excision for Rectal Cancer

Transanal perirectal access or perineal NOTES access allows access to the mesorectal fascia and the retroperitoneal space. This procedure makes possible the excision of the full mesorectum in those patients in whom, due to technical difficulties [40] (obese, narrow pelvic, etc.), this would be difficult via the abdominal approach and put the patient at a risk of amputation. It is clear that this is a very novel approach that needs greater evaluation.

Multimodal Rehabilitation, Enhanced Recovery After Surgery, or Fast-Track Surgery

Appearing on the scene in the late 1990s thanks to the Kehlet studies, the multimodal rehabilitation programs (fast-track programs) are aimed at improving patient recovery by reducing surgical stress [41].

According to the basic ERAS (Enhanced Recovery After Surgery) principles, the patient's operation is planned only after adequate preparation. Once in the hospital, the patient is assigned to a specific pathway and is permanently monitored. The clinical pathway is composed of different steps, all of them evidence-based. Soon after surgery, the patient is mobilized and put on an oral liquid diet.

ERAS programs started in colorectal surgery, but today it is difficult to find a surgical field that does not have any of these clinical pathways.

From its inception onwards, many studies have appeared (including well-designed, randomized controlled studies), and the great majority of them have shown benefits not only for the patient (less morbidity and better quality of life) but also for the health care system (shorter hospital stay).

However, multimodal rehabilitation programs are difficult to implement. On the one hand, they go against well-established surgical traditions, and on the other hand they need a multidisciplinary team in which surgeons, anesthesiologists, nurses, and dietitians work together. Moreover, the patient that is fully informed about the clinical pathway must actively participate in the decision-making process, and no one can make decisions in his/her name.

For colorectal surgery, all clinical protocols include full information, no bowel preparation (except if a protective ileostomy is planned), epidural analgesia, laparoscopic surgery when possible, goal-directed peri-operatory fluid therapy, early postoperative mobilization, and early postoperative oral intake.

References

1. Altomare DF, Giuratrabocchetta S. Conservative and surgical treatment of haemorrhoids. Nat Rev Gastroenterol Hepatol. 2013;10(9):513–21.
2. Moult HP, Aubert M, De Parades V. Classical treatment of hemorrhoids. J Visc Surg. 2014. doi:10.1016/j.jviscsurg.2014.09.012. pii: S1878-7886(14)00139-8. [Epub ahead of print].
3. Talha A, Bessa S, Abdel WM. Ligasure, Harmonic Scalpel versus conventional diathermy in excisional haemorrhoidectomy: a randomized controlled trial. ANZ J Surg. 2014. doi:10.1111/ans.12838.
4. Dong XN, Tang YC. Comparison of anorectal pressure after procedure for prolapse and hemorrhoids versus doppler-guided hemorrhoidal artery ligation for grade III (hemorrhoids). Zhonghua Wei Chang Wai Ke Za Zhi. 2013;16(12):1183–6.
5. Ratto C, de Parades V. Doppler-guided ligation of hemorrhoidal arteries with mucopexy: a technique for the future. J Visc Surg. 2014. doi:10.1016/j.jviscsurg.2014.08.003. pii: S1878-7886(14)00109-X. [Epub ahead of print].
6. Elmér SE, Nygren JO, Lenander CE. A randomized trial of transanal hemorrhoidal dearterialization with anopexy compared with open hemorrhoidectomy in the treatment of hemorrhoids. Dis Colon Rectum. 2013;56(4):484–90.
7. Vidal V, Louis G, Bartoli JM, Sielezneff I. Embolization of the hemorrhoidal arteries (the emborrhoid technique): a new concept and challenge for interventional radiology. Diagn Interv Imaging. 2014; 95(3):307–15.
8. Van Onkelen RS, Gosselink MP, Schouten WR. Treatment of anal fistulas with high intersphincteric extension. Dis Colon Rectum. 2013;56(8):987–91.
9. Göttgens KW, Vening W, van der Hagen SJ, van Gemert WG, Smeets RR, Stassen LP, Baeten CG, Breukink SO. Long-term results of mucosal advancement flap combined with platelet-rich plasma for high cryptoglandular perianal fistulas. Dis Colon Rectum. 2014;57(2):223–7.
10. Adamina M, Ross T, Guenin MO, Warschkow R, Rodger C, Cohen Z, Burnstein M. Anal fistula plug: a prospective evaluation of success, continence and quality of life in the treatment of complex fistulae. Colorectal Dis. 2014;16(7):547–54.
11. Haim N, Neufeld D, Ziv Y, Tulchinsky H, Koller M, Khaikin M, Zmora O. Long-term results of fibrin glue treatment for cryptogenic perianal fistulas: a multicenter study. Dis Colon Rectum. 2011;54(10): 1279–83.
12. Prosst RL, Ehni W, Joos AK. The OTSC® Proctology clip system for anal fistula closure: first prospective clinical data. Minim Invasive Ther Allied Technol. 2013;22(5):255–9.
13. Rojanasakul A, Pattanaarun J, Sahakitrungruang C, Tantiphlachiva K. Total anal sphincter saving technique for fistula-in-ano; the ligation of intersphincteric fistula tract. J Med Assoc Thai. 2007;90(3):581–6.
14. Sileri P, Giarratano G, Franceschilli L, Limura E, Perrone F, Stazi A, Toscana C, Gaspari AL. Ligation of the intersphincteric fistula tract (LIFT): a minimally invasive procedure for complex anal fistula: two-year results of a prospective multicentric study. Surg Innov. 2014;21(5):476–80.
15. Hong KD, Kang S, Kalaskar S, Wexner SD. Ligation of intersphincteric fistula tract (LIFT) to treat anal fistula: systematic review and meta-analysis. Tech Coloproctol. 2014;18(8):685–91.
16. De la Portilla F, Alba F, García-Olmo D, Herrerías JM, González FX, Galindo A. Expanded allogeneic adipose-derived stem cells (eASCs) for the treatment of complex perianal fistula in Crohn's disease: results from a multicenter phase I/IIa clinical trial. Int J Colorectal Dis. 2013;28(3):313–23.
17. Beggs AD, Irukulla S, Sultan AH, Ness W, Abulafi AM. A pilot study of ultrasound guided Durasphere injection in the treatment of faecal incontinence. Colorectal Dis. 2010;12(9):935–40.
18. Maeda Y, Laurberg S, Norton C. Perianal injectable bulking agents as treatment for faecal incontinence in adults. Cochrane Database Syst Rev. 2010;5, CD007959.
19. Matzel KE, Stadelmaier U, Hohenfellner M, Gall FP. [Permanent electrostimulation of sacral spinal nerves with an implantable neurostimulator in treatment of fecal incontinence]. Chirurg. 1995;66(8):813–7.
20. Melzack R. Prolonged relief of pain by brief, intense transcutaneous somatic stimulation. Pain. 1975;1(4): 357–73.
21. Nakamura M, Sakurai T, Tsujimoto Y, Tada Y. [Transcutaneous electrical stimulation for the control of frequency and urge incontinence]. Hinyokika Kiyo. 1983;29(9):1053–9.
22. Shafik A, Ahmed I, El-Sibai O, Mostafa RM. Percutaneous peripheral neuromodulation in the treatment of fecal incontinence. Eur Surg Res. 2003;35(2):103–7.
23. Queralto M, Portier G, Cabarrot PH, Bonnaud G, Chotard JP, Nadrigny M, Lazorthes F. Preliminary results of peripheral transcutaneous neuromodulation in the treatment of idiopathic fecal incontinence. Int J Colorectal Dis. 2006;21(7):670–2.
24. Heald RJ, Husband EM, Ryall RD. The mesorectum in rectal cancer surgery: the clue to pelvic recurrence? Br J Surg. 1982;613:6.
25. Jarry J, Faucheron JL, Moreno W, Bellera CA, Evrard S. Delayed colo-anal anastomosis is an alternative to prophylactic diverting stoma after total mesorectal excision for middle and low rectal carcinomas. Eur J Surg Oncol. 2011;37:127–33.
26. Kang J, Park MG, Hur H, Min BS, Lee KY, Kim NK. Safety and efficacy of the NiTi Shape Memory Compression Anastomosis Ring (CAR/ColonRing) for end-to-end compression anastomosis in anterior resection or low anterior resection. Surg Innov. 2013;20(2):164–70.
27. Liang JT, Lai HS, Lee PH, Huang KC. Comparison of functional and surgical outcomes of laparoscopic-assisted colonic J-pouch versus straight reconstruction

after total mesorectal excision for lower rectal cancer. Ann Surg Oncol. 2007;14(7):1972–9.
28. Parray FQ, Magray JA, Dar MA, Chowdri NA, Wani RA, Thakur N. Coloplasty neorectum versus straight anastomosis in low rectal cancers. ISRN Surg. 2014;2014:382371.
29. Fürst A, Burghofer K, Hutzel L, Jauch KW. Neorectal reservoir is not the functional principle of the colonic J-pouch: the volume of a short colonic J-pouch does not differ from a straight coloanal anastomosis. Dis Colon Rectum. 2002;45(5):660–7.
30. Sailer M, Fuchs KH, Fein M, Thiede A. Randomized clinical trial comparing quality of life after straight and pouch coloanal reconstruction. Br J Surg. 2002;89(9):1108–17.
31. Arumugam PJ, Bevan L, Macdonald L, Watkins AJ, Morgan AR, Beynon J, Carr ND. A prospective audit of stomas–analysis of risk factors and complications and their management. Colorectal Dis. 2003;5(1):49–52.
32. Mari FS, Di Cesare T, Novi L, Gasparrini M, Berardi G, Laracca GG, Liverani A, Brescia A. Does ghost ileostomy have a role in the laparoscopic rectal surgery era? A randomized controlled trial. Surg Endosc. 2014 Dec 5. [Epub ahead of print]
33. Menegaux F, Jordi-Galais P, Turrin N, Chigot JP. Closure of small bowel stomas on postoperative day 10. Eur J Surg. 2002;168(12):713–5.
34. Pachler J, Wille-Jørgensen P. Quality of life after rectal resection for cancer, with or without permanent colostomy. Cochrane Database of Systematic Reviews 2012; Issue 12. Art. No.: CD004323.
35. Wibe A, Syse A, Andersen E, Tretli S, Myrvold HE, Søreide O, Norwegian Rectal Cancer Group. Oncological outcomes after total mesorectal excision for cure for cancer of the lower rectum: anterior vs. abdominoperineal resection. Dis Colon Rectum. 2004;47(1):48–58.
36. West NP, Anderin C, Smith KJ, Holm T, Quirke P, European Extralevator Abdominoperineal Excision Study Group. Multicentre experience with extralevator abdominoperineal excision for low rectal cancer. Br J Surg. 2010;97:588–99.
37. Buess G, Theiss R, Günther M, Hutterer F, Pichlmaier H. Endoscopic surgery in the rectum. Endoscopy. 1985;17(1):31–5.
38. Rimonda R, Arezzo A, Arolfo S, Salvai A, Morino M. TransAnal Minimally Invasive Surgery (TAMIS) with SILSTM Port versus Transanal Endoscopic Microsurgery (TEM): a comparative experimental study. Surg Endosc. 2013;27(10):3762–8.
39. Lolle I, Rosenstock S, Bulut O. Single-port laparoscopic rectal surgery - a systematic review. Dan Med J. 2014;61(7):A4878.
40. Brown CJ, Fenech D, McLeod RS. Reconstructive techniques after rectal resection for rectal cancer. Cochrane Database of Systematic Reviews 2008; Issue 2. Art. No.: CD006040.
41. Kehlet H, Wilmore DW. Evidence-based surgical care and the evolution of fast-track surgery. Ann Surg. 2008;248:189–98.

Part VII

Advances in Organ Transplantation

Technological Advances in Heart and Lung Transplantation: Concomitant Cardiac Valve Surgery

39

Yoshiya Toyoda, Yasuhiro Toyoda,
Masako Toyoda, and Yoshiko Toyoda

Valve Surgery in Heart Transplantation

Over the last decades, heart transplantation has become a viable treatment for end-stage heart disease with the major limiting factor being the shortage of donor organs [1]. To maximize the utilization of donor organs in heart transplantation, recommendations have been made to expand the donor selection criteria, stating that in some cases, bench repair can be performed on a donor heart with mild to moderate mitral or tricuspid valve regurgitation [2].

Y. Toyoda, M.D., Ph.D. (✉)
Department of Surgery, Temple University Hospital, Philadelphia, PA, USA
e-mail: Yoshiya.toyoda@tuhs.temple.edu

Y. Toyoda
University of Pittsburgh, Pittsburgh, PA, USA
e-mail: Yasuhiro.toyoda3@gmail.com

M. Toyoda
Princeton University, Princeton, NJ, USA
e-mail: mtoyoda@princeton.edu

Y. Toyoda, B.A.
Weill Cornell Medical College, New York, NY, USA
e-mail: yot2003@med.cornell.edu

Tricuspid Valve Surgery in Heart Transplantation

Prophylactic Tricuspid Valve Surgery at the Time of Heart Transplantation

Despite the improvement in survival after heart transplantation with the transplant half-life currently 10 years, there remains the steep fall in survival at the beginning following heart transplantation [1]. Graft failure accounts for 40 % of early death within 30 days [1]. In the immediate postoperative allograft dysfunction, right ventricular dysfunction is particularly common, presumably due to elevated recipient pulmonary vascular resistance, poor right ventricular protection, increased pulmonary vascular resistance from blood transfusion and administration of protamine and other drugs, and kinking of the pulmonary arterial anastomosis [3, 4]. Functional tricuspid regurgitation has been shown to be a reliable marker of right ventricular dysfunction [5], and its severity has been shown to predict late survival following heart transplantation [6]. In order to reduce post-transplant tricuspid regurgitation, the bi-caval technique seems to be at least equal to or possibly better than the bi-atrial technique [7–9]. Furthermore, donor tricuspid valve repair is a reasonable way of thinking to reduce tricuspid regurgitation and to improve survival after heart transplantation. In fact, a group from

R. Latifi et al. (eds.), *Technological Advances in Surgery, Trauma and Critical Care*,
DOI 10.1007/978-1-4939-2671-8_39

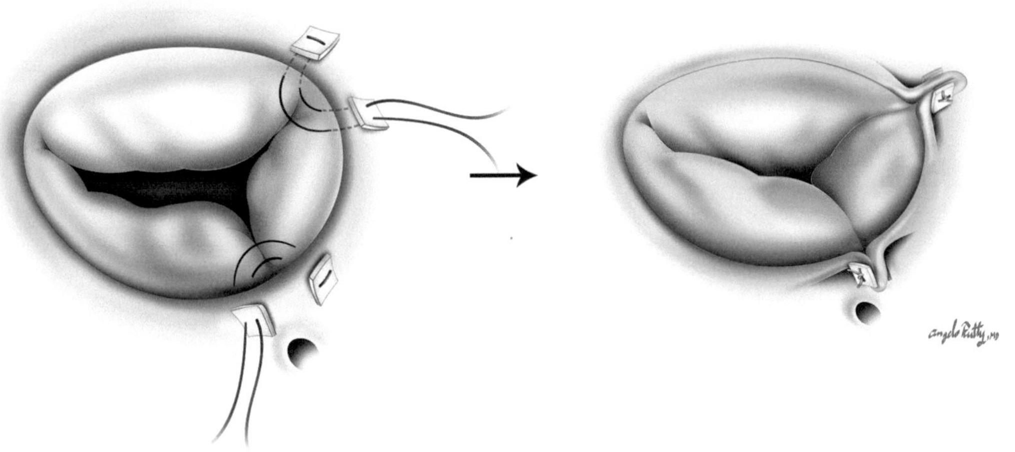

Fig. 39.1 Toyoda's commissuro-annuloplasty technique for performing bench tricuspid annuloplasty for donor hearts at the back table (courtesy of Angelo Rutty, MD.)

Temple University randomized 60 patients, and demonstrated better immediate postoperative right ventricular performance and lower perioperative mortality in bi-caval heart transplantation together with prophylactic DeVega tricuspid annuloplasty [10]. The same group also showed decreased incidence of cardiac-related mortality and tricuspid regurgitation in the long term [11]. Others also showed that prophylactic tricuspid annuloplasty with either DeVega or ring technique reduced the incidence of early postoperative tricuspid regurgitation after bi-atrial heart transplantation [12]. Despite these reports, prophylactic tricuspid annuloplasty has not become a standard care in heart transplantation probably because 80 % of patients have either no or trace tricuspid regurgitation following heart transplantation [6] and there is a linear correlation between the cardiac graft ischemic time and mortality [13]. We developed a novel, simple, effective surgical technique, "Toyoda's commissuro-annuloplasty" (Fig. 39.1), to perform bench tricuspid annuloplasty for donor hearts at the back table similar to the concept of Kay-Reed annuloplasty [14, 15]. We routinely perform this annuloplasty for almost all heart transplants, especially when the echocardiography at the donor hospital shows mild or greater tricuspid regurgitation before procurement of the heart and/or if the recipient has significantly elevated pulmonary vascular resistance, e.g., transpulmonary gradient greater than 15 mmHg.

Primary graft failure remains the most common cause of death within 30 days following heart transplantation and accounts for approximately 40 % of the 30-day mortality. Right ventricular failure is the most common type of primary graft failure after heart transplantation because of the unique circumstances after heart transplantation. These circumstances include high afterload for the right ventricle and myocardial injury. Heart transplant recipients tend to have high pulmonary vascular resistance due to long-standing heart failure. The majority of the patients have risk for bleeding such as multiple sternotomy, standing anticoagulation medication such as warfarin, clopidogrel, and aspirin, mechanical circulatory support causing coagulopathy, and severe heart failure. Increased usage of blood products, platelets, red blood cells, etc. and medications such as protamine and vasoconstrictors such as norepinephrine and phenylephrine can elevate pulmonary vascular resistance. The allograft ischemic time usually ranges between 1 and 6 h and ischemia/reperfusion injury causes myocardial damage leading to

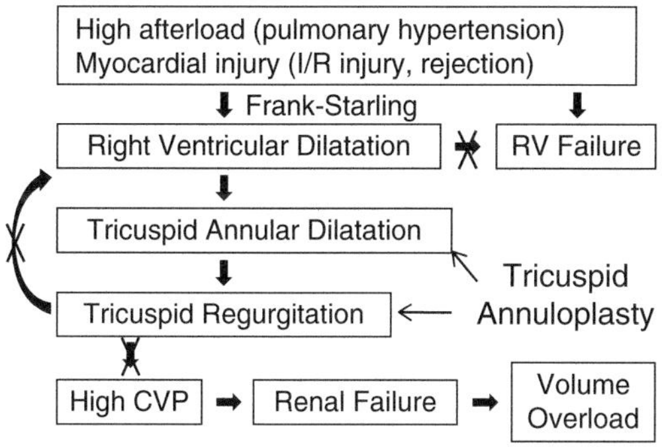

Fig. 39.2 Mechanism of right ventricular failure and effect of tricuspid annuloplasty after heart transplant

ventricular failure. In addition, acute/hyper acute rejection, air embolization, etc. can also cause ventricular dysfunction. In such situations, the right ventricle dilates according to the Frank-Starling law in order to maintain cardiac output. The right ventricular dilation results in tricuspid valve annular dilatation leading to significant tricuspid valve regurgitation. Severe tricuspid regurgitation can further dilate the right ventricle. Thus, the vicious cycle starts and eventually results in right ventricular failure. Moreover, high central venous pressure caused by tricuspid valve regurgitation can cause renal failure leading to volume overload. The prophylactic "commissuro-annuloplasty" prevents development of right ventricular failure because of the mechanism shown in Fig. 39.2. This effectively reduces the tricuspid annular size by 2–4 cm, preventing annular dilatation in the setting of right ventricular dilatation and improving coaptation of the leaflets preventing significant tricuspid regurgitation.

Case 1

The recipient is a 63-year-old male with ischemic cardiomyopathy. The donor was a 25-year-old male with transportation time of 3 h and 15 min. The donor died of head trauma. The echocardiography showed mild to moderate tricuspid valve regurgitation without evidence of leaflet or chordal disease. Orthotropic bi-caval heart transplantation with a donor tricuspid annuloplasty at the back table was performed with total allograft ischemic time of 4 h and 15 min and cardiopulmonary bypass time of 2 h and 20 min. A tricuspid annuloplasty was performed using two pledgeted 3-0 Prolene to plicate the posterior annulus. The recipient had uneventful postoperative course. Postoperative echocardiography at weeks 1 and 2 showed no tricuspid regurgitation and at 4 months, there was trace tricuspid valve regurgitation.

Tricuspid Valve Surgery After Heart Transplantation

There are two structural mechanisms of tricuspid regurgitation, namely normal leaflet motion with annular/ventricular dilation and excessive leaflet motion [3, 4]. Possible mechanisms include right ventricular dilatation due to elevated pulmonary vascular resistance [3, 4], acute allograft edema, which diminishes with time [16], papillary muscle dysfunction [17], disturbed geometry of the right atrial anastomosis with subsequent impairment of the functional integrity of the valvular apparatus, cyclic torsion of the atria during ventricular systole and diastole, asynchronous contraction of the donor and recipient atrial compartment in the bi-atrial technique [18], and biopsy-induced flail tricuspid valve [19]. The indication for tricuspid surgery is severe tricuspid valve regurgitation and clinical signs of right heart failure with fatigue, decreased exercise tolerance, hepatomegaly, and lower extremity edema [20, 21]. Common repair techniques include annuloplasty with bicuspidization, DeVega and ring and bands, artificial chordoplasty for prolapse, valve excision for endocarditis, and patch-plasty for perforation of the leaflet. Valve replacement is performed with bioprosthesis; mechanical prosthesis should be avoided due to necessity of endomyocardial biopsies.

Authors' Recommendations

1. Bench tricuspid annuloplasty should be considered under the following situations:
   (a) Preoperative echocardiography at the donor hospital shows mild or greater tricuspid regurgitation.

(b) The recipient's pulmonary vascular resistance is markedly elevated, e.g., trans-pulmonary gradient greater than 15 mmHg.

2. Suture annuloplasty with the author's technique is the preferred method for bench annuloplasty because it can be done very quickly without significantly prolonging allograft ischemic time and the annuloplasty needs to be effective only during immediate postoperative period when the recipient pulmonary vascular resistance remains high and the tricuspid regurgitation is most prevalent.
3. When the patient comes off cardiopulmonary bypass, annuloplasty should be considered for cases with moderate to severe tricuspid regurgitation. In this situation, the allograft is already reperfused and repair needs to be performed through a right atriotomy; therefore, appropriate surgical techniques such as ring annuloplasty should be chosen for a durable repair.
4. Late tricuspid regurgitation: Tricuspid valve repair utilizing ring annuloplasty and/or artificial chordoplasty is indicated for moderate to severe tricuspid regurgitation with hemodynamic compromise and symptoms of right heart failure.

Mitral Valve Surgery in Heart Transplantation

Mitral Valve Surgery at the Time of Heart Transplantation

To expand the cardiac donor pool, mitral valve surgery has been performed to repair significant donor mitral valve disease at the time of heart transplant [22–24]. Bench ring annuloplasty has been reported for tricuspid regurgitation with normal leaflet motion and annular dilation [22, 23]. Bench commissurotomy and DeVega annuloplasty have also been reported for organic mitral valve disease due to rheumatic process [24]. This author prefers to perform bench mitral annuloplasty for donor hearts at the back table using Kay-Reed annuloplasty [14, 15] only when the echocardiography at the donor hospital shows mild or greater mitral regurgitation before procurement of the heart.

Case 2

The recipient was a 56-year-old male with ischemic cardiomyopathy. He was in UNOS I-A with 0.75 mcg/kg/min of milrinone and 3 mcg/kg/min of dopamine and supported by the intra-aortic balloon pump in the intensive care unit. His right heart catheterization showed pulmonary artery pressure of 77/40(54), pulmonary artery wedge pressure of 41 mmHg, and trans-pulmonary gradient of 13 mmHg. The donor was a 23-year-old male with the transportation time of 1 h and 45 min. He died of a motor vehicle accident and suffered from severe blunt chest trauma with elevated myocardial enzyme level. The echocardiography showed mild to moderate mitral valve regurgitation without evidence of leaflet or chordal disease. An orthotopic bi-caval heart transplantation with a donor mitral annuloplasty at the back table was performed with total allograft ischemic time of 2 h and 44 min and cardiopulmonary bypass time of 2 h and 17 min. The mitral valve was tested with injection of cold saline in the left ventricle, which showed leakage through the posteromedial commissural. A mitral annuloplasty was performed in Reed's technique using 1 pledgeted 3-0 Prolene to plicate the posteromedial commissure. The patient had uneventful postoperative course and is doing well. Postoperative echocardiography at week 2 showed trace mitral valve regurgitation. Right heart catheterization 8 months postoperatively showed pulmonary artery pressure of 25/4 (15) mmHg, and pulmonary artery wedge pressure of 9 mmHg with cardiac index of 3.30 l/min/m2.

Mitral Valve Surgery After Heart Transplantation

Although significant mitral valve disease after heart transplantation is rare, the need of mitral valve surgery upon transplanted hearts is predicted to become more common with increasing longevity of heart transplant recipients and with efforts aimed at preserving cardiac allograft function to avoid cardiac re-transplantation since the donor shortage is the major limiting factor of heart transplantation [25, 26]. Unlike coronary arteries, the long-term function and structure of mitral valve has been shown to be preserved [27]; however, mitral valve repair and replacement have been reported upon transplanted hearts. Mechanisms of mitral insufficiency include left-sided endomyocardial biopsy, endocarditis, myxomatous degeneration, fibrosis of papillary muscles, and chordae tendineae due to rejection, allograft coronary artery disease leading to ventricular dysfunction with mitral annular dilation, and potential distortion of the mitral valve structure due to left atrium-to-atrium anastomosis [25–27]. Mitral valve surgery after heart transplantation can be performed with conventional techniques, indications, and outcomes.

Aortic Valve Surgery in Heart Transplantation

Aortic valve surgery is rare in relation to heart transplantation; however, in efforts to expand the donor pool, donor hearts with significant aortic valve disease can be utilized. Bench repair of donor aortic valve with sub-commissural annular plication has been performed for moderate central aortic insufficiency with normal valve structure [28]. Others reported aortic valve replacement for significant aortic insufficiency and valve-sparing aortic root replacement with reimplantation technique for type A aortic dissection with significant aortic insufficiency after heart transplantation [29, 30]. Unique to heart transplantation, distortion of the donor ascending aorta can cause severe aortic regurgitation requiring aortic valve replacement [31]. Thus, aortic valve surgery can be performed using conventional techniques, indications, and outcomes in relation to heart transplantation.

Valve Surgery in Lung Transplantation

Valve Surgery at the Time of Lung Transplantation

Over the last decades, lung transplantation has become a viable treatment for a variety of end-stage lung disease with improved outcome due to better surgical techniques, organ preservation against ischemia/reperfusion injury, immunosuppression against rejection, and infection prophylaxis [32]. Currently, the major limiting factor is the shortage of donor organs. To maximize utilization of donor organs for lung transplantation, this author has recently reported how to harvest the donor lungs from patients who had undergone cardiac valve surgery [33]. Traditionally, patients with other significant comorbidities including cardiac diseases have been denied for lung transplant candidacy [3]. With the improved outcome in lung transplantation, however, a few centers have performed lung transplantation concomitant with cardiac surgery including coronary artery bypass, patent foramen ovale closure, atrial septal defect repair, ventricular septal defect repair, patent ductus arteriosus repair, replacement of the ascending aorta, and DeVega tricuspid valve repair [34–36]. Thus, in selected cases, cardiac problems including valvular heart diseases can be repaired at the time of lung transplantation.

Tricuspid regurgitation is the most common valvular disease in lung transplant recipients because patients frequently have pulmonary hypertension due to end-stage lung disease, and this elevated afterload makes the right ventricle dilated, resulting in tricuspid annular dilatation. However, whether we should operate on the tricuspid valve or not and when we should repair it are unknown at the time of lung transplantation. A group from Austria has reported that tricuspid regurgitation disappeared 3 months after double-lung transplantation in patients with primary pulmonary hypertension due to reverse remodeling of the right ventricle with normalized or reduced pulmonary vascular resistance [37]. Another group has also reported similar results after single-lung transplantation for pulmonary hypertension [38]. However, the mortality rate at 3 months after lung transplantation was 17.5 % [37], and the most recent International Society of Heart and Lung Transplantation Registry data show that primary pulmonary hypertension has the lowest survival immediately after lung transplantation in the major diagnostic categories with initial evident separation in survival between primary pulmonary hypertension and chronic obstructive lung disease and cystic fibrosis [32].

The registry speculates that this initial difference in survival may be related to differences in the complexity of the surgery and the frequency and severity of early complications [32]. This author speculates that this high early mortality in primary pulmonary hypertension is related to heart failure, predominantly right heart failure with tricuspid regurgitation leading to multiple organ failure. It is well documented that right heart failure manifests as enlarged right atrial size due to high right atrial pressure and the severity of tricuspid regurgitation predicts mortality in primary pulmonary hypertension [39]. Severe tricuspid regurgitation is the indication for repair or replacement to improve survival either as an isolated disease or as functional tricuspid regurgitation associated with left-sided valvular diseases [40]. In this author's institution, tricuspid valve repair concomitant with double-lung transplantation is the procedure of choice for patients with primary pulmonary hypertension with severe tricuspid regurgitation, and with this strategy for primary pulmonary hypertension, from 1994 to 2006, the institution's survival rate is 86 % at 1 year, 75 % at 5 years, and 66 % at 10 years, which is better by 20–39 % compared to the 23rd official report from the registry of the International Society of Heart and Lung Transplantation data from 1994 to 2004, which is 66 % at 1 year, 39 % at 5 years, and 27 % at 10 years [41]. This author believes the importance of tricuspid valve repair at the time of lung transplant for severe tricuspid regurgitation in improving early survival after lung transplantation.

Case 3

The recipient was a 51-year-old female with primary pulmonary hypertension. Her right heart catheterization showed right atrial pressure of 18 mmHg, pulmonary artery pressure of 107/46(68) mmHg, pulmonary artery wedge pressure of 10 mmHg, and trans-pulmonary gradient of 58 mmHg. She was on sildenafil citrate, bosentan, and treprostinil sodium for her severe pulmonary hypertension. The donor was a 45-year-old female who died of stroke. Transesophageal echocardiography showed severe tricuspid regurgitation due to massive enlargement of the annulus and severely decreased right ventricular function and patent foramen ovale. First, tricuspid ring annuloplasty and closure of the patent foramen ovale were performed under cardiopulmonary bypass with arterial cannulation in the ascending aorta and bi-caval venous drainage. Then, bilateral pneumonectomies followed by double-lung transplantation were performed under cardiopulmonary bypass. The ischemic time of the right lung was 4 h and 39 min and that of the left lung 5 h and 21 min. The patient had uneventful postoperative course with extubation on postoperative day 1 and was discharged home on postoperative day 17. Postoperative echocardiography at week 2 showed mild tricuspid valve regurgitation with still moderately decreased right ventricular function. She is doing well 1 year postoperatively.

Case 4

The recipient was a 66-year-old male with idiopathic pulmonary fibrosis with severe pulmonary hypertension. His right heart catheterization showed pulmonary artery pressure of 86/40(57) mmHg, pulmonary artery wedge pressure of 18 mmHg, and trans-pulmonary gradient of 39 mmHg. His left heart catheterization showed totally occluded circumflex and right coronary artery with left ventricular ejection fraction of 50 %. The donor was a 50-year-old female, who died of stroke. Transesophageal echocardiography showed severe tricuspid regurgitation and severely dilated right ventricle. Intraoperative Swan-Ganz catheter showed severe pulmonary hypertension equivalent to systemic blood pressure with markedly elevated right atrial pressure of 30 mmHg. First, off-pump coronary artery bypass grafting was performed with a reversed saphenous vein graft from the ascending aorta to acute marginal branch to posterior descending artery and another reversed saphenous vein graft from ascending aorta to obtuse marginal branch. Next, tricuspid ring annuloplasty was performed under cardiopulmonary bypass with arterial cannulation in the ascending aorta and bi-caval venous drainage. Then, bilateral pneumonectomies followed by double-lung transplantation were performed under cardiopulmonary bypass. The ischemic time of the right lung was 8 h and

32 min and 6 h and 42 min for the left lung. The patient required tracheostomy, but eventually de-cannulated and was discharged to rehabilitation 2 months postoperatively. Postoperative echocardiography at week 1 showed mild tricuspid valve regurgitation with mildly decreased right ventricular function. He is currently doing well at home 4 months postoperatively.

Author's Recommendation

Despite expected reverse remodeling of the right ventricle after lung transplantation, the process takes some time and immediate postoperative period is the most critical time for patients with pulmonary hypertension who require lung transplantation. Therefore, severe tricuspid regurgitation should be repaired at the same time of lung transplantation to reduce tricuspid regurgitation immediately postoperatively so that patients can avoid heart failure, be managed with lower right atrial pressure to achieve adequate cardiac output, and have easier control of volume status, resulting in avoidance of multiple organ failure. The aortic and mitral valve disease will not be affected by lung transplantation; therefore, aortic and mitral valve surgery should be performed using conventional techniques, and indications in relation to lung transplantation. This author prefers to perform intracardiac repair before pneumonectomy to avoid intracardiac contamination from the exposed airway.

Valve Surgery after Lung Transplantation

Although cardiac valvular disease after lung transplantation is rare, the need for valve surgery in lung transplant recipients will become more common due to the increasing number and longevity of lung transplant recipients. Infective endocarditis is not uncommon, nor is life-threatening complications after heart, lung, and heart-lung transplantation because life-long immunosuppression continues to leave the recipients susceptible to infection including sepsis and endocarditis with very high mortality [42, 43]. *Staphylococcus aureus* seems to be the most common organism in infective endocarditis after thoracic transplantation [44, 45]. However, other organisms can be the cause of endocarditis because of the immunocompromised status of the recipients. A successful aortic valve replacement has been reported for late bacterial infective endocarditis of the aortic valve due to enterococcus species after heart-lung transplantation for cystic fibrosis [42]. A successful mitral valve replacement has been reported for aspergillus endocarditis of the mitral valve in a lung transplant patient [46]. Fungal infection remains a significant cause of morbidity and mortality following lung transplantation, and the increased risk of fungal infection for lung transplant recipients compared to other solid-organ transplant recipients can be explained by host and environmental factors because the lung is the most common site for invasive aspergillosis, and from the lung it can disseminate to other organs [47]. Thus, valve surgery should be performed using conventional techniques and indications in relation to lung transplantation although the risk of surgery for infective endocarditis seems to be high due to recipients' immunosuppressed status.

References

1. Taylorn DO, Edwards LB, Boucek MM, Trulock EP, Aurora P, Christie J, Dobbels F, Rahmel AO, Keck BM, Hertz MI. Registry of the International Society for Heart and Lung Transplantation: Twenty-fourth official adult heart transplant report – 2007. J Heart Lung Transplant. 2007;26:769–81.
2. Zaroff JG, Rosengard BR, Armstrong WF, Babcock WD, D'Alessandro A, Dec GW, Edwards NM, Higgins RS, Jeevanandum V, Kauffman M, Kirklin JK, Large SR, Marelli D, Peterson TS, Ring WS, Robbins RC, Russell SD, Taylor DO, Van Bakel A, Wallwork J, Young JB. Consensus conference report: maximizing use of organs recovered from the cadaver donor: cardiac recommendations: March 28–29, 2001, Crystal City, VA. Circulation. 2002;106:836–41.
3. Bethea BT, Yuh DD, Conte JV, Baumgartner WA. Heart transplantation. In: Cohn LH, Edmunds Jr LH, editors. Adult cardiac surgery in the adult. New York: McGraw-Hill; 2003. p. 1427–59.
4. Kouchoukos NT, Blackstone EH, Doty DB, Hanley FL, Karp RB. Heart failure. Kirklin/Barratt–Boyes

cardiac surgery. 3rd ed. London: Churchill Livingstone; 2003. p. 1724–77.
5. Hung J, Koelling T, Semigran MJ, Dec JW, Levine RA, Di Salvo TG. Usefulness of echocardiographic determined tricuspid regurgitation in predicting event-free survival in severe heart failure secondary to idiopathic-dilated cardiomyopathy or to ischemic cardiomyopathy. Am J Cardiol. 1998;82:1301–3.
6. Anderson CA, Shernan SK, Leacche M, Rawn JD, Paul S, Mihaljevic T, Jarcho JA, Stevenson LW, Fang JCT, Lewis EF, Couper GS, Mudge GH, Byrne JG. Severity of intraoperative tricuspid regurgitation predicts poor late survival following cardiac transplantation. Ann Thorac Surg. 2004;78:1635–43.
7. Baldwin JC. Valve surgery in the transplanted heart. Curr Opin Cardiol. 2003;18:124–6.
8. Copeland JG. Heart transplantation: the standard versus bicaval technique controversy. Transplant Proc. 2000;32:1519–20.
9. Aziz TM, Burgess MI, Rahman AN, Campbell CS, Deiraniya AK, Yonan NA. Risk factors for tricuspid valve regurgitation after orthotopic heart transplantation. Ann Thorac Surg. 1999;68:1247–51.
10. Jeevanandam V, Russell H, Mather P, Furukawa S, Anderson A, Grzywacz F, Raman J. A one-year comparison of prophylactic donor tricuspid annuloplasty in heart transplantation. Ann Thorac Surg. 2004; 78:759–66.
11. Jeevanandam V, Russell H, Mather P, Furukawa S, Anderson A, Raman J. Donor tricuspid annuloplasty during orthotopic heart transplantation: long-term results of a prospective controlled study. Ann Thorac Surg. 2006;82:2089–95.
12. Brown NE, Muehlebach GF, Jones P, Gorton M, Stuart RS, Borkon AM. Tricuspid annuloplasty reduces early tricuspid regurgitation after biatrial heart transplantation. J Heart Lung Transplant. 2004; 23:1160–2.
13. UNOS data for cardiac ischemic time vs. mortality. www.unos.org.
14. Kay JH, Maselli-Campagna G, Tsuji KK. Surgical treatment of tricuspid insufficiency. Ann Surg. 1965;162:53–8.
15. Reed GE, Tice DA, Clauss RH. Asymmetric exaggerated mitral annuloplasty: repair of mitral insufficiency with hemodynamic predictability. J Thorac Cardiovasc Surg. 1965;49:752–61.
16. Cladellas M, Abdal ML, Pons-Llado G, et al. Early transient multivalvular regurgitation detected by pulsed Doppler in cardiac transplantation. Am J Cardiol. 1986;58:1122–4.
17. Akasaka T, Lythall DA, Kushawaha SS, Yoshida K, Yoshikawa J, Yacoub MH. Valvular regurgitation in heart-lung transplant recipients. A Doppler color flow study. J Am Coll Cardiol. 1990;15:576–81.
18. Angerman CE, Spes CH, Tammen A, et al. Anatomic characteristics and valvular function of the transplanted heart: transthoracic versus transesophageal echocardiographic findings. J Heart Transplant. 1990; 9:331–8.
19. Williams MAJ, Lee MY, Di Salvo TG, et al. Biopsy-induced flail tricuspid leaflets and tricuspid regurgitation following orthotopic cardiac transplantation. Am J Cardiol. 1996;77:1339–44.
20. Yankah AC, Musci M, Weng Y, Loebe M, Zurbruegg RZ, Siniawski H, Mueller J, Hetzer R. Tricuspid valve dysfunction and surgery after orthotopic cardiac transplantation. Eur J Cardiothorac Surg. 2000;17: 343–8.
21. Filsoufi F, Salzberg SP, Anderson CA, Couper GS, Cohn LH, Adams DH. Optimal surgical management of severe tricuspid regurgitation in cardiac transplant patients. J Heart Lung Transplant. 2006;25:289–93.
22. Massad MG, Smedira NG, Hobbs RE, Hoercher K, Vandervoort P, McCarthy PM. Bench repair of donor mitral valve before heart transplantation. Ann Thorac Surg. 1996;61:1833–5.
23. Michler RE, Camacho DR. Ex-vivo mitral valve repair prior to orthotopic cardiac transplantation. Ann Thorac Surg. 2002;73:962–3.
24. Antunes PE, Prieto D, Eugenio L, Antunes MJ. Donor mitral valve repair in cardiac transplantation. J Thorac Cardiovasc Surg. 2005;129:227–8.
25. Aleksic I, Piotrowski JA, Kamler M, Massoudy P, Jakob HG. Heart transplantation and consecutive mitral valve replacement. Thorac Cardiovasc Surg. 2005;53:176–90.
26. Ladowski JS. Mitral valve repair in a transplanted heart via right thoracotomy. Ann Thorac Surg. 2000; 70:1723–5.
27. Vaturi M, Aravot D, Ben-Gal T, Shapira Y, Adler Y, Sahar G, Vidne B, Sagie A. Natural history of left-sided valves after heart transplantation. Transplant Proc. 2000;32:735–6.
28. Navia JL, Atik FA, Marullo A, Starling RC, Garcia M, Vega PR, Smedira NG, McCarthy PM. Bench repair of donor aortic valve with minimal access orthotopic heart transplantation. Ann Thorac Surg. 2005; 80:313–5.
29. Kpodonu J, Massad MG, Geha AS. Surgical considerations in the correction of valve dysfunction following heart transplantation. Clin Transplant. 2005;19: 694–7.
30. Teebken OE, Pethig K, Krieg P, Haverich A, Harringer W. Valve-sparing repair after aortic root dissection following heart transplantation. J Heart Lung Transplant. 1999;18:807–9.
31. Rao JN, Prendergast B, Dark JH. Orthotopic heart transplantation with concurrent aortic valve replacement and coronary artery bypass grafting. J Heart Lung Transplant. 2000;19:897–9.
32. Trulock EP, Christie JD, Edwards LB, Boucek MM, Aurora P, Taylor DO, Dobbels F, Rahmel AO, Keck BM, Hertz MI. Registry of the International Society for Heart and Lung Transplantation: Twenty-fourth official adult lung and heart-lung transplant report – 2007. J Heart Lung Transplant. 2007;26:782–95.
33. Toyoda Y, McCurry KR. Prior cardiac surgery is not a contraindication for lung donor. Ann Thorac Surg. 2007;84:314–6.

34. Parekh K, Meyers BF, Patterson GA, Guthrie TJ, Trulock EP, Damiano RJ, Moazami N. Outcome of lung transplantation for patients requiring concomitant cardiac surgery. J Thorac Cardiovasc Surg. 2005; 130:859–63.
35. Patel VS, Palmer SM, Messier RH, Davis RD. Clinical outcome after coronary artery revascularization and lung transplantation. Ann Thorac Surg. 2003;75: 372–7.
36. Pigula FA, Gandhi SK, Ristich J, Stukus D, McCurry K, Webber SA, Keenan R, Grifith BP, Kormos R. Cardiopulmonary transplantation for congenital heart disease in the adult. J Heart Lung Transplant. 2001;20:297–303.
37. Kasimir MT, Seebacher G, Jaksch P, Winkler G, Schmid K, Marta GM, Simon P, Klepetko W. Reverse cardiac remodeling in patients with primary pulmonary hypertension after isolated lung transplantation. Eur J Cardiothorac Surg. 2004;26:776–81.
38. Kramer MR, Valantine HA, Marshall SE, Starnes VA, Theodore J. Recovery of the right ventricle after single-lung transplantation in pulmonary hypertension. Am J Cardiol. 1994;73:494–500.
39. Bustamante-Labarta M, Perrone S, De La Fuente RL, Stutzbach P, De La Hoz RP, Torino A, Favaloro R. Right atrial size and tricuspid regurgitation severity predict mortality or transplantation in primary pulmonary hypertension. J Am Soc Echocardiogr. 2002; 15:1160–4.
40. Kouchoukos NT, Blackstone EH, Doty DB, Hanley FL, Karp RB. Tricuspid valve disease. Kirklin/Barratt–Boyes cardiac surgery. 3rd ed. London: Churchill Livingstone; 2003. p. 671–88.
41. Trulock EP, Edwards LB, Taylor DO, Boucek MM, Keck BM, Hertz MI. Registry of the International Society for Heart and Lung Transplantation: Twenty-third Official Adult Lung and Heart–Lung Transplantation Report—2006. J Heart Lung Transplant. 2006;25:880–92.
42. Sayeed R, Drain AJ, Sivasothy PS, Large SR, Wallwork J. Aortic valve replacement for late infective endocarditis after heart-lung transplantation. Transplant Proc. 2005;37:4537–9.
43. Uip DE, Neto VA, Strabelli TM, Bocchi EA, Pileqqi F, Jatene AD, Stolf N, Fiorelli A, Bellotti G. Infective endocarditis in 100 patients subjected to heart transplantation. Arq Bras Cardiol. 1996;66:1–3.
44. Khoo DE, Zebro TJ, English TA. Bacterial endocarditis in a transplanted heart. Pathol Res Pract. 1989; 185:445–7.
45. Kunst H, Paruchuru PK, Madden B. Bacterial endocarditis: a rare complication following orthotopic cardiac transplantation. J Heart Lung Transplant. 2001;20:483–5.
46. Saxena P, Clarke B, Dunning J. Aspergillus endocarditis of the mitral valve in a lung transplant patient. Tex Heart Inst J. 2007;34:95–7.
47. Scherer M, Fieguth HG, Aybek T, Ujvari Z, Moritz A, Wimmer-Greinecker G. Disseminated *Aspergillus fumigatus* infection with consecutive mitral valve endocarditis in a lung transplant recipient. J Heart Lung Transplant. 2005;24:2297–300.

Abdominal Organ Transplantation: An Overview

40

Jan P.M. Lerut, Laurent Coubeau, Robert J. Stratta, and Giuseppe Orlando

Kidney Transplantation

The Beginnings: From the 1950s to the End of Twentieth Century

Kidney transplantation (KT) has become the standard of care for end-stage renal disease in the past three decades. Since the first experimental attempts performed in dogs by Emerich Ullmann in 1902, the introduction of the extra-peritoneal renal transplant procedure by Rene Kuss in 1951 [1], and the pioneering efforts of Joseph Murray et al. with both living donor and then deceased donor KT during the period 1954–1959, the application of KT has evolved tremendously and indications have grown such that the organ supply is dramatically outpaced by an overwhelming kidney demand [2].

J.P.M. Lerut, M.D., Ph.D., F.A.C.S. (✉)
L. Coubeau, M.D.
Department of Abdominal and Transplantation Surgery, Starzl Unit of Abdominal Transplantation University Hospitals Saint Luc, Université catholique de Louvain - UCL Brussels, Belgium
e-mail: Jan.lerut@uclouvain.be; Laurent.coubeau@uclouvain.be

R.J. Stratta, M.D.
Department of General Surgery, Wake Forest School of Medicine, Winston-Salem, NC, USA
e-mail: rstratta@wakehealth.edu

G. Orlando, M.D., Ph.D.
Section of Transplantation, Department of General Surgery, Wake Forest Baptist Health, Wake Forest Institute for Regenerative Medicine, Wake Forest School of Medicine, Winston-Salem, NC, USA

The Kuss Procedure

The kidney graft is generally implanted heterotopically in the iliac fossa (Fig. 40.1). Although it is preferable to implant the kidney on the contralateral side (because of anatomical location of the vessels and to ensure that the renal pelvis is anterior), the right iliac fossa is more often the first choice secondary to anatomical characteristics rendering implantation more convenient. The most commonly used incision is the extended Gibson incision, which can be modified further based on patient habitus and surgeon preference. For the standard approach, the relevant anatomical landmarks are two fingerbreadths superior to the symphysis pubis and two fingerbreadths medial to the anterior superior iliac spine. In obese patients, the incision tends to be more transverse than vertical and may start several fingerbreadths above the symphysis pubis in order to stay above the fat pad. The abdominal muscles are transected down to the level of the peritoneum. Many surgeons prefer the more medial and vertical "hockey-stick," muscle-sparing, incision. This incision allows access to the retroperitoneal space by splitting the insertion of the oblique and transverse abdominal muscles at the lateral margin of the rectus muscle sheath. The splitting of this less vascularized area may reduce blood loss

R. Latifi et al. (eds.), *Technological Advances in Surgery, Trauma and Critical Care*,
DOI 10.1007/978-1-4939-2671-8_40

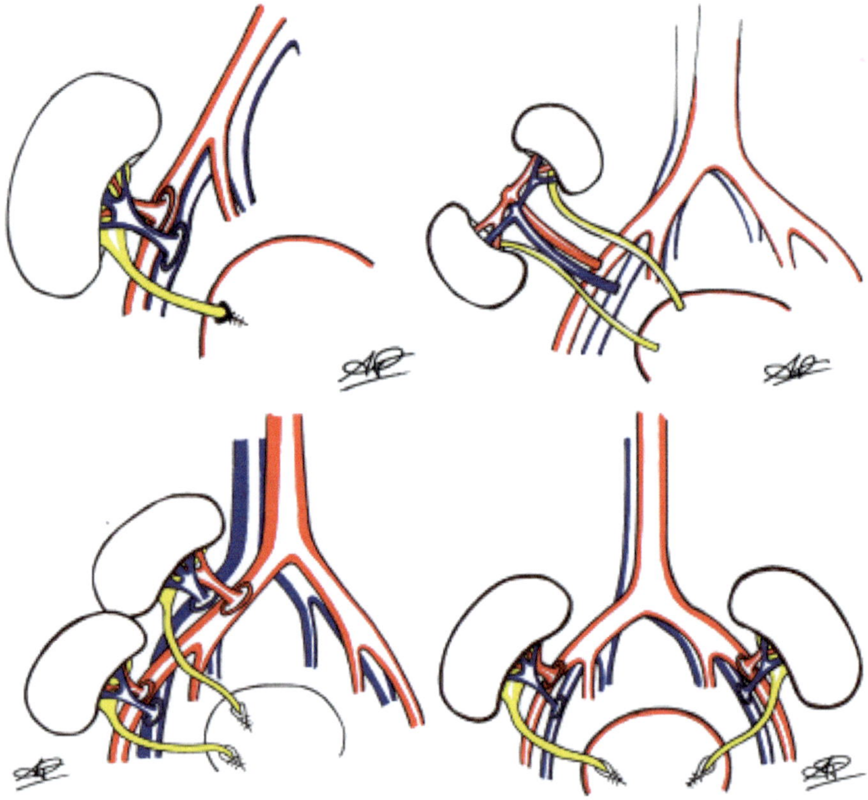

Fig. 40.1 Possible sites of implantation for single-kidney transplantation (KT) (*top left*), pediatric dual en bloc (*top right*), and double (two for one) KT. Normally, single and dual en bloc kidney are implanted onto the external iliac vessels. In the case of double KT, both kidneys can be implanted on the same side, on the external and the common axis. This allows sparing of the contralateral fossa, where a new kidney can be implanted, shall the first fail (used with permission of Andrea Peloso, MD)

and postoperative pain. During the course of this dissection, the inferior epigastric vessels are usually identified and eventually ligated and divided. Once the transversal fascia is opened, the peritoneum is prudently displaced medially by a combination of careful sharp and blunt dissection. Round ligament and spermatic cord and surrounding structures are identified, freed, and dislocated medially. The round ligament is usually sacrificed whereas the spermatic cord is usually spared. In some cases, it may be necessary to ligate and divide the cord structures to permit access to the bladder and distal iliac vessels; this option should be discussed with the patient prior to surgery. The external iliac vessels are dissected and prepared for the anastomoses, which are generally performed end to side with the vessels of the renal graft. The extent of the dissection is determined by the choice of the site of implantation. Next the more medially located external iliac vein (EIV) is dissected. It is preferred not to free completely the posterior aspect of the vessels, in order to minimize bleeding, lymphatic disruption, and postoperative thrombosis.

The kidney allograft is brought into the operative field and kept cold by wrapping in iced slush. The end-to-side venous anastomosis is usually performed first under lateral clamping of the iliac vein and irrigation of the lumen with heparinized saline solution. Upon completion of this anastomosis, a small clamp can be placed on the renal vein just above the anastomosis in order to restore native venous return by removing the clamp(s) from the EIV. The arterial anastomosis is usually performed just cephalad to the venous anastomosis on the EIA using the same principles. When the kidney is from a deceased donor, a Carrel aortic patch is usually fashioned around the renal artery orifices to simplify the anastomosis. Reperfusion is performed by retrograde perfusion through the vein first followed by anterograde arterial perfusion. Once hemostasis is achieved and the optimal kidney position determined, the bladder is distended through the bladder catheter and the dome is exposed. The ureteral reconstruction is usually done using a modified Lich-Gregoir extra-vesical anterior uretero-neocystostomy. The anterolateral detrusor muscle is carefully transected to expose the underlying bladder mucosa. The ureter is trimmed to an appropriate length, the peri-ureteral tissue carefully ligated to achieve hemostasis, and the distal part spatulated. The bladder mucosa is opened sharply and a uretero-neocystostomy is performed using fine-running monofilament suture between bladder and ureteral mucosa either with or without a ureteral stent. After completion of the mucosal anastomosis, the detrusor muscle is re-approximated with absorbable or nonabsorbable monofilament suture in an interrupted fashion to loosely recreate an anti-reflux submucosal tunnel; thereby avoiding stenosis of the anastomosis the transplant procedure is completed with confirmation of the optimal position of the kidney, patency and integrity of all anastomoses, and careful wound closure in layers.

The Kuss Procedure Challenged

The extension of inclusion criteria to elderly, obese, and/or diabetic patients as well as to patients with compromised vascular and urologic conditions has been responsible for technically more demanding KT procedures.

The Compromised Vascular Patient

Nowadays, pre-transplant investigations often include duplex ultrasonography or angio-CT scan in order to delineate the status of the aorto-iliaco-femoral vessels. If severely compromised, the surgical strategy needs to be adapted by either pre-transplant or simultaneously performed endarterectomy or vessel replacement using prosthetic grafts [3, 4]. The simultaneous vascular and transplant procedures have the disadvantage of an increased risk for infection, thrombosis, bleeding, stenosis, or aneurysm formation at the site of implantation. The venous dissection is often also more difficult because of scarring and distortion of the normal anatomy. Several (small) series have reported successful outcomes with KT performed either simultaneously with or following aorto-iliaco/aorto-femoral prosthetic replacement surgery, as well as the successful implantation of the allograft renal artery on a prosthetic graft.

In the case of pre-existing vascular procedures, anticoagulation and antiplatelet aggregation therapy must be monitored carefully in order to avoid supplementary complications.

The Compromised Urologic Patient

Presently patients with untreatable lower urinary tract disease and small-volume, poorly compliant bladder with inadequate emptying do not represent an absolute contraindication to KT anymore provided that the lower urinary tract dysfunction is either adequately corrected or managed [5]. Medical therapy (using anticholinergic, alpha-adrenergic blocking drugs) and clean intermittent self-catheterization are the first-line treatments. When insufficient, surgical intervention such as augmentation cystoplasty, intermittent catheterization mechanisms (Mitrofanoff principle), or creation of a neo-bladder with bowel or ureter may become necessary. Patients with a history of recurrent urinary tract infections, vesico-ureteral reflux, and uretero-hydronephrosis can benefit from pre-transplant or simultaneous nephrectomy or nephro-ureterectomy.

When the bladder is absent or when a reconstructive procedure becomes necessary, it is preferable to reconstruct the lower urinary tract before performing the KT. Small series indicate that KT can be safely performed in patients with reconstructed bladders, as graft survival and function are comparable to patients with normal function of the lower urinary tract that have not undergone reconstructive surgery [6].

Developments During the End of the Twentieth and the Beginning of the Twenty-First Centuries

The Expansion of the Deceased Donor Organ Pool

The burgeoning crisis in organ supply challenges the transplant community to maximize and optimize the use of organs from all consented deceased donors. The persistent scarcity of deceased donor kidneys in the face of a growing wait list mandates an ongoing reappraisal of the limits of acceptability when considering whether or not to transplant a recovered kidney.

The Expanded Criteria Donor

Over the past decade, there has been an increasing shift towards increasing numbers of older donors and recipients in KT, with cerebrovascular events now being the leading cause of brain death in deceased organ donation [7]. The value of transplanting such kidneys has been questioned because of concerns over decreased graft survival, diminished longevity, and poorer predicted outcomes when compared to KT from younger donors. In October 2002, the United Network of Organ Sharing (UNOS) defined expanded criteria donation (ECD) as donor age >60 years, or age 50–59 years with at least two of the following: history of hypertension, terminal serum creatinine >1.5 mg/dl, or cerebrovascular cause of death. There is now a more and more general agreement that these kidneys should be used to improve access to transplantation for patients whose life expectancy is less than their predicted waiting time for a kidney, particularly older patients and diabetics. Despite reports of inferior graft survival and poorer intermediate-term results, Stratta et al. have contended that ECD kidneys are defined by suboptimal nephron mass, so appropriate donor and recipient selection may optimize outcomes. Rather than transplanting ECD kidneys indiscriminately, ECD kidneys should preferentially be transplanted into "low-risk" and "low-functional-need" recipients, specifically older patients with low body mass index and low immunologic risk. This strategy of profiling ECD kidneys with appropriate recipients may result in acceptable medium-term graft survival comparable to concurrently transplanted standard criteria donor (SCD) kidneys. In addition to matching strategies, ECD kidney graft survival has also improved in the most recent era secondary to advances in donor management and selection, organ preservation and assessment, recipient management, immunosuppression, and clinical experience.

The Cardiac Death Donor

Although donation rates have not changed significantly in the past decade, the percentage of transplants performed from donation after cardiac death (DCD) has increased steadily from 1.4 % in 1998 to 15.8 % in 2011 [8]. Compared with kidneys recovered from brain-dead donors (DBD), DCD kidneys are subjected to variable periods of warm ischemia after withdrawal of life support followed by declaration of death by cardiocirculatory arrest. Warm ischemia is known to be associated with acute tubular necrosis, irreversible cell damage, and reduced graft survival after KT. Despite the warm ischemia inherent with DCD recovery, numerous studies have shown comparable short- and intermediate-term graft survival rates between DBD and DCD non-ECD kidneys, although delayed graft function (DGF) is more common with DCD kidneys, with an incidence ranging from 25 to 90 %. It has been shown that older donor age and, more specifically, ECD status negatively impact on graft survival; yet, utilizing DCD-ECD kidneys as dual transplants could potentially improve outcomes. Interestingly, several studies have shown that the presence of DGF does not have the same detrimental effect on graft survival after transplantation of DCD donor kidneys as it does after transplantation of DBD donor kidneys. Two recent randomized prospective studies reported opposite conclusions regarding the efficacy of machine preservation in reducing the incidence of DGF after DCD donor kidney transplantation. However, the incidence of DGF was >50 % in both studies irrespective of the method of preservation. Early experience with extracorporeal support to reduce ischemic injury and DGF is promising, although more widespread application of this technology is limited to date.

The Dual-Kidney Transplantation

Concerns over the limited life-span of ECD or other "marginal" kidneys have resulted in an increased prevalence of simultaneous transplantation of both kidneys from a deceased donor into a single recipient. Dual-kidney transplantation (DKT) is performed to optimize outcomes by providing adequate nephron mass using kidneys thought to be unsuitable for single use, which might otherwise result in the kidneys being discarded. DKT has been shown to have comparable outcomes to single KT, including similar rates of DGF and graft survival. Criteria for allocating kidneys for DKT vary, although primary considerations include donor age, pre-existing hypertension or diabetes, donor creatinine clearance, rising serum creatinine, machine preservation characteristics, cold ischemia time, and preimplantation donor biopsy characteristics. A recent multicenter prospective analysis showed excellent short- and long-term results after allocation of kidneys from donors older than 60 years of age based on a preimplantation histologic scoring system. While DKT graft survival was similar to solitary KT graft survival in this study, it is possible that some DKTs could have had comparable results had they been transplanted as single kidneys, since the histologic scoring system allocates kidneys with only mild chronic changes to DKT. Furthermore, while donor arteriosclerosis was included in the allocation criteria, the severity and extent of these lesions were not well defined. A recent report from Kayler examined outcomes of donor kidneys with moderate (>25 %) arteriosclerosis on preimplantation biopsy when transplanted as single transplants or DKT. Single KT from donors with moderate arteriosclerosis resulted in poor 1-year graft survival (71 %) when compared to DKT (95 %), despite the use of older and more ECD kidneys in the DKT group. Appropriate recipient selection is critical to achieving good outcomes with DKT. The ideal recipient should be older than age 50 years, have adequate cardiac reserve and a low burden of iliac atherosclerosis, weight less than 80–90 kg with a BMI <30 kg/m^2, and have adequate bladder capacitance. Reserving DKT for smaller individuals permits easier implantation of a technically more challenging procedure and favors functional outcomes by matching nephron mass with lower muscle mass and decreased metabolic demand. From a technical standpoint, DKT has evolved from a bilateral iliac fossa approach (either intra- or extra-peritoneal) to an extra-peritoneal unilateral approach (Fig. 40.1). This shortens operating time by limiting iliac artery and vein dissection to one side and preserves the contralateral iliac vessels should future re-transplantation be required.

The Pediatric Donor

Kidneys from pediatric donors (Fig. 40.1) are still regarded controversially with respect to long-term graft survival and function, particularly if originating from donors younger than 12 months of age. There is also a reluctance to separate pediatric kidneys for KT into two recipients. Recent studies have demonstrated excellent results with pediatric en bloc KT. A recent UNOS analysis demonstrated that long-term outcomes of pediatric en bloc KT from donors less than 5 years of age were superior to matched recipients of solitary, same age, pediatric KT, and SCD adult kidney recipients. The ongoing shortage of organs has prompted to explore the limits of acceptability of single KT from small pediatric donors into two recipients. Laurence et al. constructed a decision analysis model to predict the outcome in life years for patients with ESRD on the waiting list, depending on whether they received en bloc or solitary KT. Interestingly, at all recipient ages, the projected life years of both recipients of a solitary KT exceeded the projected life years of a recipient of an en bloc KT. Only recipients of solitary KT from donors weighing less than 10 kg had an estimated net loss of life years. Another UNOS review by Sureshkumar showed that the graft failure risk of solitary pediatric kidneys was consistently lower when the donor weight exceeded 10 kg. However, in this study, pediatric en bloc kidneys outperformed solitary pediatric kidneys for all donor weight groups. The Keyler review of UNOS data from 1995 to 2007 showed that the graft failure risk of solitary pediatric KT from donors weighing more than 35 kg was similar to ideal SCD KT from donors aged 18–39 without other risk factors, whereas solitary kidneys from pediatric donors weighing 10–35 kg performed more like non-ideal SCD KT. Overall, these studies indicate that more liberal transplantation of kidneys from pediatric donors may expand the donor pool. Solitary, rather than en bloc KT from donors weighing more than 10 kg offers more cumulative graft years and maximizes organ utilization without compromising outcomes and en bloc KT from donors weighing <5 kg has been favorable.

The Acute Renal Failure Donor

The rationale for using acute renal failure (ARF) kidneys is based on the observation that mechanisms of repair and regeneration do take place in the recipient. In 2006, Kumar et al. reported a series of 55 KT from ARF donors. Outcomes were compared with 55 concurrent and matched recipients of SCD kidneys and 55 concurrent and matched recipients of ECD kidneys. ARF kidneys were accepted from donors aged <50 years with no history of kidney disease and no chronic changes on pre-transplant biopsy. Three-year patient and graft survival was 90 and 90 % in the ARF group, 100 and 89 % in the SCD group, and 83 and 66 % in the ECD group. Biopsy-proven acute rejection rates were comparable among groups, although chronic allograft nephropathy (CAN) was significantly higher in the ECD group. Mean serum creatinine levels were 1.9, 1.9, and 2.2 mg/dl in the ARF, SCD, and ECD groups (SCD and ARF vs. ECD, $p=0.04$). Kidneys from selected donors with ARF had comparable graft survival and function to non-ARF kidneys, despite a higher DGF rate; so transplantation of kidneys from ARF donors may help to safely expand the donor pool. In 2009, Kayler reviewed the 1995–2007 UNOS data to study the outcome and utilization of kidneys from deceased donors with ARF. For ECD recipients, the relative risk for graft failure significantly increased with rising serum creatinine level. Among potential SCDs, elevated serum creatinine level was a strong independent risk factor for kidney discard. However, when KT was performed, elevated donor terminal serum creatinine level was not a risk factor for graft loss. This study clearly underscores the fact that potentially transplantable kidneys are being discarded on the basis of elevated serum creatinine levels and that a more aggressive approach to transplanting kidneys from ARF donors may safely increase the number of deceased donor kidneys.

Living Donor and Paired Living Donor Kidney Transplantation

Many significant innovations and advances over the past decade have increased access to living donor KT. Technical progress in laparoscopic and, more recently, robotic donor surgery played a critical role for obvious reasons. From an immunological perspective, barriers represented by highly sensitized recipients and even ABO-incompatible donor-recipient pairs can be currently overcome by sophisticated desensitization protocols, which allow effective modulation of the immune response. Desensitization regimens, including high-dose intravenous immune globulin (IVIG), plasmapheresis, and rituximab, in highly sensitized recipients provide a significant survival advantage, more than doubling survival at 8 years. Although these protocols permit satisfactory early- to intermediate-term graft survival, both acute and chronic antibody-mediated rejection (AMR) remain significant issues, occurring in 20–50 % of HLA-incompatible KT and having a significant impact on graft survival and longevity. Emerging therapies to prevent and treat AMR include proteosome inhibitors aimed at plasma cells and modifiers of complement-mediated injury.

ABO-incompatible KT can nowadays also be performed successfully without high-intensity immunomodulation [9]. Current protocols involve a brief escalation in immunosuppression using plasmapheresis and IVIG with or without long-term B-cell suppression from splenectomy or anti-CD20 treatment with rituximab.

A newer development has been the growth of paired kidney donation as an alternative for KT candidates with willing and medically suitable live donors who cannot donate to their intended recipient secondary to an incompatibility of blood type or cross-match or both. In the most basic form of paired donation, the incompatibility problems with two donor-recipient pairs can be solved by exchanging donors. Using advanced software, several organizations have successfully completed paired kidney donations involving three or more pairs. Another permutation of paired kidney donor protocols is the "non-directed" or non-simultaneous, extended, altruistic donor chain, which is initiated by an altruistic donor and completed when the last paired donor in the chain donates to an unpaired recipient on the deceased donor waiting list. The proliferation of living donor exchange programs has increased transportation of live donor kidneys and has reduced geographic barriers to live donor KT. In spite of these exciting developments, however, the number of live donor KTs performed in the USA has actually declined in the past decade, in contrast to the experience in Eurotransplant. The more widespread application of living donation also has promoted the concept of preemptive kidney transplantation. Such approach has not only a great social advantage but even more an immunologic value allowing to markedly extent graft survival [10].

Robot-Assisted Transplantation

The Universities of Pisa and Chicago have recently shown that KT and also pancreas transplantation (PT) are feasible either by laparoscopy or laparoscopic aided robotic assistance. The rationale behind these initial experiences lay in that, when compared with conventional laparoscopy, the robot offers three-dimensional high-definition view, uses wristed instruments with seven degrees of freedom, and eliminates hand tremor. The surgical manipulative ability is further enhanced by the binocular stereoscopic steady viewing and by toggling among three operative arms to eventually improve the overall surgeon's ability to operate within deep and narrow spaces. Although some of these advantages remain speculative, initial results already provide the rationale for further studies. Should this approach prove to be safe and effective in larger series, it may become an alternative to conventional open (maximally invasive) transplantation technique.

Organ Recovery and Regenerative Medicine

The marked extension of donor criteria recently renewed the interest for organ recovery/resuscitation laboratories aiming at improving the function of the "at-risk" recovered kidney grafts. Two major tendencies are under investigation, the hypothermic or normothermic perfusion. The judge is still out which method is best.

Indirectly the shortage of organs and the extension of donor criteria lead to a renewed interest for regenerative medicine. Many advances have already been made in the "kidney field." The "creation and modulation" of allografts slowly but surely becomes a realistic approach allowing not only to expand in the future the donor pool but also to reach the final goal of transplantation, the "holy grail" of clinical operational tolerance [2].

Pancreas Transplantation

The Beginnings: From the 1960s to the End of Twentieth Century

Vascularized pancreas transplantation (PT) is currently the only definitive long-term treatment for selected patients with complicated type 1 or 2 diabetes (or those rendered diabetic by total pancreatectomy) that reliably restores normal glucose homeostasis without the need either for exogenous insulin therapy or close glucose monitoring. In addition, by achieving euglycemia, PT may not only eliminate the risk of either severe hypo/hyperglycemia but also prevent, stabilize, or even reverse progressive diabetic complications. PT can be performed either simultaneously with a kidney transplant (SPKT), following a successful KT (pancreas after kidney, PAKT) or prior to a KT as a pancreas transplant alone (PTA). The latter two categories are usually combined as solitary pancreas transplantation (SPT) because of similar outcomes. In the USA, 75 % of PT are performed as SPKT, 16 % as PAKT, and 9 % as PTA [11, 12]. The total number of PT steadily increased in the USA until 2004 but has since declined, particularly in the PAKT category. In contrast, the number of PTs performed outside of the USA has steadily increased in recent years and now accounts for the majority of PTs performed worldwide.

During the last decade, era analyses in the USA have demonstrated that deceased donor recovery rates and additions to the waiting list decreased; organ discard rates and waiting times increased; and the proportion of recipients who are older, black, have a higher BMI or are characterized as having type 2 diabetes all increased. Importantly, success rates for PT have steadily improved over time as a consequence of significant reductions in technical and immunologic failures. Appropriate donor and recipient selection, minimization of cold ischemia, and use of depleting antibody induction coupled with robust maintenance, usually tacrolimus-mycophenolate-based immunosuppression, are all of paramount importance to achieve success in PT. US recipients of primary deceased donor PT have a 1-year patient survival rate of more than 95 % in all three categories; unadjusted 5-year patient survival rates are 87 % in SPKT, 83 % in PAKT, and 89 % in PTA recipients; more than 70 % of patients are alive at 10 years post-transplant. One-year pancreas (insulin-free) graft survival rates are 85.5 % in SPKT (93 % kidney graft survival), 80 % in PAKT, and 78 % in PTA recipients, which translates to pancreas graft half-lives approaching 14 years in SPKT and 10 years in SPT recipients [11, 12].

The Standard Surgical Technique

The first PT, performed on December 16, 1966, at the University of Minnesota by Lillehei, was a segmental pancreas graft performed with duct ligation as an SPKT. The next 12 PTs performed at the same institute were whole-organ pancreatico-duodenal grafts with exocrine drainage diverted to a Roux-en-Y jejunal limb. After this initial experience, segmental pancreatic grafts were predominant in the late 1970s and early 1980s until newer techniques were introduced to safely manage the exocrine secretions. Since then, the vast majority of PTs have been performed as whole-organ grafts with a variable length of donor duodenum, while segmental pancreas grafts are now rarely used from deceased donors. However, this technique remains the only possibility in PT from living donors [13, 14]. According to Registry data, the majority of whole-organ PT has been performed with systemic venous delivery of insulin and either bladder (systemic-bladder) or enteric (systemic-enteric) drainage of the exocrine secretions.

Prior to 1995, more than 90 % of PTs were performed by the standard technique of systemic-bladder drainage, usually using a short donor duodenal segment conduit for exocrine drainage. Since 1995, the number of PTs performed with primary enteric exocrine drainage has increased dramatically and currently accounts for 91 % of SPKT, 89 % of PAKT, and 85 % of PTA cases in the USA. Over 80 % of enteric drained PTs are performed with systemic (iliac or vena cava) venous delivery of insulin, resulting in peripheral hyperinsulinemia. To improve the physiology, an innovative technique of intraperitoneal portal venous drainage using the superior mesenteric vein (SMV) was developed by Gaber et al. [15] and subsequently refined to a "retroperitoneal" approach by Boggi et al. combining portal venous delivery of insulin with enteric drainage of the exocrine secretions (portal-enteric technique (PET)) [16]. At present, however, portal-enteric drainage accounts for only 18 % of SPKT and PAKT and 10 % of PTA with enteric drainage [11]. Recent studies have reported excellent outcomes using either the recipient duodenum or stomach as the site for exocrine allograft drainage.

Although all techniques are similar in terms of long-term outcome, current philosophy dictates that the most appropriate technique to be performed is defined by both donor and recipient anatomy as well as the surgical team's comfort level and experience. All PT techniques share common ground with respect to donor and recipient selection, organ recovery and preservation, bench preparation, and post-transplant management including immunosuppression. Most PTs are performed through a vertical midline abdominal incision, which preserves all possible options for transplantation of the pancreas, as well as eventual simultaneous placement of the kidney. Currently, the most common technique for arterial reconstruction of the dual-artery blood supply of the pancreas uses the bifurcating iliac artery from the donor as an interposition arterial "Y" graft. This graft can easily be anastomosed to the superior mesenteric (SMA) and splenic arteries. In the case of SPT, preemptive SPKT, history of thrombophilia or clotting disorder in the recipient, small or diseased donor or recipient vessels, prolonged cold ischemia, extended donor criteria, history of prior pancreas graft thrombosis, or abnormal intraoperative monitoring of coagulation status, perioperative systemic anticoagulation is warranted.

Advances in immunosuppression have played a pivotal role in the steadily improving results in PT. At present, 85–90 % of PT recipients receive antibody induction (70 % receive depleting antibody); nearly 80 % receive maintenance therapy with the tacrolimus/mycophenolate combination, and 40–50 % undergo steroid withdrawal without adverse consequences. Limited data with tacrolimus/sirolimus reveal excellent outcomes, whereas initial attempts with calcineurin inhibitor avoidance or minimization are less promising. One-year acute rejection rates have steadily decreased to the 5–20 % range depending on transplant category, case mix, and immunosuppressive regimen. Current 1-year rates of immunological pancreas graft loss are 6 % in PTA, 3.7 % in PAKT, and 1.8 % in SPKT recipients.

The Surgical Technique Refined: The Search for the Optimal Technique

During recent years there has been a continuous search towards the optimal endocrine and exocrine drainage technique.

Systemic Venous-Bladder Exocrine Drainage [or Systemic-Bladder Technique]

The introduction of the systemic-bladder technique (SBT) into clinical practice is regarded as a milestone in the history of PT because it dramatically lowered the exocrine complication rate and permitted a transition from the experimental to the clinical phase of PT. The graft is placed "head-down" in the pelvis. The vascular anastomoses are usually performed in an end-to-side fashion to the right external iliac vessels. The venous allograft outflow drains into the systemic venous system, thereby bypassing the portal system, thus causing systemic hyper-insulinemia and portal hypo-insulinemia. The donor duodenum (or pancreatic duct) is next anastomosed to the vesical dome (Fig. 40.2).

Safety and monitoring are the main advantages of the bladder diversion technique because exocrine leaks or pancreatitis can usually be diagnosed with standard imaging (including cystography) and managed with prolonged urethral catheter drainage. In fact, bacteria cultured from the graft duodenum are rarely involved in infections. Duodenal graft complications can be often managed conservatively with a low risk of graft loss or patient death. In addition, rejection can be more easily and timely diagnosed with monitoring of the urinary amylase concentration analysis and cystoscopy. The latter examination allows direct visualization of the duodeno-cystostomy and provides access for needle biopsy of either the duodenum or the pancreas allograft. The drainage of pancreatic enzymes into the bladder as well as systemic venous delivery of insulin have also disadvantages because it creates a non-physiologic condition associated with unique urologic and metabolic complications. These include hyperchloremic metabolic acidosis secondary to bicarbonate loss, dehydration secondary to fluid losses through the urine, recurrent urinary tract infections, dysuria, hematuria, cystitis/urethritis, and recurrent episodes of graft pancreatitis secondary to reflux of urine into the ductal system of the graft. In about 20–25 % of cases, enteric conversion is performed to eliminate persistent or recurrent urologic, metabolic, or infectious complications. Currently, SBT is used selectively but has not been abandoned because it is a time-honored technique with excellent long-term outcomes. It is used more commonly in SPT in order to allow monitoring of urine amylase levels and when there are concerns about the preservation or perfusion of the duodenal

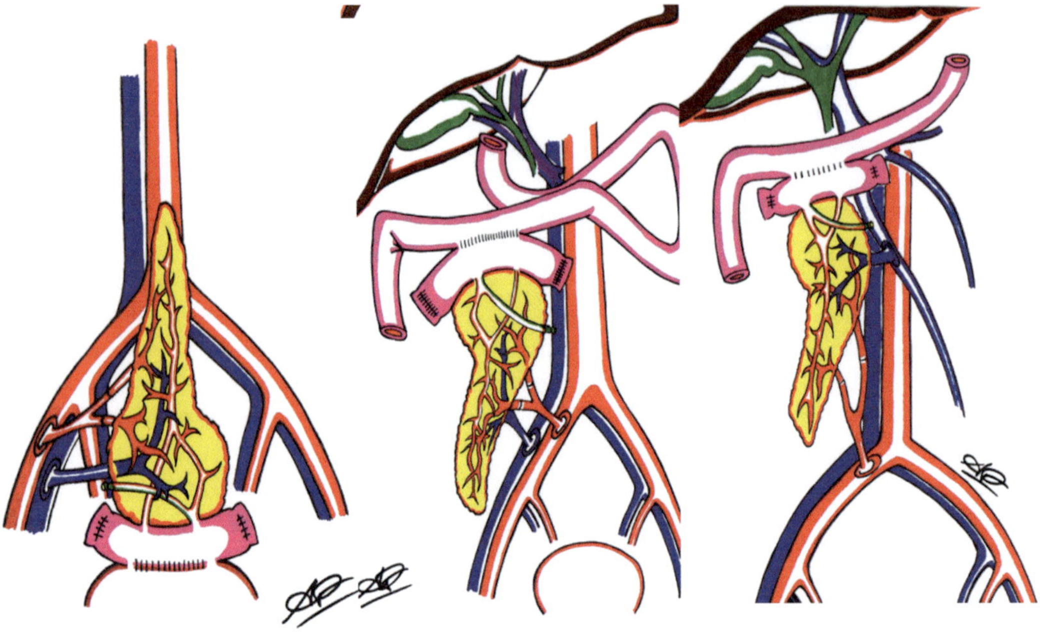

Fig. 40.2 Pancreas transplantation with bladder (*left*) or enteric drainage (*mid and right*). In the latter case, the portal vein can be implanted either on the iliac axis (*mid cartoon*) or on the SMV (*right*) (used with permission of Andrea Peloso, MD)

segment because leaks are easier to manage and have lower morbidity and a better chance to heal with bladder drainage.

Systemic Venous-Enteric Exocrine Drainage [or Systemic-Enteric Technique]

Because of the success of enteric conversion coupled with advances in donor management, organ preservation, immunosuppression, diagnostic methodology, antibiotic strategies, and overall medical management, a transformation in PT occurred from SBT to systemic-enteric technique (SET) in the mid-1990s. Since then the majority of PTs are performed using the SET with a variable length of duodenum. The SET is the most versatile technique because it permits either cephalad or caudal orientation of the pancreas with exocrine drainage into virtually any part of the mid-gastrointestinal (GI) tract (stomach, duodenum, jejunum, or ileum). The vascular anastomoses are similar as in SBT (end-to-side anastomoses to the iliac vessels or inferior vena cava/aorta). A number of techniques of performing the enteric anastomosis have been described either with or without a diverting Roux-en-Y limb including side-to-side or end-to-side anastomoses. The enteric anastomosis can be stapled or hand-sewn. Some surgeons prefer the hand-sewn anastomosis secondary to a higher bleeding risk of the stapled enteric anastomosis, especially when localized more proximal in the GI tract.

Portal Venous-Enteric Exocrine Drainage [or Portal-Enteric Technique]

The portal vein of the pancreas graft is anastomosed end to side to a major tributary of the SMV using a standard vascular running technique with polypropylene sutures. The dissection of the SMV can be performed with either an anterior, intraperitoneal, or a lateral, retroperitoneal, approach. In the former, the donor iliac artery bifurcation graft is brought through a window created in the distal ileal mesentery and anastomosed end to side to the right common iliac artery. In the latter, no window is necessary for the artery whereas a window may be needed in the right colon mesentery for the enteric anastomosis.

The pancreas will be oriented vertically with the head of the pancreas directed cephalad either in the mid-abdomen or right para-colic region depending on the approach to the SMV (Fig. 40.2). The enteric anastomosis is more commonly created directly into an adjacent bowel loop that is not excluded from the transit of intestinal contents or to a Roux-en-Y limb that is diverted from the enteric stream with or without a venting jejunostomy. Less frequently, the enteric anastomosis can also be created in an omega loop or directly into the native duodenum or stomach, which may allow easier access for endoscopic surveillance and biopsy. Complications of enteric drainage (SET or PET) include prolonged ileus, small bowel obstruction, enteric leak, infected peri-pancreatic fluid collections, GI bleeding, and intra-abdominal abscess formation.

Simultaneous Kidney Pancreas (SPKT) and Solitary Pancreas Transplantation

Because the pancreas is more sensitive to prolonged cold ischemia than the kidney, the pancreatic graft is usually implanted first in SPKT. Thereafter, the renal graft can be implanted either ipsilaterally on the right external iliac vessels or contralaterally on the left side. Generally, the ipsilateral technique reduces operating time and leaves the left side available for future transplantation. When exposing the iliac vessels for kidney implantation, care must be taken with retracting the viscera to avoid excessive traction on the revascularized pancreas graft in SPKT [17].

SPT is performed similar to SPKT. In cases in which PAKT is being performed with a prior KT on the right side, the pancreas can usually be placed "above" the kidney using either the right common iliac vessels or distal vena cava and aorta for vascular inflow. Following completion of the transplant, nasogastric tubes and peri-pancreatic drains can be avoided, employed selectively, or used routinely. In comparison to SPKT, SPT is usually associated with the more liberal use of systemic anticoagulation, more ideal donor selection, shorter cold ischemia, and better human leukocyte antigen matching to reduce the risks of early vascular thrombosis and acute rejection.

The Living Donor

PT using a segmental graft from a living donor started at the University of Minnesota in 1979 and, ever since, more than 160 cases have been performed worldwide, mainly in specialized centers where actually the technical failure rate of the procedure is now even lower than in deceased donor PT. At present, very few living donor PTs are being performed, the most active center being the Tokyo center, led by Kenmochi. Importantly, the surgical complication rate in the living donor is less than 5 %. Morbidity includes pancreatitis, splenectomy, pancreatic exocrine leak, pseudocyst formation, as well as the risk for developing diabetes or glucose intolerance post-donation. This type of PT may be a valuable alternative strategy to deceased donor PT in the case of long waiting times or in highly sensitized patients.

Liver Transplantation

The Beginnings: From the 1960s to the 1980s

Fifty years ago Starzl, the "father of modern transplantation," realized the first successful liver transplantation (LT) in a child suffering from biliary atresia. After nine worldwide attempts, a long-term (400 days) survivor could be produced in 1967; this 1.5-year young child died 400 days later due to tumor recurrence [18]. The stage was now set to possibly bringing this so-called impossible operation to the clinical arena. LT was called at that time a 100-h-long operation, using 100 U of blood and finally ending up in a 100 % mortality. This definition clearly reflected the difficulty of this procedure. In order to avoid the "deadly" recipient hepatectomy, the concept of heterotopic, full-size, LT was developed and advocated especially by the Rotterdam group [19, 20]. Indeed when looking back at the first LT experiences, most patients died of bleeding, sepsis, allograft failure, and last but not least rejection. These three events reflected a suboptimal surgical technique (causing uncontrollable bleeding), an insufficient intra- and perioperative management (putting on a par with rejection every liver dysfunction, leading thereby to an inappropriately reinforced immunosuppression causing different kinds of lethal infections), and an inappropriate cold storage organ preservation (explaining the high incidence of primary or early non-function of the allograft). This high morbidity and mortality rates triggered huge research projects in experimental surgery, intensive care, anesthesiology, immunology, and pharmacology [21].

The most breakthroughs in LT were developed during the 1980s. Firstly, the Denver team that had in between moved to Pittsburgh standardized the multi-organ procurement technique as well as the implantation technique. The biggest steps forward in the refinement of the "unfinished product" consisted in the introduction of the intraluminal vascular suture technique and the active veno-venous bypass (VVB) [22] (Fig. 40.3). Especially the VVB allowed not only to refine technique but also to improve perioperative care by eliminating venous splanchnic and renal congestion, improving intraoperative hemodynamic stability, and avoiding intra- and perioperative fluid overfilling. The biggest merit of the VVB was probably that it allowed surgeons not only to implant the organ

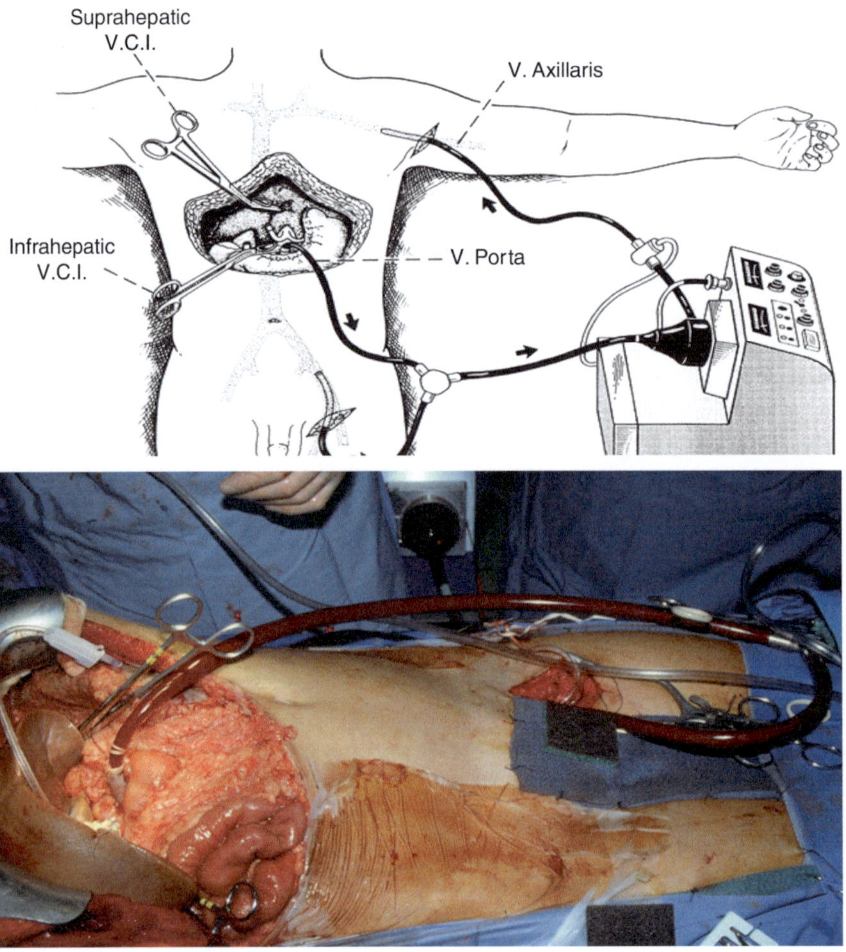

Fig. 40.3 Veno-venous bypass during the an-hepatic stage of liver transplantation with drainage of portal and cava flows into the left axillary or internal jugular veins. The centripetal bio-pump can be seen in between the two surgeon-assistants

under less stressful conditions but most of all that it allowed surgeons from all over the world to learn how to perform the hepatectomy and the implantation of the liver. When VVB was used during the an-hepatic phase of LT, this included drainage of the portal vein and the lower part of the vena cava via the greater saphenous vein into the axillary or jugular vein.

The development of LT was further boosted by the almost simultaneous introduction in clinical practice of the selective immunosuppressive drug Cyclosporin A. This CNI, discovered by Borel and Stahelin at the Swiss pharmaceutical concern Novartis and introduced in 1983 in clinical transplantation by Calne, led to an unprecedented "explosion" of KT as well as LT [23]. Some years later Belzer introduced the University of Wisconsin (UW) solution, allowing now to transform LT into a (semi-)elective procedure [24]. All these developments culminated in the 1983 NIH LT Consensus Conference (CC). This CC concluded, based on 540 LT performed at 4 centers (Denver-Pittsburgh, Groningen, Hannover, and Cambridge), that LT would be a promising alternative "to current therapy in the management of the late phase of several forms of serious liver diseases" to be applied to very selective patients [25]. The following developments have been tremendous as shown by the fact that only one from the ten absolute and five relative contraindications stated at the CC remains valid today, namely active sepsis at the moment of LT. All progress is best exemplified by the UNOS and (audited) European liver transplant registry (ELTR), founded by bismuth, containing each more than 120,000 LT [26].

Further Developments: From the 1990s to the End of the Twentieth Century

Based on an ever-increasing, worldwide experience, several technical variants to the original standard procedure have been developed mostly aiming at overcoming, technically related, contraindications, as well as shortage of organs.

The Standard Procedure Refined

The Portal and Caval Veins

Splanchnic venous thrombosis, a part of the natural evolution of chronic liver diseases, was initially seen as a huge obstacle to perform LT successfully. The identification of splanchnic and caval vein acquired or congenital anomalies taught surgeons to take care of these conditions [27]. Translation of carotid endarterectomy technique to LT into venous eversion thrombectomy allows nowadays transplanting safely most recipients presenting with, even extended, splanchnic thrombosis [28] (Fig. 40.4). If judged impossible, the liver graft can still be implanted using venous interposition grafts between donor portal vain (PV) and SMV or by connection of the donor PV to choledochal or gastric varices. The cavo-portal hemi-transposition and finally the combined liver-intestinal transplantation represent the rare solutions to these challenging situations.

The introduction of the inferior vena cava (IVC)-sparing hepatectomy technique was another technical progress [29]. Compared with the classical technique with resection of the IVC, this technique allows one to do a precise dissection during hepatectomy, reducing thereby transfusion and fluid administration needs, the preserved IVC serving in fact as an "internal VVB." The allograft is next implanted using the piggyback technique connecting the suprahepatic cuff of the liver to the common orifice of the middle and left HV (end-to-end anastomosis) or performing a large, side-to-side, cavo-caval suture anastomosing the posterior side of donor IVC to the anterior side of the recipient IVC: side-to-side cavo-cavostomy [30, 31]. This technique avoids cross-clamping of the vena cava by using a large adapted Satinsky-Lerut clamp (Ulrich, Sankt-Gallen, CH) (Fig. 40.5).

The cornerstone of LT is also the management of portal hypertension and its bleeding that can greatly complicate the surgical procedure. For this reasons, some centers perform a temporary porto-systemic shunt at the beginning of the surgery.

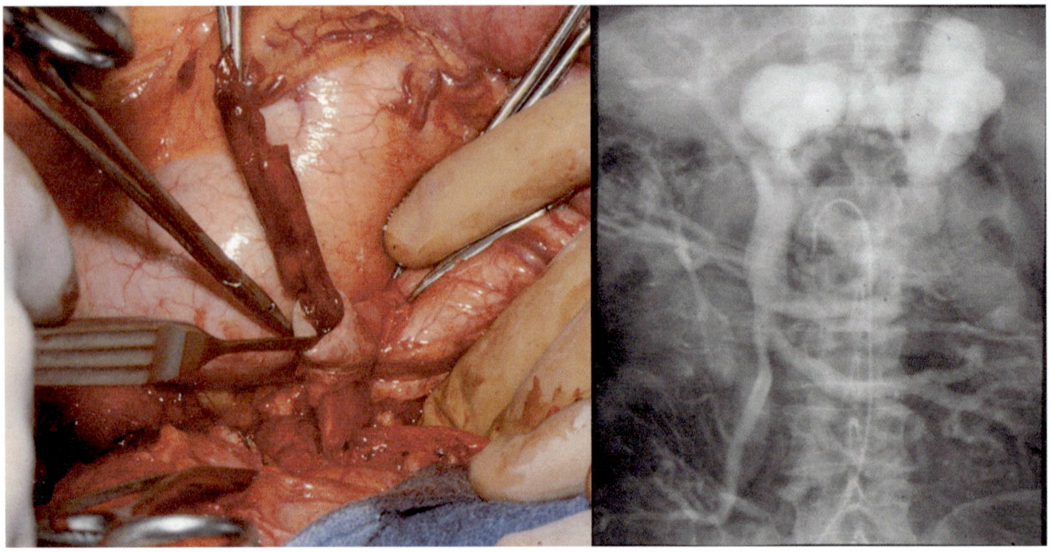

Fig. 40.4 Recanalization of the porto-mesenteric axis using extended eversion thrombectomy

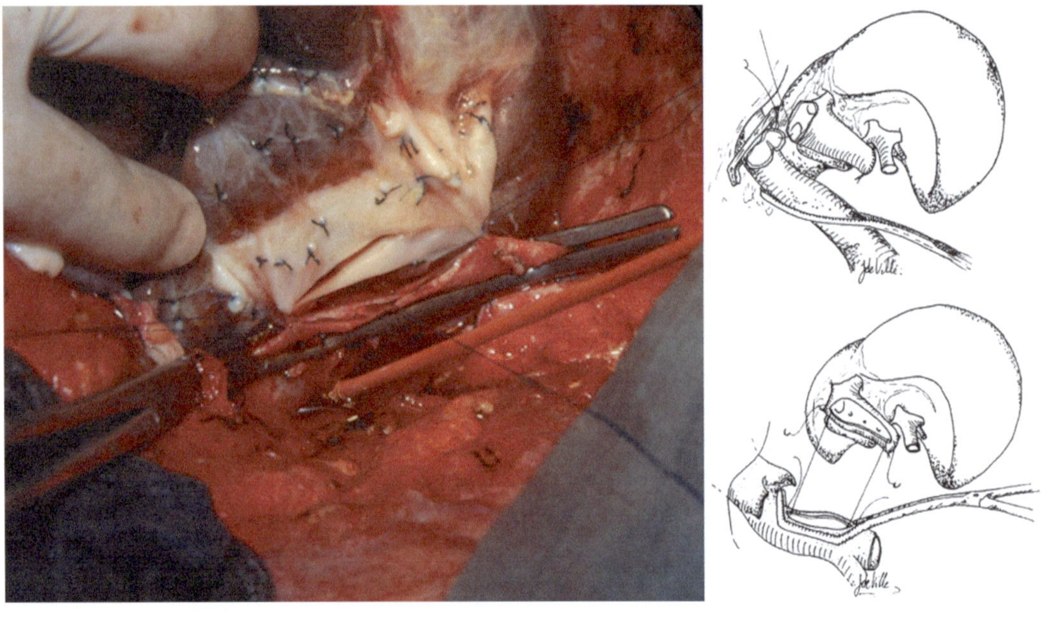

Fig. 40.5 The inferior vena cava (IVC)-sparing hepatectomy technique allowing a wide side-to-side cavo-caval anastomosis. The partial clamping of the IVC using the Satinsky-Lerut clamp allows venous return to the cardiopulmonary circulation (used with permission of Professor Jean de Ville de Goyet)

The Biliary Tract

The biliary tract still remains the Achilles heel of the procedure. Systematic retrograde or transhepatic cholangiography reveals that 15–20 % of all recipients present some biliary tract problem in the absence of hepatic artery thrombosis [32, 33]. The most difficult complications to treat are the non-anastomotic ones (better known as ischemic type biliary tract lesions—ITBL). Shortening of ischemic times and adequate rinsing of the biliary tract at procurement are important measures to take in order to reduce the incidence of biliary complications. Anastomotic strictures are more prone to be taken care of by redo-biliary surgery.

The biliary tract reconstruction has gone through different periods and "schools" navigating between systematic, selective, and nonuse of T-tube or biliary drainage [34]. The recent trend seems to favor biliary stenting, this related to the more frequent use of ECD and DC donors. Some Asiatic teams introduced microsurgical techniques using nonabsorbable polypropylene suture in order to reduce the fibrotic process during suture healing reducing thereby the complication rates [35].

Biliary tract reconstruction in patients with inflammatory bile ducts as seen in primary sclerosing cholangitis or after intra-arterial chemotherapy has also been revised. End-to-end biliary anastomosis and even bilio-duodenostomy have been realized successfully; the latter approach also allows avoiding the necessity to make a Roux-Y loop in a sometimes difficult intraoperative abdominal condition [36].

The Hepatic Artery

There is currently almost no hepatic arterial abnormality that may indicate against transplantation. The huge experience obtained in the field of living donor LT (LDLT) has shown that hepatic artery thrombosis is nearly always a surgical problem. Different reconstructions, including the use of free arterial interposition grafts between allograft arterial tree and infra-renal abdominal aorta usually allow solving difficult intraoperative situations. As more and more older recipients (presenting with coeliac trunk stenosis) and cancer patients (presenting arteritis due to repeated transarterial chemo-embolization) present with a compromised arterial tree, collaboration with the interventional radiologist becomes more and more important in order to optimize the arterialization of the allograft. Embolization of the (stealing) splenic artery and stenting of the celiac trunk are good examples of this [37]. The same holds for the frequent venous and biliary problems observed during or after LT. The interventional radiologist indeed must nowadays be a mandatory "part" of the LT team.

The Expansion of the Deceased Donor Organ Pool

Split Liver Grafting

The initial success of LT rapidly extended the indications not only to small children but also to many adults, especially those presenting with oncologic diseases. Indeed 30–50 % of patients are transplanted because of hepatocellular cancer (HCC) [26]. It has to be anticipated that these oncologic indications will be extended towards cholangiocellular cancer (CCC), rare vascular tumors such as hemangioendothelioma, and finally neuroendocrine and even colorectal metastases.

These widening of indications triggered the development of first reduced-size LT followed by split liver transplantation (SPLT). SPLT was initially developed for the adult-child pair (right lobe-left lobe); later on technical expertise was extended to develop adult-adult splitting (right liver-left liver also termed as full right-full left split LT). Undoubtedly the split LT has a huge potential; its development is however hampered by many technical as well as logistic problems. The Hamburg, Lyon, Birmingham, and Los Angeles groups and especially the NIT program in Italy have shown that excellent results can be obtained on the condition that expertise is centralized [38]. Broering showed that full right-full left splitting including splitting of the middle hepatic vein could solve the problem of small-for-size grafting in this situation [39].

The application of SPLT in very small babies remains problematic now related to a "too-large-for-size" liver syndrome. The Tokyo pediatric group developed a technique of hyper-reduction of the left liver lobe (the so-called hamburger graft) based on precise anatomical knowledge [40].

Domino or Sequential or Liver Grafting

In 1984 the procedure of domino grafting (DLT) was introduced to the transplant community by the Coimbra team of Furtado. This procedure is based

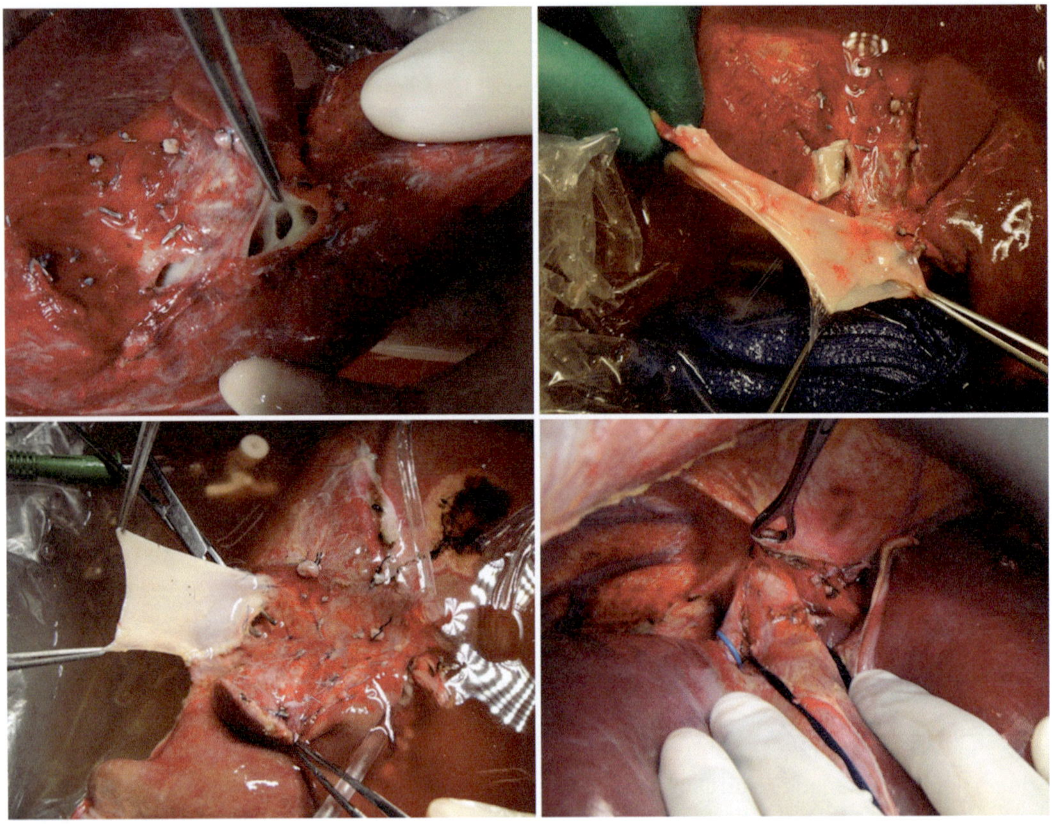

Fig. 40.6 Hepatic outflow reconstruction of a domino liver graft—harvested using IVC-sparing hepatectomy—using free venous iliaco-cava graft

on the knowledge that the non-cirrhogenic metabolic diseases (maple syrup disease and familial amyloidotic polyneuropathy (FAP)), located in the liver, are not or only very rarely (and slowly) transmitted to a recipient which does not have this inherited treat. In contrast primary hyper-oxalosis is a contraindication to DLT as the recipients rapidly develop a renal insufficiency.

In order to not compromise the "FAP liver donor," techniques have been developed by the Barroso team in Lisbon to realize in this setting the IVC-sparing hepatectomy. This modality implies a reconstruction of the suprahepatic venous outflow tract using free venous grafts [41] (Fig. 40.6).

Auxiliary Partial Liver Grafting

Auxiliary partial LT (APOLT) was much promoted by the teams of Boudjema in Strasbourg and Heaton in London in case of acute liver failure and in metabolic disease [42]. This procedure has later been taken over by the Paris and Leeds groups again for the same indication [43, 44]. Ultimate analyses showed that however results were less good than for total liver replacement; selection of the recipient is fundamental looking thereby at the potential regenerative potential of the recipient liver. This procedure remains however appealing as it allows, after repair of the original liver function, to withdraw all immunosuppressive treatment [45]. This procedure has gained renewed interest in the field of LT for liver-based inherited metabolic diseases such as Crigler-Najjar, OTC deficiency, citrullinemia, propionic acidemia, primary hypercholesterolemia, and hemophilia and in the field of combined liver-kidney transplantation (CLKT) for hypersensitized renal patients. In this situation the partial liver graft serves as "an absorber" of harmful antibodies.

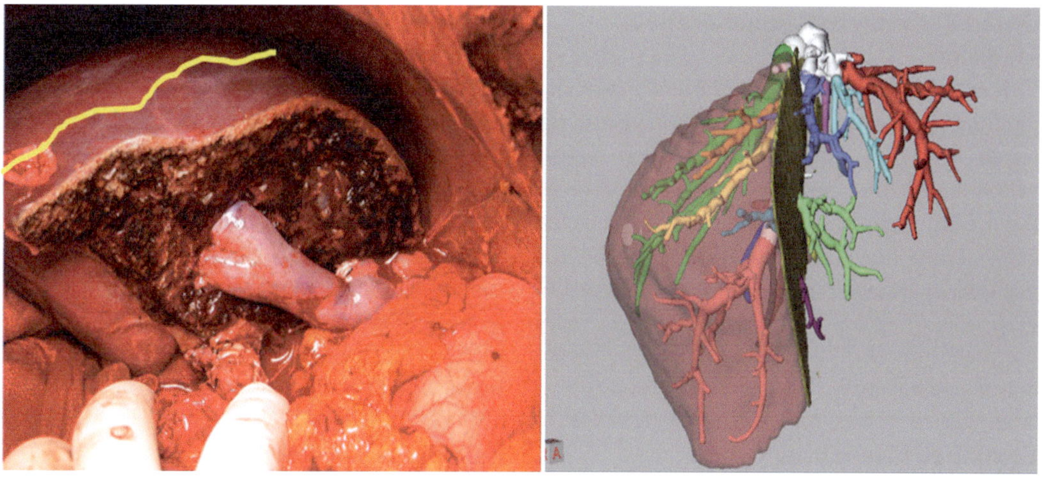

Fig. 40.7 Right liver living donor LT with drainage of the anterior sector using a free venous interposition graft between the segment 5 and 8 allograft hepatic veins and recipient IVC. Three-dimensional liver reconstruction using the MEVIS software allowing to define precisely liver allograft volume and vascularization

Further Developments: From the End of the Twentieth to the Beginning of the Twenty-First Centuries

The "Tsunami" of Living Donor Liver Transplantation

Most technical problems of LT have nowadays been resolved, but the ever-present problem of organ shortage remains. This matter has been addressed, largely, in the eastern world by the development of living donor LT (LDLT). The shortage of pediatric livers could easily be resolved by doing adult-child splitting; the split LT will however not be able to solve the shortage problem in adults. The centers of Kyoto, Tokyo, Kaohshiung, and Hong Kong and especially the five top centers in Seoul have put tremendous efforts to make LDLT a feasible and safe, although complex, undertaking. Many technical problems had to be solved besides the problem of the SFSS. Indeed safety matters must be prioritized in the donor, so the maximal amount of liver mass to be procured must be limited to 70 % of the donor liver volume. Conversely the recipient must receive a liver mass equal to 0.6–1.00 % of his body weight or 0.3–0.5 of his liver standard volume. "Modulation" of (the partial) allografts' inflow as well as outflow is of utmost importance to obtain success. Reduction of portal venous pressure by splenic artery ligation and optimization of liver segmental outflow using interposition grafts between segmental allograft hepatic veins (HV) and the IVC have solved these problems [46, 47] (Fig. 40.7). It requires a complete preoperative assessment with often a three-dimensional liver reconstruction. This method allows one to define all different hepatectomy procedures, focusing especially on the remnant-liver volume.

The ultimate solution for the SFSS has been developed by the Seoul Asan group. Lee introduced successfully the technique of "dual-liver grafting" [48]. In this technique two smaller grafts, consisting of all different right and left anatomical variants, allow to obtain a sufficient liver mass even in very sick (high MELD score) patients.

As LDLT eliminates the factor time in oncologic indications, this technical variant of LT has also been at the basis of the important extension of indications for LT in case of hepatobiliary cancer. LDLT indeed led to the continuous expansion of use of LT in case of HCC and also CCC, as shown by the Mayo Group. Use of LDLT combined with the use of tumor behavior based on m-RECIST criteria and tumor marker dynamics is a major condition to further develop and especially justify the role of LT in transplant oncology [49].

Organ Recovery and Regenerative Medicine

The extension of donor criteria and especially the frequent use of DCD livers (reaching already up to 50 % in some countries such as the Netherlands) have fostered research projects in the field of organ recovery. The shift from static cold storage to ex vivo machine perfusion has been made undoubtedly. The optimal method of perfusion, oxygenated or non-oxygenated, (sub) normothermic or hypothermic, has to be sorted out in a near future.

Combined Liver-Other Organ Transplantation

Combined Liver-Kidney Transplantation

Progresses in all different fields of organ transplantation recently moved the combined transplantation procedure from an exceptional to a more frequent undertaking. Today multi-organ transplantation including the liver represents 2 % of all LT performed in Europe. CLKT is the most frequent form of such transplantation reaching in several organ exchange organizations already up to 15 % of indications. Since the first clinical application by Margreiter in 1983, CLKT indeed became a fast-growing indication for LT [50]. This has a threefold explanation: (a) the improved surgical and medical care have rendered easier the decision to simultaneously deal with both organic end-stage liver and renal failure; (b) several chronic liver-diseased patients slide from an originally functional (e.g., hepato-renal syndrome) to a protracted, irreversible failure, probably also triggered by a, many times, hidden presence of an underlying renal disease; and (c) finally many liver recipients presenting a recurrent allograft disease have destroyed their kidney function due to prolonged intake of the nephrotoxic CNI. The introduction of the MELD-based liver allocation system, which is based on the values of bilirubin, INR, and creatinine as well as necessity for renal replacement therapy, further boosted the application of CLKT. The impact of the MELD system was so important that it really dislocated the liver allocation. Many useless CLKT were indeed done; the bad outcomes moreover were responsible for waste of valuable organs. A Consensus Conference became therefore rapidly necessary in order to "regulate" the indications for CLKT. Conversely this CC also refined the indication for renal transplantation in liver-diseased patients.

The immunosuppressive treatment of CLKT remains still protean, this despite the growing experience in this field of liver transplantation. Indeed immunosuppressive treatment varies from a "minimalistic" (including CNI monotherapy) to a very "aggressive" approach (including up to four immunosuppressant drugs and plasmapheresis). This is surprising has it had been shown both experimentally and clinically since 1985 that the liver immunologically protects the kidney (read the "canary" theory of Starzl) [51]. This is especially important in case of cross-match positivity and in case of highly sensitized kidney recipients. A larger UNOS study clearly showed that CLKT significantly reduced the incidence of chronic renal rejection and most interestingly that the half-life of the kidney allograft could be doubled. This protective effect can be explained by the facts that the liver (mass) absorbs antibodies and soluble HLA antigens. The proof of this protective "liver effect" concept has been shown by Olausson from Gothenburg [52]. Simultaneous grafting of an auxiliary orthotopic left liver graft (segments II and III) and kidney from a same donor allowed to transplant successfully 75 % of highly sensitized kidney recipients. These patients would otherwise have been denied the chance to a renal transplantation because of immunologic contraindications; see also auxiliary liver transplantation.

Combined Liver-Heart and Liver-Lung Transplantations

These surgeries remain seldom procedures. The first CHLT procedure was successfully done by Starzl for familial hypercholesterolemia in 1983 [53]; since then about 200 such operations have been done in Europe and the USA. The results are very encouraging reaching similar 5-year survival rates as for cardiac transplantation (around 70 %). Combined liver-heart transplantation (CLHT) is nowadays most frequently indicated in FAP (about 25 %) and idiopathic dilated cardiomyopathy (about 15 %).

The even much rarer combined liver-lung transplantation (CLLT) is most frequently indicated in case of cystic fibrosis alpha-1 antitrypsin deficiency and porto-pulmonary hypertension [54]. Sixty cases have been reported. In the cystic fibrosis group it can also be necessary to perform a combined heart-lung-liver transplantation. Care of these patients is indeed complex as shown by the bigger Cambridge, Paris, and Pittsburgh experiences. Five-year survival rate of around 55 % is obtained. All obtained results are also partly attributable to the protective immunologic effect of the accompanying liver graft.

Combined Liver-Pancreas (Islet or Vascularized) Transplantation

In end-stage liver-diseased patients presenting with a very unstable insulin-dependent diabetes combined islet or vascularized liver-pancreas transplantation (LPAT) has been advocated. Of course the intervention is much less invasive in case of intraportal islet injection. Unfortunately the late islet graft function is still very poor (less than 10 %). Combined en bloc or separated LPAT has been reported rarely; 42 cases have been collected in the ELTR; their 5-year survival rate is 55 %. The procedure has been shown to be feasible but has been rarely advocated in comparison with the multivisceral transplantation (MVT) procedure.

Combined Liver-Intestine and Multi-visceral Transplantation

The concept of MVT has been introduced in clinical practice by Starzl in 1993 initially for malignant and later on for benign congenital and acquired diseases [55]. The basis for the MVT was the embryologic development of the human being with foregut, mid-gut, and hind-gut, the three cornerstones. The main indications are diffuse splanchnic venous thrombosis and intestinal failure with development of cirrhosis. The MVT was defined as a graft including more than two organs including the liver; the modified MVT is defined as a graft without donor liver. The beginnings of these procedures were compromised by a high morbidity, infection rate, and development of post-transplant lymphoproliferative disease (PTLD), all problems related to "overimmunosuppression." Besides these medical problems, it took a long time to find out the "better" surgical techniques. The Pittsburgh, Miami, and Indianapolis groups produced high numbers of such MVT [56]. Finally, the concepts of combined liver-intestine transplantation (CLIT), isolated small bowel transplantation (SBT), and MVT (up to seven organs) were developed. Results have now become acceptable after refining immunologic and nutritional care as well as surgical technique. The 3-year graft survival rate now reaches 50 %; the results being better in case of combined liver-small bowel transplantation, this related to the protective liver effect.

The development of intestinal transplantation has been plagued by many difficulties and deceptions. This utmost demanding part of transplantation and medicine has also boosted the research in nutritional care and in the development of intestinal surgery. Intestinal "lengthening procedures" such as the "step" and the Bianchi procedures, based on the dual mesenteric blood supply of the intestine, have indeed allowed to multiple patients "to escape" from the intestinal transplantation.

Growing experiences also led to a constant evolution with the design of grafts adapted to the individual need of the intestinal failure patient. So combined liver-intestine, multi-visceral, and modified multi-visceral grafts eventually completed with colon, kidney, and even abdominal wall have all been applied successfully during the recent years.

Parietal Transplantation

Due to the frequently too large "intestinal" allograft implanted in recipients presenting frequently with a "small" peritoneal cavity, the concept of parietal transplantation was developed by the Miami and Bologna groups [57]. The development of small bowel and parietal transplantation have had as a corollary the development of ex situ resections and reconstructions of large, otherwise inoperable intra-abdominal tumors as shown by Kato.

Uterus Transplantation

Recently the combined effort of the Gothenburg and Miami groups launched a real program of uterus transplantation, after a very extensive experimental setup in baboons. The technical feasibility has been proven. Lots of hurdles, including ethical ones, have still to be taken before really to proceed to larger clinical application [58].

Conclusion

Since the start of clinical transplantation in 1951 by the French pioneers Kuss, Dubost, and Servelle followed by Murray in 1954, tremendous progress has been made within more than half a century both in the field of transplantation medicine and transplantation surgery. The visionary ideas of Starzl—the human being becoming a puzzle man, constituted of different organs, artificial tissues, and very probably soon of engineered organs or organ parts—become slowly but surely a reality. The ingenious ideas and dare of the transplant surgeon will be continuously fostered by technological progresses. Finally, all such achievements will have to be (re-)considered in the context of the very diverse ethical and cultural constraints of our globalized world.

References

References Kidney Transplantation

1. Küss R, Teinturier J, Milliez P. Quelques essais de greffe rein chez l'homme. Mem Acad Chir. 1951;77:755–64.
2. Rogers J. Current status of renal transplantation. In: Orlando G, Lerut JP, Soker S, Stratta RJ, editors. Regenerative medicine technologies applied to organ transplantation. Waltham, MA: Academic; 2015.
3. Coosemans W, Nevelsteen A, Pirenne J, Vanrenterghem Y. Renal transplantation in patients with a vascular aortoiliac prosthesis. Transplant Proc. 1999;31:1925–7.
4. Pfeiffer T, Sandmann W, Luther B, Böhner H, Voiculescu A, Grabensee B, Hollenbeck M. Vascular surgery for recipient preparation, improvement of graft quality and acceptability, and therapy of ischemic graft damage in kidney transplantation. Transplant Proc. 2002;34:2219–21.
5. Coosemans W, Baert L, Kuypers D, Maes B, Messiaen T, Vanrenterghem Y, Pirenne J. Renal transplantation onto abnormal urinary tract: ileal conduit urinary diversion. Transplant Proc. 2001;33:2493–4.
6. Sager C, Burek C, Durán V, Corbetta JP, Weller S, Paz E, López JC. Outcome of renal transplant in patients with abnormal urinary tract. Pediatr Surg Int. 2011;27:423–30.
7. Stratta RJ, Rohr MS, Sundberg AK, Farney AC, Hartmann EL, Moore PS, Rogers J, Iskandar SS, Gautreaux MD, Kiger DF, et al. Intermediate-term outcomes with expanded criteria deceased donors in kidney transplantation: a spectrum or specter of quality? Ann Surg. 2006;243:594–601. discussion 601–603.
8. Matas AJ, Smith JM, Skeans MA, Lamb KE, Gustafson SK, Samana CJ, Stewart DE, Snyder JJ, Israni AK, Kasiske BL. OPTN/SRTR 2011 Annual Data Report: kidney. Am J Transplant. 2013;13 Suppl 1:11–46.
9. Montgomery RA, Lonze BE, King KE, Kraus ES, Kucirka LM, Locke JE, et al. Desensitization in HLA-incompatible kidney recipients and survival. N Engl J Med. 2011;365:318–26.
10. Liem YS, Weimar W. Early living-donor kidney transplantation: a review of the associated survival benefit. Transplantation. 2009;87:317–8.

References Pancreas Transplantation

11. Gruessner AC. 2011 Update on Pancreas Transplantation: comprehensive trend analysis of 25,000 cases followed up over the course of twenty-four years at the International Pancreas Transplant Registry (IPTR). Rev Diab Stud. 2011;8:6–16.
12. Kandaswamy R, Stock PG, Skeans MA, et al. OPTN/SRTR 2011 Annual Data Report: pancreas. Am J Transplant. 2013;13(S1):47–72.
13. Sutherland DER, Gruessner RWG, Dunn DL, et al. Lessons learned from more than 1,000 pancreas transplants at a single institution. Ann Surg. 2001;233: 463–501.
14. Gruessner RW, Kendall DM, Drangstveit MB, et al. Simultaneous pancreas-kidney transplantation from live donors. Ann Surg. 1997;226:471–82.
15. Gaber AO, Shokouth-Amiri H, Grewal HP, et al. A technique for portal pancreatic transplantation with enteric drainage. Surg Gynecol Obstet. 1993;177: 417–9.
16. Boggi U, Vistoli F, Signori S, et al. A technique for retroperitoneal pancreas transplantation with portal-enteric drainage. Transplantation. 2005;79:1137–42.
17. Stratta RJ, Shokouh-Amiri MH, Egidi MF, et al. A prospective comparison of simultaneous kidney-pancreas transplantation with systemic-enteric versus portal-enteric drainage. Ann Surg. 2001;233:740–51.

References Liver Transplantation

18. Starzl T, Demetris J. Liver transplantation. Chicago: Year Book Medical Publishers; 1990.
19. Terpstra OT, Reuvers CB, Schalm SW. Auxiliary heterotopic liver transplantation. Transplantation. 1988;45:1003–7.
20. Terpstra OT, Schalm SW, Weimar W, et al. Auxiliary partial liver transplantation for end-stage chronic liver disease. N Engl J Med. 1988;8(319):1507–11.
21. Starzl T. The saga of liver replacement, with particular reference to the reciprocal influence of liver and kidney transplantation (1955–1967). J Am Coll Surg. 2002;195:587–610.
22. Calne RY, McMaster P, et al. Use of partial cardiopulmonary bypass during the anhepatic phase of orthotopic liver grafting. Lancet. 1979;2:612–4.
23. Calne RY, White DJ. The use of cyclosporin A in clinical organ grafting. Ann Surg. 1982;196:330–7.
24. Belzer FO. Clinical organ preservation with UW solution. Transplantation. 1989;47:1097–8.
25. Van Thiel DH, Schade RR, Starzl T, et al. Medical aspects of liver transplantation. Hepatology. 1984;4:79S–83.
26. Adam R, Karam V, Burroughs A, et al. Evolution of indications and results of liver transplantation in Europe. A report from the European Liver Transplant Registry (ELTR). J Hepatol. 2012;57:675–88.
27. Lerut J, Tzakis AG, Bron K, et al. Complications of venous reconstruction in human orthotopic liver transplantation. Ann Surg. 1987;205:404–14.
28. Lerut J, Mazza D, van Leeuw V, et al. Adult liver transplantation and abnormalities of splanchnic veins: experience in 53 patients. Transpl Int. 1997; 10:125–32.
29. Tzakis A, Todo S, Starzl TE. Orthotopic liver transplantation with preservation of the inferior vena cava. Ann Surg. 1989;210:649–52.
30. Lerut J, Gertsch P. Side-to-side cavo-cavostomy: a useful aid in "complicated" piggy-back liver transplantation. Transpl Int. 1993;6:299–301.
31. Belghiti J, Panis Y, Sauvanet A, et al. A new technique of side to side caval anastomosis during orthotopic hepatic transplantation without inferior vena caval occlusion. Surg Gynecol Obstet. 1992; 175:270–2.
32. Lerut J, Gordon RD, Starzl TE, et al. Biliary tract complications in human orthotopic liver transplantation. Transplantation. 1987;43:47–51.
33. Urdazpal L, Gores G, Ward E, et al. Diagnostic features and clinical outcome of ischemic-type biliary complications after liver transplantation. Hepatology. 1993;17:605–9.
34. Zalinski S, Soubrane O, Scatton O. Reducing biliary morbidity in full graft deceased donor liver transplantation: is it really a matter of T-tube? Ann Surg. 2010;252:570–1.
35. Lin TS, Concejero AM, Chen CL, et al. Routine microsurgical biliary reconstruction decreases early anastomotic complications in living donor liver transplantation. Liver Transpl. 2009;15:1766–75.
36. Sutcliffe R, Maguire D, Heaton N, et al. Bile duct strictures after adult liver transplantation: a role for biliary reconstructive surgery? Liver Transpl. 2004;10:928–34.
37. Kim JH, Kim KW, Lee SG, et al. Effect of splenic artery embolization for splenic artery steal syndrome in liver transplant recipients: estimation at computed tomography based on changes in caliber of related arteries. Transplant Proc. 2011;43:1790–3.
38. Yersiz H, Renz JF, Busuttil RW. One hundred in situ split-liver transplantations: a single-center experience. Ann Surg. 2003;238:496–505.
39. Gundlach M, Broering D, Topp S, et al. Split-cava technique: liver splitting for two adult recipients. Liver Transpl. 2000;6:703–6.
40. Kasahara M, Sakamoto S, Shigeta T, et al. Reducing the thickness of left lateral segment grafts in neonatal living donor liver transplantation. Liver Transpl. 2013;19:226–8.
41. Pinheiro RS, Lai Q, Lerut J, et al. Complex hepatic outflow reconstruction in domino liver transplantation. Hepatobiliary Pancreat Dis Int. 2014;13:98–100.
42. Boudjema K, Jaeck D, Siméoni U, et al. Temporary auxiliary liver transplantation for subacute liver failure in a child. Lancet. 1993;25(342):778–9.
43. Bismuth H, Azoulay D, Castaing D, et al. Auxiliary partial orthotopic liver transplantation for fulminant hepatitis. The Paul Brousse experience. Ann Surg. 1996;224:712–24.
44. Lodge JP, Prasad KR, Toogood GJ, et al. Auxiliary orthotopic liver transplantation: new technique and results in toxic liver injury. Transplant Proc. 2001;33:1403–4.
45. Azoulay D, Samuel D, Bismuth H, et al. Auxiliary partial orthotopic versus standard orthotopic whole liver transplantation for acute liver failure: a reappraisal from a single center by a case-control study. Ann Surg. 2001;234:723–31.
46. Makuuchi M, Sugawara Y. Living-donor liver transplantation using the left liver, with special reference to vein reconstruction. Transplantation. 2003;75:S23–4.
47. Hwang S, Lee SG, Ahn CS, et al. Outflow vein reconstruction of extended right lobe graft using quilt venoplasty technique. Liver Transpl. 2006;12:156–8.
48. Lee S, Hwang S, Park K, et al. An adult-to-adult living donor liver transplant using dual left lobe grafts. Surgery. 2001;129:647–50.
49. Lai Q, Avolio AW, Lerut J, et al. Alpha-fetoprotein and modified response evaluation criteria in solid tumors progression after locoregional therapy as predictors of hepatocellular cancer recurrence and death after transplantation. Liver Transpl. 2013;19:1108–18.
50. Margreiter R, Kramar R, Huber C, et al. Combined liver and kidney transplantation. Lancet. 1984;12(1):1077–8.
51. Starzl TE. Immunosuppressive therapy and tolerance of organ allografts. N Engl J Med. 2008;24(358): 407–11.

References Combined Transplantation

52. Olausson M, Mjörnstedt L, Nordén G, et al. Successful combined partial auxiliary liver and kidney transplantation in highly sensitized cross-match positive recipients. Am J Transplant. 2007;7:130–6.
53. Starzl TE, Bilheimer DW, Bahnson HT, et al. Heart-liver transplantation in a patient with familial hypercholesterolaemia. Lancet. 1984;23(1):1382–3.
54. Corno V, Dezza MC, Colledan M, et al. Combined double lung-liver transplantation for cystic fibrosis without cardio-pulmonary by-pass. Am J Transplant. 2007;7:2433–8.
55. Starzl TE, Todo S, Tzakis A, et al. The many faces of multivisceral transplantation. Surg Gynecol Obstet. 1991;172:335–44.
56. Abu-Elmagd KM, Kosmach-Park B, Costa G, et al. Long-term survival, nutritional autonomy, and quality of life after intestinal and multivisceral transplantation. Ann Surg. 2012;256:494–508.

Reference Abdominal Wall Transplantation

57. Selvaggi G, Pinna AD, Tzakis AG, et al. Abdominal wall transplantation: surgical and immunologic aspects. Transplant Proc. 2009;41:521–2.

Reference Uterus Transplantation

58. Brännström M, Johannesson L, Dahm-Kähler P, et al. First clinical uterus transplantation trial: a six-month report. Fertil Steril. 2014;101:1228–36.

41 Small Bowel Transplantation: Is There a Hope on the Horizon?

Baris Dogu Yildiz

Introduction

The small intestine is the major site for the absorption of nutrients. The minimum length of intestine necessary to maintain nutritional status has not been established, but approximately 10–20 cm of small intestine with an ileocecal valve and approximately 40 cm without an ileocecal valve are considered adequate [1]. Function of the intestine is also dependent on the morphology of the intestinal mucosa and other factors such as gut motility, gut hormones, biliary and fat metabolism, and intestinal microflora.

Intestinal failure (IF) can be defined as the critical reduction of functional gut mass below the minimal amount necessary for adequate digestion and absorption to satisfy body nutrient and fluid requirements in adults or children. IF itself is a general term used in combination with short bowel syndrome (SBS) which is characterized by a state of malabsorption following extensive resection of the small bowel.

SBS may occur after resection of more than 50 % and is certain after resection of more than 70 % of the small intestine, or if less than 100 cm of small bowel is left [2]. It is particularly severe after resection of the ileocecal region or if the colon has been removed. Function is not dependent on length alone, since 150 cm of diseased bowel might function worse than 75 cm of healthy intestine. For this reason, some definitions of SBS and IF have been based on measurements of the functional capacity of the remaining bowel. Intestinal failure prevents oral nutrition and may be associated with mortality and morbidity.

Symptoms of intestinal failure include persistent diarrhea, dehydration, muscle wasting, poor growth, frequent infections, weight loss, and fatigue which significantly affect the quality of life of the patient. After the insult on the gastrointestinal system, intestines show an adaptation process. This intestinal adaptation process in SBS has three phases. The acute phase serves for the patient's stabilization and starts directly after resection and generally lasts less than 4 weeks. The second phase is the adaptation phase, which lasts 1–2 years and represents maximal stimulation of intestinal adaptation achieved by gradually increasing intestinal nutrient exposure. The last phase is the maintenance phase, which requires permanent individualized dietetic treatment [3].

Several conditions requiring intestinal resection lead to SBS in adults. In a reported series of 210 cases, these conditions included 52

B.D. Yildiz, M.D. (✉)
Department of General Surgery and Transplant Surgery, Ankara Numune Teaching Hospital, Ankara, Turkey
e-mail: baris104@yahoo.com

R. Latifi et al. (eds.), *Technological Advances in Surgery, Trauma and Critical Care*,
DOI 10.1007/978-1-4939-2671-8_41

postoperative (25 %), 51 irradiation/cancer (24 %), 46 mesenteric vascular disease (22 %), 34 Crohn's disease (16 %), and 27 other benign causes (13 %) [4].

Causes of IF in children include SBS, congenital diseases of enterocyte development, and severe motility disorders (total or subtotal aganglionosis or chronic intestinal pseudo-obstruction syndrome).

Small Bowel Transplantation for the Treatment of Intestinal Failure

Small bowel transplantation (SBTx) is the transplantation of an intestinal allograft for the purpose of restoring intestinal function in patients with irreversible intestinal failure. Several features of the small bowel make it unique among transplantable organs: (1) the large amount of lymphoid tissue (mesenteric lymph nodes, Peyer's patches, and lamina propria) (2) heavy colonization with microorganisms, and (3) expression of large quantities of class II antigens on the surface of epithelial cells. Difficulties in transplanting small bowel in humans were first recognized in the 1960s [5].

In 1987, a 3½-year-old girl lived for more than 6 months after receiving a multiorgan transplant for short-gut syndrome which is considered to be the first extended survival of an intestinal transplant [6]. But the first successful isolated intestinal transplant was performed in 1988 by Deltz and coworkers in Germany. After that, successful outcomes were reported by Goulet from France and Grant from Canada. Between 1985 and 1990 a total of 15 small intestine transplantations were performed using cyclosporine but unfortunately graft survival time in these cases ranged from 10 days to 49 months [7].

Further efforts involving seven adults with SBS who had small bowel transplantation did not survive more than 76 days after the operation despite anti-lymphoglobulins, corticosteroids, and azathioprine [8].

The development of tacrolimus and combination of SBTx with liver transplantation have made SBTx a promising option for the treatment of end-stage intestinal failure. Indications for SBTx in children and adults are shown in Table 41.1 [3].

Table 41.1 Indications for bowel transplantation in children and adults in descending order

Children	Adults
Gastroschisis	Ischemia
Volvulus	Crohn's disease
Necrotizing enterocolitis	Trauma
Pseudo-obstruction	Volvulus
Intestinal atresia	Motility disorders
Aganglionosis/Hirschsprung	Desmoids
Retransplant	Retransplant
Microvillus inclusion	Miscellaneous
Malabsorption	Gardner's syndrome
Tumors	

Used with permission from Yildiz BD.Where are we at with short bowel syndrome and small bowel transplant. World J Transplant. 2012 Dec 24;2(6):95–103

Table 41.2 Contraindications to small bowel transplant

Absolute contraindications
Neurological disabilities
Life-threatening disease unrelated to the digestive system
Non-resectable malignancy
Relative contraindications
Severe immunological deficiencies
Multisystem autoimmune diseases
Inadequate vascular anatomy to warrant long-term patency
Prematurity with lung disease

Used with permission from Yildiz BD.Where are we at with short bowel syndrome and small bowel transplant. World J Transplant. 2012 Dec 24;2(6):95–103

Contraindications

Contraindications to SBTx include non-resectable or disseminated malignancy, unreconstructable vascular anatomy, diseases that are likely to recur after transplantation, profound disabilities that will not be corrected by transplantation, loss of vascular access sufficient to allow transplantation, or an inability or unwillingness to comply with the post-transplant management plan (Table 41.2) [3].

Techniques in Small Bowel Transplantation

Operative Technique Summary

Initial step is to assess the patients to ensure that the selection criteria are met (Table 41.3) and to rule out potential contraindications to the transplant procedure.

Cadaveric donors are used in most SBTx, although successful procedures have been performed with an allograft from living related donors.

Intestinal grafts are obtained from blood group compatible donors. Selection criteria for cadaveric donors include blood group ABO match, hemodynamic stability without excessive inotropic requirements, and compatible size match enabling placement of the graft within the peritoneal cavity. Some SBTx centers require a negative lymphocytotoxic cross-match and cytomegalovirus serology match.

During procurement intestinal decontamination is done in all donors with amphotericin B, an aminoglycoside, polymyxin, and broad-spectrum antibiotics. In situ perfusion with University of Wisconsin preservation solution is performed with venous bed decompression.

A cold ischemia time of less than 10 h is recommended to avoid preservation injury of the intestinal allograft. Ischemia of the intestinal graft increases the risk of bacterial translocation by disruption of the mucosal barrier and the risk of early rejection. The procurement method and intraluminal washing technique vary among surgical teams [9, 10]. Intraluminal washing at +4 °C with a storage solution containing antibacterial and antifungal agent is useful. Although University of Wisconsin solution is the most widely used solution during procurement, satisfactory preservation of intestinal morphology and enzyme activities after 8 h of cold ischemia was shown in experimental studies using Ringer's and Euro-Collins solutions. The author of this chapter personally prefers University of solution for all multivisceral organ procurements including small bowel.

The size of the allograft also has to be taken into account. In cases where the recipient has undergone extensive resection of the small bowel, the reduced volume of the abdominal cavity implies the use of allografts from donors with a lower body weight. Length can be reduced according to the size of the abdominal cavity, although the entire small bowel is often transplanted.

Transplant Procedure

Different techniques are required for the vascular reconstruction of each type of intestinal transplant. For isolated SBTx, the arterial supply is established by an end to side anastomosis to the infrarenal aorta; the superior mesenteric vein is anastomosed to the recipient superior mesenteric vein or the inferior vena cava. Routing the venous outflow via portal drainage provides first-pass delivery of hepatotropic substances to the recipient liver and filtering of translocated organisms by the native liver. It is also postulated that portal drainage provides protection from rejection [11].

Combined small bowel-liver grafts are removed en bloc, connected by the portal vein, superior mesenteric vein, and an aortic segment containing the celiac artery and the superior mesenteric artery [12]. The duodenum and the head of the pancreas are included with the graft to avoid the need for biliary reconstruction. The aortic segment is anastomosed to the infrarenal aorta of the recipient. The end of the native portal vein is anastomosed to the side of the donor portal vein or to the inferior vena cava.

Table 41.3 Selection criteria for small bowel transplantation

Absence of acute or chronic active infections that are not effectively treated
Adequate cardiovascular function (ejection fraction greater than or equal to 40 %)
No active alcohol or chemical dependency that interferes with compliance to a strict treatment regimen
No uncontrolled and/or untreated psychiatric disorders that interfere with compliance to a strict treatment regimen
Absence of inadequately controlled HIV/AIDS

There are many variants of intestinal anastomosis [13]. However, two principles must be followed: (1) exteriorization of the graft, (2) permanent flow of gastric and biliopancreatic secretions through the graft which prevent intraluminal stasis and bacterial proliferation/translocation. The proximal end of the intestinal graft is anastomosed to the native bowel. The distal end of the small bowel graft is exteriorized as a stoma or anastomosed to the native colon. A loop ileostomy (i.e., chimney) is created to divert the stool away from the intestinal anastomosis and provide access for biopsies. The ileostomy is closed after 3–6 months. The donor colon is usually removed because it appears to increase the incidence of rejection and sepsis. If recipient has nonfunctional colon due to a primary disease such as intestinal pseudo-obstruction or had a colectomy, it is preferable to limit colon grafting to the cecum and ascending colon only.

Isolated SBTx is done with or without the large intestine and is more commonly performed in adults [14]. With isolated SBTx the entire jejunum and ileum are transplanted in the majority of cases. If the intestine is donated by a living donor or when reduction of the size of the graft is required, a 200 cm segment is usually transplanted. In order to close the abdomen properly, it is important to match sizes of donor and recipient. Native bowel and allograft bowel must be preserved as much as possible because this provides protection from parenteral nutrition associated injury. The rationale behind this is the fact that these patients will need parenteral nutrition until allograft becomes functional. When SBTx is performed en bloc, duodenum with pancreas may be included (Omaha technique) to avoid the need for biliary reconstruction [13].

Multivisceral Transplantation

Multivisceral transplantation (MTx) is the removal and replacement of both native foregut and midgut. In MTx, the native abdominal viscera are resected and the composite graft including the stomach, pancreaticoduodenal complex, and small intestine are transplanted en bloc. The donors for MTx are cadaveric only. The liver, kidneys, and large intestine of the donor may or may not be included depending on the primary disease process.

The use of MTx is increasing and the 1-year graft and patient survival is at least as good as the other forms of SBTx [15].

Combined Liver and Small Bowel Transplantation

Combined small bowel-liver (SLTx) transplantation is recommended for patients with irreversible failure of both the small bowel and the liver [16]. SLTx is more commonly performed in children. The two organs can be transplanted at the same session or sequentially from the same or a different donor. Concomitant liver failure induced by parenteral nutrition is the usual reason for this type of transplant.

Living and Non-heart-Beating Donors

The technical aspects of living donor intestinal transplantation (LDIT) were standardized by Gruessner [17]. The donor operation consists of harvesting 200 cm (150 cm for pediatric recipients) of distal ileum, preserving at least 20 cm of terminal ileum and ileocecal valve. The vascular pedicle of the graft is formed by the distal branches of the superior mesenteric artery and vein and is anastomosed to the infrarenal aorta and cava of the recipient. LDIT has several potential advantages, such as elimination of waiting time, the elective nature of the procedure, better human leukocyte antigen (HLA) matching, and a short cold ischemia time. LDIT is usually performed with well HLA-matched grafts. The significance of HLA matching in SBTx is still to be determined. In fact, experienced programs have obtained good outcomes and low rates of rejection with poorly matched deceased SBTx. A significant risk of antibody-mediated graft injury in settings of positive cross-match has been demonstrated. A significant reduction of ischemia time has been achieved in the settings of LDIT.

When the intestinal graft is harvested from non-heart beating donors (NHBD), the infection-related mortality was higher and the absorptive function was lower secondary to the fact that intestinal mucosa is sensitive to ischemic injury. Histological examinations confirmed a higher grade of ischemic injury in the NHBD grafts that correlated with the clinical data. Experimental studies suggest that non-heart-beating donation may not be indicated for small bowel transplantation [18].

Classical Immunosuppression (IS) in Small Bowel Transplantation

As with other types of solid organ transplants, IS regimens for SBTx vary from center to center [19]. Many therapies and combinations of IS have been used for SBTx, but what remains undefined are the optimal IS regimens to achieve the required goals while preserving graft function and not predisposing the recipient to increased infections or malignancy. Tacrolimus is the drug that allowed the development of a consistently successful intestinal transplant series and today it is the maintenance IS drug of choice.

Most centers manage patients with a triple regimen for baseline IS including a calcineurin inhibitor (tacrolimus), corticosteroids (usually methylprednisolone), and an antiproliferative agent (usually mycophenolate mofetil) [20, 21].

After SBTx, tacrolimus can be administered immediately as a continuous intravenous infusion, at a dose of 0.05–0.1 mg/kg per day and dose is adjusted with blood levels daily. Tacrolimus is administered orally at a dose of 0.2–0.3 mg/kg twice daily after intestines start functioning. Methylprednisolone is always simultaneously prescribed but in variable doses. Mycophenolate mofetil dose is usually given at 1,000 mg twice daily or its counterpart mycophenolic acid with less gastrointestinal side effects at equivalent doses (i.e., 720 mg twice daily).

Newer Immunosuppression Drugs

The most significant difference of IS in SBTx is the prompt use of induction IS therapy in almost 90 % of cases as part of the overall regimen. The most common induction IS agents are anti-IL2-receptor antibody (*daclizumab*, *basiliximab*) and monoclonal antibody (*alemtuzumab*). Their use has been associated with a reduction in the incidence and severity of rejection episodes and an improvement of survival, which allowed use of lower levels of tacrolimus. This latter issue has become important because there is now increasing evidence of calcineurin-inhibitor toxicities in patients receiving non-renal transplants. Conversion to non-calcineurin-inhibitor drugs such as rapamycin, use of steroid sparing protocols, and determination as to which IS therapy best maintains graft acceptance still need explanation.

Sirolimus (rapamycin) was also studied as an additional IS in SBTx. In a study, authors compared 21 patients with SBTx who received daclizumab, tacrolimus, and steroid with 16 SBTx patients who received sirolimus in addition to sirolimus, basiliximab, tacrolimus, and steroids. The addition of sirolimus to the immunosuppressive regimen after SBTx resulted in fewer early rejections (17 % vs. 68 % in the first 30 days) and no exfoliative rejection. Thus sirolimus did not increase morbidity but improved 1-year patient and graft survival [22].

Bone Marrow Infusion and Ex Vivo Radiation

It was shown in 1990s that bone marrow infusion (BMI) was beneficial in augmenting chimerism in both clinical and experimental SBTx studies [23, 24].

Abu-Elmagd et al. recovered bone marrow cells from the thoracolumbar vertebrae of small bowel donors and gave a single intravenous dose of $3–5 \times 10^8$ donor cells/kg to the recipients over 20 min within the first 12 h after revascularization. The 1- and 5-year recipient and graft survival rates in the BMI group were 79 % and 74 %, and 68 % and 62 % respectively. Post-transplant lymphoproliferative disease risk in 1 year was also low in BMI group [7].

Recent experimental data suggested that low-dose graft irradiation when combined with donor-specific bone marrow transfusions may have a beneficial effect on graft outcome. In an attempt to prevent graft versus host disease (GVHD), ex vivo intestinal allograft irradiation was also tested at the Pittsburgh program. The intestine of 11 allografts for 10 primary recipients was irradiated with a single dose of 750 cGy prior to the transplant [25].

Post-transplant Care

Postoperative management of intestinal transplant recipients includes three important steps: (a) immunosuppression, (b) anti-infective prophylaxis, and (c) assessment of the graft.

After the initial 2 weeks, it is possible to initiate oral feeding with an isotonic dipeptide solution enriched with medium chain triglycerides and glutamine, changing to a gluten- and lactose-free diet within 2–4 weeks, and eventually progressing to a normal diet [26].

The mean length of stay in hospital for intestinal transplant was reported to be 59.5 ± 56 days for isolated intestinal transplant, 81.8 ± 79 days for intestine-liver transplant, and 83.5 ± 56 days for multivisceral transplant.

After discharge, patients need regular follow-up at transplant clinics and close monitoring. They may need hospital readmission for treatment of complications associated with intestinal transplantation.

Infection After Small Bowel Transplantation

Despite the use of prophylactic antimicrobial agents, infection with uncontrolled sepsis is still the leading cause of morbidity and mortality following intestinal transplant. Intestinal transplant recipients are predisposed to severe bacterial, viral, and fungal infections because of the high levels of immunosuppression, presence of pre-existing infection, and the potential for bacterial translocation from the graft during periods of stress such as ischemia, reperfusion, and rejection. The Intestinal Transplant Registry identified sepsis as the leading cause of post-intestinal transplant deaths worldwide (51.3 %) [27]. This is five times as high as the mortality rate due to rejection, the second most common cause of death. Bacterial and fungal infections are the most common infections with an incidence of 93 %. The most common organisms identified are pseudomonas and candida.

Translocation of microorganisms from the gastrointestinal tract has been demonstrated in human studies and has been suggested to be the mechanism responsible for the high rate of infection occurring after small bowel transplantation. Cicalese et al. studied the correlation of bacterial translocation and various factors in 50 pediatric small bowel transplant recipients with a mean follow-up of 30 ± 10 months (range: 20 days–6 years). Blood, stool, liver biopsies, and peritoneal fluid were collected and cultured using standard microbiologic techniques as part of follow-up or when infection was clinically suspected. A bacteria translocation episode is determined when microorganisms are found simultaneously in blood or liver biopsy and feces. Approximately 4,000 cultures were evaluated in the study. The results showed that acute rejection was not accompanied by an increased bacteria translocation rate. The inclusion of colon in the allograft significantly increased fecal bacterial count (100 % cultures vs. 84.6 % cultures $>1\times10^6$ CFU) and bacterial translocation rate (75 % of patients vs 33 % of patients) compared to transplants without the colon. Bacteria translocation was observed in a significantly higher number when cold ischemia time is longer than 9 h compared to cold ischemia time of less than 9 h (76 % vs. 20.8 %, $p=0.002$) [28].

Viral Infections

Cytomegalovirus (CMV) is the most common viral infections in intestinal transplant recipients

[29]. The allograft is more susceptible than other organs to viral infections because of the aberrant immune response within the allograft, local graft versus host reaction, or host versus graft reaction. Besides, the intestine contains a large number of donor leukocytes that might contain latent CMV. The 1997 report of the Intestinal Transplant Registry [27] showed that CMV infection rates for ISB, SB-L, and MV transplants were 24 %, 18 %, and 40 %, respectively. It was shown that CMV disease was associated with a significant increase in mortality and shorter survival among SBTx recipients. Time to death was shorter in patients with CMV enteritis and allograft rejection, while CMV prophylaxis with antiviral drug ganciclovir showed a trend to longer time to death. But prophylaxis with antiviral drugs is associated with the potential threat of nephrotoxicity, myelotoxicity, or development of resistance. Thus, it was suggested that low viral infection rates could be achieved without aggressive antiviral prophylaxis.

Epstein–Barr viral (EBV) infection is one of the most serious consequences of immunosuppressive management in transplantation [30]. EBV often leads to potentially life-threatening ß-cell PTLD. Diverse incidences between 11 and 48 % of EBV infections have been reported in literature. PTLD is the most common cause of late graft loss in intestinal transplantation with a greater incidence than in any other type of solid organ transplantation and with a different time of onset. Virological monitoring of EBV infection must be continued in SBTx patients to prevent EBV-related PTLD.

Several studies have suggested that human herpes virus-6 (HHV-6) has significant indirect immunomodulatory effects that outweigh direct clinical effects in SBTx [31, 32]. These effects may result in further opportunistic infections and promote CMV replication. More significant disease among patients co-infected with CMV can be anticipated. As HHV-6 infection usually occurs earlier than CMV or EBV, it may serve as an indicator for more intense virological surveillance, and regular HHV-6 monitoring is recommended during the first 2 months after transplantation.

Strategies for Controlling CMV and EBV Infections in Patients with Small Bowel Transplantation

Ganciclovir has been used as a prophylactic antiviral agent program. A dose of 5 mg/kg is administered twice per day for 14 days, followed by 6 mg/kg IV daily [33]. Thereafter, patients can be switched to oral acyclovir at a dose of 40 mg/kg per day until 2 years after transplant. As an adjunct to ganciclovir, CMV-specific hyperimmune globulin has also been added to the early postoperative antiviral prophylaxis for high-risk patients.

Over the last 5 years, surveillance for CMV and EBV has improved with the development of more sensitive polymerase chain reaction (PCR) assays of peripheral blood to detect virus-specific DNA, allowing for preemptive treatment prior to the development of the infection [34]. The CMV structural protein, pp65 antigenemia test has been used for early detection of reactivation or de novo CMV and has improved the preemptive treatment of the virus. The surveillance protocol includes PCR assay weekly during hospitalization, monthly during the first outpatient year, and every 4 months thereafter [35]. Positive PCR prompts preemptive therapy with ganciclovir. Persistent viremia or intolerance to therapy is treated with CMV IV immunoglobulin. Patients also undergo periodic physical examination, endoscopy, and biopsy. More effective antiviral agents against CMV are now available. Serologic status of recipients and donor is important although some programs are less restrictive about CMV status mismatches between donor and recipient.

Rejection

Risk factors identified for acute rejection were use of small bowel grafts alone when compared with composite grafts, and positive lymphocytotoxic cross-match [36]. The incidence of rejection in the liver of composite grafts is less than half the incidence in the intestine. The diagnosis of intestinal acute cellular rejection (ACR) requires close correlation of clinical, endoscopic, and pathologic findings [37]. The clinical symptoms of intestinal ACR include fever, nausea, vomiting, increased stomal output, abdominal pain, and distension. In severe cases, acute rejection may manifest as septic shock, with metabolic acidosis, hypotension, and adult respiratory distress syndrome, which likely results from loss of mucosal integrity and bacterial translocation across the intestinal wall.

The ileum is the most commonly involved site. However, graft involvement can be patchy and involvement of proximal small bowel without affecting the ileum occurs in 20–25 % of rejection episodes [38].

Most transplant programs monitor and diagnose rejection in the intestinal allograft by twice weekly serial surveillance endoscopy and endoscopy-guided multiple mucosal biopsies [7]. General endoscopic signs of rejection include mucosal edema, erythema, friability, and focal ulceration. Signs of severe rejection are a granular mucosal pattern with diffuse ulceration, mucosal sloughing, and absence of peristalsis. Chronic rejection is diagnosed on the basis of histologic examination of full-thickness enteric specimens [39].

Acute rejection is usually treated with a steroid bolus and increasing the daily tacrolimus dose to achieve higher trough levels. OKT3 or thymoglobulin is reserved for the treatment of steroid-resistant and severe rejections. About 12–25 % of rejections are reported to be refractory to these treatments, resulting in enterectomy (12–20 %) [40].

Chronic rejection occurs as a consequence of persistent episodes of refractory acute rejections and manifests clinically with persistent abdominal pain and intestinal dysmotility. Cumulated risk of graft loss from acute and chronic rejection of isolated small bowel allografts is significantly greater than that of small bowel-liver and multivisceral transplants and the risk is not significantly reduced by the use of IL-2 receptor antibodies.

Graft vs. Host Disease

Graft vs. host disease (GVHD) has the highest occurrence after small intestine transplantation (7–13 %) [41]. The amount of lymphoid tissue in the small bowel is much higher compared with other solid organ transplants, and this may explain the fact that the rate of GVHD in the recipients of small bowel transplants is increased. The organs mainly involved are skin, native gastrointestinal tract, bone marrow, lungs, and liver.

Therapy consists mainly of increasing IS, support of hematopoiesis with cytokines, and discontinuation of antibiotics or any drugs that might be myelosuppressive. However, it is difficult to determine whether this is effective, as mortality normally exceeds more than 75 %. Approximately 86 cases have been reported in the literature since 1987, and among them only 18 patients survived [42]. In 13 of the survivors, IS had been increased, while in 5 other cases, IS had been withdrawn. It could be argued that reducing IS and allowing the patient's immune system to have the opportunity to reject the engrafting donor lymphocytes as well as helping the patient to respond to infections could be an effective method of treatment. Any treatment is more likely to work if it is begun before the onset of severe pancytopenia. Other than modifying immunosuppression, currently there are no other new therapies.

Post-transplant Lymphoproliferative Disorder

The vast majority of PTLDs are EBV driven and arise either as a consequence of the reactivation of latent infection or, more commonly, infection of the host by latent virus from donor B cells. The particularly high incidence of PTLD reported after ITx is a consequence of the high levels of IS traditionally used to prevent GVHD and rejection, along with the fact that a large load of donor lymphocytes is transplanted with the graft. The gastrointestinal tract is frequently affected and it is important to distinguish between PTLD and other causes of graft infiltration, including rejection. In situ hybridization of tumor tissue for EBV RNA is a quick and sensitive way of confirming the diagnosis. It is crucial to distinguish PTLD from rejection because many patients will respond to a reduction in IS alone. If this fails, second-line treatment includes antivirals, chemotherapy, or interferon-α.

Experimental treatment using immunotherapy with donor leukocytes or specific anti-EBV-specific cytotoxic T lymphocytes may be effective in aggressive cases.

Patient Survival and Graft Survival

There has been a striking improvement in patient and graft survival in SBTx over the last decade. In 2001 Intestinal Transplant Registry data showed that actuarial graft survival rates of the total international experience at 5 years post-transplantation were 45 % for isolated SBTx, 43 % for combined intestine-liver transplants, and 30 % for multivisceral transplantation.

In a recent article published in 2009 by Mazariegos et al. 1-, 3-, and 5-year patient survival rates were 95 %, 84 %, and 77 % and corresponding graft survival rates were 88 %, 74 %, and 58 % in SBTx [43].

The improvement in patient and graft survival is associated with recipients not needing care at a facility prior to transplantation, use of induction chemotherapy, and transplantation at a high volume center (>10 transplants/year). High volume centers have standardized pre-transplantation evaluation and preparation protocols. Improved immunosuppression regimens have led to decreased rates of ACR and the use of surveillance protocols for opportunistic infections, including blood monitoring of cytomegalovirus and Epstein–Barr virus viral loads, has led to better titration of immunosuppression with decreased incidence of infections.

Quality of Life After Small Bowel Transplantation

The successful emergence of small bowel transplantation as a curative alternative has provided many patients with bowel failure to have an improved QOL, better nutrition, and a reduction in PN-associated complications. Since the initial small bowel transplants first performed in the 1980s, there have been technical improvements, novel immunosuppressive agents, better understanding of immune and gastrointestinal physiology, and increased clinical program experience. All of these factors have contributed to a remarkable improvement in bowel transplant, 1-year graft, and patient survival (estimated 80 % and 80 %, respectively), compared with only several years ago [44].

Intestinal transplant can pose challenges to patients. For approximately 6–12 months post-transplantation, care routines for patients may include 7–15 daily medications, tube feedings, intravenous fluids, and maintenance of the gastrostomy tube, jejunostomy tube, ostomy, and other catheters. The most common reasons for readmission after SBTx are infection, surgical procedures, and acute rejection. Almost 90 % of all recipients are free of ileostomy and median time to ostomy closure rarely exceeds 12 months [45].

Rovera et al. compared quality of life in a group of patients receiving home parenteral nutrition (HPN) to a group that had undergone SBTx. A significant improvement in quality of life was noted in the transplantation group compared to their pre-transplantation status when ill and receiving HPN. Of greater importance, when comparing transplantation patients with a group of patients who were stable and receiving HPN, the quality of life was similar between the two groups in spite of frequent complications in the early post-transplant period [46].

Clinicians from Pittsburgh studied the effect of transplantation on nutritional autonomy, organ function, and quality of life using a validated self-administered questionnaire containing 26 domains and 130 questions. They had 46 consecutively transplanted patients between June 2003 and July 2004. Their mean follow-up was 21 months. There was a significant improvement in the overall assessment of quality of life indicators in 13 of 26 specific domains examined leading to a conclusion that SBTx has a potential to become an alternative to home parenteral nutrition rather than a last resort [47].

Overall, 71–100 % of surviving small bowel transplant recipients were able to wean from parenteral nutrition at 20–39 days after transplant. Most patients were able to meet all caloric needs enterally, with enteral or parenteral supplementation during periods of illness [1].

Growth and Development

Sudan et al. reported that growth appeared normal in 50 % of 27 children with greater than 1-year graft survival. An additional 11 % maintained pre-transplant growth at <10th percentile and 15 % demonstrated catch-up growth. Sixty-three percent of children required special education services, speech therapy, or physical therapy. Eighty-four percent of children have been able to return to preschool, day care, or school at the appropriate level for their development and many report participation in extracurricular activities including sports, dance, and scouts [45].

Parents of pediatric SBTx recipients report significant limitations in the physical and psychological well-being of their children compared with normal school children. The pediatric SBTx recipients themselves report a quality of life similar to other school children.

Conclusion

Intestinal transplant is a high cost and low volume procedure. For patients who can no longer continue home parenteral nutrition due to life-threatening complications associated with this therapy, SBTx offers the only viable alternative. The majority of patients who survived SBTx were able to discontinue total parenteral nutrition and receive the required nutrients enterally. Limited evidence suggests that the quality of life of these patients is equivalent to that of patients on home parenteral nutrition.

Although much improvement in patient outcomes has been observed since 1995 and better outcomes were reported at more experienced centers, SBTx is still associated with significant patient mortality (overall 37–45 % in the first year) and morbidity as a result of infection, rejection, and PTLD. The procedure is also associated with high rates (45–66 %) of reoperations after transplant. These outcomes are inferior to those reported for home enteral nutrition. For the above reasons, home enteral nutrition remains the treatment of choice for individuals with intestinal failure who can tolerate this treatment.

There has been no head-to-head comparison between small bowel transplant and home enteral nutrition because small bowel transplant has only been performed in patients with intestinal failure who could no longer continue total parenteral nutrition. There is no evidence to support small bowel transplantation in patients with intestinal failure who can be treated with parenteral nutrition.

The evidence can only be obtained from case series and international registry. Since intestinal transplant has been used as a last-resort life-saving therapy, it is not likely that randomized controlled trials would be conducted on this procedure due to ethical concerns about randomization.

References

1. Health Quality Ontario. Small bowel transplant: an evidence-based analysis. Ont Health Technol Assess Ser. 2003;3(1):1–72.
2. Dudrick SJ, Latifi R, Fosnocht DE. Management of the short-bowel syndrome. Surg Clin North Am. 1991;71(3):625–43.
3. Yildiz BD. Where are we at with short bowel syndrome and small bowel transplant. World J Transplant. 2012;2(6):95–103.
4. Thompson JS, DiBaise JK, Iyer KR, Yeats M, Sudan DL. Postoperative short bowel syndrome. J Am Coll Surg. 2005;201:85–9.
5. Kocoshis SA. Small bowel transplantation in infants and children. Gastroenterol Clin North Am. 1994;23(4):727–42.
6. Starzl TE, Rowe MI, Todo S, Jaffe R, Tzakis A, Hoffman AL, Esquivel C, Porter KA, Venkataramanan R, Makowka L. Transplantation of multiple abdominal viscera. JAMA. 1989;261(10):1449–57.
7. Abu-Elmagd K, Reyes J, Bond G, Mazariegos G, Wu T, Murase N, Sindhi R, Martin D, Colangelo J, Zak M, Janson D, Ezzelarab M, Dvorchik I, Parizhskaya M, Deutsch M, Demetris A, Fung J, Starzl TE. Clinical intestinal transplantation: a decade of experience at a single center. Ann Surg. 2001;234(3):404–17.
8. Schraut WH. Current status of small-bowel transplantation. Gastroenterology. 1988;94(2):525–38.
9. Todo S, Tzakis AG, Abu-Elmagd K, Reyes J, Fung JJ, Casavilla A, Nakamura K, Yagihashi A, Jain A, Murase N, Iwaki Y, Demetris AJ, Thiel DV, Starzl TE. Cadaveric small bowel and small bowel–liver transplantation in humans. Transplantation. 1992;53(2):369–76.
10. Margot A, Roskott C, Nieuwenhuijs VB, Dijkstra G, Koudstaal LG, Leuvenink HGD, Ploeg RJ. Small bowel preservation for intestinal transplantation: a review. Transpl Int. 2011;24:107–31.

11. Qian SK, Gao L-H, He H-S, Zhu XF. Vascular anastomosis and two-stage reconstruction of the gut in a living-related small bowel transplant recipient: a case report. Transplant Proc. 2007;39:3547–50.
12. Gondolesi G, Fauda M. Technical refinements in small bowel transplantation. Curr Opin Organ Transplant. 2008;13:259–65.
13. Ruiz P, Kato T, Tzakis A. Current status of transplantation of the small intestine. Transplantation. 2007; 83(1):1–6.
14. Nickkholgh A, Contin P, Abu-Elmagd K, Golriz M, Gotthardt D, Morath C, Schemmer P, Mehrabi A. Intestinal transplantation: review of operative techniques. Clin Transplant. 2013;27 Suppl 25:56–65.
15. Tzakis AG, Kato T, Levi DM, Defaria W, Selvaggi G, Weppler D, Nishida S, Moon J, Madariaga JR, David AI, Gaynor JJ, Thompson J, Hernandez E, Martinez E, Cantwell GP, Augenstein JS, Gyamfi A, Pretto EA, Dowdy L, Tryphonopoulos P, Ruiz P. 100 multivisceral transplants at a single center. Ann Surg. 2005;242(4):480–90. discussion 491–3.
16. Bhatnagar V. Current status of small bowel transplantation in children. Indian J Pediatr. 1996;63(6):761–7.
17. Gruessner RW, Sharp HL. Living-related intestinal transplantation: first report of a standardized surgical technique. Transplantation. 1997;64(11):1605–7.
18. Cobianchi L, Zonta S, Vigano J, Dominioni T, Ciccocioppo R, Morbini P, Bottazzi A, Mazzilli M, De Martino M, Vicini E, Filisetti C, Botrugno I, Dionigi P, Alessiani M. Experimental small bowel transplantation from non-heart-beating donors: a large-animal study. Transplant Proc. 2009;41(1):55–6.
19. Yandza T, Schneider SM, Canioni D, Saint-Paul MC, Gugenheim J, Chevalier P, Goubaux B, Benchimol D, Hébuterne X. Intestinal transplantation. Gastroenterol Clin Biol. 2007;31(5):469–79.
20. Al-Hussaini A, Tredger JM, Dhawan A. Immunosuppression in pediatric liver and intestinal transplantation: a closer look at the arsenal. J Pediatr Gastroenterol Nutr. 2005;41(2):152–65.
21. Trevizol AP, David AI, Dias ER, Mantovani D, Pécora R, D'Albuquerque LA. Intestinal and multivisceral transplantation immunosuppression protocols–literature review. Transplant Proc. 2012;44(8):2445–8.
22. Florman S, Gondolesi G, Schiano T, Tschernia A, LeLeiko N, Kaufman SS, Fishbein T. Improved results in small bowel transplantation using sirolimus. Transplant Proc. 2002;34(3):936.
23. Fontes P, Rao AS, Reyes J, Furukawa H, Abu-Elmagd K, Jabbour N, Zeevi A, Iyengar A, Todo S, Fung JJ, Starzl TE. Concomitant infusion of unmodified donor bone marrow into unconditioned recipients of intestinal allografts. Transplant Proc. 1996;28(5):2757–8.
24. Alessiani M, Spada M, Bonfichi M, Ferrari P, Abbiati F, Arbustini E, Morbini P, Regazzi M, Iacona I, Noli S, Scandone M, Dionigi P, Zonta A. Effect of perioperative donor bone marrow infusion after small bowel transplantation in swine: preliminary results. Transplant Proc. 1998;30(6):2577–8.
25. Ishikawa T, Iwanami K, Okuda T, Zhu Y, Fukuda A, Zhang S, Ou J, Nalesnik MA, Venkataramanan R, Murase N. Intestinal function and morphology after ex vivo irradiated small bowel transplantation. Transplant Proc. 2002;34:988–9.
26. Prasad KR, Pollard S. Small bowel transplantation. Curr Opin Gastroenterol. 2000;16(2):126–33.
27. Grant D. Intestinal transplantation: 1997 Report of the international registry. Transplantation. 1999;67:1061–4.
28. Cicalese L, Sileri P, Green M, Abu-Elmagd K, Fung JJ, Starzl TE, et al. Bacterial translocation in clinical intestinal transplantation. Transplant Proc. 2000;32:1210.
29. Péter A, Telkes G, Varga M, Járay J. Gastrointestinal cytomegalovirus infections in organ transplant patients. Orv Hetil. 2008;149(52):2463–70.
30. Green M, Michaels MG. Epstein-Barr virus infection and posttransplant lymphoproliferative disorder. Am J Transplant. 2013;13 Suppl 3:41–54.
31. Razonable RR, Rivero A, Brown RA, Hart GD, Espy MJ, van Cruijsen H, Wilson J, Groettum C, Kremers W, Smith TF, Paya CV. Detection of simultaneous beta herpesvirus infections in clinical syndromes due to defined cytomegalovirus infection. Clin Transplant. 2003;17(2):114–20.
32. American Society of Transplantation Infectious Diseases Guidelines: Other herpesviruses: HHV-6, HHV-7, HHV-8, HSV-1 and-2, VZV. Am J Transplant 2004;4 (Suppl 10):66.
33. Farmer DG, McDiarmid SV, Winston D, Yersiz H, Cortina G, Dry S, et al. Effectiveness of aggressive prophylactic and preemptive therapies targeted against cytomegaloviral and Epstein-Barr viral disease after human intestinal transplantation. Transplant Proc. 2002;34:948–9.
34. Gunson RN, Maclean AR, Shepherd SJ, Carman WF. Simultaneous detection and quantitation of cytomegalovirus, Epstein-Barr virus, and adenovirus by use of real-time PCR and pooled standards. J Clin Microbiol. 2009;47(3):765–70.
35. Florescu DF, Langnas AN, Grant W, Mercer DF, Botha J, Qiu F, Shafer L, Kalil AC. Incidence, risk factors, and outcomes associated with cytomegalovirus disease in small bowel transplant recipients. Pediatr Transplant. 2012;16:294–301.
36. Abu-Elmagd KM, Reyes J, Fung JJ, Mazariegos G, Bueno J, Martin D, Colangelo J, Rao A, Demetris A, Starzl TE. Clinical intestinal transplantation in 1998: Pittsburgh experience. Acta Gastroenterol Belg. 1999;62(2):244–7.
37. Waye JD. Small-bowel endoscopy. Endoscopy. 2003; 35(1):15–21.
38. Sigurdsson L, Reyes J, Putnam PE, del Rosario JF, Di Lorenzo C, Orenstein SR, Todo S, Kocoshis SA. Endoscopies in pediatric small intestinal transplant recipients: five years experience. Am J Gastroenterol. 1998;93:207–11.
39. Lee RG, Nakamura K, Tsamandas AC, et al. Pathology of human intestinal transplantation. Gastroenterology. 1996;110:2009–12.
40. The Intestinal Transplant Registry. Report 2001. [http://www. intestinal transplant.org/ITR_Reports/Report_2001/Report2001_slide0002. htm]. 2003.

41. Zhang Y, Ruiz P. Solid organ transplant-associated acute graft-versus-host disease. Arch Pathol Lab Med. 2010;134(8):1220–4.
42. Taylor AL, Gibbs P, Sudhindran S, Key T, Goodman RS, Morgan CH, Watson CJ, Delriviere L, Alexander GJ, Jamieson NV, et al. Monitoring systemic donor lymphocyte macrochimerism to aid the diagnosis of graft-versus-host disease after liver transplantation. Transplantation. 2004;77:441–6.
43. Mazariegos GV, Squires RH, Sindhi RK. Current perspectives on pediatric intestinal transplantation. Curr Gastroenterol Rep. 2009;11:226–33.
44. Pritchard TJ, Kirkman RL. Small bowel transplantation. World J Surg. 1985;9:860–7.
45. Sudan DL, Iverson A, Weseman RA, Kaufman S, Horslen S, Fox IJ, Shaw Jr BW, Langnas AN. Assessment of function, growth and development, and long-term quality of life after small bowel transplantation. Transplant Proc. 2000;32:1211–2.
46. Rovera GM, DiMartini A, Schoen RE, Rakela J, Abu-Elmagd K, Graham TO. Quality of life of patients after intestinal transplantation. Transplantation. 1998; 66(9):1141–5.
47. O'Keefe SJ, Emerling M, Koritsky D, Martin D, Stamos J, Kandil H, Matarese L, Bond G, Abu-Elmagd K. Nutrition and quality of life following small intestinal transplantation. Am J Gastroenterol. 2007;102(5):1093–100.

Islet Cell Transplantation: New Techniques for an Old Disease

42

Shinichi Matsumoto and Masayuki Shimoda

Introduction: Islet Cell Transplantation as a Treatment for Diabetes

Diabetes is a group of metabolic diseases characterized by hyperglycemia resulting from defects in insulin secretion, insulin action, or both [1]. Pancreatic islets consist of beta cells, alpha cells, delta cells, and PP cells, and beta cells are the only cells producing insulin. Beta-cell replacement therapy is a straightforward treatment for the diabetes caused by insulin secretory deficiency. Both whole pancreas transplantation and islet transplantation are considered as beta-cell replacement therapy. Between the two beta-cell replacement therapies, the islet transplantation is more sophisticated because only necessary cells are transplanted which leads to fewer complications related to transplantation procedures. On the other hand, the islet transplantation requires islet isolation technology which is complicated and difficult; therefore, only limited institutes can perform it. In addition, the immune suppression protocol for islet transplantation had not been well standardized. The efficacy of islet transplantation has been inferior to whole pancreas transplantation until the University of Alberta group published their protocol (Edmonton Protocol).

S. Matsumoto, M.D., Ph.D. (✉)
M. Shimoda, M.D., Ph.D.
Department of Pancreatic Islet Cell Transplantation, Research Institute, National Center for Global Health and Medicine, Tokyo, Japan
e-mail: Shinichi41@mac.com; mshimoda@hosp.ncgm.go.jp

Edmonton Protocol: Prologue of Clinical Islet Cell Transplantation

In 2000, Shapiro et al. reported that seven out of seven patients achieved insulin independence after allogeneic islet transplantation using their new protocol [2]. The protocol is called Edmonton protocol. The Edmonton protocol includes (1) multiple (2–4) islet infusions, (2) steroid-free immunosuppressants, (3) immediate transplantation without culture, and (4) Edmonton islet isolation protocol based on the Ricordi islet isolation method.

After 5 years, the same group reported that after allogeneic islet transplantation using the Edmonton protocol, only less than 10 % of the patients maintained insulin independence; however, more than 80 % of the patients maintained functional islet proven by positive C-peptide [3]. The patients with positive C-peptide could decrease hypoglycemia events and maintain excellent HbA1c results. With those outcomes, the clinical goal for the efficacy of the Edmonton protocol was changed from insulin independence to avoidance of severe hypoglycemia with excellent HbA1c.

R. Latifi et al. (eds.), *Technological Advances in Surgery, Trauma and Critical Care*,
DOI 10.1007/978-1-4939-2671-8_42

An international clinical collaborative trial of the Edmonton protocol revealed that reproducibility of the protocol is possible but not easy [4]. Only experienced institutes could demonstrate the reproducible outcomes. Ability to isolate high quality and quantity of human islets and experiences of using immune suppressants for clinical islet transplantation were considered important factors for the success of clinical islet transplantation. Human islet isolation is notoriously difficult, and even the top center could achieve the success rate of islet isolation for clinical use at a rate of approximately 50 % [5]. In addition, necessity of multiple infusions of islets exaggerates the donor shortage.

New technologies and protocols have been implemented to improve the success rate of islet isolation and efficacy of islet transplantation.

Significant Improvement of Clinical Outcome: Donor Selection, Islet Isolation Technology, and New Immunosuppression Protocol

After the success of the Edmonton protocol, the Collaborative Islet Transplant Registry (CITR) has been established to monitor the progress and safety of islet transplantation by using the data from the USA, Canada, Europe, and Australia [6]. Clinical outcomes of allogeneic islet transplantation were reported for the following time periods: 1999–2002, 2003–2006, and 2007–2010; the rates of insulin independence at 3 years after allogeneic islet infusion were 27 %, 37 %, and 44 % respectively [6]. Factors predictive of insulin independence after islet transplantation were recipient age (odds ratio, 1.04; $P<0.001$), total number of infusions (odds ratio, 1.44; $P=0.02$), islet culture period equal to or longer than 6 h (odds ratio, 1.82; $P=0.03$), stimulation index equal to or higher than 1.5 (odds ratio, 1.83; $P=0.05$), and T cell depletion and TNF-alpha inhibitor (odds ratio, 2.38; $P<0.06$). In terms of hypoglycemic events, more than 90 % of all subjects in all eras had no severe hypoglycemia. Irrespective of previous graft loss (C-peptide, <0.3 ng/mL), more than 90 % of recipients remained free of severe hypoglycemic events in all eras [6]. On the other hand, concurrent C-peptide is a strong correlate of all other outcomes: the higher the C-peptide, the greater the likelihood of HbA1c<6.5 %, fasting blood glucose in the range of 60–140 mg/dl, and the insulin independence [6]. Adequate donor pancreas and improvement of islet isolation technology have contributed greatly to this improvement.

Pancreas Donor and Preservation

Donors with stable hemodynamic have been selected as pancreas donors [2]. Recently, the University of Illinois group analyzed their 276 cases of islet isolations and found that high body mass index of donor and short cold ischemic time of a pancreas were significant factors to obtain high islet yield [7].

A heart-beating brain-dead donor is mainly used for islet transplantation; however, a donor after cardiac death (deceased cardiac death: DCD) is also used [8]. A warm ischemic injury after cardiac arrest is the major concern for using the DCD donors, and minimizing the warm ischemic time is the key for successful islet isolation.

Living-donor islet transplantation is also conducted from mother to daughter, and a half pancreas islet preparation was sufficient to achieve a sustained period of insulin independence with excellent glycemic control [9]. However, a donor faces a major surgery and possible surgical diabetes, which are concerns for the living-donor islet transplantation.

In terms of pancreas preservation before islet isolation, the UW solution has been traditionally used (Table 42.1). It was demonstrated that the two-layer pancreas preservation which consists of oxygenated perfluorocarbon and the UW solution provided the higher islet yield after islet isolation [10]. During the two-layer pancreas preservation, pancreas is oxygenated by oxygenated-perfluorocarbon, which allows generation of ATP used for maintaining the viability of preserved pancreas. More recently, a modified two-layer method, which consisted of oxygenated perfluorocarbon and the ET-Kyoto solution, was introduced before islet isolation and provided excellent clinical outcomes [11]. On the other hand, the HTK solution was shown to be equal to the UW solution in efficacy, which could save the cost for pancreas preservation [12].

Pancreatic ductal preservation could improve the success rate of clinical islet isolation [13]. The pancreatic ductal preservation is performed immediately after pancreas procurement. The ET-Kyoto solution (approximately 1 ml/g pancreas) is directly injected into the main pancreatic duct. This method improved distribution of collagenase at the time of pancreas distention with collagenase [14].

Table 42.1 Technologies for islet isolation

1. Pancreas preservation method and solution:
a. Cold storage: UW solution, HTK solution, ET-Kyoto solution
b. The two-layer method: UW/oxygenated PFC, ET-Kyoto/oxygenated PFC
c. Ductal preservation: ET-Kyoto solution
2. Clinically used collagenase for distention and Ricordi method:
a. Liberase MTF, Serva Nb1, CIzyme
3. Islet purification method:
a. Continuous density gradient using COBE 2991 cell processor
b. Continuous density gradient using large bottle method

Islet Isolation Technology

The islet isolation technology consists of pancreas distention with collagenase solution, pancreas digestion, and islet purification (Table 42.1, Fig. 42.1a–c). Selection of collagenase is one of the important factors for successful islet isolation. Previously, Liberase HI (Roche, Basel, Switzerland) was widely used. However, due to safety issues, it is no longer used. New Liberase MTF (Roche), CIzyme™ (Viacyte, San Diego, CA), and NB1 (Serva Electrophoresis, Heidelberg, Germany) are currently used.

The Ricordi method has been widely used for pancreas digestion [15]. Distended pancreas is cut into 7–10 pieces and put into Ricordi chamber. During the digestion phase, collagenase solution is recirculated in the close-loop system connected to Ricordi chamber. Once pancreas is digested and free islets are released, the digested pancreas is collected in the massive amount of dilution solution using peristaltic pump at a rate of 300 ml/min. This immediate and massive dilution can prevent over-digestion of isolated islets.

Islets are purified from the digested pancreas using the density gradient and centrifugation method. A continuous density gradient with Ficoll® (VWR, Radnor, PA) solution or iodixanol solution in the COBE® 2991 cell processor (Terumo BCT, Lakewood, CO) is widely used. Recently, it was demonstrated that a continuous

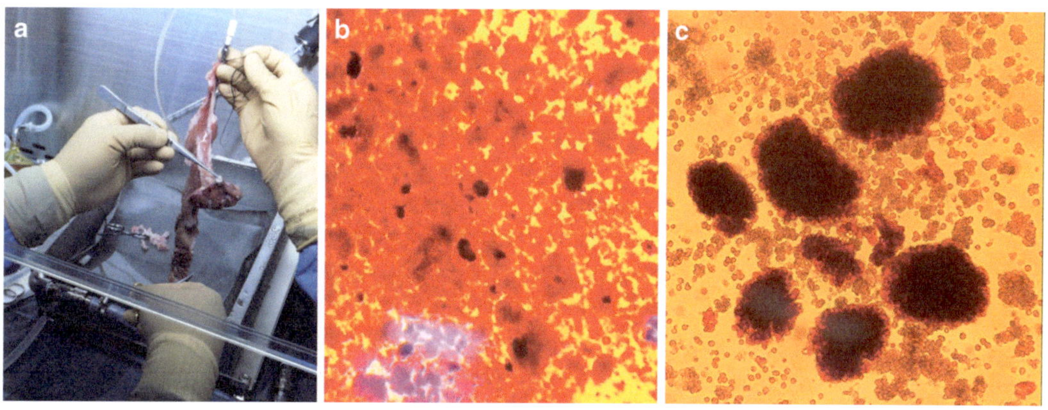

Fig. 42.1 Porcine islet isolation process. (**a**) Distended pancreas with collagenase solution. (**b**) Digested pancreas using Ricordi method. (**c**) Purified islets after the bottle purification method

Table 42.2 Published successful single-donor islet transplantation

Center	Year	Induction	Maintenance	Donor	Insulin free
Minnesota	2004	Anti-CD3	Sirolimus, Tacrolimus	Single donor	4/6
Minnesota	2005	ATC, Daclizumab, Etanercept	MMF, Sirolimus, Tacrolimus	Single donor	8/8
Miami	2005	Daclizumab	Sirolimus, Tacrolimus	1 or 2 donors	7/8
Miami	2005	Daclizumab, Infliximab	Sirolimus, Tacrolimus	1 or 2 donors	7/8
Kyoto	2005	Daclizumab	Sirolimus, Tacrolimus	Single living donor	1/1
Illinois	2008	Daclizumab, Etanercept, Exenatide	Sirolimus, Tacrolimus	Single donor	6/6
San Francisco	2010	ATG	Efalizumab, Sirolimus or MMF	1 or 2 donors	4/5
San Francisco	2010	ATG	Belatacept or Efalizumab, and Sirolimus or MMF	Single donor	3/5
Baylor	2011	ATG, Etanercept, Anakinra	Tacrolimus, MMF	Single donor	3/3

density gradient in a large bottle and centrifugation provided better islet yield [16]. The large bottle method is a simple method and avoids using an expensive COBE 2991 cell processor.

New Immunosuppression Protocol

The Edmonton protocol introduced a glucocorticoid-free immunosuppression regimen. Daclizumab is used for induction and tacrolimus and sirolimus are used for maintenance [2]. T cell depletion immunosuppression protocol substantially improved long-term islet function, and several groups achieved up to 50 % insulin independence beyond 5 years after islet transplantation, which is comparable to the pancreas alone transplantation [5].

Achieving insulin independence with single donor is another important target for islet transplantation to ameliorate the donor shortage. See Table 42.2. Hering et al. demonstrated that careful donor and recipient selection and T cell depletion using thymoglobulin or OKT-ala-ala antibody enabled them to achieve single-donor islet transplantation [17]. The Illinois group demonstrated that exenatide enables them to achieve insulin independence with single donor. Exenatide is a GLP1 analog which has several advantages for islet transplantation including enhancing of insulin-secretary ability, beta-cell proliferation, and loss of appetite. The San Francisco group introduced new immune suppression drugs, Efalizumab and Belatacept, which enables them to achieve insulin independence with single donor. Both Efalizumab and Belatacept are co-stimulatory blockage: Efalizumab blocks anti-LFA-1 and Belatacept blocks CD80-CD86 pathways. Finally, T cell depletion and potent anti-inflammation using the double blockade with IL-1 beta and TNF alpha enabled us to achieve insulin independence with single-donor islet transplantation [11]. Notably, this protocol did not use sirolimus which has notorious side effects including oral ulcer, peripheral edema, hyper lipidemia, and so on.

Next Target of Islet Cell Transplantation

Even though allogeneic islet transplantation continuously improves the clinical outcomes, this therapy never cures majority of type 1 diabetic patients due to insufficient donors. Insulin-producing cells from nonhuman donor are required to fulfill the goal. The possible nonhuman donor sources are xenografts, embryonic stem (ES) cells, and induced pluripotent stem (iPS) cells. Among the cells, xenografts derived from porcine pancreas have been clinically used since 1994 [18]. However, possible infection with porcine endogenous retrovirus (PERV) after islet xenotransplantation in SCID mice was reported, and PERV became the major concern for the porcine islet transplantation [19]. Furthermore, International Xenotransplantation Association published their statement that only a well-coordinated international effort aimed at harmonizing xenotransplantation procedures according to the highest ethical and regulatory standards on a global scale will enable the initiation of clinical xenotransplantation trials under the best auspices for its success and minimizing risk of failure [20]. In New Zealand, encapsulated neonatal porcine islet transplantation has been conducted under the comprehensive regulatory framework for the first time [21]. Thus, the islet transplantations using porcine xeno islets are already a clinical reality. Of note, porcine islet transplantation has several advantages over allogeneic transplantation besides solving donor shortage, such as well-characterized donor, scheduled procedure, and possible gene modification (Table 42.3).

In 2008, Kroon et al. demonstrated that it was possible to create insulin-secreting cells from ES cells [22]. Based on this paper, such cells have been prepared toward a clinical trial. However, the most difficult hurdle is that the ES cells are derived from human fertilized egg, which involves ethical issues.

Table 42.3 Advantages and disadvantages of porcine islet over allogeneic islet

Advantages
1. Unlimited supply of donor
2. Well-characterized (such as all designated pathogen free) donor
3. Donors are grown under a closed sterile environment with sterile and mammalian-protein-free diets
4. Scheduled islet isolation and transplantation
5. Pharmaceutical grade products
6. Possible gene modification which can improve efficacy
Disadvantages
1. Strong immune reaction
2. Possible porcine endogenous retrovirus and unknown virus infection
3. Necessity of lifelong monitoring even after completion of clinical trial
4. Limited clinical experiences

In 2007, Takahashi et al. reported the generation of human iPS cells [23]. Recently, it was demonstrated that human iPS cells can be converted into insulin-secreting cells [24]. The major hurdle of clinical use of iPS cells is safety issues, especially tumorigenicity and potential malignant conversion.

Conclusions

Islet transplantation has been continuously improved with new islet isolation technologies and immune suppression strategies, therefore becoming the standard therapy for type 1 diabetic patients in several countries. To expand this treatment, it is necessary to explore donor source other than human donors. A porcine pancreas is a promising donor source which has been clinically used. With advanced islet cell transplantation, we hope that diabetes can be converted from a non-curable disease to a curable disease.

Abbreviations

ATP	Adenosine triphosphate
DCD	Deceased cardiac death
ES cells	Embryonic stem cells
GLP-1	Glucagon-like peptide-1
HTK solution	Histidine-tryptophan-keto-glutarate solution
IL-1	Interleukin-1
iPS cells	Inducible pluripotent stem cells
PFC	Perfluorocarbon
TNF	Tumor necrosis factor
UW solution	University of Wisconsin solution

References

1. American Diabetes Association. Diagnosis and classification of diabetes mellitus. Diabetes Care. 2010;33(suppl1):S62–9.
2. Shapiro AM, Lakey JR, Ryan EA, et al. Islet transplantation in seven patients with type 1 diabetes mellitus using a glucocorticoid-free immunosuppressive regimen. N Engl J Med. 2000;343:280–8.

3. Ryan EA, Paty BW, Senior PA, Bigam D, Alfadhli E, Kneteman NM, Lakey JR, Shapiro AM. Five-year follow-up after clinical islet transplantation. Diabetes. 2005;54(7):2060–9.
4. Shapiro AM, Ricordi C, Hering BJ, et al. International trial of the Edmonton protocol for islet transplantation. N Engl J Med. 2006;355:1318–30.
5. Shapiro AMJ. Strategies towards single-donor islets of Langerhans transplantation. Curr Opin Organ Transplant. 2011;16:627–31.
6. Barton FB, Rickels MR, Alejandro R, et al. Improvement in outcomes of clinical islet transplantation: 1999-2010. Diabetes Care. 2012;35:1436–45.
7. Wang Y, Danielson KK, Ropski A, et al. Systematic analysis of donor and isolation factor's impact on human islet yield and size distribution. Cell Transplant. 2013;22:2323–33.
8. Matsumoto S, Okitsu T, Iwanaga Y, et al. Successful islet transplantation from non-heart-beating donor pancreata using modified Ricordi islet isolation method. Transplantation. 2006;82:460–5.
9. Matsumoto S, Okitsu T, Iwanaga Y, et al. Insulin independence after living donor distal pancreatectomy and islet allotransplantation. Lancet. 2005;365:1642–4.
10. Matsumoto S, Rigley TH, Qualley SA, et al. Efficacy of the oxygen-charged static two-layer method for short-term pancreas preservation and islet isolation from nonhuman primate and human pancreata. Cell Transplant. 2002;11:769–77.
11. Matsumoto S, Takita M, Chaussabel D, et al. Improving efficacy of clinical islet transplantation with iodixanol based islet purification thymoglobulin induction and blockage of IL-1-beta and TNF alpha. Cell Transplant. 2011;20:1641–7.
12. Paushter DH, Qi M, Danielson KK, et al. Histidine-tryptophan-ketoglutarate and University of Wisconsin solution demonstrate equal effectiveness in the preservation of human pancreata intended for islet isolation: a large-scale, single-center experience. Cell Transplant. 2013;22:1113–21.
13. Matsumoto S, Noguchi H, Shimoda M, et al. Seven consecutive successful clinical islet isolations with pancreatic ductal injection. Cell Transplant. 2010; 19:291–7.
14. Shimoda M, Itoh T, Sugimoto K, et al. Improvement of collagenase distribution with the ductal preservation for human islet isolation. Islets. 2012;4:130–7.
15. Ricordi C, Lacy PE, Finke EH, Olack BJ, Scharp DW. Automated method for isolation of human pancreatic islets. Diabetes. 1988;37:413–20.
16. Shimoda M, Itoh T, Iwahashi S, et al. An effective purification method using large bottles for human pancreatic isolation. Islets. 2012;4:380–404.
17. Hering BJ, Kandaswamy R, Ansite JD, et al. Single-donor, marginal-dose islet transplantation in patients with type 1 diabetes. JAMA. 2005;293:830–5.
18. Groth CG, Korsgren O, Tibell A, et al. Transplantation of porcine fetal pancreas to diabetic patients. Lancet. 1994;344:1402–4.
19. Van der Laan LJ, Lockey C, Griffeth BC, et al. Infection by porcine endogenous retrovirus after islet xenotransplantation in SCID mice. Nature. 2000; 407:90–4.
20. Cozzi E, Tallacchini M, Flanagan EB, et al. The International Xenotransplantation Association consensus statement on conditions for undertaking clinical trials of porcine islet products in type 1 diabetes – Chapter 1: Key ethical requirements and progress toward the definition of international regulatory framework. Xenotransplantation. 2009;16:203–14.
21. Matsumoto S, Tan P, Baker J, et al. Clinical porcine islet xenotransplantation under comprehensive regulation. Transplant Proc. 2014;46:1992–5.
22. Kroon E, Martinson LA, Kadoya K, et al. Pancreatic endoderm derived from human embryonic stem cells generates glucose-responsive insulin-secreting cells in vivo. Nat Biotechnol. 2008;26:443–52.
23. Takahashi K, Tanabe K, Ohnuki M, et al. Induction of pluripotent stem cells from adult human fibroblasts by defined factors. Cell. 2007;131:861–72.
24. Takeuchi H, Nakatsuji N, Suemori H. Endodermal differentiation of human pluripotent stem cells to insulin-producing cells in 3D culture. Sci Rep. 2014;4:4488. doi:10.1038/srep04488. Article number: 4488.

43 Face Transplant: The Future Is Better Than Current Concepts

Juan P. Barret

Introduction and Background

Modern history of vascularised composite tissue allotransplantation began in 1998, when the first human hand transplantation became a reality [1]. A few years later, in 2005, the first human face transplantation was attempted with success by Devauchelle and Dubernard in France [2].

Facial transplantation is a new achievement of transplantation medicine and microvascular reconstructive plastic surgery. The not-so-old dream of restorative surgery, namely the replacement of damaged parts of the body by new unharmed pre-formed tissues, has become a reality. The development of techniques aimed to transplantation of vascularised composite tissues (composite vascularised allografts, CVA) has provided clinicians with a new robust tool for the reconstruction of deformities that were, not so long ago, impossible to achieve. History of, development of, and classical attempts for CVA are not new. More than four decades ago, doctors in Ecuador attempted the transplantation of a hand limb. The transplant failed, but the dream survived. Pioneering laboratory work in experimental animals showed the path to clinicians for the achievement of human CVA. To date, there have been reports of successful transplantations of the knee joint, hand (unilateral and bilateral), arms (uni- and bilateral), face (partial and total), abdominal wall, larynx, penis, digits, and lower limbs. All recipients presented with deformities and/or amputations that were not amenable to being reconstructed by means of classical or traditional techniques. Such deformities affected non-vital parts and/or organs, and all of them had in common the impossibility to restore form, function, and cosmesis by means of conventional techniques and reconstructive surgery. The results of facial transplantation in humans demonstrate that facial transplantation is no longer an abstraction but a clinical reality. It has been implemented in the latest years with increasing interest and great success. The limits of indications are still, though, desperate catastrophic facial disfigurement.

Similarly to that learned in many other transplant and plastic surgery disciplines, the development of facial transplantation programs calls for a strong team approach, building a multidisciplinary team that involves all necessary and diverse specialists to make a robust protocol and an experienced team that warrants excellence in outcomes. This multidisciplinary team is formed by all transplant disciplines usually involved in transplant medicine (surgeons, immunologists, infectious disease specialists, renal disease

J.P. Barret, M.D., Ph.D. (✉)
Department of Plastic Surgery and Burn Center, Hospital Universitari Vall d'Hebron, Barcelona, Spain
e-mail: jpbarret@vhebron.net

R. Latifi et al. (eds.), *Technological Advances in Surgery, Trauma and Critical Care*, DOI 10.1007/978-1-4939-2671-8_43

specialists), but should include also experienced health professionals more involved in the plastic and reconstructive scenario, namely rehabilitation specialists, physiotherapists, occupational therapists, psychologists, psychiatrists, and social workers. CVA procedures must be organised in tertiary centres with a strong commitment to transplant surgery and medicine. Such institutions have in common the required laboratory, clinical services, and research units that are necessary to perform this new clinical discipline.

Patient Selection: Indications and Contraindications

An important number of patients referred to plastic surgery clinics worldwide present with facial deformities of diverse aetiologies. They include tumors, postoncologic deformities, trauma, burns, congenital abnormalities, and atrophic/involutive/aging deformities. Classic and traditional techniques (flaps, grafts, biomaterials, etc.) and more novel techniques (lipostructure, stem cell, and mesenchymal cell transfer) solve the majority of deformities producing excellent outcomes. Some patients, though, present with facial deformities difficult, if not impossible, to reconstruct. They represent a minority of patients (less than 1 %), and only a few of them will have a true indication for facial transplantation. The usual aetiologies considered for facial transplantation are listed in Table 43.1.

The indication of facial transplantation is performed in patients with important deformities that affect different structures of the human face. They normally involve muscle sphincters (oral, ocular sphincter) and exhibit an important functional impact (impossibilities to speak, feed normally, or breathe). The psychosocial impact of the deformity is extremely high, preventing them from functioning as normal human beings. Patients normally experience the facial deformity as a health status worse than being dead. The motivation of patients concentrates on becoming "normal" again, and being able to resume their premorbid lifestyle. However, when patients are considered for facial transplantation, the benefits of the procedure should surpass the risks of the proposed treatment and the toxic side effects of the immunosuppressant therapy.

Similarly, the expected result of the proposed technique must be superior to that obtained with traditional techniques. Functional and aesthetic outcomes of facial transplantation must be by far much better than those obtained with any other technique that is also available. Otherwise, the transplant should not be indicated and the reconstruction should proceed without reconstructive allotransplantation.

In our clinical series, only 25 % of patients that entered our face transplantation program ended up with an indication for facial allotransplantation. Informed consent is a must, and some patients decide to stop the process after being informed about the therapy; however, most of the contraindications are based on medical problems that contraindicate immunosuppression and psychosocial contraindications. Experienced psychiatrists, psychologists, and social workers are core members of the facial transplantation team. A thorough compulsory psychological and psychiatric evaluation must be performed in order to certify that the patient is a good candidate for face transplantation. A negative outcome of this evaluation is a formal contraindication for facial transplantation.

Table 43.1 Usual aetiologies considered for facial transplantation

1.	Gunshot injuries (ballistic trauma)
2.	Other posttraumatic injuries
3.	Burn deformity
4.	Benign tumours (i.e., neurofibromatosis)
5.	Post-oncological deformities (tumour free and risk free)

On the Ethics of Facial Allotransplantation

The success of facial transplantation throughout the world has positioned this technique as a new option for patients presenting with severe facial deformities. However, the transplantation of a cadaver's donor face still poses important psychological, social, and ethical issues into medical community. A decade ago, Siemionow and Ogich pointed out that patients affected from severe facial deformity would improve dramatically their quality of life with facial transplantation. Thus, they signalled that patients should be involved in the decision-making process of facial transplantation. Patients' informed consent is necessary, and a legally binding document and process are necessary for every single medical and surgical procedure. The patient is the person responsible for the decision to perform surgery, and therefore accepts the results and consequences of such a decision and the risks of the operation. The surgeon performs a player's role, provided that patients are informed correctly and that the surgical procedure was performed properly and according to accepted standard clinical practice. Still, in 2004 the French National Ethics Advisory Committee affirmed that it was too soon for facial transplantation accreditation, and it did not grant permission for total facial transplantation, since it considered that the discipline could not answer positively to the risk-benefit ratio dilemma. In November 2005, though, the same French committee granted permission for the first partial human transplantation. Organ transplantation carries with it a series of psychosocial problems. They are exacerbated in the case of facial transplantation, especially as related to questions of identity, communication, psychological vulnerability, aesthetic results, possibility of death, treatment compliance, and the patient's and relatives' reactions to a new identity. These are scientific and ethical issues that need to be addressed by any facial transplantation protocol. The first human transplantation protocol approved ever by an ethics or IRB Committee occurred in 2004 in the Cleveland Clinic (Dr. Siemionow, USA). The accreditation of a human protocol must include the inclusion and exclusion criteria, patient screening, informed consents for recipients and donors, and multidisciplinary team to develop the program. Only under theses auspices—the "Facial Transplant Protocol"—may patients with severe facial deformity be evaluated for facial transplantation indication.

The surgical team must maintain the patient's autonomy (inform and accept the patient's decisions), which is more important and superior to the decision to operate and the surgical procedure itself. However, the patient's autonomy is not absolute. The patient's decisions and wishes to go through with a surgical procedure may have severe risks. Composite tissue allotransplantation carries significant risks, such as immunological rejection (acute and chronic) and drug-related side effects. The medical team is not obliged whatsoever to follow and perform a surgical intervention unless they are convinced that the outcomes and results are superior to the potential risks and possible complications and that they are proportionate. Autonomy, therefore, has to be universal (applying to all parties: patients, medical teams, surgeons) and in general and optimal terms be collaborative. Any new technology, though, has to be implemented through a well-supervised and audited process that preserves the dignity and safety of all parties, although it is patient centred. All protocols, processes, and indications are to be overseen by external ethics committees that will oversee that autonomy, safety, and all ethical questions are maintained and answered. The Research Ethics Committee (REC) or IRB in the USA has the mandate to warrant that any proposed research study conforms to the ethics recognised in the Helsinki Declaration. REC examines the research protocol and shall accept it if it protects the dignity, the legal rights, clinical safety, and well-being of all individuals participating in clinical research. It will allow participation in clinical research provided that patients have received all information and they have been offered the opportunity to express all their concerns and all questions have been properly answered in a timely fashion that allows unrushed decisions.

Facial Transplantation: Technical Aspects

Face transplantation consists in the extirpation of facial tissues of a donor with the diagnosis of brain death (solid organ donor) and its transplantation to a patient to reconstruct his/her facial defect. All deformed and scarred recipient facial tissues are removed and replaced by normal tissues, which restore anatomy and function. In general terms, facial CVA procedures utilise a two teams technique approach: a donor's team and a recipient's team, similarly to that employed in SOT, especially in heart and lung allotransplantation. The fabrication of a facial prosthesis must precede any CVA procedure (limbs, face, etc.). Maintaining the dignity of the patient during the whole donation process is mandatory, and bioethics during procurement call for excellence in the care of the donor. Similarly to many other facial CVA transplantation teams, we recommend a heart-beating donation. It shortens the ischemia time, reduces the impact of ischemia-reperfusion injury, and allows for correct haemostasis during the facial procurement operation [3]. The donor operation starts by securing a patent and safe airway. If tracheotomy is selected, it should be performed in the first tracheal rings to allow for a long tracheal segment if a double-lung transplant is also planned. Major vessels are cannulated in the usual manner, which must include the carotid circulation to perfuse the graft when the in situ dissection is finished. The operation begins with the cervical incision and undermining under the platysma muscle. The external carotid artery is identified and dissected. Major external carotid artery branches are identified and preserved if necessary for the type of facial graft planned. In general terms, only the facial artery is necessary for nearly all facial transplants. Lingual artery is to be preserved if the tongue is included in the facial transplant. Similarly, the hypoglossal nerve is identified, dissected, and included in the transplant (face and tongue transplantation). A bicoronal incision is performed next. Dissection proceeds in the subperiosteal plane up to the level of the orbit. The supraorbital nerve is identified and dissected inside the orbit in order to lengthen it and allow for a tension-free neurorrhaphy. Attention is directed to the lateral aspect of the face next. An incision is made at the appropriate level. If the ears are not included, a rhytidectomy incision is chosen. When the ears are transplanted, the incision is more posterior. The soft tissues are lifted and undermined. A deep dissection plane is employed, in order to include all facial muscles and nerves; a more superficial plane is employed if only skin and soft tissues are transplanted. All five facial nerve branches are identified at the anterior margin of the parotid gland, cut, and included in the graft. The dissection approaches the infraorbital nerve and it is freed of adhesions. It is severed at the appropriate level for each individual case. If necessary, the mucosa and submucosa layers of the cheek are included with a full-thickness dissection of the lips. Inferiorly, the dissection connects with the cervical flap. The dental nerve is identified at the mental foramen and severed and included in the flap. The final step during procurement consists of dissection and inclusion of the soft tissues and cartilages of the nose and section of the eyelids at the desired level. Current evidence supports good vascularisation of an entire face graft by the facial vascular pedicle. However, the temporal vessels may be included in the flap if necessary, and they may be dissected in continuity with the facial arteries down to the external carotid. It adds difficulty in the dissection with uncertain benefits in blood flow; however, it is still our first choice in full-face grafts. If a facial transplant including bone is planned, bone osteotomies are performed at this stage, leaving them attached to the soft tissues; good periosteal vascularisation does exist. The entire face graft is then left pedicled on arteries and veins (retromandibular veins, facial veins, and external jugular veins). The graft is perfused with preservation fluid at 4 °C simultaneously with the rest of solid organs.

After transportation to the recipient operation theatre, the second part of the operation starts. The recipient neck has been prepared and major vessels dissected. Depending on the type of facial deformity, the deformed structures have been resected, creating a defect on the recipient's face to be restored by the face transplant. Other teams prefer performing the resection of the recipient's face after revascularisation. Arteries and veins are anastomosed in the standard fashion. Before reperfusion, one gram of prednisone is infused i.v. to prevent any immunological reaction during this phase of the operation; immunosuppression induction therapy starts when the patient arrives to the operation theatre. The reconstructive phase of the operation begins with bone osteotomies and osteosynthesis with titanium miniplates, intraoral insetting, nerve neurorraphies—dental nerve and infraorbital nerve are performed before the final miniplating—and the suture of soft tissues and skin.

An Overview of Current Outcomes

To date, 29 face transplantations have been performed worldwide. Medicine is an ever-evolving science, and as such, since the time of this writing, it is certain that new and novel facial transplantations have been attempted and will continue to be attempted. The reader is therefore advised to keep updated with CVA literature and reports from the international society of hand and composite tissue allotransplantation.

Worldwide Experience on Facial Transplantation

Twenty-nine face transplants have been performed in seven countries. The longest follow-up period accounts for 9 years (Isabelle Dinoire, Amiens Team) with a total published survival rate of 89.6 %. Three patients have died: one patient in China, one patient in France-Paris team, and one patient in Spain-Valencia team. Table 43.2 depicts transplant characteristics. Fourteen different transplant teams have performed in total 18 partial face transplants and 11 full-face transplants for a variety of aetiologies that include 10 postburn deformities, 9 gunshot injuries, 3 animal attacks, 4 type 1 neurofibromatosis, 2 post-traumatic deformities, and 1 post-oncological/radiotherapy deformities. After the transplantation of the first full-face transplant in 2010 [4], the indications have expanded; however, a robust team approach and specific face CVA protocols are necessary to warrant correct outcomes. The indications for facial transplantation vary among different CVA teams. In general terms, destruction of facial sphincters (orbital and/or oral muscle sphincters) is a common indication for facial transplantation. Most of the patients have undergone previous reconstruction by traditional techniques, although there is intense debate so as to whether facial transplantation should be performed early in the hospital course to leave intact other traditional techniques and donor sites should the transplanted graft failed. Most of the teams performed procurement on a brain-dead heart-beating donor. Some teams advocate procuring the face before the rest of the solid organs are approached, although synchronous procurement is feasible, as has been reported by our team. It is imperative to reduce cold ischemia time during CVA transplantation. Some teams procured the facial CVA at the end of the procedure (i.e., China's, Valencia's, and Seville's teams); this approach, though, may lead to a massive haemorrhage after revascularisation and increase the risk of ischemia-reperfusion injury.

The composition of the different facial CVA graft varies and depends on the recipient's requirements. In half of the cases, bone has been transplanted as part of the facial transplant graft, most of which included the maxilla and mandible (especially in gunshot injuries and trauma cases). Open rigid miniplate fixation, similarly to that utilised in craniomaxillary surgery, has been employed with excellent results. Survival of all tissues included in the transplanted specimen has been observed.

Good perfusion and face viability have been observed in all cases. The whole face can be successfully revascularised by one facial artery (including the maxilla and mandible through network connections and periosteal feeders), although all teams advocate for a bilateral arterial anastomosis to ensure safety. In general terms, large arterial vessels are employed (external carotid artery). Some teams have performed extensive anatomic clinical research which shows that correct vascularisation does occur through the facial artery system. A consensus does exist that temporal vessels may not be necessary in most of the facial transplants and should be considered only in cases with large portions of the scalp and external auricle. The preferred imaging method to study the recipient's vascular status

Table 43.2 World experience with face CVA to date

Number	Date	Team	Type	Aetiology	Outcome
1.	11/2005	Amiens, France	Partial	Animal attack	Alive
2.	04/2006	Xian, China	Partial + bone	Animal attack	Patient died
3.	01/2007	Paris, France	Partial	Neurofibromatosis	Alive
4.	12/2008	Cleveland, USA	Partial + bone	Gunshot injury	Alive
5.	03/2009	Paris, France	Partial + bone	Gunshot injury	Alive
6.	04/2009	Paris, France	Partial	Burn	Patient died
7.	08/2009	Boston, USA	Partial + bone	Burn	Alive
8.	08/2009	Paris, France	Partial + bone	Gunshot injury	Alive
9.	08/2009	Valencia, Spain	Partial + bone	Post-oncological + radiotherapy	Patient died
10.	11/2009	Amiens, France	Partial + bone	Burn	Alive
11.	01/2010	Seville, Spain	Partial	Neurofibromatosis	Alive
12.	03/2010	Barcelona, Spain	Full + bone	Gunshot injury	Alive
13.	07/2010	Paris, France	Full	Neurofibromatosis	Alive
14.	03/2011	Boston, USA	Full	Burn	Alive
15.	04/2011	Paris, France	Partial + bone	Gunshot injury	Alive
16.	04/2011	Paris, France	Partial + bone	Gunshot injury	Alive
17.	04/2011	Boston, USA	Full	Burn	Alive
18.	05/2011	Boston, USA	Full	Animal attack	Alive
19.	01/2012	Antalya, Turkey	Full + bone	Burn	Alive
20.	01/2012	Gent, Belgium	Partial + bone	Trauma	Alive
21.	02/2012	Ankara, Turkey	Full	Burn	Alive
22.	03/2012	Ankara, Turkey	Partial	Burn	Alive
23.	03/2012	Baltimore, USA	Full + bone	Gunshot injury	Alive
24.	05/2012	Antalya, Turkey	Full	Burn	Alive
25.	01/2013	Boston, USA	Full	Burn	Alive
26.	05/2013	Antalya, Turkey	Partial + bone	Gunshot injury	Alive
27.	07/2013	Gliwice, Poland	Partial + bone	Trauma	Alive
28.	12/2013	Gliwice, Poland	Full	Neurofibromatosis	Alive
29.	03/2014	Boston, USA	Partial + bone	Gunshot injury	Alive

includes angio CT scan, which provides not only information of the arterial and venous network but also a good exploration of the facial skeleton and the bone-soft tissue relationship.

The main objective of facial transplantation is improvement of function and quality of life and reintegration into society as full individuals. Therefore, sensation and motor function play a central role to achieve the main goal of face CVA. Motor nerve reinnervation is necessary to achieve correct function when facial transplantation is indicated for improvement in function, and facial muscles, masticator muscles, or tongue are transplanted. End-to-end neurorraphies are performed by all transplant teams between facial nerve branches, motor branches of trigeminal nerve, and hypoglossal nerve. As soon as 3 months after surgery, patients may experience fasciculations and a progressive improvement in muscle tone, although it is not until 6–12 months after transplantation that active movements are apparent. Complete recovery of all facial muscle movement seldom does occur, and a progressive recovery of function is observed that extends more than 24 months post-transplant. Sensation appears earlier in the postoperative course. As early as 2–3 months post-transplant, patients may have feeling in their new faces, and complete sensory recovery is apparent 12 months after transplant.

Current survival rate is 89.3 %. Three out of 28 recipients have died by direct complications from their facial transplantation. It is worth noting that only one patient has died in the early postoperative period. Patient number 4 (Paris, France) died few days after a face transplant and simultaneous double-hand transplantation due to sepsis and a cardiac arrest during a salvage operation. This experience depicts the difficulties that teams may experience when major CVA procedures are planned. Burn patients have received during their hospital course large amounts of blood products and may have been treated with skin homografts. Consequently, burn survivors may have been sensitised against the HLA antigens. Crossing the major histocompatibility complex may induce acquired allo-antibodies, making correct tissue typing somehow difficult. Severe rejection episodes should be expected in this situation.

Deaths of patient number 2 (China) and patient number 10 (Valencia) teach us another important lesson: patient selection. Patient number 2 died after stopping his immunosuppressant medication and implementation of alternative medicine. Patient number 10 died approximately 4 years after his facial CVA transplantation by complications of his premorbid conditions (post-oncological and radiotherapy deformity). Good selection and excellent team approach is a must in CVA transplantation. The risks and possible complications that this type of transplantation carry with them, in addition to the immunosuppression complications and side effects common to transplantation medicine, make patient compliance and psychological stability absolutely necessary.

Similarly to SOT, CVA recipients may experience different types of complications and side effects from the immunosuppressant regime. So far, complications include hip necrosis, lymphoma, endometrial dysplasia, opportunistic viral infections, CVA reactivations or de novo infections, hypertension, renal failure, and hyperglycemia. Nevertheless, despite the intense immunosuppressant regimen that is commonly used in this type of transplant, good outcomes are observed with few complications. All but one patient have returned to normal life.

Allograft rejection is a serious issue in organ transplantation. Skin and mucosa are well known to have a high immunogenic capacity; thus, CVA allograft rejection is always expected to be particularly intense and problematic. Acute rejection is reported in the CVA population (hand, face, and other composite tissues) to be as high as 85 %, although most of the patients experience only one rejection episode. Chronic rejection, normally estimated somehow between 30 and 50 % at 5 years, has not been proven so far. However, the longest survival in face CVA is 9 years, and patients should be still followed and checked for signs of chronic rejection. All teams follow similar immunosuppressant regime: an induction therapy with corticoids and some type of lymphocyte-depleting agent (polyclonal antithymocyte globulin—ATG, anti-interleukin 2 receptor monoclonal antibodies such as daclizumab and basiliximab) and a three-drug maintenance regime (calcineurin inhibitor, steroids, and mycophenolate mofetil). Some groups have developed programs for immune tolerance with bone marrow infusion and cell therapy with diverse effects. Rejection episodes are corticoid sensitive in the majority of cases. They normally resolve with boluses of prednisone with quick taper. Some teams have utilised lymphocyte-depleting agents but this type of treatment has some important implications for the immune and infectious disease homeostasis. Patients that receive such treatments require good antifungal and viral prophylaxis and surveillance.

Despite the initial intense debate and the fears for potential psychological distress and identity crisis, the overall experience is extremely positive.

Several reports indicate that patients show excellent psychological outcomes. Recipients express a rapid acceptance of their new facial appearance accompanied by good and quick social reintegration. Quantitative psychological tests find improvement in quality of life and physical and mental health based on the MOS-SF 12. Other tests such as SF-36 and DAS-59 produced similar results, with patients returning to work-related activities and correct social reintegration.

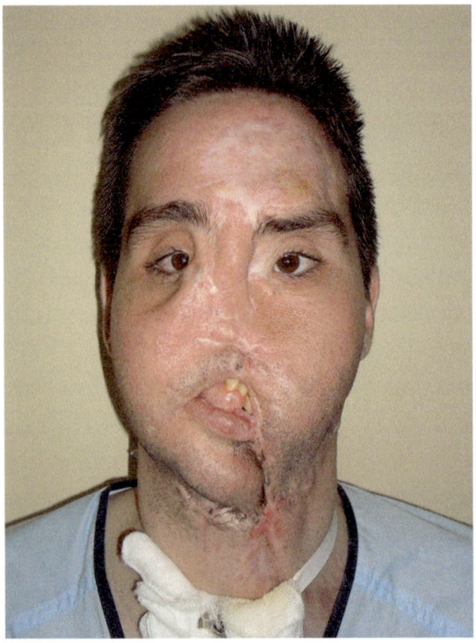

Fig. 43.1 Patient appearance after sustaining a gunshot injury to the face. Patient was unable to speak, eat, and function properly, necessitating tracheostomy and gastrostomy tube feeding

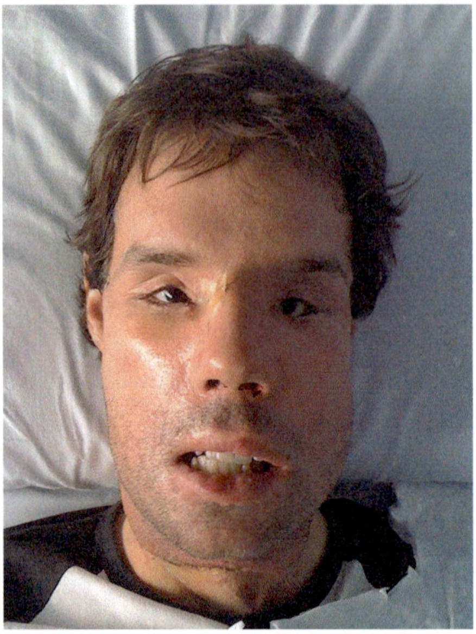

Fig. 43.2 Early appearance after full-face transplantation including intraoral structures and the whole facial skeleton

In fact, patients affected of severe facial deformities value the procedure and risks and benefits in terms of function recovery and social reintegration. When all these items are well regained, and patients may return to their premorbid life condition, a significant improvement in quality of life offsets the risks and side effects of immunosuppression and all possible complications.

Our first facial transplant patient integrated quickly his new appearance: as early as day 7, the patient was able to see and inspect his new appearance with good psychological effects (Figs. 43.1 and 43.2). During the first months after his transplant, the patient valued his experience as a significant improvement in quality of life, worth accepting all risks and side effects. Long-term outcome has provided the strong evidence that a robust team approach and good indication for facial transplantation produce excellent functional results and correct social reintegration. Significant improvement of quality of life may offset the risks and side effects of immunosuppression, although further and longer follow-up is still necessary to define the real role of facial transplantation in facial reconstructive surgery.

References

1. Dubernard JM, Owen E, Herzberg G, et al. Human hand allograft: report on first 6 months. Lancet. 1999;353:1315–20.
2. Devauchelle B, Badet L, Lengelé B, et al. First human face allograft: early report. Lancet. 2006;368(9531):203–9.
3. Bueno J, Barret JP, Serracanta J, et al. Logistics and strategy of multiorgan procurement involving total face allograft. Am J Transplant. 2011;11:1091–7.
4. Barret JP, Gavaldà J, Bueno J, et al. Full face transplant: the first case report. Ann Surg. 2011;254:252–6.

Limb Transplantation

44

Jaimie T. Shores, Gerald Brandacher,
and W.P. Andrew Lee

Introduction

Vascularized composite allotransplantation (VCA) is the transplantation of vascularized tissues from one human to another human outside the spectrum of traditional organ transplantation. This has previously been referred to as composite tissue allotransplantation (CTA) and can also be referred to more descriptively as "reconstructive transplantation." This is allotransplantation for the reconstruction of physical defects or tissue losses that may result from limb injury or loss, facial injury, loss of external genitals and/or abdominal wall tissue, larynx/trachea, uterus, and other potential deficits. It has been most commonly put into clinical practice throughout the world as hand and upper limb transplantation, with face transplantation being the second most commonly performed VCA.

J.T. Shores, M.D. (✉)
Department of Plastic and Reconstructive Surgery, The Johns Hopkins University School of Medicine, Baltimore, MD, USA
e-mail: jshores3@jhmi.edu

G. Brandacher, M.D. • W.P.A. Lee, M.D.
Reconstructive Transplantation Program, Department of Plastic and Reconstructive Surgery, The Johns Hopkins University School of Medicine, Baltimore, MD, USA
e-mail: brandacher@jhmi.edu; wpal@jhmi.edu

Overview of History and World Experience

The first hand transplant was performed in Ecuador in 1964 and was lost within 2 weeks due to rejection and the lack of understanding of immune responses to such tissues at the time [1]. However, with the advent of modern immunosuppression, the next known transplant was performed in Lyon, France, in 1998, followed shortly by a second transplant performed in Louisville, Kentucky, in 1999 [2]. Utilizing more "modern" immunosuppression, consisting of steroids, calcineurin inhibitors, and mycophenolate mofetil, these transplants were considered successes and the Kentucky patient currently has the longest surviving VCA in the world today as the patient from Lyon ultimately lost his hand due to noncompliance with medication and ultimately immunological rejection [3]. Since then, VCA has been performed for reconstruction of upper limb loss and severe facial deformity most commonly. Leg transplants have been "successfully" performed twice, once between identical twins, and once for an adult with leg loss from a traditional unrelated cadaveric donor, though outcomes here will be discussed later.

In regard to limb transplantation specifically, very little is known about outcomes in lower extremity transplantation due to the extreme rarity of this procedure, but hand and upper extremity

R. Latifi et al. (eds.), *Technological Advances in Surgery, Trauma and Critical Care*,
DOI 10.1007/978-1-4939-2671-8_44

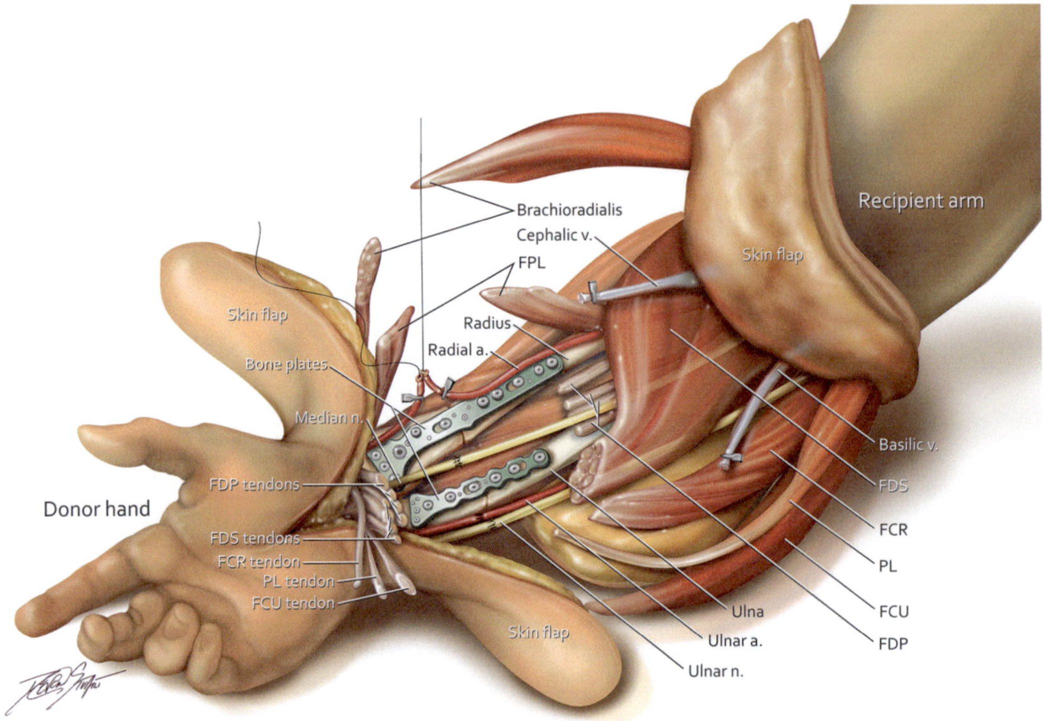

Fig. 44.1 Distal forearm level upper limb transplant (hand transplant) (used with permission. Copyright © The Johns Hopkins Health System and the authors)

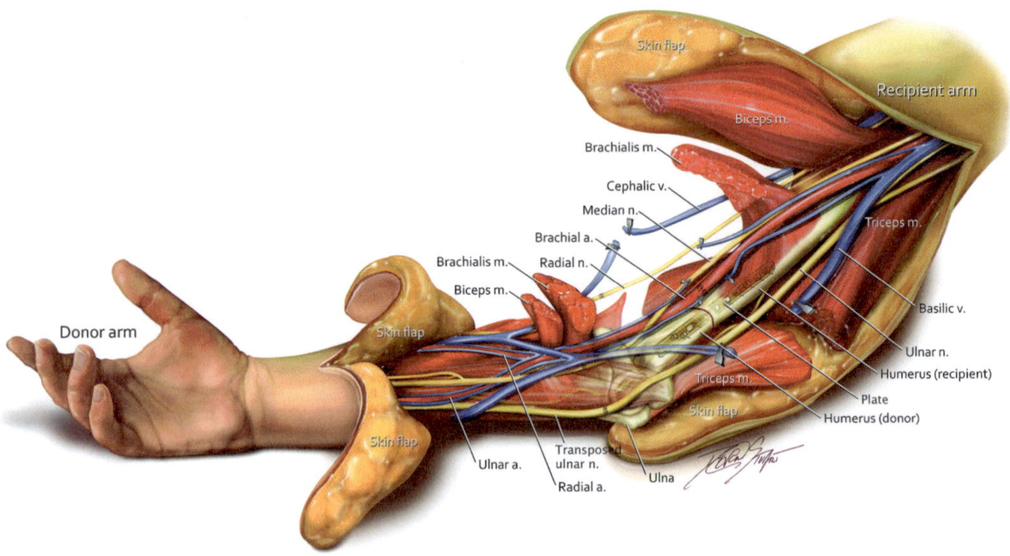

Fig. 44.2 Above-elbow upper limb transplant (used with permission. Copyright © The Johns Hopkins Health System and the authors)

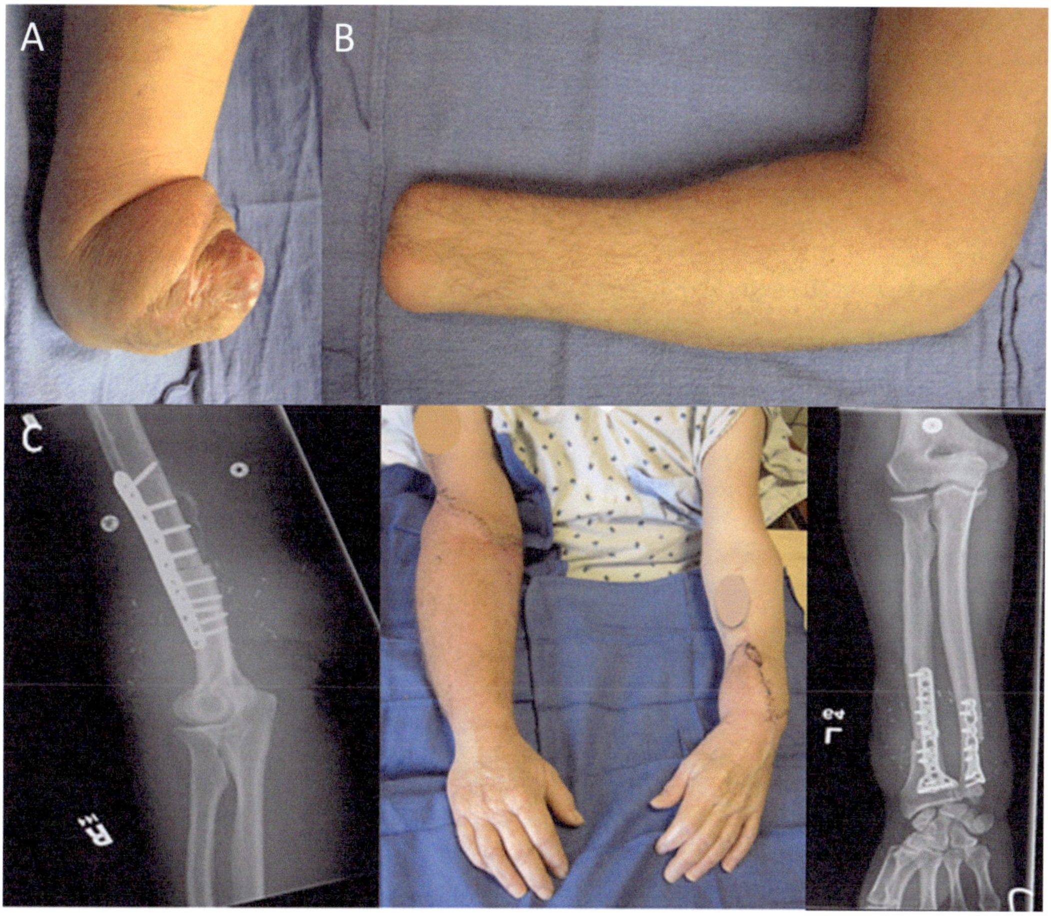

Fig. 44.3 (**a**) Right proximal forearm (just below elbow) amputation. (**b**) Left wrist amputation level. (**c**) Post right above elbow and left distal forearm upper limb transplantations with radiographs of osteosyntheses (**a–c**: Used with permission. Copyright © The Johns Hopkins Health System and the authors)

transplantation has been performed on at least 72 patients for a total of 107 limbs transplanted (at the time of writing of this chapter) [3]. Thus, much more is known in regard to outcomes, technique, and immunotherapy for this modality than any other (Figs. 44.1, 44.2, and 44.3a–c).

Theoretical Benefits and Obstacles to Limb Transplantation

The benefits and obstacles to limb transplantation while in theory are the same, in practice they have been different for upper and lower extremity applications. In theory, both upper and lower limb transplantation provide recipients with improved function by providing a missing limb that will have SOME level of function (certainly not the same level of function as a native limb), an improved or restored body image, likely improvement in phantom or stump pain, and a more comfortable limb replacement than prosthetic devices which are frequently rated to be heavy, painful, uncomfortable, and not as functional as desired by amputees. All transplants require some level of immunosuppression or immunotherapy, require significant amounts of rehabilitation, require nerve regeneration for function, are ultimately limited by nerve regeneration outcomes, and require large and potentially risk-filled surgeries for attachment of the transplanted limbs.

However, in practice, the application of these benefits and obstacles has been more supportive of upper limb than lower limb transplantation. This is partly due to the nature of the tasks required of the upper limb (fine and dexterous manipulation of the surrounding environment, physical sensing of the surrounding environment, communication, etc.) versus the lower limb (weight bearing, ambulation) [4]. For the lower limb, because fine and manipulative tasks are not typically required, the sensation requirement is much less important. Thus, an insensate prosthesis is less of an impediment than in the upper extremity, where the inability to feel objects being manipulated is a functional limitation. In addition, the lower extremity is not usually used in speech for both an aid to verbal communication and in nonverbal communication the way the hands are used. Because the hand is more visible to the patient and those surrounding the patient, there may be more psychological weight placed on upper than lower extremities in regard to body image and "wholeness." For these reasons, the threshold for amputation of an injured, painful, or nonfunctional hand is very different than the threshold for amputation of an injured, painful, or nonfunctional lower limb [5]. Every possible effort is made to avoid amputation of hands and upper limbs in typical practice due to poorer functional outcomes with an amputation and prosthesis while as it is known that many patients will immediately do better with an amputated lower limb and prosthesis. Thus, prosthetic acceptance is higher in the lower limb amputee than in the upper limb amputee, likely due to a combination of all of the discussed factors [5].

Functional outcomes after reinnervation between upper and lower extremities may be different as well. The limits of motor recovery in nerve regeneration are partially limited by the amount of time necessary to achieve motor end-plate reinnervation before permanent motor end-plate degeneration and muscle loss occur. The distance a nerve must regenerate to achieve motor reinnervation in the foot is longer than that of the hand in most human upper and lower extremities. Thus, the reinnervation potential may be greater in the upper extremity. In addition, most lower extremities tend to carry more muscle mass than upper extremities. Theoretical concerns for ischemia-reperfusion injury to the transplanted limb translating to intra- and immediate postoperative risk to the recipient as well as discussions around the increased antigen load of a lower versus upper extremity also exist. However, the actual influence of these factors in outcome has not truly been compared in a controlled and elective scenario such as a transplant, like it has been observed in more emergent scenarios such as major limb replantation.

World Experience in Limb Transplantation

As previously stated, very little is known about lower limb transplantation in the world experience. The first and only long-term successful transplant currently known involved the transplant of a unilateral leg from a conjoined twin with a fatal cardiac anomaly to the twin that would survive separation [6]. A report of 6-year outcome demonstrated growth and survival of the leg and acceptable, albeit, significantly inferior motor and sensory recovery compared to the contralateral "normal" leg. The second known leg transplant (and the first bilateral leg transplant) was performed in Spain for a 21-year-old man with bilateral above-knee amputations [7]. He had reportedly recovered some active knee flexion and extension and ankle motion, and had begun ambulation training in rehabilitation utilizing parallel bars, but suffered major a setback. He has reportedly had them amputated to stop his immunosuppression due to development of a high-grade malignancy. Two further patients have had unsuccessful attempts at leg transplants combined with hand transplants and are discussed below.

The world experience in hand and upper extremity is much more robust, however. In total, 72 patients with 107 known upper limb transplants have been reported since the first successful hand transplant in 1998 was performed [3]. This includes 37 unilateral upper limb transplants and

35 bilateral upper limb transplants, of which 4 were also combined with either face or leg transplantation. Of these 107 transplants, 24 known losses have occurred, including 4 mortalities. Of these, eight of the transplant losses and three of the four mortalities all occurred in patients undergoing simultaneous hand and face (two patients) or simultaneous hand and leg (two patients transplantation). A single patient survived this surgery and the face transplant also survived, though both hands did not and required removal. The only mortality known involving only hand transplantation occurred in a bilateral transplant attempt which was the first performed in Mexico. The same center has subsequently performed a successful transplant [3]. Of the remaining hand transplant patients that underwent only isolated unilateral or bilateral hand transplantation, 3 of the remaining 14 lost limbs were acute losses (immediate perioperative period) and 7 occurred in a single group's experience in China where access to immunosuppression was questionable and losses were blamed on noncompliance. The remaining losses come from three patients in the USA and France where noncompliance [3] and transplant vasculopathy [1], possibly, as a sign of chronic rejection, in a compliant patient, were the documented causes.

Functional outcomes have been harder to measure than transplant and patient survival data as there has not been tremendous uniformity in outcome measures used from center to center. The International Registry of Hand and Composite Tissue Transplantation (IRHCTT) has published data from member institutions that demonstrated that DASH (Disability of the Arm, Shoulder, and Hand) scores improved and HTSS (Hand Transplant Scoring System) scores improved in all 31 recipients reported with 12-month follow-up or more [8, 9]. In addition, 90 % had regained at least "protective sensation" and 84 % demonstrated "discriminative sensibility." They also reported that the "majority" of patients demonstrated some level of intrinsic muscle reinnervation. Quality of life was improved in >75 % of patients and the majority of patients had returned to some level of occupation.

In general, the more distal an upper extremity transplant is performed, the better the functional outcome. This means that motor outcomes and sensory recovery will be better and more reliable in more distal transplants, and the potential for intrinsic muscle reinnervation will be better in more distal transplants owing to the fact that nerve regeneration will require less distance and time to be completed. However, patients with more distal amputations also have less overall disability than those with above-elbow amputations as prosthetics and adaptive devices are better accepted and more functional for distal transplants. Therefore, even though proximal transplants may be expected to have inferior outcomes compared to distal transplants, the magnitude of functional improvement experienced by the recipient may be the same if not greater, even if the absolute score on an outcome measurement tool may seem lower.

Alternatives to Transplantation

The three major drawbacks to transplantation are the current need for lifelong immunotherapy, limitations in nerve regeneration, and need for a large operation combined with prolonged rehabilitation. Because of these current limitations, not all, if not most, upper extremity amputees and certainly very few lower extremity amputees have been considered ideal or good candidates for transplantation. Thus, alternative strategies for dealing with limb loss must be used. The most traditional strategy has been the use of traditional body-powered prosthetics. These are typically powered, in the upper limb, by cables that are pulled through flexion or extension of more proximal joints that translate to the opening and closing of a hook or a hand at the distal prosthesis. For lower extremities, standard below-knee prosthetics have not typically had reactive ankle joints. For both upper and lower extremity amputations more proximally, such as above the elbow or knee, these older prosthetics have been very problematic and not very functional. The advent of the myoelectric prosthesis with powered joints that work by sensing contraction of muscle groups in the remaining limb has improved this function somewhat. They can be used for more distal amputations as well, such as below-elbow amputations where forearm muscle activation can be sensed and translated into motorized digit and/or wrist motion. For proximal amputations above the elbow, this can be complicated to operate as the user must be able to signal the device that motor groups of the upper arm are intended to move either the elbow or the hand. This is accomplished by either contracting muscles in a pattern that signals the myoelectric prosthesis to "switch" from elbow mode to hand mode and activates the appropriate portion of the device to react to muscle contraction sensed through electromyography electrodes, or by an external switch hit, for instance, by the patient's chin that is mounted on the shoulder. For lower extremity prosthetics, computerized motor-driven ankle and knee joints have also been developed that react to sensed leg movements and muscle contractions. However, even further refinement has been gained by the advent of targeted muscle reinnervation or "TMR," coupled with advanced myoelectric prosthesis systems capable of much more than standard systems previously. In TMR, recognition that more than one muscle, or more than one individually innervated portion of a muscle, may exist in the shoulder area (for shoulder disarticulation amputees) or upper arm (for above-elbow amputees) or forearm (for below-elbow amputees) that can be used to signal the device to perform a set function. Nerves that normally proceed to a more downstream muscle target, which is no longer present due to amputation, can be re-routed proximally and used to reinnervate these redundant muscles or parts of muscles, to provide a more complex pattern of muscle activation that can be sensed and decoded by advanced pattern recognition algorithms within advanced prosthetics and ultimately provide simultaneous, independent, intuitive improvements in prosthesis controls [10]. This advancement in prosthetics design coupled with targeted nerve transfers has the potential to offer significant functional improvement over traditional prosthetics, especially for more proximal amputees for which prosthetics are historically rejected for poor performance. The weaknesses of such protocols are that they are still reliant upon prosthetics with limited power sources and limited if any ability to provide sensory feedback (though this is interesting and advancing) and are extremely expensive. The nerve transfers required are substantially smaller operations than transplant operations, but may also "burn bridges" in regard to allowing the patient to be considered for future transplantation if they so desired. However, for a great many amputees, this technology, along with other advancing technology in implantable muscle sensors and direct nerve interfaces, which are at more experimental levels currently, still offers significant improvements in what have been, traditionally, very limited outcomes with prosthetics.

Future Directions

The future of limb transplantation revolves around the development of strategies to significantly reduce or eliminate the need for immunotherapy as well as the enhancement of nerve regeneration. Most patients who are not candidates for transplantation, or decide not to pursue transplantation, do not receive limb transplantations because of concerns over immunotherapy. Compliance to immunotherapy is the single biggest factor in long-term transplant loss. Reasons for noncompliance may be that immunotherapy regimens are complicated with multiple medications and difficult to adhere to, or because of side effects of the medication, or because of lack of appropriate concern for the maintenance of the transplant. Likewise, many patients who choose not to pursue transplant do so out of concern for side effects of immunosuppression such as increased risks of infection, malignancy, avascular necrosis of bones/joints, metabolic complications such as diabetes, and chronic kidney disease/renal toxicity. Advancements to limit or eliminate these risks would make transplantation available to many more candidates. For this reason, some transplant centers have offered novel, nonsteroid single-drug protocols using donor bone marrow cell therapy to help recipients maintain their transplants with lower amounts of fewer medications and ultimately lower the risks to themselves and increase the likelihood of compliance [11]. At the same time, many centers are actively pursuing “tolerance” protocols that will altogether eliminate the need for immunosuppression and thus the deleterious side effects of these medications [12]. This single advancement stands to make transplantation available to most amputees with surgically reconstructable limb loss.

In addition to immunotherapy advancements, improvements in the speed and quality of motor and sensory fiber nerve regeneration would also help candidates who are already acceptable candidates have better outcomes, and help some who are not candidates due to the proximal nature of their injuries and poorer anticipated functional recoveries become better candidates. Since nerve regeneration drives all functional recovery in every kind of limb transplant, improvements here would help all recipients. Indeed, many therapeutic trials are under way testing stem cell-based augmentation of nerve regeneration, newer cell and growth factor/cytokine-impregnated scaffolds, and other neurotherapeutic strategies. However, historically, significant advancements in nerve regeneration have been difficult to demonstrate in clinical trials.

The biggest future direction, however, will be in regenerative therapies. The ability to grow isografts ex vivo, that are then surgically attached, or in situ, with no need for surgical attachment, to treat limb loss, are the long-range future for all types or organ, tissue, or limb reconstruction.

References

1. Gilbert R. Transplant is successful with a cadaver forearm. Med Trib Med News. 1964;5:20–3.
2. Shores JT, Brandacher G, Schneeberger S, Gorantla VS, Lee WP. Composite tissue allotransplantation: hand transplantation and beyond. J Am Acad Orthop Surg. 2010;18(3):127–31.
3. Shores J, Brandacher G, Lee WP. Hand and upper extremity transplantation: an update of outcomes in the worldwide experience. Plastic Reconstruct Surg. 2015;135(2):351e–60e.
4. Thorne C, Chung KC, Gosain A, Guntner GC, Mehrara BJ. Grabb and Smith's plastic surgery, 7th ed. In Charles H. Thorne (editor-in-chief), Kevin C Chung, Arun Gosain, Geoffrey C Gurtner, Babak Joseph Mehrara, J Peter Rubin, Scott L Spear (editors). Philadelphia: Lippincott Williams & WIlkins, a Wolters Kluwer Business; 2014. xbiii:1030.
5. Shores JT, Lee W. Management of mutilating injuries of the upper extremity. In: Thorne CH, Chung K, Gosain AK, Mehrara BJ, Rubin JP, Spear SL, editors. Grabb and Smith's plastic surgery. 7th ed. Philadelphia: Lippincott Williams & Wilkins; 2014. p. 833–8.
6. Fattah A, Cypel T, Donner EJ, Wang F, Alman BA, Zuker RM. The first successful lower extremity transplantation: 6-year follow-up and implications for cortical plasticity. Am J Transplant. 2011;11(12): 2762–7.
7. Cavadas PC, Thione A, Carballeira A, Blanes M. Bilateral transfemoral lower extremity transplantation: result at 1 year. Am J Transplant. 2013;13(5): 1343–9.
8. Petruzzo P, Dubernard JM. The international registry on hand and composite tissue allotransplantation. Clin Transpl. 2011;247–53.
9. Petruzzo P, Lanzetta M, Dubernard JM, Landin L, Cavadas P, Margreiter R, et al. The international registry on hand and composite tissue transplantation. Transplantation. 2010;90(12):1590–4.
10. Kuiken TA, Li G, Lock BA, Lipschutz RD, Miller LA, Stubblefield KA, et al. Targeted muscle reinnervation for real-time myoelectric control of multifunction artificial arms. JAMA. 2009;301(6):619–28.
11. Schneeberger S, Gorantla VS, Brandacher G, Zeevi A, Demetris AJ, Lunz JG, et al. Upper-extremity transplantation using a cell-based protocol to minimize immunosuppression. Ann Surg. 2013;257(2): 345–51.
12. Ibrahim Z, Cooney DS, Shores JT, Sacks JM, Wimmers EG, Bonawitz SC, et al. A modified heterotopic swine hind limb transplant model for translational vascularized composite allotransplantation (VCA) research. J Vis Exp (80); 2013.

Advances in Immunosuppressive Therapy

45

Napoleon E. Cieza, Marian Porubsky, and Tun Jie

Introduction

In the early 1900s, the surgical technique of the vascular anastomosis was described by French surgeon Alexis Carrel [1]. Experimental transplants followed, especially in animal models. Russian surgeon Yu Yu Voronoy was the first to report a series of human-to-human kidney transplants in the 1940s [2]. Outcomes were dismal and it was learned that not only the surgical technique was crucial for a successful transplant. The early rapid destruction of allografts was due to an immune process termed rejection. The work of Sir Peter B. Medawar with skin grafts in animal models and in human burn patients led to a better understanding of the important role of the immune system in the failure of skin grafts [3]. It was not until 1954 that the first human transplant with long-term success was performed by Joseph Murray [4]; however, no immunosuppression was required since it was a living related kidney transplant between identical twins. Attempts were made to perform kidney transplants between nonidentical individuals; however, results were discouraging. A breakthrough was achieved in the early 1960s with the introduction of maintenance immunosuppression [5]. In addition to the development in surgical techniques and immunosuppression protocols, progress in tissue typing and crossmatching and in preservation and transportation of harvested organs has played major roles in the rapid development of organ transplantation. While it has been considerable success in developing immunosuppressive therapy in preventing and treating graft rejection, current therapy has a number of serious complications. The aim of this chapter is to review both their use and potential complications of immunosuppressive therapy.

Rejection

The immune system protects the body from foreign pathogens. The adaptive branch of immunity is an advanced, specific and versatile host defense mechanism against invasion of pathogens. By recognition of foreign antigens, this ability of the host immune system results in rejection of the "nonself" antigens/tissue.

Transplants between genetically nonidentical persons lead to recognition and rejection of

N.E. Cieza, M.D.
General Surgery Residency Program,
University of Arizona, 1501 N. Campbell Avenue,
PO BOX 245058, 85724, USA

M. Porubsky, M.D., F.A.C.S. • T. Jie, M.D.,
M.S., F.A.C.S. (✉)
Abdominal Transplant and HPB,
Department of Surgery, School of Medicine,
University of Arizona, 1501 N Campbell Avenue,
PO Box 245066, Tucson, AZ 85724, USA
e-mail: tjie@surgery.arizona.edu

R. Latifi et al. (eds.), *Technological Advances in Surgery, Trauma and Critical Care*,
DOI 10.1007/978-1-4939-2671-8_45

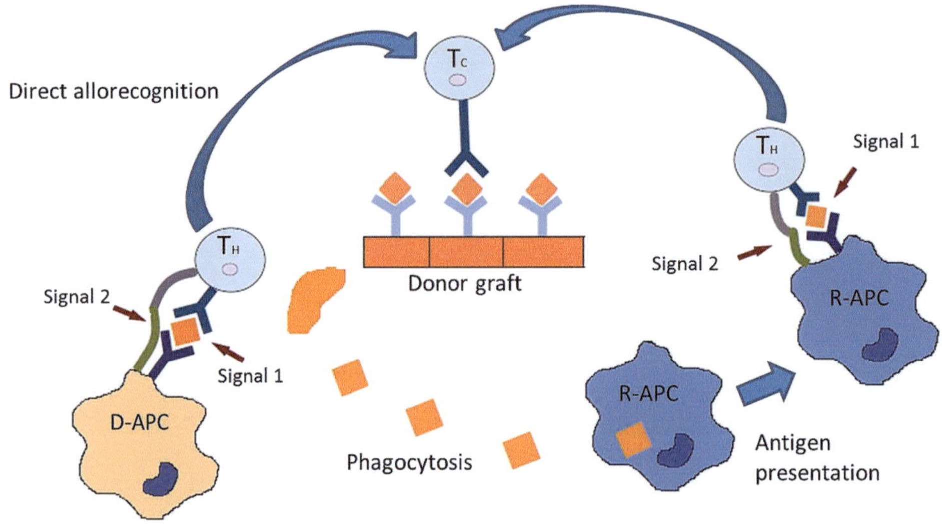

Fig. 45.1 Direct and indirect pathways of allorecognition. Signal 1 is delivered by a peptide-HLA complex. Signal 2, also known as costimulatory sign, is delivered by an array of cell surface molecules on the T-helper cell and the antigen-presenting cell (APC). *D-APC* donor APC, *R-APC* recipient APC, *TH* T-helper lymphocyte, *TC* cytotoxic T lymphocytes

the organ by the recipient's immune system. This immunologic disparity among members of the same species is based on the differences in cell surface molecules. In humans, these antigens were first identified in leukocytes and termed human leukocyte antigens (HLAs). HLAs are subdivided in two major classes that differ in structure, function, and tissue distribution. Class I (HLA-A, -B, and -C) are expressed by all nucleated cells, and class II (HLA -DR, -DQ, and -DP) are expressed on the surface of antigen-presenting cells (APCs) such as activated macrophages, dendritic cells, and B lymphocytes. The recognition of nonself tissue occurs via two distinct pathways: *direct and indirect allorecognition.* Direct allorecognition consists of recipient T-helper cells (CD4+ lymphocytes) recognizing donor HLA disparity expressed on the donor cell surface. Indirect allorecognition consists of recipient APCs phagocytosing donor cellular debris, which are then processed and re-presented on the APC surface to be recognized by recipient T-helper cells (Fig. 45.1).

As outlined before, graft rejection is due to a complex interaction of different parts of the immune system, including B and T lymphocytes, APCs, and cytokines. Interleukin 2 (IL-2) is secreted by activated CD4+ T-helper lymphocytes and acts as a pivotal, early signal in immune activation. Among its functions, IL-2 engenders increased T-cell responsiveness, clonal expansion of alloreactive T lymphocytes, B lymphocytes, and acquisition of the cytolytic phenotype by host T lymphocytes. Cellular-mediated rejection is the result of an attack of activated T cells on the transplanted organ. Activated B lymphocytes further differentiate into plasma cells and producing antigen-specific antibodies. Antibody-mediated rejection is the result of binding of these antibodies on the transplant organ. According to its onset and pathogenesis, graft rejection is classified into three main types: hyperacute, acute, and chronic.

Hyperacute Rejection

Hyperacute rejection (HAR) occurs within a few minutes to a few hours after the reperfusion of the organ and results in irreversible graft loss. It is triggered by preformed antibodies (donor's HLA or ABO blood group antigens) directed against antigens presented by the graft. These antibodies activate a series of events that result in diffuse formation of microvascular thrombi, causing ischemic necrosis of the graft [6]. Currently, no treatment is available; however, tissue crossmatching of donor and potential transplant recipients should prevent nearly all HAR.

The panel-reactive antibody (PRA) assay is a screening test that examines the ability of serum from potential transplant recipients to lyse lymphocytes from a panel of HLA-typed donors. A numerical value, expressed as a percentage, indicates the likelihood of a positive crossmatch to the donor population. The finding of a higher PRA identifies patients at high risk for a positive crossmatch and thus for HAR and subsequent graft loss.

Fortunately, pretransplant blood group typing and crossmatching have virtually eliminated the incidence of hyperacute rejection.

Acute Rejection

AR is the most common form of graft rejection. It may develop at any time, but is most frequent during the first several months posttransplant. If it occurs within the first several days posttransplant, the rejection is most likely a combination of amnestic immune response driven by sensitized memory B lymphocytes and activation of the direct allorecognition pathway. This constitutes a rare process termed *accelerated acute rejection* (AAR) in which the donor antigen exposure often occurred in the distant past. Once the host's immune systems are challenged by the same donor antigens introduced by the organ transplant, dormant memory lymphocytes reactivate, replicate, and differentiate resulting in graft rejection.

According to the mechanism involved, AR is further divided into cellular (T-cell mediated) rejection, humoral (antibody mediated) rejection, or a combination of both. Unless the host immune system is suppressed pharmacologically, a transplant inevitably leads to acute rejection.

The diagnosis is based on the results of biopsies, special immunologic stains, and laboratory tests (elevated creatinine levels in kidney transplant patients, elevated liver function values in liver transplant recipients, and elevated levels of amylase, and lipase in pancreas transplant hosts).

A variety of immunosuppressive agents are used to prevent AR that will be discussed in the next section.

Chronic Rejection

CR constitutes a slow type of rejection resulting in fibrosis and loss of graft function. The mechanism is not well understood; however, contribution of immune and nonimmune factors is likely. The observation that AR episodes significantly increase the likelihood of CR [7], as well as the correlation observed in renal transplant recipients between poor response to AR treatment and the subsequent development of CR, is evidence of immune factors contributing to this type of rejection. Nonimmune factors include the toxic effects of immunosuppressive agents and cumulative injury from infection (i.e., CMV and polyomavirus) [8, 9]. With advances in immunosuppression, this relatively rare form of rejection is becoming more common.

Immunosuppression Therapy

Balance between the recipient's immune response, the donor's allograft, and adequate pharmacologic immunosuppression is necessary for a successful transplant. The initial attempts to establish an effective immunosuppression involved use of total body radiation and 6-mercaptopurine. Results were discouraging, and toxicity was profound. In the early 1960s, the introduction of maintenance immunosuppression through a combination of corticosteroids and azathioprine (a less toxic derivate of 6-mercaptopurine) [10] and the development of cyclosporine, in the 1980s, increased allograft survival [11, 12]. Finally, the introduction of mycophenolate mofetil (MMF) [13] and the calcineurin inhibitor tacrolimus [14] in the 1990s changed the field, enabling a variety of combinations to be used for immunosuppression. Immunosuppressive drugs by groupings are shown in Table 45.1.

Table 45.1 Immunosuppressive drugs by grouping

Immunophilin binders
• Calcineurin inhibitors
Cyclosporine
Tacrolimus
• Noninhibitors of calcineurin
Sirolimus
Antimetabolites
• Inhibitors of de novo purine synthesis
Azathioprine
Mycophenolate mofetil
Biologic immunosuppression
• Polyclonal antibodies
ATGAM
Antithymocyte immunoglobulin
• Monoclonal antibodies
Muromonab-CD3 (OKT3)
Basiliximab
Alemtuzumab
Rituximab
Eculizumab
Bortezomib
Fusion proteins
Costimulation-based agents
Belatacept
Other agents
Leflunomide and malononitrilamide (FK778)
Janus Kinase 3 inhibitors
Corticosteroids

Immunosuppressive Strategies

Immunosuppressive agents can be categorized according to their use:

- Induction—those used for a limited interval at the time of transplant.
- Maintenance—those used for long term for maintenance of immunosuppression.
- Antirejection—those used for a short time or in high doses to reverse an acute rejection episode.

Considerably overlap exists among these categories and no single approach applies uniformly. These strategies must take into account the risk of an acute rejection episode, the consequences of an acute rejection episode, and the consequences of a graft loss. The relative importance of each factor varies depending on the organ transplanted.

Pharmacologic Immunosuppression

Immunophilin Binders

Calcineurin Inhibitors

Cyclosporine (CSA) and Tacrolimus (TAC) interfere with the cellular pathway for cytokine production and proliferation. The protein calcineurin has been validated as part of the calcium-dependent signal transduction pathway of interleukin-2 (IL-2) production in T cells. Cyclosporine and Tacrolimus bind to two different intracellular receptors. The resulting receptor complex binds to calcineurin, blocking its phosphatase ability and thereby stopping the production of IL-2 [15].

Cyclosporine

CSA was isolated from a soil sample in Norway and produced by the fungus *Tolypocladium inflatum*. The introduction of cyclosporine in the early 1980s dramatically altered the field of transplantation by significantly improving outcomes after kidney transplants. CSA binds to its cytoplasmic receptor protein, cyclophilin A (CypA), which subsequently inhibits the activity of calcineurin. T-cell suppression is a result of a decreased expression of several critical T-cell activation genes, the most important being for IL-2 [16]. The first formulation approved by the US Food and Drug Administration (FDA) was Sandimmune® (Novartis, Basel, Switzerland), an oil-based formulation, with poor bioavailability and variable absorption. Newer formulations, Gengraf® (Abbott Laboratories, North Chicago, IL) and Neoral® (Novartis, Basel, Switzerland), are microemulsified making absorption much more reliable. CSA can be given both intravenously or orally to maintain trough levels of 250–350 ng/mL for the first 3 months posttransplant; it can be then tapered to 150–250 ng/mL [17].

CSA is metabolized by the cytochrome P450 3A4 enzyme system that is not only in the liver

Table 45.2 Side effects and drug interactions of the main immunosuppressive drugs

	Common side effects	Other medications that increase blood levels	Other medications that decrease blood levels	Other medications that potentiate toxicity
Cyclosporine (CSA)	Hypertension, nephrotoxicity, hirsutism, neurotoxicity, gingival hyperplasia, hypomagnesemia, hyperkalemia	Verapamil, diltiazem, clarithromycin, azithromycin, erythromycin, azole antifungals, protease inhibitors, grapefruit juice	Isoniazid, carbamazepine, phenobarbital, phenytoin, rifampin, St. John's Wort	Nephrotoxicity: ganciclovir, aminoglycosides, NSAIDs, ACE-Is, and ARBs
Tacrolimus (FK 506)	Hypertension, nephrotoxicity, alopecia, hyperglycemia, neurotoxicity, hypomagnesemia, hyperkalemia	Verapamil, diltiazem, clarithromycin, azithromycin, erythromycin, azole antifungals, protease inhibitors, grapefruit juice	Isoniazid, carbamazepine, phenobarbital, phenytoin, rifampin, St. John's Wort	Nephrotoxicity: ganciclovir, aminoglycosides, NSAIDs, ACE-Is, and ARBs
Sirolimus	Thrombocytopenia and neutropenia, elevated cholesterol, extremity edema, impaired wound healing	Verapamil, diltiazem, clarithromycin, azithromycin, erythromycin, azole antifungals, protease inhibitors, grapefruit juice	Isoniazid, carbamazepine, phenobarbital, phenytoin, rifampin, St. John's Wort	—
Mycophenolate mofetil	Leukopenia, thrombocytopenia, GI upset	—	Cholestyramine, antacids	Bone marrow suppression: valganciclovir ganciclovir, TMP/SMX
Corticosteroids	Hyperglycemia, osteoporosis, cataracts, myopathy, weight gain	—	—	—
Azathioprine	Leukopenia, anemia, thrombocytopenia, neoplasia, hepatitis, cholestasis	—	—	Bone marrow suppression: allopurinol, sulfonamides

but also in the cells lining the intestine, so CSA levels can be increased or decreased by changes in gut absorption or in liver metabolism. The extensive side effect profile of CSA has long been a reason for attempts at minimizing drug exposure. Drug interactions and side effects are summarized in Table 45.2. Of most concern is its acute and chronic nephrotoxicity. Acute nephrotoxicity from CSA initially is characterized by vasoconstriction of the afferent arteriole in a dose-dependent, reversible manner. Other side effects include hyperkalemia, hypomagnesemia, hypertension, and neurotoxicity [18]. Cosmetic effects, including hirsutism and gingival hyperplasia, are also observed with the use of CSA.

Tacrolimus

With the success of CSA, researchers studied soil samples from around the world, looking for another compound that might turn out to display immunosuppressive properties. Tacrolimus (TAC), previously known as FK-506, was isolated from a soil sample in Japan in 1984 and produced by the fungus *Streptomyces tsukubaensis* [19]. Its effect on the lymphocyte is remarkably similar to CSA even though TAC has a completely different chemical structure. TAC acts by binding to FK-binding protein 12(FKBP12) causing inhibition of IL-2 production. The FKP12-TAC complex is 10–100 times more potent than CSA, possibly due to greater affinity for its binding protein [20]. TCA was approved by the FDA in 1994 for the use in liver transplantation. This has been extended to include kidney, heart, small bowel, pancreas, lung, trachea, skin, cornea, bone marrow, and limb transplants, making this drug the backbone of immunosuppressive regimens. TAC can be given intravenously, orally, or sublingually to maintain trough levels of 8–12 ng/mL for the first 3 months posttransplant; then it can be tapered to 6–10 ng/mL.

TAC metabolism is similar to CSA, via the cytochrome P450 34A system. Drug interactions are summarized in Table 45.2. Side effects include alopecia, nephrotoxicity, neurotoxicity, hypertension, hyperkalemia, hypomagnesemia, and new-onset diabetes posttransplant [21].

Noninhibitors of Calcineurin

Sirolimus

Sirolimus (SRL) belongs to a class of compounds known as the mammalian target of rapamycin (mTOR) inhibitors. It is produced by *Streptomyces hygroscopicus*, a fungus isolated from a soil sample found on Easter Island. SRL, formerly known as rapamycin, was approved in 1999 by the FDA. A derivative of sirolimus, everolimus, was approved by the FDA in 2004. In response to proliferation signals provided by cytokines like IL-2, mTOR, a key regulatory kinase, changes cells from the G1 to S phase in the cell cycle [22]. The mTOR inhibitors bind to FKBP12 (same binding protein as TAC) and this complex causes inhibition of mTOR preventing the cell cycle progression from G1 to S in lymphocytes. The primary pathway for metabolism is the cytochrome P450 34A enzyme system. SRL has been used in a variety of combinations for maintenance of immunosuppression, to help withdraw, or completely avoid, the use of steroids and also as an alternative in calcineurin-sparing protocols. Drug interactions are summarized in Table 45.2. Hypertriglyceridemia is one of the most significant side effects; impaired wound healing, thrombocytopenia, leukopenia, and anemia are also associated with SRL [23, 24].

Antiproliferative Agents

Antiproliferative agents have been part of transplant protocols since the infancy of immunosuppression.

Inhibitors of De Novo Purine Synthesis

Azathioprine

Azathioprine (AZA), a prodrug of 6-mercaptopurine, was developed in the early 1960s and was part of the first successful transplant series. AZA inhibits the purine synthesis in the de novo pathway. Purine inhibition leads to inhibition of the mixed lymphocyte reaction, and to a lesser extent, the antigen antibody reaction [25]. The use of AZA has decreased significantly with the development of new agents such as mycophenolate mofetil (MMF). However, AZA is still preferred in recipients who are considering conceiving a child, because of the teratogenic effects of MMF. The most common side effect is myelosuppression due to suppression of purine synthesis. Most patients can tolerate this effect by reducing the daily dosage, although some need to discontinue the drug entirely. Other significant side effects include hepatotoxicity, pancreatitis, neoplasia, anemia, and pulmonary fibrosis. Severe pancytopenia has been reported when AZA and allopurinol are used together. It is recommended that AZA doses be reduced by 75 % if allopurinol is added to the patient's drug regimen [25, 26].

Mycophenolate Mofetil

MMF was approved by the FDA in 1995 to prevent acute rejection in kidney recipients. It has been a major addition to the immunosuppressive arsenal and has been incorporated into routine maintenance regimens after many solid organ transplants. MMF is the prodrug of mycophenolic acid (MPA), derived from *Penicillium* fungi. Mycophenolic acid acts as a noncompetitive inhibitor of inosine monophosphate dehydrogenase, thereby blocking de novo purine synthesis and proliferation in the T and B lymphocytes [13].

MFF is available in capsules; the oral bioavailability approaches 100 %. MPA is glucuronidated in the liver to inactive metabolic mycophenolic acid glucuronide. The most commons side effects of MMF are GI in nature; these include nausea, vomiting, diarrhea, abdominal pain, and gastroesophageal reflux. Neutropenia and thrombocytopenia can also occur with MMF, requiring a dosage reduction. Since MMF is not metabolized by the cytochrome P450 system, interactions only affect its absorption, enterohepatic cycling, or renal excretion [27].

Biologic Immunosuppression

Polyclonal antibodies directed against lymphocytes have been used in transplantation since the 1960s. Monoclonal antibody techniques were discovered later and, in turn, allowed for the development of biologic agents such as OKT3, which target specific subsets of cells. One disadvantage of early murine-based antibody preparations such as OKT3 is the potential for the development of anti-mouse antibodies by the recipient, which may then limit further use of the agent. To address this problem, efforts have focused on the development of *humanized* versions of monoclonal antibodies (mAbs). These humanized mAbs have a very long half-life, reduced immunogenicity, and the possibility for repeated use [28].

Polyclonal Antibodies

Polyclonal antibodies are produced by immunizing animals, such as horses or rabbits, with human lymphoid tissue, allowing for an immune response, removing the resulting immune sera, and purifying the sera in an effort to remove unwanted antibodies. What remain are antibodies that recognize human lymphocytes. After administration of these antibodies, the transplant recipient's total lymphocyte count should fall and hence these are known as depleting antibodies.

ATGAM

ATGAM is a purified gamma globulin obtained by immunizing horses with human thymocytes. Infusion into a peripheral vein is often associated with thrombophlebitis; thus, infusion into a central vein is recommended. Side effects, which are more likely related to the release of pyrogenic cytokines, include fever, chills, arthralgia, thrombocytopenia, leukopenia, and serum-like sickness [29]. To avoid the cytokine release syndrome, recipients should be premedicated with methylprednisolone (MP) and diphenhydramine hydrochloride.

Thymoglobulin (ATG-R)

Thymoglobulin is obtained by immunizing rabbits with human thymocytes. Initial kidney transplant studies show ATG-R to be statistically superior to ATGAM in preventing and reversing acute rejection episodes [30]. Administration before reperfusion is advocated to maximize antiadhesion molecules effects. Medications should be given to prevent cytokine release syndrome. Side effects include fever, chills, arthralgias, infections, thrombocytopenia, and leukopenia [29, 31].

Monoclonal Antibodies

Hybridization of murine antibody—secreting B lymphocytes with a nonsecreting myeloma cell line—produces mAbs. Monoclonal antibodies have monovalent affinity, in that they bind to the same epitope.

Muromonab-CD3 (OKT3)

On binding to CD3, OKT3 mediates complement-dependent cell lysis and antibody-dependent cell cytotoxicity leading to rapid clearance of T cells from peripheral circulation [28]. Along with T cell depletion, the overall effect of OKT3 is likely to be due to interrupted T cell receptor binding and internalization, disrupted trafficking, and cytokine-mediated regulatory changes. If OKT3 is effective, the percentage of CD3-positive cells in the circulation should fall to, and stay below, 5 %. Side effects may occur when cytokines (e.g., TNF, IL-2, and interferon) are released by T cells into the circulation. Premedication with MP and diphenhydramine hydrochloride is important to minimize these side effects. The most serious side effect with OKT3 is a rapidly developing, noncardiogenic pulmonary edema that can be life threatening [32]. Other side effects include neurotoxicity, nephrotoxicity, and allograft thrombosis.

Anti-Interleukin-2 Monoclonal Antibodies (Basiliximab)

Basiliximab is an anti-CD25 monoclonal antibody. The alpha subunit of the IL-2 receptor, also known as Tac or CD25, is found exclusively on activated T cells. Binding of these agents to the IL-2 receptor results in blockade of IL-2-mediated responses. Because major portions of these agents are of human origin, they tend to have much longer half-lives than does OKT3. No lymphocyte depletion occurs with basiliximab; it is not designed to treat acute rejection. Its selectivity in blocking IL-2-mediated responses makes it a powerful induction agent without the added risks of infections, malignancies, or other major side effects [33, 34].

Alemtuzumab

Alemtuzumab is a CD52-specific humanized monoclonal antibody, initially used to treat chronic lymphocytic leukemia. It rapidly depletes CD52 expressing lymphocytes centrally and peripherally resulting from bulk T cell depletion with lesser depletion of B cells and monocytes. Alemtuzumab facilitates reduced maintenance immunosuppression requirements without an increase in infections or malignant complications in solid organ transplantations as compared to historical controls. Alemtuzumab causes a significant cytokine release reaction and often requires premedication [35, 36].

Rituximab

Rituximab is a chimeric monoclonal antibody specific for CD20, a cell surface glycoprotein involved in B cell activation and maturation [37]. It is FDA approved for treating lymphoma; however, its use has grown to include the treatment of antibody-mediated rejection and use in desensitization protocols with plasmapheresis and/or intravenous immunoglobulin [38]. The most important indication of Rituximab in solid organ transplantation is as a primary treatment of PTLD.

Eculizumab

Eculizumab is a humanized monoclonal antibody that is a first-in-class terminal complement inhibitor, with high affinity for C5, and the first therapy approved for the treatment of paroxysmal nocturnal hemoglobinuria (PNH). It blocks the activation of terminal complement. Adverse effects include an increased risk of infections, especially from encapsulated bacteria.

Bortezomib

Bortezomib is a proteasome inhibitor, FDA approved for treating myeloma. It has been shown to cause apoptosis of normal plasma cells, thereby decreasing alloantibody production in sensitized patients. Several case reports and series have described the use of Bortezomib for the treatment of antibody-mediated rejection and in desensitization protocols [38–40].

Fusion Proteins

Fusion proteins are made by the fusion of a single receptor targeting a ligand of interest with a secondary molecule, which is typically the Fc portion of an IgG molecule.

Costimulation-Based Agents

Costimulatory molecules alter the threshold for activation of naive T lymphocytes without having a primary activating or inhibitory function. The two costimulatory receptors on T cells are CD28 and CD152; these serve reciprocal roles: CD28 facilitates a T cell response, whereas CD152 reduces it.

Belatacept

Belatacept (also known as LEA29Y) is a second-generation costimulation-blockade agent that has two amino acid substitutions. It is a high-avidity molecule with slower dissociation rates.

Belatacept is a promising, nonnephrotoxic option in kidney transplant recipients and is being developed with the aim of providing calcineurin inhibitors avoidance [41, 42].

Other Immunosuppressive Agents

Leflunomide and Malononitrilamide (FK778)

Leflunomide and its analogues have strong antiproliferative effects on T lymphocytes and B lymphocytes. This group of medications also acts through inhibition of tyrosine kinase. FK778 and Leflunomide possess antiviral effects and have been used successfully to treat cytomegalovirus and BK virus nephropathy in renal transplant patients [43, 44].

Janus Kinase 3 Inhibitors

Janus kinase 3 (JAK3) is essential for the signal transduction from the cytokine receptors of several cytokines to the nucleus. JAK3 is expressed on immune cells only, making it an important target for developing new immunosuppressants. CP-690559 is the most potent and selective JAK3 inhibitor. Its effects include reduction in natural killer cell and T cell numbers, with unchanged numbers of CD8+ effector memory T cells [45].

Corticosteroids

Steroids have been a part of transplantation since its inception. It soon became clear, however, that the toxicities of steroids could overshadow their benefits. Despite numerous attempts to limit or discontinue their use, they remain an integral component of most immunosuppressive protocols. Steroids inhibit T cell proliferation, T cell-dependent immunity, and the expression of various cytokines, especially IL-2, IL-6, and interferon-γ, and tumor necrosis factor-α (TNF-α). They also suppress antibody formation and the delayed hypersensitivity response found in allograft rejection. Steroids use is associated with a series of problems, including acne, increased appetite, mood changes, diabetes, hypertension, and impaired wound healing [46]. Many transplant centers are switching to steroid-withdrawal/steroid-free protocols for many of their recipients [47, 48].

Infections

The suppression of the host immune response is required to establish and maintain a functioning solid organ graft. Advances in immunosuppression have led to improved graft survival rates. The growing population of immunosuppressed patients, in turn, has led to an increased incidence of opportunistic infections. Up to 80 % of solid organ transplant recipients experience an infectious complication during the first year posttransplant, and infections remain a major cause of morbidity and mortality in the transplant population [49]. In considering the epidemiology of infectious complications posttransplant, the clinician must assess several factors, including the time posttransplant, the organ transplanted, the type and degree of immunosuppression, the need for antirejection therapy, and the potential occurrence of surgical complications.

The preoperative assessment of both the recipient and the donor constitutes an important component of the solid organ transplant process. For the donor, the most important evaluation is the determination of CMV and EBV status, because those two agents are most easily transmitted to a seronegative recipient [50]. For the recipient, a thorough pretransplant history and physical examination are essential to minimize the risk of infectious complications secondary to a latent or indolent infectious process. Routine viral studies should be obtained, vaccinations updated, and prophylaxis administered where indicated.

The greatest risk of infections corresponds with the period of most intense immunosuppression, which is characteristically during the first 6–12 months posttransplant and after antirejection therapy, particularly for repeated AR episodes. Infectious complications in the first month posttransplant are typically caused by endogenous or nosocomial flora that would cause disease in an immunocompetent host; these include bacterial surgical site infections, postoperative or ventilator-associated pneumonia, urinary tract infections (UTIs) associated with prolonged or indwelling urinary catheters, intra-abdominal infections related to surgical complications, and central venous catheter infections [51, 52].

The period between 1 and 6 months posttransplant is typically the time of greatest immunosuppression and, subsequently, the time most opportunistic infections occur. They are frequently caused by fungal or especially viral pathogens that may become activated after lying dormant in the host or may be transferred from the donor with the graft [53–55].

These infection patterns may be categorized into an early cluster of viral agents occurring with peak frequency between 2 and 3 months posttransplant and a late cluster more commonly occurring between 4 and 9 months posttransplant. The early cluster includes CMV, adenoviruses, hepatitis B virus (HBV), hepatitis C virus (HCV), and human herpes virus (HHV)-6 [51–53, 55–58]. The late cluster includes varicella zoster and polyoma viruses. Epstein-Barr virus (EBV) may cause disease throughout the first year posttransplant [59].

The opportunistic fungi can similarly be observed to cluster with *Candida* and *Aspergillus* species (spp), causing infections in the first 2–3 months posttransplant, whereas *Cryptococcus*, histoplasmosis, coccidioidomycosis, and *P. jiroveci* most often occur later during the first year [60–63].

In the immediate postoperative period, recipients are significantly compromised from the stress of the operation, from induction immunosuppression, and often from initially impaired graft function. Infections in this period can be devastating. Surgical infections include generalized peritonitis, intra-abdominal abscesses, and wound infections. These require immediate intervention. Surgical infections are most severe in liver and pancreas recipients; in fact, surgical infections are the second most common cause for graft loss in pancreas recipients.

Risk factors for intra-abdominal infections include long operations with significant blood loss, prolonged warm and cold ischemic times, spillage of contaminated fluid, high level of induction immunosuppression immediately posttransplant, and anastomotic leaks. Localized infections or abscesses can be treated with percutaneous drainage and antibiotics; however, a prompt return to the operating room is often required.

Medical infections include respiratory, urinary tract, and bloodstream infections. Medical treatment should also be aggressive, often including empiric antibiotics and antifungals.

Late infections are primarily due to immunosuppression, specifically due to the depression of cell-mediated immunity that renders recipients susceptible to viruses, fungi, and parasites. Viral infections are usually from the herpesvirus group, with cytomegalovirus (CMV) and Epstein-Barr virus (EBV) being the most prominent. CMV is a latent infection that reactivates under immunosuppression. Infections usually occur 3–6 months posttransplant or during treatment for rejection. The incidence of CMV has been greatly reduced with 12-week acyclovir prophylaxis [64]. CMV infections range from an asymptomatic or mild flu-like syndrome to tissue-invasive disease resulting in pneumonitis, hepatitis, and gastrointestinal ulcerations. Symptomatic infections are treated with intravenous ganciclovir or with a reduction in immunosuppression. EBV infections range from a mononucleosis syndrome to hepatitis and, at worst, posttransplant lymphoproliferative disorder (PTLD). PTLD ranges from a localized tumor to a progressive, diffuse infiltration. It results from the proliferation of EBV-positive B cells in immunosuppressed patients. The main risk factors are a high degree of immunosuppression and a predisposing EBV serostatus [65]. The first line of treatment, for patients with early lesions, is to reduce immunosuppression. For those with more advanced PTLD, rituximab is used.

Solid organ transplants are associated with a significant risk of fungal infections. In the era of broad spectrum antibacterial prophylaxis and empiric therapy, the incidence of fungi as pathogens is increasing, as the incidence of azole drug-resistant fungal infections. Fungal infections are most common after liver and pancreas transplants, for which the incidence approaches 40 %. But they are less common after renal transplants (only 5 %) [66]. Nonetheless, all fungal infections are serious, with a mortality rate of 30–50 %.

The source of most fungal pathogens is the oral cavity, the gastrointestinal tract, or the environment. The most common fungal pathogens are the *Candida* spp. [67]. Risk factors associated with invasive candidal disease include diabetes, neutropenia, intense immunosuppression, and prolonged administration of antibiotics, particularly broad spectrum. *Pneumocystis jiroveci* is ubiquitous and can cause pulmonary disease in immunocompromised patients; however, prophylaxis with trimethoprim-sulfamethoxazole (TMP-SMX) is effective and has virtually eliminated this infection among transplant recipients [68]. *Blastomyces dermatitidis* grows in moist soil in the Midwest and Southeast regions of the United States. Diagnosis is confirmed by biopsy and treatment is with intravenous amphotericin. *Coccidioides immitis* is endemic in the Southwest, Northern Mexico, and various parts of Central and South America. High-dose amphotericin is the first line of treatment. *Histoplasma capsulatum* is found in chicken and bat droppings in the Ohio River and Mississippi River valleys. Invasive disease spreads from the lungs to the skin and bone marrow. Amphotericin B or itraconazole are appropriate therapeutic agents. Other opportunistic infections with *Aspergillus*, *Cryptococcus*, and *Rhizopus* species are rare but can cause serious infections [69].

Several common parasitic infections are seen in immunosuppressed solid organ transplant recipients. *Toxoplasma gondii* presents as a brain abscess with neurologic changes. Heart transplant recipients seem to be at greatest risk, possibly due to the presence of T. gondii cysts in donor myocardial tissue. If the heart donor was seropositive for T. gondii, the recipient normally undergoes prophylactic treatment with pyrimethamine and sulfadiazine for 3–6 months posttransplant. The mortality rate is high in transplant recipients who exhibit CNS disease [70, 71].

When assessing immunosuppressed transplant recipients for infectious diseases, the clinician must maintain a high index of suspicion at all times. The typical localizing signs of infection and inflammation may be blunted, or even absent, because of the anti-inflammatory action of immunosuppressive regimens.

Malignancy

Solid organ transplant recipients have a markedly increased risk of developing malignancy posttransplant. The increased incidence of malignancy is multifactorial, probably due to a combination of the activation of latent viruses with oncogenic potential, the direct oncogenic effect of immunosuppressive drugs such as cyclosporine, and, perhaps, environmental factors. Strong but indirect evidence points to the loss of immunologic surveillance as a mechanism of increased oncogenesis. The most extensive data, from a cohort study involving more than 175,000 solid organ transplant recipients, showed that 10,656 of them developed malignancies. The standardized incidence ratio was 2.10 (as compared with the general population). Recipients had at least a fivefold increase in these types of malignancies: Kaposi sarcoma, nonmelanoma skin cancer, non-Hodgkin lymphoma, and cancer of the liver, anus, vulva, and lip. In addition, recipients had a statistically significant increase in melanoma, Hodgkin lymphoma, and cancer of the lung, kidney, colon, rectum, and pancreas [72].

Posttransplant Lymphoproliferative Disorder (PTLD)

The term PTLD encompasses a very broad range of pathologies, from simple lymphoid hyperplasia to very aggressive monoclonal B-cell lymphomas. EBV infections play a central causative role. PTLD is least common in adult kidney transplant and most common in pediatric small bowel transplant recipients [73]. The clinical presentation varies widely. Many patients experience fever, sweats, and myalgias as the only symptoms. Some, but not all patients, have lymphadenopathy. Weight loss, diarrhea, and upper respiratory symptoms are also common. CNS involvement, which occurs in up to 20 % of patients, often manifests as mental status changes [74]. GI disease may be silent or may present as abdominal pain, GI bleeding, perforation with peritonitis, or bowel obstruction. Intrathoracic PTLD has a characteristic radiographic appearance of multiple circumscribed pulmonary nodules, which may or may not be accompanied by mediastinal lymphadenopathy. Biopsy of suspected lesions is the gold standard in establishing the diagnosis of PTLD [75]. Fluorodeoxyglucose-positron emission tomography (FDG-PET)/CT scanning has been increasingly used as a diagnostic and/or staging tool and in follow-up studies of PTLD patients [76]. No optimal prophylaxis against PTLD exists [77]. Treatment of established PTLD depends on each patient's situation and histologic diagnosis. Immunosuppression is reduced to minimal levels. Surgical intervention is clearly indicated for patients with GI PTLD that manifests as aggressive disease (e.g., viscus obstruction or perforation). Medical approaches to treating PTLD include antiviral medications (e.g., acyclovir, ganciclovir) [78]; interferon α2b [79]; immunoglobulins [78]; standard, low-dose, and high-dose chemotherapy protocols [80, 81]; and most recently, monoclonal antibodies directed against B-cell surface markers, such as CD19 and CD 20 (rituximab) [82].

Skin Cancer

The most common neoplasms associated with transplants and immunosuppression are nonmelanotic skin cancers. These lesions increase in frequency with sunlight exposure and with increasing time posttransplant. Studies show a prevalence of 66 % in transplant recipients in Australia after 24 years of surveillance and 40 % after 20 years in the Netherlands [83, 84]. Most skin cancers in transplant patients are squamous cell carcinomas. The incidence of melanomas is also higher representing 4.8 % of skin cancers in kidney transplant recipients, as compared to 2.7 % in the general population [85]. Solid organ transplant recipients are instructed to avoid direct exposure to sunlight for any prolonged period and to liberally use sunblock. Close dermatologic counseling and follow-up are warranted in this patient population. On identification of skin lesions, prompt surgical extirpation should be undertaken.

Kaposi Sarcoma

Kaposi sarcoma (KS) is a multicentric, vascularized, nodular neoplasm that may affect the skin and/or visceral tissues such as the lungs and GI tract. KS is endemic in the Mediterranean region and the Middle East; it is associated with either endogenous or exogenous immunosuppression. The incidence of this disease in US transplant recipients is 0.4 %, which represents a 20-fold increase over the basal rate in the population at large [85]. Cutaneous KS is readily identified by clinical appearance and biopsy. But patients with only visceral KS often present with more advanced disease, usually GI bleeding or viscus perforation, sometimes dyspnea related to pulmonary disease. The first step in treatment is reduction of immunosuppression, after which about 30–55 % of patients will experience remission. Chemotherapy is reserved for patients with visceral KD and for those who do not experience remission after their immunosuppression is reduced.

Cervical Cancer

The incidence of cervical intraepithelial neoplasia (CIN) in solid organ transplant patients approaches 50 %, which represents a 10–14-fold increase compared to the general population [86, 87]. Cervical carcinoma was seen in 10 % of all women with posttransplant cancer in the Transplant Tumor Registry [85]. Given the increased incidence of disease, close surveillance by pelvic examination and Papanicolaou smear is essential in this population.

Transmitted and Recurrent Malignancy

Case reports have described patients who received grafts that harbored malignant cells, leading to the development of malignancy. Currently, cancer or recent history of cancer is a contraindication to organ donation, with the possible exception of some low-grade skin cancers, noninvasive CNS neoplasms, and small, limited, extirpated cancers that are not likely to recur or spread. Patients with a history of malignancy clearly are at risk for recurrent disease posttransplant, presumably due to the use of immunosuppression. Data from the Transplant Tumor Registry show a 21 % recurrence rate, with the highest rates seen in patients with multiple myeloma (67 %), nonmelanotic skin cancer (53 %), bladder cancer (29 %), soft tissue sarcoma (29 %), renal cell cancer (27 %), and breast cancer (23 %) [88]. Tumors were least likely to recur if more than 5 years had passed between cancer treatment and the transplant.

Summary

Advances in the field of organ transplantation have been significant over the past several years. The primary limitation to further expansion may be considered to be logistic, related to organ availability. Dramatic improvements in medical care and technology have broadened the pool of potential recipients to include those who would have been considered too sick, with too much comorbidity, even a few years ago. Until medical science is able to develop immunosuppression without side effects, the predominant challenges in transplantation will remain the prevention, detection, and treatment of rejection; the prophylaxis, diagnosis, and treatment of infections; and the prevention, detection, and treatment of malignancy.

References

1. Carrel A. The surgery of blood vessels, etc. Bull Johns Hopkins Hosp. 1907;18:18–29.
2. Hamilton DN, Reid WA. Yu Yu. Voronoy and the first human kidney allograft. Surg Gynecol Obstet. 1984;159:289–94.
3. Medawar PB. Immunity to homologous grafted skin; the suppression of cell division in grafts transplanted to immunized animals. Br J Exp Pathol. 1946;27:9–14.
4. Merrill JP, Murray JE, Harrison JH, Guild WR. Successful homotransplantation of the human kidney between identical twins. J Am Med Assoc. 1956; 160:277–82.
5. Murray JE, Merrill JP, Harrison JH, Wilson RE, Dammin GJ. Prolonged survival of human-kidney homografts by immunosuppressive drug therapy. N Engl J Med. 1963;268:1315–23.
6. Squifflet J-P, et al. Lessons learned from ABO-incompatible living donor kidney transplantation: 20 years later. Exp Clin Transplant. 2004;2:208–13.
7. Matas A. Chronic rejection in renal transplant recipients–risk factors and correlates. Clin Transplant. 1994;8:332–5.
8. Womer KL, Vella JP, Sayegh MH. Chronic allograft dysfunction: mechanisms and new approaches to therapy. Semin Nephrol. 2000;20:126–47.
9. Wiseman AC. Polyomavirus nephropathy: a current perspective and clinical considerations. Am J Kidney Dis. 2009;54:131–42.
10. Starzl TE, Marchioro TL, Waddell WR. The reversal of rejection in human renal homografts with subsequent development of homograft tolerance. Surg Gynecol Obstet. 1963;117:385–95.
11. Cicciarelli J. Cyclosporine and trends in kidney transplantation. In: Terasaki P, editor. Clinical transplants. Los Angeles, CA: UCLA Tissue Typing Laboratory; 1986. p. 223–30.
12. Meier-Kriesche H-U, et al. Immunosuppression: evolution in practice and trends, 1994–2004. Am J Transplant. 2006;6:1111–31.
13. Remuzzi G, et al. Mycophenolate mofetil versus azathioprine for prevention of acute rejection in renal transplantation (MYSS): a randomised trial. Lancet. 2004;364:503–12.
14. Goto T, et al. Discovery of FK-506, a novel immunosuppressant isolated from Streptomyces tsukubaensis. Transplant Proc. 1987;19:4–8.
15. Wiederrecht G, Lam E, Hung S, Martin M, Sigal N. The mechanism of action of FK-506 and cyclosporin A. Ann N Y Acad Sci. 1993;696:9–19.
16. Burke JF, et al. Long-term efficacy and safety of cyclosporine in renal-transplant recipients. N Engl J Med. 1994;31:358–63.
17. Calne RY, et al. Cyclosporin A initially as the only immunosuppressant in 34 recipients of cadaveric organs: 32 kidneys, 2 pancreases, and 2 livers. Lancet. 1979;2:1033–6.
18. Sweny P, et al. Sixteen months experience with cyclosporin-A in human kidney transplantation. Transplant Proc. 1981;13:365–7.
19. Goto T, et al. FK 506: historical perspectives. Transplant Proc. 1991;23:2713–7.
20. Scott LJ, McKeage K, Keam SJ, Plosker GL. Tacrolimus: a further update of its use in the management of organ transplantation. Drugs. 2003;63: 1247–97.
21. Mihatsch MJ, et al. The side-effects of ciclosporine-A and tacrolimus. Clin Nephrol. 1998;49:356–63.
22. Heitman J, Movva NR, Hall MN. Targets for cell cycle arrest by the immunosuppressant rapamycin in yeast. Science. 1991;253:905–9.
23. Kaplan B, et al. Effect of sirolimus withdrawal in patients with deteriorating renal function. Am J Transplant. 2004;4:1709–12.
24. Larson TS, et al. Complete avoidance of calcineurin inhibitors in renal transplantation: a randomized trial

comparing sirolimus and tacrolimus. Am J Transplant. 2006;6:514–22.
25. Chan GL, Canafax D, Johnson CA. The therapeutic use of azathioprine in renal transplantation. Pharmacotherapy. 1987;7:165–77.
26. Elion GB. The George Hitchings and Gertrude Elion Lecture. The pharmacology of azathioprine. Ann N Y Acad Sci. 1993;685:400–7.
27. Fulton B, Markham A. Mycophenolate mofetil. A review of its pharmacodynamic and pharmacokinetic properties and clinical efficacy in renal transplantation. Drugs. 1996;51:278–98.
28. Webster A, Pankhurst T, Rinaldi F, Chapman JR, Craig JC. Polyclonal and monoclonal antibodies for treating acute rejection episodes in kidney transplant recipients. Cochrane Database Syst Rev. 2006; 1:1–94.
29. Brennan DC, et al. A randomized, double-blinded comparison of Thymoglobulin versus Atgam for induction immunosuppressive therapy in adult renal transplant recipients. Transplantation. 1999;67:1011–8.
30. Gaber AO, et al. Results of the double-blind, randomized, multicenter, phase III clinical trial of Thymoglobulin versus Atgam in the treatment of acute graft rejection episodes after renal transplantation. Transplantation. 1998;66:29–37.
31. Hardinger KL, et al. Five-year follow up of thymoglobulin versus ATGAM induction in adult renal transplantation. Transplantation. 2004;78:136–41.
32. Costanzo-Nordin MR. Cardiopulmonary effects of OKT3: determinants of hypotension, pulmonary edema, and cardiac dysfunction. Transplant Proc. 1993;25:21–4.
33. Vega O, Cárdenas G, Correa-Rotter R, Alberú J, Morales-Buenrostro LE. Basiliximab vs. limited-dose daclizumab (2 mg/kg) administered in single or two separated doses in kidney transplantation. Rev Invest Clin. 2008;60:82–6.
34. Sollinger H, et al. Basiliximab versus antithymocyte globulin for prevention of acute renal allograft rejection. Transplantation. 2001;72:1915–9.
35. Kirk AD, et al. Results from a human renal allograft tolerance trial evaluating the humanized CD52-specific monoclonal antibody alemtuzumab (CAMPATH-1H). Transplantation. 2003;76:120–9.
36. Agarwal A, Shen LY, Kirk AD. The role of alemtuzumab in facilitating maintenance immunosuppression minimization following solid organ transplantation. Transpl Immunol. 2008;20:6–11.
37. Pescovitz MD. Rituximab, an anti-cd20 monoclonal antibody: history and mechanism of action. Am J Transplant. 2006;6:859–66.
38. Blume OR, Yost SE, Kaplan B. Antibody-mediated rejection: pathogenesis, prevention, treatment, and outcomes. J Transplant. 2012;2012:7. 201754.
39. Locke JE, et al. The use of antibody to complement protein C5 for salvage treatment of severe antibody-mediated rejection. Am J Transplant. 2009;9:231–5.
40. Stegall MD, et al. Terminal complement inhibition decreases antibody-mediated rejection in sensitized renal transplant recipients. Am J Transplant. 2011;1 1:2405–13.
41. Larsen CP, et al. Rational development of LEA29Y (belatacept), a high-affinity variant of CTLA4-Ig with potent immunosuppressive properties. Am J Transplant. 2005;5:443–53.
42. Vincenti F, et al. Costimulation blockade with belatacept in renal transplantation. N Engl J Med. 2005;353:770–81.
43. John GT, Manivannan J, Chandy S, Peter S, Jacob CK. Leflunomide therapy for cytomegalovirus disease in renal allograft recipients. Transplantation. 2004;77: 1460–1.
44. Josephson MA, et al. Treatment of renal allograft polyoma BK virus infection with leflunomide. Transplantation. 2006;81:704–10.
45. Wojciechowski D, Vincenti F. Targeting JAK3 in kidney transplantation: current status and future options. Curr Opin Organ Transplant. 2011;16:614–9.
46. Fryer JP, et al. Steroid-related complications in the cyclosporine era. Clin Transplant. 1994;8:224–9.
47. Humar A, et al. Steroid minimization in liver transplant recipients: impact on hepatitis C recurrence and post-transplant diabetes. Clin Transplant. 2007; 21:526–31.
48. Matas AJ, et al. Prednisone-free maintenance immunosuppression-a 5-year experience. Am J Transplant. 2005;5:2473–8.
49. Brayman KL, et al. Analysis of infectious complications occurring after solid-organ transplantation. Arch Surg. 1992;127:38–47. discussion 47–8.
50. Spees EK, Light JA, Oakes DD, Reinmuth B. Experiences with cadaver renal allograft contamination before transplantation. Br J Surg. 1982;69:482–5.
51. Rubin RH, Wolfson J, Cosimi AB, Tolkoff-Rubin NE. Infection in the renal transplant recipient. Am J Med. 1981;70:405–11.
52. Dunn DL. Problems related to immunosuppression. Infection and malignancy occurring after solid organ transplantation. Crit Care Clin. 1990;6:955–77.
53. Kusne S, et al. Infections after liver transplantation. An analysis of 101 consecutive cases. Medicine (Baltimore). 1988;67:132–43.
54. Dummer JS, Hardy A, Poorsattar A, Ho M. Early infections in kidney, heart, and liver transplant recipients on cyclosporine. Transplantation. 1983;36: 259–67.
55. Snydman DR. Epidemiology of infections after solid-organ transplantation. Clin Infect Dis. 2001;33 Suppl 1:S5–8.
56. Fryd DS, et al. Cytomegalovirus as a risk factor in renal transplantation. Transplantation. 1980;30:436–9.
57. Singh N, Carrigan DR. Human herpesvirus-6 in transplantation: an emerging pathogen. Ann Intern Med. 1996;124:1065–71.
58. McGrath D, et al. Adenovirus infection in adult orthotopic liver transplant recipients: incidence and clinical significance. J Infect Dis. 1998;177:459–62.
59. Preiksaitis JK, Diaz-Mitoma F, Mirzayans F, Roberts S, Tyrrell DL. Quantitative oropharyngeal Epstein-

Barr virus shedding in renal and cardiac transplant recipients: relationship to immunosuppressive therapy, serologic responses, and the risk of posttransplant lymphoproliferative disorder. J Infect Dis. 1992;166:986–94.
60. Lumbreras C, et al. Randomized trial of fluconazole versus nystatin for the prophylaxis of Candida infection following liver transplantation. J Infect Dis. 1996;174:583–8.
61. Kusne S, et al. Factors associated with invasive lung aspergillosis and the significance of positive Aspergillus culture after liver transplantation. J Infect Dis. 1992;166:1379–83.
62. Wheat LJ, et al. Clinical practice guidelines for the management of patients with histoplasmosis: 2007 update by the Infectious Diseases Society of America. Clin Infect Dis. 2007;45:807–25.
63. Cohen IM, Galgiani JN, Potter D, Ogden DA. Coccidioidomycosis in renal replacement therapy. Arch Intern Med. 1982;142:489–94.
64. Hodson EM, et al. Antiviral medications to prevent cytomegalovirus disease and early death in recipients of solid-organ transplants: a systematic review of randomised controlled trials. Lancet. 2005;365:2105–15.
65. Mañez R, et al. Posttransplant lymphoproliferative disease in primary Epstein-Barr virus infection after liver transplantation: the role of cytomegalovirus disease. J Infect Dis. 1997;176:1462–7.
66. Paya CV. Fungal infections in solid-organ transplantation. Clin Infect Dis. 1993;16:677–88.
67. Nieto-Rodriguez JA, et al. Factors associated with the development of candidemia and candidemia-related death among liver transplant recipients. Ann Surg. 1996;223:70–6.
68. Glück T, et al. Pneumocystis carinii pneumonia as a complication of immunosuppressive therapy. Infection. 2000;28:227–30.
69. Playford EG, Webster AC, Sorell TC, Craig JC. Antifungal agents for preventing fungal infections in solid organ transplant recipients. Cochrane Database Syst Rev. 2004;1:1–58.
70. Luft BJ, Naot Y, Araujo FG, Stinson EB, Remington JS. Primary and reactivated toxoplasma infection in patients with cardiac transplants. Clinical spectrum and problems in diagnosis in a defined population. Ann Intern Med. 1983;99:27–31.
71. Selby R, et al. Brain abscess in solid organ transplant recipients receiving cyclosporine-based immunosuppression. Arch Surg. 1997;132:304–10.
72. Engels EA, et al. Spectrum of cancer risk among US solid organ transplant recipients. JAMA. 2011;306: 1891–901.
73. Ellis D, et al. Epstein-Barr virus-related disorders in children undergoing renal transplantation with tacrolimus-based immunosuppression. Transplantation. 1999;68:997–1003.
74. Penn I, Porat G. Central nervous system lymphomas in organ allograft recipients. Transplantation. 1995;59: 240–4.
75. Harris NL, Ferry JA, Swerdlow SH. Posttransplant lymphoproliferative disorders: summary of Society for Hematopathology Workshop. Semin Diagn Pathol. 1997;14:8–14.
76. Bianchi E, Pascual M, Nicod M, Delaloye AB, Duchosal MA. Clinical usefulness of FDG-PET/CT scan imaging in the management of posttransplant lymphoproliferative disease. Transplantation. 2008; 85:707–12.
77. Green M, Reyes J, Webber S, Rowe D. The role of antiviral and immunoglobulin therapy in the prevention of Epstein-Barr virus infection and post-transplant lymphoproliferative disease following solid organ transplantation. Transpl Infect Dis. 2001;3:97–103.
78. Pirsch JD, et al. Treatment of severe Epstein-Barr virus-induced lymphoproliferative syndrome with ganciclovir: two cases after solid organ transplantation. Am J Med. 1989;86:241–4.
79. Cantarovich M, Barkun JS, Forbes RD, Kosiuk JP, Tchervenkov JI. Successful treatment of post-transplant lymphoproliferative disorder with interferon-alpha and intravenous immunoglobulin. Clin Transplant. 1998;12:109–15.
80. Garrett TJ, et al. Posttransplantation lymphoproliferative disorders treated with cyclophosphamide-doxorubicin-vincristine-prednisone chemotherapy. Cancer. 1993;72:2782–5.
81. Smets F, et al. Indications and results of chemotherapy in children with posttransplant lymphoproliferative disease after liver transplantation. Transplantation. 2000;69:982–4.
82. Schaar CG, et al. Successful outcome with a "quintuple approach" of posttransplant lymphoproliferative disorder. Transplantation. 2001;71:47–52.
83. Sheil AG, Disney AP, Mathew TH, Amiss N. De novo malignancy emerges as a major cause of morbidity and late failure in renal transplantation. Transplant Proc. 1993;25:1383–4.
84. Bouwes Bavinck JN, et al. Relation between skin cancer and HLA antigens in renal-transplant recipients. N Engl J Med. 1991;325:843–8.
85. Penn I. Cancers in renal transplant recipients. Adv Ren Replace Ther. 2000;7:147–56.
86. Busnach G, et al. Viral and neoplastic changes of the lower genital tract in women with renal allografts. Transplant Proc. 1993;25:1389–90.
87. Ozsaran AA, et al. Evaluation of the risk of cervical intraepithelial neoplasia and human papilloma virus infection in renal transplant patients receiving immunosuppressive therapy. Eur J Gynaecol Oncol. 1999;20:127–30.
88. Penn I. Evaluation of transplant candidates with pre-existing malignancies. Ann Transplant. 1997;2:14–7.

Part VIII

Tissue Repair, Wound Healing, Abdominal Wall Hernas, Biologic Grafts, Artificial Limbs for Upper Extremities, and Pediatric/Fetal Surgery

Tissue Repair and Wound Healing: A Trip Back to the Future

46

Mahmoud A.Z. Abdelaal, Nicholas A. Giovinco, Marvin J. Slepian, and David G. Armstrong

Historical Introduction: From Healers to Doctors to Nurses and Teams

Early History Until the Early 1800s

Tissue repair and wound healing is one of the longest standing and central subjects in medicine and surgery. While records from antiquity date from the Pharaonic era (1500 BC), the basis of wound care likely had its origins much earlier extending to the period of prehistoric man where hunter-gatherers noticed that simple application of pressure to a bleeding wound and subsequent caring for its hygiene increased the chances of recovery from injury.

The finding of the Ebers Papyrus (Fig. 46.1), a document from ancient Egypt, provides insight into early Egyptian approach to wound care. It outlined the use of lint, animal grease, and honey as topical treatment of wounds. Lint provided a fibrous base that promoted wound-site closure, with the animal grease serving as a barrier to environmental pathogens, and honey functioning as an anti-infective agent [1]. The Greeks promoted similar therapies, but extended our insight into wounds to include characteristics of acute and chronic subtypes.

Claudius Galenus (better known as Galen of Pergamon) was a prominent Greek physician and a surgeon who furthered the understanding of wounds [2]. Significantly, he identified the importance of maintaining wound-site moisture to ensure successful closure of the wound.

In the twelfth century Moses Maimonides in his "Surgical Aphorisms" further identified the danger of skin "boils" and possible spread from these lesions, a precursor to the issue of infectious contamination and lateral spread. Further he identified the role of cauterization, heat, and corrosive agents as means of sterilizing a wound and preventing infectious spread [3].

All of these early observations and insight were amplified in the nineteenth century with the growth of the fields of microbiology and cellular pathology. See Fig. 46.2a–d. Finally, infection was recognized as being due to microorganism spread rather than a confluence of bad humors. Further, the role of inflammation, tissue ischemia, necrosis, and response to injury were revealed. These established the basis for a mechanistic understanding and approach to therapy.

M.A.Z. Abdelaal, M.D. • N.A. Giovinco, D.P.M. • D.G. Armstrong, D.P.M., M.D., Ph.D. (✉)
Southern Arizona Limb Salvage Alliance (SALSA), Department of Surgery, University of Arizona College of Medicine, Tucson, AZ, USA
e-mail: Dr.gm@live.com; ngiovinco@gmail.com; Armstrong@usa.net

M.J. Slepian, M.D.
Department of Medicine, University of Arizona College of Medicine, Tucson, AZ, USA
e-mail: chairman.syns@gmail.com

R. Latifi et al. (eds.), *Technological Advances in Surgery, Trauma and Critical Care*,
DOI 10.1007/978-1-4939-2671-8_46

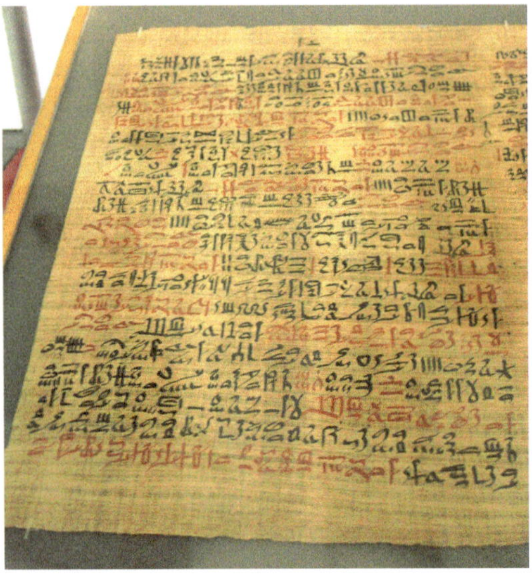

Fig. 46.1 The Ebers Papyrus (c. 1550 BC) from Ancient Egypt (*Source*: http://commons.wikimedia.org/wiki/File:PEbers_c41.jpg). By Einsamer Schütze [GFDL (http://www.gnu.org/copyleft/fdl.html) or CC BY-SA 3.0 (http://creativecommons.org/licenses/by-sa/3.0)], via Wikimedia Commons

Unfortunately, however, the same insights into the germ theory of medicine also led to physicians and surgeons literally and figuratively "washing their hands" off the problem. This perception coupled with the rise of professional societies of nurses led to much of the day-to-day management of wounds being borne on the shoulders of nurses.

1850s–1995: Poultices, Plasters, and Polymers

Much of the efforts over this period of time were focused on serving the dressing needs of nurses. Dressings were designed at best to manage drainage and to reduce pain during dressing changes. During World War I, in response to the needs of soldiers on the Western Front, Nobel Laureate Alex Carrel and chemist Henry Dakin screened more than 200 compounds and ultimately developed a wound-irrigating solution composed of sodium hypochlorite (0.45–0.5 %) in a buffered solution. This formulation, subsequently referred to as "Dakin's solution," provided excellent antimicrobial activity, combined with good irrigating properties without significant caustic, corrosive, or painful effects [4].

With the advent of synthetics and polymers in the 1950s, materials such as polyethylene, polypropylene, and polyvinyls provided constructs, in the form of gauzes and dressings, that further provided means to modulate the material properties of dressings. Some of these led to the first widely available foam/hydrocolloid-based dressings in the 1980s. More dressings such as these continued through the 1980s and into the 1990s until the next major advance: active healing technologies.

From Analog to Digital: Dressings and Supportive Care Meet Pharmaceuticals and Devices (Fig. 46.3)

In 1995, the first pharmaceutical requiring a prescription, Becaplermin (Regranex®, Smith+Nephew, Largo, FL), became available in North America. This single event led to rapid reeducation of the broader community of physicians and surgeons into chronic tissue repair and wound healing. Followed rapidly by negative pressure wound therapy (NPWT), and cell-based allografts (Dermagraft (Advanced Biohealing Ltd, La Jolla, CA), Apligraf® (Organogenesis, Inc., Canton, MA)), there emerged choices for physicians, surgeons, and nurses in therapies beyond previously available gauzes and intraoperative management/wound packing. In essence, technology further facilitated team building. This led to a dichotomy of sorts. The first of these two historical categories includes dressings and supportive care, which can now serve to manage drainage, reduce pain and frequency of dressing changes, and possibly also reduce/modulate bacterial load. The second, pharmaceuticals and devices, serves to promote angiogenesis and regeneration.

Significance of Wound Healing

Wound healing is a process via which injured tissue attempts to repair itself after injury. It is an intricate process in which the body tries to wall

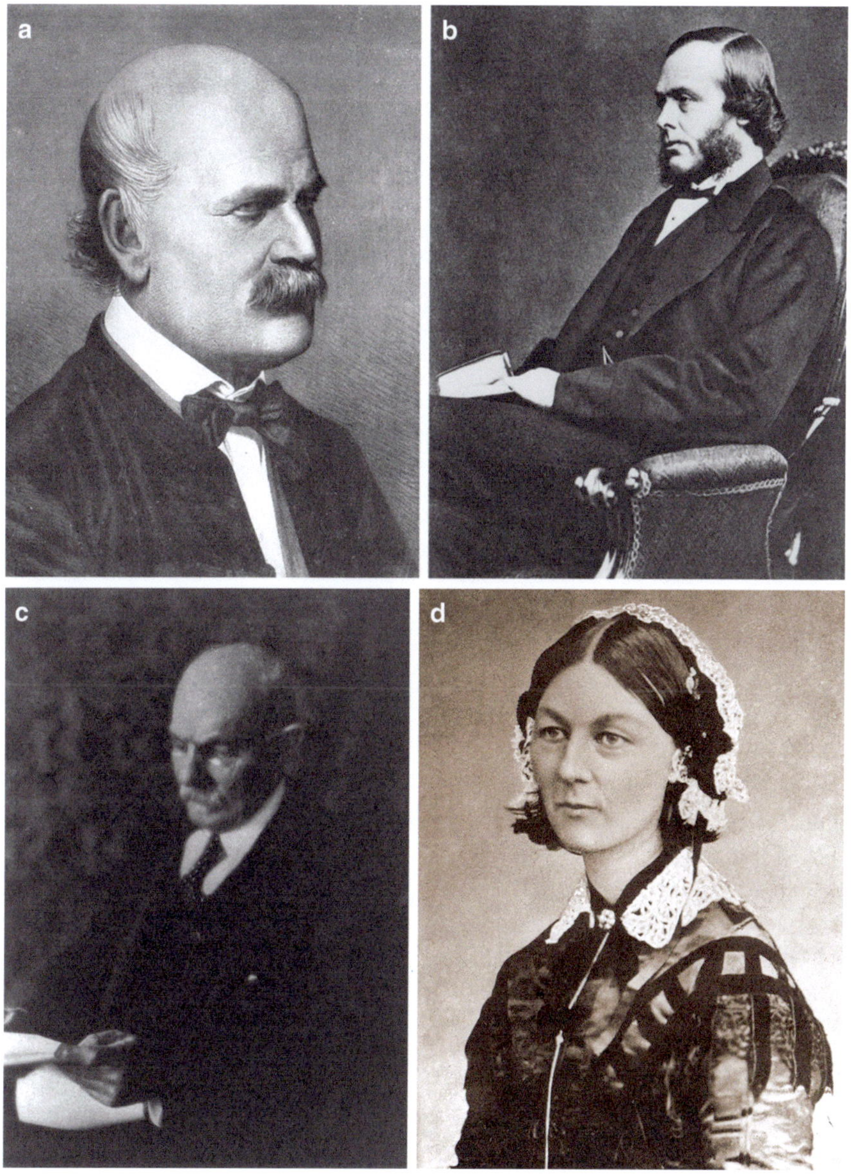

Fig. 46.2 (**a–d**) A brief timeline of wound healing. (**a**) Ignaz Philipp Semmelweis (July 1, 1818, to August 13, 1865) was a Hungarian physician now known as an early pioneer of antiseptic procedures (Ignaz Semmelweis 1860. Copper plate engraving by Jenő Doby. *Source*: http://upload.wikimedia.org/wikipedia/commons/f/f8/Ignaz_Semmelweis_1860.jpg. By Jenő Doby [Public domain], via Wikimedia Commons.); (**b**) Joseph Lister, 1st Baron Lister (April 5, 1827, to February 10, 1912). Known as Sir Joseph Lister. Between 1883 and 1897 was a British surgeon and a pioneer of antiseptic surgery (Joseph Lister, 1st Baron Lister, circa 1876: *Source*: http://commons.wikimedia.org/wiki/File%3AJoseph_Lister_c1867.jpg. Author unknown [Public domain], via Wikimedia Commons); (**c**) William Stewart Halsted (September 23, 1852 to September 7, 1922) was an American surgeon who emphasized strict aseptic technique during surgical procedures (William Stewart Halsted, 1852–1922, half-length portrait. *Source*: http://commons.wikimedia.org/wiki/File%3AWilliamHalsted.jpg. Author unknown [Public domain], via Wikimedia Commons); (**d**) Florence Nightingale (12 May 1820 to 13 August 1910) was a celebrated English social reformer and statistician, and the founder of modern nursing (Florence Nightingale from Care de Visite, circa 1850s. *Source*: http://commons.wikimedia.org/wiki/File%3AFlorence_Nightingale_CDV_by_H_Lenthall.jpg. By H. Lenthall, London [Public domain], via Wikimedia Commons)

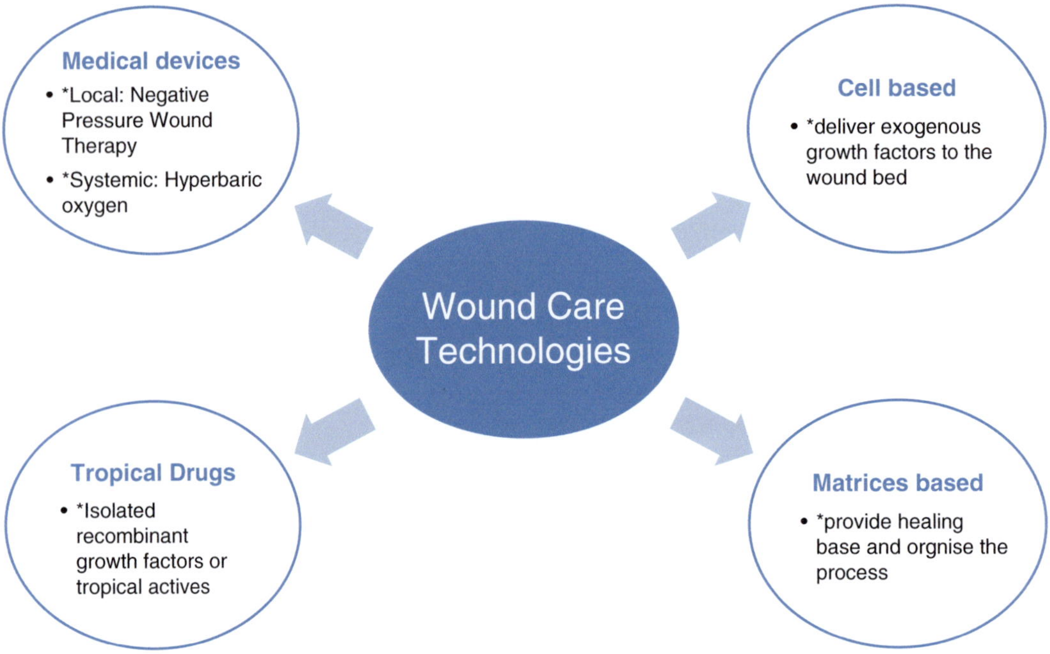

Fig. 46.3 Wound care technologies

off and eliminate infection, clear damaged and necrotic tissue, and rebuild damaged or lost tissue elements. The classic model of wound healing is divided into four sequential yet overlapping phases. These include (a) hemostasis, (b) inflammation, (c) proliferation, and (d) remodeling [5]. Under ideal conditions these phases progress synchronously. Certain pathophysiologic and metabolic conditions can alter this course of events so that healing is impaired or delayed, resulting in chronicity, i.e., chronic wounding [5, 6].

Perhaps the most common chronic wound in the developed and the developing world comes as a result of or concomitant with diabetes mellitus. According to the World health Organization, the epidemic of diabetes is affecting 285 million people (6.4 %) around the globe, and is expected to affect over 400 million adults by 2030 [7, 8]. A major cause of hospitalization and amputation among persons with diabetes is foot ulceration. It is estimated that one in four persons with diabetes in the USA will get foot ulcers at some point in their lifetimes [9]. As such, diabetic foot ulcer treatment is consuming nearly 25 % of overall cost of diabetes care, totaling around $43.5 billion [10]. Additionally, diabetes associated with ulceration increases the crude mortality rate from 6.7 to 27 % and shortens life expectancy by 3 years, relative to the average life expectancy for diabetic patients [11].

Additionally, as the world population is aging and becoming more sedentary, with an increased dependence on computers and automated manufacturing, low overall mobility results in venous obstruction or venous valvular dysfunction. This often precipitates chronic venous insufficiency which serves as yet an additional risk for foot ulceration. The annual prevalence of venous leg ulcers is estimated to be between 1.65 and 1.74 % in adults ≥65 years old, with anticipation of a substantial increase within the next several decades [12].

Wound Classification

In modern clinical practice, patients with foot ulcers present with a broad spectrum of underlying factors which contribute in the prognosis of the wound. Hence developing methods for stratification of wounds will help guide treatment decisions including the decision for amputation.

A recent advance was provided by the Society of Vascular Surgeons' Wound Ischemia Foot Infection (WIFI) classification, which was introduced in late 2013 to fill in the gaps remaining with other clinical diagnostic schemes. This classification systematically addressed individual grading of wound severity, ischemia, and presence of foot infection. Each category is graded based on specific criteria, which offers an improved and objective assessment of diabetic foot complications, and its recoverability [13].

The Strategies for Treatment: "Vertical" and "Horizontal"

There are two main strategies for treatment of ulcers, the "vertical strategy" or the "horizontal horizontal." In the vertical, the focus is aimed at trying to resolve the issue of the depth of the wound—either by filling the gap with living cells or approximating the edges using negative pressure. In the horizontal plan, the emphasis is aimed at trying to re-epithelialize the area using different techniques such as growth factors, negative pressure, stem cells, or amniotic membrane derivatives.

Modern Cell-Based Matrices: Three Examples

Grafix® (Osiris Therapeutics, Columbia, MD)

This is an example of a three-dimensional cellular matrix, designed to be directly applied to acute and chronic wounds—resulting from either burns or complications of the diabetic foot. It is a processed form of human placental membrane. With flexibility, this conforming membrane provides an excellent source of living mesenchymal stem cells (MSCs) and growth factors to the wound bed. The manufacturing process maintains the integrity of the extracellular matrix, the viability of the neonatal MSCs, and the active growth factors.

A clinical trial [14] to evaluate the safety and efficacy of Grafix for treatment of chronic foot ulcers was conducted. The trial included diabetic (both types) participants with foot ulcers which presented between 4 and 52 weeks, located around the malleoli aspects, varying in size from 1 to 15 cm^2, and age range from 18 to 80. The study protocol excluded patients with HbA1c above 12 %, active infection, osteomyelitis, cellulitis, or muscle, tendon, or joint capsule infections. Additional criteria were used to omit participants with circulatory insufficiency, which was determined using the ankle brachial index (ABI), toe brachial index (TBI), or Doppler. Participants with wound healing rates of 30 % or more during the screening period were also disqualified.

One hundred and thirty-nine patients were recruited, of which 42 were disqualified for matching the exclusion criteria. The remaining 97 were divided into two arms, 50 who received Grafix, with 47 receiving the standard wound therapy. No significant differences were observed in the baseline characteristics between the two arms. The Grafix arm revealed significant efficacy for primary and secondary endpoints when compared with the standard arm.

Thirty-one participants (62 %) of the Grafix group achieved complete wound closure, with significantly ($p=0.019$) faster median time (42 days) and probability (67.1 %) of closure, compared to ten in the standard wound therapy (21.3 %), with median time of 69.5 days and probability of 27.1 %. Grafix patients also required fewer study visits (i.e., applications) to achieve closure compared with patients in the control arm. The wound recurrence in the Grafix group, after complete closure, was 12.1 % less than the control arm.

As to safety, compared with the control arm, participants in Grafix arm experienced 22 % less adverse events, 18.2 % less wound-related infection, and 9 % fewer hospitalizations related to infection.

EpiFix® (MiMedx Group, Marietta, GA)

This is a dehydrated human amnion/chorion membrane (dHACM) allograft composed of multiple layers including a single layer of epithelial cells, a basement membrane, and an avascular connective tissue matrix. EpiFix® is a minimally manipulated, dehydrated, nonviable cellular amniotic membrane allograft that preserves and delivers multiple extracellular matrix proteins, growth factors, cytokines, and other specialty proteins present in amniotic tissue to help regenerate soft tissue.

A clinical trial with similar enrollment criteria to the Grafix study outlined above was conducted to evaluate the efficacy of the product. However, the exclusion criteria were more restrictive. The study omitted patients with active Charcot arthropathy, wounds involving bone, or patients receiving immune system modulators.

The study enrolled 25 participants following the previous criteria; they were randomized and categorized into two groups, EpiFix ($n = 13$) and standard wound care group ($n = 12$). At the 4-week point, the wound size of the EpiFix group showed threefold size reduction relative to the standard group, and at the 6-week mark, 92 % of all ulcers in the Epifix group were completely healed compared to the control group (8 %). The mean time for wound closure in the EpiFix group was 50 % less than the standard.

During the study, only one patient in the Epifix group experienced an adverse event, while four participants in the control arm encountered side effects [15].

Dermagraft® (Advanced Biohealing Ltd, La Jolla, CA): Human Fibroblast-Derived Dermal Substitute

Human fibroblast-derived dermal substitute (Dermagraft, Advanced Biohealing Ltd, La Jolla, CA) is composed of fibroblasts, extracellular matrix, and a bioabsorbable scaffold. It is produced by culturing human dermal fibroblast cells derived from newborn foreskin tissue onto a bioabsorbable polyglactin mesh scaffold. As the fibroblasts proliferate filling the interstices of this scaffold, they secrete human dermal collagen, matrix proteins, growth factors, glycosaminoglycans, and cytokines to generate a three-dimensional, allogeneic, human dermal substitute containing metabolically active, living cells with a preferred, nearly parallel alignment of the collagen fibers within human dermal substitute [16]. Unlike human skin, human fibroblast-derived dermal substitute does not contain macrophages, lymphocytes, blood vessels, or hair follicles [17]. Studies suggest that this dermal substitute encourage healing via two mechanisms. Initially, Dermagraft offers living human dermal fibroblasts that deposit matrix proteins which facilitate angiogenesis. Secondly the construct delivers a preformed collagen matrix, receptors, and bound growth factors that help the migration and colonization of the host's epithelial cells, which promote wound closure [18, 19].

Greatest efficacy with this therapy was seen in the treatment of ulcers of greater than 6-week duration, suggesting that these ulcers are deficient in many of the factors necessary for healing [20]. In a study examining risk factors related to ulcer healing it was found that initial ulcers greater than 2 cm^2 were associated with a 150 % greater incidence of closure, while females were twice likely to heal more than males [21]. However, an episode of infection during the 12 weeks of treatment was associated with 3.4 times increased risk of non-closure cases.

A precaution that should be taken with Dermagraft relates to patients with known hypersensitivity to bovine products, as the packaging medium contains traces of bovine serum. Additionally the fibroblast-derived dermal substitute cannot be used in cases of clinical infection or ulcers with sinus tracts.

Devices: Negative Pressure Wound Therapy (Fig. 46.4a–d)

The main principle of the NPWT involves the application of local subatmospheric pressure to a defect, leading to a decrease of the wound margins and promotion of granulation tissue through enhancement of the surrounding circulation within the wound bed. Continuous negative pressure stimulates cell proliferation and increases extracellular fluid, which maintain moisture

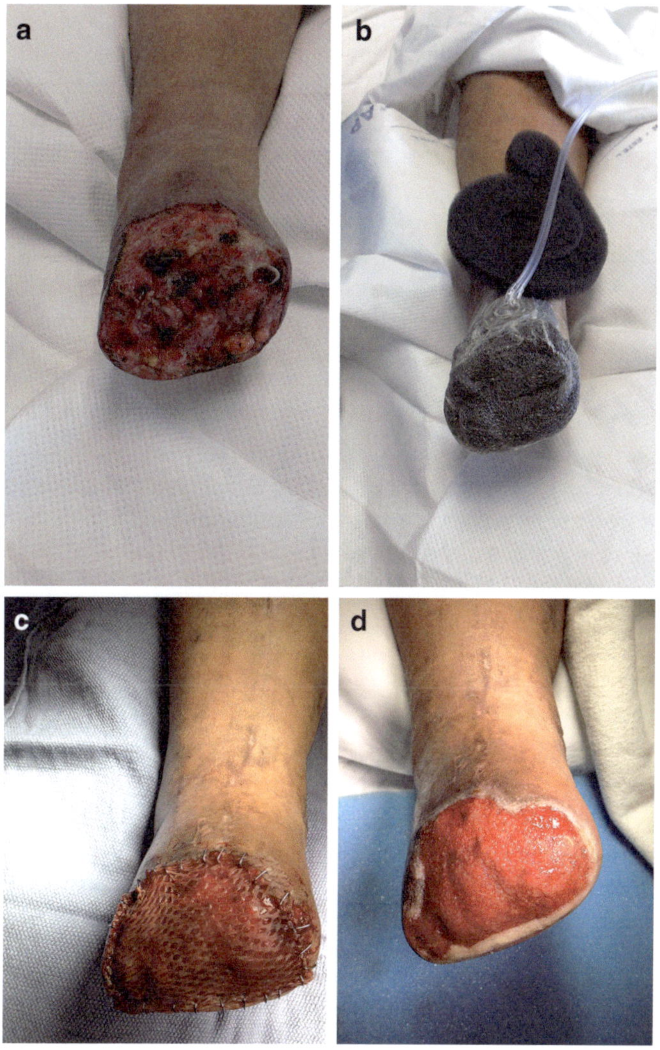

Fig. 46.4 (**a–d**) Negative pressure wound therapy (NPWT)

within the wound, as well as stimulate fibroblast migration and angiogenesis. Additionally, the system facilitates the removal of exudate and infectious material, and decreases matrix metalloproteinases (MMPs) which degrade tissue healing and block the surrounding microvascular circulation [22–27].

An early study of NPWT was conducted by Morykwas and colleagues [28], which reported a 400 % increase in the subcutaneous blood flow for tissue and muscles of Chester pigs. While they also observed a decrease of local blood flow after 5–7 min of the continuous negative pressure, they were able to reestablish high blood flow after a 2-min period of negative pressure.

Presently, there are several devices that allow for safe and effective NPWT. The most widely used system is the vacuum-assisted closure device, or VAC® (KCI, San Antonio, TX) therapy. The VAC device is offered in several forms, the black traditional and the more common, silver, and white foam. Traditionally, black GranuFoam™ (KCI, San Antonio, TX) is made of porous (400–600 mm) relatively hydrophobic, polyurethane ether. However, VAC Silver has micro-bonded metallic silver impregnated into the foam itself, whereas the WhiteFoam version has a premoistened, hydrophilic foam made from polyvinyl alcohol. This form is effective especially when used as bolster for skin grafts and when granulation tissue formation is not the desired result, as in deep-space infection.

A study in 2005 by Armstrong and Lavery [29] over a 16-week period showed that the treatment with NPWT resulted in both an increased rate and proportion of patients healing complex lower extremity diabetic wounds following partial foot amputation. An additional study in 2008, by Blume and colleagues [30], compared NPWT with advanced moist wound therapy. Similarly this study demonstrated that NPWT was more effective with 14 % more complete closure observed.

The Future: Measuring What We Manage

While many new technologies show great promise in facilitating robust angiogenic response or promoting epithelialization, tissue repair and chronic wound healing have suffered from a lack of objective criteria for success. The only hard endpoint that presently exists (healing) has become inadequate to objectively assess the potential therapeutic effects of specific agents. Point of care and near-point-of-care diagnostics such as those that can assess protease activity, pH, cell receptor vitality, and general/specific organization of the wound microbiome will all likely play a crucial role in the development of new classes of therapeutics over the coming decade [31–33].

Conclusion

Stemming from antiquity, basic aspects of wounding and wound healing—both as to cause, pathophysiologic mechanisms, response to injury, and approaches to therapy—have been revealed and increasingly appreciated. In the modern era the role of ischemia, tissue injury, release of metalloproteases, inflammation, and infection are well recognized. Further, the time course of events is increasingly appreciated and therapeutic efforts aimed at these have been developed. Significant advances have been made in all mechanistic aspects of wound treatment including the novel use of negative pressure, biomaterial substrates, and cell engraftment. In the future further advances will continue to add to both our diagnostic and therapeutic capabilities. The future remains bright for this area.

References

1. Molan PC. Honey as a topical antibacterial agent for treatment of infected wounds. Nurs Times. 2001; 49(7-8):96.
2. Peter Brain G. Galen on bloodletting: a study of the origins, development and validity of his opinions, with a translation of the three works. Cambridge: Cambridge University Press; 2009. p. 1.
3. Rosner F. The medical legacy of moses maimonides. 1st ed. Jersey City, NJ: Ktav Pub Inc; 1997.
4. Hartmann H. Classic articles in colonic and rectal surgery. New procedure for removal of cancers of the distal part of the pelvic colon. Dis Colon Rectum. 1984;27(4):273.
5. Stadelmann WK, Digenis AG, Tobin GR. Physiology and healing dynamics of chronic cutaneous wounds. Am J Surg. 1998;176(2A Suppl):26S–38.
6. Mustoe TA, O'Shaughnessy K, Kloeters O. Chronic wound pathogenesis and current treatment strategies: a unifying hypothesis. Plast Reconstr Surg. 2006; 117(7 Suppl):35S–41.
7. Guariguata L, Whiting D, Weil C, Unwin N. The International Diabetes Federation diabetes atlas methodology for estimating global and national prevalence of diabetes in adults. Diabetes Res Clin Pract. 2011;94(3):322–32.
8. The Centers for Disease Control and Prevention. Number of people with diabetes increases to 24 million. http://www.cdc.gov/media/pressrel/2008/r080624.htm. Accessed 6 Oct 2014.
9. Singh N, Armstrong DG, Lipsky BA. Preventing foot ulcers in patients with diabetes. JAMA. 2005; 293(2):217–28.
10. Kantor J, Margolis DJ. Treatment options for diabetic neuropathic foot ulcers: a cost-effectiveness analysis. Dermatol Surg. 2001;27(4):347–51.
11. Brownrigg JR, Griffin M, Hughes CO, Jones KG, Patel N, Thompson MM, Hinchliffe RJ. Influence of foot ulceration on cause-specific mortality in patients with diabetes mellitus. J Vasc Surg. 2014;60(4): 982–6. e3.

12. Charles CA, Tomic-Canic M, Vincek V, Nassiri M, Stojadinovic O, Eaglstein WH, Kirsner RS. A gene signature of nonhealing venous ulcers: potential diagnostic markers. J Am Acad Dermatol. 2008; 59(5):758–71.
13. Mills Sr JL, Conte MS, Armstrong DG, Pomposelli FB, Schanzer A, Sidawy AN, Andros G. The Society for Vascular Surgery Lower Extremity Threatened Limb Classification System: risk stratification based on wound, ischemia, and foot infection (WIfI). J Vasc Surg. 2014;59(1):220–34.e2.
14. Lavery LA, Fulmer J, Shebetka KA, Regulski M, Vayser D, Fried D, Kashefsky H, Owings TM, Nadarajah J. The efficacy and safety of Grafix® for the treatment of chronic diabetic foot ulcers: results of a multi-centre, controlled, randomised, blinded, clinical trial. Int Wound J. 2014;11(5):554–60.
15. Zelen CM, Serena TE, Denoziere G, Fetterolf DE. A prospective randomised comparative parallel study of amniotic membrane wound graft in the management of diabetic foot ulcers. Int Wound J. 2013;10(5):502–7.
16. Marston WA. Dermagraft, a bioengineered human dermal equivalent for the treatment of chronic nonhealing diabetic foot ulcer. Expert Rev Med Devices. 2004;1(1):21–31.
17. Wu SC, Marston W, Armstrong DG. Wound care: the role of advanced wound-healing technologies. J Am Podiatr Med Assoc. 2010;100(5):385–94.
18. Mansbridge J, Liu K, Patch R, Symons K, Pinney E. Three-dimensional fibroblast culture implant for the treatment of diabetic foot ulcers: metabolic activity and therapeutic range. Tissue Eng. 1998;4(4):403–14.
19. Mansbridge J. Skin substitutes to enhance wound healing. Expert Opin Investig Drugs. 1998;7(5):803–9.
20. Marston WA, Hanft J, Norwood P, Pollak R. The efficacy and safety of Dermagraft in improving the healing of chronic diabetic foot ulcers: results of a prospective randomized trial. Diabetes Care. 2003;26(6):1701–5.
21. Marston WA. Risk factors associated with healing chronic diabetic foot ulcers: the importance of hyperglycemia. Ostomy Wound Manage. 2006;52(3):26–8. 30, 32, passim.
22. Armstrong DG, Attinger CE, Boulton AJ, Frykberg RG, Kirsner RS, Lavery LA, Mills JL. Guidelines regarding negative wound therapy (NPWT) in the diabetic foot. Ostomy Wound Manage. 2004;50(4B Suppl):3S–27.
23. Dockery G, Crawford ME. Lower extremity soft tissue & cutaneous plastic surgery. 1st ed. Philadelphia: Saunders Ltd; 2006.
24. Andros G. Armstrong DG, Attinger C E, Boulton AJ, Frykberg R G, Joseph WS, Lavery LA. Morbach S, Niezgoda JA, Toursarkissian B. Consensus statement on negative pressure wound therapy (V.A.C. therapy) for the management of diabetic foot wounds. Ostomy Wound Manage 2006;Suppl:1–32.
25. Saxena V, Hwang CW, Huang S, Eichbaum Q, Ingber D, Orgill DP. Vacuum-assisted closure: microdeformations of wounds and cell proliferation. Plast Reconstr Surg. 2004;114(5):1086–96. Discussion 1097–8.
26. Olenius M, Dalsgaard CJ, Wickman M. Mitotic activity in expanded human skin. Plast Reconstr Surg. 1993;91(2):213–6.
27. Wysocki AB, Staiano-Coico L, Grinnell F. Wound fluid from chronic leg ulcers contains elevated levels of metalloproteinases MMP-2 and MMP-9. J Invest Dermatol. 1993;101(1):64–8.
28. Morykwas MJ, Argenta LC, Shelton-Brown EI, McGuirt W. Vacuum-assisted closure: a new method for wound control and treatment: animal studies and basic foundation. Ann Plast Surg. 1997;38(6): 553–62.
29. Armstrong DG, Lavery LA. Negative pressure wound therapy after partial diabetic foot amputation: a multicentre, randomised controlled trial. Lancet. 2005; 366(9498):1704–10.
30. Blume PA, Walters J, Payne W, Ayala J, Lantis J. Comparison of negative pressure wound therapy using vacuum-assisted closure with advanced moist wound therapy in the treatment of diabetic foot ulcers: a multicenter randomized controlled trial. Diabetes Care. 2008;31(4):631–6.
31. Isaac AL, Armstrong DG. Negative pressure wound therapy and other new therapies for diabetic foot ulceration: the current state of play. Med Clin North Am. 2013;97(5):899–909.
32. Armstrong DG, Giovinco NA. Diagnostics, theragnostics, and the personal health server: fundamental milestones in technology with revolutionary changes in diabetic foot and wound care to come. Foot Ankle Spec. 2011;4(1):54–60.
33. Fisher TK, Wolcott R, Wolk DM, Bharara M, Kimbriel HR, Armstrong DG. Diabetic foot infections: a need for innovative assessments. Int J Low Extrem Wounds. 2010;9(1):31–6.

Surgical Advances in the Treatment of Abdominal Wall Hernias

47

Fernando Carbonell-Tatay
and Ángel Zorraquino González

Introduction

At the end of the 1980s, the situation of abdominal wall surgery was paradoxical. While the techniques of autoplasty represented a great technological development (Albanese, Lázaro da Silva), and prosthetic materials were used to reinforce plasties, mainly polypropylene meshes in retro muscle options (Rives) or onlay (Chevrel), it was significant that at the time little attention was given to this type of surgery by the surgeons themselves, who delegated this procedure to surgeons-in-training: the opening and closing of the abdominal wall was looked upon as merely a step prior to what was then considered the main surgery on the abdominal viscera.

In the late 1990s and mainly in the last decade, we have witnessed a drastic change in this sense, due to two facts that occurred simultaneously. On the one hand, the publication of the *Component Separation Technique* by Oscar Ramirez in 1990 acted as a catalyst for the abdominal wall restorative surgery described by Albanese in 1951; and on the other hand, the development of laparoscopic surgery and the emergence of minimally invasive surgery in gastrointestinal pathology affected access to the peritoneal cavity and treatment of the abdominal wall. Both coincide in timing to polarize the attention of general surgeons regarding a surgery that was left behind, considered a complication of digestive system surgery more than a pathology by itself: the abdominal wall hernia surgery.

With the use of the laparoscopic approach, attention is on the development of prostheses that can be placed on the parietal peritoneum covering the defect without the risk of a visceral injury, and on devices to hold the prosthesis, such as helical staples, applied via trocars.

With the Component Separation Technique, the interest in abdominal wall anatomy and physiology has risen again, bringing back old techniques of autoplasty and procedures to reverse the content of large hernia sacs to a reduced abdominal cavity, adapting it to a smaller volume, such as in the case of the preoperative progressive pneumoperitoneum.

The creation of a whole arsenal of surgical techniques and prosthetic materials has led to the emergence of specific departments or sections devoted to Abdominal Wall Surgery that can be seen as a subspecialty of General Surgery in large hospitals, and to the creation of scientific societies

F. Carbonell-Tatay, M.D. (✉)
Department of Abdominal Wall Surgery, Faculty of Medicine at the University of Valencia, La Fe University Hospital, Valencia, Spain

Á. Zorraquino González, M.D.
Department of General Surgery, Abdominal Wall Surgery Unit, Faculty of Medicine at the Basque Country University, Basurto University Hospital, Bilbao, Basque Country, Spain
e-mail: zorrakino@gmail.com

R. Latifi et al. (eds.), *Technological Advances in Surgery, Trauma and Critical Care*,
DOI 10.1007/978-1-4939-2671-8_47

for the study and dissemination of the knowledge that is emerging in this surgical field still experiencing advances today.

The Preoperative Period

When we consider the surgical treatment of eventration, we must have a protocol established for the global study of the patient, for the request of preoperative tests, and for the preparation of the patient for surgery. Its implementation will allow for the best chances for a successful intervention, both in terms of a definite cure of the hernia and in terms of the reduction of complications that may arise in the postoperative period. The protocol includes:

1. Performing a Valsalva CT
2. Performing Preoperative Progressive Pneumoperitoneum
3. Use of Botulinum Toxin
4. Use of Muscle Expanders

Imaging Tests

The diagnosis of eventration and abdominal wall hernias is usually clinical, and a physical examination is sufficient in most cases. However, in cases of complicated hernias or atypical locations and in obese patients or in those with a history of previous abdominal surgery, the clinical diagnosis may be difficult.

Imaging techniques effectively establish the diagnosis in these uncertain cases, differentiating other situations that may look like hernias or eventrations, such as asymmetries, muscle atrophy and paralysis, bruising, or tumors of abdominal wall. Also, imaging allows for evaluation of related complications, abdominal volume, and hernia sac volume; helps in terms of assessing the availability of the aponeurotic muscle plane; and assists with choosing the best therapeutic options.

The development of imaging techniques in recent years has allowed us to obtain very precise and quantifiable information regarding hernia orifices, location, content, and muscle condition.

Ultrasound is a technique that has a variable sensitivity and specificity as demonstrated in published series, since it depends upon the skill and experience of the operator and also depends on the physical characteristics of the patient. It is an imaging technique that, due to its noninvasive features, is considered a technique of choice for pediatric patients.

Computerized Tomography (CT) is currently the most widely used technique in the overall assessment of the condition of the abdominal wall. It is an effective technique in the detection of hernias and allows classification with low operator variability. Also, with the current multidetector equipment, it is an extraordinarily rapid test that can be performed in just a few seconds. Although there are different imaging protocols, it is normally recommended to obtain reconstructed images with a thickness less than 3 mm, which would allow for obtaining high-quality multiplane images (sagittal, coronal, oblique) later.

In studies of abdominal wall with CT, it is not required to systematically use intravenous contrast media, although its use is indispensable for performing the test to evaluate possible complications and to study the vascularization of the abdominal wall. The positive oral contrast (iodinated or barium) can help with the identification of small bowel herniated loops and differentiate hernias from seromas or other liquid content collection.

Magnetic Resonance Imaging (MRI) is a safe imaging technique that uses magnetic properties of protons to produce high contrast resolution images. Compared to CT, MRI is less available, has lower spatial resolution, has more sensitivity to motion artifacts, and takes longer to perform; therefore, most centers use it less than CT to evaluate the abdominal wall.

It is recommended that CTs and MRIs be carried out with the *Valsalva*[1] maneuver, since the supine position reduces intra-abdominal

[1] Antonio María Valsalva (1666–1723): Italian anatomist from Imola, pupil of Malpighi and teacher of Morgagni. Valsalva published in 1704 his "De aure humana tractatus" (Human ear treatise), explaining in detail the maneuver initially designed to relieve the pressure of the Eustachian tubes and possibly to eliminate pus from the middle ear.

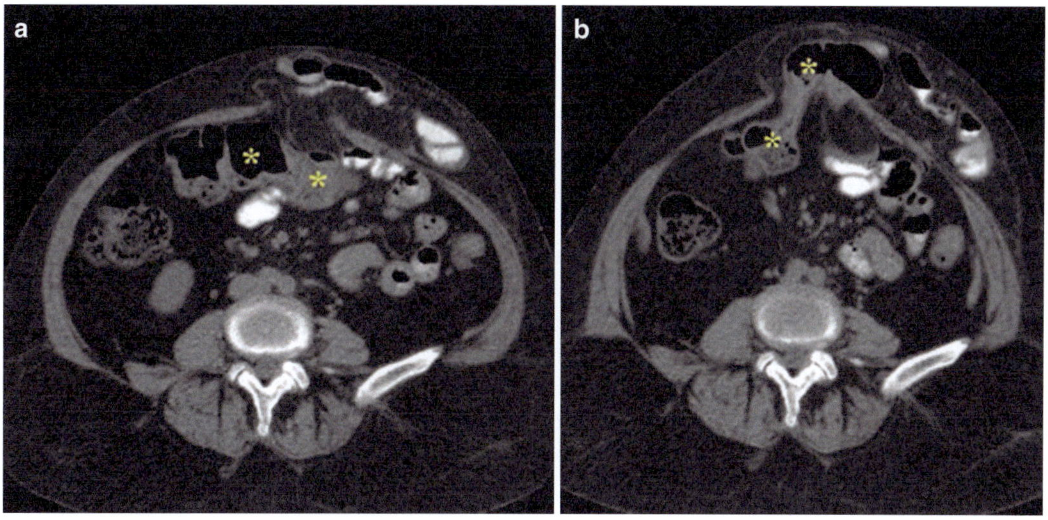

Fig. 47.1 Midline eventration with herniation of jejunal loops. Transverse CT images in apnea (**a**) and with Valsalva maneuver (**b**) where the hernia contents increased after the maneuver, including also the transverse colon (**a, b**: Used with permission from Carbonell-Tatay F, Moreno-Egea A (eds). Eventraciones. Otras hernias de pared y cavidad abdominal. Valencia (Spain): Spanish Association of Surgeons (AEC); 2012)

pressure, therefore reducing the herniated content and even decreasing the orifice diameters (see Fig. 47.1a, b).

The *Valsalva* maneuver (such as coughing and defecation) simulates abdominal pressure originating from daily life activity. When performing it during the study, it not only allows for a better evaluation of the herniated content but also minimizes false negatives. It is important to highlight that up to a 10 % of hernias are not detected in the studies performed without the Valsalva maneuver.

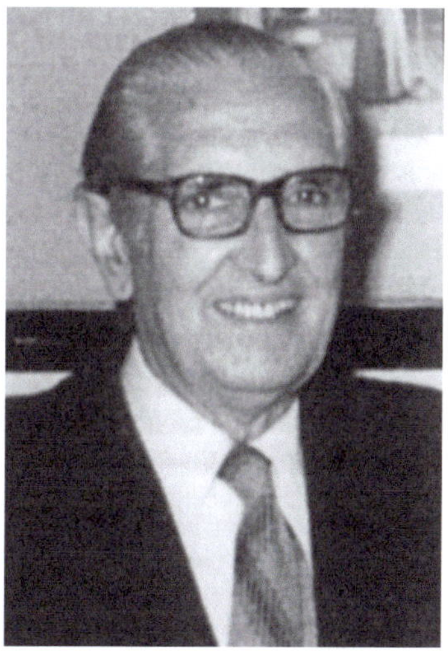

Fig. 47.2 Iván Goñi Moreno, M.D., (1905–1976) (Used with permission from Carbonell-Tatay F, Moreno-Egea A (eds). Eventraciones. Otras hernias de pared y cavidad abdominal. Valencia (Spain): Spanish Association of Surgeons (AEC); 2012)

Preoperative Progressive Pneumoperitoneum (PPP)

Surgical repair of large hernias requires the preparation of the patient to receive the visceral content from the hernia sac into an abdominal cavity reduced by the retraction of anterolateral abdominal muscles and the secondary loss of the diaphragm muscle's function that cannot find support to recover its concavity after contracting due to the loss of the abdominal wall's tone.

To make the reduction of hernia content possible without the negative consequences of the increased intra-abdominal pressure and the respiratory restriction that would cause its immediate reduction, the PPP is used.

The Argentine surgeon Iván Goñi Moreno (1905–1976) (Fig. 47.2) noticed the abdominal distension that occurred in some patients after accidental air leakage into the peritoneal cavity during the diagnostic retro-pneumoperitoneum that was performed at the time as double contrast technique to study kidneys and adrenal glands, reporting its usefulness to repair large eventrations in the XII Argentine Congress in October 1940 and publishing his experiences years later (1946). Since then, the preoperative progressive pneumoperitoneum has been used to increase the size of the abdominal cavity in the repair of large eventrations, facilitating the reduction of the hernia sac content and the closure of the abdominal wall without tension. It has avoided space conflicts, high intra-abdominal pressure, and its most severe consequence, the Abdominal Compartment Syndrome (ACS).

The way to conduct the pneumoperitoneum may vary, but it basically consists of the introduction of environment air through a catheter that is placed in the peritoneal cavity through the abdominal wall. At our hospital, an eight French catheter is introduced, with the guidance of ultrasound, into the peritoneal cavity at one of the sides of the abdomen, based on the characteristics and location of the eventration. Usually patients are admitted 7–10 days before surgical intervention in order to conduct progressive pneumoperitoneum. The preoperative progressive pneumoperitoneum is intended to stabilize the diaphragm muscle, stimulating its function, and to dissect lax adherences inside the hernia sac by the action of introduced air. To prevent the air from distending only the hernia sac, where it will usually settle itself because of its lower pressure, an abdominal binder will be placed on the patient, allowing air distribution in the abdominal cavity and increasing the efficacy of the procedure as the total volume of air required is reduced, shortening the duration of the procedure.

The increase in the abdominal cavity affecting anterolateral muscles of the abdominal wall requires the procedure to be longer, in the experience of Dr. León Herszage (Fig. 47.3), no less than 30 days.

In our experience, admitting the patient 7–10 days before the surgical intervention is sufficient to achieve the first two objectives of developing the pneumoperitoneum: give functional support to the diaphragm muscle and promote a pneumatic dissection of the hernia content, achieving its partial or complete reduction to the abdominal cavity. To increase the capacity of this cavity, we have always been confident in the use of autoplastic techniques, with good results. During the preoperative period, a functional respiratory study and chest physiotherapy should be conducted.

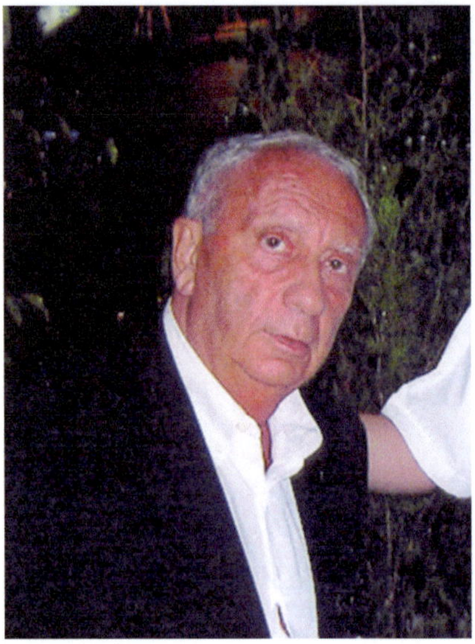

Fig. 47.3 León Herszage, M.D.

The Botulinum Toxin

Some medical schools, such as those in Mexico, combine performing the PPP with the use of Botulinum Toxin on the muscles of the abdominal wall, so that the pneumoperitoneum results are more effective due to muscle paralysis.

This is a technique described by Dr. Tomás Ibarra (Fig. 47.4) in 2007 and published in 2009. The botulinum toxin type A is used by infiltrating it in the side muscles of the abdomen (transverse and oblique of both sides) in order to cause a temporary paralysis, reducing therefore the pressures that tend to separate the rectus muscles and enlarge the hernia defects, allowing also an increase of the abdominal cavity volume up to a maximum of 20 % of its initial capacity in a period of 30 days [1].

The effect of the toxin is to block the release of acetylcholine at the motor plate of the nerve

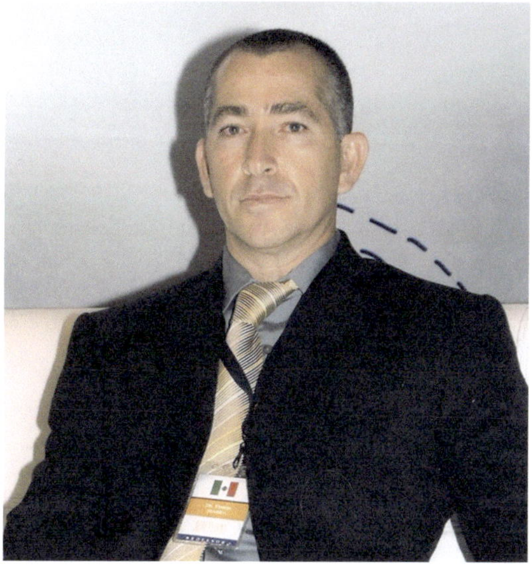

Fig. 47.4 Tomás R. Ibarra-Hurtado, M.D.

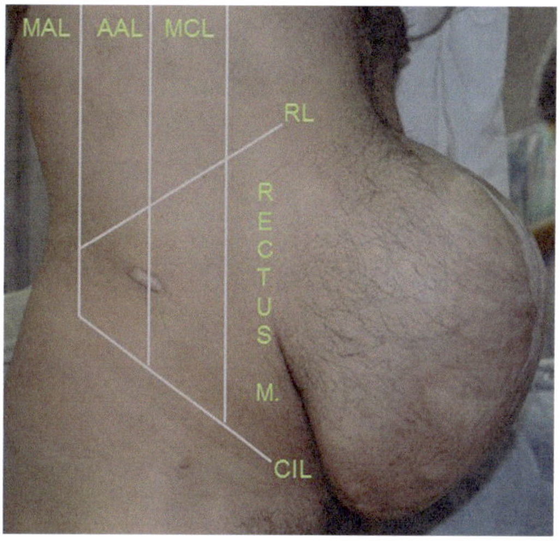

Fig. 47.5 References to locate the infiltration points of the Botulinum toxin. *MAL* medium axillary line, *AAL* anterior axillary line, *MCL* Medium clavicular line, *RL* Ribs line, *ICL* Iliac crest line, *Rectus M* Abdominal rectus muscle. Two punctures between MAL and AAL, and three between AAL and MCL; the same punctures on the *left side* (Used with permission of Dr. Tomás Ibarra-Hurtado)

ending. This effect is complete and fully reversible in a period of 5–8 months. Subsequently, the release of acetylcholine will return to its previous values with no adverse effect on muscle contractility.

The right place for the infiltration of the toxin is determined by electromyography, locating the sites with more electrical activity. There are 5 points in which, constantly and in most patients, a total paralysis of the 3 muscles can be induced with post-infiltration electromyography control. The points are located as follows: two at the midaxillary line, equidistant between the lower costal edge and the iliac crest, and another three points at the level of anterior axillary line. Nowadays Dr. Ibarra and cols. They determine these five points using anatomical references with the help of transverse CT images to measure the distance from the skin to the muscle planes in both abdominal sides (see Fig. 47.5).

For this technique, 50 U of the toxin is infiltrated in each of the five specific points of the right side and five of the left side, for a total of 500 U. The toxin is prepared by diluting the lyophilized powder in 10 ml of saline solution (1 ml = 50 U) or, if preferred, in 20 ml (2 ml = 50 U).

Total paralysis of the muscles is achieved during the first 10 days, and dilatation of the abdominal wall and the reduction of the hernia defect horizontally, without compromising the trunk movements or respiratory function, will commence. Usually, patients have no discomfort, and only some of them referred to feeling a slight flaccidness at the sides of abdomen. The maximum muscle relaxation is reached within 30 days, with an average of 20 % of volume gain, and, according to the authors' experience, there are no more volume increases afterwards (see Fig. 47.6).

It is therefore suggested that the wall repair procedure be performed after 30 days, with the advantage of still having 5–6 months of toxin effect so as to protect the suture line of the repair, which should always be reinforced with a mesh.

Muscle Expanders

Another option to achieve progressive distension of lateral muscles prior to surgical repair is placing silicone expanders between the bellies of the oblique muscles. The tissue expansion obtained provides autologous tissue, as well as vascularized, with contractile capacity for the repair of defect in the abdominal wall. This procedure can be combined with the use of Botulinum Toxin.

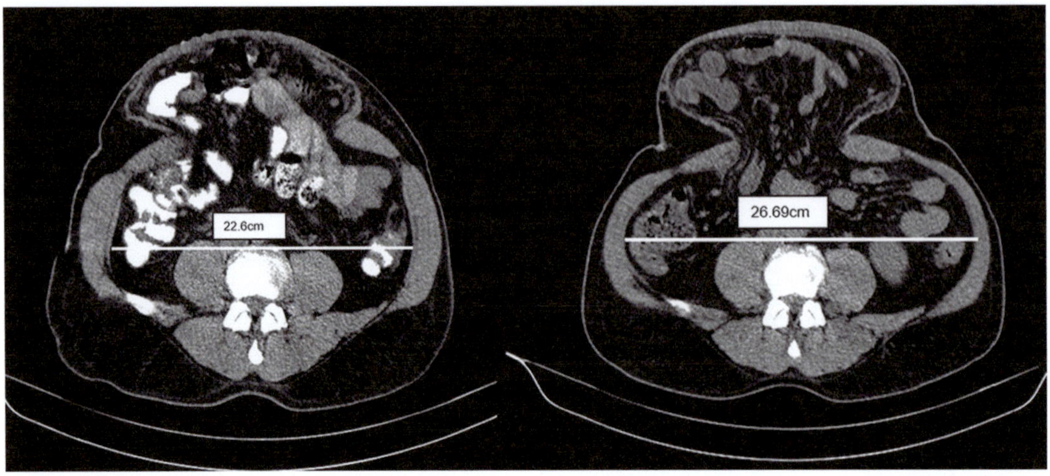

Fig. 47.6 CT images: Increased volume and abdominal muscle relaxation after injection of botulinum toxin (Used with permission of Dr. Tomás Ibarra-Hurtado)

In 1989, Henry Stephenson Byrd, a surgeon from Texas, published on the use of expanders in children with congenital abdominal abnormalities (bladder exstrophy and absence of lower half of the abdominal wall) [2]. Paul Creighton Hobar in 1994 published on the first case of abdominal wall reconstruction of an acquired defect.

The skin incision should be performed to ensure that there are no injuries in the neurovascular bundles that supply the abdominal wall, strictly respecting the anatomical planes. Normally, expanders are placed between the external oblique and the internal oblique deep complex and the fascia transversalis, this being one of the safest areas to place the expander, without interrupting blood supply or innervations of abdominal wall muscles.

A transversal incision has to be made, not a vertical one, in the costal margin, through the fascia of external oblique, so that no nerves or vessels are affected; at this plane level, between the fascia of the external oblique and the internal oblique, the pocket where the expander is placed is formed, limiting its lower edge with the inguinal ligament, medially with the lateral margin of the rectus, laterally with the midaxillary level, where the neurovascular perforating vessels of the external oblique can be found, and at superior level, with the costal margin (see Fig. 47.7).

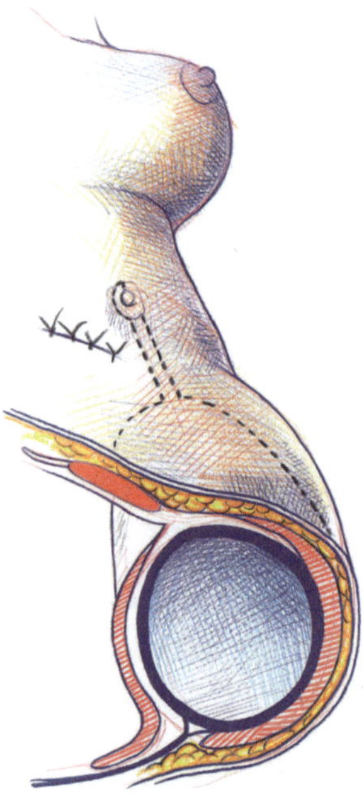

Fig. 47.7 Scheme showing the muscle expander in site (Used with permission of illustrator, Pedro Sánchez Abril. Previously published in Carbonell-Tatay F, Moreno-Egea A (eds). Eventraciones. Otras hernias de pared y cavidad abdominal. Valencia (Spain): Spanish Association of Surgeons (AEC); 2012)

The first expansion is started within 3 weeks, and the total process lasts approximately between 6 and 12 weeks until there is enough tissue; at that moment, the expander is removed and we proceed with the advance of the flap. Later, a layered closure without tension of the obtained tissue will be performed. The frequency and volume of the expansion will depend on the tolerance level of the patient, and it is normally performed every 2 weeks. The expansion at both sides of the abdominal wall defect will speed up the resolution time.

However, it is obvious that this procedure should be done in selected patients with good skin coverage.

Repair of the Abdominal Wall

The objectives of an ideal reconstruction of the abdominal wall should include prevention of acute eventration, the establishment of an adequate coverage of the abdominal content, closure without excessive tension, and adequate functional muscle support. Sometimes we must also add a fifth objective: achieving an adequate aesthetic result. Although is not always possible to achieve all these objectives, it is wise to remember them before facing a new case of eventration, as it will help with the planning of the parietal reconstruction.

Although the extremes of the defect may be brought closer with a primary closure, this usually creates quite a lot of tension at the closure line, which normally leads to poor results with a high recurrence rate.

Meshes prevent the tension, but do not achieve an adequate muscular dynamic and can present a great variety of additional complications (infection, sepsis, material extrusion, sinus formation, and fistulas).

Tissue expansion techniques and autoplasties are efficient methods of repair that, well indicated and in selected patients, could be the solution of choice, as we use the abdominal wall tissue itself, well innervated and functional, to complete the repair and restore biomechanics of the abdominal wall.

In the past decade, the dissemination of prostheses has quickly changed the way many surgeons operate, but the knowledge of these anatomical techniques below remains basic and crucial in order to be able to solve many situations successfully and combine various procedures (autoplasty plus aloplasty) into a surgery with more guarantees for the patient:

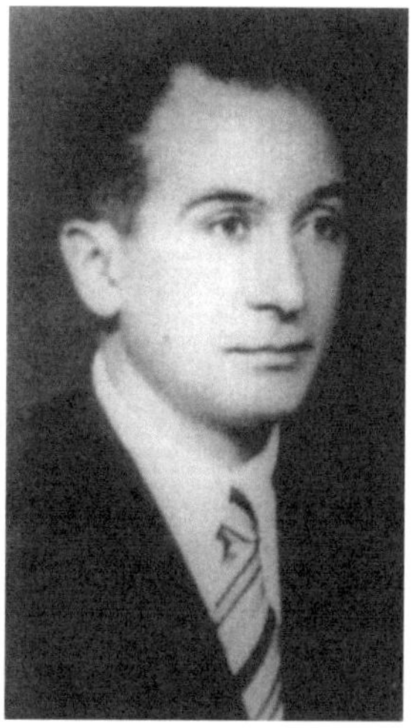

Fig. 47.8 Dr. Alfonso R. Albanese (1906–2008) (Used with permission from Carbonell-Tatay F, Moreno-Egea A (eds). Eventraciones. Otras hernias de pared y cavidad abdominal. Valencia (Spain): Spanish Association of Surgeons (AEC); 2012)

1. Autoplasty Technique described by Albanese in 1951
2. Component Separation Technique popularized by Oscar Ramírez
3. Anatomical Component Separation Technique described by Fernando Carbonell and Santiago Bonafé
4. Posterior Component Separation Technique
5. Laparoscopic Approach applied to the treatment of eventration
6. Prostheses

Autoplasties

In May 1946, Dr. Alfonso R. Albanese (1906–2008) (Fig. 47.8) operated on a 4-year-old patient who had a large midline hernia with an 8–10 cm diameter hernial ring due to a surgery done 8 months before in order to repair the obstructive symptoms that caused the peritoneal bands on the duodenum after an intestinal malrotation (Ladd's bands).

Dr. Albanese worked in the Surgery Department of the Hospital Rawson (Buenos Aires), and the

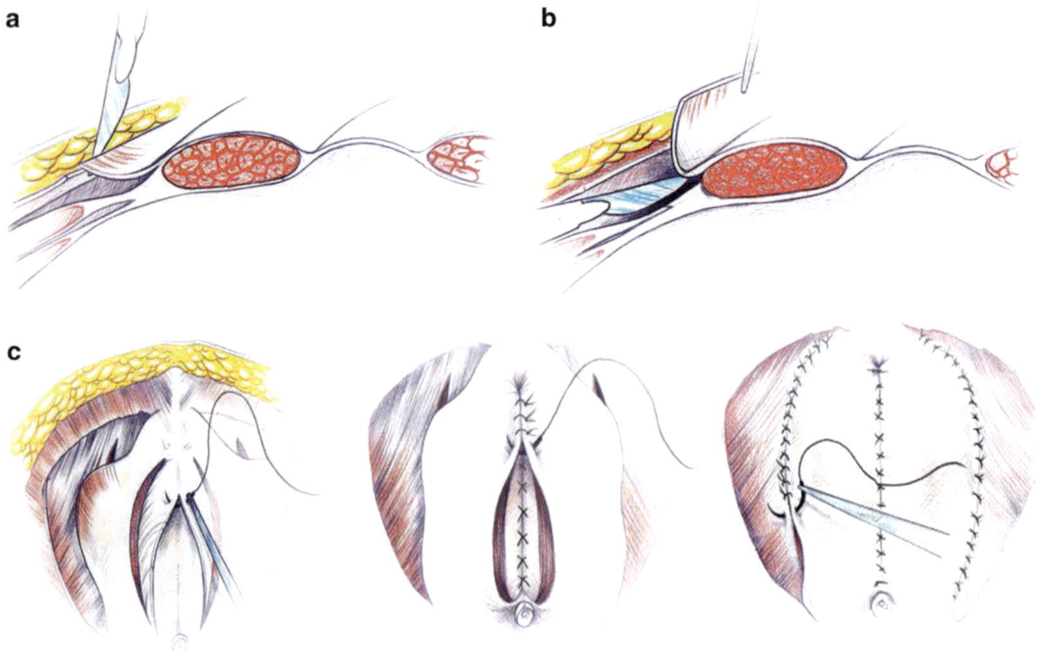

Fig. 47.9 The technique developed by Dr. Albanese and reported in 1951, designed to free the rectus muscle from the lateral traction of the oblique muscles as a result of the loss of continuity of the oblique muscles (**a–c**: Used with permission of illustrator, Pedro Sánchez Abril. Previously published in Carbonell-Tatay F, Moreno-Egea A (eds). Eventraciones. Otras hernias de pared y cavidad abdominal. Valencia (Spain): Spanish Association of Surgeons (AEC); 2012)

chief was Dr. Ricardo Finochietto. There they usually applied the Quénu-Noble technique to repair incisional hernias. Albanese also was an assistant in the Department of Topographical Anatomy of the University of Buenos Aires where he prepared anatomical materials for the classes of Professor Eugenio A. Galli. Albanese had passion for anatomy, a dedication that made him the creator of various surgical procedures, pioneering surgical repair of cardiac malformations in addition to the surgical technique for repairing large abdominal hernias.

His technique is designed to free the rectus muscle from the lateral traction of the oblique muscles as a result of the loss of continuity of the oblique muscles on each other.

With the completion of three longitudinal incisions in every hemiabdomen—one over the aponeurosis of the external oblique muscle (Fig. 47.9a), the second one in the anterior lamina of the internal oblique muscle just on the outer edge of the rectus muscle (Fig. 47.9b), and the third one on the inner third of the anterior sheath of rectus muscle (Fig. 47.9c)—this technique:

1. Expands the volume of the abdominal cavity.
2. Decreases pathological tension of the abdominal wall while restoring its function.
3. Allows anatomo-functional relocation of muscles and aesthetic reconstruction of the abdomen.

Albanese reported his procedure after the first ten cases in 1951 in the *Journal of the Argentine Medical Association* [3].

Forty years later, in 1990, Oscar Ramírez described his technique, also known as Component Separation Technique (CS), which consists of the separation of the muscular layers that form the musculature of the lateral abdominal wall so as to allow medial displacement of the rectus muscle and the set internal oblique-transversus, as Albanese did, allowing repair of large muscle aponeurotic defects. Although Ramírez described his technique without the prosthesis to reinforce the plasty—like Gibson in 1916, Albanese in 1951, and Alcino Lázaro da Silva in 1979—the introduction of new prosthesis materials refocused the interest on them.

Nowadays, the use of prosthesis reinforcement after autoplasty is required, as it was published by Ramirez in 2006, avoiding the lateral abdominal bulge and improving the recurrence rate of the hernia [4].

Autoplastic techniques based on the section of muscular aponeurosis and releasing incisions have led to more knowledge of the anatomy and physiology of the abdominal wall, so that, by the partial or complete use of these techniques, the surgeon develops technical resources to repair hernia defects of different sizes.

The great versatility of autoplasty techniques makes them the ideal resource to deal with the variability of defects of eventrations; we agree with León Herszage when he states that "in complex eventrations the adequate technique is decided intra-operatively" or when he assures that "a surgeon that knows the releasing incisions should not have any problem resolving any eventration."

The Ramirez's Technique

This surgical technique described by Oscar Ramirez (Fig. 47.10), also known as Component Separation Technique (SC), consists of the separation of the muscular planes that form the musculature of the abdominal wall in a way that allows medial displacement of the rectus and oblique minor-transverse, allowing for the repair of large aponeurotic muscle defects.

Before describing the surgical technique, we should refer to five basic principles that explain its success and effectiveness:

1. The displacement of the muscular layers of the abdominal wall, sliding one on the other, allows for increase in the tissue surface.
2. The separation of the muscular layers allows one to achieve the maximum extension with each of them.
3. This muscle extension is facilitated by the opening of the aponeurotic sheaths that cover and limit the horizontal spreading of muscles.

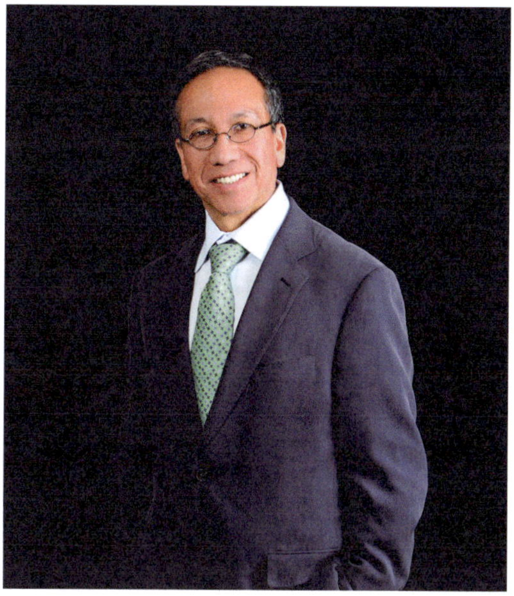

Fig. 47.10 Óscar M. Ramírez, M.D. (2011)

4. 70 % of the musculature of the abdominal wall covers hollow viscera, which can be compressed more easily than solid organs, particularly after a good bowel preparation. In the same manner, floating ribs can be moved to some degree by muscle traction action.
5. Provided that there is an integrity of the aponeurotic muscles in the abdominal wall, even with retraction or healing, performing the technique on both sides is more effective than doing so unilaterally, as it balances the strength of the abdominal musculature and centers the middle line.

A progressive mobilization must be followed, in phases, adapting the technique to the defect to be repaired (Fig. 47.11). It is recommended that a clinical exam and a radiological study be performed previously. If the absence of any component in the abdominal wall is noticed, the placement of biological prosthesis or a component separation technique or both may be required for the patient. The maximum potential with component separation technique achieves the repair of most defects in the abdominal wall; the remaining could be covered with a muscle flap or a biological matrix.

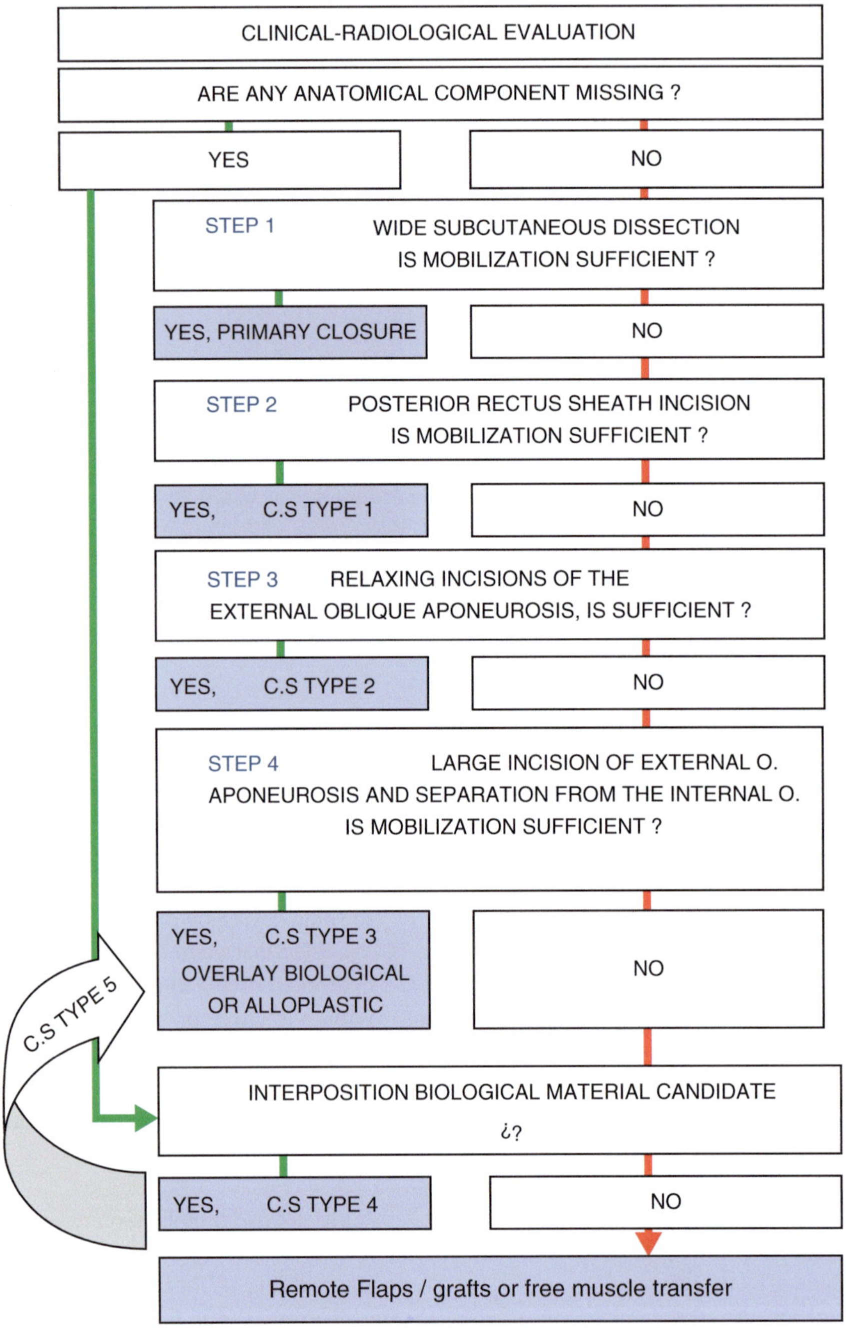

Fig. 47.11 Graduated approach to midline abdominal wall defect

If the anatomical components are present, the first step consists of performing a dissection of subcutaneous plane, separating it from the fascia to the pubis, ribs, and both iliac crests. This will allow the closure of small defects without requiring release incisions or muscle mobilization. If this maneuver does not allow closure of the defect, the next step would be opening the sheath of the rectus muscles and separating the muscle from its posterior sheath, starting from linea alba. The a

b

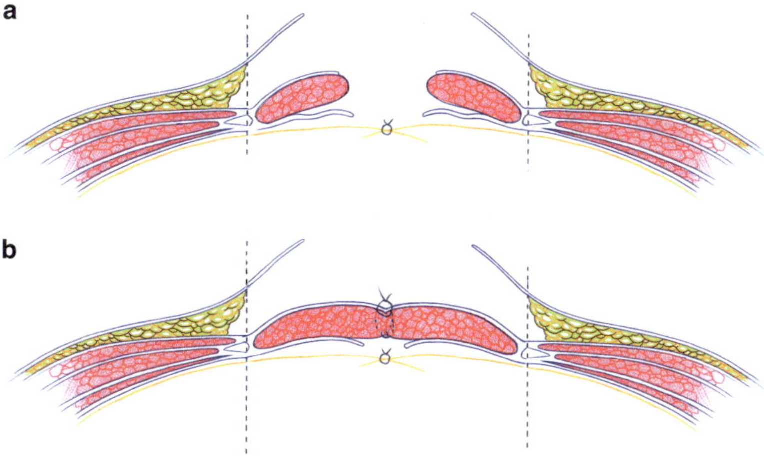

Fig. 47.12 Components Separation Type I (**a**) and Type II (**b**) (**a, b**: Used with permission of illustrator, Pedro Sánchez Abril. Previously published in Carbonell-Tatay F, Moreno-Egea A (eds). Eventraciones. Otras hernias de pared y cavidad abdominal. Valencia (Spain): Spanish Association of Surgeons (AEC); 2012)

integrity of the anterior sheath and its continuity with the aponeurosis of the external oblique are kept. The dissection of the rectus muscle on its posterior side preserves the integrity of the neurovascular bundle. This phase is called "Components Separation Type I" (Fig. 47.12a).

Average size defects require more traction towards the midline of the muscular set rectus-oblique minor-transverse. The closure of these defects requires the separation of the rectus muscle from its posterior sheath and performing release incisions over the aponeurosis of the external oblique. Occasionally, the aponeurosis of the external oblique can be moved to the closure of the side defect. This phase is called "Components Separation Type II" (Fig. 47.12b).

Major defects require more medial displacement, so a complete section of the aponeurosis of M.O. in the crescent line and a wider separation of its subjacent plane (Minor Oblique) are required. This is called "Components Separation Type III" (Fig. 47.13a). In the cases of separation Type II and III, Vicryl® (Somerville, NJ) or Polypropylene mesh can be placed in order to maintain continuity of the aponeurotic plane (O.M), avoiding weak areas and herniation, particularly in the lower lateral quadrants. As the mesh will be over muscular plane and with the subcutaneous panniculus adiposus over it, the risk of intestinal lesions or skin exposure of the mesh by decubitus is reduced. To cover small fascial defects, a resorbable Vicryl mesh may suffice, as the collagen deposition over it will provide a supporting structure similar to fascial plane. However, major defects will require permanent supporting material, such as polypropylene.

If there are doubts about the vitality or resistance of the muscular planes to close the defect, biological material can be used to reinforce the repair with autologous tissue (on-lay). In most cases, even in larger defects, the combination of the Component Separation Technique type III and a biological matrix or alloplast material will be enough to achieve stability and immediate or long-term repair of abdominal wall.

However, there will be cases where, despite performing the complete technique, mobilization of layers will not be enough to close the defect. In these cases, we must assess whether the patient is a candidate for replacement with biological material to cover a residual defect and achieve the closure of abdominal wall. This phase has been called "Component Separation Type IV" (Fig. 47.13b).

The use of prosthesis replacement (phase IV) should be considered when there is an excessive tension in the closure to avoid acute pulmonary complications or tissue necrosis. However, Dr. Ramirez does not consider this phase as the end

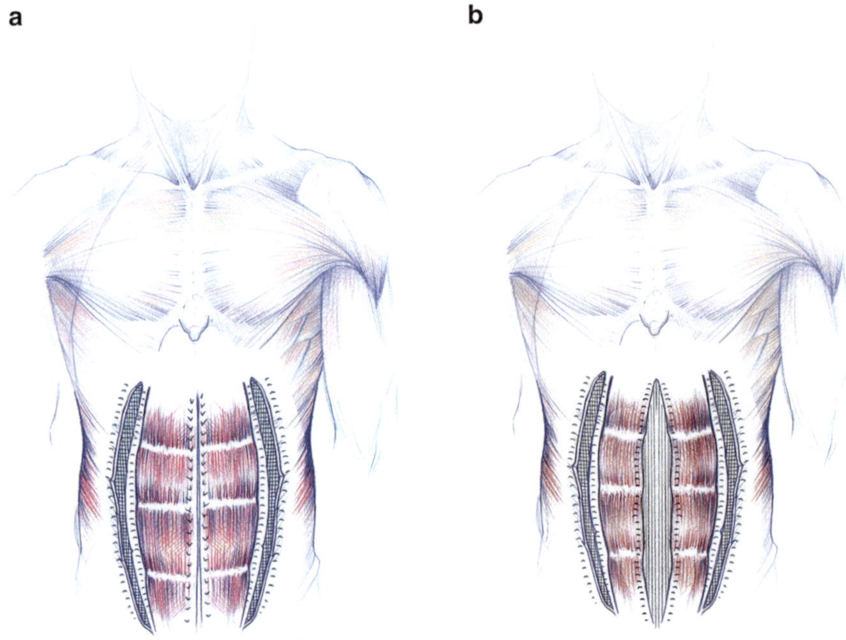

Fig. 47.13 Components Separation Type III (**a**) and Type IV (**b**) (**a, b**: Used with permission of illustrator, Pedro Sánchez Abril. Previously published in Carbonell-Tatay F, Moreno-Egea A (eds). Eventraciones. Otras hernias de pared y cavidad abdominal. Valencia (Spain): Spanish Association of Surgeons (AEC); 2012)

of the treatment. When tissue edema decreases and the tension of soft tissues is lowered, another intervention of the patient should be scheduled to convert a Type IV technique into a Type III technique, closing the abdominal defect with aponeurotic muscle tissue from the patient and using the prosthesis to reinforce. Dr. Ramirez he names to this procedure as "Component Separation Technique, Type 5".

The Carbonell and Bonafé Technique

This is a combined myoplasty, reinforced by prosthesis, pursuing anatomical and biomechanical reconstruction of abdominal wall [5].

The main differences between the *Carbonell-Bonafé* technique, Separación *Anatómica de Componentes* (SAC), and the *Component Separation* (CS) described by Óscar Ramírez are as follows:

1. Carbonell-Bonafé propose, in all suitable cases, the complete detachment of the external oblique muscle, at the entire semilunar line from the pubis to the ribs, with total dissection of the muscle flap up to the anterior superior iliac spine. They call this Level 1 (Fig. 47.14a, b).
2. Placement of a large prosthesis sized 30 × 30 to 50 × 50 cm covering the entire anterior and lateral side of abdominal wall, remaining housed and attached under the muscle flaps of the external oblique transversally and anchored to xiphoid and pubis longitudinally.
3. Reinsertion of the medial ends of the external oblique muscle flap to the prosthesis-internal oblique, more laterally, reconstructing its function (Fig. 47.15).
4. If with Level 1 the rectus muscles cannot be taken to the midline, its posterior side will be dissected, releasing it from its aponeurosis and placing prosthesis in this submuscular space after closing the midline. They call this Level 2 (Fig. 47.16).

The original idea of Drs. Carbonell and Bonafé (Fig. 47.17) is to repair the anatomy and function of the abdominal wall using the patient's

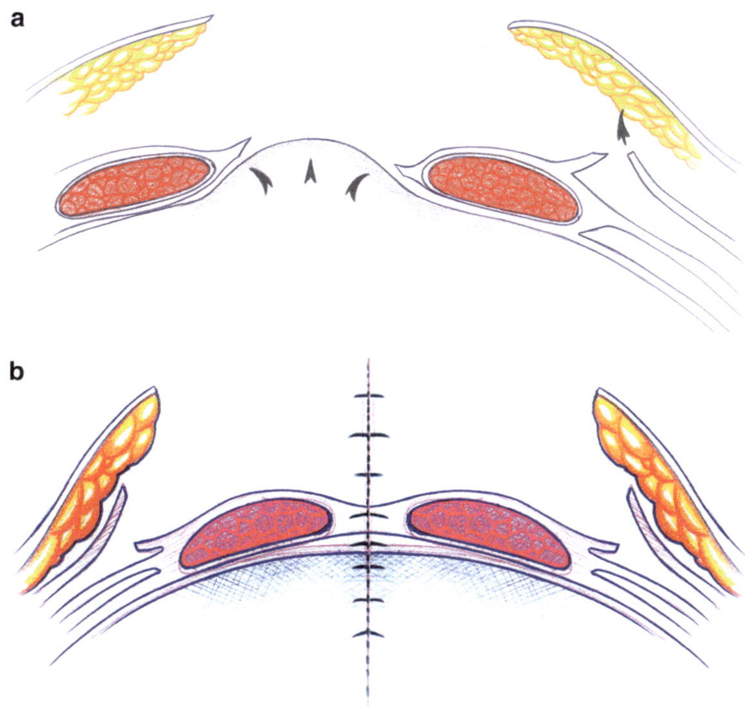

Fig. 47.14 Carbonell-Bonafé technique Level 1 (**a, b**: Used with permission of illustrator, Pedro Sánchez Abril. Previously published in Carbonell-Tatay F, Moreno-Egea A (eds). Eventraciones. Otras hernias de pared y cavidad abdominal. Valencia (Spain): Spanish Association of Surgeons (AEC); 2012)

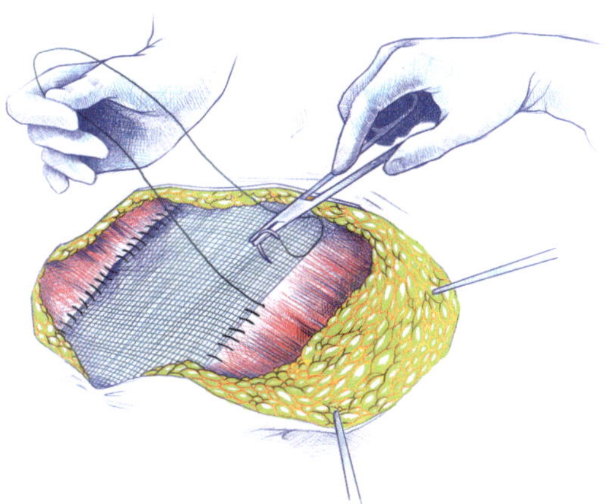

Fig. 47.15 Reinsertion of the major oblique muscles on the prosthesis (Used with permission of illustrator, Pedro Sánchez Abril. Previously published in Carbonell-Tatay F, Moreno-Egea A (eds). Eventraciones. Otras hernias de pared y cavidad abdominal. Valencia (Spain): Spanish Association of Surgeons (AEC); 2012)

own muscles and reinforcing the plastia with a prosthesis that will function like an aponeurosis; that is why the anchor of the polypropylene mesh will be at the osseous framework of the anterolateral abdominal wall: from the xiphoid process of the sternum to the pubis and from the costal arch to the anterior superior iliac spines. The flat scar, in which will turn the polypropylene mesh, will act as a containing muscular layer, much in the same way a new aponeurosis would. The reinforcement of the mesh should be provided from outside of the muscular layer, in the same way that the Chevrel and Rives techniques aim to reinforce the mid compartment, anchoring the mesh outside them in the external dihedral of the sheaths that form the aponeurosis of abdomen oblique muscles.

The Posterior Component Separation Technique

In 2008, A.M. Carbonell et al. (Fig. 47.18) published a components separation technique in the *Hernia* journal in which the dissection of the posterior rectus sheath is continued towards the sides

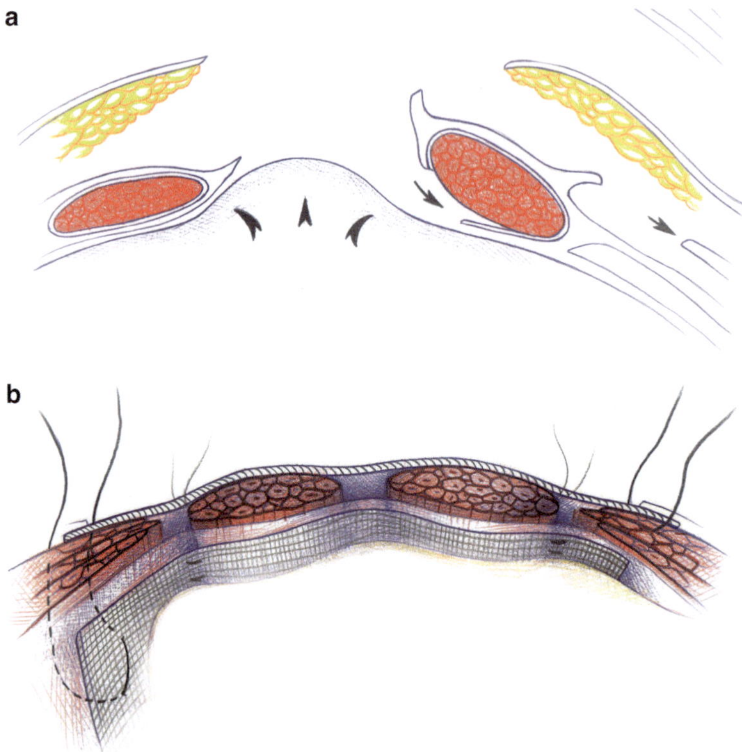

Fig. 47.16 Carbonell-Bonafé technique Level 2 (**a, b**: Used with permission of illustrator, Pedro Sánchez Abril. Previously published in Carbonell-Tatay F, Moreno-Egea A (eds). Eventraciones. Otras hernias de pared y cavidad abdominal. Valencia (Spain): Spanish Association of Surgeons (AEC); 2012)

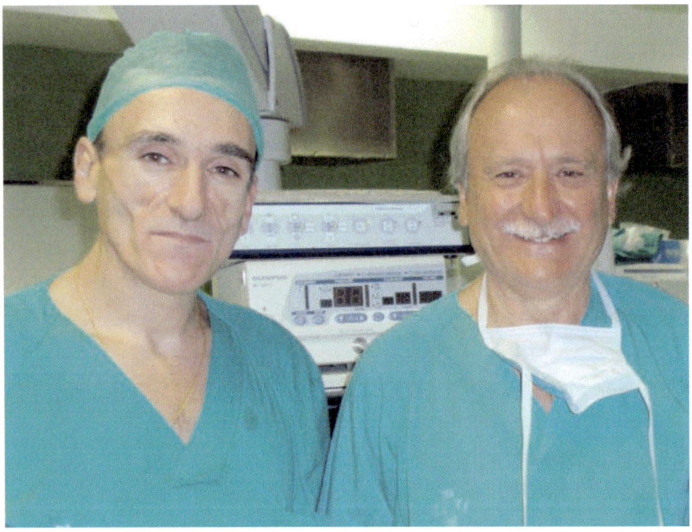

Fig. 47.17 Santiago Bonafé, M.D. (*left*), with Fernando Carbonell-Tatay, M.D. (*right*)

by the intramuscular plane between the transverse and the internal oblique: *Posterior Components Separation* (*PCS*) *Technique* (Fig. 47.19a, b) [6].

In their article, they explain the advantages of the technique related to the section and dissection of the aponeurosis of External Oblique Muscle:

- The dissection of the subcutaneous plane is not required, and, therefore, there is no sectioning of the perforating vessels, neither risk of ischemia nor skin necrosis.
- The prosthesis stays in a deep plane, with less risk of infection and exposure.

In 2012, Yuri W. Novitsky et al. (Fig. 47.20) published a new procedure of Separation of Components for the repair of the complex eventrations in the *American Journal of Surgery*, the *Transversus Abdominis Muscle Release* (*TAR*) (Fig. 47.21a, b) [7].

This is a posterior approach to the aponeurotic muscle plane that extends the dissection of the posterior sheath towards both sides, as in the PCS technique, but dissecting under the transverse muscle and over the peritoneum-fascia transversalis. Both techniques of posterior approach are like an extension of the retro muscular of Rives-Stoppa technique. Both techniques provide some advantages:

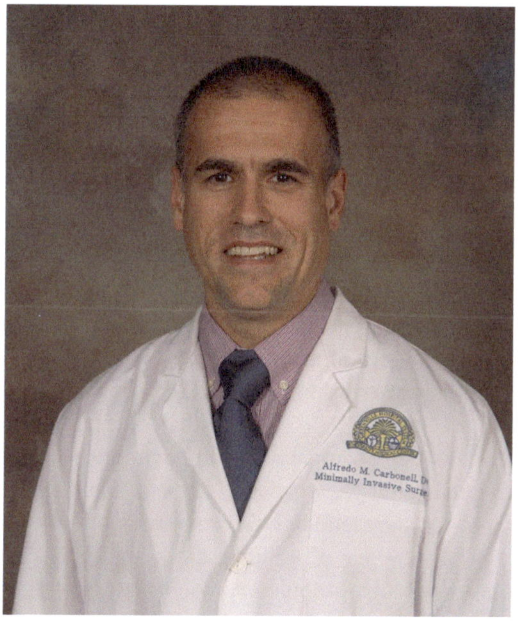

Fig. 47.18 Alfredo M. Carbonell, M.D.

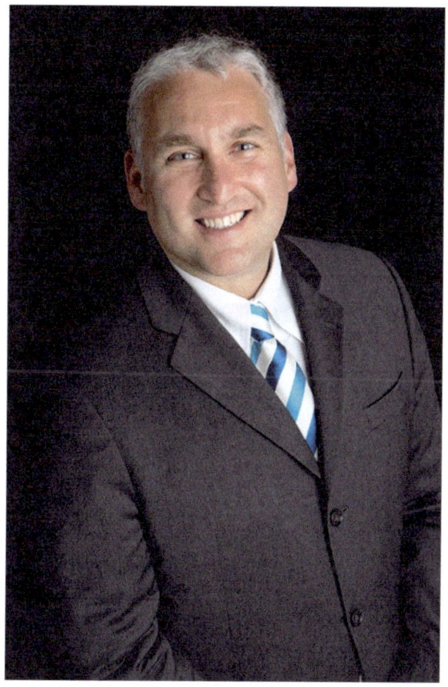

Fig. 47.20 Yuri W. Novitsky, M.D.

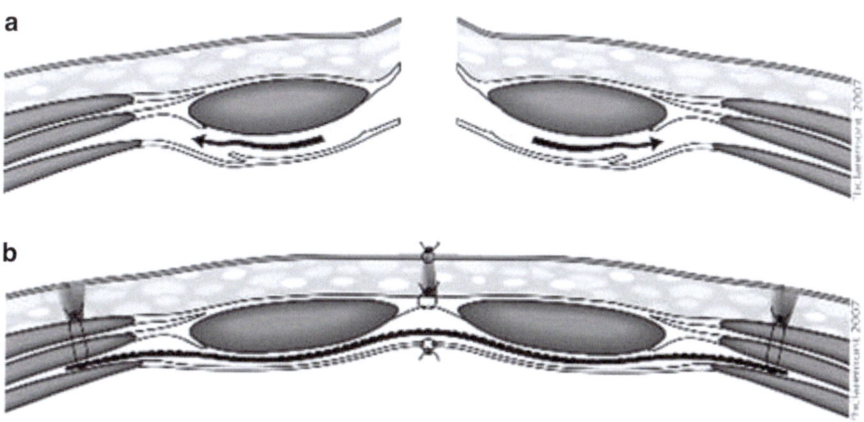

Fig. 47.19 Posterior Components Separation (PCS) Technique (**a, b**: Used with permission from Carbonell AM. Posterior components separation during retromuscular hernia repair. Hernia 2008;12(4): 359–362)

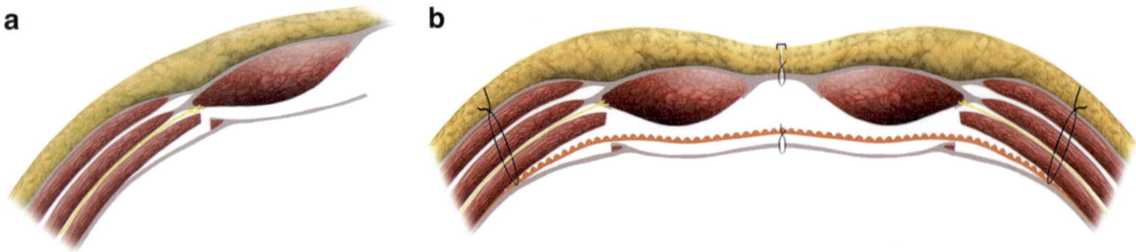

Fig. 47.21 Transversus Abdominis muscle Release (TAR) Technique (**a, b**: Used with permission from Novitsky YW et al. Transversus abdominis muscle release: a novel approach to posterior component separation during complex abdominal wall reconstruction. The American Journal of Surgery 2012;204(5):709–716)

- The disinsertion of the posterior transverse muscle of the posterior sheath allows a greater displacement of this aponeurotic sheath towards the midline.
- They avoid the extensive dissection of the subcutaneous layer over the aponeurosis that is required to section the aponeurosis of the external mayor oblique muscle along the semilunar line to place the prosthesis in the anterior access technique. As this dissection requires cutting perforating vessels, this circumstance favors abdominal skin ischemia, sometimes badly damaged as a result of pressure and distention of the hernia sac itself.
- The dissection can be extended upwards under the xiphoid process towards the diaphragm and laterally towards the subcostal plane. Going down, it is possible to access the Retzius and Bogros' spaces; in this manner, a large prosthesis can be placed in this preperitoneal plane, allowing closure of the peritoneal cavity under the fascia transversalis-peritoneum and rebuilding, above it, the aponeurotic muscle plane.
- The Components Separation Technique via posterior achieves medial displacement and the closure of the fascial layer equivalent to the anterior approach technique, and this is a very important technical resource for the repair of complex eventrations.
- With the TAR technique, dissection and possible injury of the neurovascular supply to the rectus and perforating lateral vessels as we dissect below the transversal muscle is avoided.

Laparoscopic Approach

The laparoscopic repair of eventrations is becoming increasingly popular since it was first published in 1993.

Despite of the lack of experimental tests showing that a patient improves with a laparoscopic repair, there is a general agreement that all eventrations except for the very large ones and the smallest ones are potentially operable using this technique.

Although postoperative complications are less frequent after laparoscopic surgery, when these do occur, they tend to be more serious.

The presence of multiple defects and obesity makes the laparoscopic approach a better choice in these situations. For smaller defects of 3–4 cm in diameter, it can be argued that the open approach is more suitable, especially if it can be performed with local anesthesia, while larger defects are being unanimously treated with open surgery and autoplasty.

The main strength of this repair is basically the integration of the prosthesis into the surrounding tissue with the incorporation of collagen, providing anchorage to the mesh to cover the defect and resist intra-abdominal pressure.

In the first repairs performed, nonabsorbable transfascial sutures were used. Soon afterwards, these were followed by securing devices such as staples and adhesives (see Fig. 47.22).

Staples penetrate peritoneum and fascia-muscle layers at variable depths, but they also could penetrate no further than the extraperitoneal

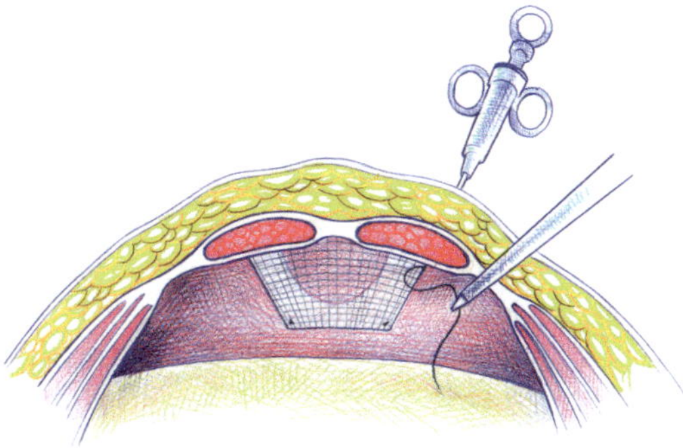

Fig. 47.22 Transfascial sutures in the laparoscopic approach (Used with permission of illustrator, Pedro Sánchez Abril. Previously published in Carbonell-Tatay F, Moreno-Egea A (eds). Eventraciones. Otras hernias de pared y cavidad abdominal. Valencia (Spain): Spanish Association of Surgeons (AEC); 2012)

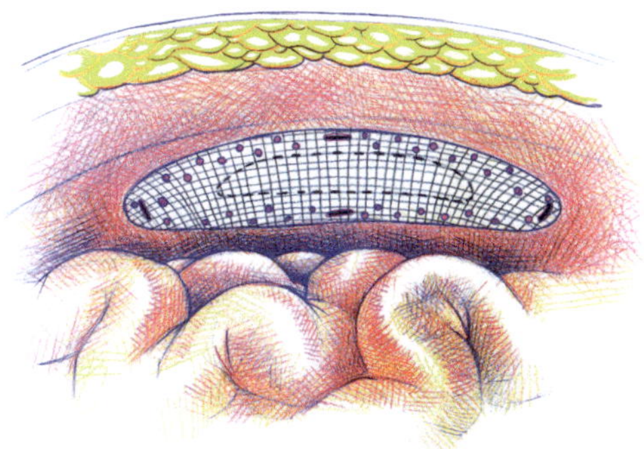

Fig. 47.23 Abdominal wall defect covered by the prosthesis (Used with permission of illustrator, Pedro Sánchez Abril. Previously published in Carbonell-Tatay F, Moreno-Egea A (eds). Eventraciones. Otras hernias de pared y cavidad abdominal. Valencia (Spain): Spanish Association of Surgeons (AEC); 2012)

fat. These staples could also damage nerves and vessels, perforate prosthesis, and erode the intestine. Absorbable staples could allow migration of the prosthesis inside the defect as a result of the same intra-abdominal pressure that caused the hernia. We are currently witnessing a revolution in terms of prosthesis fixation, from the use of permanent sutures and metal staples, to a trend towards the reduction of this permanent fixing method and replacing it with absorbable staples or glues, or a combination of both (see Fig. 47.23).

Laparoscopic surgery in most surgical procedures has represented a major achievement as it allows performing the same surgical technique as in an open approach, with the advantage of a minimally invasive intervention. In the case of abdominal wall surgery, it does not meet the essential requirement for most surgeons to repair a parietal defect, the defect closure, considered by some surgeons as essential in all hernias, even in smaller ones. Additionally, a laparoscopic approach in this field of abdominal wall surgery does not reproduce a technique corresponding to open surgery, meaning that it is not a minimally invasive approach of a repair procedure of the abdominal wall, but another surgical resource.

There is no "repair" of the default, as there is no restitution of the anatomy; most laparoscopic repairs of the abdominal wall, if not all, just cover the hernia defect without repairing it. We prevent the abdominal wall content from coming out as the prosthesis is placed, covering the defect from inside. This avoids some of the hernia consequences, and for this reason I personally (A.Z.) consider it a palliative surgery of the eventration.

This excellent resource is ideal when the hernia defect cannot be repaired, when the comorbidity and the associated pathology of the patient do not recommend a repairing surgery of the defect, or when the defect should not be repaired, as in the cases of parastomal eventrations, where currently the modified Sugarbaker technique (via laparoscope) is the most accepted technique in view of its efficacy and good results.

The laparoscopic approach has been used as a complement to open surgery in the Component Separation Technique to section the fascia of the external oblique muscle along the semilunaris line, avoiding the extensive dissection of the subcutaneous layer and the cutting of the perforating vessels, improving the incidence of skin necrosis after surgery. The optimal size of the mesh is still controversial. A minimum overlap of 5 cm around the hernia defect has been recommended, but this is an arbitrary figure, chosen because of malposition and retraction of small meshes. The latest bilamellar prosthesis, specifically designed for intraperitoneal use, has fewer adhesions but cannot be described as "not adherent" [8].

Table 47.1 Types of prostheses used in the abdominal wall repair

Polymeric/synthetic		
Reticular prosthesis (meshes)	Nonabsorbable	Polypropylene (high or low density), polyester, not expanded polytetrafluoroethylene (PTFE), polyvinylidene fluoride (PVDF)
	Partially absorbable	Polypropylene/polyglactin 910 Polypropylene/poliglecaprone
	Absorbables	Polyláctic acid, polyglactin 910
Laminar prosthesis	Nonabsorbable	Expanded polytetrafluoroethylene (PTFEe), silicon, polyurethane
Composite prosthesis	Nonabsorbable components (physical barrier)	Polypropylene/PTFEe Polypropylene/polyurethane
	Absorbable components (chemical barrier)	Polyester/polyethylene glycol Polypropylene/polyethylene glycol Polypropylene/hyaluronic acid Polypropylene/polydioxanone/cellulose

Biological/natural		
Bioprosthesis	Without covalent links (non-cross-linked)	Porcine dermis Bovine pericardium Porcine small intestinal submucosa (SIS)
	With covalent links (cross-linked)	Porcine dermis

Used with permission from Carbonell-Tatay F, Moreno-Egea A (eds). Eventraciones. Otras hernias de pared y cavidad abdominal. Valencia (Spain): Spanish Association of Surgeons (AEC); 2012

The Prosthesis

We call biomaterials to those materials of natural or synthetic origin, designed to achieve a specific function in the human body, replacing partially or totally damaged tissue.

Since the introduction by the Texas surgeon Francis Usher in 1958 of polypropylene mesh and thread to repair hernias, developing the "strainless" reparation concept, early deambulation, and checking for good integration of polypropylene, even in surgical site infection, the use of biomaterials in different surgical specialities has seen a significant increase. The field of application of biomaterials may be the most dynamic one in surgical science, and one of the many indications they have is their use to reinforce or replace abdominal wall defects.

In the last few years, the therapeutic arsenal for abdominal wall surgery has improved with the development of new materials in the search of the ideal prosthesis (see Table 47.1).

Prostheses are classified into two large groups: polymeric or synthetic and biological or natural. Polymers are, in turn, subdivided into reticular, laminar, and combined, and the biological or natural ones consist of the bioprosthesis group. The industry has developed prosthesis derived from living tissues from animals (xenografts) or human (allografts) that supposedly would offer similar repair to the ones performed with autologous tissues.

There is always a reaction of the recipient against biomaterial with the purpose of eliminating or isolating it by encapsulation.

The process of integration of the biomaterial in the tissues is directly related to its structure, namely the presence or absence of porosity of the material, which modulates tissue integration and cell penetration in the different interstices of the prosthesis and that facilitates angiogenesis.

The pore size is the main parameter to consider in prosthesis: either it is a high density or a low density one. Thus, high density prosthesis would have small pores and low density prosthesis would have large pores.

Reticular prostheses, with pores ranging between 1 and 4 mm, are mostly made from polypropylene and have optimal tissue integration. The connective tissue surrounding the filaments forms spirals over them. There is also superior angiogenesis, which is excellent for the anchorage of receiving tissues.

Reticular prostheses have been designed with absorbable material, and there are hybrid types which contain absorbable and nonabsorbable components. This prosthesis has large pores and, therefore, low density.

The objectives of the new designs are fundamentally two: first, reducing the quantity of foreign material that remains in the host, and second, leaving a smaller fibrosis in the recipient tissue.

It has been demonstrated that integration and biomechanical resistance of both low weight and partly absorbable prosthesis are similar to conventional high weight reticular prosthesis [9].

Another important innovation in the field of reticular prosthesis has been the creation of self-attachable prostheses.

These prostheses have a hook-shaped bonding system (which is also biodegradable) that allows adherence to the tissue almost immediately. These are made with polypropylene, with small pore structure.

Laminar prostheses, mainly represented by the polytetrafluorethylene (PTFEe), have differences regarding reticular ones when the biomaterial is placed in direct contact with the visceral peritoneum. Laminar prostheses allow for a good peritoneum development, and vessels do not penetrate in the interstices of the PTFEe.

To create a single prosthesis with the benefits of both the reticular and the laminar, *composite prostheses* have been developed. As proposed by Shein and colleagues in 1995, in this manner, implants could have the following qualities: (a) good tissue integration; (b) good peritoneal behavior; and (c) good mechanical resistance post-implantation. These composite prostheses or *composites* are used for the repair of large hernia defects where a total reconstruction of the abdominal wall has to be performed and where there is virtually no tissue support; therefore, the prosthesis has to be placed in contact with the visceral peritoneum.

The design of these prostheses intends that biomaterial, the first component, assumes the role of tissue integration, and the second component remains placed in direct contact with the visceral peritoneum and modules the behavior at this interface level.

The first component is usually of the reticular type, made from polypropylene or from polyester. The second component is usually of the laminar type, and it can be absorbable or nonabsorbable. The integration of these prostheses is achieved through the reticular component, while the second component allows for correct mesothelialization.

The return of biological implants to surgery, rescued by plastic surgery and introduced years ago in hernia surgery, created new revolutionary hopes with the "regeneration" concept, instead of the tissue repair concept. The objective of these biomaterials is to achieve, in addition to tissue reparation, tissue regeneration, so that once implanted they would stimulate extracellular elements of the recipient, facilitating angiogenesis involving growth factors in the creation of the new abdominal wall.

Under ideal conditions, the purpose is not only to achieve repair of the area, but also tissue regeneration, with similar properties to the ones of healthy tissue. Biological mesh started being used as a reinforcement as a result of the powerful influence of industry, which was able to raise expectations by basing these hopes on promising studies. But there has also been controversy about the purity of biological material, DNA donor fragments, incomplete bacterial clearance, and these materials activating long-lasting reactions to foreign bodies and marked immunologic responses. The main indication was its use in eventration surgery in septic-contaminated situations; however, it seems that high levels of collagenase and endotoxines in the infected wounds lead to a rapid decomposition of the nonreticulated matrices (non-cross-linked) and an alteration of reticulated ones.

When this magic of "tissue regeneration" seemed to vanish, we still had the resource of temporary protection of an open abdomen in a contaminated environment. It may seem that we are still where we were before: Just like Ulrich Dietz with a bovine patch pericardium in 1989 that was replaced later by synthetic meshes of

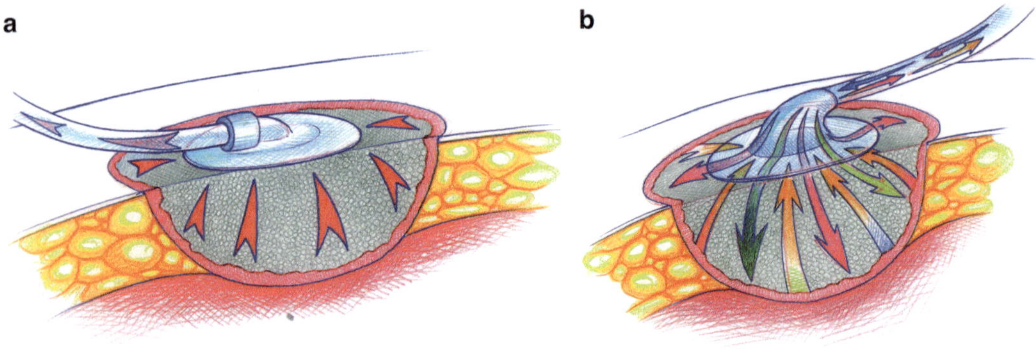

Fig. 47.24 Negative pressure therapy (NPT) (**a**) and NPT with instillation (**b**) (**a, b**: Used with permission of illustrator, Pedro Sánchez Abril. Previously published in Carbonell-Tatay F, Moreno-Egea A (eds). Eventraciones. Otras hernias de pared y cavidad abdominal. Valencia (Spain): Spanish Association of Surgeons (AEC); 2012)

polylactic acid. However, nowadays there is a wide variety of biological prostheses that can facilitate the repair/regenerating process in a way more or less desirable, although we do not have enough clinical experience and we need to conduct prospective studies with long-term monitoring to assess in detail real performance and the cost-benefit relationship of these materials [10].

Postoperative Period

Parallel to the development of techniques and prostheses to deal with large eventrations, procedures have been developed to resolve complications arising from this complex surgery.

Vacuum Assisted Cure (VAC) and Negative Pressure Therapy (NPT)

Vacuum Assisted Cure was developed to support treatment in cases of skin necrosis. Negative Pressure Therapy (NPT) or vacuum therapy is a new alternative used to manage wounds. It has had success in the treatment of acute wound infections after surgical debridement (see Fig. 47.24a).

The option of wound healing by secondary intention or deferred closures is the choice when primary closure has been tried as an option. Real evidence demonstrates that cures aided by negative topic pressure therapy, constant or intermittent, have created a revolution in treatment. The effectiveness of negative pressure therapy is documented in several studies, which found a reduction of healing time of approximately 50 % versus conventional therapies and fewer complications with less frequency in the change of cures, meaning important savings in health care.

Considering the efficacy of this procedure in many of the situations which surgeons deal with, we will describe this type of therapy.

The Negative Pressure Therapy (NPT) or vacuum therapy is a new alternative for the treatment of wounds, which has been used successfully in the treatment of acute infections after surgical debridement. It acts by maintaining a negative controlled and monitored pressure in the wound bed that allows for the removal of the existing exudates in the exposed tissue bed. An increase of the blood perfusion of the wound is achieved, and, due to the three-dimensional collapse of the reticulated foam open pore structure that causes the vacuum, it produces a reduction of tension at the edge of the wound, and this allows for an important reduction of the wound surface. Several studies prove this fact.

However, some infected or contaminated wounds in which negative pressure therapy has been applied mentioned that a satisfactory control of flora bacteria had not been achieved. The need to provide the wound with intermittent application of solutions with some antimicrobial action became the primary objective of a system combining

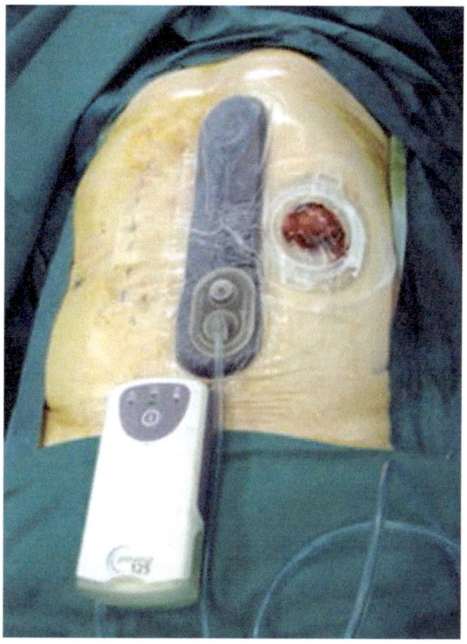

Fig. 47.25 Prophylactic use of negative pressure therapy (Used with permission from Carbonell-Tatay F, Moreno-Egea A (eds). Eventraciones. Otras hernias de pared y cavidad abdominal. Valencia (Spain): Spanish Association of Surgeons (AEC); 2012)

vacuum treatment with instillation. NPT combined with instillation developed in 1996 by Fleischmann et al. Its clinical applications were first described in 1998 (see Fig. 47.24b).

Initially, it was used when vacuum therapy was not successful with infected wounds, although clinical results have made the use of instillation therapy the first line of treatment for the infected wound.

Recently, this instillation therapy has been applied in systems that perform an automatic and controlled release of pharmacologically active solutions, or simply a saline solution.

When applying vacuum, there is a contraction in all dimensions of the foam dressing, bringing the edges closer (macro tension effect). The dressing gets pressured into the wound bed (cell micro tension effect enhancing cellular mitosis) and eliminates exudates that potentially drag microbial load, contaminating the wound (see Fig. 47.25).

To the effect of negative pressure is added the possibility of instilling pharmacologically active substances or saline solution that, after a controlled acting time in the wound bed, are removed with the exudates. Instillation cycles, therefore, are combined with negative pressure ones, and both are automatically controlled by the therapeutic unit applying the negative pressure.

Treatment and Prevention of Prosthesis Infection: The Biofilm

Currently, it can be certainly stated that the repair of abdominal wall hernias is performed in 100 % of cases using prosthesis or mesh that, as well as facilitating hernia repair, prevents recurrence. The infection of a prosthesis in hernia surgery is not, in principle, a very frequent complication; however, when it does happen, it creates a complex clinical problem, not so much for its impact but for the complex management to be resolved by the physician.

A biofilm is a microbial community that is developed and attached to an inert biological surface embedded in a self-produced exopolysaccharide matrix. The adhesion degree of microorganisms to a biomaterial (e.g., an abdominal mesh) is influenced by the material itself that constitutes the implant structure (see Fig. 47.26a).

Thus, multifilament mesh or those made of hydrophobic material (such as polytetrafluoroethylene) favor microbial adherence and the formation of a biofilm. The adhesion process is regulated by a chemical intercellular communication system called *quórum sensing*. Chronic infections where biofilms are involved have a low antimicrobial response rate, as a consequence of the physical and chemical barrier that establishes the exopolysaccharide matrix, the existence of metabolically inactive cells, the presence of microenvironments inside the biofilm that antagonize with antibiotics, and gene transmission phenomena and hyper-mutation that facilitate the development of resistance mechanisms (see Fig. 47.26b).

One potential therapeutic option is the combined use of antibiotics presenting different action targets. Beta-lactam monotherapy, active only on dividing cells, is not efficient for the infections where biofilms are involved.

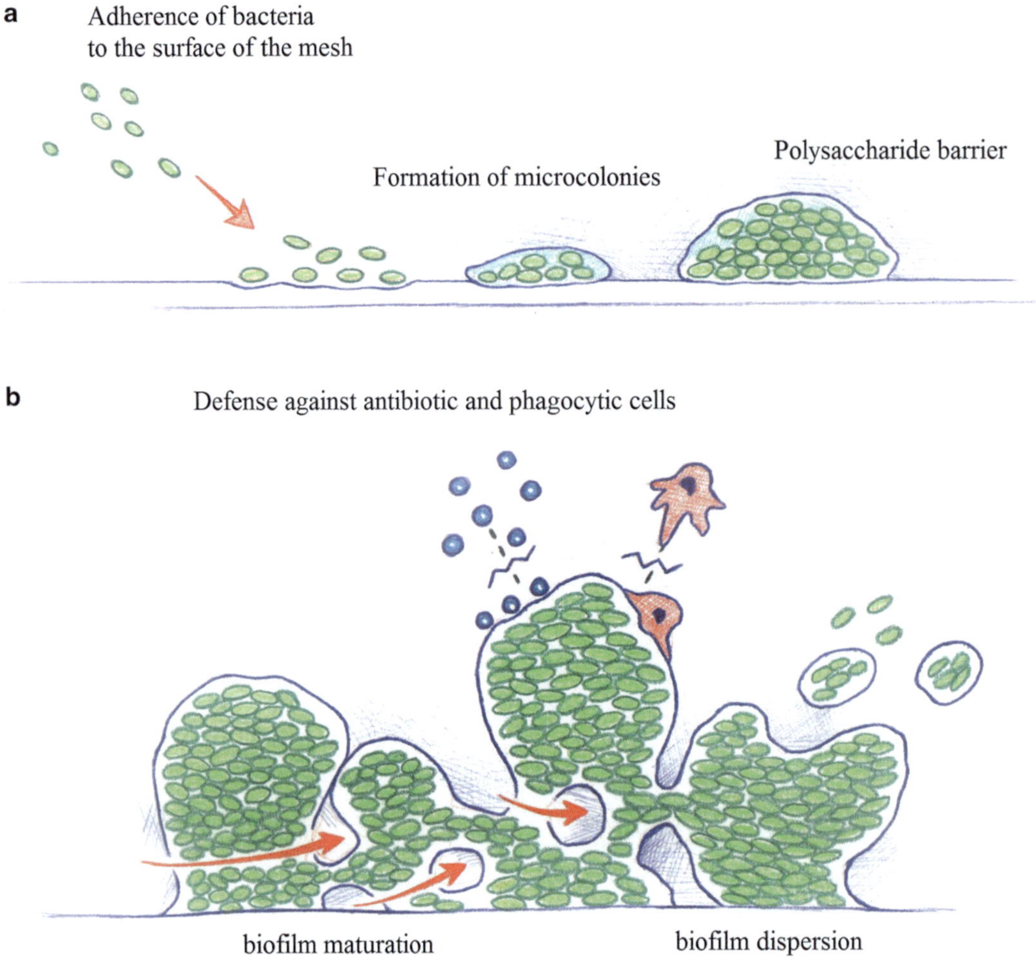

Fig. 47.26 Scheme of the formation of a Biofilm (**a**) and Biofilm growth and dispersion (**b**) (**a, b**: Used with permission of illustrator, Pedro Sánchez Abril. Previously published in Carbonell-Tatay F, Moreno-Egea A (eds). Eventraciones. Otras hernias de pared y cavidad abdominal. Valencia (Spain): Spanish Association of Surgeons (AEC); 2012)

Carbapenems, rifampicin, aminoglycosides, and fluoroquinolones, although they are more effective on dividing bacteria, have some activity on cells in the stationery phase; therefore, they could be more effective. However, rifampicin should never be administered in monotherapy due to the high frequency of resistance development. The use of daptomycin and linezolid has also shown good action against cells in the stationery phase, resulting, therefore, in efficiency over bacterial biofilms. The incorporation of antimicrobials, metals, or molecules that increase biocompatibility in implantable biomaterials is another strategy associated with lowering infection rates.

Currently, other therapeutic alternatives are being studied, such as the use of physical methods (electric fields, electromagnetic, and ultrasound), intelligent implants, depleting or destabilizing substances of the matrix, anti*quorum sensing* molecules or bacteriophages, for their possible future clinical applications to eradicate microbial biofilms.

Bacteriophages or phages are viruses that infect bacteria. They are formed with a protein coating that protects their genetic material, DNA or RNA single or double stranded. To penetrate a cell, phages bind to specific receptors of the bacterial surface, limiting the spectrum of bacteria which they are able to infect and destroy. Once inside the host, bacteriophages can develop a lytic cycle (which ends with the bacteria lysis and the release of new phages) or lysing (in which the phage genome is integrated into the bacterial chromosomal DNA they maintain in plasmid form, remaining in dormant state inside the bacteria).

Another advantage of the phage therapy compared to the antibiotic therapy in the treatment of biofilms is that the phages are effective in eradicating both antibiotic-resistant bacteria and those found in stationary phase [11].

The development of genetic engineering has also allowed for generating phages capable of expressing proteins according to their function. In this manner, T7 phages that express intracellular dispersin B protein during the infection of *E. coli* have been produced. After bacterial cell lysis, this enzyme is released into the extracellular medium and carries out its function, degrading the polysaccharides constituting the matrix; these studies make phages potentially useful tools in combination with antibiotics. However, phagotherapy also has important disadvantages, such as limited range of action and the possible appearance of bacterial strains by mutation of recipients or phages immunogenicity.

Conclusion

All these technological advancements in preparing the patient for surgery and the techniques and materials used in the surgical repair in addition to the procedures intended to treat or prevent the resulting complications make abdominal wall surgery a complex discipline that requires surgeons with a high degree of training and justifies the creation of specific working groups. This specialty requires consensual protocols and the development of national registries to guide the standardization of treatments in an activity that currently has much variability in the application of techniques and materials.

References

1. Ibarra HT, Nuño GC, Echeagaray HJ, Robles VE, González JJJ. Use of botulinum toxin type a before abdominal wall hernia reconstruction. World J Surg. 2009;33:2553–6.
2. Byrd HS, Hobar PC. Abdominal wall expansion in congenital defects. Plast Reconstr Surg. 1989; 84(2):347–52.
3. Albanese AR. Eventración media xifo-umbilical gigante: método para su tratamiento. Rev Asoc Med Argent. 1951;65:376.
4. Ramírez OM. Inception and evolution of the component separation technique: Personal recollections. Clin Plast Surg. 2006;33:241–6.
5. Carbonell Tatay F, Bonafé Diana S, García Pastor P, Gómez Gavara C, Baquero VR. Nuevo método de operar en la eventración compleja: Separación Anatómica de Componentes con Prótesis y Nuevas Inserciones Musculares. Cir Esp. 2010;86(2):87–93.
6. Carbonell AM, Cobb WS, Chen SM. Posterior components separation during retromuscular hernia repair. Hernia. 2008;12(4):359–62.
7. Novitsky YW, Elliott HL, Orenstein SB, Rosen MJ. Transversus abdominis muscle release: a novel approach to posterior component separation during complex abdominal wall reconstruction. Am J Surg. 2012;204:709–16.
8. De Beaux AC, Tulloh B. Laparoscopic ventral hernia repair. Br J Surg. 2012;99:1319–21.
9. Bellón JM, Rodríguez M, García Honduvilla N, Pascual G, Buján J. Partially absorbable meshes for hernia repair offer advantages over nonabsorbable meshes. Am J Surg. 2007;194:68–74.
10. Petter-Puchner AH, Dietz UA. Biological implants in abdominal wall repair. Br J Surg. 2013;100:987–8.
11. Del Pozo JL, Alonso M, Arciola CR, González R, Leiva J, Lasa I, et al. Biotechnological war against biofilms. could phages mean the end of device-related infections? Int J Artif Organs. 2007; 30(9):805–12.

48 Use of Biologic Grafts in Surgery

Rifat Latifi

Introduction

The ultimate advance in technologies in surgery is tissue engineering (TE), which aims to create and substitute failing or severely injured organs, by replacing them both anatomically and functionally as close as possible or entirely substituting the healthy organ. However, this is not without major issues such as scientific, technical, logistical, and ethical. Every chapter related to organ transplantation in this book has noted the lack of organ donors for patients in desperate need to replace their failed organs such as heart, lungs, liver, pancreas, intestines, and other organs. Yet there are not enough organs to fulfill this enormous need. It would be ideal if failing or injured organs could be substituted with TE organs, organs created from cell sheet engineering, or any other technique to make regenerative medicine a reality [1, 2]. Organ factories may eventually come to fruition where livers, lungs, hearts, intestines, and maybe even brains are manufactured right in our very own neighborhoods.

R. Latifi, M.D., F.A.C.S. (✉)
Department of Surgery, University of Arizona Medical Center, 1501 N. Campbell Avenue, Tucson, AZ 85724, USA
e-mail: latifi@surgery.arizona.edu

TE has contributed more advancements to general and trauma surgery than any other field currently. As general and trauma surgeons or acute care surgeons, we deal daily with large defects of the abdomen, or other parts of the body that must be sealed off with newly created tissue that eventually will become part of body and mimic fascia. This tissue has been called "biologic" and is being used to restore the functionality of abdomen. Other clinical indications have emerged also and vary from creating better cosmetics results in breast reconstruction, reconstruction after major cranioplasties, facial reconstruction or skin coverage after major burns or other musculocutaneous defects. Tissue engineering is used for new bone grafts [3], to cover major burn [4], to create new bladder or urethra [5], trachea [6], heart valves [7], fascia [8], or to cover major abdominal wall defects. All of these are already happening but at a much lower scale than we need. However, creating organs such as the liver, the heart, the kidney, the lung, the pancreas, the small bowel, and the bone poses a major challenge. Yet, I believe it is a matter of time until we will have any or all of the above organs on the "shelf." Will this be a new paradigm and will it reduce and or entirely substitute the organ transplantation process, as we know it today? The process of TE is beyond the scope of this chapter, but suffice it to say that it has undergone time development starting in the early 1900s until present day and involves cells

R. Latifi et al. (eds.), *Technological Advances in Surgery, Trauma and Critical Care*,
DOI 10.1007/978-1-4939-2671-8_48

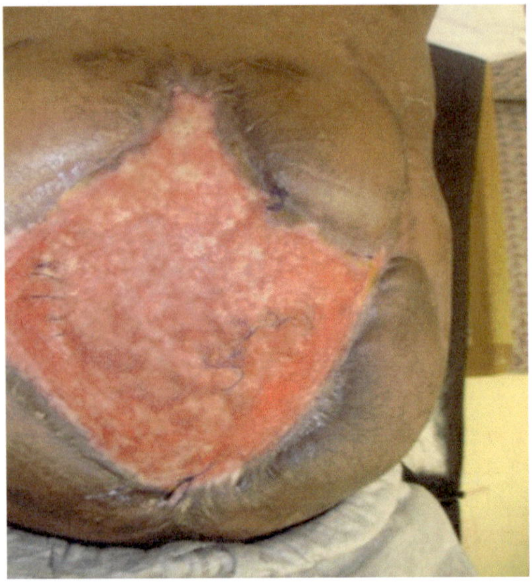

Fig. 48.1 Patient undergoing abdominal wall reconstruction with Alloderm™ (LifeCell, Branchburg, NJ) who has undergone full vascularization of the biologic graft. (Reproduced with permission from Latifi R, Peralta R, Al Thani H. Abdominal Wall Reconstruction in Patients with an Open Abdomen and Enterocutaneous Fistulas: A 9 Step Treatment Strategy. In Latifi R (ed): Surgery of Complex Abdominal Wall Defects. New York: Springer Science + Business Media; 2013)

(differentiated adult cells to undifferentiated progenitor cells and stem cells), use of scaffolds material, vascularization (Fig. 48.1), and bio-fabrication [9]. These scaffolds, composed of either natural or synthetic biomaterials, provide a spatial environment to facilitate cell proliferation, vascularization, and regeneration [10]. The complexity of TE increases dramatically as the complexity of structures being created is advanced, the simplest being for cornea and trachea, and the most challenging being for organs with metabolic functions such as kidneys, liver, and pancreas [11]. In order to have the science of tissue engineering translate into clinical arenas, clinical trials must be conducted. However, we begin the clinical applications of TE with ethical questions such as when to conduct clinical trials, how to regulate such trials, when and how to responsibly introduce these strategies into clinical practice, and how to maintain a positive public perception of the tissue engineering field. These questions have been raised and many more will come in the future as tissue engineering advances [12]. It is likely that this issue will continue to be debated in the future.

The aim of this chapter is to review current clinical application of biologic mesh used for abdominal wall reconstruction [13] and few other indications currently being used.

Abdominal Wall Defect and Enterocutaneous Fistulas

The need for major abdominal wall reconstruction has expanded. Once used mainly for trauma patient, who have undergone damage control (DC) operation, now is being used more and more in acute catastrophic abdominal conditions such as perforated viscus, grossly contaminated abdomen, when abdomen cannot or should not be closed, and whom are managed by open abdomen. However, while DC has been shown to save lives, its liberal use has it consequences and has been called an "overused procedure" [14], despite the fact that it has been accepted around the world. Higher medical cost, enterocutaneous fistulas (ECFs), and inability to be fully functional due to massive ventral hernias for long periods of time remain the most serious complications of open-abdomen management techniques and damage-control surgery, particularly in acute care and trauma surgery [15–17]. ECFs are associated with significant morbidity and mortality despite significant advances in surgical techniques and technologies for patients with complex abdominal wall hernias. Seventy-five to eighty-five percent of ECFs are postoperative and most patients with ECFs also have abdominal wall defects (through which the ECFs become evident); therefore, it is important that surgeons treat both conditions in tandem. Especially challenging is the combination of ECFs and any or all of these conditions: large abdominal defects, an open abdomen, entero-atmospheric fistulas (EAFs), or stomas. The incidence of ECFs in combination with an open abdomen on the other hand has been reported to be as high as 75 % [3]. While closing the open abdomen and establishing functional abdominal wall in these patients, especially in those with fistulas and stomas, represents a

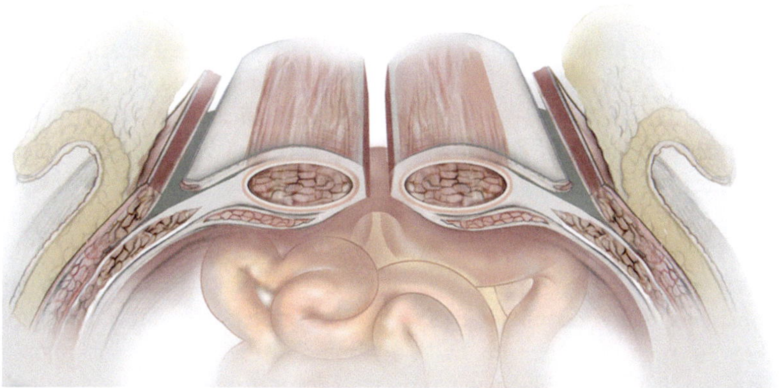

Fig. 48.2 Illustration of lateral component separation. (Used with permission from LifeCell Corporation, an Acelity Company)

major challenge and requires surgical creativity, deciding of what kind of mesh to use is also a major decision. Multidisciplinary approaches and advanced surgical techniques are required. Whatever technique is used, the goal is to create coverage of the abdominal cavity and to improve the patient's quality of life. Native abdominal wall can be used; if that is not possible, biologic or prosthetic mesh can be used instead. In most patients, some sort of combination of reconstruction techniques will be needed. If native tissue can be used without undue tension, then it should be used; but if midline tissue cannot be easily approximated or if mesh reinforcement is needed (as it is in almost all abdominal wall defects larger than 6 cm), creative techniques must be considered. In addition to the component separation technique that is based on an enlargement of the abdominal wall surface by separating and advancing the muscular layers (Fig. 48.2), there will be a need for a mesh reenforcement or entire reconstruction using a mesh.

By definition, patients with ECFs, EAFs, and/or stomas have contaminated wounds. Synthetic mesh has been used in the past, but it was associated with high rates of wound infection (often necessitating removal of infected mesh for source control of infection) as well as other complications (such as newly created fistulas). The fear of infection when using synthetic mesh has been a major facet of the decision to use biologic mesh instead.

The most common application of bioengineered tissue, created, or modified is in general surgery. Reconstruction of major abdominal walls with modified tissues that is harvested from human or pigs has become a common practice. In an experimental study examining biologic grafts in comparison to synthetic material, biologic grafts are able to clear a Staphylococcus aureus contamination; however, they do so at different rate [18]. The authors created a chronic hernia model in rats and then used various meshes (one synthetic polyester as control material ($n=12$) and four different biologic grafts ($n=24$ per material)). Biologic grafts evaluated included Surgisis® (Cook Medical, Bloomington, IN) (porcine small intestinal submucosa), Permacol™ (Covidien, Minneapolis, MN) (crosslinked porcine dermis), Xenmatrix™ (CR Bard, Murray Hill, NJ) (noncrosslinked porcine dermis), and Strattice™ (LifeCell, Branchburg, NJ) (noncrosslinked porcine dermis). Half of the repairs in each group were inoculated with Staphylococcus aureus at 104 CFU/ml and survived for 30 days without systemic antibiotic. There was a significant difference of bacterial clearance between biologic meshes. To this end, use of biologic mesh in Northern America has become standard in high-risk patients with contaminated and dirty-infected wounds, despite the very high cost associated with the use of biologic mesh.

Previously we reported our own study of 60 patients who underwent acellular dermal matrix (ADM) implantation for abdominal wall reconstruction [19]. Of the 60 patients, 56 patients had enough information on their charts and were studied retrospectively. In these patients we used two brands of ADM: AlloDerm® (LifeCell, Branchburg, NJ) in 38 patients (68 %) and Strattice™ (LifeCell, Branchburg, NJ) in 18 (32 %). A total of nine patients had concomitant ECFs and/or EAFs. For the nine patients with ECFs and/or EAFs, we used underlay placement in 4 (44 %) and interposition or bridge placement in 5 (56 %). We found that the abdominal wall reconstruction results in patients with vs. without concomitant ECFs and/or EAFs did not statistically differ, in terms of the rates of overall complications, of recurrence, and of infectious complications. However, we lack long-term data on these patients.

Others have also reported that ADM implantation can be safely used to repair large and complex ventral hernia defects in patients with clean-contaminated or dirty-infected wounds. In our study mentioned above, of the 56 patients who underwent ADM implantation with either AlloDerm or Strattice, 35 had contaminated fields as defined by the presence of intra-abdominal or soft tissue infections, stomas, or fistulas. Of those 35 patients, the majority—26 (74 %)—had Grade 4 infections, per a hernia grading system [20]. The grading system, which was recently created, is used to classify the risk for infectious complications in order to help surgeons decide on the technique and potentially on the mesh to be used. Grade 1 refers to a low risk for infections or complications in patients who have no history of wound infections; Grade 2 refers to comorbidities such as smoking, diabetes, obesity, a suppressed immune system, and chronic obstructive pulmonary disease (COPD); Grade 3 refers to previously contaminated wound infections, stomas, or intraoperative violations of the GI tract; and Grade 4 refers to infected mesh and septic foci. Obviously, Grades 3 and 4 present serious medical and surgical challenges for the patient and for the health care team, whether led by a general surgeon, trauma surgeon, or plastic surgeon but even Grade 2 means that patients may harbor a significant risk and need to be thoroughly evaluated preoperatively; otherwise a significant problem could arise. My own preference on this issue is to actually review the patient's history carefully and if possible, to use synthetic mesh unless the patient clearly is a Grade 2 with a high risk for infection and is undergoing major ventral hernia repair.

Our results suggest that biologic mesh implantation is a valid option for complex abdominal wall reconstruction in the high-risk trauma and acute care surgery population; however, long-term results are not evident yet. Other surgeons have reported abdominal wall closure in the infected field as well. In a recent study of 82 patients [21] with ventral hernia repaired predominantly with Alloderm and Strattice, 32 (39 %) had had concomitant bowel surgery. There was no difference in hernia recurrence (contaminated group—28 % vs. noncontaminated group—34 %, $P=0.58$), surgical site infections (contaminated—28 % vs. noncontaminated—20 %, $P=0.40$), or other complications when patients with and without concomitant bowel surgery were compared. One of the major complications of the biologic mesh has been hernia recurrence rate, which has been reported as high as greater than 30 % [22] or laxity that troubles both the patient and the surgeons [23]. In this study, seven of the nine patients reconstructed with component separation followed by interpositional Alloderm presented with abdominal wall laxity. Laxity was defined as a condition in which patients had clinical evidence of abdominal bulge at follow-up and required secondary reconstruction. While laxity has been common in our own patients as well, long-term data are missing [17]. In a systematic review of 25 retrospective studies performed by Slater et al. [24], the authors found that recurrence rate depended on wound class, with an overall rate of 13.8 % (95 % confidence interval [CI], 7.6–21.3). The recurrence rate in contaminated/dirty repairs was 23.1 %. Abdominal wall laxity occurred in 10.5 % of patients. The surgical morbidity rate was 46.3 %. Infection occurred in 15.9 % of patients but only led to graft removal in 4.9 % of cases. As it has been known for a while now, there is no randomized clinical trial; however, biologic grafts are associated with a high salvage rate when faced with infection. Use of biologic mesh has made possible "one operation only" as it is attempted by most surgeons who perform abdominal wall reconstruction at the time of hernia repair or at the time of takedown of ECFs and/or EAFs, even in contaminated fields, instead of series of operation. In our practice, we aim to complete the definitive procedure in a single operation. On occasion, I have used the principle of damage control, returning the next day or so to complete the operation by performing anastomosis, preparing the abdominal wall by performing lateral compartment release, and returning the next day for mesh placement and final closure.

In this study of 128 patients (76 F, 52 M) with large hernia defect (range 40–2,450 cm^2), infected mesh was present in ($n=45$), stoma ($n=24$), concomitant gastrointestinal (GI) surgery ($n=17$), enterocutaneous fistula ($n=25$), open nonhealing wound(s) ($n=6$), enterotomy/colotomy ($n=5$), and chronic draining sinus ($n=6$) [22]. Despite the high rate of wound morbidity (47.7 %) associated with single-staged reconstruction of contaminated fields, authors concluded biologic mesh can be placed without consequences. However, these authors also conclude that the long-term durability seems to be less favorable. In a similar study, this group of authors reported the simultaneous reconstruction of ECF and complex abdominal wall defects resulted in successful single-stage management of these challenging cases in nearly 70 % of patients [25]. To this end, many authors now believe that abdominal wall reconstruction (AWRs) using ADM has low rates of surgical site occurrence (SSO) and surgical site infection, despite increasing degrees of wound contamination. Most recent study of 359 patients who had AWR using ADM, with mean follow-up of 28.3 ± 19.0 months, further supports his hypothesis [26] irrespective of what kind of approach was used and despite all the advances in mesh and in techniques used, the AWR with or without biologic mesh has very high morbidity. In a report of 106 patients [27] (79 patients of whom had preoperative comorbid conditions), 67 (63 %) patients developed a postoperative complication. Skin necrosis was the most common complication ($n=21$, 19.8 %). This is similar to our experience [28]. This is particularly common with component separation and if the patient undergoes massive resuscitation. Other complications of AWRs include seroma ($n=19$, 17.9 %), cellulitis ($n=19$, 17.9 %), abscess ($n=14$ 13.2 %), pulmonary embolus/deep vein thrombosis ($n=3$, 2.8 %), small bowel obstruction ($n=2$, 1.9 %), and fistula ($n=8$, 7.5 %). Using the Methodological Index for Nonrandomized Studies and those with a score of 8 or more were combined to evaluate the end points of 16 studies from six different mesh products, a most recent study [29] analyzed 554 patients with an overall infection rate of 24 % and a recurrence rate of 20 %. The authors call for caution when using biologic mesh products in infected fields because there is a paucity of controlled data and none have US Food and Drug Administration approval for use in infected fields. When biologic mesh was compared to nonbiologic mesh in a recent meta-analysis, it was found that biologic grafts had significantly fewer infectious wound complications ($p<0.00001$); however, recurrence rates were not different. In addition, there were no differences in wound infections, and recurrence between the human and porcine-derived biologic grafts [30].

Graft Placement

Either open or laparoscopic surgical techniques can be used to repair abdominal wall defects; but, in patients with ECFs and/or EAFs, the open approach is preferred. There are three most common techniques used to place mesh during abdominal wall reconstruction, and these are *onlay* placement, *underlay* placement, and *interposition or bridge* placement.

Onlay Placement

Technically, onlay mesh placement is the easiest way to place mesh. I used this technique (Fig. 48.3) at the beginning of my practice and

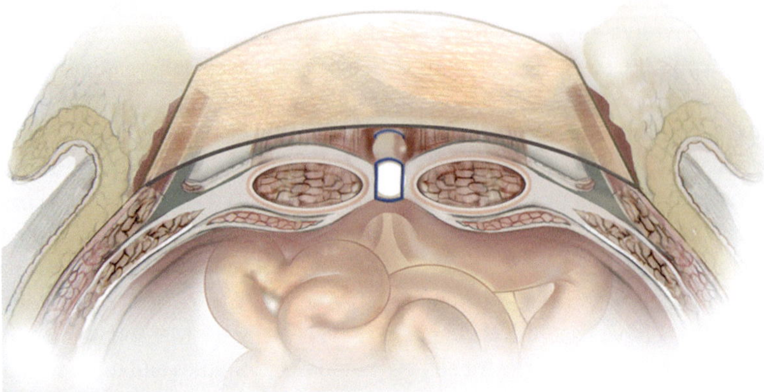

Fig. 48.3 Illustration of onlay mesh placement. (Used with permission from LifeCell Corporation, an Acelity Company)

still use it on occasions when we are able to approximate the abdominal wall edges without any major dissection or if I use synthetic mesh. The key element of this approach is fixing the mesh both laterally and over the edge of midline. I prefer fixing mesh to fascia using absorbable sutures, either interrupted or in a continuous fashion. The main objective is to reestablish tight approximation of the mesh to fascia. In addition, I use three or four large, closed suction drains (19 French [Fr]) under the subcutaneous tissue and keep them in until the individual drain output is less than 25 cc over 24 h.

Underlay Placement

In my practice, underlay graft placement (Fig. 48.4a–c) has now become the main technique of graft use in ventral major hernia defects. It is more involved but once it is learned and perfected, it does not add significant operative time. Underlay graft placement is associated with a lesser incidence of seromas. The key element of this technique is freeing the abdominal wall from any adhesions, as far laterally as possible both on the posterior and anterior aspect.

Placement of the interrupted sutures should ensure complete stretching of mesh once sutures are tight. Suture placement techniques vary, but I prefer the parachuting technique and the use of direct-vision at all times. The direct-vision parachuting technique minimizes the potential for bowel injury during fixing of graft on the abdominal wall. If lateral component release is used (which is done almost in all patients requiring major abdominal wall reconstruction: Fig. 48.5a, b), one has to place sutures in the anterior abdominal wall as far laterally as possible; clearly, the surgeon must include the medial edge of the external oblique fascia. Doing so prevents bulging laterally at the release component site; the patient might think bulging is a new hernia.

Bridge Placement

When the abdominal wall has lost its domain and the surgeon cannot bring together the medial edges of the abdominal wall (because the wall has been either removed or retracted laterally completely), then the only remaining option is to use mesh as a bridge (Fig. 48.6a, b). The surgeon must ensure that the suture bites are placed at least 2 or 3 cm into the muscles and fascia. If possible, the surgeon must avoid tacking the mesh on the edge of the fascia, given the risk of herniation or suture failure increases significantly.

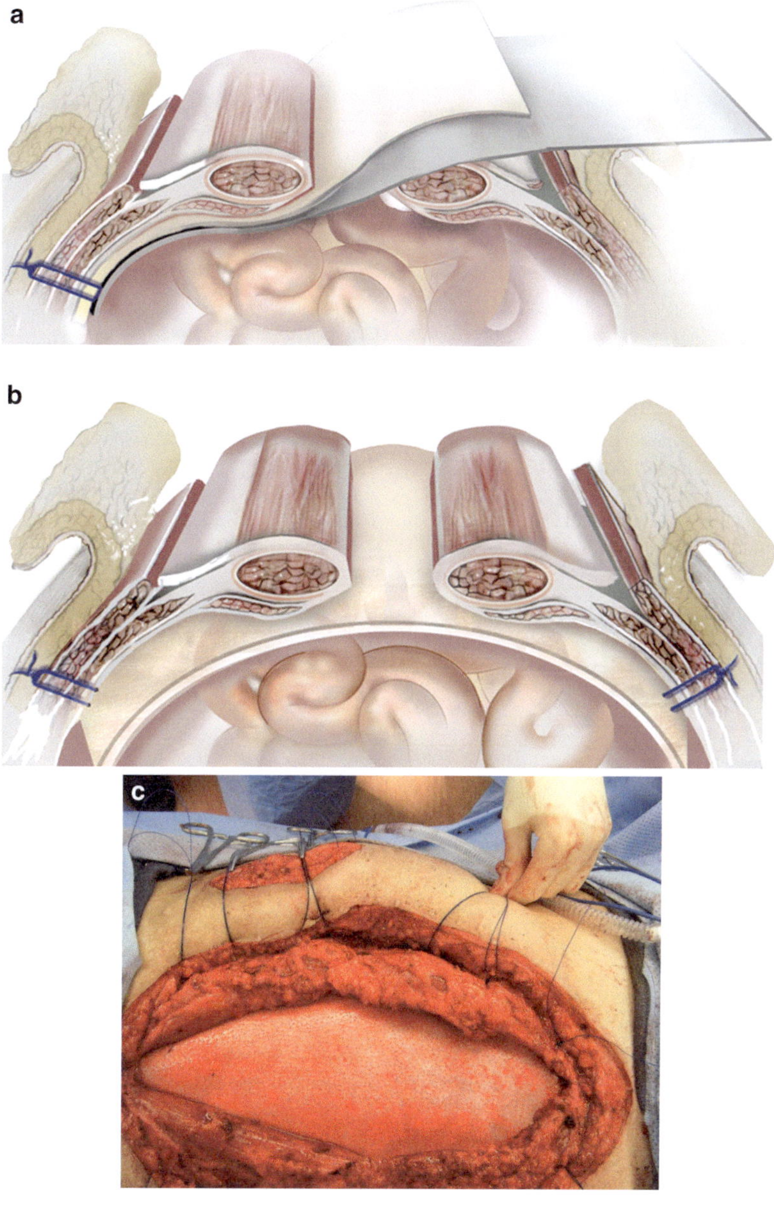

Fig. 48.4 (**a**) Illustration of underlay mesh. (**b**) Underlay mesh fixed laterally. (**c**) A patient undergoing underlay placement of Strattice™ (LifeCell, Branchburg, NJ) mesh. ((**a**, **b**) Used with permission from LifeCell Corporation, an Acelity Company; (**c**) Reproduced with permission from Latifi R, Peralta R, Al Thani H. Abdominal Wall Reconstruction in Patients with an Open Abdomen and Enterocutaneous Fistulas: A 9 Step Treatment Strategy. In Latifi R (ed): Surgery of Complex Abdominal Wall Defects. New York: Springer Science+Business Media; 2013)

Closed suction drainage to reduce or prevent seromas, which have the potential to become infected and thereby to jeopardize the integrity of the closure, is a must. When mesh is used as a bridge and there is no skin or subcutaneous tissue to cover the mesh, then use wound Vacuum Assisted Closure (VAC) with continuous irrigation, to keep the mesh moist and to speed the process of granulation for later skin grafting is very useful (Fig. 48.6).

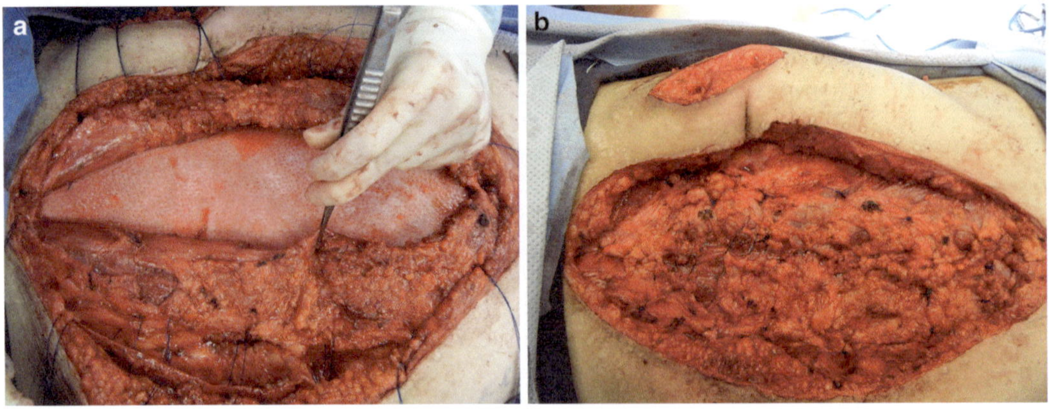

Fig. 48.5 Combination of underlay placement and bilateral lateral component separation. ((**a**, **b**) Reproduced with permission from Latifi R, Peralta R, Al Thani H. Abdominal Wall Reconstruction in Patients with an Open Abdomen and Enterocutaneous Fistulas: A 9 Step Treatment Strategy. In Latifi R (ed): Surgery of Complex Abdominal Wall Defects. New York: Springer Science+Business Media; 2013)

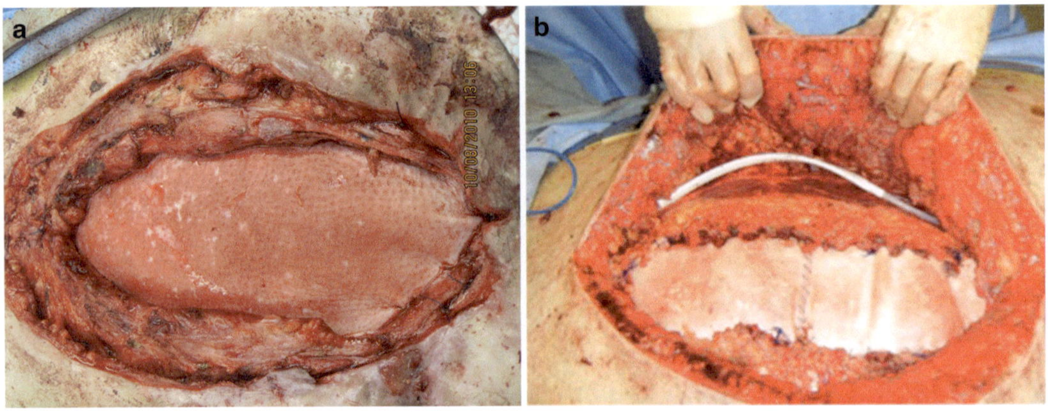

Fig. 48.6 Frozen abdomen reconstructed with bridge mesh placement. ((**a**, **b**): Reproduced with permission from Latifi R, Peralta R, Al Thani H. Abdominal Wall Reconstruction in Patients with an Open Abdomen and Enterocutaneous Fistulas: A 9 Step Treatment Strategy. In Latifi R (ed): Surgery of Complex Abdominal Wall Defects. New York: Springer Science+Business Media; 2013)

Other Clinical Applications of TE Tissue

Reconstructions of Cutaneous Soft Tissues Defects

For definitive reconstruction after excision of cutaneous and soft tissue malignancies, Acellular dermis (AlloDerm) has been reported [31]. In this study 67 patients underwent AlloDerm reconstruction. The median defect size was 42 cm(2) (range, 2–340 cm(2)), involving predominantly the lower extremity (45 %) or head and neck (32 %) was the most frequent diagnosis and the most common cause was melanoma (67 %) of the cases.

Ophthalmologic Reconstructive Surgery

Use of biologic meshes and its application to ophthalmic plastic and reconstructive surgery is less well described. However, a recent study of

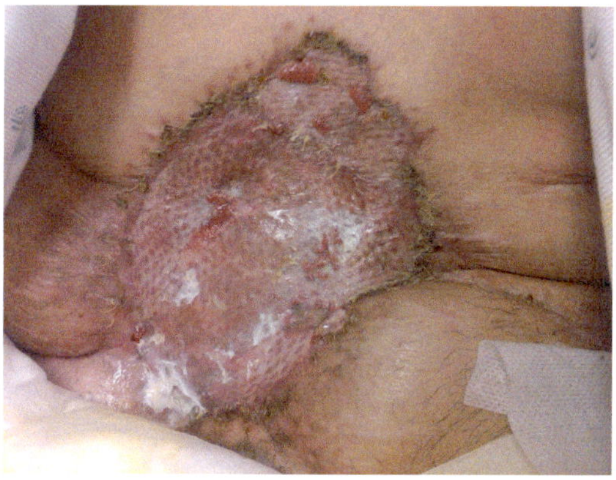

Fig. 48.7 Skin graft of patient seen in Fig. 48.6. (Reproduced with permission from Latifi R, Peralta R, Al Thani H. Abdominal Wall Reconstruction in Patients with an Open Abdomen and Enterocutaneous Fistulas: A 9 Step Treatment Strategy. In Latifi R (ed): Surgery of Complex Abdominal Wall Defects. New York: Springer Science + Business Media; 2013)

84 patients with malignancy in 26 patients (31.0 %), trauma in 19 patients (22.6 %), congenital lesions in 15 patients (17.9 %), and senile change in 11 patients (13.1 %) was reported [32]. These patients underwent lower eyelid posterior lamella elongation, socket and fornix reconstruction, scar repair, patch grafts, and filler. During the follow-up period of 530 days, authors reported that 92.8 % of patients had favorable outcomes. Factors associated with significantly worse outcomes included smoking, congenital anomaly etiologies, and previous graft/flaps in the same area ($p = 0.03$, $p = 0.029$, and $p = 0.007$, respectively).

Augmented Breast Reconstruction

After abdominal wall reconstruction using biologic mesh, augmenting breast reconstruction using biologic mesh has become the most common surgical procedure. While the indication varies and are not well defined in the literature, use of mesh to help with immediate reconstruction [33] has become most common and is being seen as a viable alternative to 2-stage expander reconstruction, presenting many advantages over expander reconstruction while offering the same risk profile and eliminating the additional risks, costs, and discomfort of a second procedure. Others [34] have reported use of biologic mesh to optimize the inframammary fold with acellular dermal matrix which they claim creates a superior aesthetic result, as its use appears to be safe and is associated with less capsular contracture and mechanical shift and improvement in the inframammary fold appearance without increasing postoperative complications. These authors reported the results of 203 patients who underwent 337 immediate expander-based breast reconstructions [with acellular dermal matrix, $n = 208$ (61.7 %); without, $n = 129$ (38.3 %)]. While the patients were similar, acellular dermal matrix use had fewer overall complications. However, incidences of seroma/hematoma, infection, and wound complications remained the same. Aesthetic outcomes were higher in the ADM group with less capsular contracture and less mechanical shift.

In a comparative cost analysis of breast reconstruction using acellular dermal matrix (ADM) and traditional tissue expander-/implant-based techniques [35], it was concluded that plastic surgeons are aware of the cost implications of using ADM products.

In summary, while the popularity of biologic mesh in breast reconstruction during the first stage of two-stage procedures continues to grow, one has to be cognizant of major cost.

Summary

Biologic meshes are derived from human dermis, porcine dermis, porcine small intestine submucosa, bovine dermis, or bovine pericardium. Their use has been rationalized by many. While their benefit has been demonstrated, although no randomized clinical trials have been conducted in the infected field, there are a number of issues with all biologic meshes. First of all, they are extremely expensive and their application has a 30 % recurrence rate of hernia. Furthermore, the biology of interaction with a host is still being studied, with particular attention being paid to mediators and the mechanism of controlling inflammatory and immune response. Nonetheless, these meshes are here to stay, and it will be up to surgeons to further study, modify, learn more about, and finally create a product that will eventually be cheaper and more effective and will become integrated fully by the scaffold through cellular and fibrovascular ingrowth tissue remodeling. Hopefully, what has happened with the expansion of biologic mesh will be followed by other organs as well. In summary, the AWR using biologic mesh has advanced this field significantly; however, the biggest challenging issue that continues to plague abdominal wall reconstruction using bioengineered materials is the extraordinary cost that simply renders it impossible to be used in the majority of the countries in the world.

References

1. Badylak SF, Weiss DJ, Caplan A, Macchiarini P. Engineered whole organs and complex tissues. Lancet. 2012;379:943–52.
2. Owaki T, Shimizu T, Yamato M, Okano T. Review. Cell sheet engineering for regenerative medicine: current challenges and strategies. Biotechnol J. 2014;7(9):904–14.
3. Burg KJL, Porter S, Kellam JF. Biomaterial developments for bone tissue engineering. Biomaterials. 2000;21(23):2347–59.
4. Pham C, Greenwood J, Cleland H, Woodruff P, Maddern G. Bioengineered skin substitutes for the management of burns: a systematic review. Burns. 2007;33:946–57.
5. Atala A, Bauer SB, Soker S, Yoo JJ, Retik AB. Tissue-engineered autologous bladders for patients needing cystoplasty. Lancet. 2006;367:1241–6.
6. Macchiarini P, Jungebluth P, Go T, Asnaghi MA, Rees LE, Cogan TA, Dodson A, Martorell J, Bellini A, Parnigotto PP, Dickinson SC, Hollander AP, Mantero S, Conconi MT, Birchall MA. Clinical transplantation of a tissue-engineered airway. Lancet. 2008;372:2023–30.
7. Kheradvar A, Groves EM, Dasi LP, Alavi SH, Tranquillo R, Grande-Allen KJ, Simmons CA, Griffith B, Falahatpisheh A, Goergen CJ, Mofrad MR, Baaijens F, Little SH, Canic S. Emerging Trends in Heart Valve Engineering: Part I. Solutions for future. Ann Biomed Eng. 2015;43(4):833–43.
8. Novitsky YW. Biology of biologic meshes used in hernia repair. Surg Clin North Am. 2013;93(5):1211–5.
9. Katari RS, Peloso A, Orlando G. Tissue engineering. Adv Surg. 2014;48(1):137–54.
10. Murphy SV, Atala A. Organ engineering: combining stem cells, biomaterials, and bioreactors to produce bioengineered organs for transplantation. Bioessays. 2013;35:163–72.
11. Atala A, Kasper FK, Mikos AG. Engineering complex tissues. Sci Transl Med. 2012;4(160):160rv12.
12. Taylor DA, Caplan AL, Macchiarini C. Ethics of bioengineering organs and tissues. Exp Opin Biol Ther. 2014;14(7):879–82.
13. Latifi R, editor. Surgery of complex abdominal wall defects. New York, NY: Springer Science+Business Media; 2013.
14. Higa G, Friese R, O'Keeffe T, Wynne J, Bowlby P, Ziemba M, Latifi R, Kulvatunyou N, Rhee P. Damage control laparotomy: a vital tool once overused. J Trauma. 2010;69(1):53–9.
15. Higa G, Latifi R. A difficult abdomen: clinical course-based management. In: Latifi R, editor. Surgery of complex abdominal wall defects. New York, NY: Springer Science+Business Media; 2013.
16. Latifi R, Leppaniemi A. Practical approach to patient with a hostile abdomen. In: Latifi R, editor. Surgery of complex abdominal wall defects. New York, NY: Springer Science+Business Media; 2013.
17. Latifi R, Peralta R, Althani H. Abdominal wall reconstruction in patients with an open abdomen and enterocutaneous fistulas: a nine-step treatment strategy. In: Latifi R, editor. Surgery of complex abdominal wall defects. New York, NY: Springer Science+Business Media; 2013.
18. Harth KC, Broome A-M, Jacobs MR, Blatnik JR, Zeinali F, Bajaksouzian S, Rosen MJ. Bacterial clearance of biologic grafts used in hernia repair: an experimental study. Surg Endosc. 2011;25(7):2224–9.
19. Latifi R, Joseph B, Kulvatunyou N, Wynne JL, O'Keeffe T, Tang A, Friese R, Rhee PM. Enterocutaneous fistulas and a hostile abdomen: reoperative surgical approaches. World J Surg. 2012;36(3):516–23.
20. The Ventral Hernia Working Group, Breuing K, Butler C, Ferzoco S, Franz M, Hultman C, Kilbridge J, Rosen M, Silverman R, Vargo D. Incisional ventral hernias: review of the literature and recommendations regarding the grading and technique of repair. Surgery. 2010;148(3):544–58.
21. Pinell-White XA, Gruszynski M, Losken A. Ventral hernia repair after bowel surgery: does gastrointestinal contamination matter in the era of biologic mesh? Ann Plast Surg. 2014;72(6):S150–2.
22. Rosen MJ, Krpata DM, Ermlich B, Blatnik JA. A 5-year clinical experience with single-staged repairs of infected and contaminated abdominal wall defects utilizing biologic mesh. Ann Surg. 2013;257(6):991–6.
23. Bluebond-Langner R, Keifa ES, Mithani S, Bochicchio GV, Scalea T, Rodriguez ED. Recurrent abdominal laxity following interpositional human acellular dermal matrix. Ann Plast Surg. 2008;60(1):76–80.
24. Slater NJ, van der Kolk M, van Hendriks T, Goor H, Bleichrodt RP. Biologic grafts for ventral hernia repair: a systematic review. Am J Surg. 2013;205(2):220–30.

25. Krpata DM, Stein SL, Eston M, Ermlich B, Blatnik JA, Novitsky YW, Rosen MJ. Outcomes of simultaneous large complex abdominal wall reconstruction and enterocutaneous fistula takedown. Am J Surg. 2013;205(3):354–8. Discussion 358–9.
26. Garvey PB, Martinez RA, Baumann DP, Liu J, Butler CE. Outcomes of abdominal wall reconstruction with acellular dermal matrix are not affected by wound contamination. J Am Coll Surg. 2014;219:853–64.
27. Satterwhite TS, Miri S, Chung C, Spain D, Lorenz HP, Lee GK. Outcomes of complex abdominal herniorrhaphy: experience with 106 cases. Ann Plast Surg. 2012;68(4):382–8.
28. Latifi R, Gustafson M. Abdominal wall reconstruction in patients with enterocutaneous fistulas. J Trauma Emerg Surg. 2011;37:241–50.
29. Cross W, Kumar A, Chandru KG. Biologic mesh in contaminated fields: overuse without data: a systematic review of their use in abdominal wall reconstruction. Am Surg. 2014;80(1):3–8.
30. Darehzereshki A, Golfarb M, Zehetner J, et al. Biologic versus nonbiologic mesh in ventral hernia repair: a systematic review and meta-analysis. World J Surg. 2014;38:40–50.
31. Deneve JL, Turaga KK, Marzban SS, Puleo CA, Sarnaik AA, Gonzalez RJ, Sondak VK, Zager JS. Single-institution outcome experience using AlloDerm® as temporary coverage or definitive reconstruction for cutaneous and soft tissue malignancy defects. Am Surg. 2013;79(5):476–82.
32. Bee YS, Alonzo B, Ng JD. Review of AlloDerm acellular human dermis regenerative tissue matrix in multiple types of oculofacial plastic and reconstructive surgery. Ophthal Plast Reconstr Surg. 2014 (in press).
33. Cassileth L, Kohanzadeh S, Amersi F. One-stage immediate breast reconstruction with implants: a new option for immediate reconstruction. Ann Plast Surg. 2012;69(2):134–8.
34. Vardanian AJ, Clayton JL, Roostaeian J, Shirvanian V, Da Lio A, Lipa JE, Crisera C, Festekjian JH. Comparison of implant-based immediate breast reconstruction with and without acellular dermal matrix. Plast Reconstr Surg. 2011;128(5):403e–10e.
35. de Blacam C, Momoh AO, Colakoglu S, Slavin SA, Tobias AM, Lee BT. Cost analysis of implant-based breast reconstruction with acellular dermal matrix. Ann Plast Surg. 2012;69(5):516–20.

Artificial Limbs for Upper Extremity Amputation

49

Paul D. Marasco, Jacqueline S. Hebert, and Beth M. Orzell

Introduction

Prosthetic limbs have been a part of human culture throughout much of our recorded history. There is archaeological evidence that functional load-bearing devices have been utilized as early as the Third Intermediate Period of ancient Egypt [1]. Interestingly, many of the design components of these early technologies, such as load-bearing rigid outer shells or sockets (950–710 BC), articulated hands (early sixteenth century), locking knees (mid-sixteenth century), moveable joints (late seventeenth century), and suspension harnesses (late seventeenth century), are still readily recognized and maintained in current standard-of-care devices [2]. While the design goals of prosthetic replacements have changed little through history, modern artificial limbs have become marvels of advanced human technology. Standard-of-care prosthetic fittings now utilize microprocessor controlled hydraulics, powered joints, powered multi-articulate digits, and advanced materials such as carbon fiber and titanium which are displayed proudly on devices that were, until very recently, only envisioned in science fiction.

Much of the recent innovation in prosthetic limbs has been spurred by advances in battery technology, motor design, composite materials, alloys, and most importantly intuitive control systems that map the intention of the user to device function. Many of these significant breakthroughs have been due in large part to US Federal investment in a number of advanced research projects focusing on expanding the function and capabilities of prosthetic limbs and interfaces. These include programs such as the Defense Advanced Research Projects Agency's (DARPA) Revolutionizing Prosthetics Initiative 2007, Revolutionizing Prosthetics Initiative 2009, the Reliable Neural Interfaces (RE-NET) family of efforts, programs within the National Institutes of Health (NIH) such as the Neural Interfaces Program, and also sponsored research

P.D. Marasco, Ph.D. (✉)
Department of Biomedical Engineering, Cleveland Clinic, 9500 Euclid Ave, ND20, Cleveland, OH 44195, USA

Advanced Platform Technology Center of Excellence, Louis Stokes Cleveland Department of Veterans Affairs Medical Center, Cleveland, OH USA
e-mail: marascp2@ccf.org; pmarasco@aptcenter.org

J.S. Hebert, M.D.
Department of Medicine, University of Alberta, 5005 Katz Group Centre, Edmonton, AB, Canada, T6G2E1

Glenrose Rehabilitation Hospital, Alberta Health Services, Edmonton, AB, Canada
e-mail: jhebert@ualberta.ca

B.M. Orzell, B.S.M.E.
Prosthetics and Sensory Aid Service, Louis Stokes Cleveland Department of Veterans Affairs Medical Center, 10701 East Blvd. Mail Stop 121(W), Cleveland, OH 44106, USA
e-mail: Beth.orzell@va.gov

R. Latifi et al. (eds.), *Technological Advances in Surgery, Trauma and Critical Care*,
DOI 10.1007/978-1-4939-2671-8_49

through the National Science Foundation (NSF). The development of advanced technologies through these programs has had the added benefit of creating innovative shifts in surgical and rehabilitation approaches for limb amputation. The importance of integrating the surgical, prosthetic, and rehabilitation treatment of a person with limb loss to optimize outcome has never been more evident.

The Surgical Approach to Amputation

A limb amputation leaves a number of critical structural challenges. With removal of the natural load-bearing and articulating functions of a limb, the terminal bone must be padded and secured to provide structural support for the prosthetic limb. One of the most important aspects to the amputation surgery itself is to appropriately stabilize the divided muscle (myodesis) and/or tendon (tenodesis) by drilling into the bone or attaching to the periosteum. Muscle stabilization can also be achieved by attaching muscle to muscle over the terminal bone (myoplasty); however, myodesis is the preferred treatment. Properly stabilized musculature lays the foundation for a residual limb that can tolerate the forces required for supporting the prosthesis. Furthermore, a secure myodesis prevents retraction of the muscle and allows a stable electromyographic (EMG) signal site for myoelectric control.

There is a certain amount of controversy over optimal management of the nerve endings. In general, aggressively proximal transection is not advised so that nerve length may be preserved for possible future reinnervation. This also helps to avoid inadvertent sensory loss or denervation of remaining muscle that might be useful for myoelectric control. The recommended current course of action is to sharply transect the nerve end and bury it in muscle tissue. Recently, there has been preliminary evidence in case series that muscle reinnervation (immediately at the time of amputation, or as a delayed procedure) may reduce painful neuroma formation and neuropathic pain [3].

Appropriate residuum length is another critical aspect of upper limb amputation. If the elbow joint cannot be preserved and a transhumeral amputation is required, the humerus length is often shortened to accommodate a prosthetic elbow. However, if enough of the humerus remains, rather than simply resecting to fit a prosthetic elbow, orthopedic techniques such as angulation osteotomy can be applied by fixing a distal fragment of the humerus with a screw or an angled (60°–70°) posterior plate to improve rotational stabilization and control of the prosthesis (Fig. 49.1a). Another potential surgical technique for increasing stabilization while allowing room

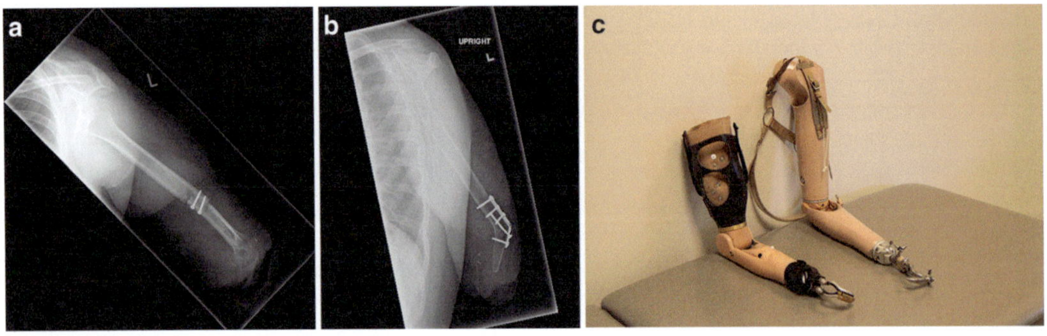

Fig. 49.1 (**a**) Humeral osteotomy: a section of humerus is removed and the remaining segments fixated (shown here with fixation screws), shortening the transhumeral limb to make room for a prosthetic elbow joint, yet retaining the epicondyles for improved socket suspension and rotational control. (**b**) Angulation osteotomy: a section of the distal humerus is fixated at an angle (with a plate as illustrated, or with a fixation screw). (**c**) Transhumeral socket with much lower proximal trimlines on the *left* is for a patient with angulation osteotomy, compared to traditional transhumeral socket with high trimlines and anterior and posterior flares for rotational control shown on the *right*

for a prosthetic elbow when the epicondyles are present is to remove a section of the humerus to shorten it at mid-level (humeral osteotomy) which retains a stable epicondylar suspension without the disadvantage of the long length of a traditional elbow disarticulation (Fig. 49.1b, c).

Recent advances in limb reconstruction for military casualties with complex injuries have also improved outcomes for prosthetic use. Limb reconstruction techniques that fix proximal fractures specifically to conserve length have allowed for longer residual limbs with better soft tissue coverage. Furthermore, advances in skin grafting techniques have improved salvage of longer residual limbs. This is particularly important for the upper limb where partial thickness grafts with less durability can tolerate socket fittings due to advanced interface materials and new socket technology.

Socket Technology

Modern prosthetic limbs utilize a rigid thermoplastic or laminated (resin impregnated carbon and nyglass) socket that surrounds the residual limb and distributes the mechanical loads through the soft tissue to the underlying bone. Because of this, the soft tissue must bear the stress of serving as a structural interface between the prosthesis and the remaining bone. The prosthetic socket is held in place on the limb through a combination of suction, silicone sleeves, and/or harnesses. While the construction of the socket has improved with modern materials such as thermoplastics and carbon fiber, the basic idea of the socket has remained essentially unchanged since the earliest documented advent of prosthetic limbs in 300 BC and perhaps as early as the ninth century BC [1, 2].

The socket is the foundation of the prosthesis and if it does not fit appropriately the wearer will have comfort issues, skin breakdown, suspension loss, and ultimately they will reject the prosthesis. Traditionally, the socket is made by taking an impression of the amputee's residual limb (negative model) with Plaster of Paris or fiberglass casting material. Then a positive model of the residuum is made and modified, creating voids or areas of relief for sensitive areas, to serve as a base to form the socket. Recently, digital laser scanning approaches have been developed that reduce the need for plaster casting. The scanner creates a 3-d image of the limb for the prosthetist to manipulate using software. Care is taken to highlight areas that can withstand more pressure, usually muscle tissue, and areas that cannot, such as bony prominences, scar tissue, and neuromas. The load tolerant areas are compressed in order to gain suspension and reduce excess movement between the socket and the residuum. If this is done digitally, the resulting computer file is then uploaded to a robotic carving machine that produces a blank of the residual limb from rigid polyurethane foam.

Modern socket designs rely on total contact with the limb while accommodating for load tolerant or intolerant areas as described above. By loading on a majority of the soft tissue surface area, the limb weight is transferred more evenly throughout the socket. However, as the bony residuum is not directly secured to the prosthesis, rotation and movement of the limb in relationship to the socket can cause loss of socket fit or poor suspension. These problems are magnified with limb atrophy, changes in volume, or physical load on the limb. High-compression socket designs came about to reduce the amount of socket motion that may occur within the prosthesis. When motion is eliminated and better suspension is achieved, the prosthesis feels "a part of the patient." The weight of the device feels less and the patient will likely tolerate wearing the device for longer amounts of time. The more the device is used and incorporated into the patient's activities of daily living, the more successful the prosthesis is deemed.

In order to maximize comfort and function with the development of new highly functional prosthetic limbs, the systems that attach the devices to the amputated limb must evolve. New high-compression or compression/release-stabilized sockets squeeze the soft tissue of the limb through longitudinal depressions or bands that compress and displace the tissue between the residual bone and the socket to reduce motion.

In effect, tolerant areas are loaded aggressively with alternating relief areas to provide the patient more comfort and control. Care must be taken with this design to ensure that compression is maintained at a safe level for the patient. One design incorporates a blood volume perfusion sensor to ensure that there is adequate/safe blood flow to the residual limb.

In addition to new compression type approaches, dynamic systems that are able to adjust to the amputee over the course of the day are beginning to be realized. A recent advanced shoulder disarticulation prosthetic system utilized inflatable socket bladders that could be adjusted to increase stability under loaded conditions, account for changes in volume, and aid donning and doffing [4]. The pneumatic inflation and deflation of the individual bladders of the system were dynamically controlled by a belt-worn unit. This type of adjustability within the socket system could potentially address concerns with fluctuations in socket fit and comfort throughout the day.

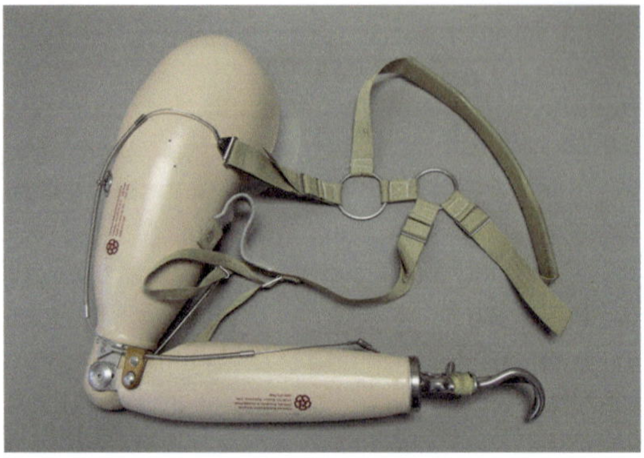

Fig. 49.2 A traditional body-powered transhumeral socket, with a "Figure of 8" harness system used for suspension and cable control of the terminal device and elbow

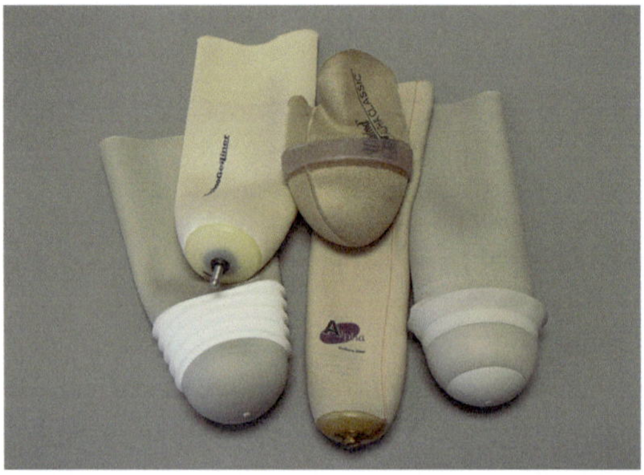

Fig. 49.3 Examples of liners typically used as an interface between the residual limb and the hard socket. Suspension can be provided by a pin affixed to the bottom of the liner matched to a shuttle lock in the socket, or by various ring seals around the outside of the liner to form a vacuum seal

Prosthetic Suspension

The rigid prosthetic socket must be suspended from the residual limb in order to functionally approximate the lost limb. Multiple modes of suspension are available for upper extremity sockets and therefore residual limb quality, patient tolerances, and prosthetist preference influence the final design choices.

Harness suspensions utilize a series of straps and buckles that attach to the socket and anchor to the trunk and contralateral limb. The straps of the harness are typically routed in the form of a figure eight across the back and this type of suspension is most commonly used in conventional body-powered style prosthetic limbs (Fig. 49.2). The harness provides both an anchor for the socket and an attachment for cables to gain excursion to operate a terminal device.

A suction fit socket attaches directly over the amputee's residual limb. An intimate airtight fit retains adhesion to the residual limb by using a one-way expulsion valve that is built into the socket. This negative pressure within the socket provides a stable attachment and prevents the limb from slipping off during use.

Silicone suction liners provide a mechanical connection to the socket by "gripping" the residual limb of the amputee (Fig. 49.3). The advent of the silicone suction socket liner in the late 1980s revolutionized the fit of prosthetic limbs [5]. The use of a gel liner against the skin greatly reduces the shear forces transferred to the residual limb in comparison to the earlier leather liner and prosthetic sock system. This has resulted in much more comfortable prosthetic limbs, better skin management, and less problematic fitting issues.

Silicone and related polyurethanes are excellent liner materials. They are more comfortable next to the skin than most materials. They are also compliant, strong, and maintain an airtight seal in both suction and traction applications. One particular advantage of these liners is that they provide comfort by creating a soft barrier between the hard socket and sensitive or scarred skin and bony prominences. These liners can also effectively have numerous adjunct suspension mechanisms incorporated into their design such as locking pins, valves, or lanyards.

Self-suspending sockets interconnect with the remaining bony anatomy of the residual limb through contours built into the socket. For example, these sockets can be used to apply medial and lateral pressure over the humeral epicondyles in transradial level amputation. In this type of fitting, the socket terminates proximal to the epicondyles to create a bony lock or anchor that helps reduce soft tissue movement and enhances suspension.

Other Attachment Strategies: Osseointegration

One strategy that has been used to overcome the above-mentioned socket limitations is direct skeletal attachment, or osseointegration. This technique for prosthetic limb attachment was pioneered in Sweden in the 1950s, with the first clinical patients treated in the 1990s [6]. This is now an accepted treatment technique in several European centers. In this approach the use of a rigid socket is eliminated entirely by attaching the prosthesis to a metal abutment that passes through the skin and is anchored within the residual limb bone. This type of approach has been used successfully for many years in dental implants, facial reconstructions, and prosthetic digits. In the modern implementation, a titanium fixture is placed down the center of the amputated limb bone and the terminal bone encapsulates the device. This bone anchored attachment then accepts a replaceable titanium abutment that transverses the skin. At the point where the percutaneous abutment traverses the skin, the skin is encouraged to adhere to the bone in a junction that is similar in rigidity to the base of the fingernail. This prevents breakdown at the percutaneous junction. The distal end of the abutment serves as the mounting point for a prosthetic limb. This type of attachment is highly robust and able to bear considerable forces beyond simple weight bearing. The main persisting complication is that of intermittent superficial skin infections that can occur at the percutaneous junction [7].

The primary advantage of osseointegration is that the weight and functional leverage of the prosthetic limb is transferred directly to the skeleton. This direct bone attachment approach has recently been applied in upper limb prosthetics with high success in individuals who have highly demanding physical occupations. There has also been described a phenomenon of "osseoperception," whereby the osseointegrated fixture is able to supply tactile or proprioceptive feedback to the individual through vibrations transmitted to the direct skeletal attachment. One of the exciting recent developments in transdermal bone-integrated upper limbs is the inclusion of an internally routed feedback and control system that will be discussed in more detail later in this chapter.

Prosthetic Power and Control Strategies

There are three current control strategies for most standard-of-care functional (active) prosthetic limbs: body-powered, externally powered (myoelectric), and hybrid design. Body-powered devices mechanically harness the movement of proximal joints through a single or dual cable linkage to actuate the joints of the prosthesis. These designs reached their zenith after World War II and were based on cable and housing technology that originally came from bicycle brakes and aircraft control systems. Body-powered limb systems with a cable-actuated split hook are highly functional and are still employed widely in the clinic today. These devices are simple, intuitive to operate, robust, and interestingly, they provide a high level of useful position and movement feedback that can be felt through the excursion of the cables.

The joints of myoelectric devices are driven by battery powered motors. These systems are controlled by electrodes that are placed on the skin to read and amplify the EMG signals that are generated from volitional contraction of the underlying muscles. These systems typically utilize preserved antagonistic muscle groups to operate up to 3 degrees of freedom: hand open/close, wrist rotation, and elbow flexion/extension. The movement at each joint is sequentially operated and the individual functions are selected by a switch strategy, for example co-contracting the muscle pairs, or pushing an externally mounted electric switch.

Hybrid prosthetic limbs combine both power and cable control systems. For instance a typical setup will utilize myoelectric componentry for the hand and wrist, with elbow function operated by body-powered cable actuation. This approach simplifies the control strategy for the user and often makes the prosthesis less heavy than a full myoelectric system, and therefore more tolerable to wear for extended use.

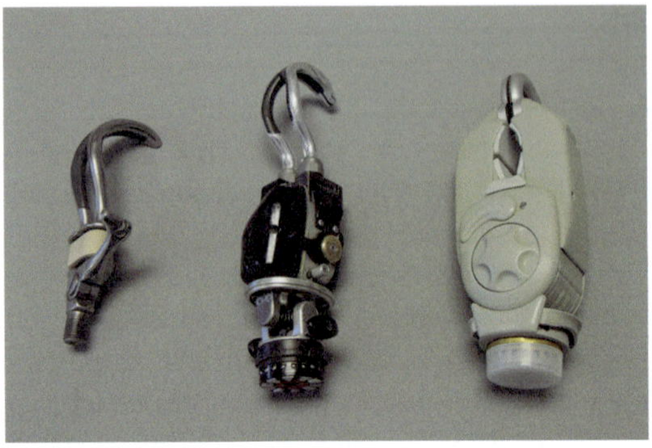

Fig. 49.4 Body-powered hook (*left*), myoelectrically powered hook (*middle*), and myoelectrically powered split hook (*right*)

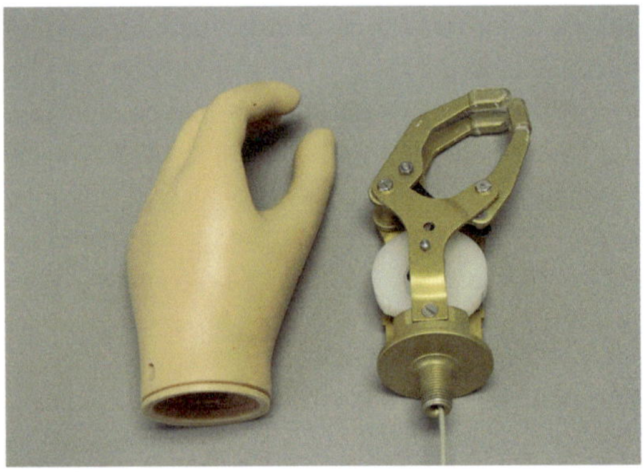

Fig. 49.5 "Three jaw chuck" hand. Both body-powered and myoelectrically powered versions are available

Terminal Device Advancements

The human hand is a sophisticated anatomical structure that is highly dexterous. It is used to manipulate a variety of objects, to interact with our environment and even to communicate. There have been limited prosthetic options for replacing even a fraction of the functionality of a human hand. However, one of the most successful and functional devices is the common body-powered hook (Fig. 49.4). This replacement for the hand provides a fine "tip-to-tip" pinch, or a canted "lateral key pinch" grip. Unfortunately, the primary drawback of this simple, robust, and highly dexterous device is its aesthetic appearance.

A somewhat less functional but more visually appealing option for some users is the mechanical 3-jaw chuck hand (Fig. 49.5). The index and middle finger of this type of device move to meet the thumb in opposition. The ring and pinky fingers are passive and not functional. These hands can be used with either body-powered (cable) devices, or they can be motorized and coupled with myoelectric control.

The most dramatic and recent advancement in terminal devices has been the advent of anthropomorphic robotic hands with individual articulating digits (Fig. 49.6). These hands are beginning to approach the dexterity of the hand they are replacing and while still in the early stages of development their technical sophistication is becoming more clinically accessible.

There are currently four available commercial multifunction hands with articulating digits and multiple grip patterns. The *Bebionic* hand by RSL Steeper (Leeds, UK) features 14 different grip patterns and hand positions. The *I-Limb*™ *Ultra* by Touch Bionics (Edinburgh, UK) has five articulating fingers that move independently, and the thumb can be manually rotated to two positions, with 13 different grip patterns and hand positions. Another version, the *I-Limb*™ *Revolution* has a powered rotating thumb. It can

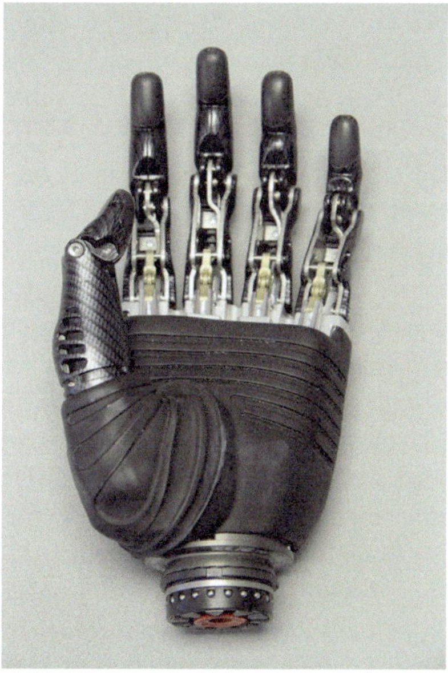

Fig. 49.6 Multifunction myoelectric hands with the capability to provide multiple grip conformations

interface with a mobile application to provide the option of 24 grip patterns to choose from. These prosthetic hands can be used with a manual rotatable quick disconnect or multifunction wrist, or in some cases an electric rotating wrist. The *Michelangelo* hand by Ottobock (Duderstadt, Germany) features seven different hand positions, and a flexible compliant wrist to assist with hand positioning.

These multifunction hands offer precision grips (key pinch, tip to tip, tripod), power grips (hook, cylindrical), active index pointing, "mouse" position, open palm, "hand shake" grip, relaxed or "natural" hand position, and in some cases a customizable hand position. Microprocessors and individual motors are used to control each of the four fingers, and maximum grip forces for the power grips can range from 70 to 140 N. However, one of the primary reasons that the standard hook configuration and 3-jaw chuck hands have continued as clinical standard of care is that they can be controlled by the limited available inputs of the user, without the need for manual or powered switching between multiple grasps. In order for multifunction hands to become fully realized for prosthetic users, the different functional grasp patterns must have equally detailed and sophisticated methods for control and feedback.

Sensory Motor Interfaces

Despite the advanced new devices available, utilization of prosthetic technology is currently limited by the human-machine interface, that is, being able to communicate with the complex neural system that governs fine motor and sensory functions. From a motor perspective, there are more available degrees of freedom in multifunction prosthetic devices than there are accessible controls sites in the residual limb of the amputee to activate the various functions. For example, after transhumeral amputation there are generally two remaining muscle signal sites in the residual limb: one in the elbow flexion group, and one in the elbow extension group. These two signal sites are drastically insufficient to adequately control a multifunction grip prosthetic hand in addition to wrist and elbow motion. In addition, the activation of these sites is physiologically matched to one function—elbow motion. To employ switching strategies and use elbow muscles to activate hand and wrist motions is nonintuitive and requires learning to associate new motor commands.

From a sensory perspective, simple sensory feedback systems can communicate states of the prosthetic device to the user in a nonphysiologic manner via sensory substitution (i.e., grip pressure from the device transmitted as force or vibration applied to the residual limb), but not in a physiologically or anatomically matched fashion. In fact, various forms of sensory substitution have been tried in prostheses for decades but none have so far been clinically accepted in the long term, likely due to the cognitive burden of having to interpret a non-matched stimulus. Along with motor control, there is a need to directly access and restore physiologically natural and matched sensation from the prosthetic device to the user if dexterous prosthetic hand function is to be attained.

Approaches to solve this dilemma of insufficient motor and sensory communication between the prosthesis and the amputee range from central to peripheral. The main approaches can be summarized as: (1) Extracting more signals from various levels of the nervous system (via implanted neural interfaces); (2) Better utilizing myoelectric signals from remaining muscles; (3) Rewiring or reconstructing the human to produce more accessible information (targeted reinnervation).

Neural Interfaces

Brain-machine interfacing (extracting signals from the motor cortex) has been shown in human subjects with severe paralysis to allow fairly complex control of a robotic arm for several weeks, with some degradation of signal strength over time [8]. Sensory cortical input has also recently been achieved although these approaches are still restricted to animal research models. While fascinating in the ability to restore movement control of a robotic arm for those with severely impaired motor function, cortical interfacing is not thought to be a clinically viable technique for restoring prosthetic function due to the invasiveness required for direct brain recordings.

In contrast, direct communication with the peripheral nervous system is less invasive than central nervous system approaches and has been investigated for several years. The ability to extract motor control signals as well as use sensory input feedback bidirectionally in real time has been demonstrated in amputee subjects using longitudinal intrafascicular electrodes (LIFEs) [9] and transversal intrafascicular multichannel electrodes (TIMEs) [10]. Recent advances also include recording motor control signals from peripheral nerves with an array of electrodes that penetrate the fiber bundles (the Utah Slant Array). The main limitation to using intraneural electrodes to provide physiologically appropriate sensory information with dexterous prosthetic control is currently the unknown long-term viability. All experiments have involved short time frames (4 weeks or less), with general degradation of the small neural signals over time.

Nerve cuff approaches, which surround the nerve rather than penetrate it, such as the Flat Interface Nerve Electrode (FINE) have progressed into long-term first human trials in amputee subjects [11]. This system has been successfully employed for sensory feedback in human amputees for over 2 years. In addition, this approach has pushed beyond the paraesthetic sensations of tingling normally associated with direct electrical stimulation of the nerve by altering the input parameters of stimulation so that the amputee interprets the tunable perception of functional pressure and texture. Ongoing research to improve signal quality and longevity for long-term implantation, focusing on wireless transmission to avoid the risk of percutaneous wires, is being actively investigated in several centers. These investigations will likely lead to significant changes in the approach to sensory motor restoration in the future.

Focused EMG Interfaces

In these approaches, the motor control signals are accessed directly from the muscles themselves. The limitations of surface EMG recordings typically used for myoelectric prosthetic control are not only the limited number of muscle sites but also the inconsistency of using a surface electrode within a prosthetic socket. Muscle contraction, sweat, and socket displacement can all cause misalignment of the sensors and subsequent inconsistency of activation of the prosthesis. Some of these difficulties have been addressed through approaches that are less sensitive to EMG electrode placement. One currently commercially available approach is that of pattern recognition. Pattern recognition systems have an advantage over conventional direct myoelectric control as the approach uses physiologically natural motor commands, is less discriminating in the requirement for exact electrode placement, and allows detection of multiple movement patterns without the concern over cross-talk or need for mode switching. In addition, the commercially available pattern recognition system has a "retraining" function that allows the user to recalibrate the prosthesis as needed throughout the day to adjust to current state. Pattern recognition systems can increase the number of motor commands that can be detected at any level of amputation with remaining muscle signals.

Another possible future option for reliably extracting muscle signals is that of wireless implantable EMG recording electrodes that are injected directly into the muscle belly, the so-called Implantable Myoelectric Sensors (IMES), which are currently undergoing first human trials [12]. With more distal amputation at the transradial level, the vast amount of motor control information still present in the forearm muscles that used to control the hand and fingers is difficult to separate with surface EMG, so the IMES approach may be a promising technique to translate signals for multifunction dexterous hand control. However, for more proximal levels of amputation, the insufficient motor commands remaining due to loss of forearm muscles would be an issue, and sensory feedback for true dexterous hand function would still need to be addressed by another mechanism.

Rewiring of the Human: Targeted Reinnervation

Of the approaches developed to address the human-machine interface challenge, one currently available clinical technique is Targeted Reinnervation (TR) [13]. TR surgically redirects the amputated nerve endings that used to innervate the hand and wrist muscles to new more proximal biomechanically nonfunctional muscle sites, to provide physiologically natural motor command signals for myoelectric control. The surgically redirected nerves are used to reinnervate purposely denervated muscles which then act as biological amplifiers for the new neural signals. The TR procedure is typically performed as a secondary revision procedure, with an extremely high rate of muscle reinnervation success and ability to use these sites for myoelectric control. Patients are able to operate multiple degrees of freedom of advanced prosthetic devices with increased ease following TR surgery and appropriate rehabilitation. This technique may also reduce neuroma-related pain [3], an otherwise common post-amputation complication. One drawback to TR is the need for many EMG electrode sites to represent each of the controllable joints of the prosthesis. Maintaining effective control with multiple surface electrodes is difficult and is easily disrupted if control sites are misaligned during socket donning or as the socket fit changes with limb volume and sweating. However, the pattern recognition approach mentioned above, in combination with TR, may allow even more signals to be extracted for prosthetic control. Recently, in subjects with upper limb amputation having undergone TR, simultaneous pattern recognition control was found to be superior in preference and performance to both sequential pattern recognition and conventional myoelectric control [14].

In addition to improved motor control, targeted reinnervation can provide a potential portal for sensory feedback. Redirection of the amputated sensory nerves to denervated skin has been shown to restore the sensation of the hand and fingers on the new target area of skin [15, 16]. This "transfer sensation" from reinnervation of the sensory afferents is being investigated as a possible access point to provide physiologically natural and appropriate avenues of cutaneous touch and proprioception feedback through robotic devices. These techniques have been applied in the lab through engineered perception where feedback is used to generate cognitive illusionary perceptions of limb ownership through appropriately actuated touch arising from the prosthesis.

There are three main surgical techniques that have been reported with sensory reinnervation: (1) traditional TR with motor branch coaptation, and associated denervation of overlying skin to allow sensory afferents to reinnervate the skin; (2) TR with the addition of end-to-side coaptation of a cutaneous sensory nerve to a main nerve trunk, and (3) an end-to-end targeted fascicular sensory reinnervation technique using intraoperative nerve stimulation to aid in fascicle selection [17]. Although there has been limited ability to control the territory of the sensory reinnervation, there is some evidence that the sensory maps can be better directed with specific microsurgical sensory nerve handling. The promising preliminary results on the use of sensory reinnervation to provide somatotopically matched sensory feedback with physiological control of devices currently involve a small number of subjects, and further study is needed to ascertain the constancy and reliability of the approaches. The technical challenges of providing sensory feedback to these areas in a clinical prosthetic socket through haptic devices are also being actively investigated.

A Combination of Approaches

One of the most significant advances to occur recently has been the assemblage of a number of the most promising approaches described above into one cohesive prosthetic intervention called the osseointegrated human-machine gateway [18]. As of the writing of this chapter, researchers in Sweden have implemented an upper limb prosthetic system that is integrated into the skeleton and communicates directly with the residual muscles and nervous system for control and sensory feedback. This system uses the osseointegration approach described above to anchor the abutment fixture to the amputated humeral bone. A control and feedback pathway is established through a special connection in the abutment, where wires connect the function of the external prosthetic limb to muscular and neural interfaces that are internally implanted within the upper arm. The movement of the elbow and hand is controlled through epimysial EMG electrodes placed internally directly on the muscle. Signals from these electrodes are processed through pattern recognition approaches and are used to predict elbow and hand control with high accuracy. A cuff electrode placed on the ulnar nerve is able to provide percepts of sensation from the hand through electrical stimulation, although this feedback is not currently linked to the prosthesis. In all, this approach has yielded a prosthetic limb that can be instantly attached to the skeleton and controlled intuitively. The device can be used in many positions, including overhead tasks, and is robust enough to allow for return to normal strenuous activity.

Conclusions

Great strides are being made in sensory motor interfaces for prosthetic control. Current clinically viable solutions such as targeted reinnervation, in combination with simultaneous control pattern recognition techniques and physiologically relevant multimodal sensory feedback, promise to afford vastly improved seamless coordinated control of several degrees of freedom of advanced devices. Surgical implications for amputated limbs necessitate preserving muscle viability and maximizing muscle stability in the residual limb through secure distal myodesis. Handling of nerves should now be done so with the very serious consideration for possible future use of those nerves for neural interface approaches with avoidance of overly zealous proximal transection. Other approaches in research development such as peripheral nerve interfaces and implantable wireless EMG recording devices should be watched closely as they are arriving in the clinic now and as clinical trials proceed, they hold promising potential to further address the human-machine interface challenges in prosthetic restoration.

Acknowledgment Thank you to David Home, CPO, Glenrose Rehabilitation Hospital, Alberta Health Services, Edmonton, Alberta, Canada, for photography.

References

1. Finch J. The ancient origins of prosthetic medicine. Lancet. 2011;377(9765):548–9.
2. Thurston AJ. Paré and prosthetics: the early history of artificial limbs. ANZ J Surg. 2007;77(12):1114–9.
3. Souza JM, Cheesborough JE, Ko JH, Cho MS, Kuiken TA, Dumanian GA. Targeted muscle reinnervation: a novel approach to postamputation neuroma pain. Clin Orthop Relat Res. 2014;472(2):1–7.
4. Resnik L, Klinger SL, Etter K. The DEKA arm: its features, functionality, and evolution during the veterans affairs study to optimize the DEKA arm. Prosthet Orthot Int. 2014;38(6):492–504.
5. Fillauer CE, Pritham CH, Fillauer KD. Evolution and development of the silicone suction socket (3S) for below-knee prostheses. J Prosthet Orthot. 1989;1(2):92–103.
6. Hagberg K, Brånemark R. One hundred patients treated with osseointegrated transfemoral amputation

prostheses: rehabilitation perspective. J Rehabil Res Dev. 2009;46(3):331–44.
7. Tikandylakis G, Berlin O, Branemark R. Implant survival, adverse events, and bone remodeling of osseointegrated, percutaneous implants for transhumeral amputees. Clin Orthop Relat Res. 2014;472(10): 2947–56.
8. Collinger JL, Wodlinger B, Downey JE, Wang W, Tyler-Kabara EC, Weber DJ, McMorland AJC, Velliste M, Boninger ML, Schwartz AB. High-performance neuroprosthetic control by an individual with tetraplegia. Lancet. 2013;381:557–64.
9. Rossini PM, Micera S, Benvenuto A, Carpaneto J, Cavallo G, Citi L, Cipriani C, Denaro L, Denaro V, Di Pino G, Ferrari F, Guglielmelli E, Hoffmann KP, Raspopovic S, Rigosa J, Rossini L, Tombini M, Dario P. Double nerve intraneural interface implant on a human amputee for robotic hand control. Clin Neurophysiol. 2010;121:777–83.
10. Raspopovic S, Capogrosso M, Petrini FM, Bonizzato M, Rigosa J, Di Pino G, Carpaneto J, Controzzi M, Boretius T, Fernandez E, Granata G, Oddo CM, Citi L, Ciancio AL, Cipriani C, Carrozza MC, Jensen W, Guglielmelli E, Stieglitz T, Rossini PM, Micera S. Restoring natural sensory feedback in real-time bidirectional hand prostheses. Sci Transl Med. 2014;6(222):222ra19.
11. Tan DW, Schiefer MA, Keith MW, Anderson JR, Tyler J, Tyler DJ. A neural interface provides long-term stable natural touch perception. Sci Transl Med. 2014;6(257):257ra138.
12. Weir RF, Troyk PR, Schorsch JF, Maas H. Implantable myoelectric sensors (IMESs) for intramuscular electromyogram recording. IEEE Trans Biomed Eng. 2009;56(1):159–71.
13. Kuiken TA, Schultz Feuser AE, Barlow AK, editors. Targeted muscle reinnervation: a neural interface for artificial limbs. Boca Raton, FL: Tayor & Francis; 2013.
14. Young AJ, Smith LH, Rouse EJ, Hargrove LJ. A comparison of the real-time controllability of pattern recognition to conventional myoelectric control for discrete and simultaneous movements. J Neuro Eng Rehabil. 2014;11(1):5.
15. Kuiken TA, Miller LA, Lipschutz RD, Lock BA, Stubblefield K, Marasco PD, Zhou P, Dumanian GA. Targeted reinnervation for enhanced prosthetic arm function in a woman with a proximal amputation: a case study. Lancet. 2007;369(9559):371–80.
16. Marasco PD, Schultz AE, Kuiken TA. Sensory capacity of reinnervated skin after redirection of amputated upper limb nerves to the chest. Brain. 2009;132: 1441–8.
17. Hebert JS, Olson JL, Morhart MJ, Dawson MR, Marasco PD, Kuiken TA, Chan KM. Novel targeted sensory reinnervation technique to restore functional hand sensation after transhumeral amputation. IEEE Trans Neural Syst Rehabil Eng. 2014;22(4):765–73.
18. Ortiz-Catalan M, Håkansson B, Brånemark R. An osseointegrated human-machine gateway for long-term sensory feedback and motor control of artificial limbs. Sci Transl Med. 2014;6(257):257re6.

Advanced Technologies in Pediatric Critical Care/Surgery and Fetal Surgery

50

John M. Draus Jr.

Introduction

Pediatric surgery continues to be a broad field. The pediatric surgeon specializes in the surgical care of children and is trained to operate in all body cavities. The scope of operative practice ranges from the correction of congenital anomalies to the resection of malignant tumors and to the management of injured trauma patients. Patient sizes range from premature neonates, weighing several hundred grams, to morbidly obese adolescents, weighing upwards of 150 kg. The surgeon must appreciate the physiologic differences and anatomic consideration of infants and children. Furthermore, the psychosocial stressors which affect sick children and their families cannot be overlooked. As in all of medicine, the data and knowledge in the field of pediatric surgery continue to evolve. New discoveries and technologic advancements are occurring constantly. Many of these contributions have dramatically improved the care of pediatric patients.

J.M. Draus Jr., M.D. (✉)
Division of Pediatric Surgery, Department of Surgery, Kentucky Children's Hospital, Lexington, KY, USA
e-mail: john.draus@uky.edu; Jmdr226@uky.edu

Critical Care

Much of the improved survival of pediatric surgical patients can be attributed to advancements in critical care. In the USA, it is widely agreed that modern neonatology began in the 1960s when Dr. Lewis Gluck established the first neonatal unit at Yale University. In 1975, neonatology became a subspecialty of pediatric medicine recognized by the American Board of Pediatrics. Although technologies such as incubators, ventilators, intravenous lines, and monitors are commonplace in modern ICUs, their profound impact on patient survival cannot be overlooked. Similarly, advancements in infant nutrition and advanced respiratory support have vastly contributed to the care of critically ill children.

Parenteral Nutrition

Parenteral nutrition (PN) is the sterile infusion of water, protein, fat, carbohydrates, electrolytes, vitamins, minerals, and trace elements via the venous system. TPN, introduced to clinical practice by Stanley J. Dudrick in 1968, is a life-saving therapy for patients with intestinal failure. Surgical patients with congenital anomalies, such as gastroschisis and intestinal atresias, and acquired anomalies, such as necrotizing enterocolitis and

R. Latifi et al. (eds.), *Technological Advances in Surgery, Trauma and Critical Care*,
DOI 10.1007/978-1-4939-2671-8_50

short-bowel syndrome, are dependent on PN to meet their high nutritional needs. Prolonged PN is associated with several complications including bloodstream infections, metabolic abnormalities, and hepatobiliary dysfunction. The most serious complication is parenteral nutrition-associated liver disease (PNALD) which may progress to liver failure and death. The pathophysiology is poorly understood, and the etiology is multifactorial. Risk factors include prematurity, poor gut motility, prolonged administration of PN, sepsis, and short bowel syndrome.

Lipid emulsions currently approved for use in the USA are derived from soybean or safflower oils which are rich in omega-6 fatty acids. In 2006, Mark Pruder described the use of Omegaven® (Fresenius Kabi AG, Bad Homburg, Germany) to successfully reverse severe PN-associated cholestasis in two infants [1]. Omegaven is an omega-3 fatty acid emulsion which is derived from fish oil. He postulated that standard intralipid may contribute to liver disease because of proinflammatory metabolites of the omega-6 fatty acids. A subsequent study reported the outcome of 18 patients on Omegaven monotherapy compared to a group of 21 historical controls who received conventional soybean oil-based lipid emulsions [2]. Patients who received Omegaven experienced reversal of cholestasis approximately seven times faster than the historical controls, effectively halting the progression of PNALD and providing a chance for the children to develop enteral tolerance and PN independence. A prospective, randomized trial is currently under way at Boston Children's Hospital to objectively determine the role of fish oil monotherapy in the prevention of PNALD.

Mechanical Ventilation

Acute lung injury (ALI) and acute respiratory distress syndrome (ARDS) are life-threatening conditions of acute pulmonary inflammation, alveolar edema, and hypoxemia that often lead to respiratory failure. The management of acute respiratory failure has dramatically changed since positive-pressure mechanical ventilation was first introduced over 40 years ago. Today, we recognize that high-peak airway pressures and high-inspired oxygen concentrations cause barotrauma and pulmonary oxygen toxicity. The resultant epithelial and endothelial damages lead to protein leak and pulmonary edema. Advanced strategies have been developed to minimize the trauma of conventional ventilation, including low-volume protective ventilation, inhaled nitric oxide (iNO), surfactant replacement therapy, and high-frequency oscillatory ventilation (HFOV).

Conventional neonatal and pediatric mechanical ventilators provide physiologic tidal volumes at physiologic rates. Modern microprocessor-controlled ventilators are able to provide multiple modes of ventilation. A protective lung ventilation strategy should be employed to avoid high-peak inspiratory pressures and maximize lung recruitment. Lower tidal volumes (4–8 ml/kg) with optimized positive end-expiratory pressure (PEEP) are used to prevent ventilator-induced lung injury. "Permissive hypercapnia" allows the $PaCO_2$ to rise to levels as high as 100 mmHg as long as the blood pH is maintained above 7.2 by means of intravenous bicarbonate. Inspiratory airway pressures should be limited below 35 cm water.

Inhaled nitric oxide is a selective pulmonary vasodilator that is approved for use in term and near-term newborns with hypoxic respiratory failure. iNO reduces pulmonary vascular resistance and improves oxygenation secondary to improvements in ventilation-perfusion matching. Furthermore, iNO is used in babies with pulmonary hypertension to increase blood flow without causing systemic hypotension. iNO has been shown to safely improve oxygen levels and decrease the need for extracorporeal membrane oxygenation (ECMO) therapy in infants with persistent pulmonary hypertension of the newborn [3].

Pulmonary surfactant is a phospholipoprotein produced by type II pneumatocytes. Surfactant reduces the alveolar surface tension, thereby increasing pulmonary compliance and allowing the lungs to inflate more easily. Animal-derived and synthetic surfactants are commercially available for replacement therapy. Natural surfactants are derived from bovine or porcine sources. Synthetic formulations differ most notably in their protein composition. Both have been shown to reduce the incidence of death, air leak syndromes, and intraventricular hemorrhage in premature infants with respiratory distress syndrome [4]. The use of surfactant in babies with ARDS secondary to meconium aspiration reduces the need for ECMO [5]. The role of surfactant replacement therapy outside the newborn period is less clear. Pediatric ALI patients who are treated with surfactant replacement early in the course of their illness have shown the most promising results.

The high-frequency oscillatory ventilator generates tidal volumes less than or equal to dead space by means of an oscillating diaphragm or piston. HFOV is an unconventional form of mechanical ventilation that produces active inspiration and exhalation to maintain constant lung recruitment. HFOV is indicated when conventional ventilation produces inadequate ventilation and inadequate oxygenation, or requires very high airway pressures. Best results are seen when parenchymal disease is homogeneous and increased airway resistance is not dominant lung pathology. Some clinicians advocate that HFOV should be the primary method of assisted ventilation in newborns with respiratory distress syndrome. Furthermore, HFOV has proven efficacious as a rescue therapy in older children with acute respiratory failure complicated by barotrauma. Air trapping is a potential threat with this type of mechanical ventilation. Frequent assessment of lung expansion and adequate gas exchange are necessary.

Extracorporeal Membrane Oxygenation

ECMO is used in critically ill pediatric patients with reversible pulmonary and/or cardiac processes who have failed ventilator support, iNO, volume expansion, and ionotropic/vasopressor support. ECMO provides oxygen delivery, carbon dioxide removal, and cardiac support to patients with respiratory and/or cardiac failure (Fig. 50.1).

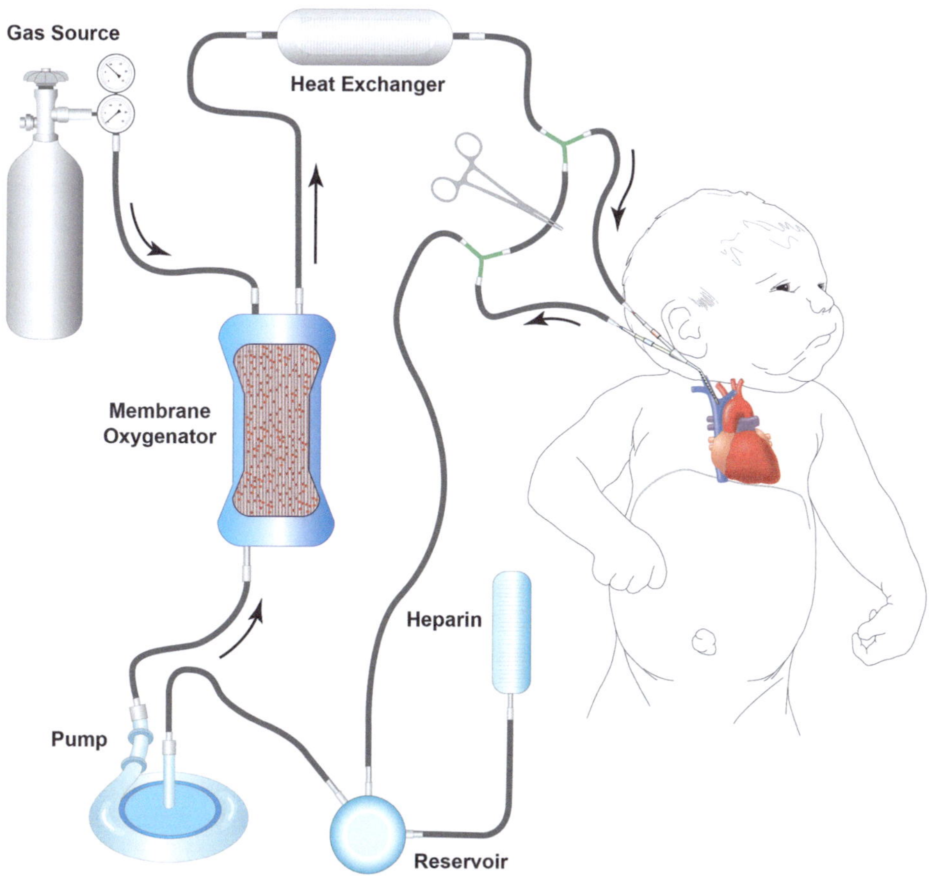

Fig. 50.1 Neonatal extracorporeal membrane oxygenation (ECMO) circuit. The *arrows* show the direction of blood flow

Deoxygenated blood is drained from the right atrium via a cannula. A pump device propels the blood across a membrane oxygenator where gas exchange occurs. Oxygenated blood is then returned to the patient via the aorta (venoarterial [VA]) or the right atrium (venovenous [VV]). ECMO has reduced infant mortality from 80 to 25 % for critically ill infants with acute reversible respiratory and cardiac failure in conditions such as persistent pulmonary hypertension, meconium aspiration, and sepsis [6].

There have been substantial technological improvements in contemporary ECMO support devices. Modern hollow-fiber oxygenators provide much lower resistance across the oxygenator membrane, allowing for the use of centrifugal pumps in the ECMO circuit. Centrifugal blood pumps are being used with increased frequency over traditional roller pumps. Both magnetically driven and magnetically suspended centrifugal pumps are available and are designed to reduce mechanically induced hemolysis. Some of the newest pumps can even provide pulsatile blood flow. Newer cannula designs, such as the double-lumen Avalon cannula (Avalon Elite®; Avalon Laboratories, Rancho Dominguez, CA), allow for more effective circuit flow and decrease recirculation during VV-ECMO support. Ongoing research efforts are directed toward improving the biocompatibility of circuit surface-blood interfaces in hopes of reducing the need for anticoagulation.

Minimally Invasive Surgery

Minimally invasive surgical (MIS) techniques have proven safe and efficacious in infants, children, and adolescents. Their main advantages relate to decreased postoperative pain, reduced hospital stay, faster return to normal activities, and superior cosmetic results when compared to conventional open techniques. Disadvantages include loss of haptic feedback, steeper learning curves, and increased operative costs for many procedures. Driven by numerous influences, MIS has quickly become the standard of care for many pediatric surgical conditions.

Laparoscopy

In 1987, Philippe Mouret reported the first laparoscopic cholecystectomy in Lyon, France. Since that historic event, the use of laparoscopy in general surgery has grown exponentially. This worldwide revolution has been driven by patient demand, surgeon ingenuity, and advances in medical technology. Initially, pediatric surgeons were slow to embrace laparoscopic techniques. Many believed that they were already performing most procedures through small incisions, and their patients recovered quickly. Optics and instruments were designed for adult patients, and their use in children was often cumbersome.

In the past two decades, technological advances have produced progressively smaller laparoscopic instruments and higher quality imaging. Smaller, lightweight trocars have been specifically designed for pediatric patients. Rigid laparoscopes (3 and 5 mm diameters) with angled lenses (30°, 45°, and 70°) foster the ability to work in confined spaces. Complete 3 and 5 mm instrument sets with shorter lengths have been engineered to suit the needs of pediatric surgeons. Advanced energy devices, such as the LigaSure™ vessel sealing system (Covidien, Mansfield, MA) and the Harmonic ACE® (Ethicon Endo-Surgery, Cincinnati, OH), achieve hemostasis and tissue dissection with minimal lateral thermal spread or tissue damage.

Today, advanced pediatric laparoscopic techniques have been applied to virtually every general and thoracic procedure in children. Laparoscopy is routinely used for cholecystectomy, appendectomy, pyloromyotomy, splenectomy, adrenalectomy, small bowel resections, exploration, and more. Advanced procedures include ileocolectomy for Crohn's disease, endorectal pull-through for Hirschsprung's disease, resection of choledochal cyst, and Roux-en-Y gastric bypass. Thoracoscopy has become standard for decortication, wedge resections, and minimally invasive repair of pectus excavatum. More advanced procedures include lobectomy, tracheoesophageal fistula repair, and congenital diaphragmatic hernia repair (Fig. 50.2).

Recently, there has been increasing enthusiasm about decreasing the number of ports used for

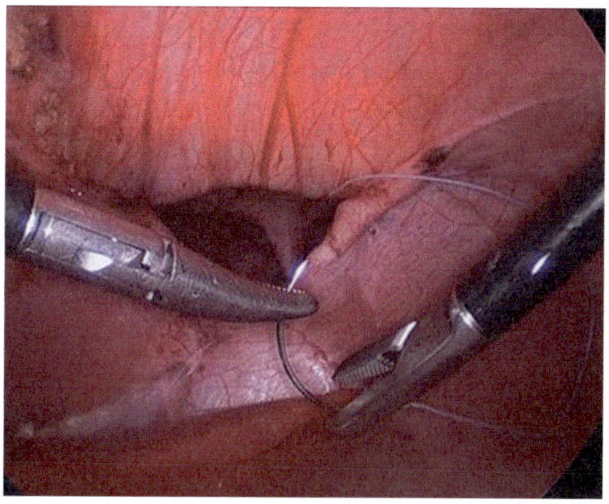

Fig. 50.2 Minimally invasive repair of a Morgagni diaphragmatic hernia in an infant

laparoscopic and thoracoscopic surgery. The most common techniques are single-port and single-incision laparoscopic surgery (SILS). The development of articulating cameras and instruments has made these techniques more plausible by allowing spatial separation and improved optics. Modified single ports are available which measure a few centimeters in diameter and allow the introduction of the scope and two instruments. In SILS, two or three small trocars are placed through an umbilical incision. There are successful reports of cholecystectomy, appendectomy, splenectomy, intussusception reduction, gastrostomy tube placement, thoracoscopic lung biopsy, decortications, and other pediatric procedures. The main advantage of these techniques is improved cosmetic results. Disadvantages include increased postoperative pain and incisional hernias.

Robotic Surgery

Robotic surgery is an emerging technology that may expand the variety of MIS procedures that can be accomplished in pediatric patients. Advantages of robotic surgery are its greater surgical precision, articulating instruments with increased range of motion, enhanced 3-D high-definition visualization of the operative field, reduced tremor, and improved ergonomics for the surgeon. Disadvantages include extended operative times, prolonged exposure to anesthesia, and significant expense of new devices, software upgrades, and operating room costs. Because of loss of domain, robotic surgery is difficult to perform in infants weighing less than 4 kg.

Essentially, any procedure can be done robotically. It is debated as to which procedures should be performed robotically and which procedures are more appropriate for other MIS techniques. Robotic techniques are best suited for complex operations which require fine dissection and suturing. Abdominal procedures include fundoplication, gastric bypass, resection of tumors, colectomy, and repair of congenital defects such as duodenal atresia, gastric duplications, and diaphragmatic hernia. Thoracic procedures include lobectomy, segmentectomy, tracheoesophageal fistula repair, and resection of mediastinal masses. Genitourinary and pelvic procedures include pyeloplasty, extramucosal ureteral reimplantation, and ovarian teratoma resection.

Fetal Surgery

Fetal surgery is a developing field. In the past three decades, it has evolved from a fanciful idea to a dedicated medical subspecialty. Fetal surgery is conducted in specialized centers throughout the USA and Europe. The fetal surgeon is an integral part of a collaborative, multidisciplinary fetal care team. Health care professionals from the fields of obstetrics, perinatology, genetics, neonatology, anesthesiology, radiology, and surgery must be readily available. Advances in fetal imaging and diagnosis have allowed clinicians to accurately classify congenital anomalies and stratify patients into appropriate risk groups. Each family must undergo extensive counseling that includes a detailed discussion of the maternal and fetal risks and potential benefits of a fetal intervention. Complications from fetal interventions include fetal demise, preterm labor, premature rupture of membranes, chorioamnionitis, and bleeding. Open fetal surgeries can cause uterine rupture in the current pregnancy and any future pregnancies. Procedures should only be offered when there is clear benefit to the fetus.

Congenital Lung Lesions

Congenital lung lesions (CLL) are a diverse group of malformations. Their antenatal detection has increased with the liberalized use of screening ultrasonography. These lesions are thought to exist across a spectrum of developmental pathways. Follow-up assessment with high-resolution ultrasound or ultrafast MRI is encouraged to better assess theses masses. The prenatal diagnosis and management of these lesions can be challenging, and urgent fetal intervention may be warranted in some cases.

Congenital cystic adenomatoid malformation (CCAM) is the most common CLL. A CCAM is a multicystic mass of nonfunctional pulmonary tissue that is usually confined to one lobe of the lung. The cysts can range in size from <1 mm to >10 cm. CCAMs can be classified as being macrocystic (>5 mm diameter for single or multiple cysts) or microcystic. However, prognosis depends on the size of the CCAM and its growth characteristics. CCAMs display unpredictable growth patterns between 18- and 26-week gestation. Thereafter, the growth rates plateau and may even regress.

Bronchopulmonary sequestration (BPS) is an area of nonfunctional lung tissue that does not communicate with the bronchial tree. It has a systemic arterial blood supply and variable venous drainage. An intralobar sequestration is located within the lung parenchyma. An extralobar sequestration is enveloped in its own pleura and may be located above or below the diaphragm.

Fetal hydrops is defined as the accumulation of fluid in two body cavities (pleural effusion, ascites, skin/scalp edema). Hydrops is often a harbinger of poor fetal or postnatal outcomes. The CCAM volume ratio (CVR) has emerged as a reliable way of predicting outcomes in a fetus with a CLL. CVR is calculated by measuring three tumor dimensions (length, width, height), multiplied by a constant (0.52), and divided by head circumference (to correct for gestational age). In a recent study, 56 % of fetuses with a CVR >2 required a fetal intervention, whereas only 3 % of fetuses with a CVR <2 required intervention [7]. Smaller CLLs and larger CLLs without hydrops can be followed with weekly or bimonthly ultrasound studies.

Fetal interventions are reserved for only the most severe CLLs. Prenatal steroids should be considered in patients with large, symptomatic solid or microcystic lung masses. Lesion regression and hydrops reversal have been reported from multiple centers. Ultrasound-guided thoraco-amniotic shunting can be attempted in fetuses with large macrocysts or BPS-related severe pulmonary effusions (Fig. 50.3). Open fetal surgery is reserved

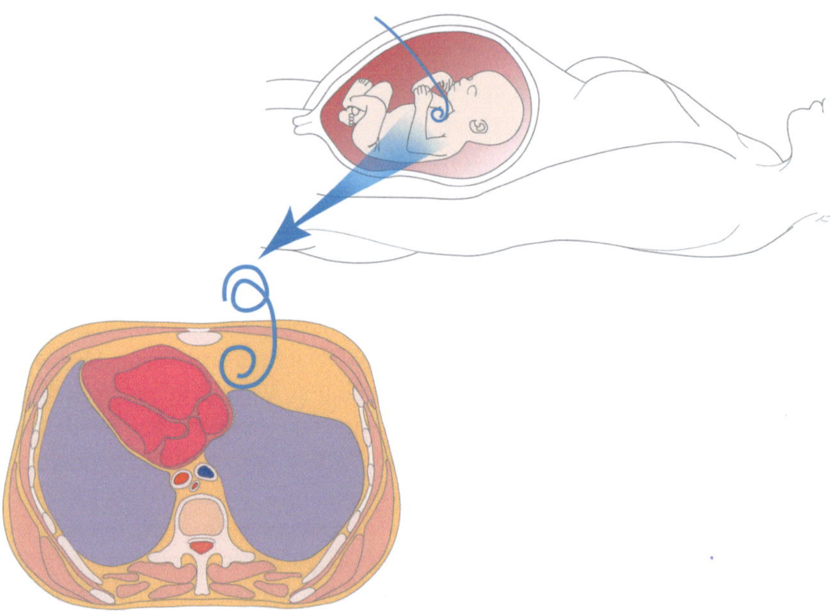

Fig. 50.3 Thoraco-amniotic shunting for a congenital lung lesion

for cases where fetal demise is imminent. These procedures are considered to patients younger than 30-week gestation with predominantly solid lesions and hydrops. Fetal lobectomy can be performed, but preterm delivery remains a challenge. In patients greater than 30 weeks, an ex utero intrapartum therapy (EXIT) procedure may be considered. An airway is secured and the lung mass is resected while the patient remains on placental bypass.

Congenital Diaphragmatic Hernia

Congenital diaphragmatic hernia (CDH) occurs when the pleuroperitoneal canals fail to fully close during the embryologic development of the diaphragm. The abdominal viscera herniate into the chest during a crucial period of lung development. CDH is associated with pulmonary hypoplasia and pulmonary hypertension. Despite advances in medical care, reported mortality rates continue to be between 50 and 75 %. Prenatal diagnosis is improving as imaging technologies become more advanced and clinicians become more adept at recognizing the associated findings. Due to the severity of illness, early detection of CDH is important so that families can be counseled appropriately and their treatment choices can be supported.

Imaging plays an important role in the evaluation of a fetus with CDH. Much work has been done to find ways which accurately predict postnatal outcomes using prenatal anatomic assessments. High-resolution ultrasound and fetal MRI are commonly utilized. It is well established that babies with right-sided CDH have a worse prognosis than those with left-sided defects—the need for ECMO support is higher and overall survival is lower. Furthermore, the presence of liver herniation reliably predicts worse outcomes in CHD patients, as does the identification of additional congenital anomalies.

Antenatal imaging parameters are frequently used to assess the degree of pulmonary hypoplasia. The lung-to-head ratio (LHR) is used to estimate lung volumes and is calculated by measuring the size of the contralateral lung and dividing by head circumference. Sonographic measurements are obtained between 23- and 26-week gestation. In multiple studies, an LHR <0.6 was associated with 100 % mortality, and an LHR >1.35 was associated with 100 % survival [8–10]. Recently, MRI has been used to estimate total lung volumes and predict prognosis. The study is typically performed between 23- and 26-week gestation. Volumetric measurements of both lungs are calculated and compared to standardized volumes for normal fetuses. The observed-to-expected fetal lung volume (O/E FLV) ratio is relatively easy to obtain, but its interpretation is debated. In one study, 0.15 appeared to be the determinant of survival—those with an O/E FLV >0.2 had 100 % survival, while only 40 % of those with a ratio <0.15 survived [11]. In another study, 0.25 seemed to be the cutoff point—those with an O/E FLV >0.35 had an 83 % survival, while those with a ratio <0.25 had a 13 % survival [12].

The vast majority of CDH patients are not candidates for fetal interventions. Attempts at fetal CDH repair have been abandoned due to failure to prove a survival advantage, despite a higher incidence of prematurity and longer hospital stays. Current interventions are based on the observation that tracheal occlusion prevents the egress of pulmonary fluid and stimulates stretch-induced lung growth. In Europe, fetal tracheal occlusion (FeTO) is achieved with a balloon which is delivered through a single 3.3 mm port (Fig. 50.4). FeTO is performed between 26- and 28-week gestation. Early reports from the Eurofetus multicenter, prospective trial are favorable. To date, this technology has not gained FDA approval in the USA.

Twin-to-Twin Transfusion Syndrome

Twin-to-twin transfusion syndrome (TTTS) occurs when there is an abnormal communication between placental blood vessels, resulting in a steal of placental blood flow from one twin to the other. TTTS develops in 10–15 % of all monochorionic pregnancies or about 4,000 babies per year. Both fetuses are seriously

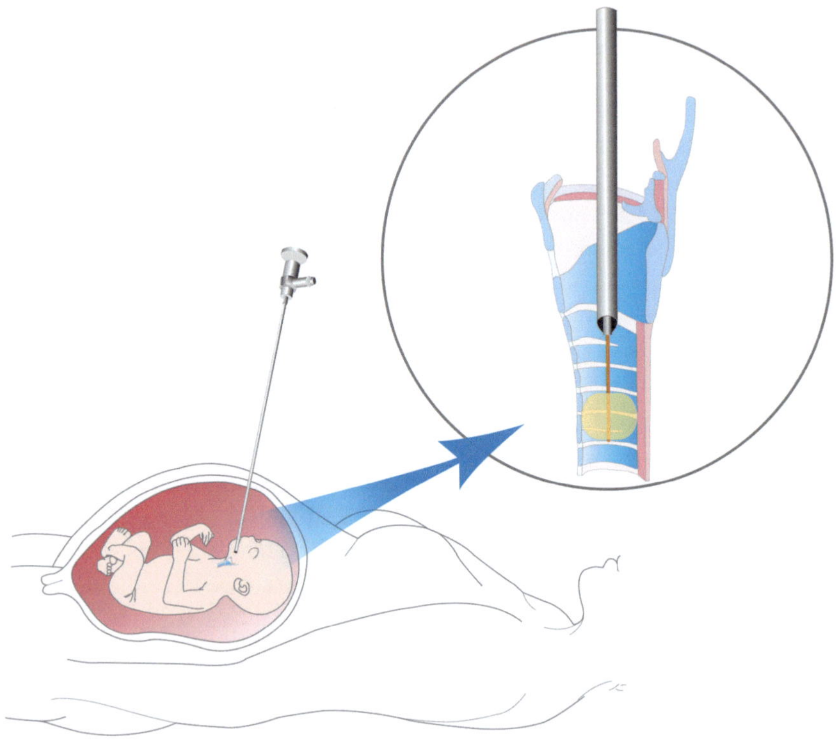

Fig. 50.4 Fetal tracheal occlusion (FeTO) for treatment of congenital diaphragmatic hernia

affected by the unbalanced transfusion. The "donor twin" experiences a chronic hypovolemia and oligohydramnios which may result in growth failure, high output cardiac failure, hydrops, and death. The "recipient twin" experiences chronic hypervolemia and polyhydramnios which can lead to cardiomegaly, tricuspid regurgitation, hydrops, and death. Mortality rates may be as high as 70 % in severe, untreated cases.

Advanced TTTS is the most common indication for operative fetoscopy. Fetoscopic laser ablation (FLA) selectively destroys the abnormal interconnecting placental vessels. It is estimated that 500 FLA procedures were performed in the USA last year. FLA has shown favorable results when compared to amnioreduction in randomized controlled trials. FLA had significantly higher likelihood of survival of at least one fetus to 28 days of age (76 % vs. 56 %) [13]. Furthermore, babies in the FLA group had an 80 % reduction in neurologic complications.

Future Perspectives

Tissue Engineering

The goal of tissue engineering is to allow organ replacement with a functional allograft which would grow with the child, minimize rejection, and not impair the patient's anatomy. Researchers are able to combine scaffolds, cells, and growth factors to create bioartificial tissues and organs. Scaffolds are constructed de novo using proteins or plastics or from decellularized organs. Recent advancements in stem cell research provide exciting opportunities for regeneration of tissues and organs. Artificial skin and cartilage are examples of engineered tissues that have been approved by the FDA. More complex tissues such as heart, lung, and liver have been successfully created in the lab but are a long way from use in medical therapies.

Artificial Placenta

Respiratory failure in extremely premature neonates contributes to significant mortality and long-term morbidity. The development of an artificial placenta would change the treatment paradigm for these fragile patients. The ideal artificial placenta would maintain fetal circulation and provide complete respiratory support without injuring the underdeveloped lungs. Current lamb models maintain the fetus in an artificial amniotic solution to provide a thermally neutral environment and maintain body metabolism. The lungs are filled with fluid and fetal breathing movements are stimulated. VV and VA circuits have used with outflow via the right jugular vein or umbilical artery, respectively, and inflow via the umbilical vein. Some experiments have shown that VV techniques are able to maintain more stable hemodynamics. Additional work is needed to balance the need for anticoagulation with the risk of intraventricular hemorrhage in the underdeveloped brain.

Summary

The limits of modern medicine are constantly challenged. In no other surgical subspecialty is this truer than in pediatric surgery. Technologic advances in critical care, minimally invasive surgery, and fetal surgery have revolutionized the field. New therapies are constantly offered to our patients—both born and unborn. Pathologic processes that were not survivable a generation ago are now being treated with newfound success. More complex procedures are being performed in less invasive ways. These advancements are due to the ideas, discoveries, and innovations of the men and women who have dedicated their lives to the surgical care of children. There is great potential to continue expanding these benefits in the future.

Abbreviations

ALI	Acute lung injury
ARDS	Acute respiratory distress syndrome
BPS	Bronchopulmonary sequestration
CCAM	Congenital cystic adenomatoid malformation
CDH	Congenital diaphragmatic hernia
CLL	Congenital lung lesion
CVR	CCAM volume ratio
ECMO	Extracorporeal membrane oxygenation
EXIT	Ex utero intrapartum therapy
FeTO	Fetal tracheal occlusion
FLA	Fetoscopic laser ablation
HFOV	High-frequency oscillatory ventilation
iNO	Inhaled nitric oxide
LHR	Lung-to-head ratio
MIS	Minimally invasive surgery
O/E FLV	Observed-to-expected fetal lung volume
PEEP	Positive end-expiratory pressure
PN	Parenteral nutrition
PNALD	Parenteral nutrition-associated liver disease
SILS	Single-incision laparoscopic surgery
TTTS	Twin-to-twin transfusion syndrome
VA	Venoarterial
VV	Venovenous

References

1. Gura KM, Duggan CP, Collier SB, Jennings RW, Folkman J, Bistrian BR, et al. Reversal of parenteral nutrition-associated liver disease in two infants with short bowel syndrome using parenteral fish oil: implications for future management. Pediatrics. 2006; 118:e197–201.
2. Gura KM, Lee S, Valim C, Zhou J, Kim S, Modi BP, et al. Safety and efficacy of a fish-oil-based fat emulsion in the treatment of parenteral nutrition-associated liver disease. Pediatrics. 2008;121:e678–86.
3. Roberts Jr JD, Fineman JR, Morin III FC, Shaul PW, Rimar S, Schreiber MD, et al. Inhaled nitric oxide and persistent pulmonary hypertension of the newborn:

the Inhaled Nitric Oxide Study Group. N Engl J Med. 1997;336:605–10.
4. Polin RA, Carlo WA. Surfactant replacement therapy for preterm and term neonates with respiratory distress. Pediatrics. 2014;133:156–63.
5. Wirbelauer J, Speer CP. The role of surfactant treatment in preterm infants and term newborns with acute respiratory distress syndrome. J Perinatol. 2009;29 Suppl 2:S18–22.
6. Gray BW, Shaffer AW, Mychaliska GB. Advances in neonatal extracorporeal support: the role of extracorporeal membrane oxygenation and the artificial placenta. Clin Perinatol. 2012;39:311–29.
7. Cass DL, Olutoye OO, Cassady CI, Zamora IJ, Ivey RT, Ayres NA, et al. Prenatal diagnosis and outcome of fetal lung masses. J Pediatr Surg. 2011;46:292–8.
8. Metkus AP, Filly RA, Stringer MD, Harrison MR, Adzick NS. Sonographic predictors of survival in fetal diaphragmatic hernia. J Pediatr Surg. 1996;31:148–51.
9. Lipshutz GS, Albanese CT, Feldstein VA, Jennings RW, Housley HT, Beech R, et al. Prospective analysis of lung-to-head ratio predicts survival for patients with prenatally diagnosed congenital diaphragmatic hernia. J Pediatr Surg. 1997;32:1634–6.
10. Yang SH, Nobuhara KK, Keller RL, Ball RH, Goldstein RB, Feldstein VA, et al. Reliability of the lung-to-head ratio as a predictor of outcome in fetuses with isolated left congenital diaphragmatic hernia at gestation outside 24–26 weeks. Am J Obstet Gynecol. 2007;197:30.e1–7.
11. Barnewolt CE, Kunisaki SM, Fauza DO, Nemes LP, Estroff JA, Jennings RW. Percent predicted lung volumes as measured on fetal magnetic resonance imaging: a useful biometric parameter for risk stratification in congenital diaphragmatic hernia. J Pediatr Surg. 2007;42:193–7.
12. Victoria T, Bebbington MW, Danzer E, Flake AW, Johnson MP, Dinan D. Use of magnetic resonance imaging in prenatal prognosis of the fetus with isolated left congenital diaphragmatic hernia. Prenat Diagn. 2012;32:715–23.
13. Rossi AC, D'Addario V. Laser therapy and serial amnioreduction as treatment for twin-twin transfusion syndrome: a metaanalysis and review of literature. Am J Obstet Gynecol. 2008;198:147–52.

Index

R. Latifi et al. (eds.), *Technological Advances in Surgery, Trauma and Critical Care*,
DOI 10.1007/978-1-4939-2671-8

C

N

O

P

S

V

W

X

FSC
www.fsc.org
MIX
Papier aus verantwortungsvollen Quellen
Paper from responsible sources
FSC® C105338

If you have any concerns about our products,
you can contact us on
ProductSafety@springernature.com

In case Publisher is established outside the EU,
the EU authorized representative is:
Springer Nature Customer Service Center GmbH
Europaplatz 3, 69115 Heidelberg, Germany

Printed by Libri Plureos GmbH
in Hamburg, Germany